THIRTEENTH EDITION

VANDER'S Human Physiology

THE MECHANISMS OF BODY FUNCTION

ERIC P. WIDMAIER
BOSTON UNIVERSITY

HERSHEL RAFF
MEDICAL COLLEGE OF WISCONSIN
AURORA ST. LUKE'S MEDICAL CENTER

KEVIN T. STRANG
UNIVERSITY OF WISCONSIN–MADISON

Mc Graw Hill
Connect Learn Succeed™

The McGraw·Hill Companies

Connect Learn Succeed™

VANDER'S HUMAN PHYSIOLOGY: THE MECHANISMS OF BODY FUNCTION, THIRTEENTH EDITION

Published by McGraw-Hill, a business unit of The McGraw-Hill Companies, Inc., 1221 Avenue of the Americas, New York, NY 10020.

This book is printed on acid-free paper.

1 2 3 4 5 6 7 8 9 0 DOW/DOW 1 0 9 8 7 6 5 4 3

ISBN 978–1–259–08082–1
MHID 1–259–08082–X

www.mhhe.com

Meet the Authors

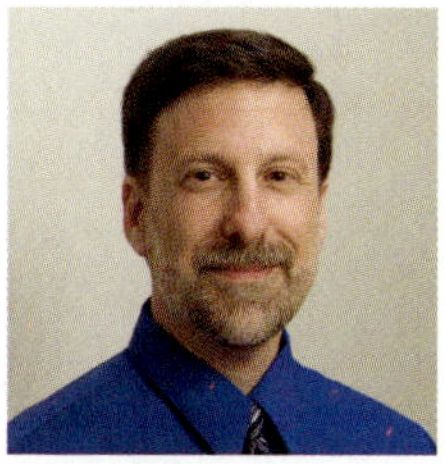

ERIC P. WIDMAIER received his Ph.D. in 1984 in Endocrinology from the *University of California at San Francisco.* His postdoctoral training was in endocrinology and physiology at the *Worcester Foundation for Experimental Biology* and *The Salk Institute* in La Jolla, California. His research is focused on the control of body mass and metabolism in mammals, the mechanisms of hormone action, and molecular mechanisms of intestinal and hypothalamic adaptation to high-fat diets. He is currently Professor of Biology at *Boston University,* where he teaches Human Physiology and has been recognized with the Gitner Award for Distinguished Teaching by the College of Arts and Sciences, and the Metcalf Prize for Excellence in Teaching by Boston University. He is the author of numerous scientific and lay publications, including books about physiology for the general reader. He lives outside Boston with his wife Maria and children Caroline and Richard.

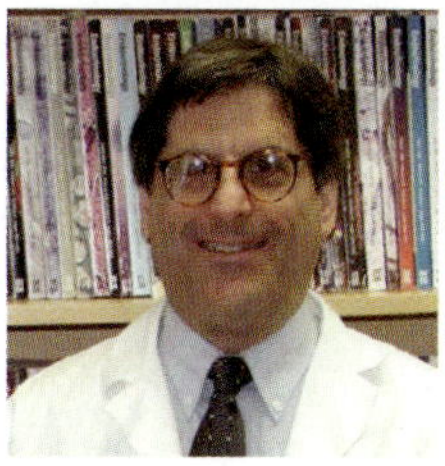

HERSHEL RAFF received his Ph.D. in Environmental Physiology from the *Johns Hopkins University* in 1981 and did postdoctoral training in Endocrinology at the *University of California at San Francisco.* He is now a Professor of Medicine (Endocrinology, Metabolism, and Clinical Nutrition), Surgery, and Physiology at the *Medical College of Wisconsin* and Director of the Endocrine Research Laboratory at *Aurora St. Luke's Medical Center.* At the *Medical College of Wisconsin,* he teaches physiology and pharmacology to medical and graduate students, and is the Endocrinology/Reproduction Unit Director for the new integrated curriculum. He was an inaugural inductee into the Society of Teaching Scholars, received the Beckman Basic Science Teaching Award three times, received the Outstanding Teacher Award from the Graduate School, and has been one of the MCW's Outstanding Medical Student Teachers for each year the award has been given. He is also an Adjunct Professor of Biomedical Sciences at *Marquette University.* He is the former Associate Editor of *Advances in Physiology Education.* Dr. Raff's basic research focuses on the adaptation to low oxygen (hypoxia). His clinical interest focuses on pituitary and adrenal diseases, with a special focus on laboratory tests for the diagnosis of Cushing's syndrome. He resides outside Milwaukee with his wife Judy and son Jonathan.

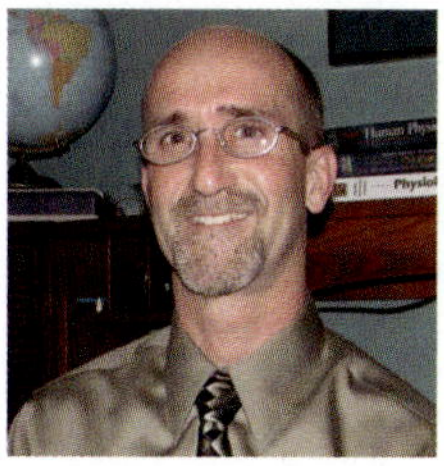

KEVIN T. STRANG received his Master's Degree in Zoology (1988) and his Ph.D. in Physiology (1994) from the *University of Wisconsin at Madison.* His research area is cellular mechanisms of contractility modulation in cardiac muscle. He teaches a large undergraduate systems physiology course as well as first-year medical physiology in the *UW-Madison School of Medicine and Public Health.* He was elected to UW-Madison's Teaching Academy and as a Fellow of the Wisconsin Initiative for Science Literacy. He is a frequent guest speaker at colleges and high schools on the physiology of alcohol consumption. He has twice been awarded the UW Medical Alumni Association's Distinguished Teaching Award for Basic Sciences, and also received the University of Wisconsin System's Underkofler/Alliant Energy Excellence in Teaching Award. In 2012 he was featured in *The Princeton Review* publication, *"The Best 300 Professors."* Interested in teaching technology, Dr. Strang has produced numerous animations of figures from *Vander's Human Physiology* available to instructors and students. He lives in Madison with his wife Sheryl and his children Jake and Amy.

TO OUR FAMILIES: MARIA, RICHARD, AND CAROLINE; JUDY AND JONATHAN; SHERYL, JAKE, AND AMY

Brief Contents

Table of Contents

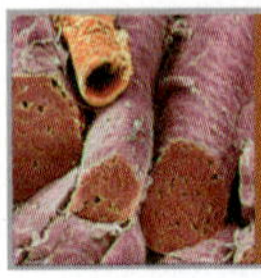

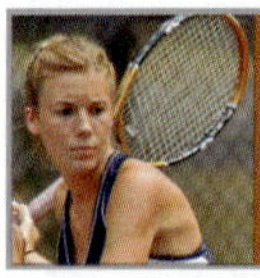

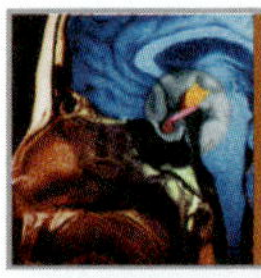

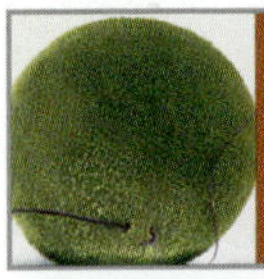

17 Reproduction 602

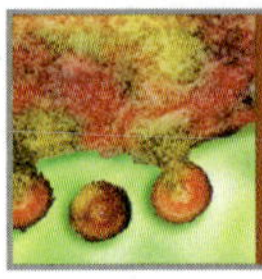

18 The Immune System 652

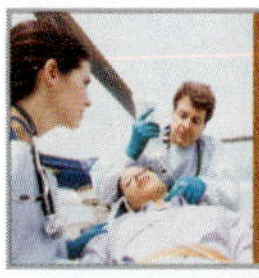

19 Medical Physiology: Integration Using Clinical Cases 692

Index of Exercise Physiology

From the Authors

It is with great pleasure that we present the thirteenth edition of *Vander's Human Physiology*. The cover of this edition reflects some of the major themes of the textbook: homeostasis, exercise, pathophysiology, and cellular and molecular mechanisms of body function. These themes and others have now been introduced in Chapter 1, called "General Principles of Physiology." These principles have been integrated throughout the remaining chapters in order to continually reinforce their importance. Each chapter opens with a preview of those principles that are particularly relevant for the material covered in that chapter. The principles are then reinforced when specific examples arise within a chapter. Finally, assessments are provided at the end of each chapter to provide immediate feedback for students to gauge their understanding of the chapter material and its relationship to physiological principles. These assessments tend to require analytical and critical thinking; answers are provided in an appendix.

Users of the book will also benefit from expanded assessments of the traditional type, such as multiple choice and thought questions, as well as additional Physiological Inquiries associated with various key figures. In total, approximately 70 new assessment questions have been added to the textbook; this is in addition to the several hundred test questions available on the McGraw-Hill Connect site associated with the book.

As in earlier editions, there is extensive coverage of exercise physiology (see the special exercise index that follows the detailed Table of Contents), and special attention to the clinical relevance of much of the basic science (see the Index of Clinical Terms in Appendix B). This index is organized according to disease; infectious or causative agents; and the treatments, diagnostics, and therapeutic drugs used to treat disease. This is a very useful resource for instructors and students interested in the extensive medical applications of human physiology that are covered in this book.

As textbooks become more integrated with digital content, we are pleased that McGraw-Hill has provided ***Vander's Human Physiology*** with cutting-edge digital content that continues to expand and develop. Students will again find a Connect Plus site associated with the text. The assessments have been updated and are now authored by one of the author team, Kevin Strang. For the first time we also have LearnSmart! McGraw-Hill LearnSmart™ is an adaptive diagnostic tool that constantly assesses student knowledge of course material.

We are always grateful to receive e-mail messages from instructors and students worldwide who are using the book and wish to offer suggestions regarding content. Finally, no textbook such as this could be written without the expert and critical eyes of our many reviewers; we are thankful to those colleagues who took time from their busy schedules to read all or a portion of a chapter (or more) and provide us with their insights and suggestions for improvements.

Guided Tour Through a Chapter

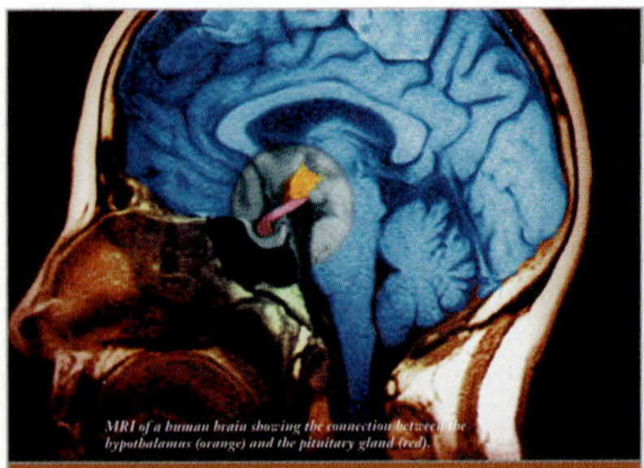

MRI of a human brain showing the connection between the hypothalamus (orange) and the pituitary gland (red).

11 The Endocrine System

319

Chapter Outline

Every chapter starts with an introduction giving the reader a brief overview of what is to be covered in that chapter. Included in the introduction for the thirteenth edition is a new feature that provides students with a preview of those General Principles of Physiology (introduced in Chapter 1) that will be covered in the chapter.

General Principles of Physiology—NEW!

General Principles of Physiology have been integrated throughout each chapter in order to continually reinforce their importance. Each chapter opens with a preview of those principles that are particularly relevant for the material covered in that chapter. The principles are then reinforced when specific examples arise within a chapter.

In Chapters 6–8 and 10, you learned that the nervous system is one of the two major control systems of the body, and now we turn our attention to the other—the endocrine system. The endocrine system consists of all those glands, called endocrine glands, that secrete hormones, as well as hormone-secreting cells located in various organs such as the heart, kidneys, liver, and stomach. Hormones are chemical messengers that enter the blood, which carries them from their site of secretion to the cells upon which they act. The cells a particular hormone influences are known as the target cells for that hormone. The aim of this chapter is to first present a detailed overview of endocrinology—that is, a structural and functional analysis of general features of hormones—followed by a more detailed analysis of several important hormonal systems. Before continuing, you should review the principles of ligand-receptor interactions and cell signaling that were described in Chapter 3 (Section C) and Chapter 5, because they pertain to the mechanisms by which hormones exert their actions.

Hormones functionally link various organ systems together. As such, several of the general principles of physiology first introduced in Chapter 1 apply to the study of the endocrine system, including the principle that the functions of organ systems are coordinated with each other. This coordination is key to the maintenance of homeostasis, another important general principle of physiology that will be covered in Sections C, D, and F. In many cases, the actions of one hormone can be potentiated, inhibited, or counterbalanced by the actions of another. This illustrates the general principle of physiology that most physiological functions are controlled by multiple regulatory systems, often working in opposition. It will be especially relevant in the sections on the endocrine control of metabolism and the control of pituitary gland function. Finally, this chapter exemplifies the general principle of physiology that information flow between cells, tissues, and organs is an essential feature of homeostasis and allows for integration of physiological processes.

Clinical Case Studies

The authors have drawn from their teaching and research experiences and the clinical experiences of colleagues to provide students with real-life applications through clinical case studies in each chapter.

CHAPTER 11

Clinical Case Study: Mouth Pain, Sleep Apnea, and Enlargement of the Hands in a 35-Year-Old Man

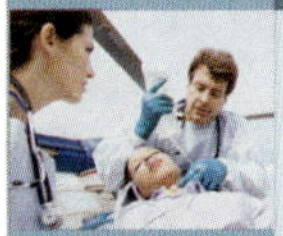

A 35-year-old man visited his dentist with a complaint of chronic mouth pain and headaches. After examining the patient, the dentist concluded that there was no dental disease but that the patient's jaw appeared enlarged and his tongue was thickened and large. The dentist referred the patient to a physician. The physician noted enlargement of the jaw and tongue, enlargement of the fingers and toes, and a very deep voice. The patient acknowledged that his voice seemed to have deepened over the past few years and that he no longer wore his wedding ring because it was too tight. The patient's height and weight were within normal ranges. His blood pressure was significantly elevated, as was his fasting plasma glucose concentration. The patient also mentioned that his wife could no longer sleep in the same room as he because of his loud snoring and sleep apnea. Based on these signs and symptoms, the physician referred the patient to an endocrinologist, who ordered a series of tests to better elucidate the cause of the diverse symptoms.

The enlarged bones and facial features suggested the possibility of ***acromegaly*** (from the Greek *akros*, "extreme" or "extremities," and *megalos*, "large"), a disease characterized by excess growth hormone and IGF-1 concentrations in the blood. This was confirmed with a blood test that revealed greatly elevated concentrations of both hormones. Based on these results, an MRI scan was ordered to look for a possible tumor of the anterior pituitary gland. A 1.5 cm mass was discovered in the sella turcica, consistent with the possibility of a growth hormone–secreting tumor. Because the patient was of normal height, it was concluded that the tumor arose at some point after puberty, when linear growth ceased because of closure of the epiphyseal plates. Had the tumor developed prior to puberty, the man would have been well above normal height because of the growth-promoting actions of growth hormone and IGF-1. Such individuals are known as pituitary giants and have a condition called ***gigantism.*** In many cases, the affected person develops both gigantism and later acromegaly, as occurred in the individual shown in **Figure 11.33**.

Acromegaly and gigantism arise when chronic, excess amounts of growth hormone are secreted into the blood. In almost all cases, acromegaly and gigantism are caused by benign (noncancerous) tumors of the anterior pituitary gland that secrete growth hormone at very high rates, which in turn results in elevated IGF-1 concentrations in the blood. Because these tumors are abnormal tissue, they are not suppressed adequately by normal negative feedback inhibitors like IGF-1, so the growth hormone concentrations remain elevated. These tumors are typically very slow growing, and, if they arise after puberty, it may be many years before a person realizes that there is something wrong. In our patient, the changes in his appearance were gradual enough that he attributed them simply to "aging," despite his relative youth.

Even when linear growth is no longer possible (after the growth plates have fused), very high plasma concentrations of

(continued)

358 Chapter 11

(continued)

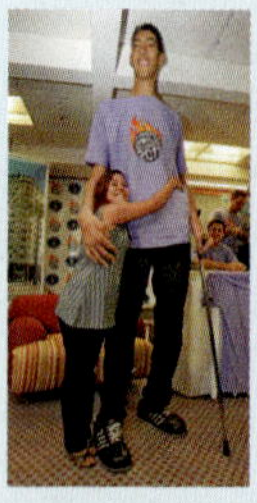

Figure 11.33 Appearance of an individual with gigantism and acromegaly.

growth hormone and IGF-1 result in the thickening of many bones in the body, most noticeably in the hands, feet, and head. The jaw, particularly, enlarges to give the characteristic facial appearance called ***prognathism*** (from the Greek *pro*, "forward," and *gnathos*, "jaw") that is associated with acromegaly. This was likely the cause of our patient's chronic mouth pain. The enlarged sinuses that resulted from the thickening of his skull bones may have been responsible in part for his headaches. In addition, many internal organs—such as the heart—also become enlarged due to growth hormone and IGF-1-induced hypertrophy, and this can interfere with their ability to function normally. In some acromegalics, the tissues comprising the larynx enlarge, resulting in a deepening of the voice as in our subject. The enlarged and deformed tongue was likely a contributor to the sleep apnea and snoring reported by the patient; this is called obstructive sleep apnea because the tongue base weakens and, consequently, the tongue obstructs the upper airway (see Chapter 13 for a discussion of sleep apnea). Finally, roughly half of all people with acromegaly have elevated blood pressure (hypertension). The cause of the hypertension is uncertain, but it is a serious medical condition that requires treatment with antihypertensive drugs.

As described earlier, adults continue to make and secrete growth hormone even after growth ceases. That is because growth hormone has metabolic actions in addition to its effects on growth. The major actions of growth hormone in metabolism are to increase the concentrations of glucose and fatty acids in the blood and decrease the sensitivity of skeletal muscle and adipose tissue to insulin. Not surprisingly, therefore, one of the stimuli that increases growth hormone concentrations in the healthy adult is a decrease in blood glucose or fatty acids. The secretion of growth hormone during these metabolic crises, however, is transient; once glucose or fatty acid concentrations are restored to normal, growth hormone concentrations decrease to baseline. In acromegaly, however, growth hormone concentrations are almost always increased. Consequently, acromegaly is often associated with increased plasma concentrations of glucose and fatty acids, in some cases even reaching the concentrations observed in diabetes mellitus. As in Cushing's syndrome (Section D), therefore, the presence of chronically increased concentrations of growth hormone may result in diabetes-like symptoms. This explains why our patient had a high fasting plasma glucose concentration.

Our subject was fortunate to have had a quick diagnosis. This case study illustrates one of the confounding features of endocrine disorders. The rarity of some endocrine diseases (e.g., acromegaly occurs in roughly 4 per million individuals), together with the fact that the symptoms of a given endocrine disease can be varied and insidious in their onset, often results in a delayed diagnosis. This means that in many cases, a patient is subjected to numerous tests for more common disorders before a diagnosis of endocrine disease is made.

Treatment of gigantism and acromegaly usually requires surgical removal of the pituitary tumor. The residual normal pituitary tissue is then sufficient to maintain baseline growth hormone concentrations. If this treatment is impossible or not successful, treatment with long-acting analogs of somatostatin is sometimes necessary. (Recall that somatostatin is the hypothalamic hormone that inhibits GH secretion.) Our patient elected to have surgery. This resulted in a reduction in his plasma growth hormone and IGF-1 concentrations. With time, several of his symptoms were reduced, including the increased plasma glucose concentrations. However, within 2 years, his growth hormone and IGF-1 concentrations were three times higher than the normal range for his age and a follow-up MRI revealed that the tumor had regrown. Not wanting a second surgery, the patient was treated with radiation therapy focused on the pituitary tumor, followed by regular administration of somatostatin analogs. This treatment decreased but did not completely normalize his hormone concentrations. His blood pressure remained elevated and was treated with two different antihypertensive drugs (see Chapter 12).

Clinical terms: acromegaly, gigantism, prognathism

See Chapter 19 for complete, integrative case studies.

Summary Tables

Summary tables are used to bring together large amounts of information that may be scattered throughout the book or to summarize small or moderate amounts of information. The tables complement the accompanying figures to provide a rapid means of reviewing the most important material in the chapter.

TABLE 11.6 Major Hormones Influencing Growth

Hormone	Principal Actions
Growth hormone	Major stimulus of postnatal growth: Induces precursor cells to differentiate and secrete insulin-like growth factor 1 (IGF-1), which stimulates cell division Stimulates liver to secrete IGF-1 Stimulates protein synthesis
Insulin	Stimulates fetal growth Stimulates postnatal growth by stimulating secretion of IGF-1 Stimulates protein synthesis
Thyroid hormone	Permissive for growth hormone's secretion and actions Permissive for development of the central nervous system
Testosterone	Stimulates growth at puberty, in large part by stimulating the secretion of growth hormone Causes eventual epiphyseal closure Stimulates protein synthesis in male
Estrogen	Stimulates the secretion of growth hormone at puberty Causes eventual epiphyseal closure
Cortisol	Inhibits growth Stimulates protein catabolism

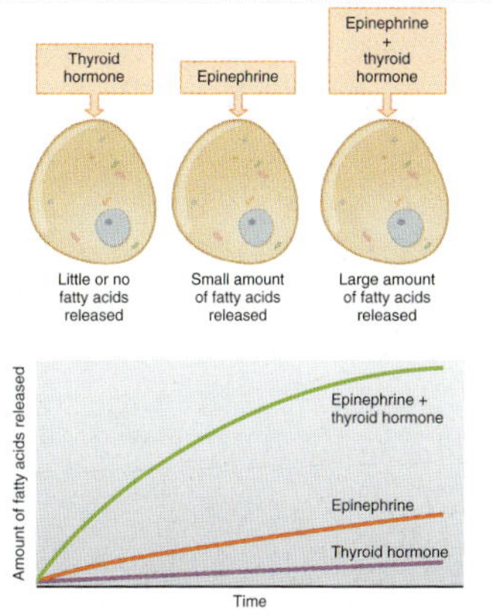

Figure 11.9 The ability of thyroid hormone to "permit" epinephrine-induced release of fatty acids from adipose tissue cells. Thyroid hormone exerts this effect by causing an increased number of beta-adrenergic receptors on the cell. Thyroid hormone by itself stimulates only a small amount of fatty acid release.

PHYSIOLOGICAL INQUIRY

- A patient is observed to have symptoms that are consistent with elevated concentrations of epinephrine in the blood, including a rapid heart rate, anxiety, and elevated fatty acid concentrations. However, the circulating epinephrine concentrations are tested and found to be in the normal range. What might explain this?

Answer can be found at end of chapter.

Physiological Inquiries

The authors have continued to refine and expand the number of critical-thinking questions based on many figures from all chapters. These concept checks were introduced in the eleventh edition and continue to prove extremely popular with users of the textbook. They are designed to help students become more engaged in learning a concept or process depicted in the art. These questions challenge a student to analyze the content of the figure, and occasionally to recall information from previous chapters. Many of the questions also require quantitative skills. Many instructors find that these Physiological Inquiries make great exam questions.

Anatomy and Physiology Revealed (APR) Icon—NEW!

APR icons are found in figure legends. These icons indicate that there is a direct link to APR available in the eBook provided with Connect Plus for this title!

Descriptive Art Style

A realistic three-dimensional perspective is included in many of the figures for greater clarity and understanding of concepts presented.

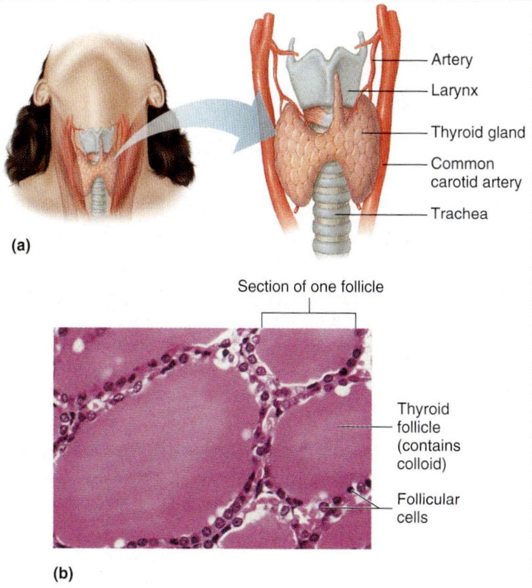

Figure 11.20 APR (a) Location of the bilobed thyroid gland. (b) A cross section through several adjoining follicles filled with colloid. (b): © Biophoto Associates/Photo Researchers

Guided Tour Through a Chapter

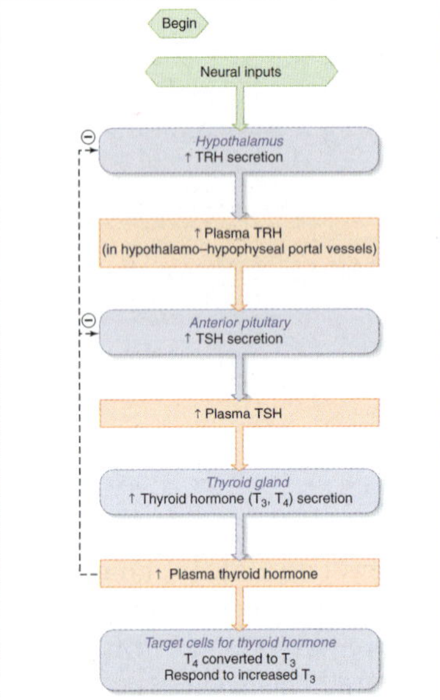

Figure 11.22 TRH-TSH-thyroid hormone sequence. T_3 and T_4 inhibit secretion of TSH and TRH by negative feedback, indicated by the ⊖ symbol.

Flow Diagrams

Long a hallmark of this book, extensive use of flow diagrams is continued in this edition. They have been updated to assist in learning.

Key to Flow Diagrams

- The beginning boxes of the diagrams are color-coded green.
- Other boxes are consistently color-coded throughout the book.
- Structures are always shown in three-dimensional form.

Uniform Color-Coded Illustrations

Color-coding is effectively used to promote learning. For example, there are specific colors for extracellular fluid, the intracellular fluid, muscle filaments, and transporter molecules.

Multilevel Perspective

Illustrations depicting complex structures or processes combine macroscopic and microscopic views to help students see the relationships between increasingly detailed drawings.

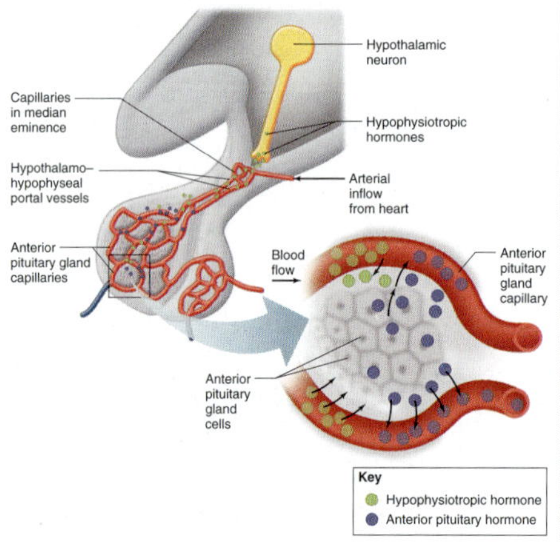

Figure 11.16 APR Hormone secretion by the anterior pituitary gland is controlled by hypophysiotropic hormones released by hypothalamic neurons and reaching the anterior pituitary gland by way of the hypothalamo–hypophyseal portal vessels.

End of Section

At the end of sections throughout the book, you will find a summary, review questions, key terms, and clinical terms.

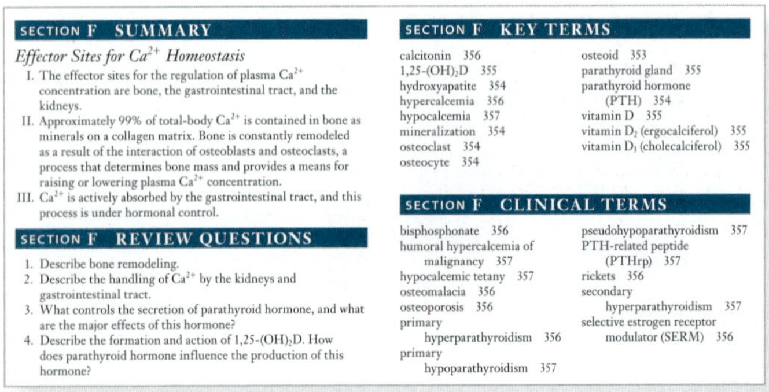

SECTION F SUMMARY

Effector Sites for Ca^{2+} Homeostasis

I. The effector sites for the regulation of plasma Ca^{2+} concentration are bone, the gastrointestinal tract, and the kidneys.

II. Approximately 99% of total-body Ca^{2+} is contained in bone as minerals on a collagen matrix. Bone is constantly remodeled as a result of the interaction of osteoblasts and osteoclasts, a process that determines bone mass and provides a means for raising or lowering plasma Ca^{2+} concentration.

III. Ca^{2+} is actively absorbed by the gastrointestinal tract, and this process is under hormonal control.

SECTION F REVIEW QUESTIONS

1. Describe bone remodeling.
2. Describe the handling of Ca^{2+} by the kidneys and gastrointestinal tract.
3. What controls the secretion of parathyroid hormone, and what are the major effects of this hormone?
4. Describe the formation and action of 1,25-$(OH)_2D$. How does parathyroid hormone influence the production of this hormone?

SECTION F KEY TERMS

calcitonin 356
1,25-$(OH)_2D$ 355
hydroxyapatite 354
hypercalcemia 356
hypocalcemia 357
mineralization 354
osteoclast 354
osteocyte 354
osteoid 353
parathyroid gland 355
parathyroid hormone (PTH) 354
vitamin D 355
vitamin D_2 (ergocalciferol) 355
vitamin D_3 (cholecalciferol) 355

SECTION F CLINICAL TERMS

bisphosphonate 356
humoral hypercalcemia of malignancy 357
hypocalcemic tetany 357
osteomalacia 356
osteoporosis 356
primary hyperparathyroidism 356
primary hypoparathyroidism 357
pseudohypoparathyroidism 357
PTH-related peptide (PTHrp) 357
rickets 356
secondary hyperparathyroidism 357
selective estrogen receptor modulator (SERM) 356

End of Chapter

At the end of the chapters, you will find

- Test Questions that are designed to test student comprehension of key concepts.
- *NEW!*—General Principles Assessment questions that test the student's ability to relate the material covered in a given chapter to one or more of the General Principles of Physiology described in Chapter 1. This provides a powerful unifying theme to understanding all of physiology, and is also an excellent gauge of a student's progress from the beginning to the end of a semester.
- Quantitative and Thought Questions that challenge the student to go beyond the memorization of facts, to solve problems and to encourage thinking about the meaning or broader significance of what has just been read.
- Answers to the Physiological Inquiries in that chapter.

CHAPTER 11 TEST QUESTIONS

Answers found in Appendix A.

1–5: Match the hormone with the function or feature (choices a–e).

Hormone:

1. vasopressin
2. ACTH
3. oxytocin
4. prolactin
5. luteinizing hormone

Function:

a. tropic for the adrenal cortex
b. is controlled by an amine-derived hormone of the hypothalamus
c. antidiuresis
d. stimulation of testosterone production
e. stimulation of uterine contractions during labor

6. In the following figure, which hormone (A or B) binds to receptor X with higher affinity?

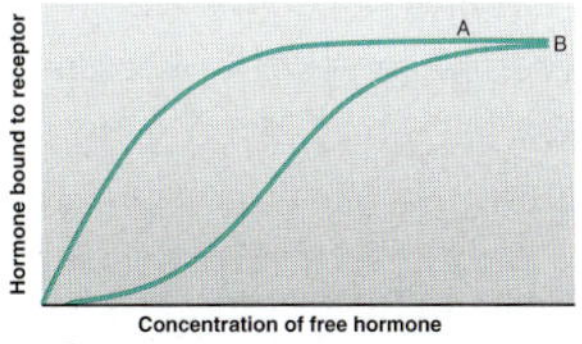

7. Which is *not* a symptom of Cushing's disease?
   a. high blood pressure
   b. bone loss
   c. suppressed immune function
   d. goiter
   e. hyperglycemia (increased blood glucose)
8. Tremors, nervousness, and increased heart rate can all be symptoms of
   a. increased activation of the sympathetic nervous system.
   b. excessive secretion of epinephrine from the adrenal medulla.
   c. hyperthyroidism.
   d. hypothyroidism.
   e. answers a, b, and c (all are correct).
9. Which of the following could theoretically result in short stature?
   a. pituitary tumor making excess thyroid-stimulating hormone
   b. mutations that result in inactive IGF-1 receptors
   c. delayed onset of puberty
   d. decreased hypothalamic concentrations of somatostatin
   e. normal plasma GH but decreased feedback of GH on GHRH
10. Choose the correct statement.
    a. During times of stress, cortisol acts as an anabolic hormone in muscle and adipose tissue.
    b. A deficiency of thyroid hormone would result in increased cellular concentrations of Na^+/K^+-ATPase pumps in target tissues.
    c. The posterior pituitary is connected to the hypothalamus by long portal vessels.
    d. Adrenal insufficiency often results in increased blood pressure and increased plasma glucose concentrations.
    e. A lack of iodide in the diet will have no significant effect on the concentration of circulating thyroid hormone for at least several weeks.
11. A lower-than-normal concentration of plasma Ca^{2+} causes
    a. a PTH-mediated increase in 25-OH D.
    b. a decrease in renal 1-hydroxylase activity.
    c. a decrease in the urinary excretion of Ca^{2+}.
    d. a decrease in bone resorption.
    e. an increase in vitamin D release from the skin.
12. Which of the following is *not* consistent with primary hyperparathyroidism?
    a. hypercalcemia
    b. elevated plasma 1,25-$(OH)_2D$
    c. increased urinary excretion of phosphate ions
    d. a decrease in Ca^{2+} resorption from bone
    e. an increase in Ca^{2+} reabsorption in the kidney

True or False

13. T_4 is the chief circulating form of thyroid hormone but is less active than T_3.
14. Acromegaly is usually associated with hypoglycemia and hypotension.
15. Thyroid hormone and cortisol are both permissive for the actions of epinephrine.

CHAPTER 11 GENERAL PRINCIPLES ASSESSMENT

Answers found in Appendix A.

1. Referring back to Tables 11.3, 11.4, and 11.5, explain how certain of the actions of epinephrine, cortisol, and growth hormone illustrate in part the general principle of physiology that *most physiological functions are controlled by multiple regulatory systems, often working in opposition.*
2. Another general principle of physiology is that *structure is a determinant of—and has coevolved with—function.* The structure of the thyroid gland is very unlike other endocrine glands. How is the structure of this gland related to its function?
3. *Homeostasis is essential for health and survival.* How do parathyroid hormone, ADH, and thyroid hormone contribute to homeostasis? What might be the consequence of having too little of each of those hormones?

CHAPTER 11 QUANTITATIVE AND THOUGHT QUESTIONS

Answers found at www.mhhe.com/widmaier13.

1. In an experimental animal, the sympathetic preganglionic fibers to the adrenal medulla are cut. What happens to the plasma concentration of epinephrine at rest and during stress?
2. During pregnancy, there is an increase in the liver's production and, consequently, the plasma concentration of the major plasma binding protein for thyroid hormone. This causes a sequence of events involving feedback that results in an increase in the plasma concentrations of T_3 but no evidence of hyperthyroidism. Describe the sequence of events.
3. A child shows the following symptoms: deficient growth, failure to show sexual development, decreased ability to respond to stress. What is the most likely cause of all these symptoms?
4. If all the neural connections between the hypothalamus and pituitary gland below the median eminence were severed, the secretion of which pituitary gland hormones would be affected? Which pituitary gland hormones would not be affected?
5. Typically, an antibody to a peptide combines with the peptide and renders it nonfunctional. If an animal were given an antibody to somatostatin, the secretion of which anterior pituitary gland hormone would change and in what direction?
6. A drug that blocks the action of norepinephrine is injected directly into the hypothalamus of an experimental animal, and the secretion rates of several anterior pituitary gland hormones are observed to change. How is this possible, given the fact that norepinephrine is not a hypophysiotropic hormone?

CHAPTER 11 ANSWERS TO PHYSIOLOGICAL INQUIRIES

Figure 11.3 By storing large amounts of hormone in an endocrine cell, the plasma concentration of the hormone can be increased within seconds when the cell is stimulated. Such rapid responses may be critical for an appropriate response to a challenge to homeostasis. Packaging peptides in this way also prevents intracellular degradation.

Figure 11.5 Because steroid hormones are derived from cholesterol, they are lipophilic. Consequently, they can freely diffuse through lipid bilayers, including those that constitute secretory vesicles. Therefore, once a steroid hormone is synthesized, it diffuses out of the cell.

Figure 11.9 One explanation for this patient's symptoms may be that his or her circulating concentration of thyroid hormone was elevated. This might occur if the person's thyroid was overstimulated due, for example, to thyroid disease. The control of the anterior pituitary gland by a very small number of discrete neurons within the hypothalamus.

Figure 11.21 Iodine is not widely found in foods; in the absence of iodized salt, an acute or chronic deficiency in dietary iodine is possible. The colloid permits a long-term store of iodinated thyroglobulin that can be used during times when dietary iodine intake is reduced or absent.

Figure 11.24 Plasma cortisol concentrations would increase. This would result in decreased ACTH concentrations in the systemic blood, and CRH concentrations in the portal vein blood, due to increased negative feedback at the pituitary gland and hypothalamus, respectively. The right adrenal gland would shrink in size (atrophy) as a consequence of the decreased ACTH concentrations (decreased "trophic" stimulation of the adrenal cortex).

Figure 11.28 Note from the figure that a decrease in plasma glucose concentrations results in an increase in growth hormone concentrations. This makes sense, because one of the metabolic actions of growth hormone is to increase the concentrations will decrease. This is a form of secondary hypoparathyroidism.

Visit this book's website at **www.mhhe.com/widmaier13** for chapter quizzes, interactive learning exercises, and other study tools.

connect | HUMAN PHYSIOLOGY

Anatomy & Physiology REVEALED aprevealed.com

Updates and Additions

In addition to updating material throughout the text to reflect cutting-edge changes in physiology and medicine, the authors have introduced the following:

- A new unifying theme has been integrated into all chapters based on fundamental, key principles of physiology. These are outlined in Chapter 1 in a new section called General Principles of Physiology, and include such things as homeostasis, structure/function relationships, information flow, and several others. Beginning with Chapter 2, the introduction to each chapter provides a preview for the student of the general principles that will be covered in that chapter. Within the chapter, the principles are reinforced where appropriate. At the end of each chapter, one or more assessments are provided that enable the student to relate the material in that chapter to an understanding of unifying physiological themes.
- The number of Test Questions and Quantitative and Thought Questions has been expanded. These assessments complement the many test questions available free of charge to students on the McGraw-Hill website that accompanies the textbook.
- The Physiological Inquiries feature has been retained and expanded. Continued positive feedback from users of the text indicated that this learning tool is extremely valuable, and thus we have added additional inquiries associated with key figures.

In addition to new assessments, and the usual editing to make sure the text remains even more reader-friendly, up-to-date, and accurate, approximately 25 new pieces of art have been added, and another 25 existing pieces of art have been considerably modified to provide updated information. A sampling of substantive changes to each chapter follows.

Chapter 1 Homeostasis: A Framework for Human Physiology

New section introducing and describing the important General Principles of Physiology, providing an instructional framework that unifies all the chapters.

Chapter 2 Chemical Composition of the Body

Increased emphasis on the physiological relevance of chemical principles; expanded discussion of the use of isotopes in physiology with a new PET scan figure; ionic bonds treated in a new section.

Chapter 3 Cellular Structure, Proteins, and Metabolism

Importance of cholesterol in determining membrane fluidity is now discussed and illustrated.

Chapter 4 Movement of Molecules Across Cell Membranes

Compensatory endocytosis now discussed.

Chapter 5 Control of Cells by Chemical Messengers

Illustrations of receptor conformations with and without bound ligand are now depicted to emphasize binding-induced shape changes linked to receptor activation; IP_3 receptor/ion channel now depicted in illustration of cell signaling.

Chapter 6 Neuronal Signaling and the Structure of the Nervous System

New discussion about the use of adult stem cells to treat neurological diseases; new figure illustrating the way in which synapses that increase chloride conductance stabilize the membrane potential.

Chapter 7 Sensory Physiology

A new table has been added summarizing the general principles of sensory stimulus processing; discussion of Müller cells added to section on retinal function; expanded discussion and illustration of the mechanism by which retinal dissociates from its opsin and is enzymatically reassociated.

Chapter 8 Consciousness, the Brain, and Behavior

A comparison between PET, MRI, and EEG as effective tools for assessing tumors, clots, or hemorrhages in the brain has been added; new discussion of high-frequency gamma-wave patterns; updated the NREM designations to the new Phase N1–N3 nomenclature; discussion of hypnic jerk movements added; new section added describing the neural basis of the conscious state, including the role of RAS monoamine, orexins/hypocretins, and the "sleep center" of the brain; discussion of narcolepsy; new discussion regarding the role of the right cerebral hemisphere in the emotional context of language; new figure illustrating brain regions involved in consciousness; a new figure showing a model of the regulation of sleep/wake transitions; new figure of a CT scan of the brain of a person with an epidural hemorrhage.

Chapter 9 Muscle

A new figure illustrating cardiac muscle excitation–contraction coupling; reorganization of the first two sections of the chapter such that events are described in the order in which they occur: excitation, E–C coupling, sliding filament mechanism; updated discussion about muscle fatigue; new discussion about myostatin and its role in muscle mass; new discussion about caldesmon's role in smooth muscle function.

Chapter 10 Control of Body Movement

Interconnections of structures participating in the motor control hierarchy have been updated; new example demonstrating the importance of association areas in motor control.

Chapter 11 The Endocrine System

Role of pendrin in thyroid hormone synthesis now introduced and illustrated; steroid synthetic pathway simplified to illustrate major events; improved illustration of anatomical relationship between hypothalamus and anterior pituitary gland; addition of numerous specific examples to highlight general principles, such as hyporesponsiveness; new figure showing production of insulin from proinsulin.

Chapter 12 Cardiovascular Physiology

Numerous figures have been updated or improved for clarity, or modified to include additional important information; discussion added about internodal pathways between the SA and AV nodes; new description about transient outward K^+ channels in myocytes; new table added comparing hemodynamics of systemic and pulmonary circuits; new discussion about VEGF antibodies and angiogenesis; section on hypertension has been updated to include the latest information about the effects of a high-salt diet, the findings of the DASH diet study, and other environmental causes or links to hypertension.

Chapter 13 Respiratory Physiology

New information about the cystic fibrosis channel mutation and treatment of cystic fibrosis; new figure showing the muscles of respiration; new improved illustration of respiratory cycle; enhanced illustration of the factors that change the shape of the O_2 dissociation curve including a panel on fetal hemoglobin; new figure on brainstem respiratory control centers and simplification of the description of respiratory control.

Chapter 14 The Kidneys and Regulation of Water and Inorganic Ions

New figure showing major anatomical structures of the kidney; new figure and text describing the effects of vasopressin on the volume and osmolarity of the filtrate along the length of the nephron; revised and expanded discussion of the local and central control of micturition.

Chapter 15 The Digestion and Absorption of Food

New figure and text updating the control of bicarbonate secretion in the pancreatic duct cells and the role of the cystic fibrosis transmembrane conductance regulator (CFTR) in this process; reorganization of portions of the text to improve the flow of the chapter.

Chapter 16 Regulation of Organic Metabolism and Energy Balance

New figure on energy expenditure during common activities; streamlined text with greater emphasis on general principles of physiology.

Chapter 17 Reproduction

Reorganization of first two sections into a single new section entitled Gametogenesis, Sex Determination, and Sex Differentiation; General Principles of Reproductive Endocrinology; several new figures illustrating the events of gametogenesis, embryonic development of the male and female reproductive tracts, development of external genitalia in males and females, and synthesis of gonadal steroids; new section on anabolic steroid use.

Chapter 18 The Immune System

Additional artwork and photographs including a new micrograph of a human blood smear, a new micrograph of a leukocyte undergoing diapedesis, and a computer model of an immunoglobulin.

Chapter 19 Medical Physiology: Integration Using Clinical Cases

This chapter reinforces the General Physiological Principles introduced in Chapter 1 by demonstrating how these principles relate to human disease.

Teaching and Learning Supplements

NEW! McGraw-Hill LearnSmart™

McGraw-Hill LearnSmart™ is an online diagnostic learning system that determines the level of student knowledge, and feeds the students suitable content for their physiology course. Students learn faster and study more effectively. As a student works within the system, LearnSmart develops a personal learning path adapted to what the student has learned and retained. LearnSmart is able to recommend additional study resources to help the student master topics. This innovative and outstanding study tool also has features for instructors where they can see exactly what students have accomplished, and a built-in assessment tool for graded assignments.

For more information, go to www.mhlearnsmart.com.

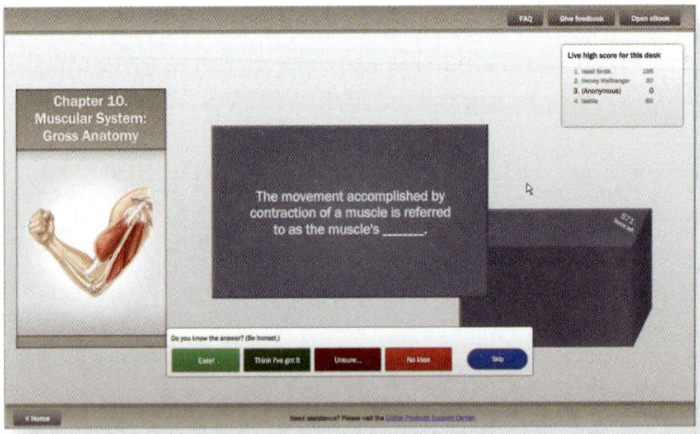

McGraw-Hill Connect™ Anatomy & Physiology

This Web-based assignment and assessment platform that gives students the means to better connect with their coursework, with their instructors, and with the important concepts that they will need to know for success now and in the future.

With Connect, instructors can deliver assignments, quizzes, and tests online. Questions are presented in an auto-gradable format and tied to the organization of the textbook. Instructors can edit existing questions and author entirely new problems; track individual student performance—by question, assignment, or in relation to the class overall—with detailed grade reports; integrate grade reports easily with learning management systems (LMS) such as WebCT and Blackboard; and much more. By choosing Connect, instructors are providing their students with a powerful tool for improving academic performance and truly mastering course material. Connect allows students to practice important skills at their own pace and on their own schedule.

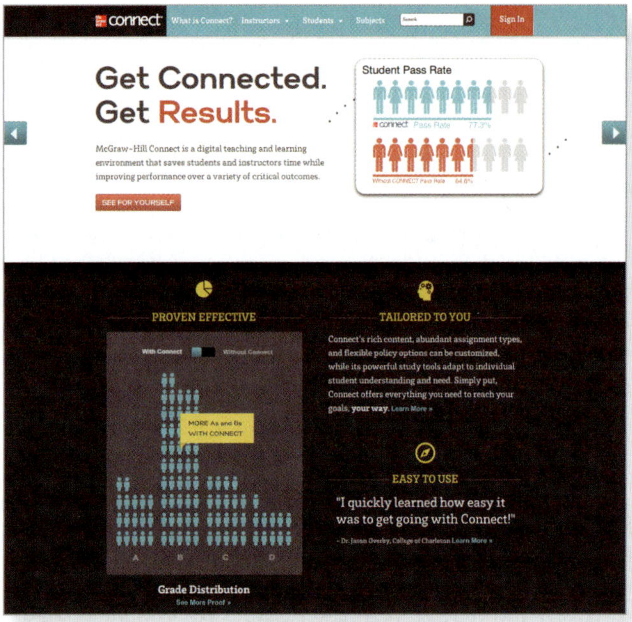

Importantly, students' assessment results and instructors' feedback are all saved online—so students can continually review their progress and plot their course to success.

Some instructors may also choose ConnectPlus™ for their students. Like Connect, ConnectPlus provides students with online assignments and assessments, plus 24/7 online access to an eBook—an online edition of the text—to aid them in successfully completing their work, wherever and whenever they choose.

Physiology Interactive Lab Simulations (Ph.I.L.S.)

NEW! Ph.I.L.S. 4.0 has been updated! Users have requested and we are providing ***five new exercises*** (Respiratory Quotient, Weight & Contraction, Insulin and Glucose Tolerance, Blood Typing, and Anti-Diuretic Hormone).

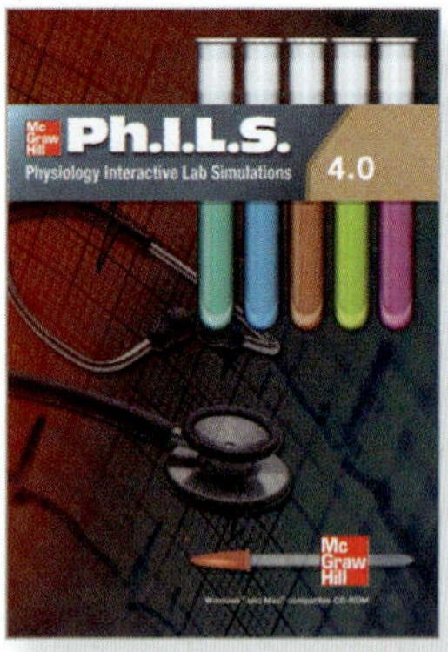

Ph.I.L.S. 4.0 is the perfect way to reinforce key physiology concepts with powerful lab experiments. Created by Dr. Phil Stephens at Villanova University, this program offers ***42 laboratory simulations*** that may be used to supplement or substitute for wet labs. All 42 labs are self-contained experiments—no lengthy instruction manual required. Users can adjust variables, view outcomes, make predictions, draw conclusions, and print lab reports. This easy-to-use software offers the flexibility to change the parameters of the lab experiment. There is no limit!

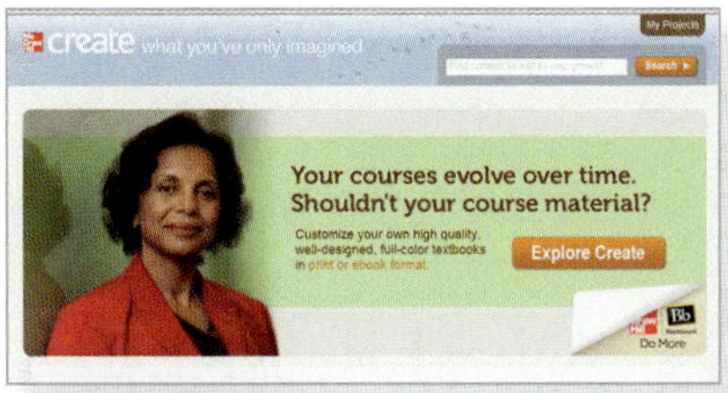

Craft your teaching resources to match the way you teach! With McGraw-Hill Create™, www.mcgrawhillcreate.com, you can easily rearrange chapters, combine material from other content sources, and quickly upload content you have written, like your course syllabus or teaching notes. Find the content you need in Create by searching through thousands of leading McGraw-Hill textbooks. Arrange your book to fit your teaching style. Create even allows you to personalize your book's appearance by selecting the cover and adding your name, school, and course information. Order a Create book and you'll receive a complimentary print review copy in 3–5 business days or a complimentary electronic review copy (eComp) via e-mail in minutes. Go to www.mcgrawhillcreate.com today and register to experience how McGraw-Hill Create™ empowers you to teach *your* students *your* way.

Text Website—www.mhhe.com/widmaier13

The text website that accompanies this text offers an extensive array of learning and teaching tools.

- Interactive Activities—Fun and exciting learning experiences await the student at *Vander's Human Physiology* text website. Chapters offer a series of interactive activities like art labeling, animations, vocabulary flashcards, and more!
- Practice Quizzes at the *Vander's Human Physiology* text website contain hundreds of test questions that gauge student mastery of chapter content. Each chapter quiz is specifically constructed to test student comprehension of key concepts. Immediate feedback to student responses explains why an answer is correct or incorrect.
- Presentation Center is an online digital library containing assets such as photos, artwork, animations, and PowerPoints that can be used to create customized lectures, visually enhanced tests and quizzes, compelling course website, or attractive printed support materials.

Test Bank

Written by the textbook authors, a computerized test bank that uses testing software to quickly create customized exams is available for this text. The user-friendly program allows instructors to search for questions by topic or format, edit existing questions or add new ones, and scramble questions for multiple versions of the same test. Word files of the test bank questions are provided for those instructors who prefer to work outside the test-generator software.

Instructor's Manual

The Instructor's Manual is available on the text website (www.mhhe.com/widmaier13). It contains teaching/learning objectives, sample lecture outlines, and the answers to Review Questions for each chapter.

The Best of Both Worlds

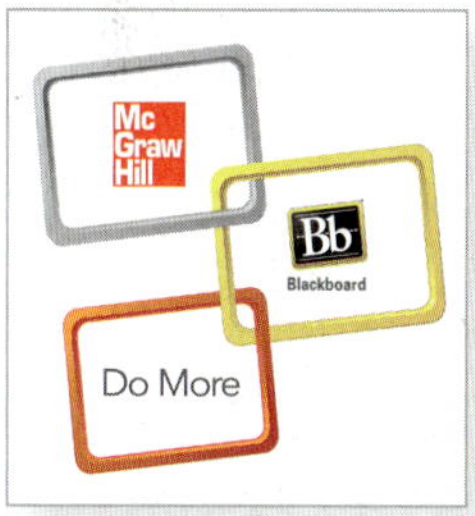

McGraw-Hill and Blackboard®

McGraw-Hill Higher Education and Blackboard have teamed up. What does this partnership mean for you? Blackboard users will find the single sign-on and deep Integration of ConnectPlus within their Blackboard course an invaluable benefit. Even if your school is not using Blackboard, we have a solution for you. Learn more at www.domorenow.com.

Acknowledgments

The authors are deeply indebted to the following individuals for their contributions to the thirteenth edition of *Vander's Human Physiology*. Their feedback on the twelfth edition or their critique of the revised text provided invaluable assistance and greatly improved the final product. Any errors that may remain are solely the responsibility of the authors.

Allan Albig, *Indiana State University*
Lisa Carney Anderson, *University of Minnesota*
Heather Wilson-Ashworth, *Utah Valley University*
Kim Barrett, *University of California, San Diego*
Daniel Bergman, *Grand Valley State University*
Nicole Berthelemy, *Weber State University*
Robert W. Blair, *University of Oklahoma Health Sciences Center*
Eric Blough, *Marshall University*
Carol A. Britson, *University of Mississippi*
George A. Brooks, *University of California–Berkeley*
Martin G. Burg, *Grand Valley State University*
Patricia Cai, *Brooklyn College of CUNY*
Edwin R. Chapman, *University of Wisconsin–Madison*
Pat Clark, *IUPUI*
Maria Elena de Bellard, *CSUN*
Lee D. Faucher, *University of Wisconsin–Madison SMPH*
James S. Ferraro, *Southern Illinois University–School of Medicine*
Margaret Flanigan Skinner, *University of Wyoming*
Kennon M. Garrett, *University of Oklahoma Health Sciences Center*
Nicholas Geist, *Sonoma State University*
Brian Geraghty, *CUNY @ Brooklyn College & Kingsborough Community College*
Chaya Gopalan, *St. Louis College of Pharmacy*
Marion Greaser, *University of Wisconsin–Madison*
Eric Green, *Salt Lake Community College*
Chi-Ming Hai, *Brown University*
Janet L. Haynes, *Long Island University*
Steve Henderson, *California State University*
David W. Johnson, *University of New England*
Kelly Johnson, *Kansas University*
Tim Juergens, *University of Wisconsin–Madison SMPH*
Kenneth Kaloustian, *Quinnipiac University*
David King, *Nova Southeastern University*
Brian H. Kipp, *Grand Valley State University*
Sumana Koduri, *Medical College of Wisconsin*
Dean V. Lauritzen, *City College of San Francisco*
Mingyu Liang, *Medical College of Wisconsin*
Christian Lytle, *University of California, Riverside*
Steven Magill, *Medical College of Wisconsin*
David L. Mattson, *Medical College of Wisconsin*
Donald W. Michielli, *Brooklyn College of the City University of New York*
Kevin Middleton, *California State University*
Paul Nealen, *Indiana University of PA*
Lisa Parks, *North Carolina State University*
Mark Paternostro, *West Virginia University*
Timothy Plagge, *San Diego Mesa College*
Jocelyn Parks Ramos, *Ivy Tech Community College*
Laurel B. Roberts, *University of Pittsburgh*
Angela M. Seliga, *Boston University*
Virginia K. Shea, *University of North Carolina*
Mark Smith, *Santiago Canyon College*
Andrea Sobieraj, *Brown University*
Nadja Spitzer, *Marshall University*
Ruy Tchao, *University of the Sciences*
Dana K. Vaughan, *University of Wisconsin–Oshkosh*
Gordon M. Wahler, *Midwestern University*
R. Douglas Watson, *University of Alabama at Birmingham*
Eliot Williams, *University of Wisconsin–Madison SMPH*
Loren E. Wold, *The Research Institute at Nationwide Children's Hospital/The Ohio State University*
Yuri Zagvazdin, *Nova Southeastern University*

The authors are indebted to the many individuals who assisted with the numerous digital and ancillary products associated with these text. Thank you to Beth Altschafl, Patti Atkins, Janet Casagrand, Patricia Clark, Mike Griffin, David Johnson, Tami Mau, Carla Reinstadtl, Laurel Bridges Roberts, Rebecca Sheller, Andrea Jeanne Sobieraj, Nadja Spitzer, and Melanie Waite-Wright.

The authors are also indebted to the editors and staff at McGraw-Hill Higher Education who contributed to the development and publication of this text, particularly Developmental Editor Fran Simon, Brand Manager Marija Magner, Project Manager Sherry Kane, Production Supervisor Sandy Ludovissy, Designer Tara McDermott, and Photo Researcher John Leland. We also thank freelance copy editor C. Jeanne Patterson and freelance proofreader Beatrice Sussman. As always, we are grateful to the many students and faculty who have provided us with critiques and suggestions for improvement.

Eric P. Widmaier
Hershel Raff
Kevin T. Strang

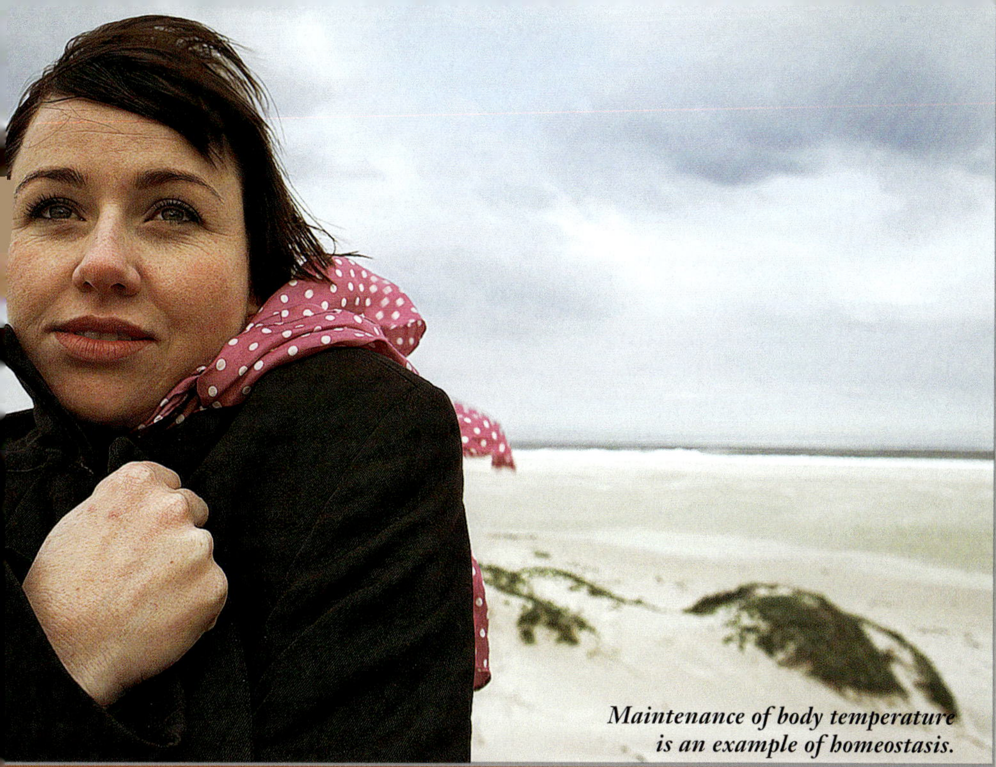

Maintenance of body temperature is an example of homeostasis.

1 Homeostasis:

A FRAMEWORK FOR HUMAN PHYSIOLOGY

The purpose of this chapter is to provide an orientation to the subject of human physiology and the central role of homeostasis in the study of this science. An understanding of the functions of the body also requires knowledge of the structures and relationships of the body parts. For this reason, this chapter also introduces the way the body is organized into cells, tissues, organs, and organ systems. Lastly, several "General Principles of Physiology" are introduced. These serve as unifying themes throughout the textbook, and the student is encouraged to return to them often to see how they apply to the material covered in subsequent chapters.

1.1 The Scope of Human Physiology

Physiology is the study of how living organisms function. As applied to human beings, its scope is extremely broad. At one end of the spectrum, it includes the study of individual molecules—for example, how a particular protein's shape and electrical properties allow it to function as a channel for ions to move into or out of a cell. At the other end, it is concerned with complex processes that depend on the integrated functions of many organs in the body—for example, how the heart, kidneys, and several glands all work together to cause the excretion of more sodium ions in the urine when a person has eaten salty food.

Physiologists are interested in function and integration—how parts of the body work together at various levels of organization and, most importantly, in the entire organism. Even when physiologists study parts of organisms, all the way down to individual molecules, the intention is ultimately to apply the information they gain to understanding the function of the whole body. As the nineteenth-century physiologist Claude Bernard put it, "After carrying out an analysis of phenomena, we must . . . always reconstruct our physiological synthesis, so as to see the *joint action* of all the parts we have isolated. . . ."

In this regard, a very important point must be made about the present and future status of physiology. It is easy for a student to gain the impression from a textbook that almost everything is known about the subject, but nothing could be farther from the truth for physiology. Many areas of function are still only poorly understood, such as how the workings of the brain produce conscious thought and memory.

Finally, in many areas of this text, we will relate physiology to medicine. Some disease states can be viewed as physiology "gone wrong," or **pathophysiology,** which makes an understanding of physiology essential for the study and practice of medicine. Indeed, many physiologists are actively engaged in research on the physiological bases of a wide range of diseases. In this text, we will give many examples of pathophysiology to illustrate the basic physiology that underlies the disease. A handy index of all the diseases and medical conditions discussed in this text appears in Appendix B. We begin our study of physiology by describing the organization of the structures of the human body.

1.2 How Is the Body Organized?

Before exploring how the human body works, it is necessary to understand the components of the body and their anatomical relationships to each other. The simplest structural units into which a complex multicellular organism can be divided and still retain the functions characteristic of life are called **cells** (**Figure 1.1**). Each human being begins as a single cell, a fertilized egg, which divides to create two cells, each of which divides in turn to result in four cells, and so on. If cell multiplication were the only event occurring, the end result would be a spherical mass of identical cells. During development, however, each cell

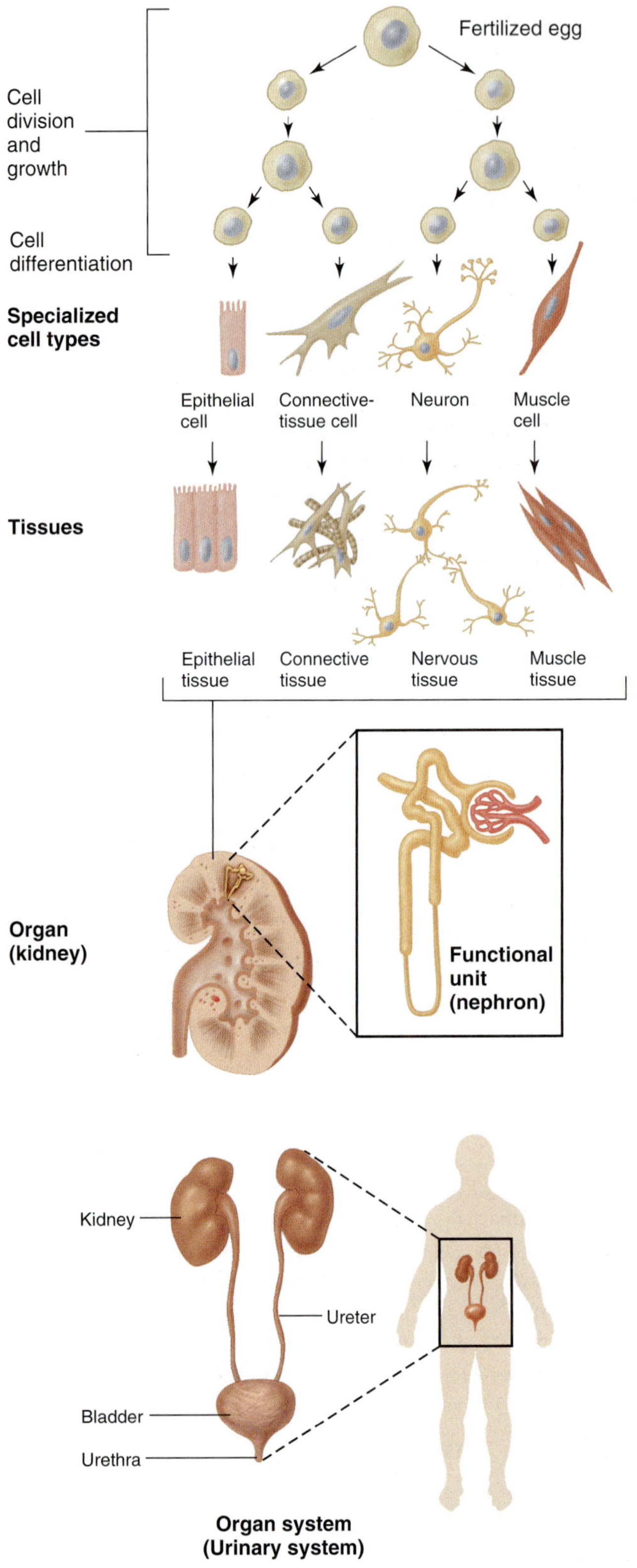

Figure 1.1 Levels of cellular organization. The nephron is not drawn to scale.

becomes specialized for the performance of a particular function, such as producing force and movement or generating electrical signals. The process of transforming an unspecialized cell into a specialized cell is known as **cell**

differentiation, the study of which is one of the most exciting areas in biology today. About 200 distinct kinds of cells can be identified in the body in terms of differences in structure and function. When cells are classified according to the broad types of function they perform, however, four major categories emerge: (1) muscle cells, (2) neurons, (3) epithelial cells, and (4) connective-tissue cells. In each of these functional categories, several cell types perform variations of the specialized function. For example, there are three types of muscle cells—skeletal, cardiac, and smooth. These cells differ from each other in shape, in the mechanisms controlling their contractile activity, and in their location in the various organs of the body, but each of them is a muscle cell.

In addition to differentiating, cells migrate to new locations during development and form selective adhesions with other cells to produce multicellular structures. In this manner, the cells of the body arrange themselves in various combinations to form a hierarchy of organized structures. Differentiated cells with similar properties aggregate to form **tissues.** Corresponding to the four general categories of differentiated cells, there are four general types of tissues: (1) **muscle tissue,** (2) **nervous tissue,** (3) **epithelial tissue,** and (4) **connective tissue.** The term *tissue* is used in different ways. It is formally defined as an aggregate of a single type of specialized cell. However, it is also commonly used to denote the general cellular fabric of any organ or structure—for example, kidney tissue or lung tissue, each of which in fact usually contains all four types of tissue.

One type of tissue combines with other types of tissues to form **organs,** such as the heart, lungs, and kidneys. Organs, in turn, work together as **organ systems,** such as the urinary system (see Figure 1.1). We turn now to a brief discussion of each of the four general types of cells and tissues that make up the organs of the human body.

Muscle Cells and Tissue

As noted earlier, there are three types of muscle cells. These cells form skeletal, cardiac, or smooth muscle tissue. All **muscle cells** are specialized to generate mechanical force. Skeletal muscle cells are attached through other structures to bones and produce movements of the limbs or trunk. They are also attached to skin, such as the muscles producing facial expressions. Contraction of skeletal muscle is under voluntary control, which simply means that you can choose to contract a skeletal muscle whenever you wish. Cardiac muscle cells are found only in the heart. When cardiac muscle cells generate force, the heart contracts and consequently pumps blood into the circulation. Smooth muscle cells surround many of the tubes in the body—blood vessels, for example, or the tubes of the gastrointestinal tract—and their contraction decreases the diameter or shortens the length of these tubes. For example, contraction of smooth muscle cells along the esophagus—the tube leading from the pharynx to the stomach—helps "squeeze" swallowed food down to the stomach. Cardiac and smooth muscle tissues are said to be "involuntary" muscle, because you cannot consciously alter the activity of these types of muscle. You will learn about the structure and function of each of the three types of muscle cells in Chapter 9.

Neurons and Nervous Tissue

A **neuron** is a cell of the nervous system that is specialized to initiate, integrate, and conduct electrical signals to other cells, sometimes over long distances. A signal may initiate new electrical signals in other neurons, or it may stimulate a gland cell to secrete substances or a muscle cell to contract. Thus, neurons provide a major means of controlling the activities of other cells. The incredible complexity of connections between neurons underlies such phenomena as consciousness and perception. A collection of neurons forms nervous tissue, such as that of the brain or spinal cord. In some parts of the body, cellular extensions from many neurons are packaged together along with connective tissue (described shortly); these neuron extensions form a nerve, which carries the signals from many neurons between the nervous system and other parts of the body. Neurons, nervous tissue, and the nervous system will be covered in Chapter 6.

Epithelial Cells and Epithelial Tissue

Epithelial cells are specialized for the selective secretion and absorption of ions and organic molecules, and for protection. These cells are characterized and named according to their unique shapes, including cuboidal (cube-shaped), columnar (elongated), squamous (flattened), and ciliated. Epithelial tissue (known as an epithelium) may form from any type of epithelial cell. Epithelia may be arranged in single-cell-thick tissue, called a simple epithelium, or a thicker tissue consisting of numerous layers of cells, called a stratified epithelium. The type of epithelium that forms in a given region of the body reflects the function of that particular epithelium. For example, the epithelium that lines the inner surface of the main airway, the trachea, consists of ciliated epithelial cells (see Chapter 13). The beating of these cilia helps propel mucus up the trachea and into the mouth, which aids in preventing airborne particles and pollutants from reaching the sensitive lung tissue.

Epithelia are located at the surfaces that cover the body or individual organs, and they line the inner surfaces of the tubular and hollow structures within the body, such as the trachea just mentioned. Epithelial cells rest on an extracellular protein layer called the **basement membrane,** which (among other functions) anchors the tissue (**Figure 1.2**). The side of the cell anchored to the basement membrane is called the basolateral side; the opposite side, which typically faces the interior (called the lumen) of a structure such as the trachea or the tubules of the kidney (see Figure 1.1), is called the apical side. A defining feature of many epithelia is that the two sides of all the epithelial cells in the tissue may perform different physiological functions. In addition, the cells are held together along their lateral surfaces by extracellular barriers called tight junctions (look ahead to Figure 3.9, b and c, for a depiction of tight junctions). Tight junctions enable epithelia to form boundaries between body compartments and to function as selective barriers regulating the exchange of molecules. For

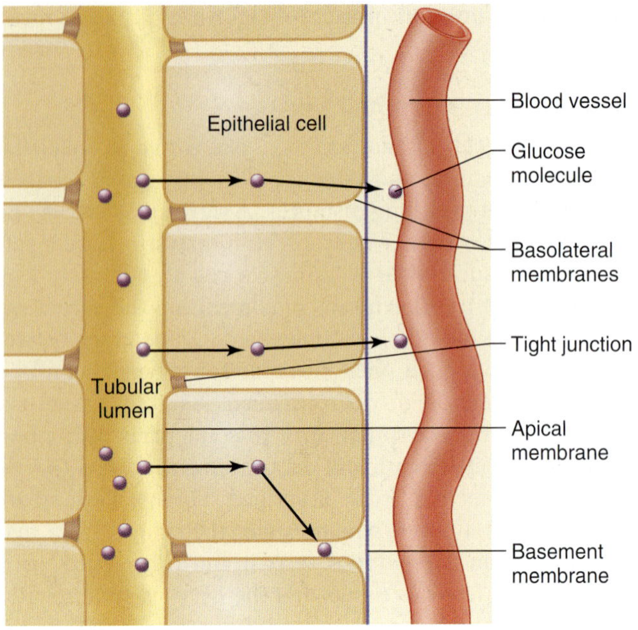

Figure 1.2 Epithelial tissue lining the inside of a structure such as a kidney tubule. The basolateral side of the cell is attached to a basement membrane. Each side of the cell can perform different functions, as in this example in which glucose is moved across the epithelium, first directed into the cell, and then directed out of the cell.

example, the epithelial cells at the surface of the skin form a barrier that prevents most substances in the external environment from entering the body through the skin. In the kidney tubules, the apical membranes transport useful solutes such as the sugar glucose from the tubule lumen into the epithelial cell; the basolateral sides of the cells transport glucose out of the cell and into the surrounding fluid where it can reach the bloodstream. The tight junctions prevent glucose from leaking "backward."

Connective-Tissue Cells and Connective Tissue

Connective-tissue cells, as their name implies, connect, anchor, and support the structures of the body. Some connective-tissue cells are found in the loose meshwork of cells and fibers underlying most epithelial layers; this is called loose connective tissue. Another type called dense connective tissue includes the tough, rigid tissue that makes up tendons and ligaments. Other types of connective tissue include bone, cartilage, and adipose (fat-storing) tissue. Finally, blood is a type of fluid connective tissue. This is because the cells in the blood have the same embryonic origin as other connective tissue, and because the blood connects the various organs and tissues of the body through the delivery of nutrients, removal of wastes, and transport of chemical signals from one part of the body to another.

An important function of some connective tissue is to form the **extracellular matrix** (ECM) around cells. The immediate environment that surrounds each individual cell in the body is the **extracellular fluid.** Actually, this fluid is interspersed within a complex ECM consisting of a mixture of proteins; polysaccharides (chains of sugar molecules); and, in some cases, minerals, specific for any given tissue. The matrix serves two general functions: (1) it provides a scaffold for cellular attachments; and (2) it transmits information in the form of chemical messengers to the cells to help regulate their activity, migration, growth, and differentiation.

The proteins of the extracellular matrix consist of proteins called **fibers**—ropelike **collagen fibers** and rubberband-like **elastin fibers**—and a mixture of nonfibrous proteins that contain carbohydrate. In some ways, the extracellular matrix is analogous to reinforced concrete. The fibers of the matrix, particularly collagen, which constitutes as much as one-third of all bodily proteins, are like the reinforcing iron mesh or rods in the concrete. The carbohydrate-containing protein molecules are analogous to the surrounding cement. However, these latter molecules are not merely inert packing material, as in concrete, but function as adhesion or recognition molecules between cells. Thus, they are links in the communication between extracellular messenger molecules and cells.

Organs and Organ Systems

Organs are composed of two or more of the four kinds of tissues arranged in various proportions and patterns, such as sheets, tubes, layers, bundles, and strips. For example, the kidneys consist of (1) a series of small tubes, each composed of a simple epithelium; (2) blood vessels, whose walls contain varying quantities of smooth muscle and connective tissue; (3) extensions from neurons that end near the muscle and epithelial cells; (4) a loose network of connective-tissue elements that are interspersed throughout the kidneys and include the protective capsule that surrounds the organ.

Many organs are organized into small, similar subunits often referred to as **functional units,** each performing the function of the organ. For example, the functional unit of the kidney, the nephron, contains the small tubes mentioned in the previous paragraph. The total production of urine by the kidneys is the sum of the amounts produced by the 2 million or so individual nephrons.

Finally, we have the organ system, a collection of organs that together perform an overall function. For example, the kidneys; the urinary bladder; the ureters, the tubes leading from the kidneys to the bladder; and the urethra, the tube leading from the bladder to the exterior, constitute the urinary system. **Table 1.1** lists the components and functions of the organ systems in the body.

To sum up, the human body can be viewed as a complex society of differentiated cells that combine structurally and functionally to carry out the functions essential to the survival of the entire organism. The individual cells constitute the basic units of this society, and almost all of these cells individually exhibit the fundamental activities common to all forms of life, such as metabolism and replication. Key to the survival of all body cells is the **internal environment** of the body; this refers to the fluids that surround cells and exist in the blood. These fluid compartments and one other—that which exists inside cells—are described next.

TABLE 1.1	Organ Systems of the Body	
System	**Major Organs or Tissues**	**Primary Functions**
Circulatory	Heart, blood vessels, blood	Transport of blood throughout the body
Digestive	Mouth, salivary glands, pharynx, esophagus, stomach, small and large intestines, anus, pancreas, liver, gallbladder	Digestion and absorption of nutrients and water; elimination of wastes
Endocrine	All glands or organs secreting hormones: Pancreas, testes, ovaries, hypothalamus, kidneys, pituitary, thyroid, parathyroids, adrenals, stomach, small intestine, liver, adipose tissue, heart, and pineal gland; and endocrine cells in other organs	Regulation and coordination of many activities in the body, including growth, metabolism, reproduction, blood pressure, water and electrolyte balance, and others
Immune	White blood cells and their organs of production	Defense against pathogens
Integumentary	Skin	Protection against injury and dehydration; defense against pathogens; regulation of body temperature
Lymphatic	Lymph vessels, lymph nodes	Collection of extracellular fluid for return to blood; participation in immune defenses; absorption of fats from digestive system
Musculoskeletal	Cartilage, bone, ligaments, tendons, joints, skeletal muscle	Support, protection, and movement of the body; production of blood cells
Nervous	Brain, spinal cord, peripheral nerves and ganglia, sense organs	Regulation and coordination of many activities in the body; detection of and response to changes in the internal and external environments; states of consciousness; learning; memory; emotion; others
Reproductive	Male: Testes, penis, and associated ducts and glands Female: Ovaries, fallopian tubes, uterus, vagina, mammary glands	Male: Production of sperm; transfer of sperm to female Female: Production of eggs; provision of a nutritive environment for the developing embryo and fetus; nutrition of the infant
Respiratory	Nose, pharynx, larynx, trachea, bronchi, lungs	Exchange of carbon dioxide and oxygen; regulation of hydrogen ion concentration in the body fluids
Urinary	Kidneys, ureters, bladder, urethra	Regulation of plasma composition through controlled excretion of salts, water, and organic wastes

1.3 Body Fluid Compartments

Water is present within and around the cells of the body, and within all the blood vessels. When we refer to "body fluids," we are referring to a watery solution of dissolved substances such as oxygen, nutrients, and wastes. Body fluids exist in two major compartments, intracellular fluid and extracellular fluid. **Intracellular fluid** is the fluid contained within all the cells of the body and accounts for about 67% of all the fluid in the body. Collectively, the fluid present in the blood and in the spaces surrounding cells is called **extracellular fluid,** that is, all the fluid that is outside of cells. Of this, only about 20%–25% is in the fluid portion of blood, which is called the **plasma,** in which the various blood cells are suspended. The remaining 75%–80% of the extracellular fluid, which lies around and between cells, is known as the **interstitial fluid.** The space containing interstitial fluid is called the **interstitium.** Therefore, the total volume of extracellular fluid is the sum of the plasma and interstitial volumes. **Figure 1.3** summarizes the relative volumes of water in the different fluid compartments of the body. Water accounts for about 55%–60% of body weight in an adult.

As the blood flows through the smallest of blood vessels in all parts of the body, the plasma exchanges oxygen, nutrients, wastes, and other substances with the interstitial fluid. Because of these exchanges, concentrations of dissolved substances are virtually identical in the plasma and interstitial fluid, except for protein concentration (which, as you will learn in Chapter 12, remains higher in plasma than in interstitial fluid). With this major exception, the entire extracellular fluid may be considered to have a homogeneous solute composition. In contrast, the composition of the extracellular

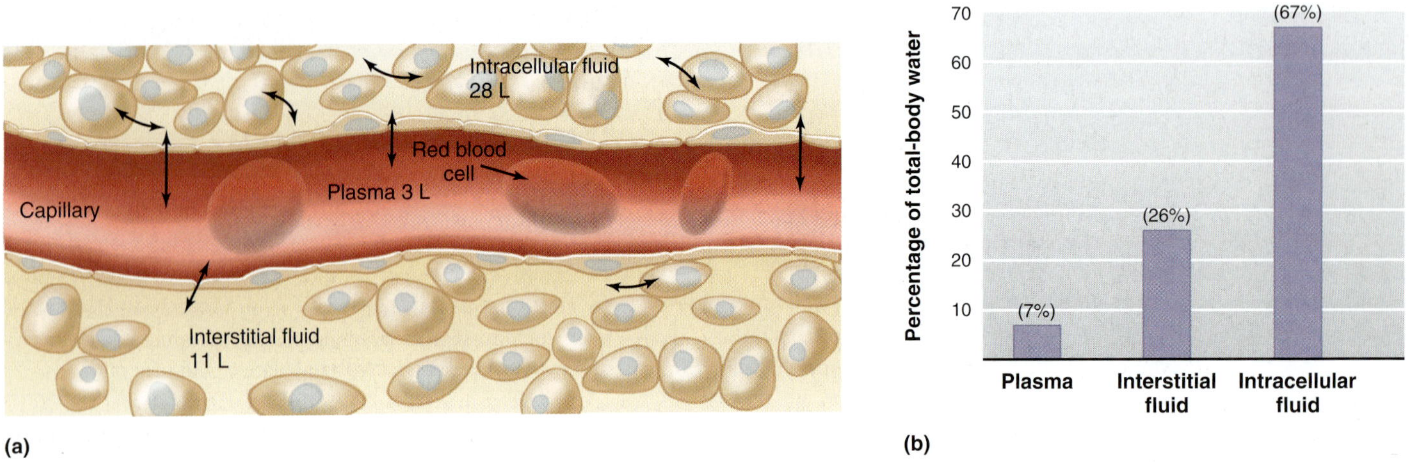

Figure 1.3 Fluid compartments of the body. Volumes are for an average 70-kilogram (kg) (154-pound [lb]) person. (a) The bidirectional arrows indicate that fluid can move between any two adjacent compartments. Total-body water is about 42 liters (L), which makes up about 55%–60% of body weight. (b) The approximate percentage of total-body water normally found in each compartment.

PHYSIOLOGICAL INQUIRY

- What fraction of total-body water is extracellular? Assume that water constitutes 60% of a person's body weight. What fraction of this person's body weight is due to extracellular body water?

Answer can be found at end of chapter.

fluid is very different from that of the intracellular fluid. Maintaining differences in fluid composition across the cell membrane is an important way in which cells regulate their own activity. For example, intracellular fluid contains many different proteins that are important in regulating cellular events such as growth and metabolism. These proteins must be retained within the intracellular fluid and are not required in the extracellular fluid.

Compartmentalization is an important feature of physiology and is achieved by barriers between the compartments. The properties of the barriers determine which substances can move between compartments. These movements, in turn, account for the differences in composition of the different compartments. In the case of the body fluid compartments, plasma membranes that surround each cell separate the intracellular fluid from the extracellular fluid. Chapters 3 and 4 describe the properties of plasma membranes and how they account for the profound differences between intracellular and extracellular fluid. In contrast, the two components of extracellular fluid—the interstitial fluid and the plasma—are separated by the wall of the blood vessels. Chapter 12 discusses how this barrier normally keeps 75%–80% of the extracellular fluid in the interstitial compartment and restricts proteins mainly to the plasma.

With this understanding of the structural organization of the body, we turn to a description of how balance is achieved in the internal environment of the body.

1.4 Homeostasis: A Defining Feature of Physiology

From the earliest days of physiology—at least as early as the time of Aristotle—physicians recognized that good health was somehow associated with a balance among the multiple life-sustaining forces ("humours") in the body. It would take millennia, however, for scientists to determine what it was that was being balanced and how this balance was achieved. The advent of modern tools of science, including the ordinary microscope, led to the discovery that the human body is composed of trillions of cells, each of which can permit movement of certain substances—but not others—across the cell membrane. Over the course of the nineteenth and twentieth centuries, it became clear that most cells are in contact with the interstitial fluid. The interstitial fluid, in turn, was found to be in a state of flux, with water and solutes such as ions and gases moving back and forth through it between the cell interiors and the blood in nearby capillaries (see Figure 1.3).

It was further determined by careful observation that most of the common physiological variables found in healthy organisms such as humans—blood pressure; body temperature; and blood-borne factors such as oxygen, glucose, and sodium ions, for example—are maintained within a predictable range. This is true despite external environmental conditions that may be far from constant. Thus was born the idea, first put forth by Claude Bernard, of a constant internal environment that is a prerequisite for good health, a concept later refined by the American physiologist Walter Cannon, who coined the term *homeostasis*.

Originally, **homeostasis** was defined as a state of reasonably stable balance between physiological variables such as those just described. However, this simple definition cannot give one a complete appreciation of what homeostasis entails. There probably is no such thing as a physiological variable that is constant over long periods of time. In fact, some variables undergo fairly dramatic swings around an average value during the course of a day, yet are still considered to be in balance. That is because homeostasis is a *dynamic*, not a static, process.

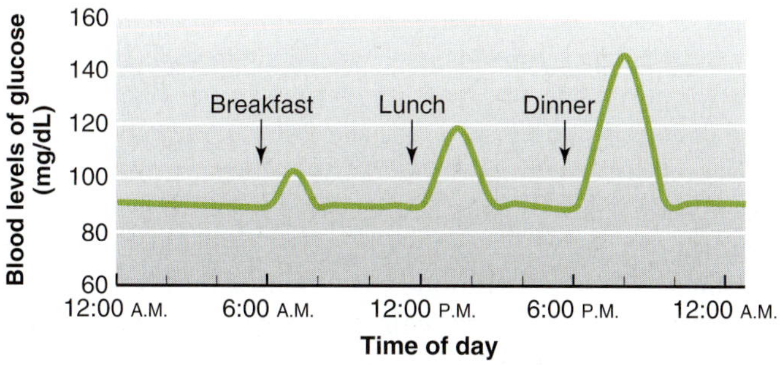

Figure 1.4 Changes in blood glucose concentrations during a typical 24 h period. Note that glucose concentration increases after each meal, more so after larger meals, and then returns to the premeal concentration in a short while. The profile shown here is that of a person who is homeostatic for blood glucose, even though concentrations of this sugar vary considerably throughout the day.

Consider swings in the concentration of glucose in the blood over the course of a day (**Figure 1.4**). After a typical meal, carbohydrates in food are broken down in the intestines into glucose molecules, which are then absorbed across the intestinal epithelium and released into the blood. As a consequence, blood glucose concentrations increase considerably within a short time after eating. Clearly, such a large change in the blood concentration of glucose is not consistent with the idea of a stable or static internal environment. What is important is that once the concentration of glucose in the blood increases, compensatory mechanisms restore it toward the concentration it was before the meal. These homeostatic compensatory mechanisms do not, however, overshoot to any significant degree in the opposite direction. That is, the blood glucose usually does not decrease below the premeal concentration, or does so only slightly. In the case of glucose, the endocrine system is primarily responsible for this adjustment, but a wide variety of control systems may be initiated to regulate other processes. In later chapters, we will see how every organ and tissue of the human body contributes to homeostasis, sometimes in multiple ways, and usually in concert with each other.

Homeostasis, therefore, does not imply that a given physiological function or variable is rigidly constant with respect to time but that it fluctuates within a predictable and often narrow range. When disturbed above or below the normal range, it is restored to normal.

What do we mean when we say that something varies within a normal range? This depends on just what we are monitoring. If the oxygen level in the blood of a healthy person breathing air at sea level is measured, it barely changes over the course of time, even if the person exercises. Such a system is said to be tightly controlled and to demonstrate very little variability or scatter around an average value. Blood glucose concentrations, as we have seen, may vary considerably over the course of a day. Yet, if the daily average glucose concentration was determined in the same person on many consecutive days, it would be much more predictable over days or even years than random, individual measurements of glucose over the course of a single day. In other words, there may be considerable variation in glucose values over short time periods, but less when they are averaged over long periods of time. This has led to the concept that homeostasis is a state of **dynamic constancy.** In such a state, a given variable like blood glucose may vary in the short term but is stable and predictable when averaged over the long term.

It is also important to realize that a person may be homeostatic for one variable but not homeostatic for another. Homeostasis must be described differently, therefore, for each variable. For example, as long as the concentration of sodium ions in the blood remains within a few percentage points of its normal range, sodium homeostasis exists. However, a person whose sodium ion concentrations are homeostatic may suffer from other disturbances, such as abnormally high carbon dioxide levels in the blood resulting from lung disease, a condition that could be fatal. Just one nonhomeostatic variable, among the many that can be described, can have life-threatening consequences. Often, when one variable becomes dramatically out of balance, other variables in the body become nonhomeostatic as a consequence. For example, when you exercise strenuously and begin to get warm, you perspire to help maintain body temperature homeostasis. This is important, because many cells (notably neurons) malfunction at elevated temperatures. However, the water that is lost in perspiration creates a situation in which total-body water is no longer in balance. In general, if all the major organ systems are operating in a homeostatic manner, a person is in good health. Certain kinds of disease, in fact, can be defined as the loss of homeostasis in one or more systems in the body. To elaborate on our earlier definition of *physiology*, therefore, when homeostasis is maintained, we refer to physiology; when it is not, we refer to pathophysiology (from the Greek *pathos*, meaning "suffering" or "disease").

1.5 General Characteristics of Homeostatic Control Systems

The activities of cells, tissues, and organs must be regulated and integrated with each other so that any change in the extracellular fluid initiates a reaction to correct the change. The compensating mechanisms that mediate such responses are performed by **homeostatic control systems.**

Consider again an example of the regulation of body temperature. This time, our subject is a resting, lightly clad man in a room having a temperature of 20°C and moderate humidity. His internal body temperature is 37°C, and he is losing heat to the external environment because it is at a lower temperature. However, the chemical reactions occurring within the cells of his body are producing heat at a rate equal to the rate of heat loss. Under these conditions, the body undergoes no *net* gain or loss of heat, and the body temperature remains constant. The system is in a **steady state,** defined as a system in which a particular variable—temperature, in this case—is not changing but in which energy—in this case, heat—must be added continuously to maintain a constant condition. (Steady state differs from **equilibrium,** in which a particular variable is not changing but no input of energy is required to maintain the constancy.) The steady-state temperature in our example is known as the **set point** of the thermoregulatory system.

This example illustrates a crucial generalization about homeostasis. Stability of an internal environmental variable is achieved by the balancing of inputs and outputs. In the previous example, the variable (body temperature) remains constant because metabolic heat production (input) equals heat loss from the body (output).

Now imagine that we rapidly reduce the temperature of the room, say to 5°C, and keep it there. This immediately increases the loss of heat from our subject's warm skin, upsetting the balance between heat gain and loss. The body temperature therefore starts to decrease. Very rapidly, however, a variety of homeostatic responses occur to limit the decrease. **Figure 1.5** summarizes these responses. *The reader is urged to study Figure 1.5 and its legend carefully because the figure is typical of those used throughout the remainder of the book to illustrate homeostatic systems, and the legend emphasizes several conventions common to such figures.*

The first homeostatic response is that blood vessels to the skin become constricted (narrowed), reducing the amount of blood flowing through the skin. This reduces heat loss from the blood to the environment and helps maintain body temperature. At a room temperature of 5°C, however, blood vessel constriction cannot completely eliminate the extra heat loss

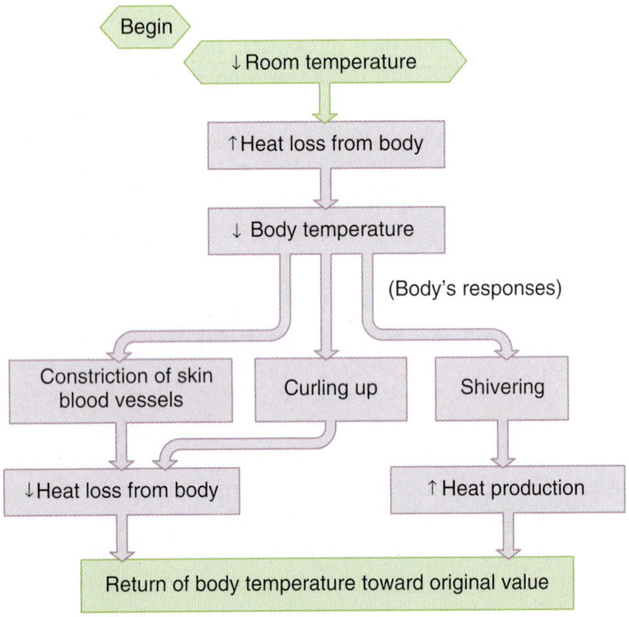

Figure 1.5 A homeostatic control system maintains body temperature when room temperature decreases. This flow diagram is typical of those used throughout this book to illustrate homeostatic systems, and several conventions should be noted. The "Begin" sign indicates where to start. The arrows next to each term within the boxes denote increases or decreases. The arrows connecting any two boxes in the figure denote cause and effect; that is, an arrow can be read as "causes" or "leads to." (For example, decreased room temperature "leads to" increased heat loss from the body.) In general, you should add the words "tends to" in thinking about these cause-and-effect relationships. For example, decreased room temperature tends to cause an increase in heat loss from the body, and curling up tends to cause a decrease in heat loss from the body. Qualifying the relationship in this way is necessary because variables like heat production and heat loss are under the influence of many factors, some of which oppose each other.

from the skin. Like the person shown in the chapter opening photo, our subject hunches his shoulders and folds his arms in order to reduce the surface area of the skin available for heat loss. This helps somewhat, but excessive heat loss still continues, and body temperature keeps decreasing, although at a slower rate. Clearly, then, if excessive heat loss (output) cannot be prevented, the only way of restoring the balance between heat input and output is to increase input, and this is precisely what occurs. Our subject begins to shiver, and the chemical reactions responsible for the skeletal muscle contractions that constitute shivering produce large quantities of heat.

Feedback Systems

The thermoregulatory system just described is an example of a **negative feedback** system, in which an increase or decrease in the variable being regulated brings about responses that tend to move the variable in the direction opposite ("negative" to) the direction of the original change. Thus, in our example, a decrease in body temperature led to responses that tended to increase the body temperature—that is, move it toward its original value.

Without negative feedback, oscillations like some of those described in this chapter would be much greater and, therefore, the variability in a given system would increase. Negative feedback also prevents the compensatory responses to a loss of homeostasis from continuing unabated. Details of the mechanisms and characteristics of negative feedback in different systems will be addressed in later chapters. For now, it is important to recognize that negative feedback plays a vital part in the checks and balances on most physiological variables.

Negative feedback may occur at the organ, cellular, or molecular level. For instance, negative feedback regulates many enzymatic processes, as shown in schematic form in **Figure 1.6.** (An enzyme is a protein that catalyzes chemical reactions.) In this example, the product formed from a substrate by an enzyme negatively feeds back to inhibit further action of the enzyme. This may occur by several processes, such as chemical modification of the enzyme by the product of the reaction. The production of adenosine triphosphate (ATP) within cells is a good example of a chemical process regulated by feedback. Normally, glucose molecules are enzymatically broken down inside cells to release some of the chemical energy that was contained in the bonds of the molecule. This energy is then stored in the bonds of ATP. The energy from ATP can later be tapped by cells to power such functions as muscle contraction, cellular secretions, and transport of molecules across cell membranes. As ATP accumulates in the cell, however, it inhibits the activity of some of the enzymes involved in the breakdown of glucose. Therefore, as ATP concentrations increase within a cell, further production of ATP slows down due to negative feedback. Conversely, if ATP concentrations decrease within a cell, negative feedback is removed and more glucose is broken down so that more ATP can be produced.

Not all forms of feedback are negative. In some cases, **positive feedback** accelerates a process, leading to an "explosive" system. This is counter to the principle of homeostasis, because positive feedback has no obvious means of stopping. Not surprisingly, therefore, positive feedback is much less

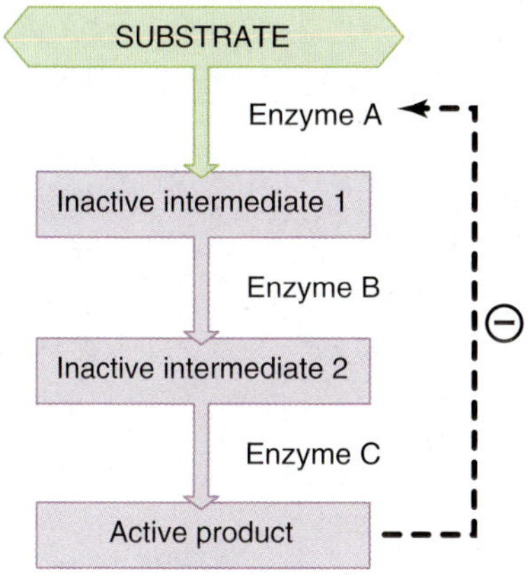

Figure 1.6 Hypothetical example of negative feedback (as denoted by the circled minus sign and dashed feedback line) occurring within a set of sequential chemical reactions. By inhibiting the activity of the first enzyme involved in the formation of a product, the product can regulate the rate of its own formation.

PHYSIOLOGICAL INQUIRY

- What would be the effect on this pathway if negative feedback was removed?

Answer can be found at end of chapter.

common in nature than negative feedback. Nonetheless, there are examples in physiology in which positive feedback is very important. One well-described example, which you will learn about in Chapter 17, is the process of parturition (birth). As the uterine muscles contract and a baby's head is pressed against the mother's cervix during labor, signals are relayed via nerves from the cervix to the mother's brain. The brain initiates the secretion into the blood of a molecule called oxytocin from the mother's pituitary gland. Oxytocin is a potent stimulator of further uterine contractions. As the uterus contracts even harder in response to oxytocin, the baby's head is pushed harder against the cervix, causing it to stretch more; this stimulates yet more nerve signals to the mother's brain, resulting in yet more oxytocin secretion. This self-perpetuating cycle continues until finally the baby pushes through the stretched cervix and is born.

Resetting of Set Points

As we have seen, changes in the external environment can displace a variable from its set point. In addition, the set points for many regulated variables can be physiologically reset to a new value. A common example is fever, the increase in body temperature that occurs in response to infection and that is somewhat analogous to raising the setting of a thermostat in a room. The homeostatic control systems regulating body temperature are still functioning during a fever, but they maintain the temperature at an increased value. This regulated increase in body temperature is adaptive for fighting the infection, because elevated temperature inhibits proliferation of some pathogens. In fact, this is why a fever is often preceded by chills and shivering. The set point for body temperature has been reset to a higher value, and the body responds by shivering to generate heat.

The example of fever may have left the impression that set points are reset only in response to external stimuli, such as the presence of pathogens, but this is not the case. Indeed, the set points for many regulated variables change on a rhythmic basis every day. For example, the set point for body temperature is higher during the day than at night.

Although the resetting of a set point is adaptive in some cases, in others it simply reflects the clashing demands of different regulatory systems. This brings us to one more generalization. It is not possible for everything to be held constant by homeostatic control systems. In our earlier example, body temperature was maintained despite large swings in ambient temperature, but only because the homeostatic control system brought about large changes in skin blood flow and skeletal muscle contraction. Moreover, because so many properties of the internal environment are closely interrelated, it is often possible to keep one property relatively stable only by moving others away from their usual set point. This is what we mean by "clashing demands," which explains the phenomenon mentioned earlier about the interplay between body temperature and water balance during exercise.

The generalizations we have given about homeostatic control systems are summarized in **Table 1.2**. One additional point is that, as is illustrated by the regulation of body temperature, multiple systems usually control a single parameter. The adaptive value of such redundancy is that it provides much greater fine-tuning and also permits regulation to occur even when one of the systems is not functioning properly because of disease.

Feedforward Regulation

Another type of regulatory process often used in conjunction with feedback systems is *feedforward*. Let us give an example of feedforward and then define it. The temperature-sensitive neurons that trigger negative feedback regulation of body temperature when

TABLE 1.2 Some Important Generalizations About Homeostatic Control Systems
Stability of an internal environmental variable is achieved by balancing inputs and outputs. It is not the absolute magnitudes of the inputs and outputs that matter but the balance between them.
In negative feedback, a change in the variable being regulated brings about responses that tend to move the variable in the direction opposite the original change—that is, back toward the initial value (set point).
Homeostatic control systems cannot maintain complete constancy of any given feature of the internal environment. Therefore, any regulated variable will have a more or less narrow range of normal values depending on the external environmental conditions.
The set point of some variables regulated by homeostatic control systems can be reset—that is, physiologically raised or lowered.
It is not always possible for homeostatic control systems to maintain every variable within a narrow normal range in response to an environmental challenge. There is a hierarchy of importance, so that certain variables may be altered markedly to maintain others within their normal range.

it begins to decrease are located inside the body. In addition, there are temperature-sensitive neurons in the skin; these cells, in effect, monitor outside temperature. When outside temperature decreases, as in our example, these neurons immediately detect the change and relay this information to the brain. The brain then sends out signals to the blood vessels and muscles, resulting in heat conservation and increased heat production. In this manner, compensatory thermoregulatory responses are activated *before* the colder outside temperature can cause the internal body temperature to decrease. In another familiar example, the smell of food triggers nerve responses from odor receptors in the nose to the cells of the digestive system. The effect is to prepare the digestive system for the arrival of food before we even consume it, for example by inducing saliva to be secreted in the mouth and causing the stomach to churn and produce acid. Thus, **feedforward** regulation anticipates changes in regulated variables such as internal body temperature or energy availability, improves the speed of the body's homeostatic responses, and minimizes fluctuations in the level of the variable being regulated—that is, it reduces the amount of deviation from the set point.

In our examples, feedforward regulation utilizes a set of external or internal environmental detectors. It is likely, however, that many examples of feedforward regulation are the result of a different phenomenon—learning. The first times they occur, early in life, perturbations in the external environment probably cause relatively large changes in regulated internal environmental factors, and in responding to these changes the central nervous system learns to anticipate them and resist them more effectively. A familiar form of this is the increased heart rate that occurs in an athlete just before a competition begins.

1.6 Components of Homeostatic Control Systems

Reflexes

The thermoregulatory system we used as an example in the previous section and many of the other homeostatic control systems belong to the general category of stimulus–response sequences known as *reflexes.* Although in some reflexes we are aware of the stimulus and/or the response, many reflexes regulating the internal environment occur without our conscious awareness.

In the narrowest sense of the word, a **reflex** is a specific, involuntary, unpremeditated, "built-in" response to a particular stimulus. Examples of such reflexes include pulling your hand away from a hot object or shutting your eyes as an object rapidly approaches your face. Many responses, however, appear automatic and stereotyped but are actually the result of learning and practice. For example, an experienced driver performs many complicated acts in operating a car. To the driver, these motions are, in large part, automatic, stereotyped, and unpremeditated, but they occur only because a great deal of conscious effort was spent learning them. We term such reflexes **learned** or **acquired reflexes.** In general, most reflexes, no matter how simple they may appear to be, are subject to alteration by learning.

The pathway mediating a reflex is known as the **reflex arc,** and its components are shown in Figure 1.7. A **stimulus** is defined as a detectable change in the internal or external environment, such as a change in temperature, plasma potassium concentration, or blood pressure. A **receptor** detects the environmental change. A stimulus acts upon a receptor to produce a signal that is relayed to an **integrating center.** The signal travels between the receptor and the integrating center along the **afferent pathway** (the general term *afferent* means "to carry to," in this case, to the integrating center).

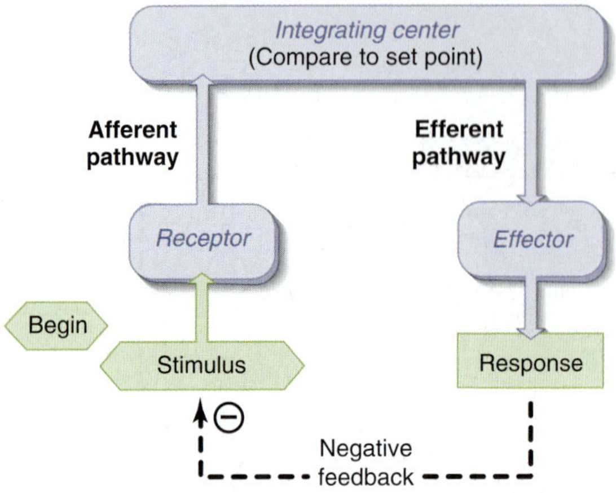

Figure 1.7 General components of a reflex arc that functions as a negative feedback control system. The response of the system has the effect of counteracting or eliminating the stimulus. This phenomenon of negative feedback is emphasized by the minus sign in the dashed feedback loop.

An integrating center often receives signals from many receptors, some of which may respond to quite different types of stimuli. Thus, the output of an integrating center reflects the net effect of the total afferent input; that is, it represents an integration of numerous bits of information.

The output of an integrating center is sent to the last component of the system, whose change in activity constitutes the overall response of the system. This component is known as an **effector.** The information going from an integrating center to an effector is like a command directing the effector to alter its activity. This information travels along the **efferent pathway** (the general term *efferent* means "to carry away from," in this case, away from the integrating center).

Thus far, we have described the reflex arc as the sequence of events linking a stimulus to a response. If the response produced by the effector causes a decrease in the magnitude of the stimulus that triggered the sequence of events, then the reflex leads to negative feedback and we have a typical homeostatic control system. Not all reflexes are associated with such feedback. For example, the smell of food stimulates the stomach to secrete molecules that are important for digestion, but these molecules do not eliminate the smell of food (the stimulus).

Figure 1.8 demonstrates the components of a negative feedback homeostatic reflex arc in the process of thermoregulation. The temperature receptors are the endings of certain neurons in various parts of the body. They generate electrical signals in the neurons at a rate determined by the temperature. These electrical signals are conducted by nerves containing processes from the neurons—the afferent pathway—to the brain, where the integrating center for temperature regulation is located. The

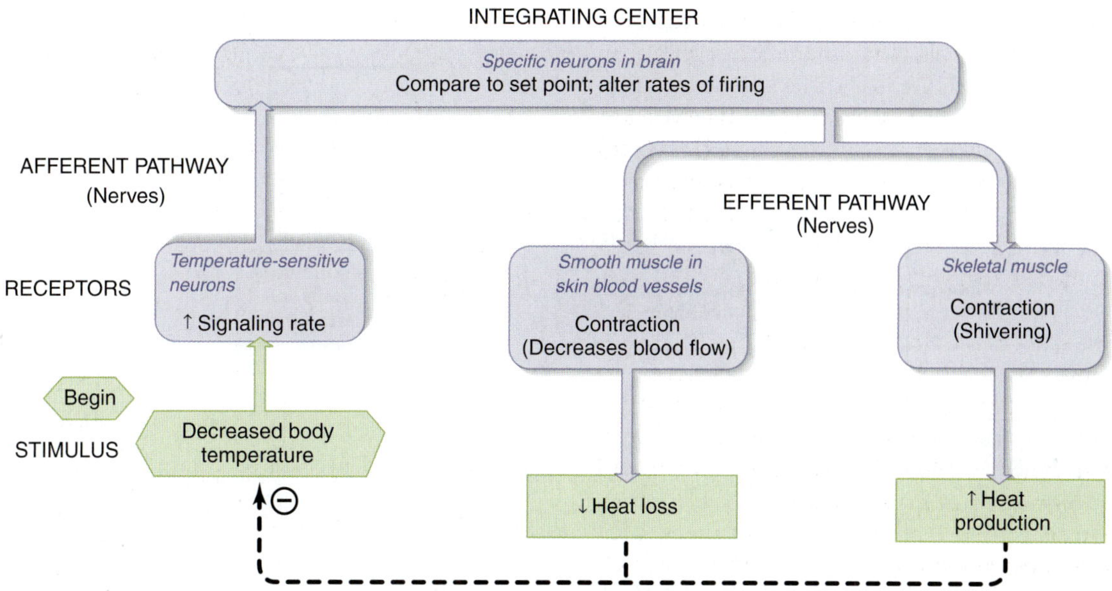

Figure 1.8 Reflex for minimizing the decrease in body temperature that occurs on exposure to a reduced external environmental temperature. This figure provides the internal components for the reflex shown in Figure 1.5. The dashed arrow and the ⊖ indicate the negative feedback nature of the reflex, denoting that the reflex responses cause the decreased body temperature to return toward normal. An additional flow-diagram convention is shown in this figure: blue boxes always denote events that are occurring in anatomical structures (labeled in blue italic type in the upper portion of the box).

PHYSIOLOGICAL INQUIRY

- What might happen to the efferent pathway in this control system if body temperature *increased* above normal?

Answer can be found at end of chapter.

integrating center, in turn, sends signals out along neurons that cause skeletal muscles and the muscles in skin blood vessels to contract. The neurons to the muscles are the efferent pathway, and the muscles are the effectors. The dashed arrow and the negative sign indicate the negative feedback nature of the reflex.

Almost all body cells can act as effectors in homeostatic reflexes. Muscles and glands, however, are the major effectors of biological control systems. In the case of glands, for example, the effector may be a hormone secreted into the blood. A **hormone** is a type of chemical messenger secreted into the blood by cells of the endocrine system (see Table 1.1). Hormones may act on many different cells simultaneously because they circulate throughout the body.

Traditionally, the term *reflex* was restricted to situations in which the receptors, afferent pathway, integrating center, and efferent pathway were all parts of the nervous system, as in the thermoregulatory reflex. However, the principles are essentially the same when a blood-borne chemical messenger, rather than a nerve, serves as the efferent pathway, or when a hormone-secreting gland serves as the integrating center.

In our use of the term *reflex*, therefore, we include hormones as reflex components. Moreover, depending on the specific nature of the reflex, the integrating center may reside either in the nervous system or in a gland. In addition, a gland may act as both receptor and integrating center in a reflex. For example, the gland cells that secrete the hormone insulin, which *decreases* plasma glucose concentration, also detect *increases* in the plasma glucose concentration.

Local Homeostatic Responses

In addition to reflexes, another group of biological responses, called **local homeostatic responses,** is of great importance for homeostasis. These responses are initiated by a change in the external or internal environment (that is, a stimulus), and they induce an alteration of cell activity with the net effect of counteracting the stimulus. Like a reflex, therefore, a local response is the result of a sequence of events proceeding from a stimulus. Unlike a reflex, however, the entire sequence occurs only in the area of the stimulus. For example, when cells of a tissue become very metabolically active, they secrete substances into the interstitial fluid that dilate (widen) local blood vessels. The resulting increased blood flow increases the rate at which nutrients and oxygen are delivered to that area, and the rate at which wastes are removed. The significance of local responses is that they provide individual areas of the body with mechanisms for local self-regulation.

1.7 The Role of Intercellular Chemical Messengers in Homeostasis

Essential to reflexes and local homeostatic responses—and therefore to homeostasis—is the ability of cells to communicate with one another. In this way, cells in the brain, for example, can be made aware of the status of activities of structures outside the brain, such as the heart, and help regulate those activities to meet new homeostatic challenges. In the majority of cases, intercellular

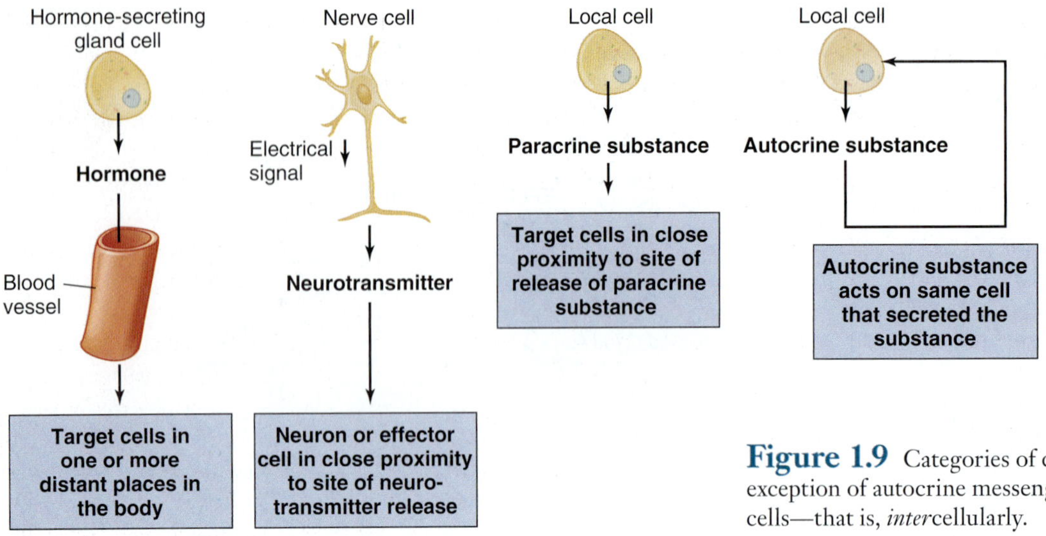

Figure 1.9 Categories of chemical messengers. With the exception of autocrine messengers, all messengers act between cells—that is, *inter*cellularly.

communication is performed by chemical messengers. There are three categories of such messengers: hormones, neurotransmitters, and paracrine or autocrine substances (**Figure 1.9**).

As noted earlier, a hormone functions as a chemical messenger that enables the hormone-secreting cell to communicate with cells acted upon by the hormone—its **target cells**—with the blood acting as the delivery system. Hormones are produced in and secreted from **endocrine glands** or in scattered cells that are distributed throughout another organ. They play key roles in essentially all physiological processes, including growth, reproduction, metabolism, mineral balance, and blood pressure, and are often produced whenever homeostasis is threatened.

In contrast to hormones, **neurotransmitters** are chemical messengers that are released from the endings of neurons onto other neurons, muscle cells, or gland cells. A neurotransmitter diffuses through the extracellular fluid separating the neuron and its target cell; it is not released into the blood like a hormone. Neurotransmitters and their roles in neuronal signaling and brain function will be covered in Chapter 6. In the context of homeostasis, they form the signaling basis of some reflexes, as well as playing a vital role in the compensatory responses to a wide variety of challenges, such as the requirement for increased heart and lung function during exercise.

Chemical messengers participate not only in reflexes but also in local responses. Chemical messengers involved in local communication between cells are known as **paracrine substances** (or agents). Paracrine substances are synthesized by cells and released, once given the appropriate stimulus, into the extracellular fluid. They then diffuse to neighboring cells, some of which are their target cells. Given this broad definition, neurotransmitters could be classified as a subgroup of paracrine substances, but by convention they are not. Once they have performed their functions, paracrine substances are generally inactivated by locally existing enzymes and therefore they do not enter the bloodstream in large quantities. Paracrine substances are produced throughout the body; an example of their key role in homeostasis that you will learn about in Chapter 15 is their ability to fine-tune the amount of acid produced by cells of the stomach in response to eating food.

There is one category of local chemical messengers that are not *inter*cellular messengers—that is, they do not communicate *between* cells. Rather, the chemical is secreted by a cell into the extracellular fluid and then acts upon the very cell that secreted it. Such messengers are called **autocrine substances** (or agents) (see Figure 1.9). Frequently, a messenger may serve both paracrine and autocrine functions simultaneously—that is, molecules of the messenger released by a cell may act locally on adjacent cells as well as on the same cell that released the messenger.

A point of great importance must be emphasized here to avoid later confusion. A neuron, endocrine gland cell, and other cell type may all secrete the same chemical messenger. In some cases, a particular messenger may sometimes function as a neurotransmitter, a hormone, or a paracrine or autocrine substance. Norepinephrine, for example, is not only a neurotransmitter in the brain; it is also produced as a hormone by cells of the adrenal glands.

All types of intercellular communication described thus far in this section involve secretion of a chemical messenger into the extracellular fluid. However, there are two important types of chemical communication between cells that do not require such secretion. In the first type, which occurs via gap junctions (physical linkages connecting the cytosol between two cells; see Chapter 3), molecules move from one cell to an adjacent cell without entering the extracellular fluid. In the second type, the chemical messenger is not actually released from the cell producing it but rather is located in the plasma membrane of that cell. When the cell encounters another cell type capable of responding to the message, the two cells link up via the membrane-bound messenger. This type of signaling, sometimes termed *juxtacrine*, is of particular importance in the growth and differentiation of tissues as well as in the functioning of cells that protect the body against pathogens (Chapter 18).

1.8 Processes Related to Homeostasis

Adaptation and Acclimatization

The term **adaptation** denotes a characteristic that favors survival in specific environments. Homeostatic control systems are inherited biological adaptations. The ability to respond to a particular environmental stress is not fixed, however, but can be enhanced by prolonged exposure to that stress. This type of adaptation—the improved functioning of an already existing homeostatic system—is known as **acclimatization.**

Let us take sweating in response to heat exposure as an example and perform a simple experiment. On day 1, we expose a person for 30 minutes (min) to an elevated temperature and ask her to do a standardized exercise test. Body temperature increases, and sweating begins after a certain period of time. The sweating provides a mechanism for increasing heat loss from the body and therefore tends to minimize the increase in body temperature in a hot environment. The volume of sweat produced under these conditions is measured. Then, for a week, our subject enters the heat chamber for 1 or 2 hours (h) per day and exercises. On day 8, her body temperature and sweating rate are again measured during the same exercise test performed on day 1. The striking finding is that the subject begins to sweat sooner and much more profusely than she did on day 1. As a consequence, her body temperature does not increase to nearly the same degree. The subject has become acclimatized to the heat. She has undergone an adaptive change induced by repeated exposure to the heat and is now better able to respond to heat exposure.

Acclimatizations are usually reversible. If, in the example just described, the daily exposures to heat are discontinued, our subject's sweating rate will revert to the preacclimatized value within a relatively short time.

The precise anatomical and physiological changes that bring about increased capacity to withstand change during acclimatization are highly varied. Typically, they involve an increase in the number, size, or sensitivity of one or more of the cell types in the homeostatic control system that mediates the basic response.

Biological Rhythms

As noted earlier, a striking characteristic of many body functions is the rhythmic changes they manifest. The most common type is the **circadian rhythm,** which cycles approximately once every 24 h. Waking and sleeping, body temperature, hormone concentrations in the blood, the excretion of ions into the urine, and many other functions undergo circadian variation; an example of one type of rhythm is shown in **Figure 1.10**.

What do biological rhythms have to do with homeostasis? They add an anticipatory component to homeostatic control systems, in effect, a feedforward system operating without detectors. The negative feedback homeostatic responses we described earlier in this chapter are *corrective* responses. They are initiated *after* the steady state of the individual has been perturbed. In contrast, biological rhythms enable homeostatic mechanisms to be utilized immediately and automatically by activating them at times when a challenge is *likely* to occur but before it actually does occur. For example, body temperature increases prior to waking in a person on a typical sleep–wake cycle. This allows the metabolic machinery of the body to operate most efficiently immediately upon waking, because metabolism (chemical reactions) is to some extent temperature dependent. During sleep, metabolism is slower than during the active hours, and therefore body temperature decreases at that time. A crucial point concerning most body rhythms is that they are internally driven. Environmental factors do not drive the rhythm but rather provide the timing cues important for **entrainment,** or setting of the actual hours of the rhythm. A classic experiment will clarify this distinction.

Subjects were put in experimental chambers that completely isolated them from their usual external environment, including knowledge of the time of day. For the first few days, they were exposed to a 24 h rest–activity cycle in which the room lights were turned on and off at the same times each day. Under these conditions, their sleep–wake cycles were 24 h long. Then, all environmental time cues were eliminated, and the subjects were allowed to control the lights themselves. Immediately, their sleep–wake patterns began to change. On average, bedtime began about 30 min later each day, and so did wake-up time. Thus, a sleep–wake cycle persisted in the complete absence of environmental cues. Such a rhythm is called a **free-running rhythm.** In this case, it was approximately 24.5 h rather than 24. This indicates that cues are required to entrain or set a circadian rhythm to 24 h.

The light–dark cycle is the most important environmental time cue in our lives—but not the only one. Others include external environmental temperature, meal timing, and many social cues. Thus, if several people were undergoing the experiment just described in isolation from each other, their free-running rhythms would be somewhat different, but if they were all in the same room, social cues would entrain all of them to the same rhythm.

Environmental time cues also function to **phase-shift** rhythms—in other words, to reset the internal clock. Thus, if you fly west or east to a different time zone, your sleep–wake cycle and other circadian rhythms slowly shift to the new light–dark cycle. These shifts take time, however, and the disparity between external time and internal time is one of the causes of the symptoms of jet lag—a disruption of homeostasis that leads to gastrointestinal disturbances, decreased vigilance and attention span, sleep problems, and a general feeling of malaise.

Similar symptoms occur in workers on permanent or rotating night shifts. These people generally do not adapt

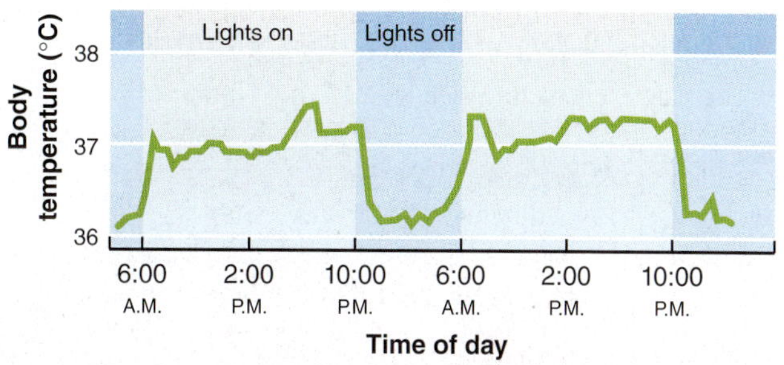

Figure 1.10 Circadian rhythm of body temperature in a human subject with room lights on (open bars at top) for 16 h, and off (blue bars at top) for 8 h. Note the increase in body temperature that occurs just prior to lights on, in anticipation of the increased activity and metabolism that occur during waking hours.
Adapted from Moore-Ede and Sulzman.

to their schedules even after several years because they are exposed to the usual outdoor light–dark cycle (normal indoor lighting is too dim to function as a good entrainer). In recent experiments, night-shift workers were exposed to extremely bright indoor lighting while they worked and they were exposed to 8 h of total darkness during the day when they slept. This schedule produced total adaptation to night-shift work within 5 days.

What is the neural basis of body rhythms? In the part of the brain called the hypothalamus, a specific collection of neurons (the suprachiasmatic nucleus) functions as the principal **pacemaker,** or time clock, for circadian rhythms. How it keeps time independent of any external environmental cues is not fully understood, but it appears to involve the rhythmic turning on and off of critical genes in the pacemaker cells.

The pacemaker receives input from the eyes and many other parts of the nervous system, and these inputs mediate the entrainment effects exerted by the external environment. In turn, the pacemaker sends out neural signals to other parts of the brain, which then influence the various body systems, activating some and inhibiting others. One output of the pacemaker goes to the **pineal gland,** a gland within the brain that secretes the hormone **melatonin.** These neural signals from the pacemaker cause the pineal gland to secrete melatonin during darkness but not during daylight. It has been hypothesized, therefore, that melatonin may act as an important mediator to influence other organs either directly or by altering the activity of the parts of the brain that control these organs.

Balance of Chemical Substances in the Body

Many homeostatic systems regulate the balance between addition and removal of a chemical substance from the body. **Figure 1.11** is a generalized schema of the possible pathways involved in maintaining such balance. The **pool** occupies a position of central importance in the balance sheet. It is the body's readily available quantity of the substance and is often identical to the amount present in the extracellular fluid. The pool receives substances and redistributes them to all the pathways.

The pathways on the left of Figure 1.11 are sources of net gain to the body. A substance may enter the body through the gastrointestinal (GI) tract or the lungs. Alternatively, a substance may be synthesized within the body from other materials.

The pathways on the right of the figure are causes of net loss from the body. A substance may be lost in the urine, feces, expired air, or menstrual fluid, as well as from the surface of the body as skin, hair, nails, sweat, or tears. The substance may also be chemically altered by enzymes and thus removed by metabolism.

The central portion of the figure illustrates the distribution of the substance within the body. The substance may be taken from the pool and accumulated in storage depots—such as the accumulation of fat in adipose tissue. Conversely, it may leave the storage depots to reenter the pool. Finally, the substance may be incorporated reversibly into some other molecular structure, such as fatty acids into plasma membranes. Incorporation is reversible because the substance is liberated again whenever the more complex structure is broken down. This pathway is distinguished from storage in that the incorporation of the substance into other molecules produces new molecules with specific functions.

Substances do not necessarily follow all pathways of this generalized schema. For example, minerals such as Na^+ cannot be synthesized, do not normally enter through the lungs, and cannot be removed by metabolism.

The orientation of Figure 1.11 illustrates two important generalizations concerning the balance concept: (1) during any period of time, total-body balance depends upon the relative rates of net gain and net loss to the body; and (2) the pool concentration depends not only upon the total amount of the substance in the body but also upon exchanges of the substance *within* the body.

For any substance, three states of total-body balance are possible: (1) loss exceeds gain, so that the total amount of the substance in the body is decreasing, and the person is in **negative balance;** (2) gain exceeds loss, so that the total amount of the substance in the body is increasing, and the person is in **positive balance;** and (3) gain equals loss, and the person is in **stable balance.**

Clearly, a stable balance can be upset by a change in the amount being gained or lost in any single pathway in the schema. For example, increased sweating can cause severe negative water balance. Conversely, stable balance can be restored by homeostatic control of water intake and output.

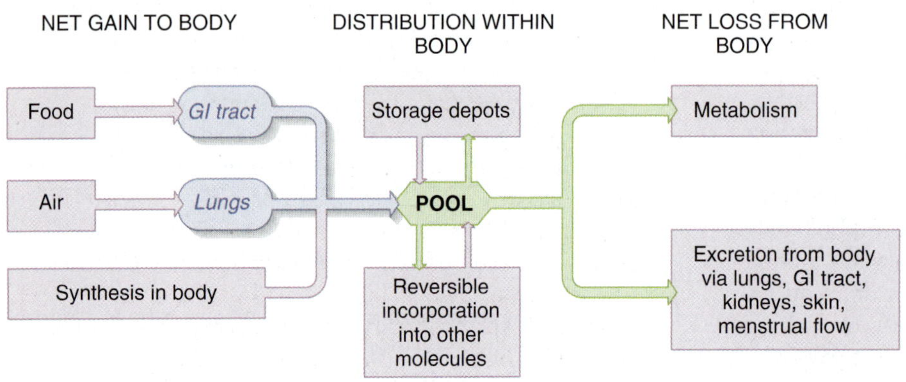

Figure 1.11 Balance diagram for a chemical substance.

Let us take the balance of calcium ions as another example. The concentration of calcium ions (Ca^{2+}) in the extracellular fluid is critical for normal cellular functioning, notably muscle cells and neurons, but also for the formation and maintenance of the skeleton. The vast majority of the body's Ca^{2+} is present in bone. The control systems for Ca^{2+} balance target the intestines and kidneys such that the amount of Ca^{2+} absorbed from the diet is balanced with the amount excreted in the urine. During infancy and childhood, however, the net balance of Ca^{2+} is positive, and Ca^{2+} is deposited in growing bone. In later life, especially in women after menopause (see Chapter 17), Ca^{2+} is released from bones faster than it can be deposited, and that extra Ca^{2+} is lost in the urine. Consequently, the bone pool of Ca^{2+} becomes smaller, the rate of Ca^{2+} loss from the body exceeds the rate of intake, and Ca^{2+} balance is negative.

In summary, homeostasis is a complex, dynamic process that regulates the adaptive responses of the body to changes in the external and internal environments. To work properly, homeostatic systems require a sensor to detect the environmental change, and a means to produce a compensatory response. Because compensatory responses require muscle activity, behavioral changes, or synthesis of chemical messengers such as hormones, homeostasis is achieved by the expenditure of energy. The nutrients that provide this energy, as well as the cellular structures and chemical reactions that release the energy stored in the chemical bonds of the nutrients, are described in the following two chapters.

1.9 General Principles of Physiology

When you undertake a detailed study of the functions of the human body, several fundamental, general principles are repeatedly observed. Recognizing these principles and how they manifest in the different organ systems can provide a deeper understanding of the integrated function of the human body. To help you gain this insight, beginning with Chapter 2, the introduction to each chapter will highlight the general principles demonstrated in that chapter. Your understanding of how to apply the following general principles of physiology to a given chapter's content will then be tested with assessments at the end of the chapter.

1. ***Homeostasis is essential for health and survival.*** The ability to maintain physiological variables such as body temperature and blood sugar concentrations within normal ranges is the underlying principle upon which all physiology is based. Keys to this principle are the processes of feedback and feedforward, first introduced in this chapter. Challenges to homeostasis may result from disease or from environmental factors such as famine or exposure to extremes of temperature.
2. ***The functions of organ systems are coordinated with each other.*** Physiological mechanisms operate and interact at the level of cells, tissues, organs, and organ systems. Furthermore, the different organ systems in the human body do not function independently of each other. Each system typically interacts with one or more others to control a homeostatic variable. A good example that you will learn about in Chapters 12 and 14 is the coordinated activity of the circulatory and urinary systems in regulating blood pressure. This type of coordination is often referred to as "integration" in physiological contexts.
3. ***Most physiological functions are controlled by multiple regulatory systems, often working in opposition.*** Typically, control systems in the human body operate such that a given variable, such as heart rate, receives both stimulatory and inhibitory signals. As you will learn in detail in Chapter 6, for example, the autonomic nervous system sends both types of signals to the heart; adjusting the ratio of stimulatory to inhibitory signals allows for fine-tuning of the heart rate under changing conditions such as rest or exercise.
4. ***Information flow between cells, tissues, and organs is an essential feature of homeostasis and allows for integration of physiological processes.*** Cells can communicate with nearby cells via locally secreted chemical signals; a good example of this is the signaling between cells of the stomach that results in acid production, a key feature of the digestion of proteins (see Chapter 15). Cells in one structure can also communicate long distances using electrical signals or chemical messengers such as hormones. Electrical and hormonal signaling will be discussed throughout the textbook and particularly in Chapters 6, 7, and 11.
5. ***Controlled exchange of materials occurs between compartments and across cellular membranes.*** The movement of water and solutes—such as ions, sugars, and other molecules—between the extracellular and intracellular fluid is critical for the survival of all cells, tissues, and organs. In this way, important biological molecules are delivered to cells and wastes are removed and eliminated from the body. In addition, regulation of ion movements creates the electrical properties that are crucial to the function of many cell types. These exchanges occur via several different mechanisms, which are introduced in Chapter 4 and are reinforced where appropriate for each organ system throughout the book.
6. ***Physiological processes are dictated by the laws of chemistry and physics.*** Throughout this textbook, you will encounter some simple chemical reactions, such as the reversible binding of oxygen to the protein hemoglobin in red blood cells (Chapter 13). The basic mechanisms that regulate such reactions are reviewed in Chapter 3. Physical laws, too, such as gravity, electromagnetism, and the relation between the diameter of a tube and the flow of liquid through the tube, help explain things like why we may feel lightheaded upon standing too suddenly (Chapter 12, but also see the Clinical Case Study that follows in this chapter), how our eyes detect light (Chapter 7), and how we inflate our lungs with air (Chapter 13).
7. ***Physiological processes require the transfer and balance of matter and energy.*** Growth and the maintenance of homeostasis require regulation of the movement and transformation of energy-yielding nutrients and molecular building blocks between the body and the environment and between different regions of the body. Nutrients are ingested (Chapter 15), stored in various forms (Chapter 16), and ultimately metabolized to provide energy that can be stored in the bonds of ATP (Chapters 2, 3, and 16). The concentrations of many inorganic molecules must also be regulated to maintain body structure and function,

for example, the calcium found in bones (Chapter 11). One of the most important functions of the body is to respond to changing demands, such as the increased requirement for nutrients and oxygen in exercising muscle. This requires a coordinated allocation of resources to regions that most require them at a particular time. The mechanisms by which the organ systems of the body recognize and respond to changing demands is a theme you will encounter repeatedly in Chapters 6 through 19.

8. ***Structure is a determinant of—and has coevolved with—function.*** The form and composition of cells, tissues, organs, and organ systems determine how they interact with each other and with the physical world. Throughout the text, you will see examples of how different body parts converge in their structure to accomplish similar functions. For example, enormous elaborations of surface areas to facilitate membrane transport and diffusion can be observed in the circulatory (Chapter 12), respiratory (Chapter 13), urinary (Chapter 14), digestive (Chapter 15), and reproductive (Chapter 17) systems.

SUMMARY

The Scope of Human Physiology

I. Physiology is the study of how living organisms work. Physiologists are interested in the regulation of body function.

II. Disease states are physiology "gone wrong" (pathophysiology).

How Is the Body Organized?

I. Cells are the simplest structural units into which a complex multicellular organism can be divided and still retain the functions characteristic of life.

II. Cell differentiation results in the formation of four general categories of specialized cells:
   a. Muscle cells generate the mechanical activities that produce force and movement.
   b. Neurons initiate and conduct electrical signals.
   c. Epithelial cells form barriers and selectively secrete and absorb ions and organic molecules.
   d. Connective-tissue cells connect, anchor, and support the structures of the body.

III. Specialized cells associate with similar cells to form tissues: muscle tissue, nervous tissue, epithelial tissue, and connective tissue.

IV. Organs are composed of two or more of the four kinds of tissues arranged in various proportions and patterns. Many organs contain multiple, small, similar functional units.

V. An organ system is a collection of organs that together perform an overall function.

Body Fluid Compartments

I. The body fluids are enclosed in compartments.
   a. The extracellular fluid is composed of the interstitial fluid (the fluid between cells) and the blood plasma. Of the extracellular fluid, 75%–80% is interstitial fluid, and 20%–25% is plasma.
   b. Interstitial fluid and plasma have essentially the same composition except that plasma contains a much greater concentration of protein.
   c. Extracellular fluid differs markedly in composition from the fluid inside cells—the intracellular fluid.
   d. Approximately one-third of body water is in the extracellular compartment, and two-thirds is intracellular.

II. The differing compositions of the compartments reflect the activities of the barriers separating them.

Homeostasis: A Defining Feature of Physiology

I. The body's internal environment is the extracellular fluid.

II. The function of organ systems is to maintain a stable internal environment—this is called homeostasis.

III. Numerous variables within the body must be maintained homeostatically. When homeostasis is lost for one variable, it may trigger a series of changes in other variables.

General Characteristics of Homeostatic Control Systems

I. Homeostasis denotes the stable condition of the internal environment that results from the operation of compensatory homeostatic control systems.
   a. In a negative feedback control system, a change in the variable being regulated brings about responses that tend to push the variable in the direction opposite to the original change. Negative feedback minimizes changes from the set point of the system, leading to stability.
   b. Homeostatic control systems minimize changes in the internal environment but cannot maintain complete constancy.
   c. Feedforward regulation anticipates changes in a regulated variable, improves the speed of the body's homeostatic responses, and minimizes fluctuations in the level of the variable being regulated.

Components of Homeostatic Control Systems

I. The components of a reflex arc are the receptor, afferent pathway, integrating center, efferent pathway, and effector. The pathways may be neural or hormonal.

II. Local homeostatic responses are also stimulus–response sequences, but they occur only in the area of the stimulus, with neither nerves nor hormones involved.

The Role of Intercellular Chemical Messengers in Homeostasis

I. Intercellular communication is essential to reflexes and local responses and is achieved by neurotransmitters, hormones, and paracrine or autocrine substances. Less common is intercellular communication through either gap junctions or cell-bound messengers.

Processes Related to Homeostasis

I. Acclimatization is an improved ability to respond to an environmental stress. The improvement is induced by prolonged exposure to the stress with no change in genetic endowment.

II. Biological rhythms provide a feedforward component to homeostatic control systems.
   a. The rhythms are internally driven by brain pacemakers but are entrained by environmental cues, such as light, which also serve to phase-shift (reset) the rhythms when necessary.
   b. In the absence of cues, rhythms free-run.

III. The balance of substances in the body is achieved by matching inputs and outputs. Total-body balance of a substance may be negative, positive, or stable.

General Principles of Physiology

I. Several fundamental, general principles of physiology are important in understanding how the human body functions at all levels of structure, from cells to organ systems. These include, among others, such things as homeostasis, information flow, coordination between the function of different organ systems, and the balance of matter and energy.

REVIEW QUESTIONS

1. Describe the levels of cellular organization and state the four types of specialized cells and tissues.
2. List the organ systems of the body and give one-sentence descriptions of their functions.
3. Name the two fluids that constitute the extracellular fluid. What are their relative proportions in the body, and how do they differ from each other in composition?
4. State the relative volumes of water in the body fluid compartments.
5. Describe several important generalizations about homeostatic control systems.
6. Contrast feedforward and negative feedback.
7. List the components of a reflex arc.
8. What is the basic difference between a local homeostatic response and a reflex?
9. List the general categories of intercellular messengers.
10. Describe the conditions under which acclimatization occurs. Are acclimatizations passed on to a person's offspring?
11. Under what conditions do circadian rhythms become free running?
12. How do phase shifts occur?
13. What is the most important environmental cue for entrainment of body rhythms?
14. Draw a figure illustrating the balance concept in homeostasis.
15. Make a list of the General Principles of Physiology, without the paragraphs that accompany each one. See if you can explain what is meant by each principle. To really see how well you've learned physiology at the end of your course, remember to return to the list you've made and try this exercise again at that time.

KEY TERMS

acclimatization 13
acquired reflex 10
adaptation 12
afferent pathway 10
autocrine substance 12
basement membrane 3
cell 2
cell differentiation 2
circadian rhythm 13
collagen fiber 4
connective tissue 3
connective-tissue cell 4
dynamic constancy 7
effector 10
efferent pathway 10
elastin fiber 4
endocrine gland 12
entrainment 13
epithelial cell 3
epithelial tissue 2
equilibrium 7
extracellular fluid 5
extracellular matrix 4
feedforward 10
fiber 4
free-running rhythm 13
functional unit 4
homeostasis 6
homeostatic control system 7
hormone 11
integrating center 10
internal environment 4
interstitial fluid 5
interstitium 5
intracellular fluid 5
learned reflex 10
local homeostatic response 11
melatonin 14
muscle cell 3
muscle tissue 3
negative balance 14
negative feedback 8
nervous tissue 3
neuron 3
neurotransmitter 12
organ 3
organ system 3
pacemaker 14
paracrine substance 12
pathophysiology 2
phase-shift 13
physiology 2
pineal gland 14
plasma 5
pool 14
positive balance 14
positive feedback 8
receptor 10
reflex 10
reflex arc 10
set point 7
stable balance 14
steady state 7
stimulus 10
target cell 12
tissue 3

CHAPTER 1 Clinical Case Study: Loss of Consciousness in a 64-Year-Old Man While Gardening on a Hot Day

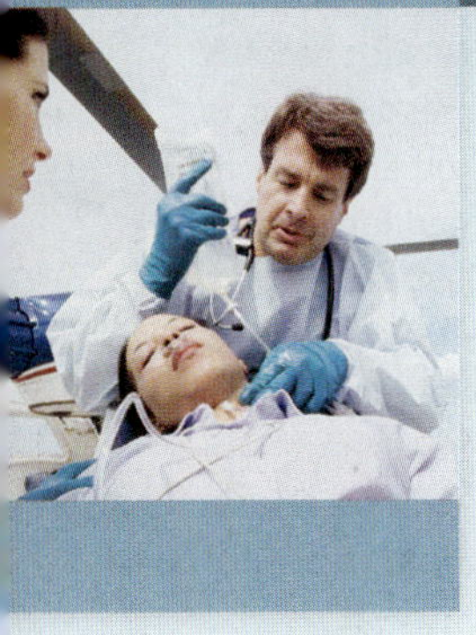

Throughout this text, you will find a feature at the end of each chapter called the "Clinical Case Study." These segments reinforce what you have learned in that chapter by applying it to real-life examples of different medical conditions. The clinical case studies will increase in complexity as you progress through the text and will enable you to integrate recent material from a given chapter with information learned in previous chapters. In this first clinical case study, we examine a serious and potentially life-threatening condition that can occur in individuals in whom body temperature homeostasis is disrupted. All of the material presented in this clinical case study will be explored in depth in subsequent chapters, as you learn the mechanisms that underlie the pathologies and compensatory responses illustrated here in brief. Notice as you read that the first two general principles of physiology described earlier are particularly relevant to this case. *It is highly recommended that you return to this case study as a benchmark at the end of your semester; we are certain that you will be amazed at how your understanding of physiology has grown in that time.*

A 64-year-old, fair-skinned man in good overall health spent a very hot, humid summer day gardening in his backyard. After several hours in the sun, he began to feel light-headed and

(continued)

(continued)

confused as he knelt over his vegetable garden. Although earlier he had been perspiring profusely, his sweating had eventually stopped. Because he also felt confused and disoriented, he could not recall for how long he had not been perspiring, or even how long it had been since he had taken a drink of water. He called to his wife, who was alarmed to see that his skin had turned a pale-blue color. She asked her husband to come indoors, but he fainted as soon as he tried to stand. The wife called for an ambulance, and the man was taken to a hospital and diagnosed with a condition called heatstroke. What happened to this man that would explain his condition? How does it relate to homeostasis?

As you learned in this chapter, body temperature is a physiological function that is under homeostatic control. If body temperature decreases, heat production increases and heat loss decreases, as illustrated in Figures 1.5 and 1.8. Conversely, as in our example here, if body temperature increases, heat production decreases and heat loss increases. When our patient began gardening on a hot, humid day, his body temperature began to increase. At first, he perspired heavily. As you will learn in Chapter 16, perspiration is an important mechanism by which the body loses heat; it takes considerable heat to evaporate water from the surface of the skin, and the source of that heat is from the body. However, as you likely know from personal experience, evaporation of water from the body is less effective in humid environments, which makes it more dangerous to exercise when it is not only hot but also humid.

The sources of perspiration are the sweat glands, which are located beneath the skin and which secrete a salty solution through ducts to the surface of the skin. The fluid in sweat comes from the extracellular fluid compartment, which, as you have learned, consists of the plasma and interstitial fluid compartments (see Figure 1.3). Consequently, the profuse sweating that initially occurred in this man caused his extracellular fluid levels to decrease. In fact, the fluid levels decreased so severely that the amount of blood available to be pumped out of his heart with each heartbeat also decreased. The relationship between fluid volume and blood pressure is an important one that you will learn about in detail in Chapter 12. Generally speaking, if extracellular fluid levels decrease, blood pressure decreases as a consequence. This explains why our patient felt light-headed, particularly when he suddenly tried to stand up. As his blood pressure decreased, the ability of his heart to pump sufficient blood against gravity up to his brain also decreased; when brain cells are deprived of blood flow, they begin to malfunction. Standing suddenly only made matters worse. Perhaps you have occasionally experienced a little of this light-headed feeling when you have jumped out of a chair or bed and stood up too quickly. Normally, your nervous system quickly compensates for the effects of gravity on blood flowing up to the brain, as will be described in Chapters 6 and 12. In a person with decreased blood volume and pressure, however, this compensation may not happen and the person can lose consciousness. After fainting and falling, the man's head and heart were at the same horizontal level; consequently, blood could more easily reach his brain.

Another concern is that the salt concentrations in the body fluids changed. If you have ever tasted the sweat on your upper lip on a hot day, you know that it is somewhat salty. That is because sweat is derived from extracellular fluid, which as you have learned is a watery solution of ions (derived from salts, such as NaCl) and other substances. Sweat, however, is slightly more dilute than extracellular fluid because more water than ions is secreted from sweat glands. Consequently, the more heavily one perspires, the more concentrated the extracellular fluid becomes. In other words, the total amount of water and ions in the extracellular fluid decreases with perspiration, but the remaining fluid is "saltier." Heavy perspiration, therefore, not only disrupts fluid balance and blood pressure homeostasis but also has an impact on the balance of the ions in the body fluids, notably Na^+, K^+, and Cl^-. A homeostatic balance of ion concentrations in the body fluids is absolutely essential for normal heart and brain function, as you will learn in Chapters 4 and 6. As the man's ion concentrations changed, therefore, the change affected the activity of the cells of his brain.

Why did the man stop perspiring and why did his skin turn pale? To understand this, we must consider that several homeostatic variables were disrupted by his activities. His body temperature increased, which initially resulted in heavy sweating. As the sweating continued, it resulted in an imbalance in fluid levels and ion concentrations in his body; this contributed to a decrease in mental function, and he became confused. As his body fluid levels continued to decrease, his blood pressure also decreased, further endangering brain function. At this point, the homeostatic control systems were essentially in competition. Though it is potentially life threatening for body temperature to increase too much, it is also life threatening for blood pressure to decrease too much. Eventually, many of the blood vessels in regions of the body that are not immediately required for survival, such as the skin, began to close off. By doing so, the more vital organs of the body—such as the brain—could receive sufficient blood. This is why the man's skin turned a pale blue, because the amount of oxygen-rich blood flowing to the surface of his skin was decreased. Unfortunately, although this compensatory mechanism helped save the man's brain and other vital organs, reducing the amount of blood flowing to the skin made it impossible for the sweat glands under the skin to extract extracellular fluid and make more sweat. The man stopped perspiring, therefore, and a key mechanism to controlling his body temperature was lost. At that point, his body temperature spiraled out of control and he was hospitalized.

This case illustrates a critical feature of homeostasis that you will encounter throughout this textbook and that was emphasized in this chapter. Often, when one physiological variable such as body temperature is disrupted, the compensatory responses initiated to correct that disruption cause, in turn, imbalances in other variables. These secondary imbalances must also be compensated for, and the significance of each imbalance must be "weighed" against the others. In this example, the man was treated with intravenous fluids made up of a salt solution to restore his fluid levels and concentrations, and he was immersed in a cool bath and given cool compresses to help reduce his body temperature. Although he recovered, many people do not survive heatstroke because of its profound impact on homeostasis.

See Chapter 19 for complete, integrative case studies.

CHAPTER 1 TEST QUESTIONS

Answers found in Appendix A.

1. Which of the following is one of the four basic cell types in the body?
   a. respiratory
   b. epithelial
   c. endocrine
   d. integumentary
   e. immune
2. Which of the following is incorrect?
   a. Equilibrium requires a constant input of energy.
   b. Positive feedback is less common in nature than negative feedback.
   c. Homeostasis does not imply that a given variable is unchanging.
   d. Fever is an example of resetting a set point.
   e. Efferent pathways carry information away from the integrating center of a reflex arc.
3. In a reflex arc initiated by touching a hand to a hot stove, the effector belongs to which class of tissue?
   a. nervous
   b. connective
   c. muscle
   d. epithelial
4. In the absence of any environmental cues, a circadian rhythm is said to be
   a. entrained.
   b. in phase.
   c. free running.
   d. phase-shifted.
   e. no longer present.
5. Most of the water in the human body is found in
   a. the interstitial fluid compartment.
   b. the intracellular fluid compartment.
   c. the plasma compartment.
   d. the total extracellular fluid compartment.

CHAPTER 1 QUANTITATIVE AND THOUGHT QUESTIONS

Answers found at www.mhhe.com/widmaier13.

1. The Inuit of Alaska and Canada have a remarkable ability to work in the cold without gloves and not suffer decreased skin blood flow. Does this prove that there is a genetic difference between the Inuit and other people with regard to this characteristic?
2. Explain how an imbalance in any given physiological variable may produce a change in one or more *other* variables.

CHAPTER 1 ANSWERS TO PHYSIOLOGICAL INQUIRIES

Figure 1.3 Approximately one-third of total-body water is in the extracellular compartments. If water makes up 60% of a person's body weight, then the water in extracellular fluid makes up approximately 20% of body weight (because $0.33 \times 0.60 = 0.20$).

Figure 1.6 Removing negative feedback in this example would result in an increase in the amount of active product formed, and eventually the amount of available substrate would be greatly depleted.

Figure 1.8 If body temperature were to increase, the efferent pathway shown in this diagram would either turn off or become reversed. For example, shivering would not occur (muscles may even become more relaxed than usual), and blood vessels in the skin would not constrict. Indeed, in such a scenario, skin blood vessels would dilate to bring warm blood to the skin surface, where the heat could leave the body across the skin. Heat loss, therefore, would be increased.

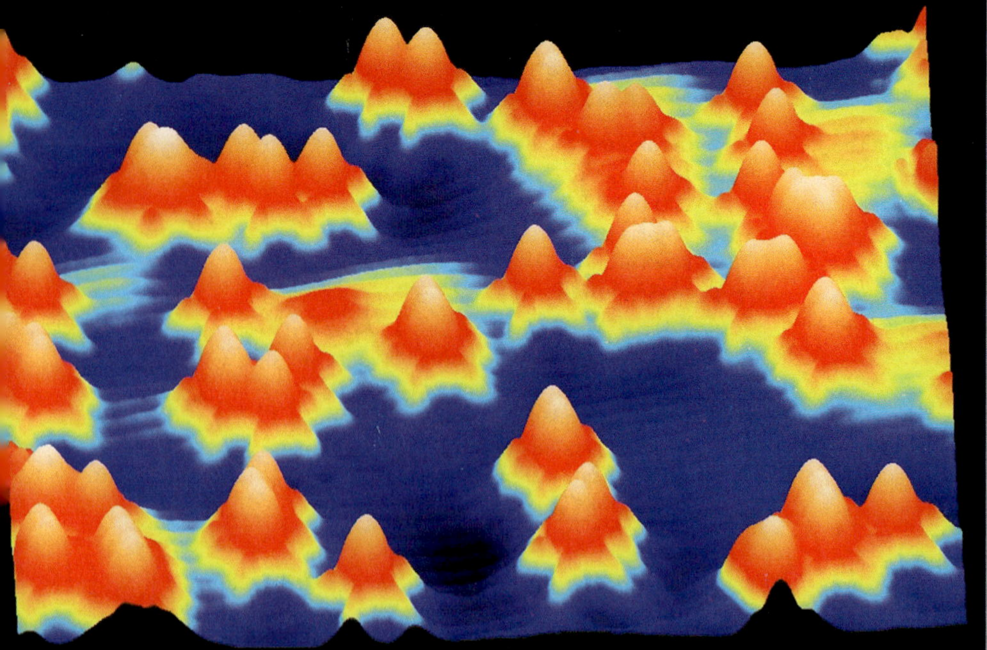

Colorized scanning tunneling micrograph of individual manganese atoms; clouds of orbiting electrons are shown in red and yellow.

2 Chemical Composition of the Body

In Chapter 1, you were introduced to the concept of homeostasis, and how chemistry plays an important role in the maintenance of homeostasis, particularly at the cellular level. To fully appreciate the importance of chemistry to physiology, it is necessary to briefly review some of the key features of atoms and molecules that contribute to their ability to interact with one another. Such interactions form the basis for processes as diverse as maintaining a healthy pH of the body fluids, determining which molecules will bind to or otherwise influence the function of other molecules, forming functional proteins that mediate numerous physiological processes, and maintaining energy homeostasis.

In this chapter, we describe the distinguishing characteristics of some of the major molecules in the human body. The specific roles of these substances in physiology will be introduced here and discussed more fully in subsequent chapters where appropriate. This chapter will provide you with the knowledge required to best appreciate the significance of one of the general principles of physiology introduced in Chapter 1, namely that physiological processes are dictated by the laws of chemistry and physics.

2.1 Atoms

The units of matter that form all chemical substances are called **atoms.** Each type of atom—carbon, hydrogen, oxygen, and so on—is called a **chemical element.** A one- or two-letter symbol is used as an abbreviated identification for each element. Although more than 100 elements occur naturally or have been synthesized in the laboratory, only 24 (**Table 2.1**) are known to be essential for the structure and function of the human body and are therefore of particular interest to physiologists.

Components of Atoms

The chemical properties of atoms can be described in terms of three subatomic particles—**protons, neutrons,** and **electrons.** The protons and neutrons are confined to a very small volume at the center of an atom called the **atomic nucleus.** The electrons revolve in orbitals at various distances from the nucleus. Each orbital can hold up to two electrons and no more. The larger the atom, the more electrons it contains, and therefore the more orbitals that exist around the nucleus. Orbitals are found in regions known as electron shells; additional shells exist at greater and greater distances from the nucleus as atoms get bigger. An atom such as carbon has more shells than does hydrogen with its lone electron, but fewer than an atom such as iron, which has a greater number of electrons. The first, innermost shell of any atom can hold up to two electrons in a single, spherical ("*s*") orbital (**Figure 2.1a**). Once the innermost shell is filled, electrons begin to fill the second shell. The second shell can hold up to eight electrons; the first two electrons fill a spherical orbital, and subsequent electrons fill three additional, propeller-shaped ("*p*") orbitals. Additional shells can accommodate further orbitals; this will happen once the inner shells are filled. For simplicity, we will ignore the distinction between *s* and *p* orbitals and represent the shells of an atom in two dimensions as shown in **Figure 2.1b** for nitrogen.

An atom is most stable when all of the orbitals in its outermost shell are filled with two electrons each. If one or more orbitals do not have their capacity of electrons, the atom can react with other atoms and form molecules, as described later. For many of the atoms that are most important for physiology, the outer shell requires eight electrons in its orbitals in order to be filled to capacity.

TABLE 2.1 Essential Chemical Elements in the Body (neo-Latin terms in italics)

Element	Symbol
Major Elements: 99.3% of Total Atoms in the Body	
Hydrogen	H (63%)
Oxygen	O (26%)
Carbon	C (9%)
Nitrogen	N (1%)
Mineral Elements: 0.7% of Total Atoms in the Body	
Calcium	Ca
Phosphorus	P
Potassium	K (*kalium*)
Sulfur	S
Sodium	Na (*natrium*)
Chlorine	Cl
Magnesium	Mg
Trace Elements: Less than 0.01% of Total Atoms in the Body	
Iron	Fe (*ferrum*)
Iodine	I
Copper	Cu (*cuprum*)
Zinc	Zn
Manganese	Mn
Cobalt	Co
Chromium	Cr
Selenium	Se
Molybdenum	Mo
Fluorine	F
Tin	Sn (*stannum*)
Silicon	Si
Vanadium	V

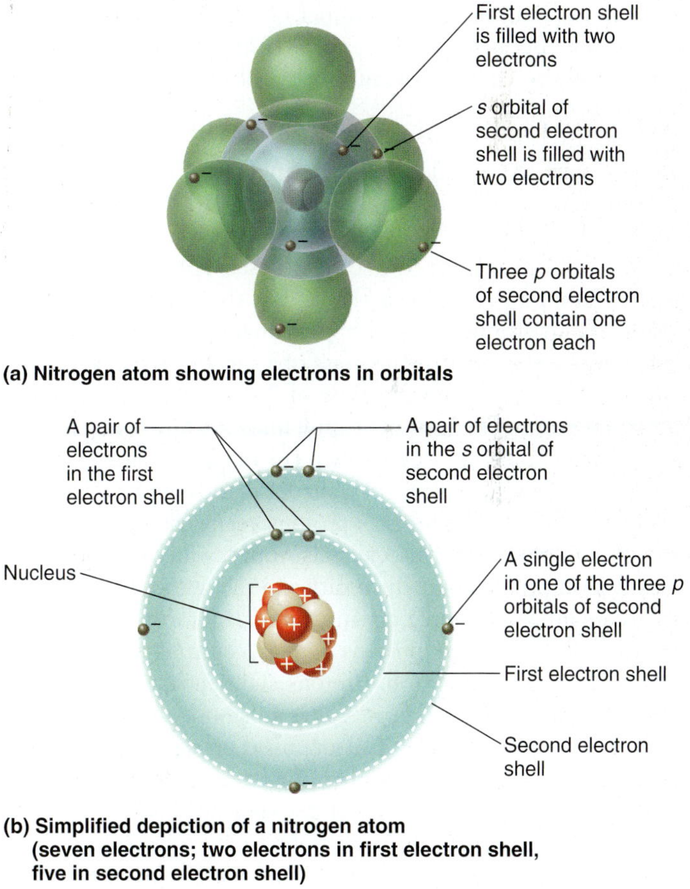

Figure 2.1 APIR Arrangement of subatomic particles in an atom, shown here for nitrogen. (a) Negatively charged electrons orbit around a nucleus consisting of positively charged protons and (except for hydrogen) uncharged neutrons. Up to two electrons may occupy an orbital, shown here as regions in which an electron is likely to be found. The orbitals exist within electron shells at progressively greater distances from the nucleus as atoms get bigger. Different shells may contain a different number of orbitals. (b) Simplified, two-dimensional depiction of a nitrogen atom, showing a full complement of two electrons in its innermost shell and five electrons in its second, outermost shell. Orbitals are not depicted using this simplified means of illustrating an atom.

Each of the subatomic particles has a different electrical charge. Protons have one unit of positive charge, electrons have one unit of negative charge, and neutrons are electrically neutral. Because the protons are located in the atomic nucleus, the nucleus has a net positive charge equal to the number of protons it contains. One of the fundamental principles of physics is that opposite electrical charges attract each other and like charges repel each other. It is the attraction between the positively charged protons and the negatively charged electrons that serves as a major force that forms an atom. The entire atom has no net electrical charge, however, because the number of negatively charged electrons orbiting the nucleus equals the number of positively charged protons in the nucleus.

Atomic Number

Each chemical element contains a unique and specific number of protons, and it is this number, known as the **atomic number,** that distinguishes one type of atom from another. For example, hydrogen, the simplest atom, has an atomic number of 1, corresponding to its single proton. As another example, calcium has an atomic number of 20, corresponding to its 20 protons. Because an atom is electrically neutral, the atomic number is also equal to the number of electrons in the atom.

Atomic Mass

Atoms have very little mass. A single hydrogen atom, for example, has a mass of only 1.67×10^{-24} g. The **atomic mass** scale indicates an atom's mass relative to the mass of other atoms. By convention, this scale is based upon assigning the carbon atom a mass of exactly 12. On this scale, a hydrogen atom has an atomic mass of approximately 1, indicating that it has about one-twelfth the mass of a carbon atom. A magnesium atom, with an atomic mass of 24, has twice the mass of a carbon atom. The unit of atomic mass is known as a dalton. One dalton (d) equals one-twelfth the mass of a carbon atom.

Although the number of neutrons in the nucleus of an atom is often equal to the number of protons, many chemical elements can exist in multiple forms, called **isotopes,** which have identical numbers of protons but which differ in the number of neutrons they contain. For example, the most abundant form of the carbon atom, ^{12}C, contains six protons and six neutrons and therefore has an atomic number of 6. Protons and neutrons are approximately equal in mass, and so ^{12}C has an atomic mass of 12. The radioactive carbon isotope ^{14}C contains six protons and eight neutrons, giving it an atomic number of 6 but an atomic mass of 14. The value of atomic mass given in the standard Periodic Table of the Elements is actually an average mass that reflects the relative abundance in nature of the different isotopes of a given element.

Many isotopes are unstable; they will spontaneously emit energy or even release components of the atom itself, such as part of the nucleus. This process is known as radiation, and such isotopes are called **radioisotopes.** The special qualities of radioisotopes are of great practical benefit in the practice of medicine and the study of physiology. In one example, high-energy radiation can be focused onto cancerous areas of the body to kill cancer cells. Radioisotopes may also be useful in making diagnoses. In one common method, the sugar glucose can be chemically modified so that it contains a radioactive isotope of fluorine. When injected into the blood, all of the organs of the body take up the radioactive glucose just as they would ordinary glucose. Special imaging techniques such as ***PET (positron emission tomography) scans*** can then be used to detect how much of the radioactive glucose appears in different organs (**Figure 2.2**); because glucose is a key source of energy used by all cells, this information can be used to determine if a given organ is functioning normally or at an increased or decreased rate. For example, a PET scan that revealed decreased uptake of radioactive glucose into the heart might indicate that the blood vessels of the heart were diseased, thereby depriving the heart of nutrients. PET scans can also reveal the presence of cancer—a disease characterized by uncontrolled cell growth and increased glucose uptake.

The **gram atomic mass** of a chemical element is the amount of the element, in grams, equal to the numerical value of its atomic mass. Thus, 12 g of carbon (assuming it is all ^{12}C) is 1 gram atomic mass of carbon, and 1 g of hydrogen is 1 gram atomic mass of hydrogen. *One gram atomic mass of any element contains the same number of atoms.* For example, 1 g of hydrogen contains 6×10^{23} atoms; likewise, 12 g of carbon, whose atoms have 12 times the mass of a hydrogen atom, also has 6×10^{23} atoms (this value is often called Avogadro's constant, or Avogadro's number, after the nineteenth-century Italian scientist Amedeo Avogadro).

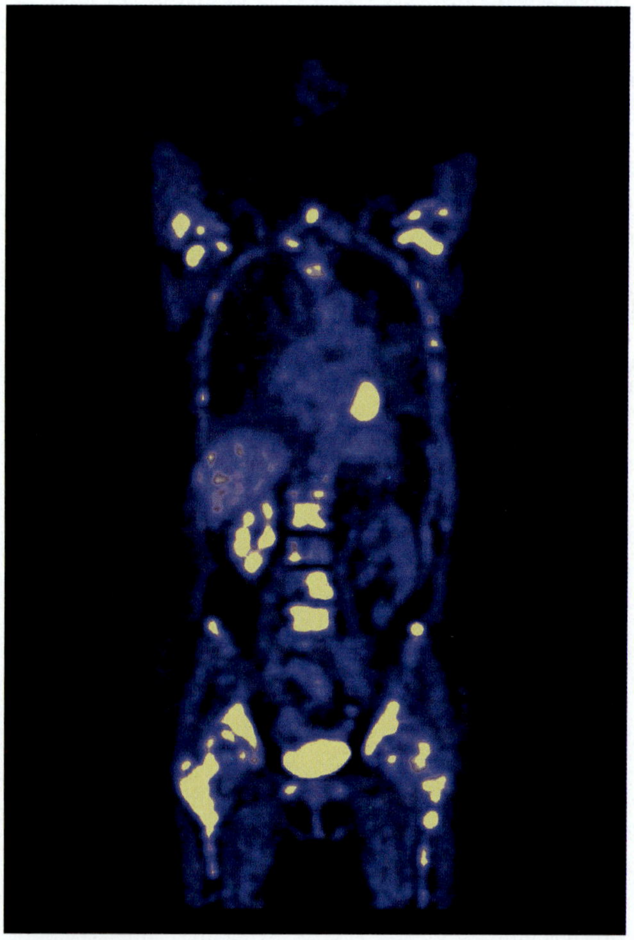

Figure 2.2 Positron emission tomography (PET) scan of a human body. In this image, radioactive glucose that has been taken up by the body's organs appears as a false color; the greater the uptake, the more intense the color. The brightest regions were found to be areas of cancer in this particular individual.

Ions

As mentioned earlier, a single atom is electrically neutral because it contains equal numbers of negative electrons and positive protons. There are instances, however, in which certain atoms may gain or lose one or more electrons; in such cases, they will then acquire a net electrical charge and become an **ion.** This may happen, for example, if an atom has an outer shell that contains only one or a few electrons; losing those electrons would mean that the next innermost shell would then become the outermost shell. This shell is complete with a full capacity of electrons and is therefore very stable (recall that each successive shell does not begin to acquire electrons until all the preceding inner shells are filled). For example, when a sodium atom (Na), which has 11 electrons, loses one electron, it becomes a sodium ion (Na^+) with a net positive charge; it still has 11 protons, but it now has only 10 electrons, two in its first shell and a full complement of eight in its second, outer shell. On the other hand, a chlorine atom (Cl), which has 17 electrons, is one electron shy of a full outer shell. It can gain an electron and become a chloride ion (Cl^-) with a net negative charge—it now has 18 electrons but only 17 protons. Some atoms can gain or lose more than one electron to become ions with two or even three units of net electrical charge (for example, the calcium ion Ca^{2+}).

Hydrogen and many other atoms readily form ions. Table 2.2 lists the ionic forms of some of these elements that are found in the body. Ions that have a net positive charge are called **cations,** and those that have a net negative charge are called **anions.** Because of their charge, ions are able to conduct electricity when dissolved in water; consequently, the ionic forms of mineral elements are collectively referred to as **electrolytes.** This is extremely important in physiology, because electrolytes are used to carry electrical charge across cell membranes; in this way, they serve as the source of electrical current in certain cells. You will learn in Chapters 6, 9, and 12 that such currents are critical to the ability of muscle cells and neurons to function in their characteristic ways.

Atomic Composition of the Body

Just four of the body's essential elements (see Table 2.1)—hydrogen, oxygen, carbon, and nitrogen—account for over 99% of the atoms in the body.

The seven essential **mineral elements** are the most abundant substances dissolved in the extracellular and intracellular fluids. Most of the body's calcium and phosphorus atoms, however, make up the solid matrix of bone tissue.

The 13 essential **trace elements,** so-called because they are present in extremely small quantities, are required for normal growth and function. For example, iron plays a critical role in the blood's transport of oxygen, and iodine is required for the production of thyroid hormone.

Many other elements, in addition to the 24 listed in Table 2.1, may be detected in the body. These elements enter in the foods we eat and the air we breathe but are not essential for normal body function and may even interfere with normal body chemistry. For example, ingested arsenic has poisonous effects.

2.2 Molecules

Two or more atoms bonded together make up a **molecule.** A molecule made up of two or more different elements is called a compound, but the two terms are often used interchangeably. For example, a molecule of oxygen gas consists of two atoms of oxygen bonded together. By contrast, water is a compound that contains two hydrogen atoms and one oxygen atom. For simplicity, we will simply use the term *molecule* in this textbook. Molecules can be represented by their component atoms. In the two examples just given, a molecule of oxygen can be represented as O_2 and water as H_2O. The atomic composition of glucose, a sugar, is $C_6H_{12}O_6$, indicating that the molecule contains 6 carbon atoms, 12 hydrogen atoms, and 6 oxygen atoms. Such formulas, however, do not indicate how the atoms are linked together in the molecule. This occurs by means of chemical bonds, as described next.

Covalent Chemical Bonds

Chemical bonds between atoms in a molecule form when electrons transfer from the outer electron shell of one atom to that of another, or when two atoms with partially unfilled electron orbitals share electrons. The strongest chemical bond between two atoms is called a **covalent bond,** which forms when one or more electrons in the outer electron orbitals of each atom are shared between the two atoms (**Figure 2.3**). In the example shown in Figure 2.3, a carbon atom with two electrons in its innermost shell and four in its outer shell forms covalent bonds with four hydrogen atoms. Recall that the second shell of atoms can hold up to eight electrons. Carbon has six total electrons

TABLE 2.2 Ionic Forms of Elements Most Frequently Encountered in the Body

Chemical Atom	Symbol	Ion	Chemical Symbol	Electrons Gained or Lost
Hydrogen	H	Hydrogen ion	H^+	**1 lost**
Sodium	Na	Sodium ion	Na^+	**1 lost**
Potassium	K	Potassium ion	K^+	**1 lost**
Chlorine	Cl	Chloride ion	Cl^-	**1 gained**
Magnesium	Mg	Magnesium ion	Mg^{2+}	**2 lost**
Calcium	Ca	Calcium ion	Ca^{2+}	**2 lost**

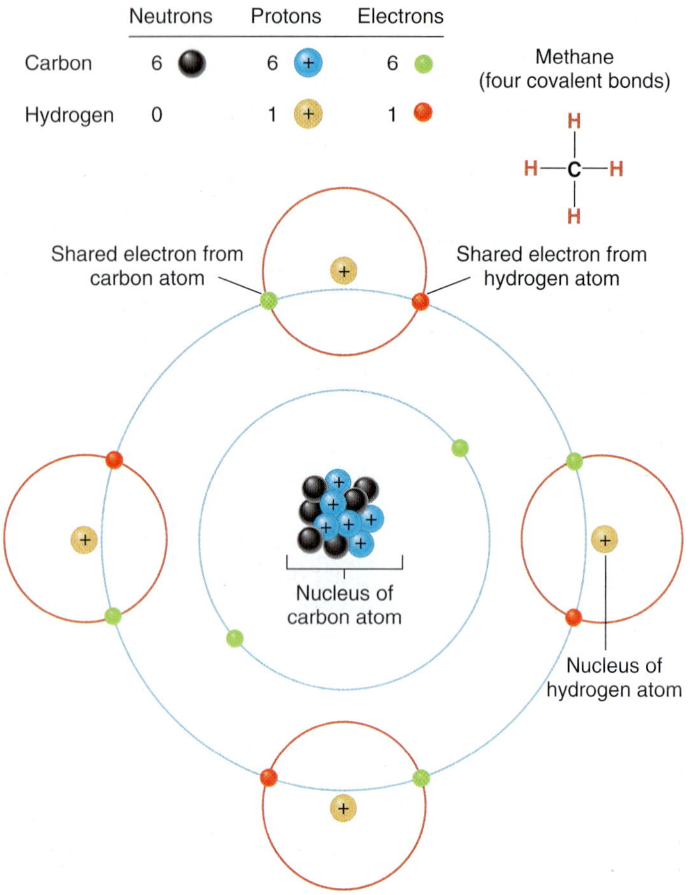

Figure 2.3 APIR A covalent bond formed by sharing electrons. Hydrogen atoms have room for one additional electron in their sole orbital; carbon atoms have four electrons in their second shell, which can accommodate up to eight electrons. Each of the four hydrogen atoms in a molecule of methane (CH_4) forms a covalent bond with the carbon atom by sharing its one electron with one of the electrons in carbon. Each shared pair of electrons—one electron from the carbon and one from a hydrogen atom—forms a covalent bond. The sizes of protons, neutrons, and electrons are not to scale.

and only four in the second shell, because two electrons are used to fill the first shell. Therefore, it has "room" to acquire four additional electrons in its outer shell. Hydrogen has only a single electron, but like all orbitals, its single orbital can hold up to two electrons. Therefore, hydrogen also has room for an additional electron. In this example, a single carbon atom shares its four electrons with four different hydrogen atoms, which in turn share their electrons with the carbon atom. The shared electrons orbit around both atoms, bonding them together into a molecule of methane (CH_4). These covalent bonds are the strongest type of bonds in the body; once formed, they usually do not break apart unless acted upon by an energy source (heat) or an enzyme (see Chapter 3 for a description of enzymes).

As mentioned, the atoms of some elements can form more than one covalent bond and thus become linked simultaneously to two or more other atoms. Each type of atom forms a characteristic number of covalent bonds, which depends on the number of electrons in its outermost orbit. The number of chemical bonds formed by the four most abundant atoms in the body are hydrogen, one; oxygen, two; nitrogen, three; and carbon, four. When the structure of a molecule is diagrammed, each covalent bond is represented by a line indicating a pair of shared electrons. The covalent bonds of the four elements just mentioned can be represented as

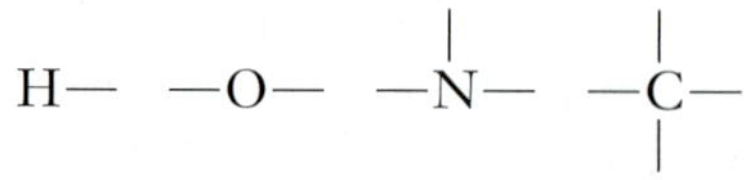

A molecule of water, H_2O, can be diagrammed as

H—O—H

In some cases, two covalent bonds—a double bond—form between two atoms when they share two electrons from each atom. Carbon dioxide (CO_2), a waste product of metabolism, contains two double bonds:

O=C=O

Note that in this molecule the carbon atom still forms four covalent bonds and each oxygen atom only two.

Polar Covalent Bonds

Not all atoms have the same ability to attract shared electrons. The measure of an atom's ability to attract electrons in a covalent bond is called its **electronegativity.** Electronegativity generally increases as the total positive charge of a nucleus increases but decreases as the distance between the shared electrons and the nucleus increases. When two atoms with different electronegativities combine to form a covalent bond, the shared electrons will tend to spend more time orbiting the atom with the higher electronegativity. This creates a polarity across the bond (think of the poles of a magnet; only in this case the polarity refers to a difference in charge).

Due to the polarity in electron distribution just described, the more electronegative atom acquires a slight negative charge, whereas the other atom, having partly lost an electron, becomes slightly positive. Such bonds are known as **polar covalent bonds** (or, simply, polar bonds) because the atoms at each end of the bond have an opposite electrical charge. For example, the bond between hydrogen and oxygen in a **hydroxyl group** (—OH) is a polar covalent bond in which the oxygen is slightly negative and the hydrogen slightly positive:

$$R—\overset{(\delta^-)}{O}—\overset{(\delta^+)}{H}$$

The δ^- and δ^+ symbols refer to atoms with a partial negative or positive charge, respectively. The R symbolizes the remainder of the molecule; in water, for example, R is simply another hydrogen atom carrying another partial positive charge. The electrical charge associated with the ends of a polar bond is considerably less than the charge on a fully ionized atom. Polar bonds do not have a *net* electrical charge, as do ions, because they contain overall equal amounts of negative and positive charge.

Atoms of oxygen, nitrogen, and sulfur, which have a relatively strong attraction for electrons, form polar bonds with hydrogen atoms (Table 2.3). One of the characteristics of polar bonds that is important in our understanding of physiology is that molecules that contain such bonds tend to be more soluble in water than molecules containing the other major type of covalent bond, described next. Consequently, these molecules—called **polar molecules**—readily dissolve in the blood, interstitial fluid,

TABLE 2.3 Examples of Nonpolar and Polar Bonds and Ionized Chemical Groups

Nonpolar Bonds	—C—H	Carbon–hydrogen bond
	—C—C—	Carbon–carbon bond
Polar Bonds	$R—\overset{(\delta^-)}{O}—\overset{(\delta^+)}{H}$	Hydroxyl group (R—OH)
	$R—\overset{(\delta^-)}{S}—\overset{(\delta^+)}{H}$	Sulfhydryl group (R—SH)
	$H^{(\delta^+)}$ bonded to $N^{(\delta^-)}$ in R—N—R	Nitrogen–hydrogen bond
Ionized Groups	R—C(=O)—O^-	Carboxyl group (R—COO^-)
	R—N^+(H_3)	Amino group (R—NH_3^+)
	R—O—P(=O)(O^-)—O^-	Phosphate group (R—PO_4^{2-})

and intracellular fluid. Indeed, water itself is the classic example of a polar molecule, with a partially negatively charged oxygen atom and two partially positively charged hydrogen atoms.

Nonpolar Covalent Bonds

In contrast to polar covalent bonds, bonds between atoms with similar electronegativities are said to be **nonpolar covalent bonds.** In such bonds, the electrons are equally or nearly equally shared by the two atoms, such that there is little or no unequal charge distribution across the bond. Bonds between carbon and hydrogen atoms and between two carbon atoms are electrically neutral, nonpolar covalent bonds (see Table 2.3). Molecules that contain high proportions of nonpolar covalent bonds are called **nonpolar molecules;** they tend to be less soluble in water than those with polar covalent bonds. Consequently, such molecules are often found in the lipid bilayers of the membranes of cells and intracellular organelles. When present in body fluids such as the blood, they may associate with a polar molecule that serves as a sort of "carrier" to prevent the nonpolar molecule from coming out of solution. The characteristics of molecules in solution will be covered later in this chapter.

Ionic Bonds

As noted earlier, some elements, such as those that make up table salt (NaCl), can form ions. NaCl is a solid crystalline substance because of the strong electrical attraction between positive sodium ions and negative chloride ions. This strong attraction between two oppositely charged ions is known as an **ionic bond.** When a crystal of sodium chloride is placed in water, the highly polar water molecules with their partial positive and negative charges are attracted to the charged sodium and chloride ions (**Figure 2.4**). Clusters of water molecules surround the ions, allowing the sodium and chloride ions to separate from each other and enter the water—that is, to dissolve.

Hydrogen Bonds

When two polar molecules are in close contact, an electrical attraction may form between them. For example, the hydrogen atom in a polar bond in one molecule and an oxygen or nitrogen atom in a polar bond of another molecule attract each other forming a type of bond called a **hydrogen bond.** Such bonds may also form between atoms within the same molecule. Hydrogen bonds are represented in diagrams by dashed or dotted lines to distinguish them from covalent bonds, as illustrated in the bonds between water molecules (**Figure 2.5**). Hydrogen bonds are very weak, having only about 4% of the strength of the polar bonds between the hydrogen and oxygen atoms in a single molecule of water. Although hydrogen bonds are weak individually, when present in large numbers, they play an extremely important role in molecular interactions and in determining the shape of large molecules. This is of great importance for physiology, because the shape of large molecules often determines their

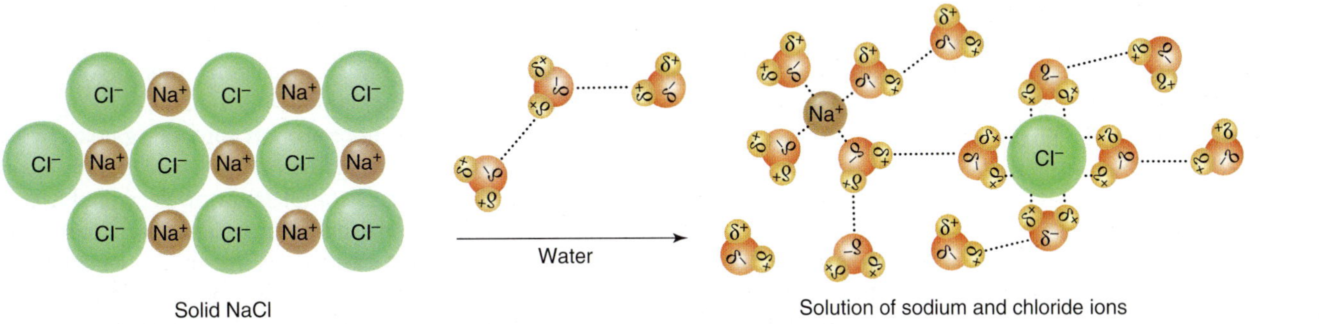

Figure 2.4 APR The electrical attraction between the charged sodium and chloride ions forms ionic bonds in solid NaCl. The attraction of the polar, partially charged regions of water molecules breaks the ionic bonds and the sodium and chloride ions dissolve.

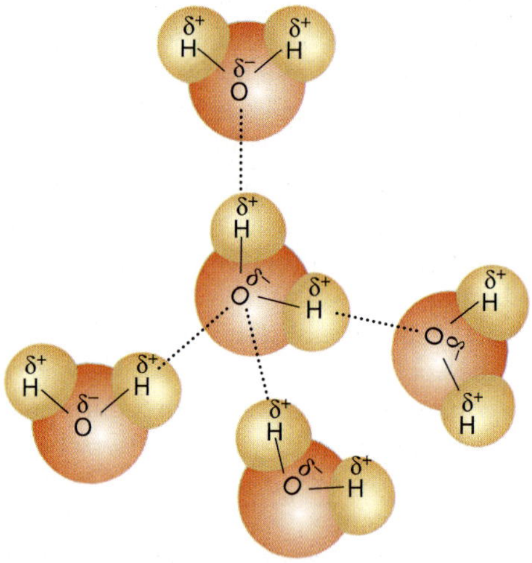

Figure 2.5 Five water molecules. Note that polar covalent bonds link the hydrogen and oxygen atoms within each molecule and that hydrogen bonds occur between adjacent molecules. Hydrogen bonds are represented in diagrams by dashed or dotted lines, and covalent bonds by solid lines.

PHYSIOLOGICAL INQUIRY

- What effect might hydrogen bonds have on the temperature at which liquid water becomes a vapor?

Answer can be found at end of chapter.

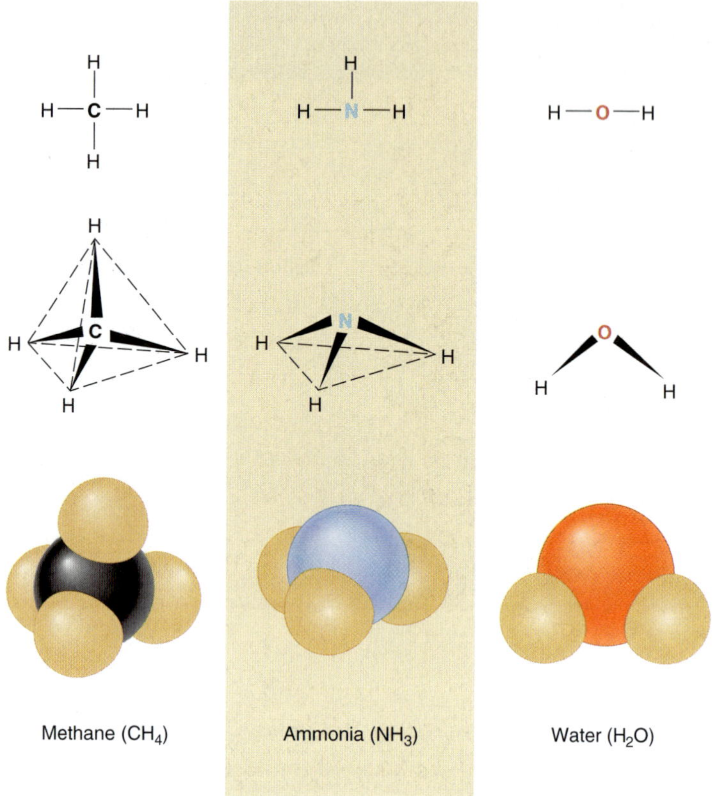

Figure 2.6 Three different ways of representing the geometric configuration of covalent bonds around the carbon, nitrogen, and oxygen atoms bonded to hydrogen atoms.

functions and their ability to interact with other molecules. For example, some molecules interact with a "lock-and-key" arrangement that can only occur if both molecules have precisely the correct shape, which in turn depends in part upon the number and location of hydrogen bonds.

Molecular Shape

As just mentioned, when atoms are linked together they form molecules with various shapes. Although we draw diagrammatic structures of molecules on flat sheets of paper, molecules are three-dimensional. When more than one covalent bond is formed with a given atom, the bonds are distributed around the atom in a pattern that may or may not be symmetrical (**Figure 2.6**).

Molecules are not rigid, inflexible structures. Within certain limits, the shape of a molecule can be changed without breaking the covalent bonds linking its atoms together. A covalent bond is like an axle around which the joined atoms can rotate. As illustrated in **Figure 2.7**, a sequence of six carbon atoms can assume a number of shapes by rotating around various covalent bonds. As we will see in subsequent chapters, the three-dimensional, flexible shape of molecules is one of the major factors governing molecular interactions.

Ionic Molecules

The process of ion formation, known as ionization, can occur not only in single atoms, as stated earlier, but also in atoms that are covalently linked in molecules. Two commonly encountered groups of atoms that undergo ionization in molecules are the **carboxyl group** (—COOH) and the **amino group** ($—NH_2$). The shorthand formula for only a portion of a molecule can be written as R—COOH or $R—NH_2$, with R being the remainder of the molecule. The carboxyl group ionizes when the oxygen linked to the hydrogen captures the hydrogen's only electron to form a carboxyl ion ($R—COO^-$), releasing a hydrogen ion (H^+):

$$R—COOH \rightleftharpoons R—COO^- + H^+$$

The amino group can bind a hydrogen ion to form an ionized amino group ($R—NH_3^+$):

$$R—NH_2 + H^+ \rightleftharpoons R—NH_3^+$$

The ionization of each of these groups can be reversed, as indicated by the double arrows; the ionized carboxyl group can combine with a hydrogen ion to form a nonionized carboxyl group, and the ionized amino group can lose a hydrogen ion and become a nonionized amino group.

Free Radicals

As described earlier, the electrons that revolve around the nucleus of an atom occupy energy shells, each of which can be occupied by one or more orbitals containing up to two electrons each. An atom is most stable when each orbital in the outer shell is occupied by its full complement of electrons. An atom containing a single (unpaired) electron in an orbital of its outer shell is known as a **free radical,** as are molecules containing such atoms. Free radicals are unstable molecules that can react with other atoms, through the process known as oxidation. When a free radical oxidizes another atom, the free radical gains an electron and the other atom usually becomes a new free radical.

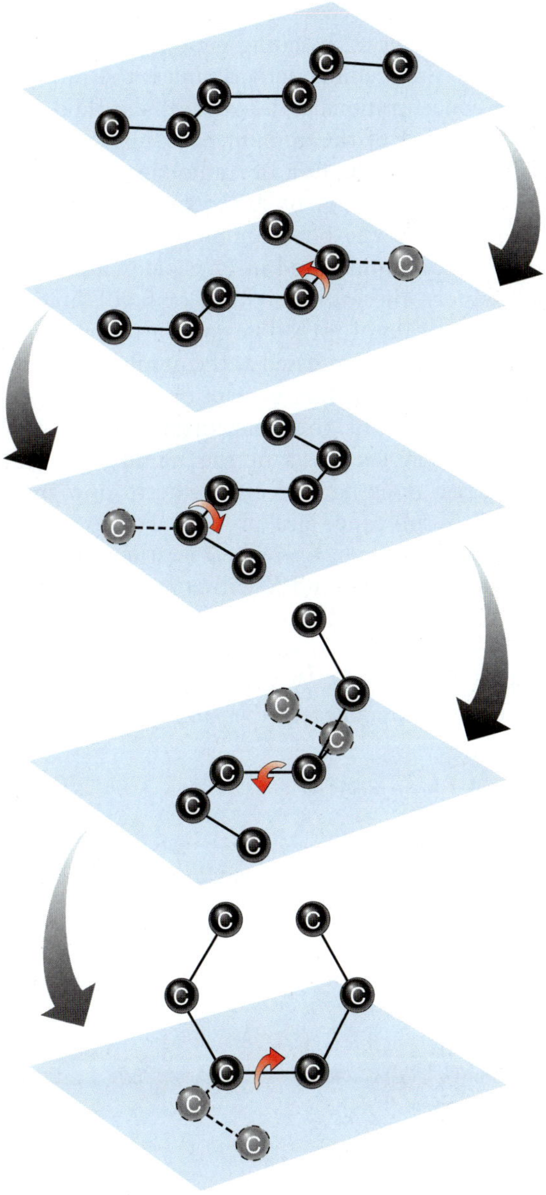

Figure 2.7 Changes in molecular shape occur as portions of a molecule rotate around different carbon-to-carbon bonds, transforming this molecule's shape, for example, from a relatively straight chain (top) into a ring (bottom).

Free radicals are formed by the actions of certain enzymes in some cells, such as types of white blood cells that destroy pathogens. The free radicals are highly reactive, removing electrons from the outer shells of atoms within molecules present in the pathogen cell wall or membrane, for example. This mechanism begins the process whereby the pathogen is destroyed.

In addition, however, free radicals can be produced in the body following exposure to radiation or toxin ingestion. These free radicals can do considerable harm to the cells of the body. For example, oxidation due to long-term buildup of free radicals has been proposed as one cause of several different human diseases, notably eye, cardiovascular, and neural diseases associated with aging. Thus, it is important that free radicals be inactivated by molecules that can donate electrons to free radicals without becoming dangerous free radicals themselves. Examples of such protective molecules are the antioxidant vitamins C and E.

Free radicals are diagrammed with a dot next to the atomic symbol. Examples of biologically important free radicals are superoxide anion, $O_2 \cdot^-$; hydroxyl radical, $OH \cdot$; and nitric oxide, $NO \cdot$. Note that a free radical configuration can occur in either an ionized (charged) or a nonionized molecule.

We turn now to a discussion of solutions and molecular solubility in water. We begin with a review of some of the properties of water that make it so suitable for life.

2.3 Solutions

Substances dissolved in a liquid are known as **solutes,** and the liquid in which they are dissolved is the **solvent.** Solutes dissolve in a solvent to form a **solution.** Water is the most abundant solvent in the body, accounting for ≈60% of total body weight. A majority of the chemical reactions that occur in the body involve molecules that are dissolved in water, either in the intracellular or extracellular fluid. However, not all molecules dissolve in water.

Water

Out of every 100 molecules in the human body, about 99 are water. The covalent bonds linking the two hydrogen atoms to the oxygen atom in a water molecule are polar. Therefore, as noted earlier, the oxygen in water has a partial negative charge, and each hydrogen has a partial positive charge. The positively polarized regions near the hydrogen atoms of one water molecule are electrically attracted to the negatively polarized regions of the oxygen atoms in adjacent water molecules by hydrogen bonds (see Figure 2.5).

At temperatures between 0°C and 100°C, water exists as a liquid; in this state, the weak hydrogen bonds between water molecules are continuously forming and breaking, and occasionally some water molecules escape the liquid phase and become a gas. If the temperature is increased, the hydrogen bonds break more readily and molecules of water escape into the gaseous state. However, if the temperature is reduced, hydrogen bonds break less frequently, so larger and larger clusters of water molecules form until at 0°C, water freezes into a solid crystalline matrix—ice. Body temperature in humans is normally close to 37°C, and therefore water exists in liquid form in the body. Nonetheless, even at this temperature, some water leaves the body as a gas (water vapor) each time we exhale during breathing. This water loss in the form of water vapor has considerable importance for total-body-water homeostasis and must be replaced with water obtained from food or drink.

Water molecules take part in many chemical reactions of the general type:

$$R_1{-}R_2 + H{-}O{-}H \rightleftharpoons R_1{-}OH + H{-}R_2$$

In this reaction, the covalent bond between R_1 and R_2 and the one between a hydrogen atom and oxygen in water are broken, and the hydroxyl group and hydrogen atom are transferred to R_1 and R_2, respectively. Reactions of this type are known as hydrolytic reactions, or **hydrolysis.** Many large molecules in the body are broken down into smaller molecular units by hydrolysis, usually with the assistance of a class of molecules called enzymes. These reactions are usually reversible, a process known as condensation or **dehydration.** In dehydration, one net water molecule is removed to combine two small molecules into one larger one. Dehydration reactions are responsible for, among other things, building proteins and other large molecules required by the body.

Other properties of water that are of importance in physiology include the colligative properties—those that depend on the *number* of dissolved substances, or solutes, in water. For example, water moves between fluid compartments by the process of osmosis, which you will learn about in detail in Chapter 4. In osmosis, water moves from regions of low solute concentrations to regions of high solute concentrations, regardless of the specific type of solute. Osmosis is the mechanism by which water is absorbed from the intestinal tract (Chapter 15) and from the kidney tubules into the blood (Chapter 14).

Having presented this brief survey of some of the physiologically relevant properties of water, we turn now to a discussion of how molecules dissolve in water. Keep in mind as you read on that most of the chemical reactions in the body take place between molecules that are in watery solution. Therefore, the relative solubilities of different molecules influence their abilities to participate in chemical reactions.

Molecular Solubility

Molecules having a number of polar bonds and/or ionized groups will dissolve in water. Such molecules are said to be **hydrophilic,** or "water-loving." Therefore, the presence of ionized groups such as carboxyl and amino groups or of polar groups such as hydroxyl groups in a molecule promotes solubility in water. In contrast, molecules composed predominantly of carbon and hydrogen are poorly or almost completely insoluble in water because their electrically neutral covalent bonds are not attracted to water molecules. These molecules are **hydrophobic,** or "water-fearing."

When hydrophobic molecules are mixed with water, two phases form, as occurs when oil is mixed with water. The strong attraction between polar molecules "squeezes" the nonpolar molecules out of the water phase. Such a separation is rarely if ever 100% complete, however, so very small amounts of nonpolar solutes remain dissolved in the water phase.

A special class of molecules has a polar or ionized region at one site and a nonpolar region at another site. Such molecules are called **amphipathic,** derived from Greek terms meaning "love both." When mixed with water, amphipathic molecules form clusters, with their polar (hydrophilic) regions at the surface of the cluster where they are attracted to the surrounding water molecules. The nonpolar (hydrophobic) ends are oriented toward the interior of the cluster (**Figure 2.8**). This arrangement provides the maximal interaction between water molecules and the polar ends of the amphipathic molecules. Nonpolar molecules can dissolve in the central nonpolar regions of these clusters and thus exist in aqueous solutions in far greater amounts than would otherwise be possible based on their decreased solubility in water. As we will see, the orientation of amphipathic molecules plays an important role in plasma membrane structure (Chapter 3) and in both the absorption of nonpolar molecules from the intestines and their transport in the blood (Chapter 15).

Concentration

Solute **concentration** is defined as the amount of the solute present in a unit volume of solution. The concentrations of solutes in a solution are key to their ability to produce physiological actions. For example, the extracellular signaling molecules described in Chapter 1, including neurotransmitters and hormones, cannot alter cellular activity unless they are present in appropriate concentrations in the extracellular fluid.

One measure of the amount of a substance is its mass expressed in grams. The unit of volume in the metric system is a liter (L). (One liter equals 1.06 quarts; see the conversion table at the back of the book for metric and English units.) Smaller units commonly used in physiology are the deciliter (dL, or 0.1 liter), the milliliter (mL, or 0.001 liter), and the microliter (μL, or 0.001 mL). The concentration of a solute in a solution can then be expressed as the number of grams of the substance present in one liter of solution (g/L).

A comparison of the concentrations of two different substances on the basis of the number of grams per liter of solution does not directly indicate how many molecules of each substance are present. For example, if the molecules of compound X are heavier than those of compound Y, 10 g of compound X will contain fewer molecules than 10 g of compound Y. Concentrations in units of grams per liter are most often used when the chemical structure of the solute is unknown. When the chemical structure of a molecule is known, concentrations are expressed based upon

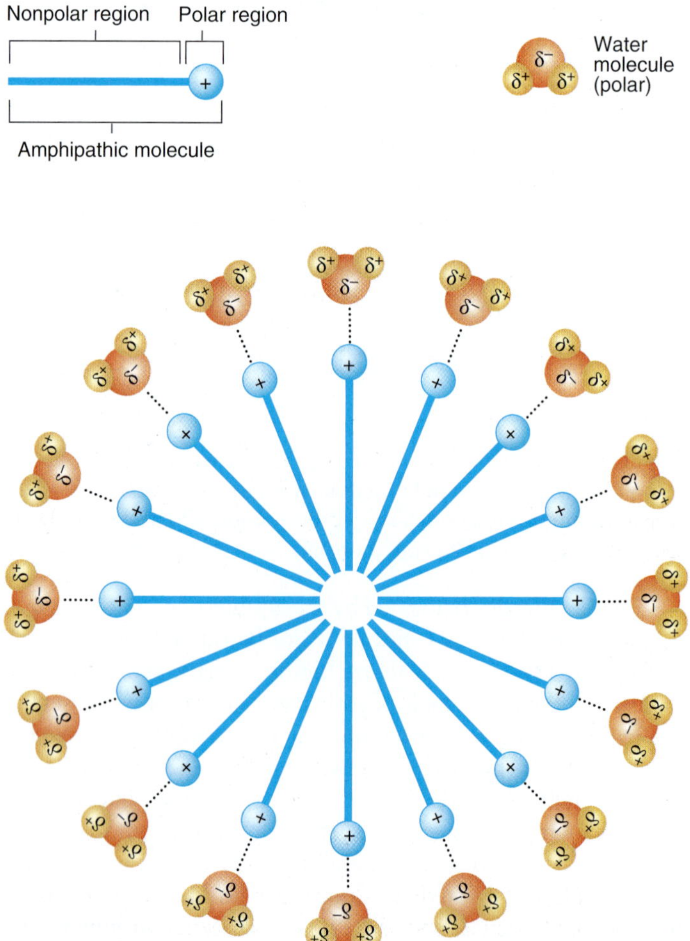

Figure 2.8 In water, amphipathic molecules aggregate into spherical clusters. Their polar regions form hydrogen bonds with water molecules at the surface of the cluster, whereas the nonpolar regions cluster together and exclude water.

the number of solute molecules in solution, using a measure of mass called the molecular weight. The **molecular weight** of a molecule is equal to the sum of the atomic masses of all the atoms in the molecule. For example, glucose ($C_6H_{12}O_6$) has a molecular weight of 180 because $[(6 \times 12) + (12 \times 1) + (6 \times 16)] = 180$. One **mole** (mol) of a compound is the amount of the compound in grams equal to its molecular weight. A solution containing 180 g glucose (1 mol) in 1 L of solution is a 1 molar solution of glucose (1 mol/L). If 90 g of glucose were dissolved in 1 L of water, the solution would have a concentration of 0.5 mol/L. Just as a 1 g atomic mass of any element contains the same number of atoms, 1 mol of any molecule will contain the same number of molecules—6×10^{23} (Avogadro's number). Thus, a 1 mol/L solution of glucose contains the same number of solute molecules per liter as a 1 mol/L solution of any other substance.

The concentrations of solutes dissolved in the body fluids are much less than 1 mol/L. Many have concentrations in the range of millimoles per liter (1 mmol/L = 0.001 mol/L), whereas others are present in even smaller concentrations—micromoles per liter (1 μmol/L = 0.000001 mol/L) or nanomoles per liter (1 mol/L = 0.000000001 mol/L). By convention, the liter (L) term is sometimes dropped when referring to concentrations. Thus, a 1 mmol/L solution is often written as 1 mM (the capital "M" stands for "molar" and is defined as mol/L).

An example of the importance of solute concentrations is related to a key homeostatic variable, that of the pH of the body fluids, as described next. Maintenance of a narrow range of pH (that is, hydrogen ion concentration) in the body fluids is absolutely critical to most physiological processes, in part because enzymes and other proteins depend on pH for their normal shape and activity.

Hydrogen Ions and Acidity

As mentioned earlier, a hydrogen atom consists of a single proton in its nucleus orbited by a single electron. The most common type of hydrogen ion (H^+) is formed by the loss of the electron and is, therefore, a single free proton. Molecules that release protons (hydrogen ions) in solution are called **acids,** for example:

$$\underset{\text{hydrochloric acid}}{HCl} \longrightarrow H^+ + \underset{\text{chloride}}{Cl^-}$$

$$\underset{\text{carbonic acid}}{H_2CO_3} \rightleftharpoons H^+ + \underset{\text{bicarbonate}}{HCO_3^-}$$

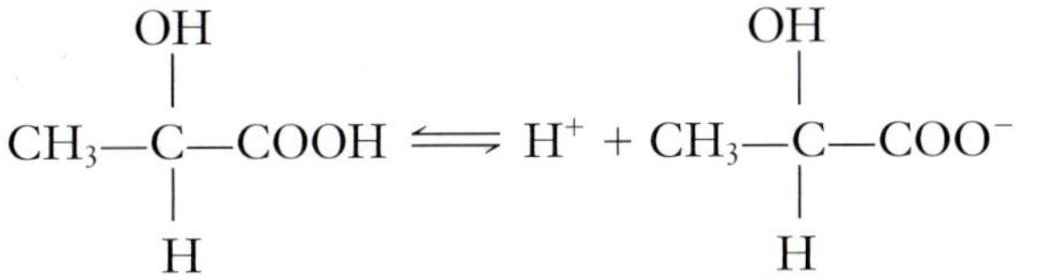

lactic acid　　　　lactate

Conversely, any substance that can accept a hydrogen ion (proton) is termed a **base.** In the reactions shown, bicarbonate and lactate are bases because they can combine with hydrogen ions (note the two-way arrows in the two reactions). Also, note that by convention, separate terms are used for the acid forms—*lactic acid* and *carbonic acid*—and the bases derived from the acids—*lactate* and *bicarbonate.* By combining with hydrogen ions, bases decrease the hydrogen ion concentration of a solution.

When hydrochloric acid is dissolved in water, 100% of its atoms separate to form hydrogen and chloride ions, and these ions do not recombine in solution (note the one-way arrow in the preceding reaction). In the case of lactic acid, however, only a fraction of the lactic acid molecules in solution release hydrogen ions at any instant. Therefore, if a 1 mol/L solution of lactic acid is compared with a 1 mol/L solution of hydrochloric acid, the hydrogen ion concentration will be lower in the lactic acid solution than in the hydrochloric acid solution. Hydrochloric acid and other acids that are completely or nearly completely ionized in solution are known as **strong acids,** whereas carbonic and lactic acids and other acids that do not completely ionize in solution are **weak acids.** The same principles apply to bases.

It is important to understand that the hydrogen ion concentration of a solution refers only to the hydrogen ions that are free in solution and not to those that may be bound, for example, to amino groups ($R—NH_3^+$). The **acidity** of a solution thus refers to the *free* (unbound) hydrogen ion concentration in the solution; the greater the hydrogen ion concentration, the greater the acidity. The hydrogen ion concentration is often expressed as the solution's **pH,** which is defined as the negative logarithm to the base 10 of the hydrogen ion concentration. The brackets around the symbol for the hydrogen ion in the following formula indicate concentration:

$$pH = -\log [H^+]$$

As an example, a solution with a hydrogen ion concentration of 10^{-7} mol/L has a pH of 7. Pure water, due to the ionization of some of the molecules into H^+ and OH^-, has hydrogen ion and hydroxyl ion concentrations of 10^{-7} mol/L (pH = 7.0) at 25°C. The product of the concentrations of H^+ and OH^- in pure water is always 10^{-14} M at 25°C. A solution of pH 7.0 is termed a **neutral solution. Alkaline solutions** have a lower hydrogen ion concentration (a pH greater than 7.0), whereas those with a greater hydrogen ion concentration (a pH lower than 7.0) are **acidic solutions.** Note that as the acidity *increases,* the pH *decreases;* a change in pH from 7 to 6 represents a 10-fold increase in the hydrogen ion concentration. The extracellular fluid of the body has a hydrogen ion concentration of about 4×10^{-8} mol/L (pH = 7.4), with a homeostatic range of about pH 7.35 to 7.45, and is thus slightly alkaline. Most intracellular fluids have a slightly greater hydrogen ion concentration (pH 7.0 to 7.2) than extracellular fluids.

As we saw earlier, the ionization of carboxyl and amino groups involves the release and uptake, respectively, of hydrogen ions. These groups behave as weak acids and bases. Changes in the acidity of solutions containing molecules with carboxyl and amino groups alter the net electrical charge on these molecules by shifting the ionization reaction to the right or left according to the general form:

$$R—COO^- + H^+ \rightleftharpoons R—COOH$$

For example, if the acidity of a solution containing lactate is increased by adding hydrochloric acid, the concentration of lactic acid will increase and that of lactate will decrease.

If the electrical charge on a molecule is altered, its interaction with other molecules or with other regions within the same molecule changes, and thus its functional characteristics change. In the extracellular fluid, *hydrogen ion concentrations beyond the 10-fold pH range of 7.8 to 6.8 are incompatible with life if maintained for more than a brief period of time.* Even small changes in the hydrogen ion concentration can produce large changes in molecular interaction. For example, many enzymes in the body operate efficiently within very narrow ranges of pH. Should pH vary from the normal homeostatic range due to disease, these enzymes work at reduced rates, creating an even worse pathological situation.

This concludes our overview of atomic and molecular structure, water, and pH. We turn now to a description of the molecules essential for life in all living organisms, including humans. These are the carbon-based molecules required for forming the building blocks of cells, tissues, and organs; providing energy; and forming the genetic blueprints of all life.

2.4 Classes of Organic Molecules

Because most naturally occurring carbon-containing molecules are found in living organisms, the study of these compounds is known as organic chemistry. (Inorganic chemistry refers to the study of non-carbon-containing molecules.) However, the chemistry of living organisms, or biochemistry, now forms only a portion of the broad field of organic chemistry.

One of the properties of the carbon atom that makes life possible is its ability to form four covalent bonds with other atoms, including with other carbon atoms. Because carbon atoms can also combine with hydrogen, oxygen, nitrogen, and sulfur atoms, a vast number of compounds can form from relatively few chemical elements. Some of these molecules are extremely large (**macromolecules**), composed of thousands of atoms. In some cases, such large molecules form when many identical smaller molecules, called subunits or monomers (literally, "one part"), link together. These large molecules are known as **polymers** ("many parts"). The structure of any polymer depends upon the structure of the subunits, the number of subunits bonded together, and the three-dimensional way in which the subunits are linked.

Most of the organic molecules in the body can be classified into one of four groups: carbohydrates, lipids, proteins, and nucleic acids (**Table 2.4**). We will consider each of these groups separately, but it is worth mentioning here that many molecules in the body are made up of two or more of these groups. For example, glycoproteins are composed of a protein covalently bonded to one or more carbohydrates.

Carbohydrates

Although carbohydrates account for only about 1% of body weight, they play a central role in the chemical reactions that provide cells with energy. As you will learn later in this chapter and in greater detail in Chapter 3, energy is stored in the chemical bonds in glucose molecules; this energy can be released within cells when required and stored in the bonds of another molecule called adenosine triphosphate (ATP). The energy stored in the bonds in ATP is used to power many different reactions in the body, including those necessary for cell survival, muscle contraction, protein synthesis, and many others.

Carbohydrates are composed of carbon, hydrogen, and oxygen atoms. Linked to most of the carbon atoms in a carbohydrate are a hydrogen atom and a hydroxyl group:

```
    |
H—C—OH
    |
```

The presence of numerous polar hydroxyl groups makes most carbohydrates readily soluble in water.

TABLE 2.4 Major Categories of Organic Molecules in the Body

Category	Percentage of Body Weight	Predominant Atoms	Subclass	Subunits
Carbohydrates	1	C, H, O	Polysaccharides (and disaccharides)	Monosaccharides
Lipids	15	C, H	Triglycerides	3 fatty acids + glycerol
			Phospholipids	2 fatty acids + glycerol + phosphate + small charged nitrogen-containing group
			Steroids	None
Proteins	17	C, H, O, N	Peptides and polypeptides	Amino acids
Nucleic acids	2	C, H, O, N	DNA	Nucleotides containing the bases adenine, cytosine, guanine, thymine; the sugar deoxyribose; and phosphate
			RNA	Nucleotides containing the bases adenine, cytosine, guanine, uracil; the sugar ribose; and phosphate

Many carbohydrates taste sweet, particularly the carbohydrates known as sugars. The simplest sugars are the monomers called **monosaccharides** (from the Greek for "single sugars"), the most abundant of which is **glucose,** a six-carbon molecule ($C_6H_{12}O_6$). Glucose is often called "blood sugar" because it is the major monosaccharide found in the blood.

Glucose may exist in an open chain form, or, more commonly, a cyclic structure as shown in **Figure 2.9**. Five carbon atoms and an oxygen atom form a ring that lies in an essentially flat plane. The hydrogen and hydroxyl groups on each carbon lie above and below the plane of this ring. If one of the hydroxyl groups below the ring is shifted to a position above the ring, a different monosaccharide is produced.

Most monosaccharides in the body contain five or six carbon atoms and are called **pentoses** and **hexoses,** respectively. Larger carbohydrates can be formed by joining a number of monosaccharides together. Carbohydrates composed of two monosaccharides are known as **disaccharides. Sucrose,** or table sugar, is composed of two monosaccharides, glucose and fructose (**Figure 2.10**). The linking together of most monosaccharides involves a dehydration reaction in which a hydroxyl group is removed from one monosaccharide and a hydrogen atom is removed from the other, giving rise to a molecule of water and covalently bonding the two sugars together through an oxygen atom. Conversely, hydrolysis of the disaccharide breaks this linkage by adding back the water and thus uncoupling the two monosaccharides. Other disaccharides frequently encountered are maltose (glucose–glucose), formed during the digestion of large carbohydrates in the intestinal tract, and lactose (glucose–galactose), present in milk.

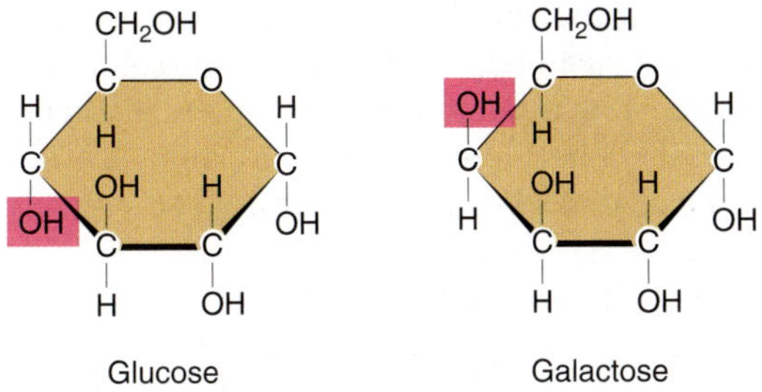

Figure 2.9 The structural difference between the monosaccharides glucose and galactose is based on whether the hydroxyl group at the position indicated lies below or above the plane of the ring.

When many monosaccharides are linked together to form polymers, the molecules are known as **polysaccharides.** Starch, found in plant cells, and **glycogen,** present in animal cells, are examples of polysaccharides (**Figure 2.11**). Both of these polysaccharides are composed of thousands of glucose molecules linked together in long chains, differing only in the degree of branching along the chain. Glycogen exists in the body as a reservoir of available energy that is stored in the chemical bonds within individual glucose monomers. Hydrolysis of glycogen, as occurs during periods of fasting, leads to release of the glucose monomers into the blood, thereby preventing blood glucose from decreasing to dangerously low concentrations.

Lipids

Lipids are molecules composed predominantly (but not exclusively) of hydrogen and carbon atoms. These atoms are linked by nonpolar covalent bonds; therefore, lipids are nonpolar and have a very low solubility in water. Lipids, which account for about 40% of the organic matter in the average body (15% of the body weight), can be divided into four subclasses: fatty

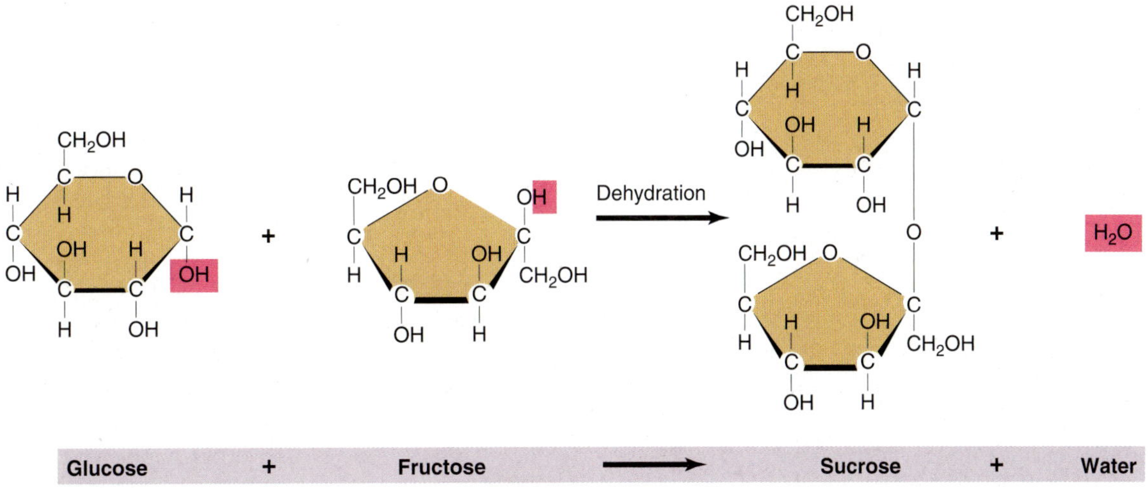

Figure 2.10 AP|R Sucrose (table sugar) is a disaccharide formed when two monosaccharides, glucose and fructose, bond together through a dehydration reaction.

PHYSIOLOGICAL INQUIRY

- What is the reverse reaction called?

Answer can be found at end of chapter.

acids, triglycerides, phospholipids, and steroids. Like carbohydrates, lipids are important in physiology partly because some of them provide a valuable source of energy. Other lipids are a major component of all cellular membranes, and still others are important signaling molecules.

Fatty Acids

A **fatty acid** consists of a chain of carbon and hydrogen atoms with an acidic carboxyl group at one end (**Figure 2.12a**). Therefore, fatty acids contain two oxygen atoms in addition to their complement of carbon and hydrogen. Fatty acids are synthesized in cells by the covalent bonding together of two-carbon fragments, resulting most commonly in fatty acids of 16 or 18 carbon atoms. When all the carbons in a fatty acid are linked by single covalent bonds, the fatty acid is said to be a **saturated fatty acid,** because both of the remaining available bonds in each carbon atom are occupied—or saturated—with covalently bound H. Some fatty acids contain one or more double bonds between carbon atoms, and these are known as **unsaturated fatty acids** (they have fewer C—H bonds than a saturated fatty acid). If one double bond is present, the fatty acid is **monounsaturated,** and if there is more than one double bond, it is **polyunsaturated** (see Figure 2.12a).

Most naturally occurring unsaturated fatty acids exist in the cis position, with both hydrogens on the same side of the double-bonded carbons (see Figure 2.12a). It is possible, however, to modify fatty acids during the processing of certain fatty foods, such that the hydrogens are on opposite sides of the double bond. These chemically altered fatty acids are known as **trans fatty acids.** The trans configuration imparts stability to the food for longer storage and alters the food's flavor and consistency. However, trans fatty acids have recently been linked with a number of serious health conditions, including elevated blood concentrations of cholesterol; current health guidelines recommend against the consumption of foods containing trans fatty acids.

Fatty acids have many important functions in the body, including but not limited to providing energy for cellular metabolism. The bonds between carbon and hydrogen atoms in a fatty acid can be broken to release chemical energy that can be stored in the chemical bonds of ATP. Like glucose, therefore, fatty acids are an extremely important source of energy. In addition, some fatty acids can be altered to produce a special class of molecules that regulate a number of cell functions by acting as cell signaling molecules. These modified fatty acids—collectively termed *eicosanoids*—are derived from the 20-carbon, polyunsaturated fatty acid arachidonic acid. They have been implicated in the control of blood pressure (Chapter 12), inflammation (Chapters 12 and 18), and smooth muscle contraction (Chapter 9), among other things. Finally, fatty acids form part of the structure of triglycerides, described next.

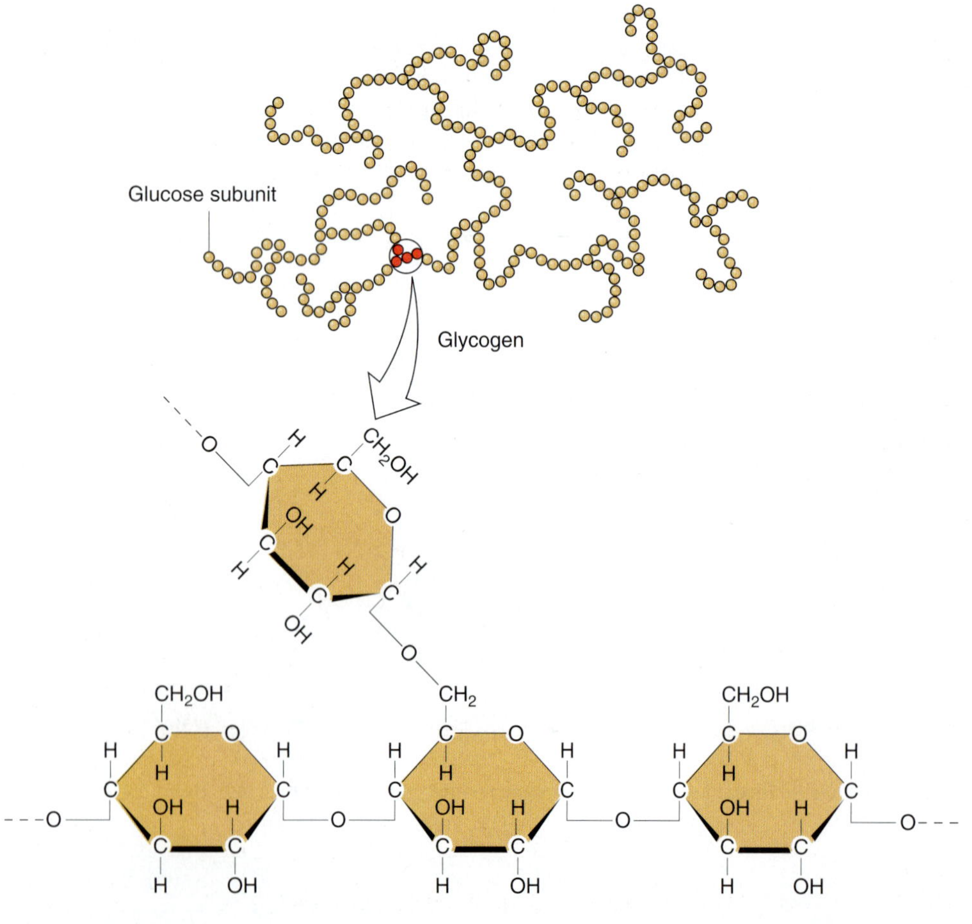

Figure 2.11 Many molecules of glucose joined end to end and at branch points form the branched-chain polysaccharide glycogen, shown here in diagrammatic form. The four red subunits in the glycogen molecule correspond to the four glucose subunits shown at the bottom.

Triglycerides

Triglycerides (also known as *triacylglycerols*) constitute the majority of the lipids in the body; these molecules are generally referred to simply as "fats." Triglycerides form when **glycerol,** a three-carbon sugar-alcohol, bonds to three fatty acids (**Figure 2.12b**). Each of the three hydroxyl groups in glycerol is bonded to the carboxyl group of a fatty acid by a dehydration reaction.

The three fatty acids in a molecule of triglyceride are usually not identical. Therefore, a variety of triglycerides can be formed with fatty acids of different chain lengths and degrees of saturation. Animal triglycerides generally contain a high proportion of saturated fatty acids, whereas vegetable triglycerides contain more unsaturated fatty acids. Saturated fats tend to be solid at low temperatures. Unsaturated fats, on the other hand, have a very low melting point, and thus they are liquids (oil) even at low temperatures. In a familiar example, heating a hamburger on the stove melts the saturated animal fats, leaving grease in the frying pan. When allowed to cool, however, the oily grease returns to its solid form.

Triglycerides are present in the blood and can be synthesized in the liver.

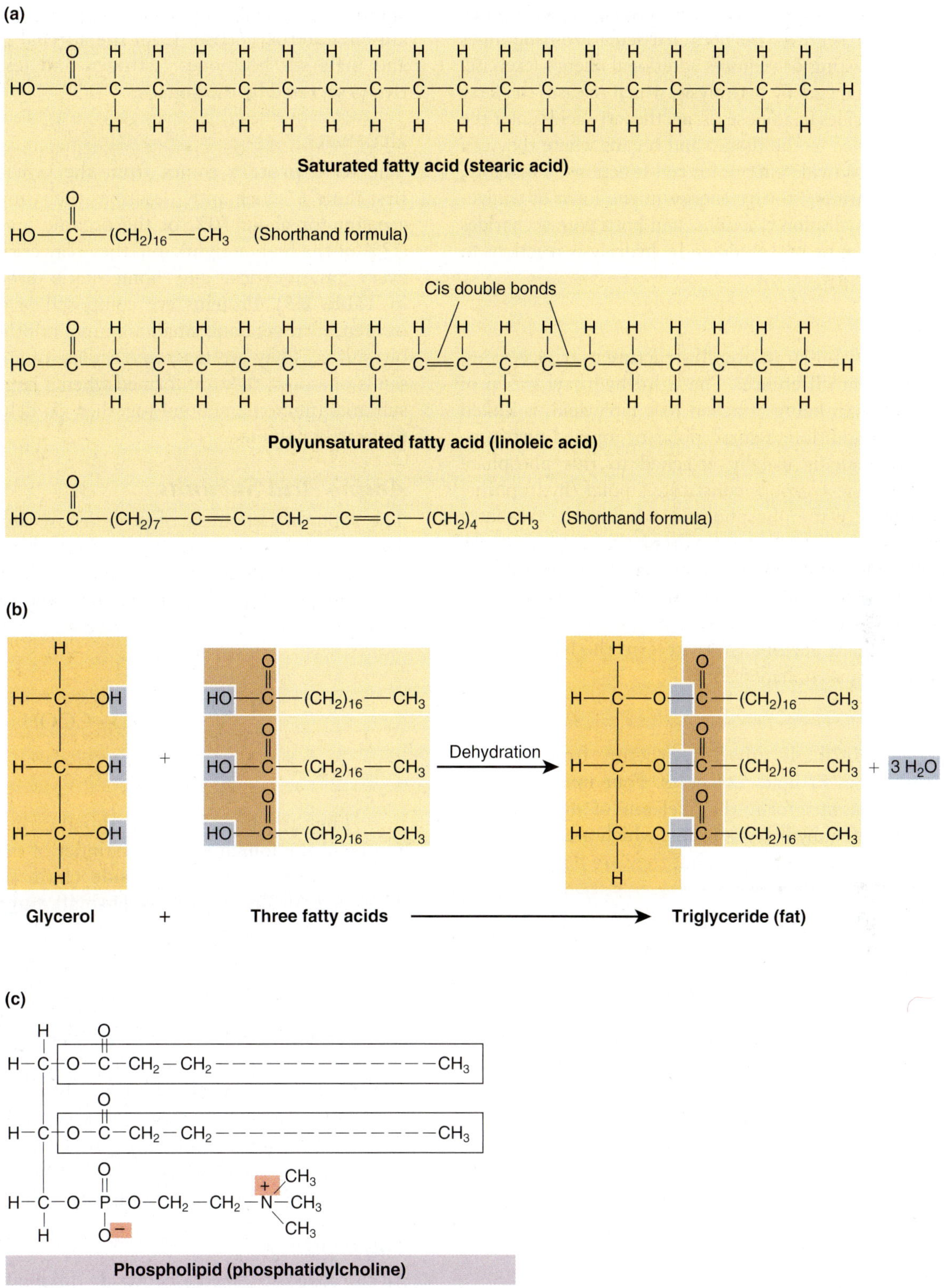

Figure 2.12 Lipids. (a) Fatty acids may be saturated or unsaturated, such as the two common ones shown here. Note the shorthand way of depicting the formula of a fatty acid. (b) Glycerol and fatty acids are the subunits that combine by a dehydration reaction to form triglycerides and water. (c) Phospholipids are formed from glycerol, two fatty acids, and one or more charged groups.

PHYSIOLOGICAL INQUIRY

- Which portion of the phospholipid depicted in Figure 2.12c would face the water molecules as shown in Figure 2.8?

Answer can be found at end of chapter.

They are stored in great quantities in adipose tissue, where they serve as an energy reserve for the body, particularly during times when a person is fasting or requires additional energy (exercise, for example). This occurs by hydrolysis, which releases the fatty acids from triglycerides in adipose tissue; the fatty acids enter the blood and are carried to the tissues and organs where they can be metabolized to provide energy for cell functions. Therefore, as with polysaccharides, storing energy in the form of triglycerides requires dehydration reactions, and both polysaccharides and triglycerides can be broken down by hydrolysis reactions to usable forms of energy.

Phospholipids

Phospholipids are similar in overall structure to triglycerides, with one important difference. The third hydroxyl group of glycerol, rather than being attached to a fatty acid, is linked to phosphate. In addition, a small polar or ionized nitrogen-containing molecule is usually attached to this phosphate (**Figure 2.12c**). These groups constitute a polar (hydrophilic) region at one end of the phospholipid, whereas the two fatty acid chains provide a nonpolar (hydrophobic) region at the opposite end. Therefore, phospholipids are amphipathic. In aqueous solution, they become organized into clusters, with their polar ends attracted to the water molecules. This property of phospholipids permits them to form the lipid bilayers of cellular membranes (Chapter 3).

Steroids

Steroids have a distinctly different structure from those of the other subclasses of lipid molecules. Four interconnected rings of carbon atoms form the skeleton of every steroid (**Figure 2.13**). A few hydroxyl groups, which are polar, may be attached to this ring structure, but they are not numerous

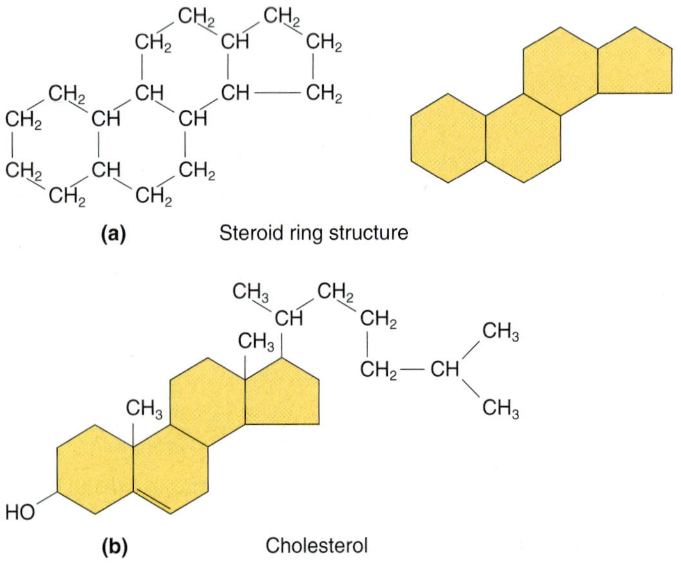

Figure 2.13 (a) Steroid ring structure, shown with all the carbon and hydrogen atoms in the rings and again without these atoms to emphasize the overall ring structure of this class of lipids. (b) Different steroids have different types and numbers of chemical groups attached at various locations on the steroid ring, as shown by the structure of cholesterol.

enough to make a steroid water-soluble. Examples of steroids are cholesterol, cortisol from the adrenal glands, and female and male sex hormones (estrogen and testosterone, respectively) secreted by the gonads.

Proteins

The term **protein** comes from the Greek *proteios* ("of the first rank"), which aptly describes their importance. Proteins account for about 50% of the organic material in the body (17% of the body weight), and they play critical roles in almost every physiological and homeostatic process (summarized in **Table 2.5**). Proteins are composed of carbon, hydrogen, oxygen, nitrogen, and small amounts of other elements, notably sulfur. They are macromolecules, often containing thousands of atoms; they are formed when a large number of small subunits (monomers) bond together via dehydration reactions to create a polymer.

Amino Acid Subunits

The subunit monomers of proteins are **amino acids;** therefore, proteins are polymers of amino acids. Every amino acid except one (proline) has an amino (—NH_2) and a carboxyl (—COOH) group bound to the terminal carbon atom in the molecule:

$$\begin{array}{c} \mathrm{H} \\ | \\ \mathrm{R{-}C{-}COOH} \\ | \\ \mathrm{NH_2} \end{array}$$

The third bond of this terminal carbon is to a hydrogen atom and the fourth to the remainder of the molecule, which is known as the **amino acid side chain** (R in the formula). These side chains are relatively small, ranging from a single hydrogen atom to nine carbon atoms with their associated hydrogen atoms.

The proteins of all living organisms are composed of the same set of 20 different amino acids, corresponding to 20 different side chains. The side chains may be nonpolar (eight amino acids), polar but not ionized (seven amino acids), or polar and ionized (five amino acids) (**Figure 2.14**). The human body can synthesize many amino acids, but several must be obtained in the diet; the latter are known as essential amino acids. This term does not imply that these amino acids are somehow more important than others, only that they must be obtained in the diet.

Polypeptides

Amino acids are joined together by linking the carboxyl group of one amino acid to the amino group of another. As in the formation of glycogen and triglycerides, a molecule of water is formed by dehydration (**Figure 2.15**). The bond formed between the amino and carboxyl group is called a **peptide bond.** Although peptide bonds are covalent, they can be enzymatically broken by hydrolysis to yield individual amino acids, as happens in the stomach and intestines, for example, when we digest protein in our diet.

Notice in Figure 2.15 that when two amino acids are linked together, one end of the resulting molecule has a

TABLE 2.5 Major Categories and Functions of Proteins		
Category	**Functions**	**Examples**
Proteins that regulate gene expression	Make RNA from DNA; synthesize polypeptides from RNA	Transcription factors activate genes; RNA polymerase transcribes genes; ribosomal proteins are required for translation of mRNA into protein.
Transporter proteins	Mediate the movement of solutes such as ions and organic molecules across plasma membranes	Ion channels in plasma membranes allow movement across the membrane of ions such as Na^+ and K^+.
Enzymes	Accelerate the rate of specific chemical reactions, such as those required for cellular metabolism	Pancreatic lipase, amylase, and proteases released into the small intestine break down macromolecules into smaller molecules that can be absorbed by the intestinal cells; protein kinases modify other proteins by the addition of phosphate groups, which changes the function of the protein.
Cell signaling proteins	Enable cells to communicate with each other, themselves, and with the external environment	Plasma membrane receptors bind to hormones or neurotransmitters in extracellular fluid.
Motor proteins	Initiate movement	Myosin, found in muscle cells, provides the contractile force that shortens a muscle.
Structural proteins	Support, connect, and strengthen cells, tissues, and organs	Collagen and elastin provide support for ligaments, tendons, and certain large blood vessels; actin makes up much of the cytoskeleton of cells.
Defense proteins	Protect against infection and disease due to pathogens	Cytokines and antibodies attack foreign cells and proteins, such as those from bacteria and viruses.

free amino group and the other has a free carboxyl group. Additional amino acids can be linked by peptide bonds to these free ends. A sequence of amino acids linked by peptide bonds is known as a **polypeptide.** The peptide bonds form the backbone of the polypeptide, and the side chain of each amino acid sticks out from the chain. Strictly speaking, the term *polypeptide* refers to a structural unit and does not necessarily suggest that the molecule is functional. By convention, if the number of amino acids in a polypeptide is about 50 or fewer and has a known biological function, the molecule is often referred to simply as a **peptide,** a term we will use throughout the text where relevant. When one or more polypeptides are folded into a characteristic shape forming a functional molecule, that molecule is called a protein.

As mentioned earlier, one or more monosaccharides may become covalently attached to the side chains of specific amino acids in a protein; such proteins are known as **glycoproteins.** These proteins are present in plasma membranes; are major components of connective tissue; and are also abundant in fluids like mucus, where they play a protective or lubricating role.

All proteins have multiple levels of structure that give each protein a unique shape; these are called the primary, secondary, tertiary, and—in some proteins—quaternary structure.

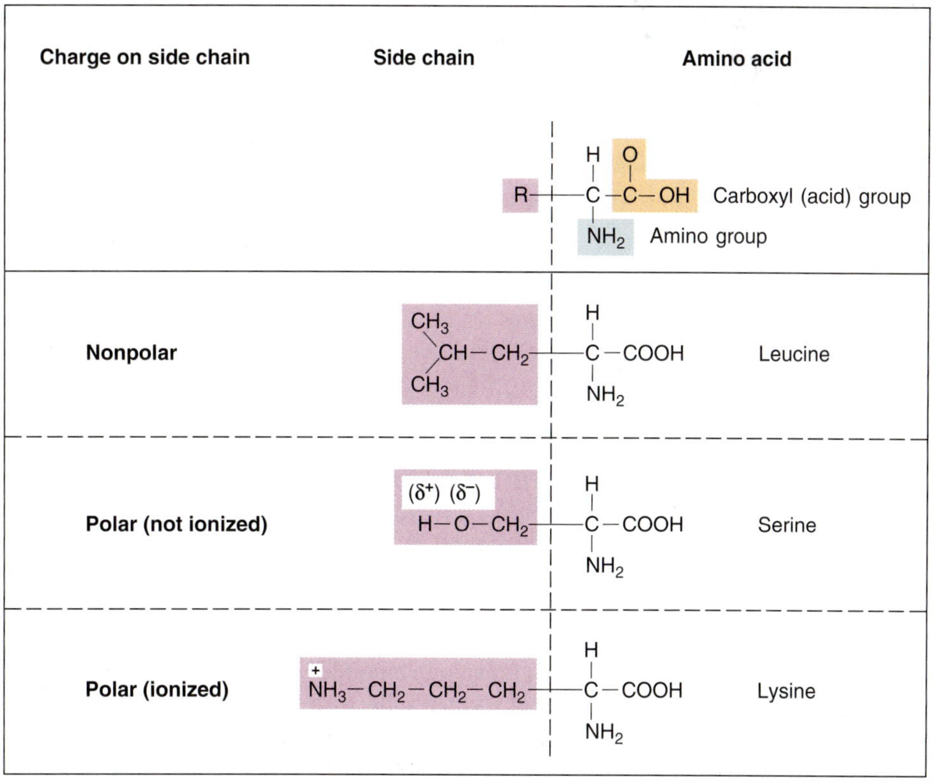

Figure 2.14 Representative structures of each class of amino acids found in proteins.

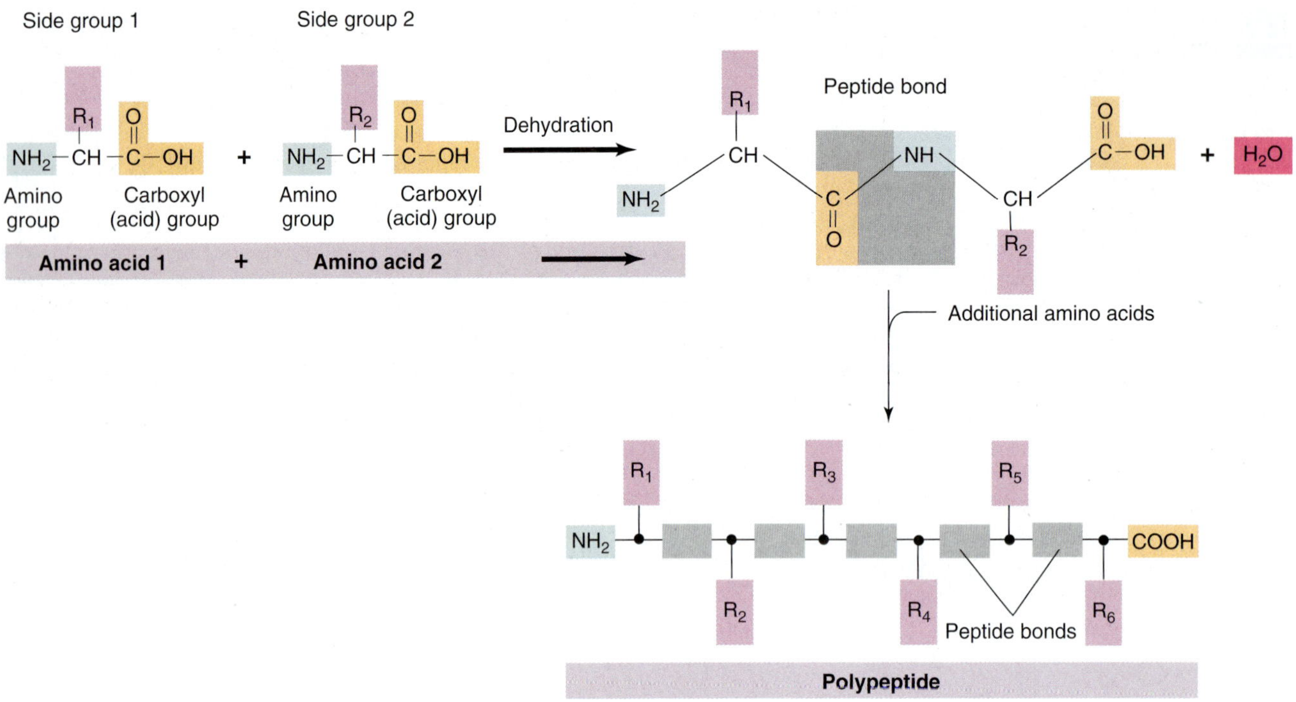

Figure 2.15 Linkage of amino acids by peptide bonds to form a polypeptide.

A general principle of physiology is that structure and function are linked. This is true even at the molecular level. The shape of a protein determines its physiological activity. In all cases, a protein's shape depends on its amino acid sequence, known as the *primary structure* of the protein.

Primary Structure

Two variables determine the **primary structure** of a protein: (1) the number of amino acids in the chain, and (2) the specific type of amino acid at each position along the chain (**Figure 2.16**). Each position along the chain can be occupied by any one of the 20 different amino acids.

Secondary Structure

A polypeptide can be envisioned as analogous to a string of beads, each bead representing one amino acid (see Figure 2.16). Moreover, because amino acids can rotate around bonds within a polypeptide chain, the chain is flexible and can bend into a number of shapes, just as a string of beads can be twisted into many configurations. Proteins do not appear in nature like a linear string of beads on a chain; interactions between side groups of each amino acid lead to bending, twisting, and folding of the chain into a more compact structure. The final shape of a protein is known as its **conformation.**

The attractions between various regions along a polypeptide chain create **secondary structure** in a protein. For example, hydrogen bonds can occur between a hydrogen linked to the nitrogen atom in one peptide bond and the double-bonded oxygen atom in another peptide bond (**Figure 2.17**). Because peptide bonds occur at regular intervals along a polypeptide chain, the hydrogen bonds between them tend to force the chain into a coiled conformation known as an **alpha helix.** Hydrogen bonds can also form between peptide bonds when extended regions of a polypeptide chain run approximately parallel to each other, forming a relatively straight, extended region known as a **beta pleated sheet** (see Figure 2.17). However, for several reasons,

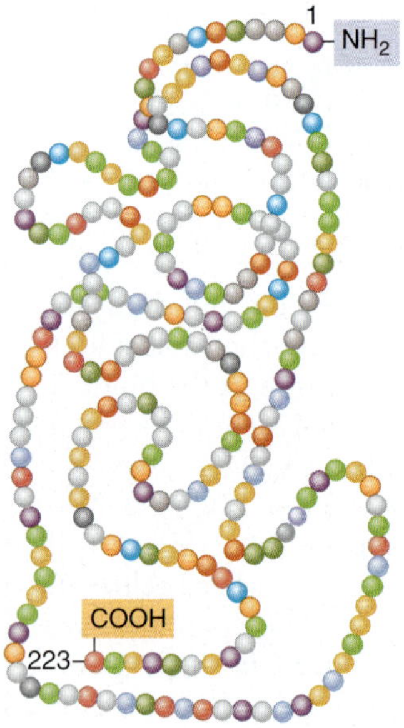

Figure 2.16 The primary structure of a polypeptide chain is the sequence of amino acids in that chain. The polypeptide illustrated contains 223 amino acids. Different amino acids are represented by different-colored circles. The numbering system begins with the amino terminal (NH_2).

PHYSIOLOGICAL INQUIRY

- What is the difference between the terms *polypeptide* and *protein?*

Answer can be found at end of chapter.

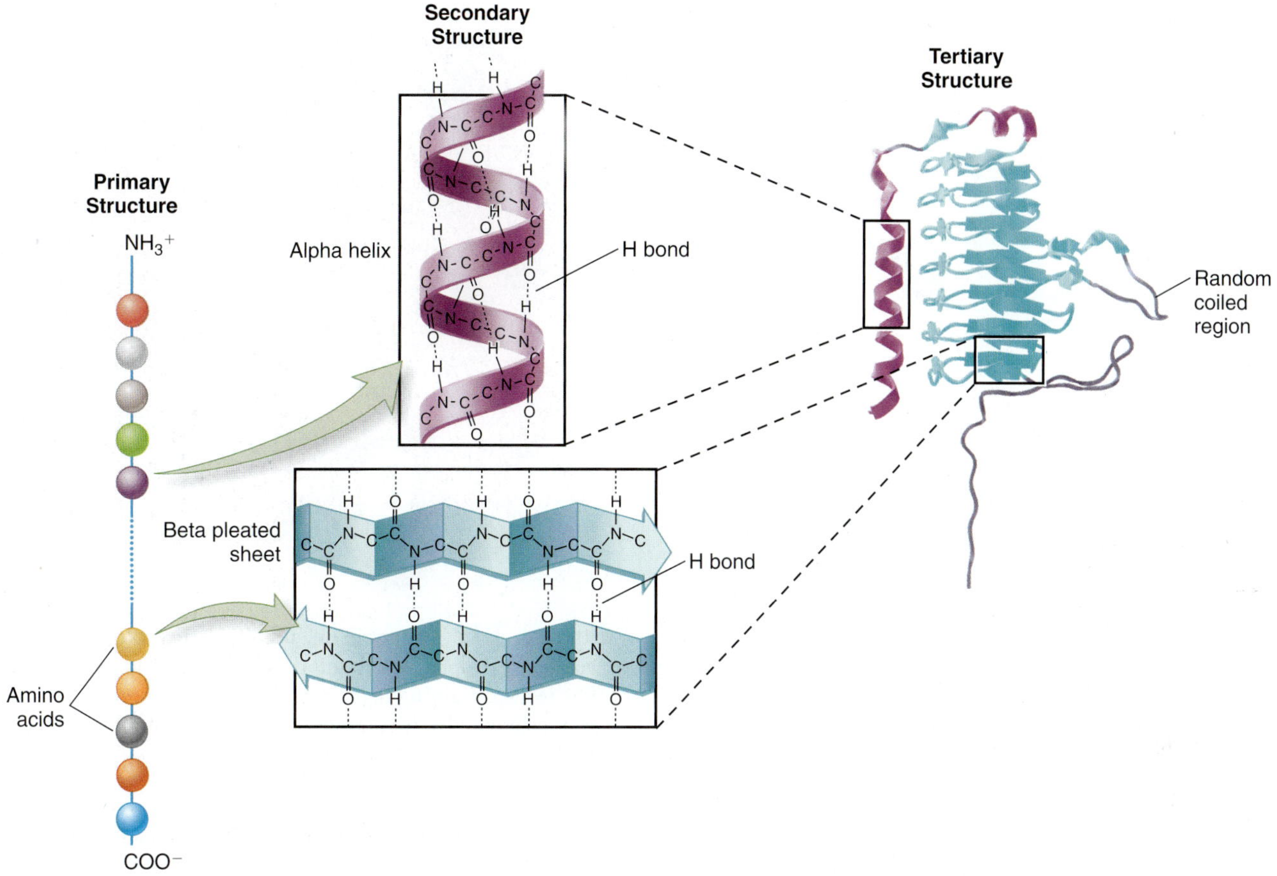

Figure 2.17 Secondary structure of a protein forms when regions of a polypeptide chain fold and twist into either an alpha-helical or beta pleated sheet conformation. The folding occurs largely through hydrogen bonds between nearby amino acid side groups. Further folding of the polypeptide chain produces tertiary structure, which is the final conformation of the protein.

a given region of a polypeptide chain may not assume either a helical or beta pleated sheet conformation. For example, the sizes of the side chains and the presence of ionic bonds between side chains with opposite charges can interfere with the repetitive hydrogen bonding required to produce these shapes. These irregular regions, known as random coil conformations, occur in regions linking the more regular helical and beta pleated sheet patterns (see Figure 2.17).

Beta pleated sheets and alpha helices tend to impart upon a protein the ability to anchor itself into a lipid bilayer, like that of a plasma membrane, because these regions of the protein usually contain amino acids with hydrophobic side chains. The hydrophobicity of the side chains makes them more likely to remain in the lipid environment of the plasma membrane.

Tertiary Structure

Once secondary structure has been formed, associations between additional amino acid side chains become possible. For example, two amino acids that may have been too far apart in the linear sequence of a polypeptide to interact with each other may become very near each other once secondary structure has changed the shape of the molecule. These interactions fold the polypeptide into its final three-dimensional conformation, making it a functional protein (see Figure 2.17). Five major factors determine the final conformation, or **tertiary structure,** of a polypeptide chain once the amino acid sequence (primary structure) has been formed: (1) hydrogen bonds between portions of the chain or with surrounding water molecules; (2) ionic bonds between polar and ionized regions along the chain; (3) attraction between nonpolar (hydrophobic) regions; (4) covalent **disulfide bonds** linking the sulfur-containing side chains of two cysteine amino acids; and (5) **van der Waals forces,** which are very weak and transient electrical interactions between the electrons in the outer shells of two atoms that are in close proximity to each other (**Figure 2.18**).

Quaternary Structure

Some proteins are composed of more than one polypeptide chain; they are said to have **quaternary structure** and are known as **multimeric** ("many parts") **proteins.** The same factors that influence the conformation of a single polypeptide also determine the interactions between the polypeptides in a multimeric protein. Therefore, the chains can be held together by interactions between various ionized, polar, and nonpolar side chains, as well as by disulfide covalent bonds between the chains.

Multimeric proteins have many diverse functions. The polypeptide chains in a multimeric protein may be

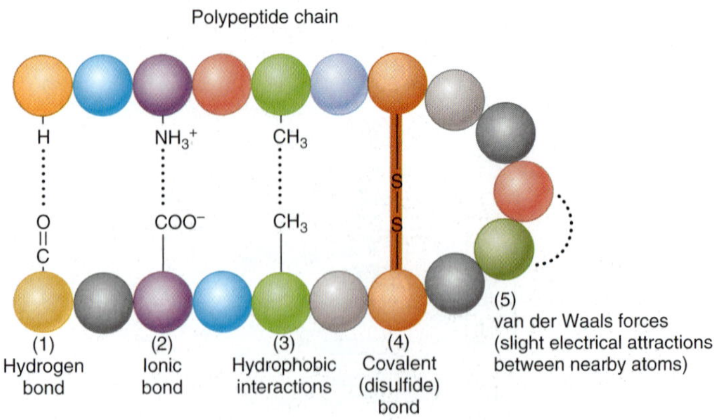

Figure 2.18 Factors that contribute to the folding of polypeptide chains and thus to their conformation are (1) hydrogen bonds between side chains or with surrounding water molecules, (2) ionic bonds between polar or ionized side chains, (3) hydrophobic attractive forces between nonpolar side chains, (4) disulfide bonds between side chains, and (5) van der Waals forces between atoms in the side chains of nearby amino acids.

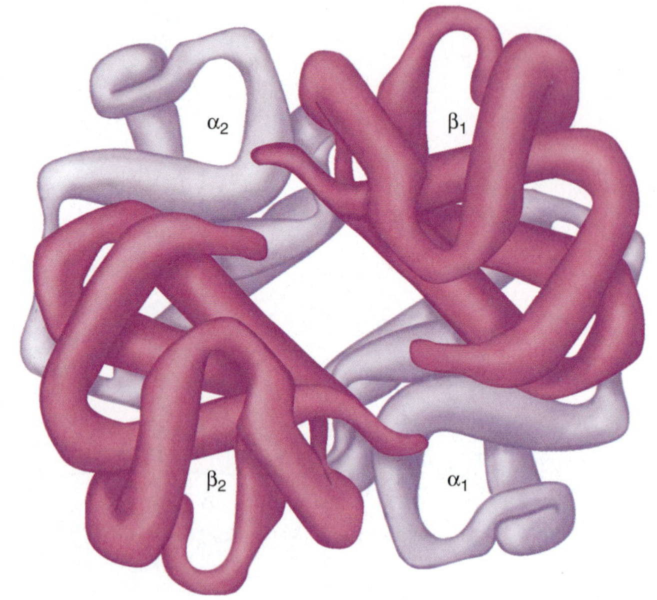

Figure 2.19 Hemoglobin, a multimeric protein composed of two identical alpha (α) subunits and two identical beta (β) subunits. (The iron-containing heme groups attached to each globin chain are not shown.) In this simplified view, the overall arrangement of subunits is shown without details of secondary structure.

identical or different. For example, hemoglobin, the protein that transports oxygen in the blood, is a multimeric protein with four polypeptide chains, two of one kind and two of another (**Figure 2.19**). Each subunit can transport one oxygen molecule. Other multimeric proteins that you will learn of in this textbook play a role in creating pores, or channels, in plasma membranes to allow movement of small solutes in and out of cells.

The primary structures (amino acid sequences) of a large number of proteins are known, but three-dimensional conformations have been determined for only a small number. Because of the multiple factors that can influence the folding of a polypeptide chain, it is not yet possible to accurately predict the conformation of a protein from its primary amino acid sequence. However, it should be clear that a change in the primary structure of a protein may alter its secondary, tertiary, and quaternary structures. Such an alteration in primary structure is called a **mutation.** Even a single amino acid change resulting from a mutation may have devastating consequences, as occurs when a molecule of valine replaces a molecule of glutamic acid in the beta chains of hemoglobin. The result of this change is a serious disease called ***sickle-cell disease*** (formerly called *sickle-cell anemia*). When red blood cells in a person with this disease are exposed to decreased oxygen levels, their hemoglobin precipitates. This contorts the red blood cells into a crescent shape, which makes the cells fragile and unable to function normally.

Nucleic Acids

Nucleic acids account for only 2% of body weight, yet these molecules are extremely important because they are responsible for the storage, expression, and transmission of genetic information. The expression of genetic information in the form of specific proteins determines whether one is a human or a mouse, or whether a cell is a muscle cell or an epithelial cell.

There are two classes of nucleic acids, **deoxyribonucleic acid (DNA)** and **ribonucleic acid (RNA)**. DNA molecules store genetic information coded in the sequence of their genes, whereas RNA molecules are involved in decoding this information into instructions for linking together a specific sequence of amino acids to form a specific polypeptide chain.

Both types of nucleic acids are polymers and are therefore composed of linear sequences of repeating subunits. Each subunit, known as a **nucleotide,** has three components: a phosphate group, a sugar, and a ring of carbon and nitrogen atoms known as a base because it can accept hydrogen ions (**Figure 2.20**). The phosphate group of one nucleotide is linked to the sugar of the adjacent nucleotide to form a chain, with the bases sticking out from the side of the phosphate–sugar backbone (**Figure 2.21**).

DNA

The nucleotides in DNA contain the five-carbon sugar **deoxyribose** (hence the name "deoxyribonucleic acid"). Four different nucleotides are present in DNA, corresponding to the four different bases that can be bound to deoxyribose. These bases are divided into two classes: (1) the **purine** bases, **adenine** (A) and **guanine** (G), which have double rings of nitrogen and carbon atoms; and (2) the **pyrimidine** bases, **cytosine** (C) and **thymine** (T), which have only a single ring (see Figure 2.21).

A DNA molecule consists of not one but two chains of nucleotides coiled around each other in the form of a double helix (**Figure 2.22**). The two chains are held together by hydrogen bonds between a purine base on one chain and a pyrimidine base on the opposite chain. The ring structure of

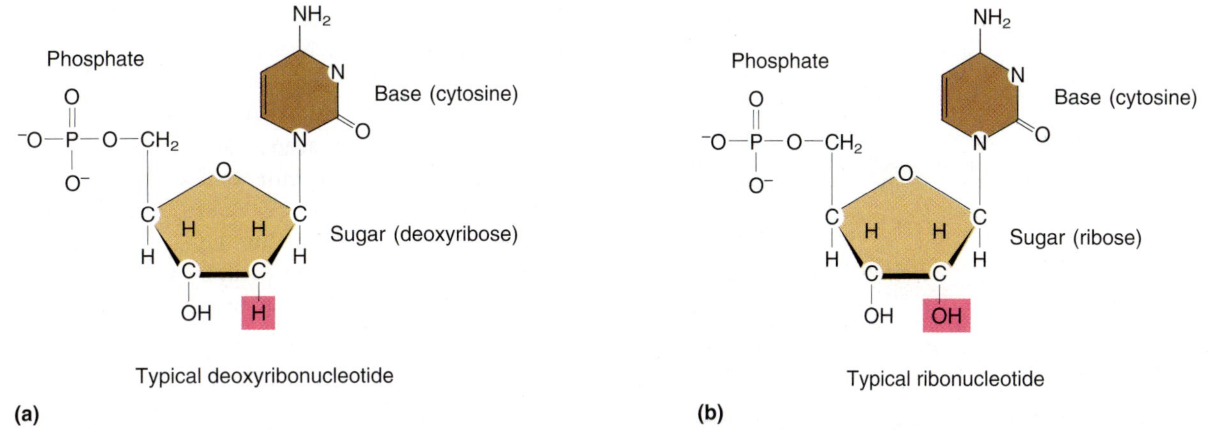

Figure 2.20 Nucleotide subunits of DNA and RNA. Nucleotides are composed of a sugar, a base, and a phosphate group. (a) Deoxyribonucleotides present in DNA contain the sugar deoxyribose. (b) The sugar in ribonucleotides, present in RNA, is ribose, which has an OH at a position in which deoxyribose has only a hydrogen atom.

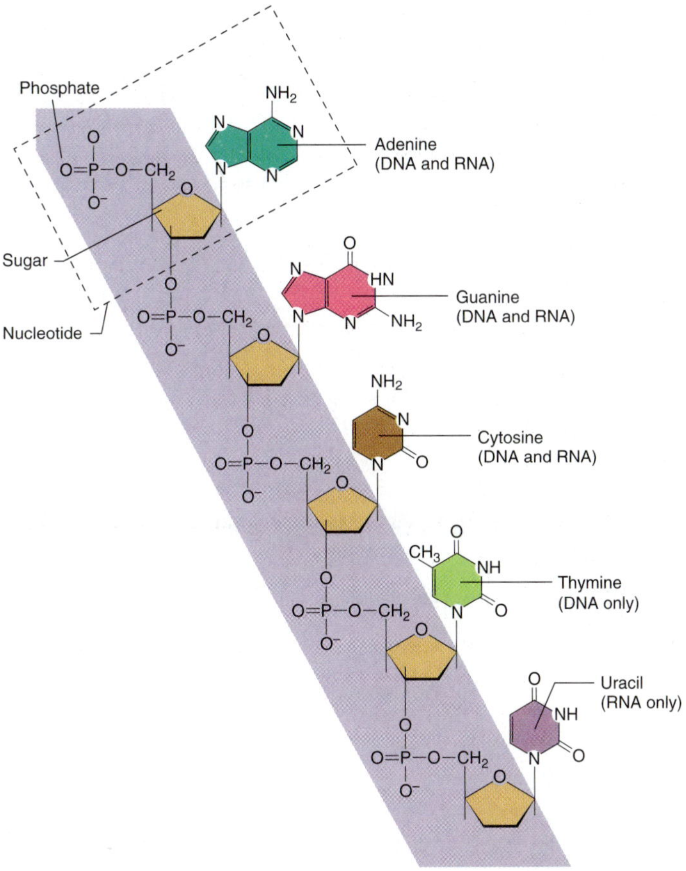

Figure 2.21 APR Phosphate–sugar bonds link nucleotides in sequence to form nucleic acids. Note that the pyrimidine base thymine is only found in DNA, and uracil is only present in RNA.

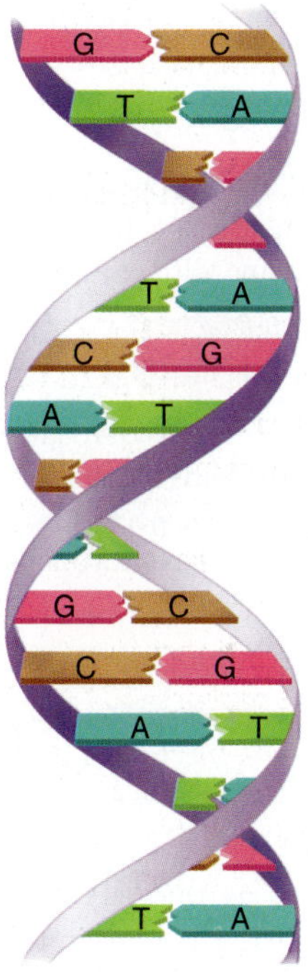

Figure 2.22 APR Base pairings between a purine and pyrimidine base link the two polynucleotide strands of the DNA double helix.

each base lies in a flat plane perpendicular to the phosphate–sugar backbone, like steps on a spiral staircase. This base pairing maintains a constant distance between the sugar–phosphate backbones of the two chains as they coil around each other.

Specificity is imposed on the base pairings by the location of the hydrogen-bonding groups in the four bases (**Figure 2.23**). Three hydrogen bonds form between the purine guanine and the pyrimidine cytosine (G–C pairing), whereas only two hydrogen bonds can form between the purine adenine and the pyrimidine thymine (A–T pairing). As a result, G is always paired with C, and A with T. This specificity provides the mechanism for duplicating and transferring genetic information.

The hydrogen bonds between the bases can be broken by enzymes. This separates the double helix into two strands; such DNA is said to be denatured. Each single strand can be replicated to form two new molecules of DNA. This occurs during cell division such that each daughter cell has a full complement of DNA. The bonds can also be broken by heating DNA in a test tube, which provides a convenient way for researchers to examine such processes as DNA replication.

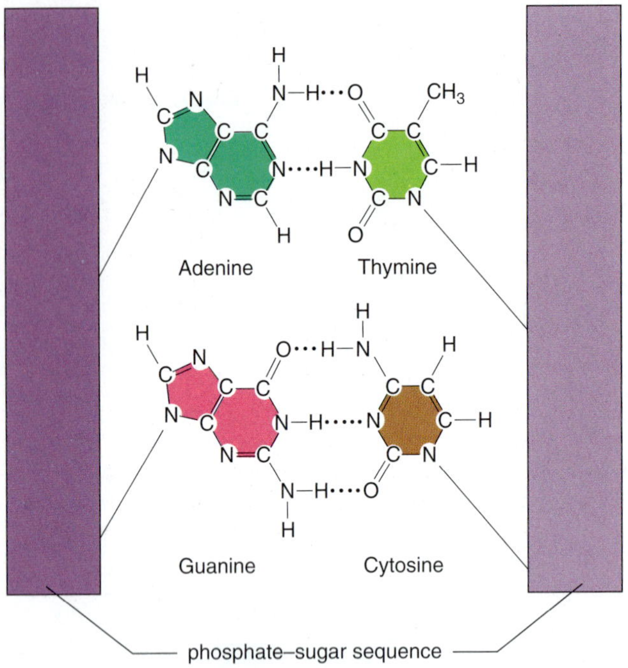

Figure 2.23 AP|R Hydrogen bonds between the nucleotide bases in DNA determine the specificity of base pairings: adenine with thymine, and guanine with cytosine.

PHYSIOLOGICAL INQUIRY

- When a DNA molecule is heated to an extreme temperature in a test tube, the two chains break apart. Which type of DNA molecule would you expect to break down at a reduced temperature, one with more G–C bonds, or one with more A–T bonds?

Answer can be found at end of chapter.

RNA

RNA molecules differ in only a few respects from DNA: (1) RNA consists of a single (rather than a double) chain of nucleotides; (2) in RNA, the sugar in each nucleotide is **ribose** rather than deoxyribose; and (3) the pyrimidine base thymine in DNA is replaced in RNA by the pyrimidine base **uracil** (U) (see Figure 2.21), which can base-pair with the purine adenine (A–U pairing). The other three bases—adenine, guanine, and cytosine—are the same in both DNA and RNA. Because RNA contains only a single chain of nucleotides, portions of this chain can bend back upon themselves and undergo base pairing with nucleotides in the same chain or in other molecules of DNA or RNA.

ATP

The purine bases are important not only in DNA and RNA synthesis but also in a molecule that serves as the molecular energy source for all cells.

The functioning of a cell depends upon its ability to extract and use the chemical energy in the organic molecules discussed in this chapter. For example, when, in the presence of oxygen, a cell breaks down glucose to carbon dioxide and water, energy is released. Some of this energy is in the form of heat, but a cell cannot use heat energy to perform its functions. The remainder of the energy is transferred to another important molecule that can in turn transfer it to yet another molecule or to energy-requiring processes. In all cells, from bacterial to human, **adenosine triphosphate (ATP)** (**Figure 2.24**) is the primary molecule that receives the transfer of energy from the breakdown of fuel molecules—carbohydrates, fats, and proteins.

Energy released from organic molecules is used to add phosphate groups to molecules of adenosine. This stored energy can then be released upon hydrolysis:

$$ATP + H_2O \longrightarrow ADP + P_i + H^+ + \text{energy}$$

The products of the reaction are **adenosine diphosphate (ADP)**, inorganic phosphate (P_i), and H^+.

Among other things, the energy derived from the hydrolysis of ATP is used by the cells for (1) the production of force and movement, as in muscle contraction; (2) active transport of molecules across membranes; and (3) synthesis of the organic molecules used in cell structures and functions. ■

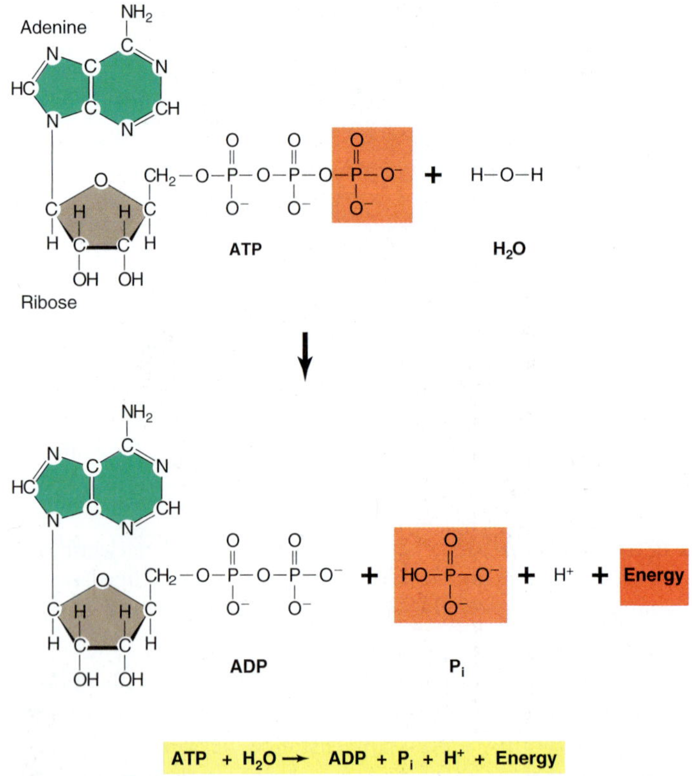

Figure 2.24 Chemical structure of ATP. Its breakdown to ADP and P_i is accompanied by the release of energy.

SUMMARY

Atoms

I. Atoms are composed of three subatomic particles: positive protons and neutral neutrons, both located in the nucleus, and negative electrons revolving around the nucleus in orbitals contained within electron shells.

II. The atomic number is the number of protons in an atom, and because atoms (except ions) are electrically neutral, it is also the number of electrons.

III. The atomic mass of an atom is the ratio of the atom's mass relative to that of a carbon-12 atom.

IV. One gram atomic mass is the number of grams of an element equal to its atomic mass. One gram atomic mass of any element contains the same number of atoms: 6×10^{23}.

V. When an atom gains or loses one or more electrons, it acquires a net electrical charge and becomes an ion.

Molecules

I. Molecules are formed by linking atoms together.

II. A covalent bond forms when two atoms share a pair of electrons. Each type of atom can form a characteristic number of covalent bonds: hydrogen forms one; oxygen, two; nitrogen, three; and carbon, four. In polar covalent bonds, one atom attracts the bonding electrons more than the other atom of the pair. Nonpolar covalent bonds are between two atoms of similar electronegativities.

III. Molecules have characteristic shapes that can be altered within limits by the rotation of their atoms around covalent bonds.

IV. The electrical attraction between hydrogen and an oxygen or nitrogen atom in a separate molecule, or between different regions of the same molecule, forms a hydrogen bond.

V. Molecules may have ionic regions within their structure.

VI. Free radicals are atoms or molecules that contain atoms having an unpaired electron in their outer electron orbital.

Solutions

I. Water, a polar molecule, is attracted to other water molecules by hydrogen bonds. Water is the solvent in which most of the chemical reactions in the body take place.

II. Substances dissolved in a liquid are solutes, and the liquid in which they are dissolved is the solvent.

III. Substances that have polar or ionized groups dissolve in water by being electrically attracted to the polar water molecules.

IV. In water, amphipathic molecules form clusters with the polar regions at the surface and the nonpolar regions in the interior of the cluster.

V. The molecular weight of a molecule is the sum of the atomic weights of all its atoms. One mole of any substance is its molecular weight in grams and contains 6×10^{23} molecules.

VI. Substances that release a hydrogen ion in solution are called acids. Those that accept a hydrogen ion are bases.
   a. The acidity of a solution is determined by its free hydrogen ion concentration; the greater the hydrogen ion concentration, the greater the acidity.
   b. The pH of a solution is the negative logarithm of the hydrogen ion concentration. As the acidity of a solution increases, the pH decreases. Acid solutions have a pH less than 7.0, whereas alkaline solutions have a pH greater than 7.0.

Classes of Organic Molecules

I. Carbohydrates are composed of carbon, hydrogen, and oxygen atoms.
   a. The presence of the polar hydroxyl groups makes carbohydrates soluble in water.
   b. The most abundant monosaccharide in the body is glucose ($C_6H_{12}O_6$), which is stored in cells in the form of the polysaccharide glycogen.

II. Most lipids have many fewer polar and ionized groups than carbohydrates, a characteristic that makes them nearly or completely insoluble in water.
   a. Triglycerides (fats) form when fatty acids are bound to each of the three hydroxyl groups in glycerol.
   b. Phospholipids contain two fatty acids bound to two of the hydroxyl groups in glycerol, with the third hydroxyl bound to phosphate, which in turn is linked to a small charged or polar compound. The polar and ionized groups at one end of phospholipids make these molecules amphipathic.
   c. Steroids are composed of four interconnected rings, often containing a few hydroxyl and other groups.
   d. One fatty acid (arachidonic acid) can be converted to a class of signaling substances called eicosanoids.

III. Proteins, macromolecules composed primarily of carbon, hydrogen, oxygen, and nitrogen, are polymers of 20 different amino acids.
   a. Amino acids have an amino ($—NH_2$) and a carboxyl ($—COOH$) group bound to their terminal carbon atom.
   b. Amino acids are bound together by peptide bonds between the carboxyl group of one amino acid and the amino group of the next.
   c. The primary structure of a polypeptide chain is determined by (1) the number of amino acids in sequence and (2) the type of amino acid at each position.
   d. Hydrogen bonds between peptide bonds along a polypeptide force much of the chain into an alpha helix or beta pleated sheet (secondary structure).
   e. Covalent disulfide bonds can form between the sulfhydryl groups of cysteine side chains to hold regions of a polypeptide chain close to each other; together with hydrogen bonds, ionic bonds, hydrophobic interactions, and van der Waals forces, this creates the final conformation of the protein (tertiary structure).
   f. Multimeric proteins have multiple polypeptide chains (quaternary structure).

IV. Nucleic acids are responsible for the storage, expression, and transmission of genetic information.
   a. Deoxyribonucleic acid (DNA) stores genetic information.
   b. Ribonucleic acid (RNA) is involved in decoding the information in DNA into instructions for linking amino acids together to form proteins.
   c. Both types of nucleic acids are polymers of nucleotides, each containing a phosphate group; a sugar; and a base of carbon, hydrogen, oxygen, and nitrogen atoms.
   d. DNA contains the sugar deoxyribose and consists of two chains of nucleotides coiled around each other in a double helix. The chains are held together by hydrogen bonds between purine and pyrimidine bases in the two chains.
   e. Base pairings in DNA always occur between guanine and cytosine and between adenine and thymine.

f. RNA consists of a single chain of nucleotides, containing the sugar ribose and three of the four bases found in DNA. The fourth base in RNA is the pyrimidine uracil rather than thymine. Uracil base-pairs with adenine.
g. In all cells, energy from the catabolism of organic molecules is transferred to ATP. Hydrolysis of ATP to ADP + P_i then transfers this energy to power cell functions. ATP consists of the purine adenine coupled by high-energy bonds to three phosphate groups.

REVIEW QUESTIONS

1. Describe the electrical charge, mass, and location of the three major subatomic particles in an atom.
2. Which four kinds of atoms are most abundant in the body?
3. Describe the distinguishing characteristics of the three classes of essential chemical elements found in the body.
4. How many covalent bonds can be formed by atoms of carbon, nitrogen, oxygen, and hydrogen?
5. What property of molecules allows them to change their three-dimensional shape?
6. Define *ion* and *ionic bond.*
7. Draw the structures of an ionized carboxyl group and an ionized amino group.
8. Define *free radical.*
9. Describe the polar characteristics of a water molecule.
10. What determines a molecule's solubility or lack of solubility in water?
11. Describe the organization of amphipathic molecules in water.
12. What is the molar concentration of 80 g of glucose dissolved in sufficient water to make 2 L of solution?
13. What distinguishes a weak acid from a strong acid?
14. What effect does increasing the pH of a solution have upon the ionization of a carboxyl group? An amino group?
15. Name the four classes of organic molecules in the body.
16. Describe the three subclasses of carbohydrate molecules.
17. What properties are characteristic of lipids?
18. Describe the subclasses of lipids.
19. Describe the linkages between amino acids that form polypeptide chains.
20. What distinguishes the terms *peptide, polypeptide,* and *protein?*
21. What two factors determine the primary structure of a polypeptide chain?
22. Describe the types of interactions that determine the conformation of a polypeptide chain.
23. Describe the structure of DNA and RNA.
24. Describe the characteristics of base pairings between nucleotide bases.

KEY TERMS

acid 29
acidic solution 29
acidity 29
adenine 38
adenosine diphosphate (ADP) 40
adenosine triphosphate (ATP) 40
alkaline solution 29
alpha helix 36
amino acid 34
amino acid side chain 34
amino group 26
amphipathic 28
anion 23
atom 21
atomic nucleus 21
atomic number 22
atomic mass 22
base 29
beta pleated sheet 36
carbohydrate 30
carboxyl group 26
cation 23
chemical element 21
concentration 28
conformation 36
covalent bond 23
cytosine 38
dehydration 27
deoxyribonucleic acid (DNA) 38
deoxyribose 38
disaccharide 31
disulfide bond 37
electrolyte 23
electron 21
electronegativity 24
fatty acid 32
free radical 26
glucose 31
glycerol 32
glycogen 31
glycoprotein 35
gram atomic mass 22
guanine 38
hexose 31
hydrogen bond 25
hydrolysis 27
hydrophilic 28
hydrophobic 28
hydroxyl group 24
ion 23
ionic bond 25
isotope 22
lipid 31
macromolecule 30
mineral element 23
mole 29
molecular weight 29
molecule 23
monosaccharide 31
monounsaturated fatty acid 32
multimeric protein 37
mutation 38
neutral solution 29
neutron 21
nonpolar covalent bond 25
nonpolar molecule 25
nucleic acid 38
nucleotide 38
pentose 31
peptide 36
peptide bond 34
pH 29
phospholipid 34
polar covalent bond 24
polar molecule 24
polymer 30
polypeptide 35
polysaccharide 31
polyunsaturated fatty acid 32
primary structure 36
protein 34
proton 21
purine 38
pyrimidine 38
quaternary structure 37
radioisotope 22
ribonucleic acid (RNA) 38
ribose 40
saturated fatty acid 32
secondary structure 36
solute 27
solution 27
solvent 27
steroid 34
strong acid 29
sucrose 31
tertiary structure 37
thymine 39
trace element 23
trans fatty acid 32
triglyceride 32
unsaturated fatty acid 32
uracil 40
van der Waals forces 37
weak acid 29

CLINICAL TERMS

PET (positron emission tomography) scan 22
sickle-cell disease 38
sickle-cell trait 41

CHAPTER 2 Clinical Case Study: A Young Man with Severe Abdominal Pain While Mountain Climbing

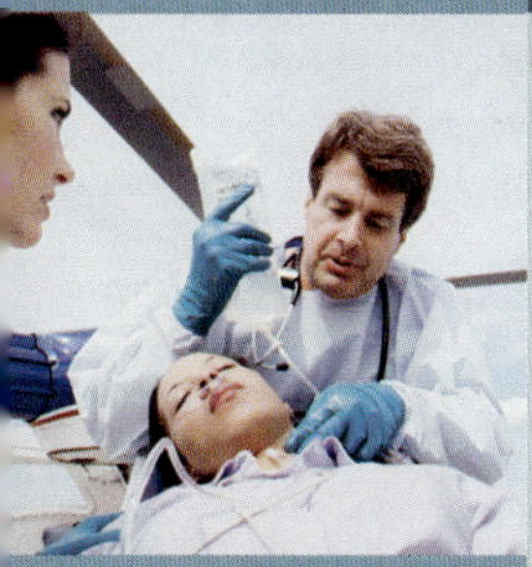

An athletic, 21-year-old African-American male in good health spent part of the summer before his senior year in college traveling with friends in the western United States. Although not an experienced mountain climber, he joined his friends in a professionally guided climb partway up Mt. Rainier in Washington. Despite his overall fitness, the rigors of the climb were far greater than he expected, and he found himself breathing heavily. At an elevation of around 6000 feet, he began to feel twinges of pain on the left side of his upper abdomen. By the time he reached 9000 feet, the pain worsened to the point that he stopped climbing and descended the mountain. However, the pain did not go away and in fact became very severe during the days after his climb. At that point, he went to a local emergency room, where he was subjected to a number of tests that revealed a disorder in his red blood cells due to an abnormal form of the protein hemoglobin.

Recall from Figure 2.19 that hemoglobin is a protein with quaternary structure. Each subunit in hemoglobin is noncovalently bound to the other subunits by the forces described in Figure 2.18. The three-dimensional (tertiary) structure of each subunit spatially aligns the individual amino acids in such a way that the bonding forces exert themselves between specific amino acid side groups. Therefore, anything that disrupts the tertiary structure of hemoglobin also disrupts the way in which subunits bond with one another. The patient described here had a condition called ***sickle-cell trait*** (SCT). Such individuals are carriers of the gene that causes sickle-cell disease (SCD), formerly called sickle-cell anemia. Individuals with SCT have one normal gene inherited from one parent and one gene with a mutation inherited from the other parent. The SCT/SCD gene is prevalent in several regions of the world, particularly in sub-Saharan Africa. In SCD, a mutation in the gene for the beta subunits of hemoglobin results in the replacement of a single glutamic acid residue with one of valine. Glutamic acid has a charged, polar side group, whereas valine has a nonpolar side group. Thus, in hemoglobin containing the mutation, one type of intermolecular bonding force is replaced with a completely different one, and this can lead to abnormal bonding of hemoglobin subunits with each other. In fact, the hydrophobic interactions created by the valine side groups cause multiple hemoglobin molecules to bond with each other, forming huge polymer-like structures that precipitate out of solution within the cytoplasm of the red blood cell resulting in a deformation of the entire cell. This happens most noticeably when the amount of oxygen in the red blood cell is decreased. Such a situation can occur at high altitude, where the atmospheric pressure is low and consequently the amount of oxygen that diffuses into the lung circulation is also low. (You will learn about the relationship between altitude, oxygen, and atmospheric pressure in Chapter 13.)

When red blood cells become deformed into the sicklelike shape characteristic of SCD, they are removed from the circulation by the spleen, an organ that lies in the upper left quadrant of the abdomen and plays an important role in eliminating dead or damaged red blood cells from the circulation. However, in the event of a sudden, large increase in the number of sickled cells, the spleen can become overfilled with damaged cells and painfully enlarged. Moreover, some of the sickled cells can block some of the small blood vessels in the spleen, which also causes pain and damage to the organ. This may begin quickly but may also continue for several days, which is why our subject's pain did not become very severe until a day or two after his climb.

Why would our patient attempt to climb a mountain to high altitude, knowing that the available amount of oxygen in the air is decreased at such altitudes? Recall that we said that the patient had sickle-cell *trait,* not sickle-cell disease. Individuals with sickle-cell trait produce enough normal hemoglobin to be symptom free their entire lives and may never know that they are carriers of a mutated gene. However, when pushed to the limits of oxygen deprivation by high altitude and exercise, as our patient was, the result is sickling of some of the red blood cells. Once the young man's condition was confirmed, he was given analgesics (painkillers) and advised to rest for the next 2 to 3 weeks until his spleen returned to normal. His spleen was carefully monitored during this time, and he recovered fully. Our patient was lucky; numerous deaths due to unrecognized SCT have occurred throughout the world as a result of situations just like the one described here. It is a striking example of how a protein's overall structure and function depend upon its primary structure, and how protein–protein interactions are critically dependent on the bonding forces described in this chapter. This theme will be explored in more detail in Sections B–D of Chapter 3.

Clinical term: sickle-cell trait (SCT)

See Chapter 19 for complete, integrative case studies.

CHAPTER 2 TEST QUESTIONS

Answers found in Appendix A.

1. A molecule that loses an electron to a free radical
   a. becomes more stable.
   b. becomes electrically neutral.
   c. becomes less reactive.
   d. is permanently destroyed.
   e. becomes a free radical itself.

2. Of the bonding forces between atoms and molecules, which are strongest?
   a. hydrogen bonds
   b. bonds between oppositely charged ionized groups
   c. bonds between nearby nonpolar groups
   d. covalent bonds
   e. bonds between polar groups

3. The process by which monomers of organic molecules are made into larger units
   a. requires hydrolysis.
   b. results in the generation of water molecules.
   c. is irreversible.
   d. occurs only with carbohydrates.
   e. results in the production of ATP.
4. Which of the following is/are not found in DNA?
   a. adenine
   b. uracil
   c. cytosine
   d. deoxyribose
   e. both b and d
5. Which of the following statements is incorrect about disulfide bonds?
   a. They form between two cysteine amino acids.
   b. They are noncovalent.
   c. They contribute to the tertiary structure of some proteins.
   d. They contribute to the quaternary structure of some proteins.
   e. They involve the loss of two hydrogen atoms.
6. Match the following compounds with choices (a) monosaccharide, (b) disaccharide, or (c) polysaccharide:
   Sucrose
   Glucose
   Glycogen
   Fructose
   Starch
7. Which of the following reactions involve/involves hydrolysis?
   a. formation of triglycerides
   b. formation of proteins
   c. breakdown of proteins
   d. formation of polysaccharides
   e. a, b, and d

CHAPTER 2 GENERAL PRINCIPLES ASSESSMENT

Answers found in Appendix A.

1. Proteins play important roles in many physiological processes. Using Figures 2.17 through 2.19 as your guide, explain how protein structure is an example of the general physiological principle that *physiological processes are dictated by the laws of chemistry and physics.*

CHAPTER 2 QUANTITATIVE AND THOUGHT QUESTIONS

Answers found at www.mhhe.com/widmaier13.

1. What is the molarity of a solution with 100 g fructose dissolved in 0.7 L water? (See Figure 2.10 for the chemical structure of fructose.)
2. The pH of the fluid in the human stomach following a meal is generally around 1.5. What is the hydrogen ion concentration in such a fluid?
3. Potassium has an atomic number of 19 and an atomic mass of 39 (ignore the possibility of isotopes for this question). How many neutrons and electrons are present in potassium in its nonionized (K) and ionized (K^+) forms?

CHAPTER 2 ANSWERS TO PHYSIOLOGICAL INQUIRIES

Figure 2.5 The presence of hydrogen bonds helps stabilize water in its liquid form such that less water escapes into the gaseous phase.

Figure 2.10 The reverse of a dehydration reaction is called hydrolysis, which is derived from Greek words for "water" and "break apart." In hydrolysis, a molecule of water is added to a complex molecule that is broken down into two smaller molecules.

Figure 2.12 The portion of the phospholipid containing the charged phosphate and nitrogen groups would face the water, and the two fatty acid tails would exclude water.

Figure 2.16 *Polypeptide* refers to a structural unit of two or more amino acids bonded together by peptide bonds and does not imply anything about function. A *protein* is a functional molecule formed by the folding of a polypeptide into a characteristic shape, or conformation.

Figure 2.23 Because adenine and thymine are bonded by two hydrogen bonds, whereas guanine and cytosine are held together by three hydrogen bonds, A–T bonds would be more easily broken by heat.

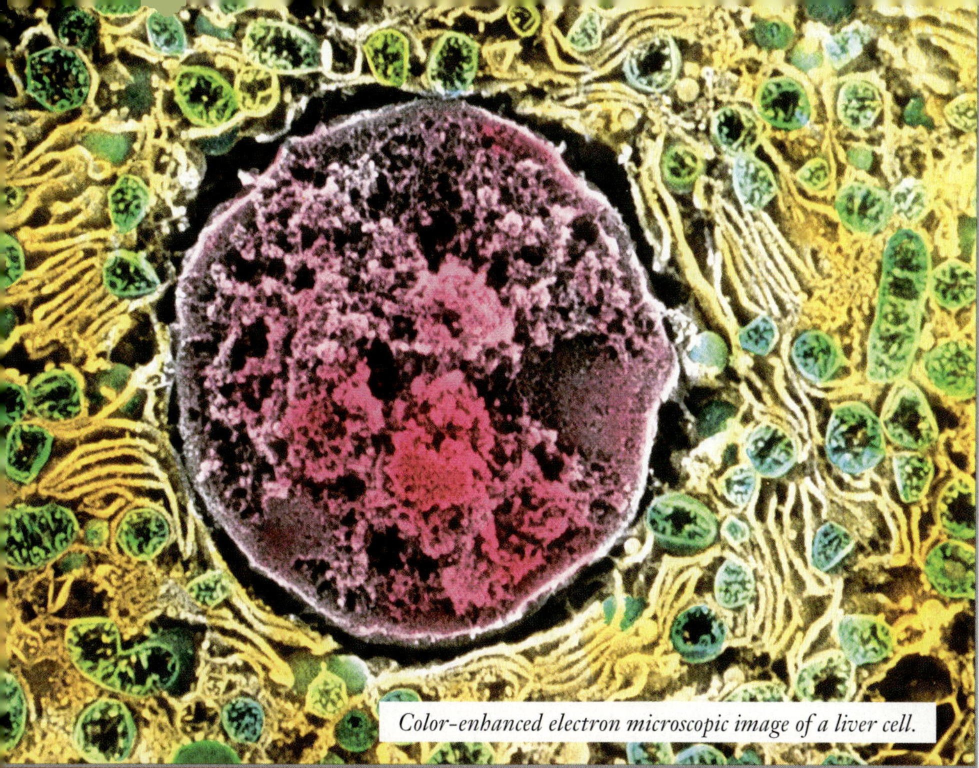

Color-enhanced electron microscopic image of a liver cell.

3 Cellular Structure, Proteins, and Metabolism

Cells are the structural and functional units of all living organisms and comprise the tissues and organs that physiologists study. The human body is composed of trillions of cells with highly specialized structures and functions, but you learned in Chapter 1 that most cells can be included in one of four major functional and morphological categories: muscle, connective, nervous and epithelial cells. In this chapter, we briefly describe the structures that are common to most of the cells of the body regardless of the category to which they belong.

Having learned the basic structures that comprise cells, we next turn our attention to how cellular proteins are synthesized, secreted, and degraded, and how proteins participate in the chemical reactions required for cells to survive. Proteins are associated with practically every function living cells perform. As described in Chapter 2, proteins have a unique shape or conformation that is established by their primary, secondary, tertiary, and—in some cases—quaternary structures. This conformation enables them to bind specific molecules on portions of their surfaces known as binding sites. This chapter includes a discussion of the properties of protein-binding sites that apply to all proteins, as well as a description of how these properties are involved in one special class of protein functions—the ability of enzymes to accelerate specific chemical reactions. We then apply this information to a description of the multitude of biochemical reactions involved in metabolism and cellular energy balance.

As you read this chapter, think about where the following general principles of physiology apply. The general principle that structure is a determinant of—and has coevolved with—function was described at the molecular level in Chapter 2; in Section A of this chapter, you will see how that principle is important at the cellular level, and in Sections C and D at the protein level. Also in Sections C and D, you will see how the general principle that physiological processes are dictated by the laws of chemistry and physics applies to protein function. The general principle that homeostasis is essential for health and survival will be explored in Sections D and E. Finally, the general principle that physiological processes require the transfer and balance of matter and energy will be explored in Section E.

SECTION **A**

Cell Structure

3.1 Microscopic Observations of Cells

The smallest object that can be resolved with a microscope depends upon the wavelength of the radiation used to illuminate the specimen—the shorter the wavelength, the smaller the object that can be seen. Whereas a light microscope can resolve objects as small as 0.2 μm in diameter, an electron microscope, which uses electron beams instead of light rays, can resolve structures as small as 0.002 μm. Typical sizes of cells and cellular components are illustrated in **Figure 3.1**.

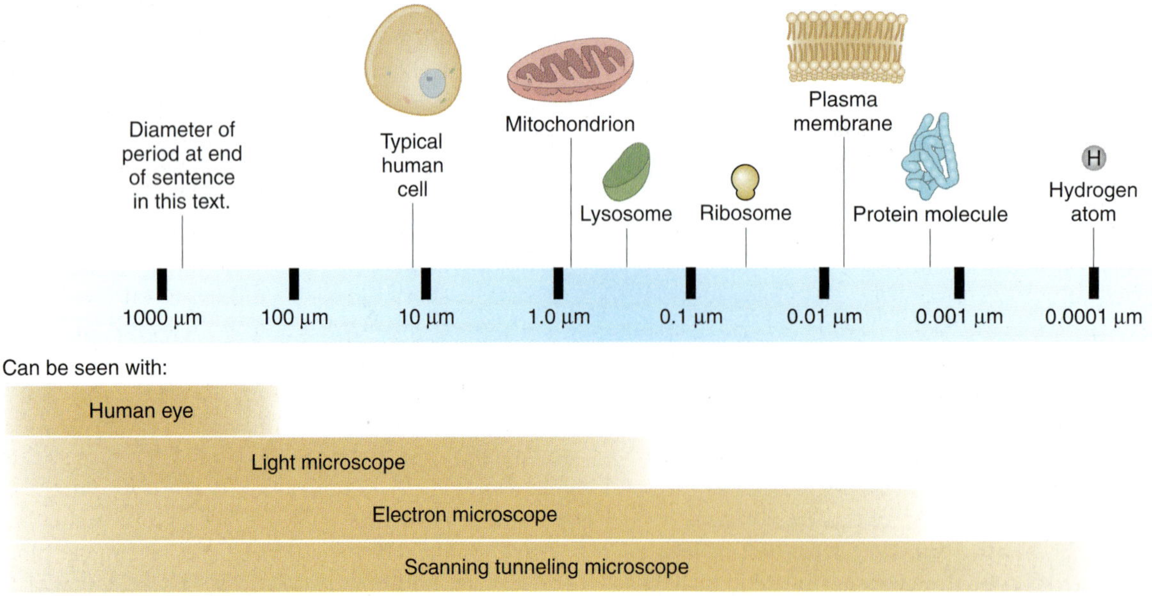

Figure 3.1 Typical sizes of cell structures, plotted on a logarithmic scale.

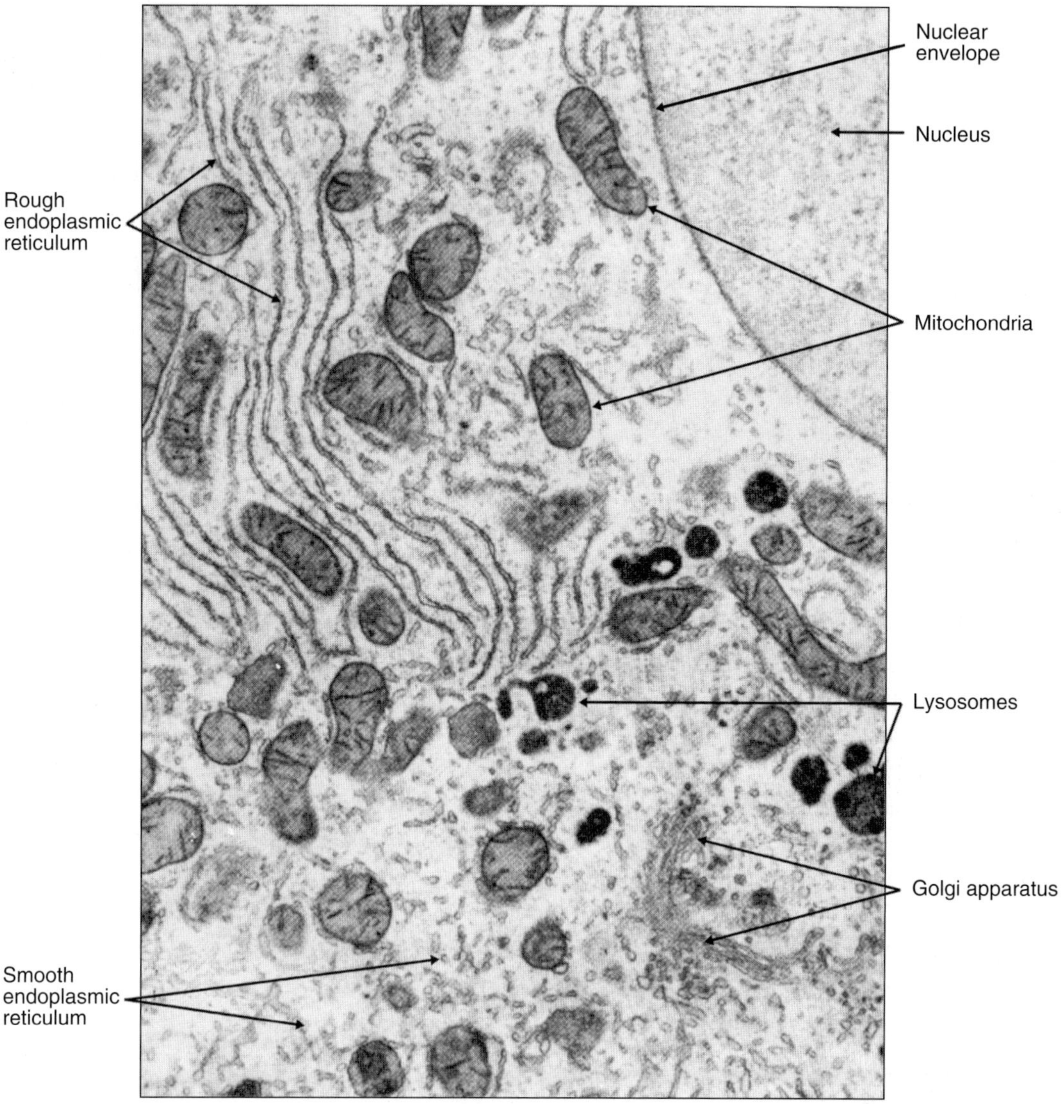

Figure 3.2 APIR Electron micrograph of a thin section through a portion of a human adrenal cell, showing the appearance of intracellular organelles.

Although living cells can be observed with a light microscope, this is not possible with an electron microscope. To form an image with an electron beam, most of the electrons must pass through the specimen, just as light passes through a specimen in a light microscope. However, electrons can penetrate only a short distance through matter; therefore, the observed specimen must be very thin. Cells to be observed with an electron microscope must be cut into sections on the order of 0.1 μm thick, which is about one-hundredth of the thickness of a typical cell.

Because electron micrographs, such as the one in **Figure 3.2**, are images of very thin sections of a cell, they can sometimes be misleading. Structures that appear as separate objects in the electron micrograph may actually be continuous structures connected through a region lying outside the plane of the section. As an analogy, a thin section through a ball of string would appear to be a collection of separate lines and disconnected dots even though the piece of string was originally continuous.

Two classes of cells, **eukaryotic cells** and **prokaryotic cells,** can be distinguished by their structure. The cells of the human body, as well as those of other multicellular animals and plants, are eukaryotic (true-nucleus) cells. These cells contain a nuclear membrane surrounding the cell nucleus and also contain numerous other membrane-bound structures. Prokaryotic cells, such as bacteria, lack these membranous structures. This chapter describes the structure of eukaryotic cells only.

Compare an electron micrograph of a section through a cell (see Figure 3.2) with a diagrammatic illustration of a typical human cell (**Figure 3.3**). What is immediately obvious from both figures is the extensive structure inside the cell. Cells are surrounded by a limiting barrier, the **plasma membrane** (also called the cell membrane), which covers the cell surface. The cell interior is divided into a number of compartments surrounded by membranes. These membrane-bound compartments, along with some particles and filaments, are known as **cell organelles.** Each cell organelle performs specific functions that contribute to the cell's survival.

The interior of a cell is divided into two regions: (1) the **nucleus,** a spherical or oval structure usually near the center of the cell, and (2) the **cytoplasm,** the region outside the nucleus (**Figure 3.4**). The cytoplasm contains cell organelles and fluid surrounding the organelles, known as the **cytosol.** As described in Chapter 1, the term **intracellular fluid** refers to *all* the fluid inside a cell—in other words, cytosol plus the fluid inside all the organelles, including the nucleus. The chemical compositions of the fluids in cell organelles may differ from that of the cytosol. The cytosol is by far the largest intracellular fluid compartment.

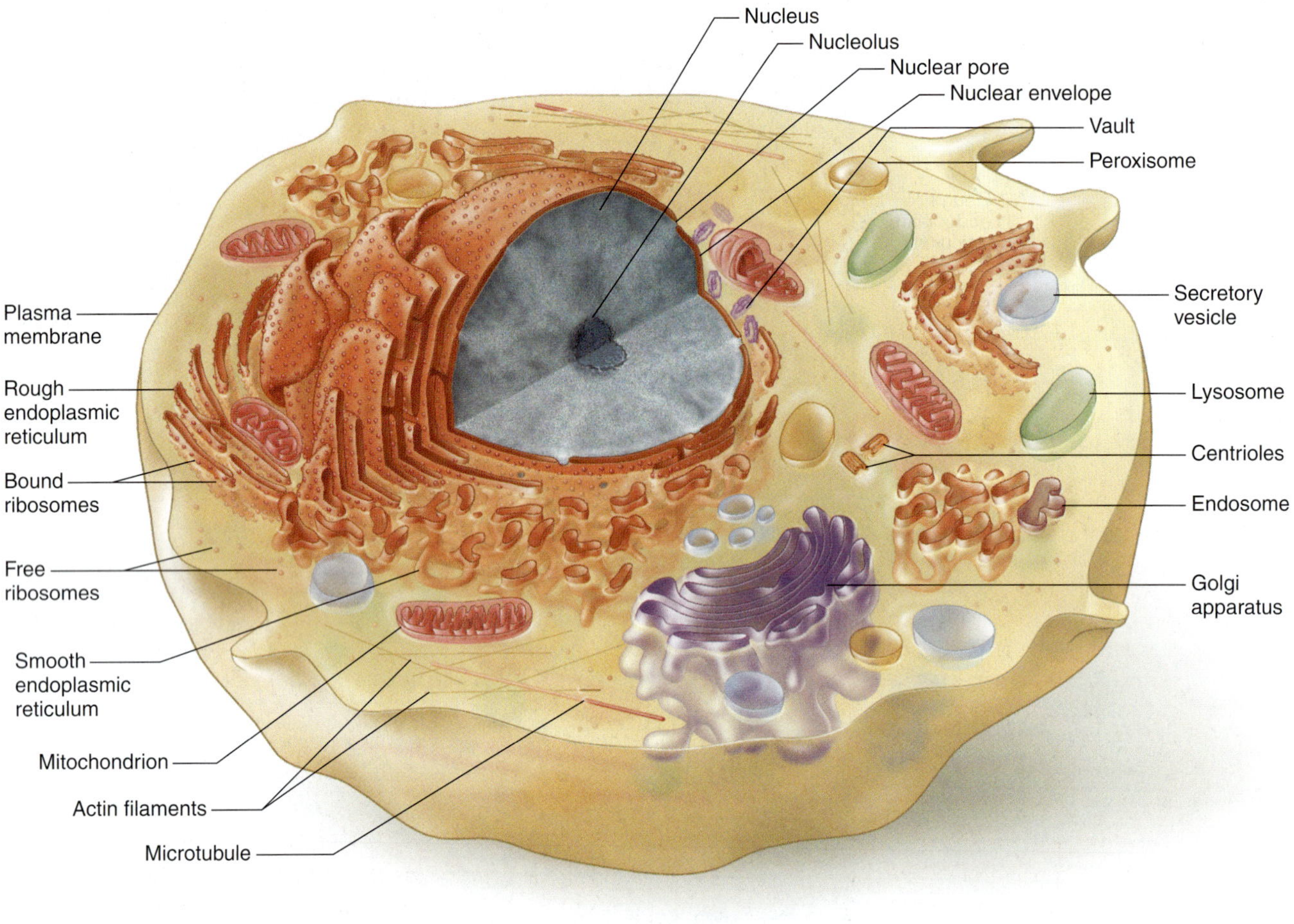

Figure 3.3 APIR Structures found in most human cells. Not all structures are drawn to scale.

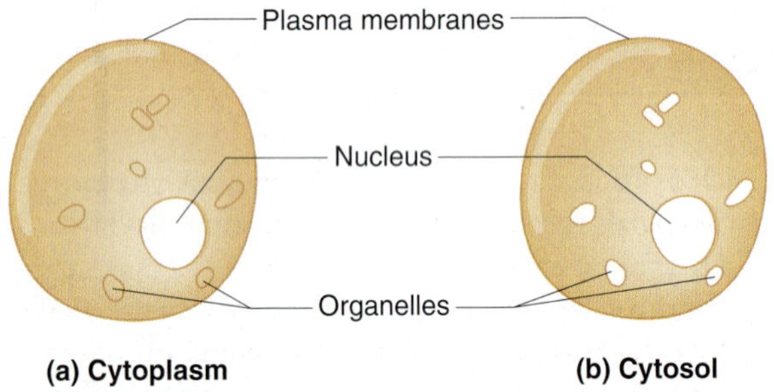

Figure 3.4 APIR Comparison of cytoplasm and cytosol. (a) Cytoplasm (shaded area) is the region of the cell outside the nucleus. (b) Cytosol (shaded area) is the fluid portion of the cytoplasm outside the cell organelles.

PHYSIOLOGICAL INQUIRY

- What compartments constitute the entire intracellular fluid?

Answer can be found at end of chapter.

3.2 Membranes

Membranes form a major structural element in cells. Although membranes perform a variety of functions that are important in physiology (**Table 3.1**), their most universal role is to act as a selective barrier to the passage of molecules, allowing some molecules to cross while excluding others. The plasma membrane regulates the passage of substances into and out of the cell, whereas the membranes surrounding cell organelles allow the selective movement of substances between the organelles and the cytosol. One of the advantages of restricting the movements of molecules across membranes is confining the products of chemical reactions to specific cell organelles. The hindrance a membrane offers to the passage of substances can be altered to allow increased or decreased flow of molecules or ions across the membrane in response to various signals.

In addition to acting as a selective barrier, the plasma membrane plays an important role in detecting chemical signals from other cells and in anchoring cells to adjacent cells and to the extracellular matrix of connective-tissue proteins.

TABLE 3.1	Functions of Plasma Membranes
Regulate the passage of substances into and out of cells and between cell organelles and cytosol.	
Detect chemical messengers arriving at the cell surface.	
Link adjacent cells together by membrane junctions.	
Anchor cells to the extracellular matrix.	

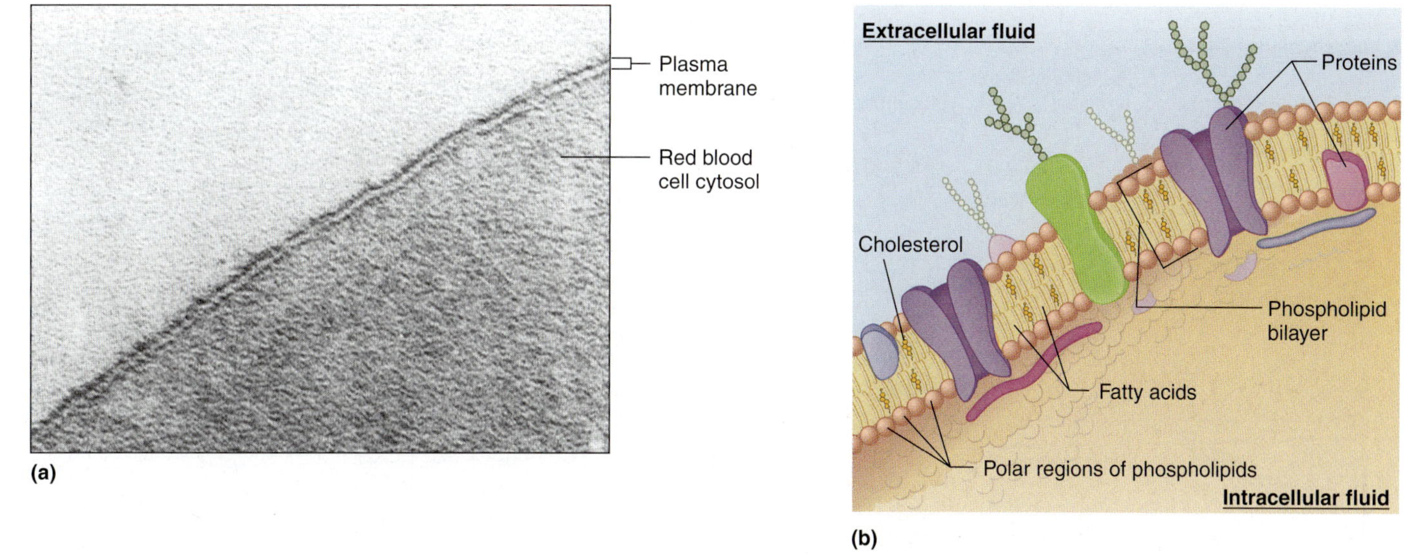

Figure 3.5 APIR (a) Electron micrograph of a human red blood cell plasma membrane. Plasma membranes are 6 to 10 nm thick, too thin to be seen without the aid of an electron microscope. In an electron micrograph, a membrane appears as two dark lines separated by a light interspace. The dark lines correspond to the polar regions of the proteins and lipids, whereas the light interspace corresponds to the nonpolar regions of these molecules. (b) Schematic arrangement of the proteins, phospholipids and cholesterol in a membrane. Some proteins have carbohydrate molecules attached to their extracellular surface. From J. D. Robertson in Michael Locke (ed.), *Cell Membranes in Development*, Academic Press, Inc., New York.

Membrane Structure

The structure of membranes determines their function. For example, all membranes consist of a double layer of lipid molecules containing embedded proteins (**Figure 3.5**). The major membrane lipids are **phospholipids.** One end of a phospholipid has a charged or polar region, and the remainder of the molecule, which consists of two long fatty acid chains, is nonpolar; therefore, phospholipids are amphipathic (see Chapter 2). The phospholipids in plasma membranes are organized into a bilayer with the nonpolar fatty acid chains in the middle. The polar regions of the phospholipids are oriented toward the surfaces of the membrane as a result of their attraction to the polar water molecules in the extracellular fluid and cytosol. The lipid bilayer acts as a barrier to the movement of polar molecules into and out of cells.

With some exceptions, chemical bonds do not link the phospholipids to each other or to the membrane proteins. Therefore, each molecule is free to move independently of the others. This results in considerable random lateral movement of both membrane lipids and proteins parallel to the surfaces of the bilayer. In addition, the long fatty acid chains can bend and wiggle back and forth. As a consequence, the lipid bilayer has the characteristics of a fluid, much like a thin layer of oil on a water surface, and this makes the membrane quite flexible. This flexibility, along with the fact that cells are filled with fluid, allows cells to undergo moderate changes in shape without disrupting their structural integrity. Like a piece of cloth, a membrane can be bent and folded but cannot be significantly stretched without being torn. As you will learn in Chapter 4, these structural features of membranes permit cells to undergo processes such as exocytosis and endocytosis, and to withstand slight changes in volume due to osmotic imbalances.

The plasma membrane also contains cholesterol, whereas intracellular membranes contain very little. Cholesterol is slightly amphipathic because of a single polar hydroxyl group (see Figure 2.13) attached to its relatively rigid, nonpolar ring structure. Like the phospholipids, therefore, cholesterol is inserted into the lipid bilayer with its polar region at the bilayer surface and its nonpolar rings in the interior in association with the fatty acid chains. The polar hydroxyl group forms hydrogen bonds with the polar regions of phospholipids. The close association of the nonpolar rings of cholesterol with the fatty acid tails of phospholipids tends to limit the ordered packing of fatty acids in the membrane. A more highly ordered, tightly packed arrangement of fatty acids tends to reduce membrane fluidity. Thus, cholesterol and phospholipids play a coordinated role in maintaining an intermediate membrane fluidity. At high temperatures, cholesterol reduces membrane fluidity, possibly by limiting lateral movement of phospholipids. At low temperatures, cholesterol minimizes the decrease in fluidity that would otherwise occur. The latter effect most likely is due to the reduced ability of fatty acid chains to form tightly packed, ordered structures. Cholesterol also may associate with certain classes of plasma membrane phospholipids and proteins, forming organized clusters that work together to pinch off portions of the plasma membrane to form vesicles that deliver their contents to various intracellular organelles, as Chapter 4 will describe.

There are two classes of membrane proteins: integral and peripheral. **Integral membrane proteins** are closely associated with the membrane lipids and cannot be extracted from the membrane without disrupting the lipid bilayer. Like the phospholipids, the integral proteins are amphipathic, having polar amino acid side chains in one region of the molecule and nonpolar side chains clustered together in a separate region. Because they are amphipathic, integral proteins are arranged in the membrane with the same orientation as amphipathic lipids—the polar regions are at the surfaces in association with polar water molecules, and the nonpolar regions are in the interior in

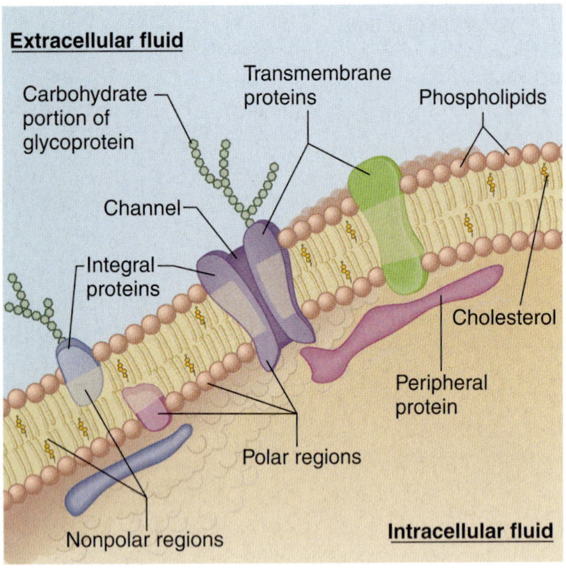

Figure 3.6 APIR Arrangement of integral and peripheral membrane proteins in association with a bimolecular layer of phospholipids.

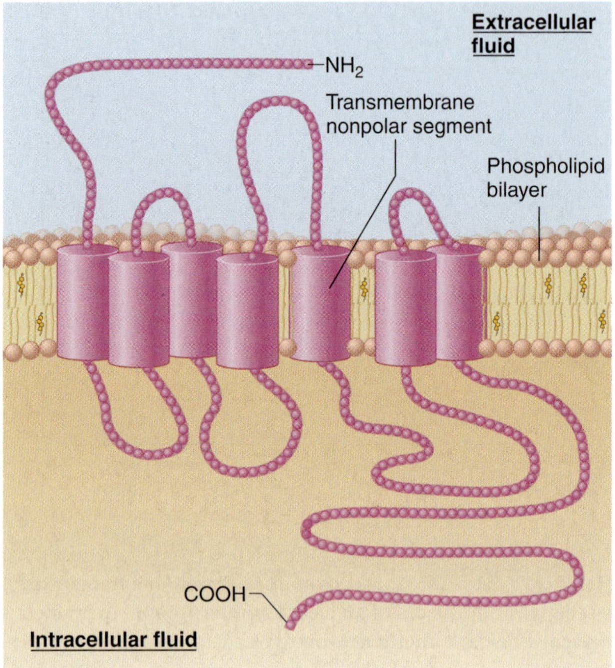

Figure 3.7 A typical transmembrane protein with multiple hydrophobic segments traversing the lipid bilayer. Each transmembrane segment is composed of nonpolar amino acids spiraled in an alpha-helical conformation (shown as cylinders).

association with nonpolar fatty acid chains (**Figure 3.6**). Like the membrane lipids, many of the integral proteins can move laterally in the plane of the membrane, but others are immobilized because they are linked to a network of peripheral proteins located primarily at the cytosolic surface of the membrane.

Most integral proteins span the entire membrane and are referred to as **transmembrane proteins.** The polypeptide chains of many of these transmembrane proteins cross the lipid bilayer several times (**Figure 3.7**). These proteins have polar regions connected by nonpolar segments that associate with the nonpolar regions of the lipids in the membrane interior. The polar regions of transmembrane proteins may extend far beyond the surfaces of the lipid bilayer. Some transmembrane proteins form channels through which ions or water can cross the membrane, whereas others are associated with the transmission of chemical signals across the membrane or the anchoring of extracellular and intracellular protein filaments to the plasma membrane.

Peripheral membrane proteins are not amphipathic and do not associate with the nonpolar regions of the lipids in the interior of the membrane. They are located at the membrane surface where they are bound to the polar regions of the integral membrane proteins (see Figure 3.6) and also in some cases to the charged polar regions of membrane phospholipids. Most of the peripheral proteins are on the cytosolic surface of the plasma membrane where they may perform one of several different types of actions. For example, some peripheral proteins are enzymes that mediate metabolism of membrane components; others are involved in local transport of small molecules along the membrane or between the membrane and cytosol. Many are associated with cytoskeletal elements that influence cell shape and motility.

The extracellular surface of the plasma membrane contains small amounts of carbohydrate covalently linked to some of the membrane lipids and proteins. These carbohydrates consist of short, branched chains of monosaccharides that extend from the cell surface into the extracellular fluid, where they form a layer known as the **glycocalyx.** These surface carbohydrates play important roles in enabling cells to identify and interact with each other.

The lipids in the outer half of the bilayer differ somewhat in kind and amount from those in the inner half, and, as we have seen, the proteins or portions of proteins on the outer surface differ from those on the inner surface. Many membrane functions are related to these asymmetries in chemical composition between the two surfaces of a membrane.

All membranes have the general structure just described, which is known as the **fluid-mosaic model** because a "mosaic" or mix of membrane proteins are free to move in a sea of lipid (**Figure 3.8**). However, the proteins and, to a lesser extent, the

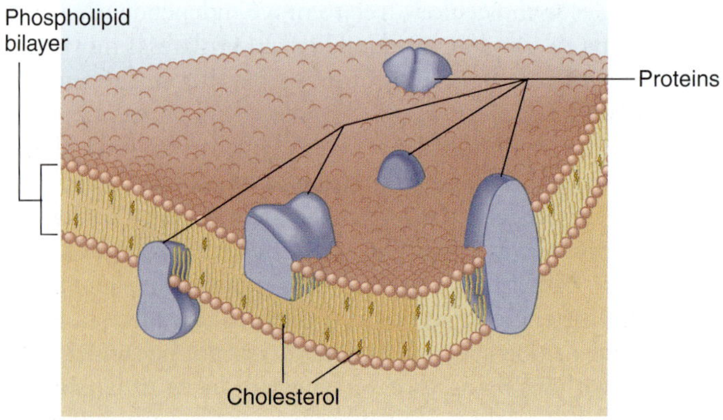

Figure 3.8 Fluid-mosaic model of plasma membrane structure. The proteins and lipids may move within the bilayer; cholesterol helps maintain an intermediate membrane fluidity through the interactions of its polar and nonpolar regions with phospholipids.

lipids in the plasma membrane differ from those in organelle membranes—for example, in the distribution of cholesterol. Therefore, the special functions of membranes, which depend primarily on the membrane proteins, may differ in the various membrane-bound organelles and in the plasma membranes of different types of cells.

The fluid-mosaic model is a useful way of visualizing cellular membranes. However, isolated regions within some cell membranes do not conform to this model. These include regions in which certain membrane proteins are anchored to cytoplasmic proteins, for example, or covalently linked with membrane lipids to form structures called "lipid rafts." **Lipid rafts** are cholesterol-rich regions of reduced membrane fluidity that are believed to serve as organizing centers for the generation of complex intracellular signals. Such signals may arise when a cell binds a hormone or paracrine molecule, for example (see Chapter 1), and lead to changes in cellular activities such as secretion, cell division, and many others. Another example in which cellular membranes do not entirely conform to the fluid-mosaic model is found when proteins in a plasma membrane are linked together to form specialized patches of membrane junctions, as described next.

Membrane Junctions

In addition to providing a barrier to the movements of molecules between the intracellular and extracellular fluids, plasma membranes are involved in the interactions between cells to form tissues. Most cells are packaged into tissues and are not free to move around the body. Even in tissues, however, there is usually a space between the plasma membranes of adjacent cells. This space, filled with extracellular (interstitial) fluid (see Figure 1.3), provides a pathway for substances to pass between cells on their way to and from the blood.

The way that cells become organized into tissues and organs depends, in part, on the ability of certain transmembrane proteins in the plasma membrane, known as **integrins,** to bind to specific proteins in the extracellular matrix and link them to membrane proteins on adjacent cells.

Many cells are physically joined at discrete locations along their membranes by specialized types of junctions, including desmosomes, tight junctions, and gap junctions. These junctions provide an excellent example of the physiological principle that structure and function are related, in this case at the cellular level. **Desmosomes** (**Figure 3.9a**) consist of a region between two adjacent cells where the apposed plasma membranes are separated by about 20 nm. Desmosomes are characterized by accumulations of protein known as "dense plaques" along the cytoplasmic surface of the plasma membrane. These proteins serve as anchoring points for cadherins. **Cadherins** are proteins that extend from the cell into the extracellular space, where they link up and bind with cadherins from an adjacent cell. In this way, two adjacent cells can be firmly attached to each other. The presence of numerous desmosomes between cells helps to provide the structural integrity of tissues in the body. In addition, other proteins such as keratin filaments anchor the cytoplasmic surface of desmosomes to interior structures of the cell. It is believed that this helps secure the desmosome in place and also provides structural support for the cell. Desmosomes hold adjacent cells firmly together in areas that are subject to considerable stretching, such as the skin. The specialized area of the membrane in the region of a desmosome is usually disk-shaped; these membrane junctions could be likened to rivets or spot welds.

A second type of membrane junction, the **tight junction** (**Figure 3.9b**), forms when the extracellular surfaces of two adjacent plasma membranes join together so that no extracellular space remains between them. Unlike the desmosome, which is limited to a disk-shaped area of the membrane, the tight junction occurs in a band around the entire circumference of the cell. Most epithelial cells are joined by tight junctions near their apical surfaces. For example, epithelial cells line the inner surface of the small intestine, where they come in contact with the digestion products in the cavity (or lumen) of the intestine. During absorption, the products of digestion move across the epithelium and enter the blood. This movement could theoretically take place either through the extracellular space between the epithelial cells or through the epithelial cells themselves. For many substances, however, movement through the extracellular space is blocked by the tight junctions; this forces organic nutrients to pass through the cells rather than between them. In this way, the selective barrier properties of the plasma membrane can control the types and amounts of substances absorbed. The ability of tight junctions to impede molecular movement between cells is not absolute. Ions and water can move through these junctions with varying degrees of ease in different epithelia. **Figure 3.9c** shows both a tight junction and a desmosome near the apical (luminal) border between two epithelial cells.

A third type of junction, the **gap junction,** consists of protein channels linking the cytosols of adjacent cells (**Figure 3.9d**). In the region of the gap junction, the two opposing plasma membranes come within 2 to 4 nm of each other, which allows specific proteins (called connexins) from the two membranes to join, forming small, protein-lined channels linking the two cells. The small diameter of these channels (about 1.5 nm) limits what can pass between the cytosols of the connected cells to small molecules and ions, such as Na^+ and K^+, and excludes the exchange of large proteins. A variety of cell types possess gap junctions, including the muscle cells of the heart, where they play a very important role in the transmission of electrical activity between the cells.

3.3 Cell Organelles

In this section, we highlight some of the major structural and functional features of the organelles found in nearly all the cells of the human body. The reader should use this brief overview as a reference to help with subsequent chapters in the textbook.

Nucleus

Almost all cells contain a single nucleus, the largest of the membrane-bound cell organelles. A few specialized cells, such as skeletal muscle cells, contain multiple nuclei, whereas mature red blood cells have none. The primary function of the nucleus is the storage and transmission of genetic information to the next generation of cells. This information, coded in molecules of DNA, is also used to synthesize the proteins that determine the structure and function of the cell, as described later in this chapter.

Surrounding the nucleus is a barrier, the **nuclear envelope,** composed of two membranes. At regular intervals

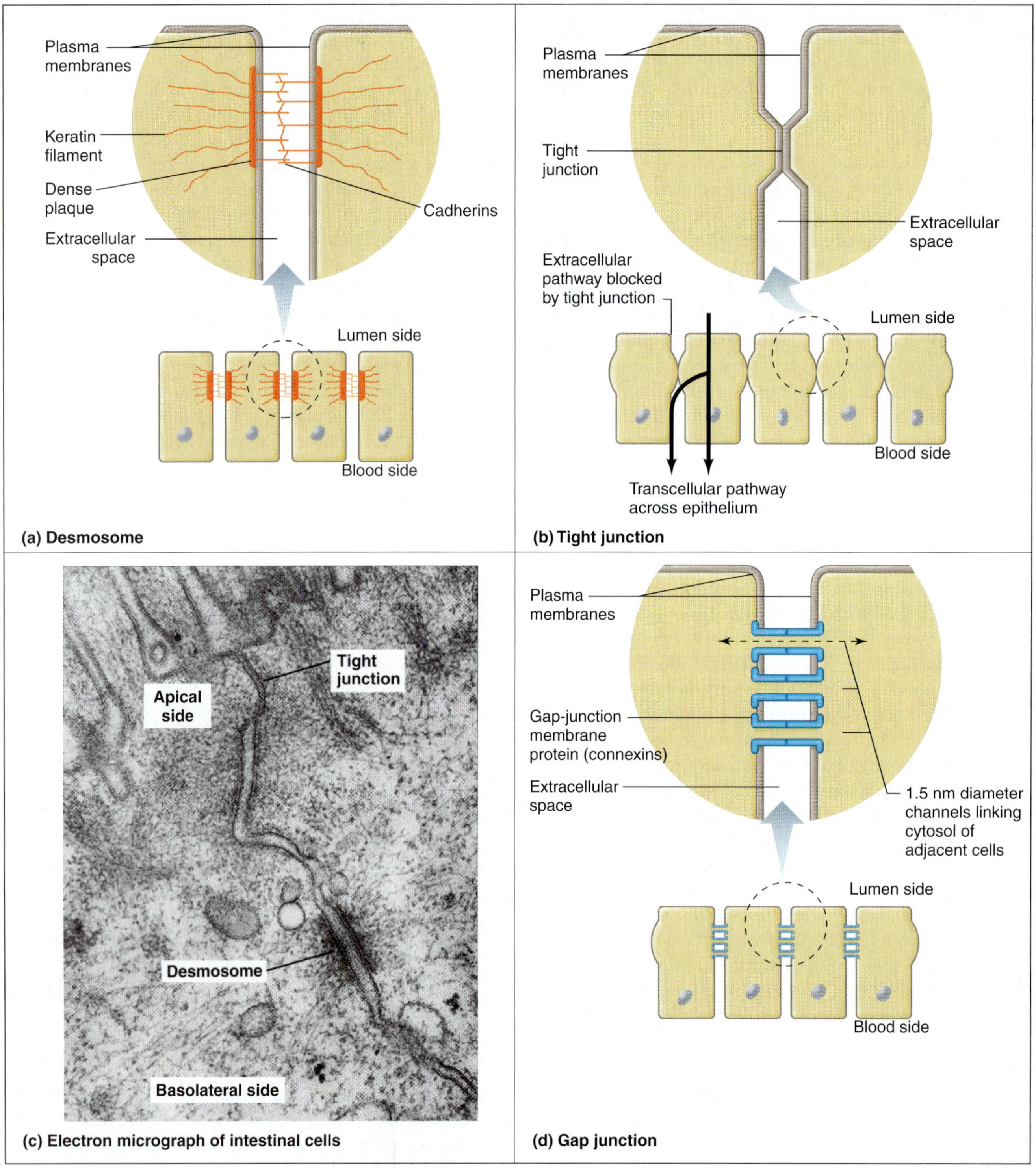

Figure 3.9 APIR Three types of specialized membrane junctions: (a) desmosome; (b) tight junction; (c) electron micrograph of two intestinal epithelial cells joined by a tight junction near the apical (luminal) surface and a desmosome below the tight junction; and (d) gap junction. Electron micrograph from M. Farquhar and G. E. Palade, *J. Cell. Biol.*, 17:375–412.

PHYSIOLOGICAL INQUIRY

- What physiological function might tight junctions serve in the epithelium of the intestine, as shown in part (c) of this figure?

Answer can be found at end of chapter.

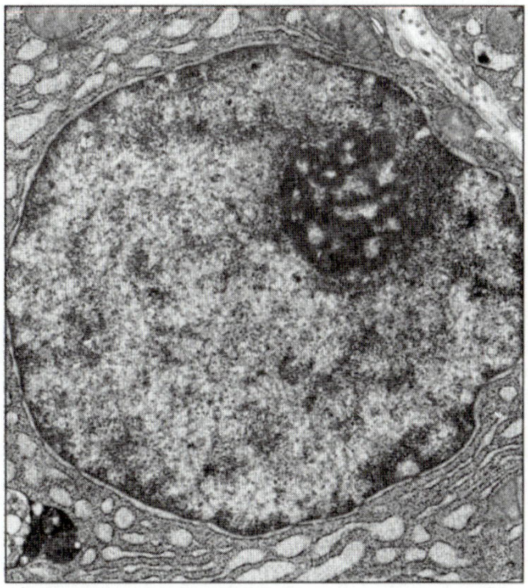

Nucleus

Structure: Largest organelle. Round or oval body located near the cell center. Surrounded by a nuclear envelope composed of two membranes. Envelope contains nuclear pores; messenger molecules pass between the nucleus and the cytoplasm through these pores. No membrane-bound organelles are present in the nucleus, which contains coiled strands of DNA known as chromatin. These condense to form chromosomes at the time of cell division.

Function: Stores and transmits genetic information in the form of DNA. Genetic information passes from the nucleus to the cytoplasm, where amino acids are assembled into proteins.

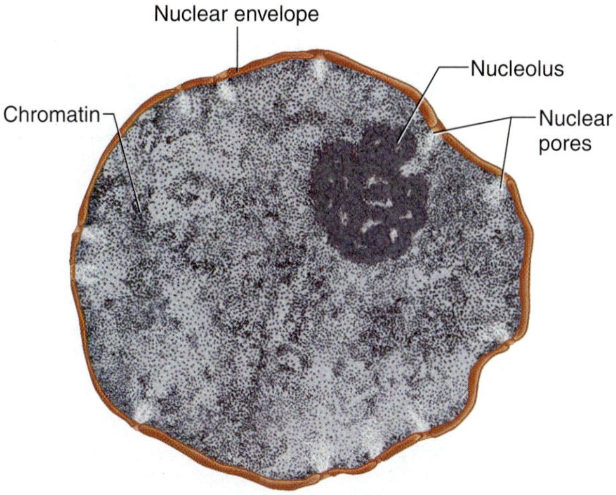

Nucleolus

Structure: Densely stained filamentous structure within the nucleus. Consists of proteins associated with DNA in regions where information concerning ribosomal proteins is being expressed.

Function: Site of ribosomal RNA synthesis. Assembles RNA and protein components of ribosomal subunits, which then move to the cytoplasm through nuclear pores.

Figure 3.10 APIR
Nucleus and nucleolus.
Electron micrograph courtesy of K. R. Porter.

along the surface of the nuclear envelope, the two membranes are joined to each other, forming the rims of circular openings known as **nuclear pores** (Figure 3.10). RNA molecules that determine the structure of proteins synthesized in the cytoplasm move between the nucleus and cytoplasm through these nuclear pores. Proteins that modulate the expression of various genes in DNA move into the nucleus through these pores.

Within the nucleus, DNA, in association with proteins, forms a fine network of threads known as **chromatin.** The threads are coiled to a greater or lesser degree, producing the variations in density seen in electron micrographs of the nucleus (see Figure 3.10). At the time of cell division, the chromatin threads become tightly condensed, forming rodlike bodies known as **chromosomes.**

The most prominent structure in the nucleus is the **nucleolus,** a densely staining filamentous region without a membrane. It is associated with specific regions of DNA that contain the genes for forming the particular type of RNA found in cytoplasmic organelles called ribosomes. This RNA and the protein components of ribosomes are assembled in the nucleolus, then transferred through the nuclear pores to the cytoplasm, where they form functional ribosomes.

Ribosomes

Ribosomes are the protein factories of a cell. On ribosomes, protein molecules are synthesized from amino acids, using genetic information carried by RNA messenger molecules from DNA in the nucleus. Ribosomes are large particles, about 20 nm in diameter, composed of about 70 to 80 proteins and several RNA molecules. As described in Section B, ribosomes consist of two subunits that either are floating free in the cytoplasm or combine during protein synthesis. In the latter case, the ribosomes bind to the organelle called rough endoplasmic reticulum (described next). A typical cell may contain as many as 10 million ribosomes.

The proteins synthesized on the free ribosomes are released into the cytosol, where they perform their varied functions. The proteins synthesized by ribosomes attached to the rough endoplasmic reticulum pass into the lumen of the reticulum and are then transferred to yet another organelle, the Golgi apparatus. They are ultimately secreted from the cell or distributed to other organelles.

Endoplasmic Reticulum

The most extensive cytoplasmic organelle is the network (or "reticulum") of membranes that form the **endoplasmic reticulum** (Figure 3.11). These membranes enclose a space that is continuous throughout the network.

Two forms of endoplasmic reticulum can be distinguished: rough, or granular, and smooth, or agranular. The rough endoplasmic reticulum has ribosomes bound to its cytosolic surface, and it has a flattened-sac appearance. Rough endoplasmic reticulum is involved in packaging proteins that, after processing in the Golgi apparatus, are secreted by the cell or distributed to other cell organelles.

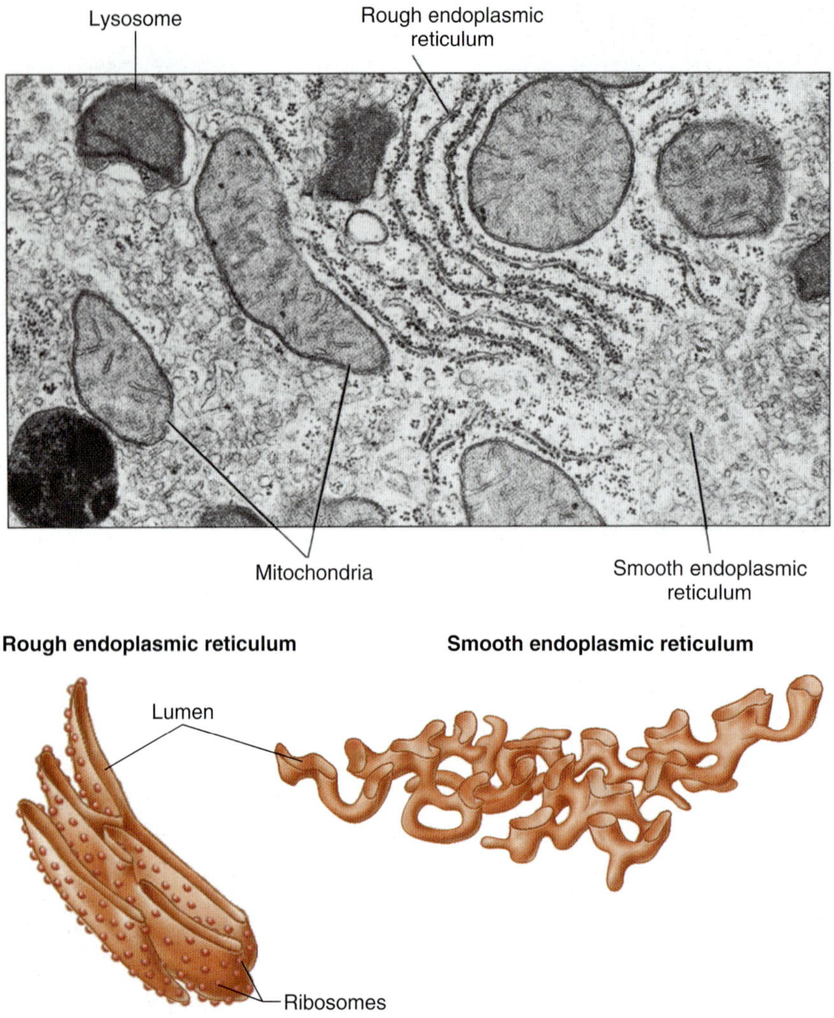

Rough endoplasmic reticulum

Structure: Extensive membranous network of flattened sacs. Encloses a space that is continuous throughout the organelle and with the space between the two nuclear-envelope membranes. Has ribosomal particles attached to its cytosolic surface.

Function: Proteins synthesized on the attached ribosomes enter the lumen of the reticulum from which they are ultimately distributed to other organelles or secreted from the cell.

Smooth endoplasmic reticulum

Structure: Highly branched tubular network that does not have attached ribosomes but may be continuous with the rough endoplasmic reticulum.

Function: Contains enzymes for fatty acid and steroid synthesis. Stores and releases calcium, which controls various cell activities.

Figure 3.11 APIR Endoplasmic reticulum. Electron micrograph from D. W. Fawcett, *The Cell, An Atlas of Fine Structure*, W. B. Saunders Company, Philadelphia.

The smooth endoplasmic reticulum has no ribosomal particles on its surface and has a branched, tubular structure. It is the site at which certain lipid molecules are synthesized, it plays a role in detoxification of certain hydrophobic molecules, and it also stores and releases calcium ions involved in controlling various cell activities.

Golgi Apparatus

The **Golgi apparatus** is a series of closely apposed, flattened membranous sacs that are slightly curved, forming a cup-shaped structure (**Figure 3.12**). Associated with this organelle, particularly near its concave surface, are a number of roughly spherical, membrane-enclosed vesicles.

Proteins arriving at the Golgi apparatus from the rough endoplasmic reticulum undergo a series of modifications as they pass from one Golgi compartment to the next. For example, carbohydrates are linked to proteins to form glycoproteins, and the length of the protein is often shortened by removing a terminal portion of the polypeptide chain. The Golgi apparatus sorts the modified proteins into discrete classes of transport vesicles that will travel to various cell organelles or to the plasma membrane, where the protein contents of the vesicle are released to the outside of the cell. Vesicles containing proteins to be secreted from the cell are known as **secretory vesicles.** Such vesicles are found, for example, in certain endocrine gland cells, where protein hormones are released into the extracellular fluid to modify the activities of other cells.

Endosomes

A number of membrane-bound vesicular and tubular structures called **endosomes** lie between the plasma membrane and the Golgi apparatus. Certain types of vesicles that pinch off the plasma membrane travel to and fuse with endosomes. In turn, the endosome can pinch off vesicles that then move to other cell organelles or return to the plasma membrane. Like the Golgi apparatus, endosomes are involved in sorting, modifying, and directing vesicular traffic in cells.

Mitochondria

Mitochondria (singular, *mitochondrion*) participate in the chemical processes that transfer energy from the chemical bonds of nutrient molecules to newly created adenosine triphosphate (ATP) molecules, which are then made available to cells. Most of the ATP that cells use is formed in the mitochondria by a process called cellular respiration, which consumes oxygen and produces carbon dioxide, heat, and water.

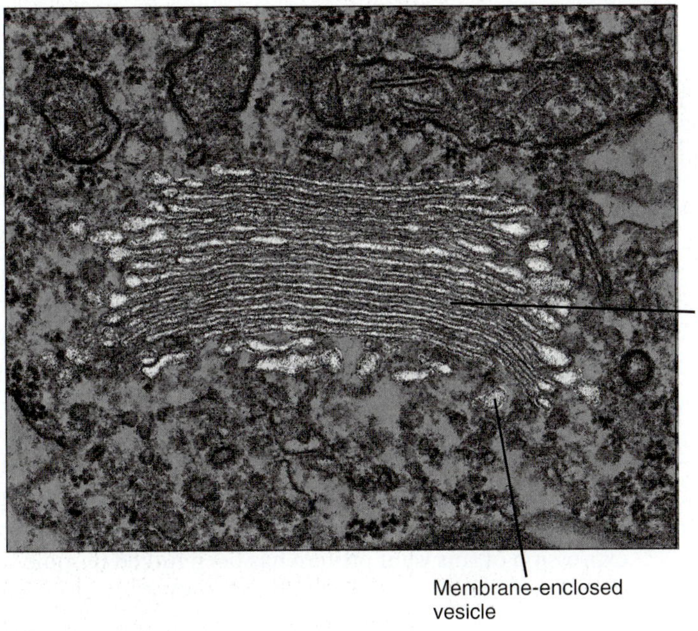

Golgi apparatus

Structure: Series of cup-shaped, closely apposed, flattened, membranous sacs; associated with numerous vesicles. Generally, a single Golgi apparatus is located in the central portion of a cell near its nucleus.

Function: Concentrates, modifies, and sorts proteins arriving from the rough endoplasmic reticulum prior to their distribution, by way of the Golgi vesicles, to other organelles or to secretion from the cell.

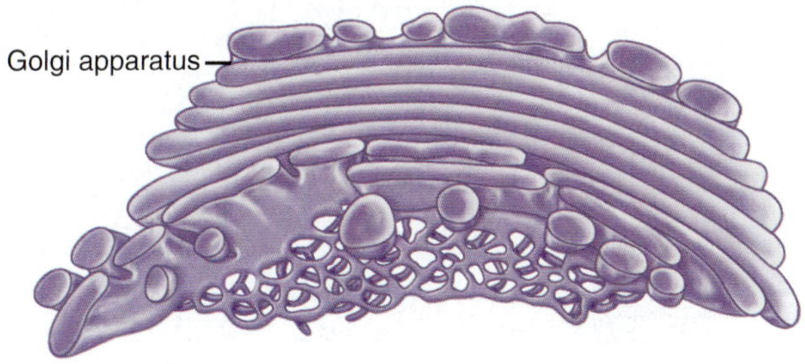

Figure 3.12 AP|R Golgi apparatus. Electron micrograph from W. Bloom and D. W. Fawcett, *Textbook of Histology*, 9th ed. W. B. Saunders Company, Philadelphia.

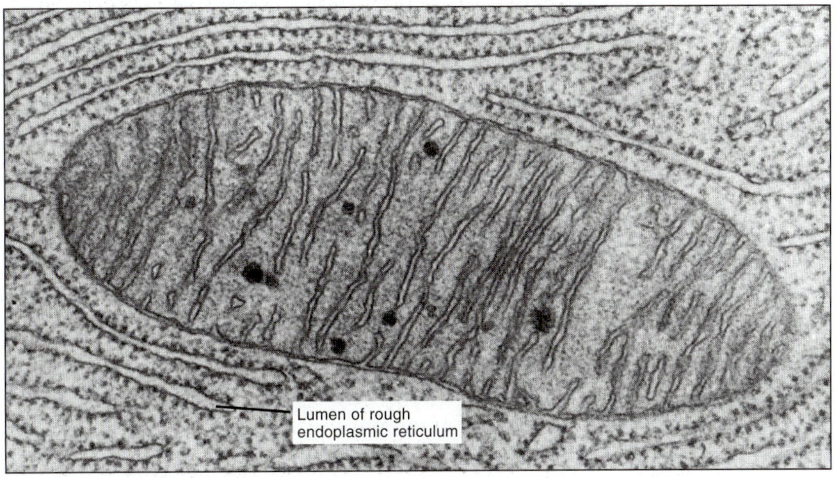

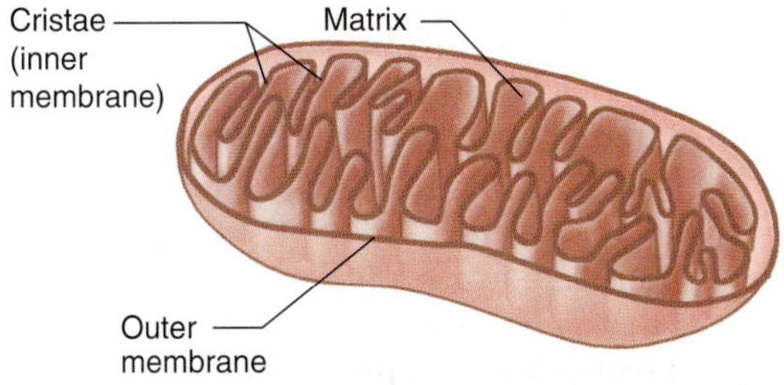

Mitochondrion

Structure: Rod- or oval-shaped body surrounded by two membranes. Inner membrane folds into matrix of the mitochondrion, forming cristae.

Function: Major site of ATP production, O_2 utilization, and CO_2 formation. Contains enzymes active in Krebs cycle and oxidative phosphorylation.

Figure 3.13 AP|R Mitochondrion. Electron micrograph courtesy of K. R. Porter.

Mitochondria are spherical or elongated, rodlike structures surrounded by an inner and an outer membrane (**Figure 3.13**). The outer membrane is smooth, whereas the inner membrane is folded into sheets or tubules known as **cristae,** which extend into the inner mitochondrial compartment, the **matrix.** Mitochondria are found throughout the cytoplasm. Large numbers of them, as many as 1000, are present in cells that utilize large amounts of energy, whereas less active cells contain fewer. Our modern understanding of mitochondrial structure and function has evolved, however, from the idea that each mitochondrion is physically and functionally isolated from others. In all cell types that have been examined, mitochondria appear to exist at least in part in a reticulum (**Figure 3.14**). This interconnected network of mitochondria may be particularly important in the distribution of oxygen and energy sources (notably, fatty acids) throughout the mitochondria within a cell. Moreover, the extent of the reticulum may change in different physiological settings; more mitochondria may fuse, or split apart, or even destroy themselves as the energetic demands of cells change.

In addition to providing most of the energy required to power physiological events such as muscle contraction, mitochondria also play a role in the synthesis of certain lipids, such as the hormones estrogen and testosterone (Chapter 11).

Lysosomes

Lysosomes are spherical or oval organelles surrounded by a single membrane (see Figure 3.3). A typical cell may contain several hundred lysosomes. The fluid within a lysosome is

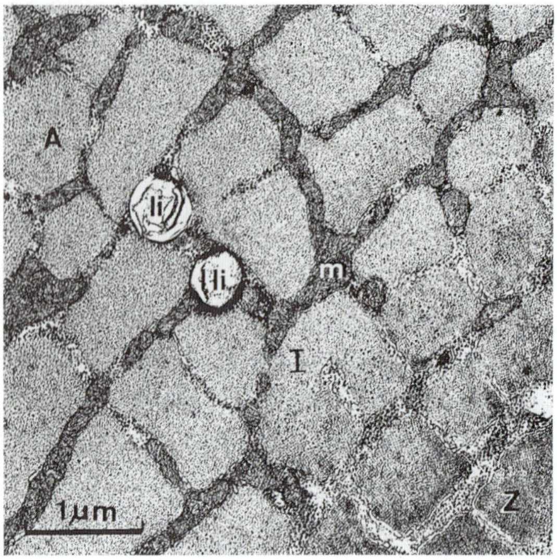

Figure 3.14 Mitochondrial reticulum in skeletal muscle cells. The mitochondria are indicated by the letter *m;* other labels refer to structures found in skeletal muscle and will be described in later chapters. Electron micrograph courtesy G. A. Brooks et al., *Exercise Physiology: Human Bioenergetics and its Applications*, McGraw-Hill Higher Education, New York.

acidic and contains a variety of digestive enzymes. Lysosomes act to break down bacteria and the debris from dead cells that have been engulfed by a cell. They may also break down cell organelles that have been damaged and no longer function normally. They play an especially important role in the various cells that make up the defense systems of the body (Chapter 18).

Peroxisomes

Like lysosomes, **peroxisomes** are moderately dense oval bodies enclosed by a single membrane. Like mitochondria, peroxisomes consume molecular oxygen, although in much smaller amounts. This oxygen is not used in the transfer of energy to ATP, however. Instead, it undergoes reactions that remove hydrogen from organic molecules including lipids, alcohol, and potentially toxic ingested substances. One of the reaction products is hydrogen peroxide, H_2O_2, thus the organelle's name. Hydrogen peroxide can be toxic to cells in high concentrations, but peroxisomes can also destroy hydrogen peroxide and thereby prevent its toxic effects. Peroxisomes are also involved in the process by which fatty acids are broken down into two-carbon fragments, which the cell can then use as a source for generating ATP.

Vaults

Vaults are cytoplasmic structures composed of protein and a type of untranslated RNA called vault RNA (vRNA). These tiny structures have been described as barrel-shaped but also as resembling vaulted cathedrals, from which they get their name. Although the functions of vaults are not certain, studies using electron microscopy and other methods have revealed that vaults tend to be associated with nuclear pores. This has led to the hypothesis that vaults are important for transport of molecules between the cytosol and the nucleus. In addition, at least one vault protein is believed to function in regulating a cell's sensitivity to certain drugs. For example, increased expression of this vault protein has been linked in some studies to drug resistance, including some drugs used in the treatment of cancer. If true, then vaults may someday provide a target for modulating the effectiveness of such drugs in human patients.

Cytoskeleton

In addition to the membrane-enclosed organelles, the cytoplasm of most cells contains a variety of protein filaments. This filamentous network is referred to as the cell's **cytoskeleton,** and, like the bony skeleton of the body, it is associated with processes that maintain and change cell shape and produce cell movements.

The three classes of cytoskeletal filaments are based on their diameter and the types of protein they contain. In order of size, starting with the thinnest, they are (1) actin filaments (also called microfilaments), (2) intermediate filaments, and (3) microtubules (**Figure 3.15**). Actin filaments and microtubules can be assembled and disassembled rapidly, allowing a cell to alter these components of its cytoskeletal framework according to changing requirements. In contrast, intermediate filaments, once assembled, are less readily disassembled.

Actin filaments are composed of monomers of the protein **G-actin** (or "globular actin"), which assemble into a

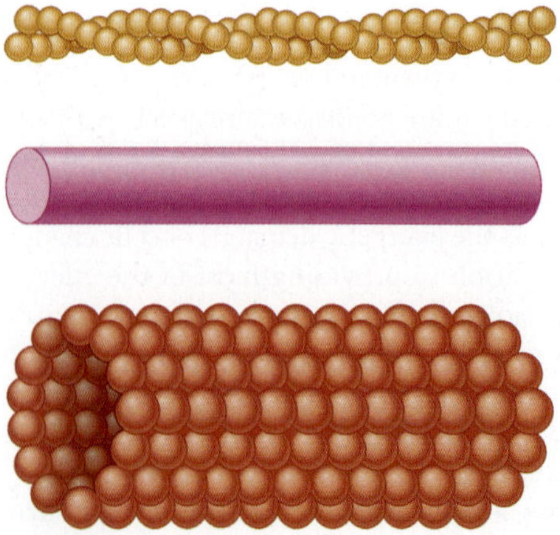

Cytoskeletal filaments	Diameter (nm)	Protein subunit
Actin filament	7	G-actin
Intermediate filament	10	Several proteins
Microtubule	25	Tubulin

Figure 3.15 AP|R Cytoskeletal filaments associated with cell shape and motility.

polymer of two twisting chains known as **F-actin** (for "filamentous"). These filaments make up a major portion of the cytoskeleton in all cells. They play important roles in determining cell shape, the ability of cells to move by amoeboid-like movements, cell division, and muscle cell contraction.

Intermediate filaments are composed of twisted strands of several different proteins, including keratin, desmin, and lamin. These filaments also contribute to cell shape and help anchor the nucleus. They provide considerable strength to cells and consequently are most extensively developed in the regions of cells subject to mechanical stress (for example, in association with desmosomes).

Microtubules are hollow tubes about 25 nm in diameter, whose subunits are composed of the protein **tubulin.** They are the most rigid of the cytoskeletal filaments and are present in the long processes of neurons, where they provide the framework that maintains the processes' cylindrical shape. Microtubules also radiate from a region of the cell known as the **centrosome,** which surrounds two small, cylindrical bodies called **centrioles,** composed of nine sets of fused microtubules. The centrosome is a cloud of amorphous material that regulates the formation and elongation of microtubules. During cell division, the centrosome generates the microtubular spindle fibers used in chromosome separation. Microtubules and actin filaments have also been implicated in the movements of organelles within the cytoplasm. These fibrous elements form tracks, and organelles are propelled along these tracks by contractile proteins attached to the surface of the organelles. **Cilia,** the hairlike motile extensions on the surfaces of some epithelial cells, have a central core of microtubules organized in a pattern similar to that found in the centrioles. These microtubules, in combination with a contractile protein, produce movements of the cilia. In hollow organs lined with ciliated epithelium, the cilia wave back and forth, propelling the luminal contents along the surface of the epithelium. An example of this is the cilia-mediated movement of mucus up the trachea, which helps remove inhaled particles that could damage the lungs.

SECTION A SUMMARY

Microscopic Observations of Cells

I. All living matter is composed of cells.

II. There are two types of cells: prokaryotic cells (bacteria) and eukaryotic cells (plant and animal cells).

Membranes

I. Every cell is surrounded by a plasma membrane.

II. Within each eukaryotic cell are numerous membrane-bound compartments, nonmembranous particles, and filaments, known collectively as cell organelles.

III. A cell is divided into two regions, the nucleus and the cytoplasm. The latter is composed of the cytosol and cell organelles other than the nucleus.

IV. The membranes that surround the cell and cell organelles regulate the movements of molecules and ions into and out of the cell and its compartments.
- a. Membranes consist of a bimolecular lipid layer, composed of phospholipids with embedded proteins.
- b. Integral membrane proteins are amphipathic proteins that often span the membrane, whereas peripheral membrane proteins are confined to the surfaces of the membrane.

V. Three types of membrane junctions link adjacent cells.
- a. Desmosomes link cells that are subject to considerable stretching.
- b. Tight junctions, found primarily in epithelial cells, limit the passage of molecules through the extracellular space between the cells.
- c. Gap junctions form channels between the cytosols of adjacent cells.

Cell Organelles

I. The nucleus transmits and expresses genetic information.
- a. Threads of chromatin, composed of DNA and protein, condense to form chromosomes when a cell divides.
- b. Ribosomal subunits are assembled in the nucleolus.

II. Ribosomes, composed of RNA and protein, are the sites of protein synthesis.

III. The endoplasmic reticulum is a network of flattened sacs and tubules in the cytoplasm.
- a. Rough endoplasmic reticulum has attached ribosomes and is primarily involved in the packaging of proteins to be secreted by the cell or distributed to other organelles.
- b. Smooth endoplasmic reticulum is tubular, lacks ribosomes, and is the site of lipid synthesis and calcium accumulation and release.

IV. The Golgi apparatus modifies and sorts the proteins that are synthesized on the rough or granular endoplasmic reticulum and packages them into secretory vesicles.

V. Endosomes are membrane-bound vesicles that fuse with vesicles derived from the plasma membrane and bud off vesicles that travel to other cell organelles.

VI. Mitochondria are the major cell sites that consume oxygen and produce carbon dioxide in chemical processes that transfer energy to ATP, which can then provide energy for cell functions.

VII. Lysosomes digest particulate matter that enters the cell.

VIII. Peroxisomes use oxygen to remove hydrogen from organic molecules and in the process form hydrogen peroxide.

IX. Vaults are cytoplasmic structures made of protein and RNA and may be involved in cytoplasmic-nuclear transport.

X. The cytoplasm contains a network of three types of filaments that form the cytoskeleton: (a) actin filaments, (b) intermediate filaments, and (c) microtubules. These filaments are involved in determining cell shape, regulating cell motility and division, and regulating cell contractility, among other functions.

SECTION A REVIEW QUESTIONS

1. Identify the location of cytoplasm, cytosol, and intracellular fluid within a cell.
2. Identify the classes of organic molecules found in plasma membranes.
3. Describe the orientation of the phospholipid molecules in a membrane.
4. Which plasma membrane components are responsible for membrane fluidity?
5. Describe the location and characteristics of integral and peripheral membrane proteins.
6. Describe the structure and function of the three types of junctions found between cells.

7. What function does the nucleolus perform?
8. Describe the location and function of ribosomes.
9. Contrast the structure and functions of the rough and smooth endoplasmic reticulum.
10. What function does the Golgi apparatus perform?
11. What functions do endosomes perform?
12. Describe the structure and primary function of mitochondria.
13. What functions do lysosomes and peroxisomes perform?
14. List the three types of filaments associated with the cytoskeleton. Identify the structures in cells that are composed of microtubules.

SECTION A KEY TERMS

SECTION **B**

Protein Synthesis, Degradation, and Secretion

3.4 Genetic Code

The importance of proteins in physiology cannot be overstated. Proteins are involved in all physiological processes, from cell signaling to tissue remodeling to organ function. This section describes how cells synthesize, degrade, and, in some cases, secrete proteins. We begin with an overview of the genetic basis of protein synthesis.

As noted previously, the nucleus of a cell contains DNA, which directs the synthesis of all proteins in the body. Molecules of DNA contain information, coded in the sequence of nucleotides, for protein synthesis. A sequence of DNA nucleotides containing the information that specifies the amino acid sequence of a single polypeptide chain is known as a **gene.** A gene is thus a unit of hereditary information. A single molecule of DNA contains many genes.

The total genetic information coded in the DNA of a typical cell in an organism is known as its **genome.** The human genome contains roughly 20,000 genes. Scientists have determined the nucleotide sequence of the entire human genome (approximately 3 billion nucleotides). This is only a first step, however, because the function and regulation of most genes in the human genome remain unknown.

It is easy to misunderstand the relationship between genes, DNA molecules, and chromosomes. In all human cells other than eggs or sperm, there are 46 separate DNA molecules in the cell nucleus, each molecule containing many genes. Each DNA molecule is packaged into a single chromosome composed of DNA and proteins, so there are 46 chromosomes in each cell. A chromosome contains not only its DNA molecule but also a special class of proteins called **histones.** The cell's nucleus is a marvel of packaging. The very long DNA molecules, with lengths a thousand times greater than the diameter of the nucleus, fit into the nucleus by coiling around clusters of histones at frequent intervals to form complexes known as **nucleosomes.** There are about 25 million of these complexes on the chromosomes, resembling beads on a string.

Although DNA contains the information specifying the amino acid sequences in proteins, it does not itself participate directly in the assembly of protein molecules. Most of a cell's DNA is in the nucleus, whereas most protein synthesis occurs in the cytoplasm. The transfer of information from DNA to the site of protein synthesis is accomplished by RNA molecules, whose synthesis is governed by the information coded in DNA. Genetic information flows from DNA to RNA and then to protein (**Figure 3.16**). The process of transferring genetic information from DNA to RNA in the nucleus is known as **transcription.** The process that uses the coded information in RNA to assemble a protein in the cytoplasm is known as **translation.**

$$\text{DNA} \xrightarrow{\text{transcription}} \text{RNA} \xrightarrow{\text{translation}} \text{Protein}$$

As described in Chapter 2, a molecule of DNA consists of two chains of nucleotides coiled around each other to form a double helix. Each DNA nucleotide contains one of four bases—adenine (A), guanine (G), cytosine (C), or thymine (T)—and each of these bases is specifically paired by hydrogen bonds with a base on the opposite chain of the double helix. In this base pairing, A and T bond together and G and C bond together. Thus, both nucleotide chains contain a specifically ordered sequence of bases, with one chain complementary to the other. This specificity of base pairing forms the basis of the transfer of information from DNA to RNA and of the duplication of DNA during cell division.

The genetic language is similar in principle to a written language, which consists of a set of symbols, such as A, B, C, D, that form an alphabet. The letters are arranged in specific sequences to form words, and the words are arranged in linear sequences to

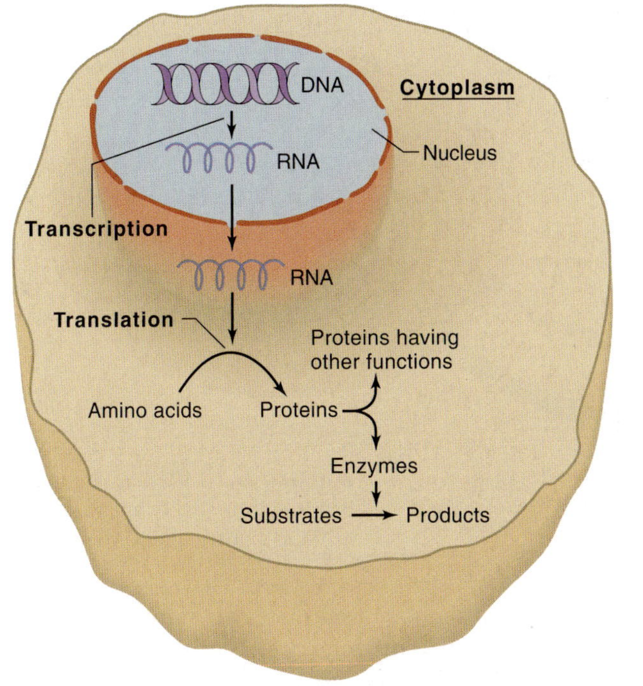

Figure 3.16 AP|R The expression of genetic information in a cell occurs through the *transcription* of coded information from DNA to RNA in the nucleus, followed by the *translation* of the RNA information into protein synthesis in the cytoplasm. The proteins then perform the functions that determine the characteristics of the cell.

form sentences. The genetic language contains only four letters, corresponding to the bases A, G, C, and T. The genetic words are three-base sequences that specify particular amino acids—that is, each word in the genetic language is only three letters long. This is termed a *triplet code.* The sequence of three-letter code words (triplets) along a gene in a single strand of DNA specifies the sequence of amino acids in a polypeptide chain (**Figure 3.17**). In this way, a gene is equivalent to a sentence, and the genetic information in the human genome is equivalent to a book containing about 20,000 sentences. Using a single letter (A, T, C, or G) to specify each of the four bases in the DNA nucleotides, it would require about 550,000 pages, each equivalent to this text page, to print the nucleotide sequence of the human genome.

The four bases in the DNA alphabet can be arranged in 64 different three-letter combinations to form 64 triplets ($4 \times 4 \times 4 = 64$). Therefore, this code actually provides more than enough words to code for the 20 different amino acids that are found in proteins. This means that a given amino acid is usually specified by more than one triplet. For example, the four DNA triplets C—C—A, C—C—G, C—C—T, and C—C—C all specify the amino acid glycine. Only 61 of the 64 possible triplets are used to specify amino acids. The triplets that do not specify amino acids are known as **stop signals.** They perform the same function as a period at the end of a sentence—they indicate that the end of a genetic message has been reached.

The genetic code is a universal language used by all living cells. For example, the triplets specifying the amino acid tryptophan are the same in the DNA of a bacterium, an amoeba, a plant, and a human being. Although the same triplets are used by all living cells, the messages they spell out—the sequences of triplets that code for a specific protein—vary from gene to gene in each organism. The universal nature of the genetic code supports the concept that all forms of life on earth evolved from a common ancestor.

Before we turn to the specific mechanisms by which the DNA code operates in protein synthesis, an important qualification is required. Although the information coded in genes is always first transcribed into RNA, there are several classes of RNA required for protein synthesis—including messenger RNA, ribosomal RNA, and transfer RNA. Only messenger RNA *directly* codes for the amino acid sequences of proteins, even though the other RNA classes participate in the overall process of protein synthesis.

3.5 Protein Synthesis

To repeat, the first step in using the genetic information in DNA to synthesize a protein is called transcription, and it involves the synthesis of an RNA molecule containing coded information that corresponds to the information in a single gene. The class of RNA molecules that specifies the amino acid sequence of a protein and carries this message from DNA to the site of protein synthesis in the cytoplasm is known as **messenger RNA (mRNA)**.

Transcription: mRNA Synthesis

Recall from Chapter 2 that ribonucleic acids are single-chain polynucleotides whose nucleotides differ from DNA because they contain the sugar ribose (rather than deoxyribose) and the base uracil (rather than thymine). The other three bases—adenine, guanine, and cytosine—occur in both DNA and RNA. The subunits used to synthesize mRNA are free (uncombined) ribonucleotide triphosphates: ATP, GTP, CTP, and UTP.

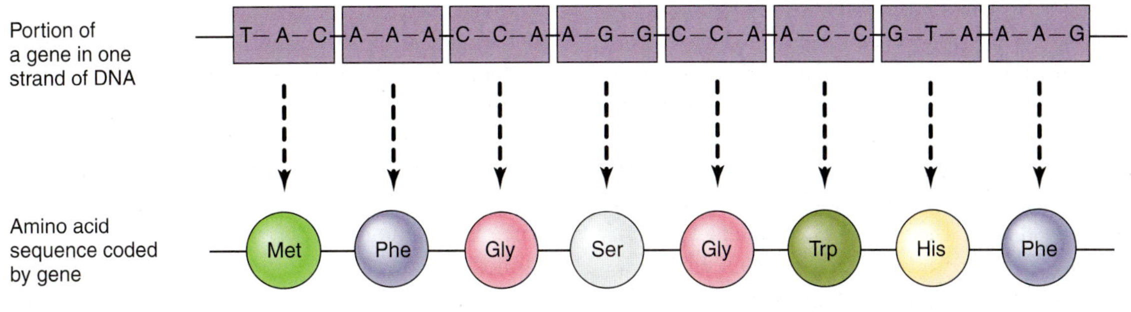

Figure 3.17 AP|R The sequence of three-letter code words in a gene determines the sequence of amino acids in a polypeptide chain. The names of the amino acids are abbreviated. Note that more than one three-letter code sequence can specify the same amino acid; for example, the amino acid phenylalanine (Phe) is coded by two triplet codes, A—A—A and A—A—G.

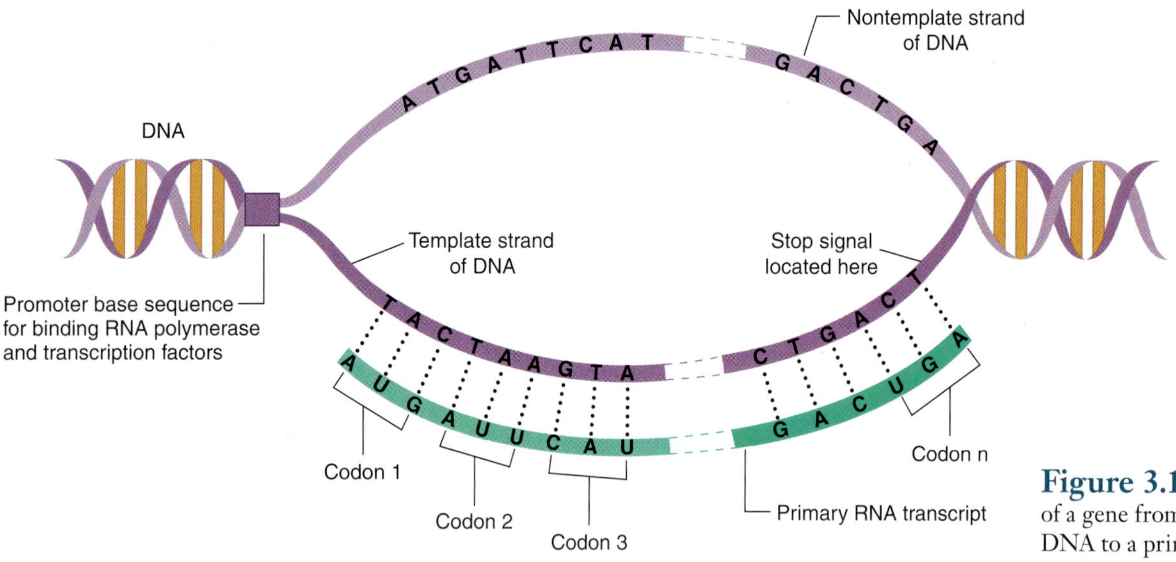

Figure 3.18 AP|R Transcription of a gene from the template strand of DNA to a primary mRNA transcript.

Recall also that the two polynucleotide chains in DNA are linked together by hydrogen bonds between specific pairs of bases: A—T and C—G. To initiate RNA synthesis, the two antiparallel strands of the DNA double helix must separate so that the bases in the exposed DNA can pair with the bases in free ribonucleotide triphosphates (**Figure 3.18**). Free ribonucleotides containing U bases pair with the exposed A bases in DNA; likewise, free ribonucleotides containing G, C, or A bases pair with the exposed DNA bases C, G, and T, respectively. Note that uracil, which is present in RNA but not DNA, pairs with the base adenine in DNA. In this way, the nucleotide sequence in one strand of DNA acts as a template that determines the sequence of nucleotides in mRNA.

The aligned ribonucleotides are joined together by the enzyme **RNA polymerase,** which hydrolyzes the nucleotide triphosphates, releasing two of the terminal phosphate groups and joining the remaining phosphate in covalent linkage to the ribose of the adjacent nucleotide.

DNA consists of two strands of polynucleotides that run antiparallel to each other based on the orientation of their phosphate–sugar backbone. Because both strands are exposed during transcription, it should theoretically be possible to form two individual RNA molecules, one complementary to each strand of DNA. However, only one of the two potential RNAs is typically formed. This is because RNA polymerase binds to DNA only at specific sites of a gene, adjacent to a sequence called the **promoter.** The promoter is a specific sequence of DNA nucleotides, including some that are common to most genes. The promoter directs RNA polymerase to proceed along a strand in only one direction that is determined by the orientation of the phosphate–sugar backbone. Thus, for a given gene, one strand, called the **template strand** or antisense strand, has the correct orientation relative to the location of the promoter to bind RNA polymerase. The location of the promoter, therefore, determines which strand will be the template strand (see Figure 3.18). Consequently, for any given gene, only one DNA strand typically is transcribed.

Thus, the transcription of a gene begins when RNA polymerase binds to the promoter region of that gene. This initiates the separation of the two strands of DNA. RNA polymerase moves along the template strand, joining one ribonucleotide at a time (at a rate of about 30 nucleotides per second) to the growing RNA chain. Upon reaching a stop signal specifying the end of the gene, the RNA polymerase releases the newly formed RNA transcript, which is then translocated out of the nucleus where it binds to ribosomes in the cytoplasm.

In a given cell, typically only 10% to 20% of the genes present in DNA are transcribed into RNA. Genes are transcribed only when RNA polymerase can bind to their promoter sites. Cells use various mechanisms to either block or make accessible the promoter region of a particular gene to RNA polymerase. Such regulation of gene transcription provides a means of controlling the synthesis of specific proteins and thereby the activities characteristic of a particular type of cell. Collectively, the specific proteins expressed in a given cell at a particular time constitute the **proteome** of the cell. The proteome determines the structure and function of the cell at that time.

Note that the base sequence in the RNA transcript is not identical to that in the template strand of DNA, because the formation of RNA depends on the pairing between *complementary*, not identical, bases (see Figure 3.18). A three-base sequence in RNA that specifies one amino acid is called a **codon.** Each codon is complementary to a three-base sequence in DNA. For example, the base sequence T—A—C in the template strand of DNA corresponds to the codon A—U—G in transcribed RNA.

Although the entire sequence of nucleotides in the template strand of a gene is transcribed into a complementary sequence of nucleotides known as the **primary RNA transcript** or **pre-mRNA,** only certain segments of most genes actually code for sequences of amino acids. These regions of the gene, known as **exons** (expression regions), are separated by noncoding sequences of nucleotides known as **introns** (from "intragenic region" and also called intervening sequences). It is estimated that as much as 98.5% of human DNA is composed of intron sequences that do not contain protein-coding information. What role, if any, such large amounts of noncoding DNA may perform is unclear, although they have been postulated to exert some transcriptional regulation. In addition, a class of very short RNA molecules called microRNAs are transcribed in some cases from noncoding DNA. MicroRNAs are not themselves translated into protein but, rather, prevent the translation of specific mRNA molecules.

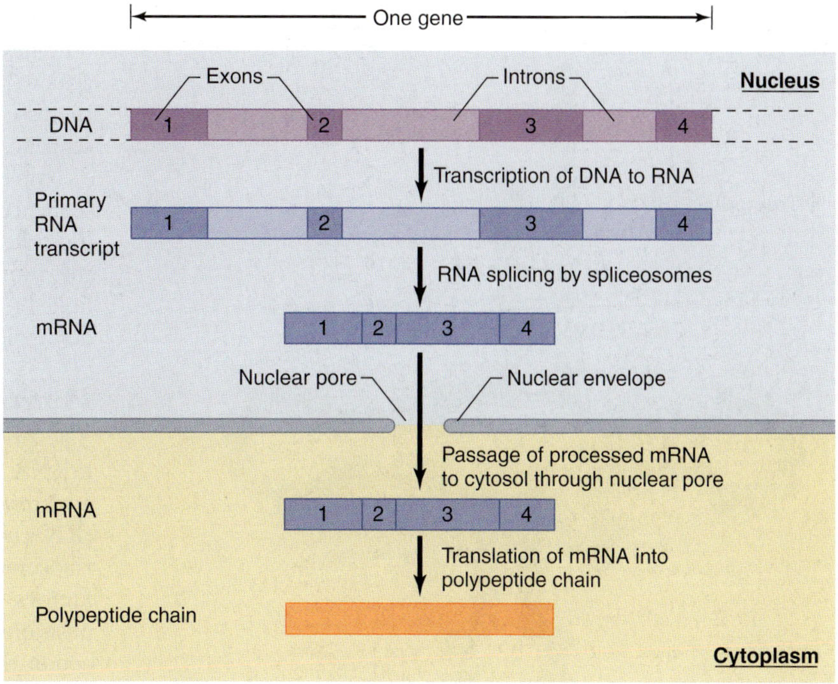

Figure 3.19 Spliceosomes remove the noncoding intron-derived segments from a primary RNA transcript (or pre-mRNA) and link the exon-derived segments together to form the mature mRNA molecule that passes through the nuclear pores to the cytosol. The lengths of the intron- and exon-derived segments represent the relative lengths of the base sequences in these regions.

PHYSIOLOGICAL INQUIRY

- Using the format of this diagram, draw an mRNA molecule that might result from alternative splicing of the primary RNA transcript.

Answer can be found at end of chapter.

Before passing to the cytoplasm, a newly formed primary RNA transcript must undergo splicing (**Figure 3.19**) to remove the sequences that correspond to the DNA introns. This allows the formation of the continuous sequence of exons that will be translated into protein. Only after this splicing occurs is the RNA termed *mature messenger RNA*, or *mature mRNA*.

Splicing occurs in the nucleus and is performed by a complex of proteins and small nuclear RNAs known as a **spliceosome.** The spliceosome identifies specific nucleotide sequences at the beginning and end of each intron-derived segment in the primary RNA transcript, removes the segment, and splices the end of one exon-derived segment to the beginning of another to form mRNA with a continuous coding sequence. In many cases during the splicing process, the exon-derived segments from a single gene can be spliced together in different sequences or some exon-derived segments can be deleted entirely; this is called alternative splicing and is estimated to occur in more than half of all genes. These processes result in the formation of different mRNA sequences from the same gene and give rise, in turn, to proteins with different amino acid sequences. Thus, there are more different proteins in the human body than there are genes.

Translation: Polypeptide Synthesis

After splicing, the mRNA moves through the pores in the nuclear envelope into the cytoplasm. Although the nuclear pores allow the diffusion of small molecules and ions between the nucleus and cytoplasm, they have specific energy-dependent mechanisms for the selective transport of large molecules such as proteins and RNA.

In the cytoplasm, mRNA binds to a ribosome, the cell organelle that contains the enzymes and other components required for the translation of mRNA into protein. Before describing this assembly process, we will examine the structure of a ribosome and the characteristics of two additional classes of RNA involved in protein synthesis.

Ribosomes and rRNA

A ribosome is a complex particle composed of about 70 to 80 different proteins in association with a class of RNA molecules known as **ribosomal RNA (rRNA)**. The genes for rRNA are transcribed from DNA in a process similar to that for mRNA except that a different RNA polymerase is used. Ribosomal RNA transcription occurs in the region of the nucleus known as the nucleolus. Ribosomal proteins, like other proteins, are synthesized in the cytoplasm from the mRNAs specific for them. These proteins then move back through nuclear pores to the nucleolus, where they combine with newly synthesized rRNA to form two ribosomal subunits, one large and one small. These subunits are then individually transported to the cytoplasm, where they combine to form a functional ribosome during protein translation.

Transfer RNA

How do individual amino acids identify the appropriate codons in mRNA during the process of translation? By themselves, free amino acids do not have the ability to bind to the bases in mRNA codons. This process of identification involves the third major class of RNA, known as **transfer RNA (tRNA)**. Transfer RNA molecules are the smallest (about 80 nucleotides long) of the major classes of RNA. The single chain of tRNA loops back upon itself, forming a structure resembling a cloverleaf with three loops (**Figure 3.20**).

Like mRNA and rRNA, tRNA molecules are synthesized in the nucleus by base-pairing with DNA nucleotides at specific tRNA genes; then they move to the cytoplasm. The key to tRNA's role in protein synthesis is its ability to combine with both a specific amino acid and a codon in ribosome-bound mRNA specific for that amino acid. This permits tRNA to act as the link between an amino acid and the mRNA codon for that amino acid.

A tRNA molecule is covalently linked to a specific amino acid by an enzyme known as aminoacyl-tRNA synthetase. There are 20 different aminoacyl-tRNA synthetases, each of which catalyzes

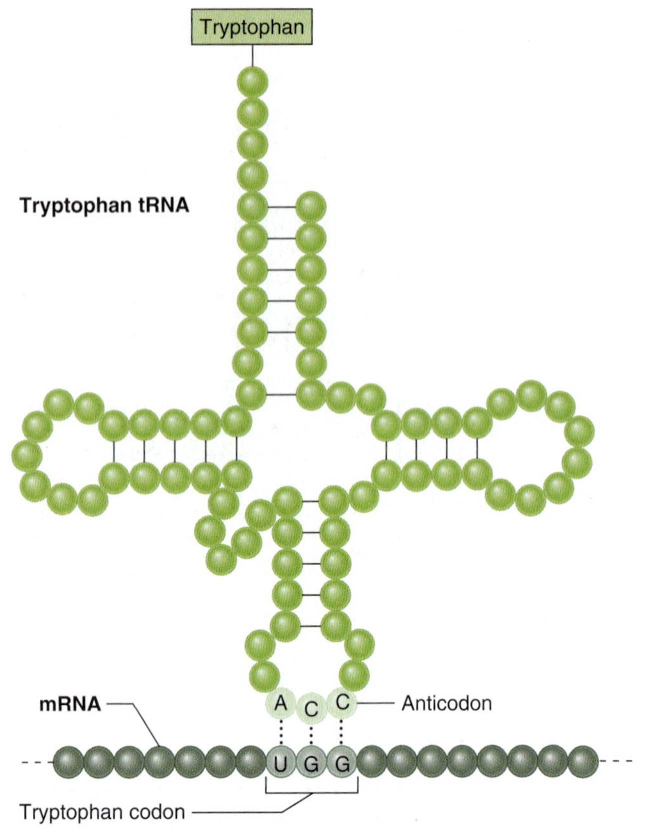

Figure 3.20 APIR Base pairing between the anticodon region of a tRNA molecule and the corresponding codon region of an mRNA molecule.

the linkage of a specific amino acid to a specific type of tRNA. The next step is to link the tRNA, bearing its attached amino acid, to the mRNA codon for that amino acid. This is achieved by the base pairing between tRNA and mRNA. A three-nucleotide sequence at the end of one of the loops of tRNA can base-pair with a complementary codon in mRNA. This tRNA three-letter code sequence is appropriately known as an **anticodon.** Figure 3.20 illustrates the binding between mRNA and a tRNA specific for the amino acid tryptophan. Note that tryptophan is covalently linked to one end of tRNA and does not bind to either the anticodon region of tRNA or the codon region of mRNA.

Protein Assembly

The process of assembling a polypeptide chain based on an mRNA message involves three stages—initiation, elongation, and termination. The initiation of synthesis occurs when a tRNA containing the amino acid methionine binds to the small ribosomal subunit. A number of proteins known as **initiation factors** are required to establish an initiation complex, which positions the methionine-containing tRNA opposite the mRNA codon that signals the start site at which assembly is to begin. The large ribosomal subunit then binds, enclosing the mRNA between the two subunits. This initiation phase is the slowest step in protein assembly, and factors that influence the activity of initiation factors can regulate the rate of protein synthesis.

Following the initiation process, the protein chain is elongated by the successive addition of amino acids (**Figure 3.21**). A ribosome has two binding sites for tRNA. Site 1 holds the tRNA linked to the portion of the protein chain that has been assembled up to this point, and site 2 holds the tRNA containing the

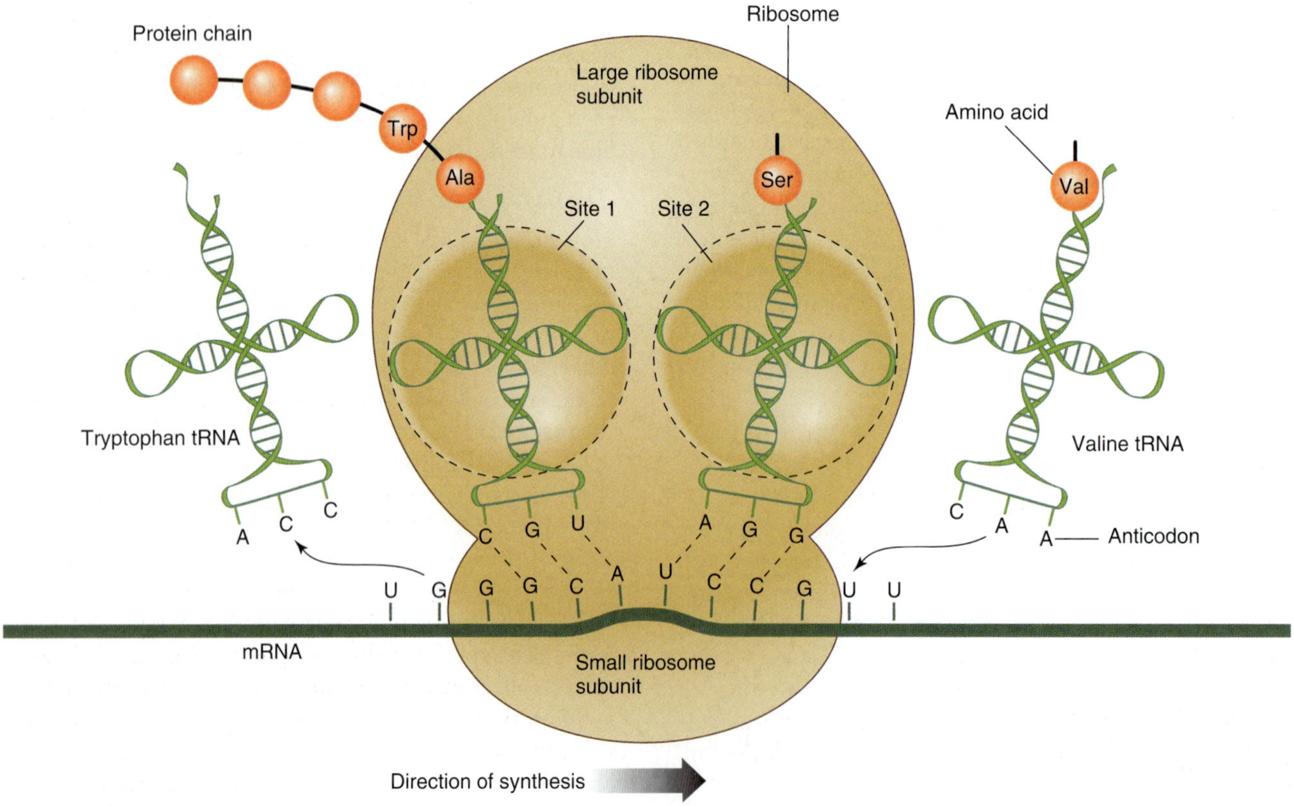

Figure 3.21 APIR Sequence of events during protein synthesis by a ribosome.

next amino acid to be added to the chain. Ribosomal enzymes catalyze the linkage of the protein chain to the newly arrived amino acid. Following the formation of the peptide bond, the tRNA at site 1 is released from the ribosome, and the tRNA at site 2—now linked to the peptide chain—is transferred to site 1. The ribosome moves down one codon along the mRNA, making room for the binding of the next amino acid–tRNA molecule. This process is repeated over and over as amino acids are added to the growing peptide chain, at an average rate of two to three per second. When the ribosome reaches a termination sequence in mRNA (called a stop codon) specifying the end of the protein, the link between the polypeptide chain and the last tRNA is broken, and the completed protein is released from the ribosome.

Messenger RNA molecules are not destroyed during protein synthesis, so they may be used to synthesize many more protein molecules. In fact, while one ribosome is moving along a particular strand of mRNA, a second ribosome may become attached to the start site on that same mRNA and begin the synthesis of a second identical protein molecule. Therefore, a number of ribosomes—as many as 70—may be moving along a single strand of mRNA, each at a different stage of the translation process (**Figure 3.22**).

Molecules of mRNA do not, however, remain in the cytoplasm indefinitely. Eventually, cytoplasmic enzymes break them down into nucleotides. Therefore, if a gene corresponding to a particular protein ceases to be transcribed into mRNA, the protein will no longer be formed after its cytoplasmic mRNA molecules have broken down.

Once a polypeptide chain has been assembled, it may undergo posttranslational modifications to its amino acid sequence. For example, the amino acid methionine that is used to identify the start site of the assembly process is cleaved from the end of most proteins. In some cases, other specific peptide bonds within the polypeptide chain are broken, producing a number of smaller peptides, each of which may perform a different function. For example, as illustrated in **Figure 3.23**, five different proteins can be derived from the same mRNA as a result of posttranslational cleavage. The same initial polypeptide may be split at different points in different cells depending on the specificity of the hydrolyzing enzymes present.

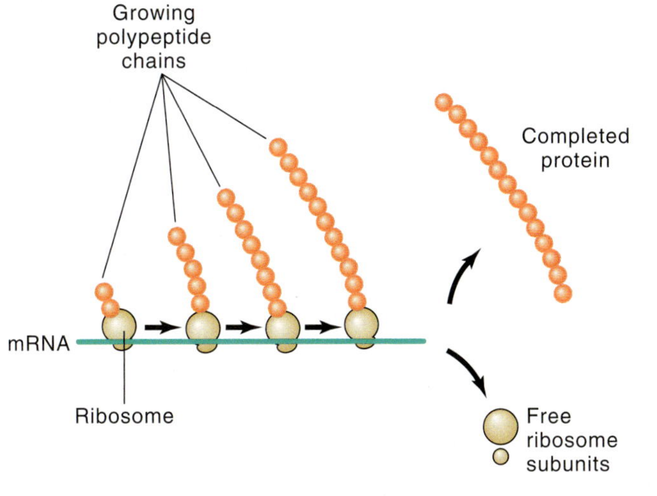

Figure 3.22 APIR Several ribosomes can simultaneously move along a strand of mRNA, producing the same protein in different stages of assembly.

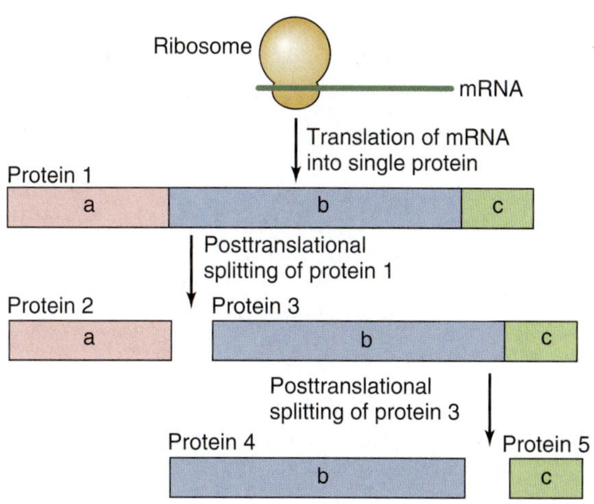

Figure 3.23 Posttranslational splitting of a protein can result in several smaller proteins, each of which may perform a different function. All these proteins are derived from the same gene.

Carbohydrates and lipid derivatives are often covalently linked to particular amino acid side chains. These additions may protect the protein from rapid degradation by proteolytic enzymes or act as signals to direct the protein to those locations in the cell where it is to function. The addition of a fatty acid to a protein, for example, can lead the protein to anchor to a membrane as the nonpolar portion of the fatty acid inserts into the lipid bilayer.

The steps leading from DNA to a functional protein are summarized in **Table 3.2**.

Regulation of Protein Synthesis

As noted earlier, in any given cell, only a small fraction of the genes in the human genome are ever transcribed into mRNA and translated into proteins. Of this fraction, a small number of genes are continuously being transcribed into mRNA. The transcription of other genes, however, is regulated and can be turned on or off in response to either signals generated within the cell or external signals the cell receives. In order for a gene to be transcribed, RNA polymerase must be able to bind to the promoter region of the gene and be in an activated configuration.

Transcription of most genes is regulated by a class of proteins known as **transcription factors,** which act as gene switches, interacting in a variety of ways to activate or repress the initiation process that takes place at the promoter region of a particular gene. The influence of a transcription factor on transcription is not necessarily all or none, on or off; it may simply slow or speed up the initiation of the transcription process. The transcription factors, along with accessory proteins, form a **preinitiation complex** at the promoter that is needed to carry out the process of separating the DNA strands, removing any blocking nucleosomes in the region of the promoter, activating the bound RNA polymerase, and moving the complex along the template strand of DNA. Some transcription factors bind to regions of DNA that are far removed from the promoter region of the gene whose transcription they regulate. In this case, the DNA containing the bound transcription factor forms a loop that brings the transcription factor into contact with the promoter region, where it may then activate or repress transcription (**Figure 3.24**).

Many genes contain regulatory sites that a common transcription factor can influence; there does not need to be a

TABLE 3.2 Events Leading from DNA to Protein Synthesis

Transcription
RNA polymerase binds to the promoter region of a gene and separates the two strands of the DNA double helix in the region of the gene to be transcribed.
Free ribonucleotide triphosphates base-pair with the deoxynucleotides in the template strand of DNA.
The ribonucleotides paired with this strand of DNA are linked by RNA polymerase to form a primary RNA transcript containing a sequence of bases complementary to the template strand of the DNA base sequence.
RNA splicing removes the intron-derived regions, which contain noncoding sequences, in the primary RNA transcript and splices together the exon-derived regions, which code for specific amino acids, producing a molecule of mature mRNA.
Translation
The mRNA passes from the nucleus to the cytoplasm, where one end of the mRNA binds to the small subunit of a ribosome.
Free amino acids are linked to their corresponding tRNAs by aminoacyl-tRNA synthetase.
The three-base anticodon in an amino acid–tRNA complex pairs with its corresponding codon in the region of the mRNA bound to the ribosome.
The amino acid on the tRNA is linked by a peptide bond to the end of the growing polypeptide chain.
The tRNA that has been freed of its amino acid is released from the ribosome.
The ribosome moves one codon step along mRNA.
The previous four steps are repeated until a termination sequence is reached, and the completed protein is released from the ribosome.
In some cases, the protein undergoes posttranslational processing in which various chemical groups are attached to specific side chains and/or the protein is split into several smaller peptide chains.

different transcription factor for every gene. In addition, more than one transcription factor may interact to control the transcription of a given gene.

Because transcription factors are proteins, the activity of a particular transcription factor—that is, its ability to bind to DNA or to other regulatory proteins—can be turned on or off by allosteric or covalent modulation in response to signals a cell either receives or generates. Thus, specific genes can be regulated in response to specific signals.

To summarize, the rate of a protein's synthesis can be regulated at various points: (1) gene transcription into mRNA; (2) the initiation of protein assembly on a ribosome; and (3) mRNA degradation in the cytoplasm.

Mutation

Any alteration in the nucleotide sequence that spells out a genetic message in DNA is known as a **mutation.** Certain chemicals and various forms of ionizing radiation, such as x-rays, cosmic rays, and atomic radiation, can break the chemical bonds in DNA. This can result in the loss of segments of DNA or the incorporation of the wrong base when the broken bonds re-form. Environmental factors that increase the rate of mutation are known as **mutagens.**

Types of Mutations

The simplest type of mutation, known as a point mutation, occurs when a single base is replaced by a different one. For example, the base sequence C—G—T is the DNA triplet for the amino acid alanine. If guanine (G) is replaced by adenine (A), the sequence becomes C—A—T, which is the code for valine. If, however, cytosine (C) replaces thymine (T), the sequence becomes C—G—C, which is another code for alanine, and the amino acid sequence transcribed from the mutated gene would not be altered. On the other hand, if an amino acid code mutates to one of the termination triplets, the translation of the mRNA message will cease when this triplet is reached, resulting in the synthesis of a shortened, typically nonfunctional protein.

Assume that a mutation has altered a single triplet code in a gene, for example, alanine C—G—T changed to valine C—A—T, so that it now codes for a protein with one different amino acid. What effect does this mutation have upon the cell? The answer depends upon where in the gene the mutation has occurred. Although proteins are composed of many amino acids, the properties of a protein often depend upon a very small region of the total molecule, such as the binding site of an enzyme. If the mutation does not alter the conformation of the binding site, there may be little or no change in the protein's properties. On the other hand, if the mutation alters the binding site, a marked change in the protein's properties may occur.

What effects do mutations have upon the functioning of a cell? If a mutated, nonfunctional protein is part of a chemical reaction supplying most of a cell's chemical energy, the loss of the protein's function could lead to the death of the cell. In contrast, if the active protein were involved in the synthesis of a particular amino acid, and if the cell could also obtain that amino acid from the extracellular fluid, the cell function would not be impaired by the absence of the protein.

To generalize, a mutation may have any one of three effects upon a cell: (1) it may cause no noticeable change in cell function; (2) it may modify cell function but still be compatible with cell growth and replication; or (3) it may lead to cell death.

Mutations and Evolution

Mutations contribute to the evolution of organisms. Although most mutations result in either no change or an impairment of cell function, a very small number may alter the activity of a protein in such a way that it is more, rather than less, active; or they may introduce an entirely new type of protein activity into a cell. If an organism carrying such a mutant gene is able to perform some function more effectively than an organism lacking the

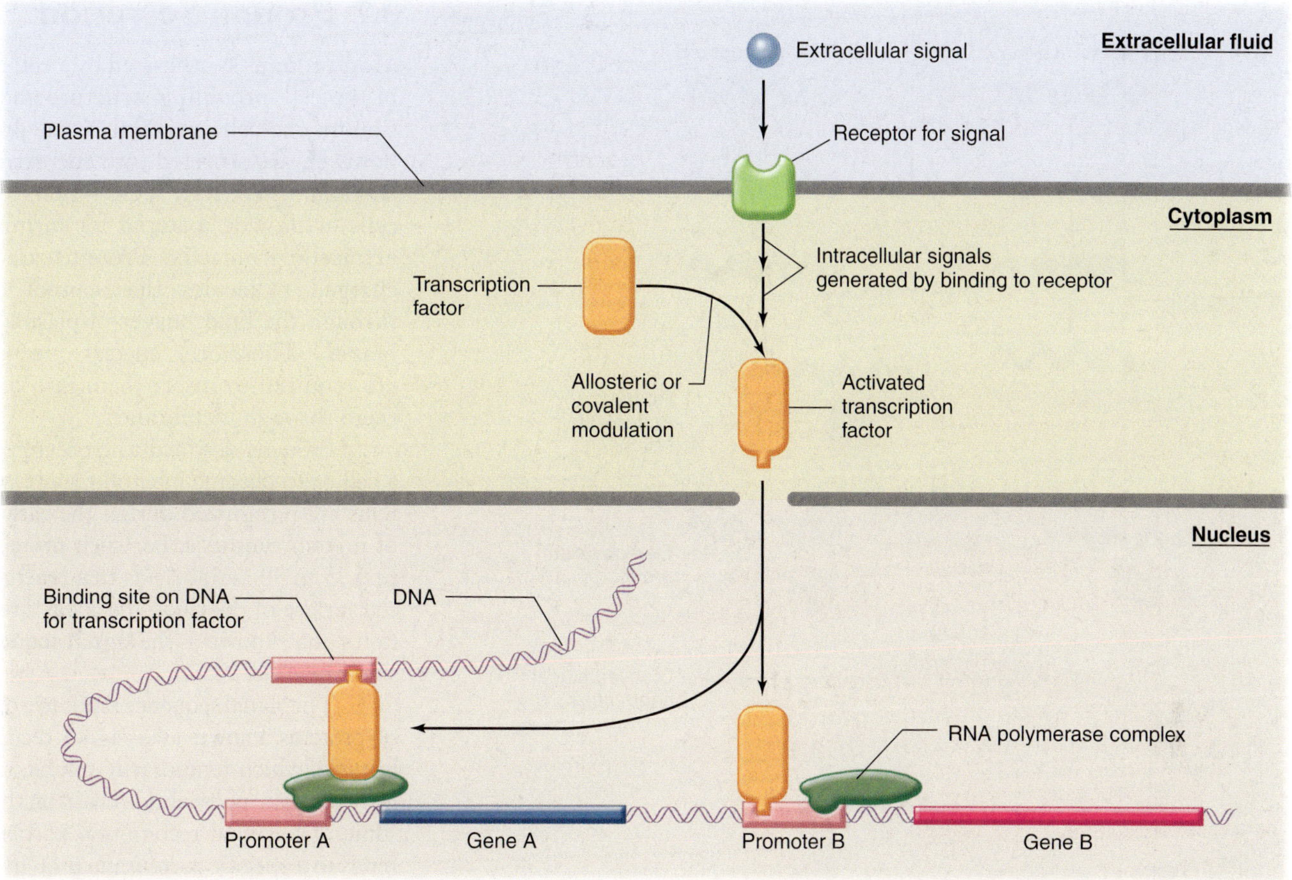

Figure 3.24 AP|R Transcription of gene B is modulated by the binding of an activated transcription factor directly to the promoter region. In contrast, transcription of gene A is modulated by the same transcription factor, which, in this case, binds to a region of DNA considerably distant from the promoter region.

mutant gene, the organism has a better chance of reproducing and passing on the mutant gene to its descendants. On the other hand, if the mutation produces an organism that functions less effectively than organisms lacking the mutation, the organism is less likely to reproduce and pass on the mutant gene. This is the principle of **natural selection.** Although any one mutation, if it is able to survive in the population, may cause only a very slight alteration in the properties of a cell, given enough time, a large number of small changes can accumulate to produce very large changes in the structure and function of an organism.

3.6 Protein Degradation

We have thus far emphasized protein synthesis, but the concentration of a particular protein in a cell at a particular time depends upon not only its rate of synthesis but also its rates of degradation and/or secretion.

Different proteins degrade at different rates. In part, this depends on the structure of the protein, with some proteins having a higher affinity for certain proteolytic enzymes than others. A denatured (unfolded) protein is more readily digested than a protein with an intact conformation. Proteins can be targeted for degradation by the attachment of a small peptide, **ubiquitin,** to the protein. This peptide directs the protein to a protein complex known as a **proteasome,** which unfolds the protein and breaks it down into small peptides. Degradation is an important mechanism for confining the activity of a given protein to a precise window of time.

In summary, there are many steps in the path from a gene in DNA to a fully active protein, which allow the rate of protein synthesis or the final active form of the protein to be altered (**Table 3.3**). By controlling these

TABLE 3.3 Factors That Alter the Amount and Activity of Specific Cell Proteins

Process Altered	Mechanism of Alteration
Transcription of DNA	Activation or inhibition by transcription factors
Splicing of RNA	Activity of enzymes in spliceosome
mRNA degradation	Activity of RNase
Translation of mRNA	Activity of initiating factors on ribosomes
Protein degradation	Activity of proteasomes
Allosteric and covalent modulation	Signal ligands, protein kinases, and phosphatases

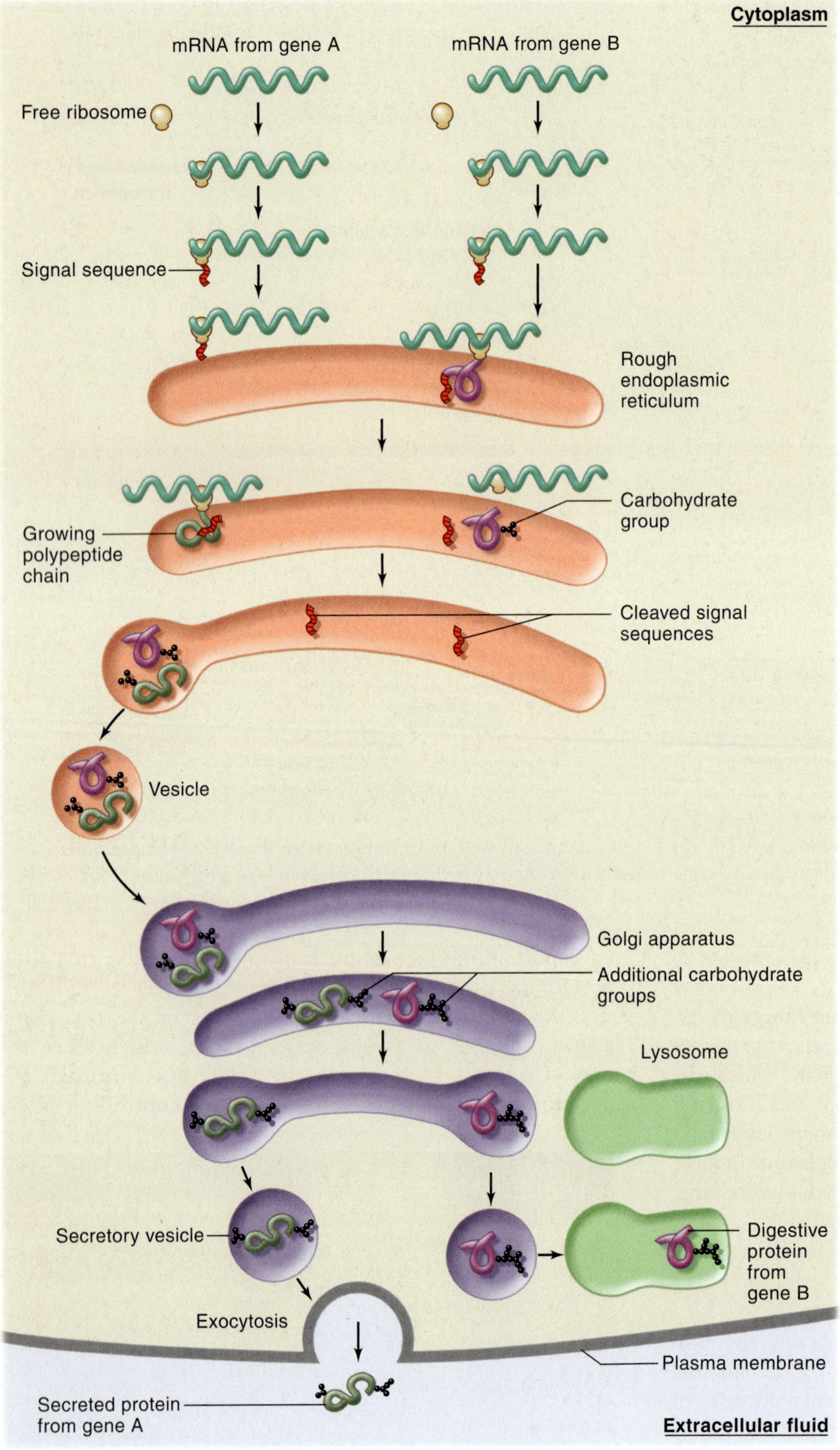

Figure 3.25 Pathway of proteins destined to be secreted by cells or transferred to lysosomes. An example of the latter might be a protein important in digestive functions in which a cell degrades other intracellular molecules.

steps, extracellular or intracellular signals, as described in Chapter 5, can regulate the total amount of a specific protein in a cell.

3.7 Protein Secretion

Most proteins synthesized by a cell remain in the cell, providing structure and function for the cell's survival. Some proteins, however, are secreted into the extracellular fluid, where they act as signals to other cells or provide material for forming the extracellular matrix. Proteins are large, charged molecules that cannot diffuse through the lipid bilayer of plasma membranes. Therefore, special mechanisms are required to insert them into or move them through membranes.

Proteins destined to be secreted from a cell or to become integral membrane proteins are recognized during the early stages of protein synthesis. For such proteins, the first 15 to 30 amino acids that emerge from the surface of the ribosome act as a recognition signal, known as the **signal sequence** or signal peptide.

The signal sequence binds to a complex of proteins known as a signal recognition particle, which temporarily inhibits further growth of the polypeptide chain on the ribosome. The signal recognition particle then binds to a specific membrane protein on the surface of the rough endoplasmic reticulum. This binding restarts the process of protein assembly, and the growing polypeptide chain is fed through a protein complex in the endoplasmic reticulum membrane into the lumen of the reticulum (**Figure 3.25**). Upon completion of protein assembly, proteins that are to be secreted end up in the lumen of the rough endoplasmic reticulum. Proteins that are destined to function as integral membrane proteins remain embedded in the reticulum membrane.

Within the lumen of the endoplasmic reticulum, enzymes remove the signal sequence from most proteins, so this portion is not present in the final protein. In addition, carbohydrate groups are sometimes linked to various side chains in the proteins.

Following these modifications, portions of the reticulum membrane bud off, forming vesicles that contain the newly synthesized proteins. These vesicles migrate to the Golgi apparatus (see Figure 3.25) and fuse with the Golgi membranes.

Within the Golgi apparatus, the protein may undergo further modifications. For example, additional carbohydrate groups may be added; these groups are typically important as recognition sites within the cell.

While in the Golgi apparatus, the many different proteins that have been funneled into this organelle are sorted out according to their final destinations. This sorting involves the binding of regions of a particular protein to specific proteins in the Golgi membrane that are destined to form vesicles targeted to a particular destination.

Following modification and sorting, the proteins are packaged into vesicles that bud off the surface of the Golgi membrane. Some of the vesicles travel to the plasma membrane, where they fuse with the membrane and release their contents to the extracellular fluid, a process known as exocytosis. Other vesicles may dock and fuse with lysosome membranes, delivering digestive enzymes to the interior of this organelle. Specific docking proteins on the surface of the membrane where the vesicle finally fuses recognize the specific proteins on the surface of the vesicle.

In contrast to this entire story, if a protein does not have a signal sequence, synthesis continues on a free ribosome until the completed protein is released into the cytosol. These proteins are not secreted but are destined to function within the cell. Many remain in the cytosol, where they function as enzymes, for example, in various metabolic pathways. Others are targeted to particular cell organelles. For example, ribosomal proteins are directed to the nucleus, where they combine with rRNA before returning to the cytosol as part of the ribosomal subunits. The specific location of a protein is determined by binding sites on the protein that bind to specific sites at the protein's destination. For example, in the case of the ribosomal proteins, they bind to sites on the nuclear pores that control access to the nucleus.

SECTION B SUMMARY

Genetic Code

I. Genetic information is coded in the nucleotide sequences of DNA molecules. A single gene contains either (a) the information that, via mRNA, determines the amino acid sequence in a specific protein; or (b) the information for forming rRNA, tRNA, or small nuclear RNAs, which assist in protein assembly.

II. Genetic information is transferred from DNA to mRNA in the nucleus (transcription); then mRNA passes to the cytoplasm, where its information is used to synthesize protein (translation).

III. The "words" in the DNA genetic code consist of a sequence of three nucleotide bases that specify a single amino acid. The sequence of three-letter codes along a gene determines the sequence of amino acids in a protein. More than one triplet can specify a given amino acid.

Protein Synthesis

I. Table 3.2 summarizes the steps leading from DNA to protein synthesis.

II. Transcription involves forming a primary RNA transcript by base-pairing with the template strand of DNA containing a single gene. Transcription also involves the removal of intron-derived segments by spliceosomes to form mRNA, which moves to the cytoplasm.

III. Translation of mRNA occurs on the ribosomes in the cytoplasm when the anticodons in tRNAs, linked to single amino acids, base-pair with the corresponding codons in mRNA.

IV. Protein transcription factors activate or repress the transcription of specific genes by binding to regions of DNA that interact with the promoter region of a gene.

V. Mutagens alter DNA molecules, resulting in the addition or deletion of nucleotides or segments of DNA. The result is an altered DNA sequence known as a mutation. A mutation may (a) cause no noticeable change in cell function, (b) modify cell function but still be compatible with cell growth and replication, or (c) lead to the death of the cell.

Protein Degradation

I. The concentration of a particular protein in a cell depends on (a) the rate of the corresponding gene's transcription; (b) the rate of initiating protein assembly on a ribosome; (c) the rate at which mRNA is degraded; (d) the rate of protein digestion by enzymes associated with proteasomes; and (e) the rate of secretion, if any, of the protein from the cell.

Protein Secretion

I. Targeting of a protein for secretion depends on the signal sequence of amino acids that first emerge from a ribosome during protein synthesis.

SECTION B REVIEW QUESTIONS

1. Describe how the genetic code in DNA specifies the amino acid sequence in a protein.
2. List the four nucleotides found in mRNA.
3. Describe the main events in the transcription of genetic information from DNA into mRNA.
4. Explain the difference between an exon and an intron.
5. What is the function of a spliceosome?
6. Identify the site of ribosomal subunit assembly.
7. Describe the role of tRNA in protein assembly.
8. Describe the events of protein translation that occur on the surface of a ribosome.
9. Describe the effects of transcription factors on gene transcription.
10. List the factors that regulate the concentration of a protein in a cell.
11. What is the function of the signal sequence of a protein? How is it formed, and where is it located?
12. Describe the pathway that leads to the secretion of proteins from cells.
13. List the three general types of effects a mutation can have on a cell's function.

SECTION B KEY TERMS

anticodon 62
codon 60
exon 60
gene 58
genome 58
histone 58
initiation factor 62
intron 60
messenger RNA (mRNA) 59
mutagen 64
mutation 64
natural selection 65
nucleosome 58
preinitiation complex 63
pre-mRNA 60
primary RNA transcript 60
promoter 60
proteasome 65
proteome 60
ribosomal RNA (rRNA) 61
RNA polymerase 60
signal sequence 66
spliceosome 61
stop signal 59
template strand 60
transcription 58
transcription factor 63
transfer RNA (tRNA) 61
translation 58
ubiquitin 65

SECTION C

Interactions Between Proteins and Ligands

3.8 Binding Site Characteristics

In the previous sections, we learned how the cellular machinery synthesizes and processes proteins. We now turn our attention to how proteins physically interact with each other and with other molecules and ions. These interactions are fundamental to nearly all physiological processes, clearly illustrating the general principle that physiological processes are dictated by the laws of chemistry and physics.

The ability of various molecules and ions to bind to specific sites on the surface of a protein forms the basis for the wide variety of protein functions (refer back to Table 2.5 for a summary of protein functions). A **ligand** is any molecule (including another protein) or ion that is bound to a protein by one of the following physical forces: (1) electrical attractions between oppositely charged ionic or polarized groups on the ligand and the protein, or (2) weaker attractions due to hydrophobic forces between nonpolar regions on the two molecules. These types of binding do not involve covalent bonds; in other words, binding is generally reversible. The region of a protein to which a ligand binds is known as a **binding site** or a ligand-binding site. A protein may contain several binding sites, each specific for a particular ligand, or it may have multiple binding sites for the same ligand. Typically, the binding of a ligand to a protein changes the conformation of the protein. When this happens, the protein's specific function may either be activated or inhibited, depending on the ligand. In the case of an enzyme, for example, the change in conformation may make the enzyme more active until the ligand is removed.

Chemical Specificity

A principle of physics states that the force of electrical attraction between oppositely charged particles decreases exponentially as the distance between them increases. This applies to charges within proteins and their ligands, as well. The even weaker hydrophobic forces act only between nonpolar groups that are very close to each other. Therefore, for a ligand to bind to a protein, the ligand must be close to the protein surface. This proximity occurs when the shape of the ligand is complementary to the shape of the protein's binding site, so that the two fit together like pieces of a jigsaw puzzle, illustrating the importance of structure to function at the molecular level (**Figure 3.26**).

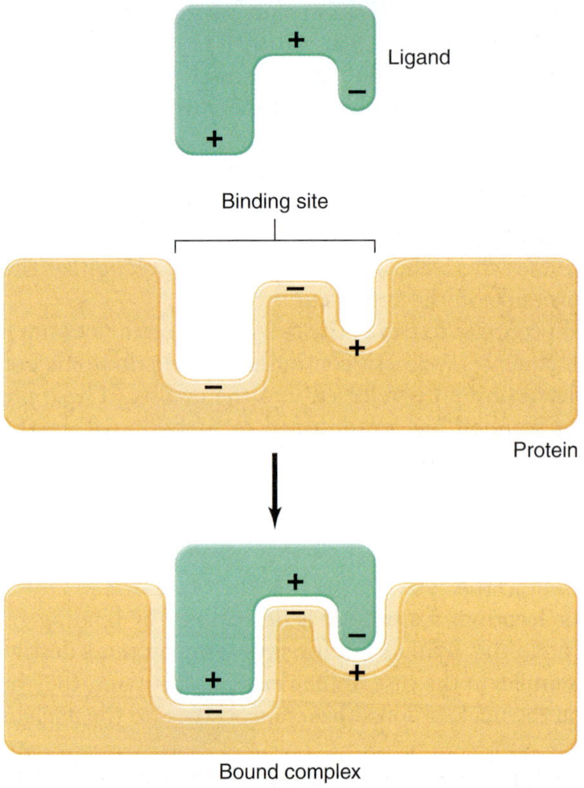

Figure 3.26 AP|R The complementary shapes of ligand and the protein-binding site determine the chemical specificity of binding.

The binding between a ligand and a protein may be so specific that a binding site can bind only one type of ligand and no other. Such selectivity allows a protein to identify (by binding) one particular molecule in a solution containing hundreds of different molecules. This ability of a protein-binding site to bind specific ligands is known as **chemical specificity,** because the binding site determines the type of chemical that is bound.

In Chapter 2, we described how the conformation of a protein is determined by the sequence of the various amino acids along the polypeptide chain. Accordingly, proteins with different amino acid sequences have different shapes and, therefore, differently shaped binding sites, each with its own chemical specificity. As illustrated in **Figure 3.27**, the amino acids that interact with a ligand at a binding site do not need to be adjacent to each other along the polypeptide chain, because the three-dimensional folding of the protein may bring various segments of the molecule into close contact.

Although some binding sites have a chemical specificity that allows them to bind only one type of ligand, others are less specific and thus can bind a number of related ligands. For example, three different ligands can combine with the binding site of protein X in **Figure 3.28**, because a portion of each ligand is complementary to the shape of the binding site. In contrast, protein Y has a greater chemical specificity and can bind only one of the three ligands. It is the degree of specificity of proteins that determines, in part, the side effects of therapeutic drugs. For example, a drug (ligand) designed to treat high blood pressure may act by binding to and thereby activating certain proteins that, in turn, help restore pressure to normal. The same drug, however, may also bind to a lesser degree to other proteins, whose functions may be completely unrelated to blood pressure. Changing the activities of these other proteins may lead to unwanted side effects of the medication.

Affinity

The strength of ligand–protein binding is a property of the binding site known as **affinity.** The affinity of a binding site for a ligand determines how likely it is that a bound ligand will

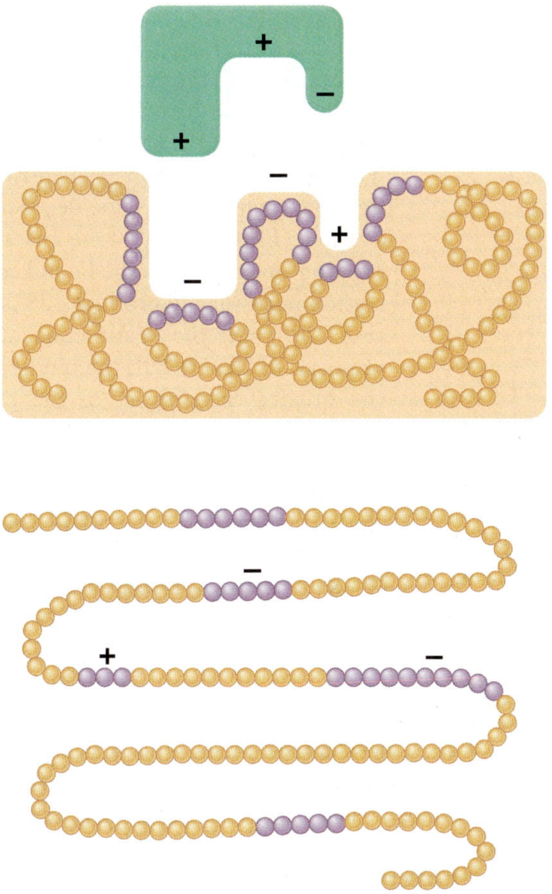

Figure 3.27 Amino acids that interact with the ligand at a binding site need not be at adjacent sites along the polypeptide chain, as indicated in this model showing the three-dimensional folding of a protein. The unfolded polypeptide chain appears at the bottom.

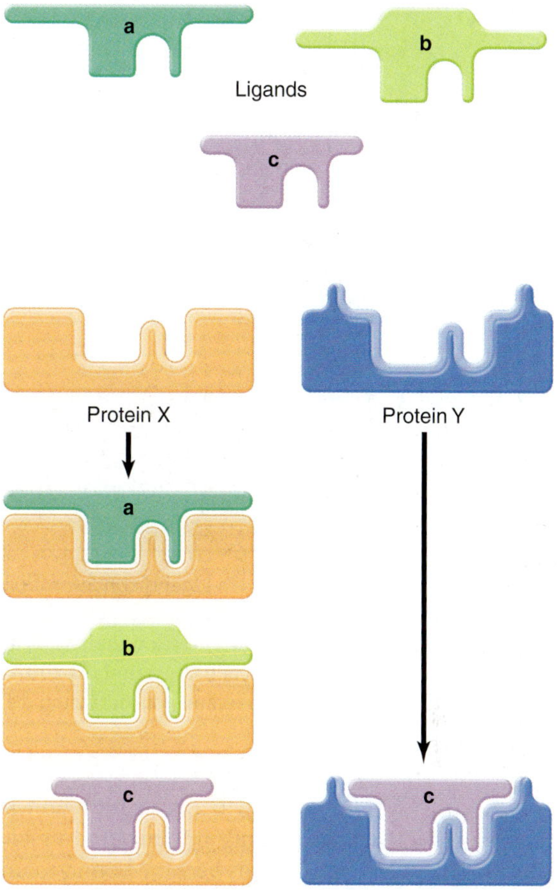

Figure 3.28 Protein X can bind all three ligands, which have similar chemical structures. Protein Y, because of the shape of its binding site, can bind only ligand c. Protein Y, therefore, has a greater chemical specificity than protein X.

leave the protein surface and return to its unbound state. Binding sites that tightly bind a ligand are called high-affinity binding sites; those that weakly bind the ligand are low-affinity binding sites.

Affinity and chemical specificity are two distinct, although closely related, properties of binding sites. Chemical specificity, as we have seen, depends only on the shape of the binding site, whereas affinity depends on the strength of the attraction between the protein and the ligand. Consequently, different proteins may be able to bind the same ligand—that is, may have the same chemical specificity—but may have different affinities for that ligand. For example, a ligand may have a negatively charged ionized group that would bind strongly to a site containing a positively charged amino acid side chain but would bind less strongly to a binding site having the same shape but no positive charge (**Figure 3.29**). In addition, the closer the surfaces of the ligand and binding site are to each other, the stronger the attractions. Thus, the more closely the ligand shape matches the binding site shape, the greater the affinity. In other words, shape can influence affinity as well as chemical specificity. Affinity has great importance in physiology and medicine, because when a protein has a high-affinity binding site for a ligand, very little of the ligand is required to bind to the protein. For example, a therapeutic drug may act by binding to a protein; if the protein has a high-affinity binding site for the drug, then only very small quantities of the drug are usually required to treat an illness. This reduces the likelihood of unwanted side effects.

PHYSIOLOGICAL INQUIRY

- Assume that both proteins X and Y have been linked with disease in humans. For which protein do you think it would be easier to design therapeutic drugs?

Answer can be found at end of chapter.

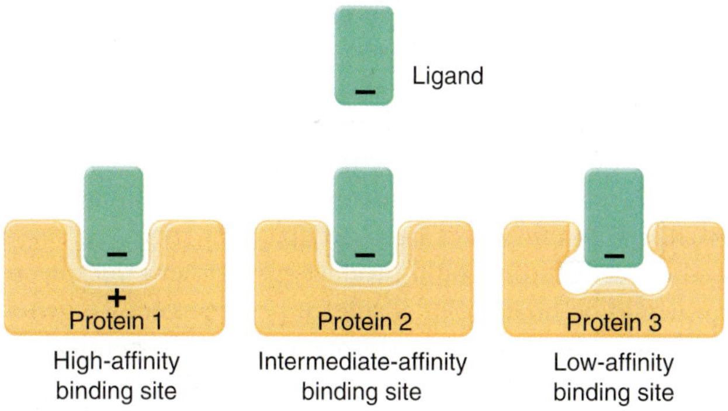

Figure 3.29 Three binding sites with the same chemical specificity but different affinities for a ligand.

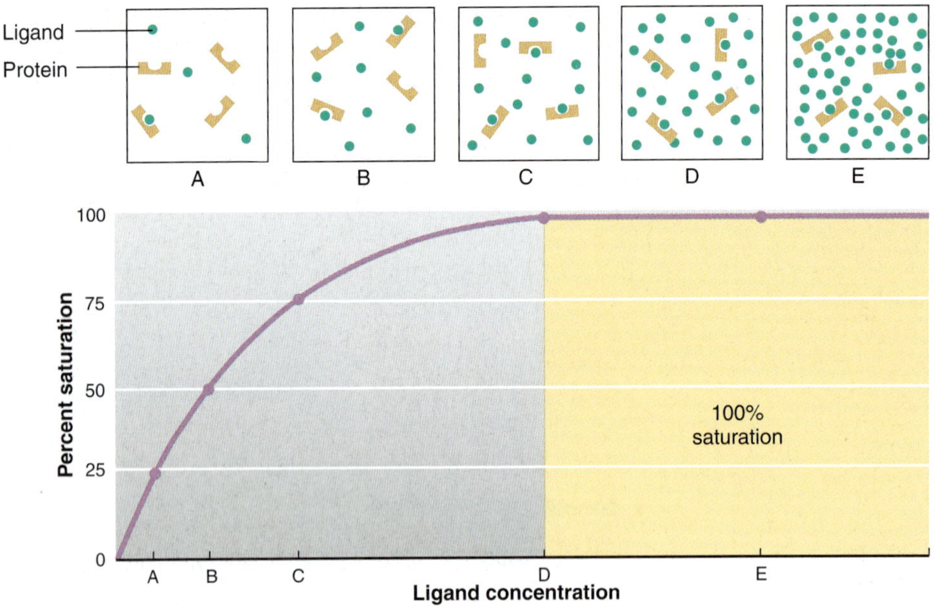

Figure 3.30 Increasing ligand concentration increases the number of binding sites occupied—that is, it increases the percent saturation. At 100% saturation, all the binding sites are occupied, and further increases in ligand concentration do not increase the number bound.

Saturation

An equilibrium is rapidly reached between unbound ligands in solution and their corresponding protein-binding sites. At any instant, some of the free ligands become bound to unoccupied binding sites, and some of the bound ligands are released back into solution. A single binding site is either occupied or unoccupied. The term **saturation** refers to the fraction of total binding sites that are occupied at any given time. When all the binding sites are occupied, the population of binding sites is 100% saturated. When half the available sites are occupied, the system is 50% saturated, and so on. A *single* binding site would also be 50% saturated if it were occupied by a ligand 50% of the time. The percent saturation of a binding site depends upon two factors: (1) the concentration of unbound ligand in the solution, and (2) the affinity of the binding site for the ligand.

The greater the ligand concentration, the greater the probability of a ligand molecule encountering an unoccupied binding site and becoming bound. Therefore, the percent saturation of binding sites increases with increasing ligand concentration until all the sites become occupied (**Figure 3.30**). Assuming that the ligand is a molecule that exerts a biological effect when it binds to a protein, the magnitude of the effect would also increase with increasing numbers of bound ligands until all the binding sites were occupied. Further increases in ligand concentration would produce no further effect because there would be no additional sites to be occupied. To generalize, a continuous increase in the magnitude of a chemical stimulus (ligand concentration) that exerts its effects by binding to proteins will produce an increased biological response until the point at which the protein-binding sites are 100% saturated.

The second factor determining the percent saturation of a binding site is the affinity of the binding site. Collisions between molecules in a solution and a protein containing a bound ligand can dislodge a loosely bound ligand, just as tackling a football player may cause a fumble. If a binding site has a high affinity for a ligand, even a reduced ligand concentration will result in a high degree of saturation because, once bound to the site, the ligand is not easily dislodged. A low-affinity site, on the other hand, requires a higher concentration of ligand to achieve the same degree of saturation (**Figure 3.31**). One measure of binding site affinity is the ligand concentration necessary to produce 50% saturation; the lower the ligand concentration required to bind to half the binding sites, the greater the affinity of the binding site (see Figure 3.31).

Competition

As we have seen, more than one type of ligand can bind to certain binding sites (see Figure 3.28). In such cases, **competition** occurs between the ligands for the same binding site. In other words, the presence of multiple ligands able to bind to the same binding site affects the percentage of binding sites occupied by any one ligand. If two competing ligands, A and B, are present, increasing the concentration of A will increase the amount of A that is bound, thereby decreasing the number of sites available to B and decreasing the amount of B that is bound.

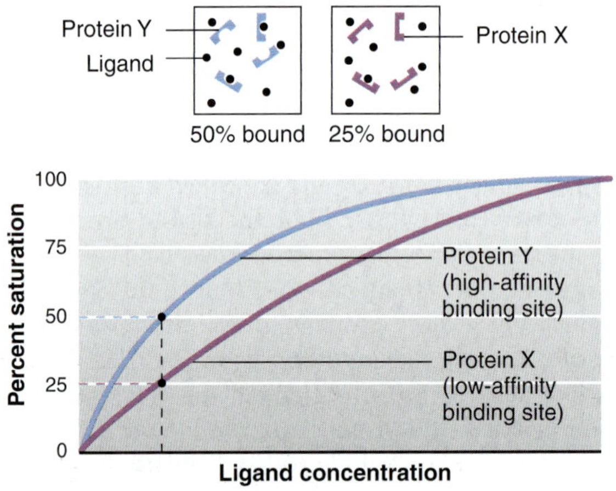

Figure 3.31 When two different proteins, X and Y, are able to bind the same ligand, the protein with the higher-affinity binding site (protein Y) has more bound sites at any given ligand concentration up to 100% saturation.

PHYSIOLOGICAL INQUIRY

- Assume that the function of protein Y in the body is to increase blood pressure by some amount and that of protein X is to decrease blood pressure by about the same amount. These effects only occur, however, if the protein binds the ligand shown in this figure. Predict what might happen if the ligand were administered to a person with normal blood pressure.

Answer can be found at end of chapter.

As a result of competition, the biological effects of one ligand may be diminished by the presence of another. For example, many drugs produce their effects by competing with the body's natural ligands for binding sites. By occupying the binding sites, the drug decreases the amount of natural ligand that can be bound.

3.9 Regulation of Binding Site Characteristics

Because proteins are associated with practically everything that occurs in a cell, the mechanisms for controlling these functions center on the control of protein activity. There are two ways of controlling protein activity: (1) changing protein shape, which alters the binding of ligands; and (2) as described earlier in this chapter, regulating protein synthesis and degradation, which determines the types and amounts of proteins in a cell.

As described in Chapter 2, a protein's shape depends partly on electrical attractions between charged or polarized groups in various regions of the protein. Therefore, a change in the charge distribution along a protein or in the polarity of the molecules immediately surrounding it will alter its shape. The two mechanisms found in cells that selectively alter protein shape are known as allosteric modulation and covalent modulation, though only certain proteins are regulated by modulation. Many proteins are not subject to either of these types of modulation.

Allosteric Modulation

Whenever a ligand binds to a protein, the attracting forces between the ligand and the protein alter the protein's shape. For example, as a ligand approaches a binding site, these attracting forces can cause the surface of the binding site to bend into a shape that more closely approximates the shape of the ligand's surface.

Moreover, as the shape of a binding site changes, it produces changes in the shape of *other* regions of the protein, just as pulling on one end of a rope (the polypeptide chain) causes the other end of the rope to move. Therefore, when a protein contains *two* binding sites, the noncovalent binding of a ligand to one site can alter the shape of the second binding site and, therefore, the binding characteristics of that site. This is termed **allosteric** (other shape) **modulation** (Figure 3.32a), and such proteins are known as **allosteric proteins.**

One binding site on an allosteric protein, known as the **functional** (or active) **site,** carries out the protein's physiological function. The other binding site is the **regulatory site.** The ligand that binds to the regulatory site is known as a **modulator molecule,** because its binding allosterically modulates the shape, and therefore the activity, of the functional site. Here again is a physiologically important example of how structure and function are related at the molecular level.

The regulatory site to which modulator molecules bind is the equivalent of a molecular switch that controls the functional site. In some allosteric proteins, the binding of the modulator molecule to the regulatory site turns on the functional site by changing its shape so that it can bind the functional ligand. In other cases, the binding of a modulator molecule turns off the functional site by preventing the functional site from binding its ligand. In still other cases, binding of the modulator molecule may decrease or increase the affinity of the functional site. For example, if the functional site is 75% saturated at a particular ligand concentration, the binding of a modulator molecule that decreases the affinity of the functional site may decrease its saturation to 50%. This concept will be especially important when we consider how carbon dioxide acts as a modulator molecule to lower the affinity of the protein hemoglobin for oxygen (Chapter 13).

To summarize, the activity of a protein can be increased without changing the concentration of either the protein or the functional ligand. By controlling the concentration of the modulator molecule, and therefore the percent saturation of the regulatory site, the functional activity of an allosterically regulated protein can be increased or decreased.

We have described thus far only those interactions between regulatory and functional binding sites. There is, however, a way that functional sites can influence each other in certain proteins. These proteins are composed of more than one polypeptide chain held together by electrical attractions between the chains. There may be only one binding site, a functional binding site, on each chain. The binding of

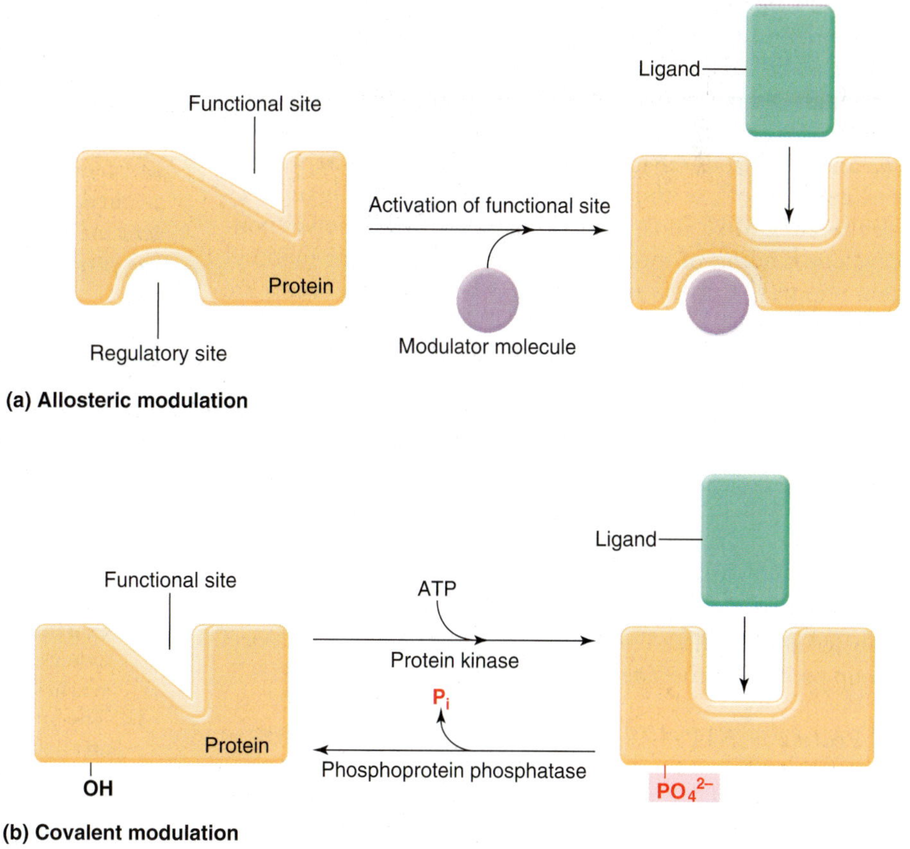

Figure 3.32 (a) Allosteric modulation and (b) covalent modulation of a protein's functional binding site.

a functional ligand to one of the chains, however, can result in an alteration of the functional binding sites in the other chains. This happens because the change in shape of the chain that holds the bound ligand induces a change in the shape of the other chains. The interaction between the functional binding sites of a multimeric (more than one polypeptide chain) protein is known as **cooperativity.** It can result in a progressive increase in the affinity for ligand binding as more and more of the sites become occupied. Hemoglobin again provides a useful example. As described in Chapter 2, hemoglobin is a protein composed of four polypeptide chains, each containing one binding site for oxygen. When oxygen binds to the first binding site, the affinity of the other sites for oxygen increases, and this continues as additional oxygen molecules bind to each polypeptide chain until all four chains have bound an oxygen molecule (see Chapter 13 for a description of this process and its physiological importance).

Covalent Modulation

The second way to alter the shape and therefore the activity of a protein is by the covalent bonding of charged chemical groups to some of the protein's side chains. This is known as **covalent modulation.** In most cases, a phosphate group, which has a net negative charge, is covalently attached by a chemical reaction called **phosphorylation,** in which a phosphate group is transferred from one molecule to another. Phosphorylation of one of the side chains of certain amino acids in a protein introduces a negative charge into that region of the protein. This charge alters the distribution of electrical forces in the protein and produces a change in protein conformation (**Figure 3.32b**). If the conformational change affects a binding site, it changes the binding site's properties. Although the mechanism is completely different, the effects produced by covalent modulation are similar to those of allosteric modulation—that is, a functional binding site may be turned on or off, or the affinity of the site for its ligand may be altered. Unlike allosteric modulation, which involves noncovalent binding of modulator molecules, covalent modulation requires chemical reactions in which covalent bonds are formed.

Most chemical reactions in the body are mediated by a special class of proteins known as enzymes, whose properties will be discussed in Section D of this chapter. For now, suffice it to say that enzymes accelerate the rate at which reactant molecules, called substrates, are converted to different molecules called products. Two enzymes control a protein's activity by covalent modulation: one adds phosphate, and one removes it. Any enzyme that mediates protein phosphorylation is called a **protein kinase.** These enzymes catalyze the transfer of phosphate from a molecule of ATP to a hydroxyl group present on the side chain of certain amino acids:

$$\text{Protein} + \text{ATP} \xrightarrow{\text{protein kinase}} \text{Protein} - PO_4^{2-} + \text{AD}$$

The protein and ATP are the substrates for protein kinase, and the phosphorylated protein and adenosine diphosphate (ADP) are the products of the reaction.

There is also a mechanism for removing the phosphate group and returning the protein to its original shape. This dephosphorylation is accomplished by a second class of enzymes known as **phosphoprotein phosphatases:**

$$\text{Protein} - PO_4^{2-} + H_2O \xrightarrow{\text{phosphoprotein phosphatase}} \text{Protein} + HPO_4^{2-}$$

The activity of the protein will depend on the relative activity of the kinase and phosphatase that controls the extent of the protein's phosphorylation. There are many protein kinases, each with specificities for different proteins, and several kinases may be present in the same cell. The chemical specificities of the phosphoprotein phosphatases are broader; a single enzyme can dephosphorylate many different phosphorylated proteins.

An important interaction between allosteric and covalent modulation results from the fact that protein kinases are themselves allosteric proteins whose activity can be controlled by modulator molecules. Therefore, the process of covalent modulation is itself indirectly regulated by allosteric mechanisms. In addition, some allosteric proteins can also be modified by covalent modulation.

In Chapter 5, we will describe how cell activities can be regulated in response to signals that alter the concentrations of various modulator molecules. These modulator molecules, in turn, alter specific protein activities via allosteric and covalent modulations. **Table 3.4** summarizes the factors influencing protein function.

TABLE 3.4 Factors That Influence Protein Function

I. Changing protein shape
  A. Allosteric modulation
  B. Covalent modulation
    1. Protein kinase activity
    2. Phosphoprotein–phosphatase activity

II. Changing protein concentration
  A. Protein synthesis
  B. Protein degradation

SECTION C SUMMARY

Binding Site Characteristics

I. Ligands bind to proteins at sites with shapes complementary to the ligand shape.
II. Protein-binding sites have the properties of chemical specificity, affinity, saturation, and competition.

Regulation of Binding Site Characteristics

I. Protein function in a cell can be controlled by regulating either the shape of the protein or the amounts of protein synthesized and degraded.
II. The binding of a modulator molecule to the regulatory site on an allosteric protein alters the shape of the functional binding site, thereby altering its binding characteristics and the activity of the protein. The activity of allosteric proteins is regulated by varying the concentrations of their modulator molecules.
III. Protein kinase enzymes catalyze the addition of a phosphate group to the side chains of certain amino acids in a protein, changing the shape of the protein's functional binding site and

thus altering the protein's activity by covalent modulation. A second enzyme is required to remove the phosphate group, returning the protein to its original state.

SECTION C REVIEW QUESTIONS

1. List the four characteristics of a protein-binding site.
2. List the types of forces that hold a ligand on a protein surface.
3. What characteristics of a binding site determine its chemical specificity?
4. Under what conditions can a single binding site have a chemical specificity for more than one type of ligand?
5. What characteristics of a binding site determine its affinity for a ligand?
6. What two factors determine the percent saturation of a binding site?
7. How is the activity of an allosteric protein modulated?
8. How does regulation of protein activity by covalent modulation differ from that by allosteric modulation?

SECTION C KEY TERMS

affinity 68
allosteric modulation 71
allosteric protein 71
binding site 68
chemical specificity 68
competition 70
cooperativity 72
covalent modulation 72
functional site 71
ligand 68
modulator molecule 71
phosphoprotein phosphatase 72
phosphorylation 72
protein kinase 72
regulatory site 71
saturation 70

SECTION **D**

Enzymes and Chemical Energy

Thus far, we have discussed the synthesis and regulation of proteins. In this section, we describe some of the major functions of proteins, specifically those that relate to facilitating chemical reactions.

Thousands of chemical reactions occur each instant throughout the body; this coordinated process of chemical change is termed *metabolism* (Greek, "change"). **Metabolism** involves the synthesis and breakdown of organic molecules required for cell structure and function and the release of chemical energy used for cell functions. The synthesis of organic molecules by cells is called **anabolism,** and their breakdown, **catabolism.** For example, the synthesis of a triglyceride is an anabolic reaction, whereas the breakdown of a triglyceride to glycerol and fatty acids is a catabolic reaction.

The organic molecules of the body undergo continuous transformation as some molecules are broken down while others of the same type are being synthesized. Molecularly, no person is the same at noon as at 8:00 A.M. because during even this short period, some of the body's structure has been broken down and replaced with newly synthesized molecules. In a healthy adult, the body's composition is in a steady state in which the anabolic and catabolic rates for the synthesis and breakdown of most molecules are equal. In other words, homeostasis is achieved as a result of a balance between anabolism and catabolism.

3.10 Chemical Reactions

Chemical reactions involve (1) the breaking of chemical bonds in reactant molecules, followed by (2) the making of new chemical bonds to form the product molecules. Take, for example, a chemical reaction that occurs in the blood in the lungs, which permits the lungs to rid the body of carbon dioxide. In the following reaction, carbonic acid is transformed into carbon dioxide and water. Two of the chemical bonds in carbonic acid are broken, and the product molecules are formed by establishing two new bonds between different pairs of atoms:

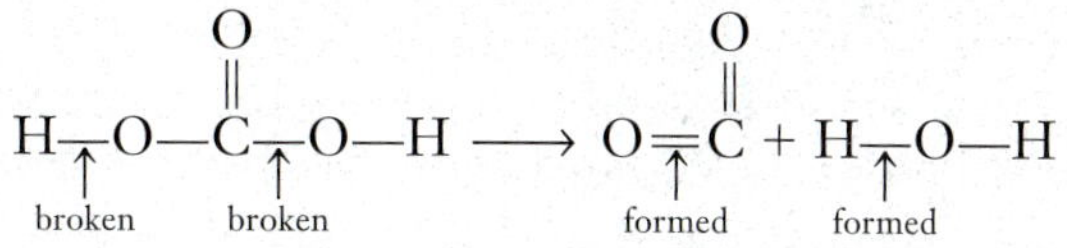

$$\underset{\text{carbonic acid}}{H_2CO_3} \longrightarrow \underset{\text{carbon dioxide}}{CO_2} + \underset{\text{water}}{H_2O} + \text{Energy}$$

Because the energy contents of the reactants and products are usually different, and because it is a fundamental law of physics that energy can neither be created nor destroyed, energy must either be added or released during most chemical reactions. For example, the breakdown of carbonic acid into carbon dioxide and water releases energy because carbonic acid has a higher energy content than the sum of the energy contents of carbon dioxide and water.

The released energy takes the form of heat, the energy of increased molecular motion, which is measured in units of calories. One **calorie** (1 cal) is the amount of heat required to raise the temperature of 1 g of water 1°C. Energies associated with most chemical reactions are several thousand calories per mole and are reported as **kilocalories** (1 kcal = 1000 cal; 1 kcal is sometimes written as 1 Calorie with a capital "C").

Determinants of Reaction Rates

The rate of a chemical reaction (in other words, how many molecules of product form per unit of time) can be determined by measuring the change in the concentration of reactants or products per unit of time. The faster the product concentration increases or the reactant concentration decreases, the greater the rate of the reaction. Four factors (**Table 3.5**) influence the reaction rate: reactant concentration, activation energy, temperature, and the presence of a catalyst.

The lower the concentration of reactants, the slower the reaction simply because there are fewer molecules available to react and the likelihood of any two reactants encountering

TABLE 3.5	Determinants of Chemical Reaction Rates
Reactant concentrations (greater concentrations: faster reaction rate)	
Activation energy (greater activation energy: slower reaction rate)	
Temperature (higher temperature: faster reaction rate)	
Catalyst (presence of catalyst: faster reaction rate)	

each other is low. Conversely, the higher the concentration of reactants, the faster the reaction rate.

Given the same initial concentrations of reactants, however, not all reactions occur at the same rate. Each type of chemical reaction has its own characteristic rate, which depends upon what is called the activation energy for the reaction. For a chemical reaction to occur, reactant molecules must acquire enough energy—the **activation energy**—to overcome the mutual repulsion of the electrons surrounding the atoms in each molecule. The activation energy does not affect the difference in energy content between the reactants and final products because the activation energy is released when the products are formed.

How do reactants acquire activation energy? In most of the metabolic reactions we will be considering, the reactants obtain activation energy when they collide with other molecules. If the activation energy required for a reaction is large, then the probability of a given reactant molecule acquiring this amount of energy will be small, and the reaction rate will be slow. Thus, the greater the activation energy required, the slower the rate of a chemical reaction.

Temperature is the third factor influencing reaction rates. The higher the temperature, the faster molecules move and the greater their impact when they collide. Therefore, one reason that increasing the temperature increases a reaction rate is that reactants have a better chance of acquiring sufficient activation energy such that when they collide, bonds can be broken or formed. In addition, faster-moving molecules collide more often.

A **catalyst** is a substance or molecule that interacts with one or more reactants by altering the distribution of energy between the chemical bonds of the reactants, resulting in a decrease in the activation energy required to transform the reactants into products. Catalysts may also bind two reactants and thereby bring them in close proximity and in an orientation that facilitates their interaction; this, too, reduces the activation energy. Because less activation energy is required, a reaction will proceed at a faster rate in the presence of a catalyst. The chemical composition of a catalyst is not altered by the reaction, so *a single catalyst molecule can act over and over again to catalyze the conversion of many reactant molecules to products.* Furthermore, a catalyst does not alter the difference in the energy contents of the reactants and products.

Reversible and Irreversible Reactions

Every chemical reaction is, in theory, reversible. Reactants are converted to products (we will call this a "forward reaction"), and products are converted to reactants (a "reverse reaction"). The overall reaction is a **reversible reaction:**

$$\text{Reactants} \underset{\text{reverse}}{\overset{\text{forward}}{\rightleftharpoons}} \text{Products}$$

As a reaction progresses, the rate of the forward reaction decreases as the concentration of reactants decreases. Simultaneously, the rate of the reverse reaction increases as the concentration of the product molecules increases. Eventually, the reaction will reach a state of **chemical equilibrium** in which the forward and reverse reaction rates are equal. At this point, there will be no further change in the concentrations of reactants or products even though reactants will continue to be converted into products and products converted into reactants.

Consider our previous example in which carbonic acid breaks down into carbon dioxide and water. The products of this reaction, carbon dioxide and water, can also recombine to form carbonic acid. This occurs outside the lungs and is a means for safely transporting CO_2 in the blood in a nongaseous state.

$$CO_2 + H_2O + \text{Energy} \rightleftharpoons H_2CO_3$$

Carbonic acid has a greater energy content than the sum of the energies contained in carbon dioxide and water; therefore, energy must be added to the latter molecules to form carbonic acid. This energy is not activation energy but is an integral part of the energy balance. This energy can be obtained, along with the activation energy, through collisions with other molecules.

When chemical equilibrium has been reached, the concentration of products does not need to be equal to the concentration of reactants even though the forward and reverse reaction rates are equal. The ratio of product concentration to reactant concentration at equilibrium depends upon the amount of energy released (or added) during the reaction. The greater the energy released, the smaller the probability that the product molecules will be able to obtain this energy and undergo the reverse reaction to re-form reactants. Therefore, in such a case, the ratio of product concentration to reactant concentration at chemical equilibrium will be large. If there is no difference in the energy contents of reactants and products, their concentrations will be equal at equilibrium.

Thus, although all chemical reactions are reversible to some extent, reactions that release large quantities of energy are said to be **irreversible reactions** because almost all of the reactant molecules are converted to product molecules when chemical equilibrium is reached. The energy released in a reaction determines the degree to which the reaction is reversible or irreversible. This energy is not the activation energy and it does not determine the reaction rate, which is governed by the four factors discussed earlier. The characteristics of reversible and irreversible reactions are summarized in **Table 3.6**.

Law of Mass Action

The concentrations of reactants and products play a very important role in determining not only the rates of the forward and reverse reactions but also the direction in which the *net* reaction proceeds—whether reactants or products are accumulating at a given time.

TABLE 3.6	Characteristics of Reversible and Irreversible Chemical Reactions
Reversible Reactions	$A + B \rightleftharpoons C + D$ + Small amount of energy At chemical equilibrium, product concentrations are only slightly higher than reactant concentrations.
Irreversible Reactions	$E + F \longrightarrow G + H$ + Large amount of energy At chemical equilibrium, almost all reactant molecules have been converted to product.

Consider the following reversible reaction that has reached chemical equilibrium:

$$\underset{\text{Reactants}}{A + B} \underset{\text{reverse}}{\overset{\text{forward}}{\rightleftharpoons}} \underset{\text{Products}}{C + D}$$

If at this point we increase the concentration of one of the reactants, the rate of the forward reaction will increase and lead to increased product formation. In contrast, increasing the concentration of one of the product molecules will drive the reaction in the reverse direction, increasing the formation of reactants. The direction in which the net reaction is proceeding can also be altered by *decreasing* the concentration of one of the participants. Therefore, decreasing the concentration of one of the products drives the net reaction in the forward direction because it decreases the rate of the reverse reaction without changing the rate of the forward reaction.

These effects of reaction and product concentrations on the direction in which the net reaction proceeds are known as the **law of mass action.** Mass action is often a major determining factor controlling the direction in which metabolic pathways proceed because reactions in the body seldom come to chemical equilibrium. More typically, new reactant molecules are added and product molecules are simultaneously removed by other reactions.

3.11 Enzymes

Most of the chemical reactions in the body, if carried out in a test tube with only reactants and products present, would proceed at very slow rates because they have large activation energies. To achieve the fast reaction rates observed in living organisms, catalysts must lower the activation energies. These particular catalysts are called **enzymes.** Enzymes are protein molecules, so an enzyme can be defined as a protein catalyst. (Although some RNA molecules possess catalytic activity, the number of reactions they catalyze is very small, so we will restrict the term *enzyme* to protein catalysts.)

To function, an enzyme must come into contact with reactants, which are called **substrates** in the case of enzyme-mediated reactions. The substrate becomes bound to the enzyme, forming an enzyme–substrate complex, which then breaks down to release products and enzyme. The reaction between enzyme and substrate can be written:

$$\underset{\text{Substrate}}{S} + \underset{\text{Enzyme}}{E} \rightleftharpoons \underset{\text{Enzyme–substrate complex}}{ES} \rightleftharpoons \underset{\text{Product}}{P} + \underset{\text{Enzyme}}{E}$$

At the end of the reaction, the enzyme is free to undergo the same reaction with additional substrate molecules. The overall effect is to accelerate the conversion of substrate into product, with the enzyme acting as a catalyst. An enzyme increases both the forward and reverse rates of a reaction and thus does not change the chemical equilibrium that is finally reached.

The interaction between substrate and enzyme has all the characteristics described previously for the binding of a ligand to a binding site on a protein—specificity, affinity, competition, and saturation. The region of the enzyme the substrate binds to is known as the enzyme's **active site** (a term equivalent to "binding site"). The shape of the enzyme in the region of the active site provides the basis for the enzyme's chemical specificity. Two models have been proposed to describe the interaction of an enzyme with its substrate(s). In one, the enzyme and substrate(s) fit together in a "lock-and-key" configuration. In another model, the substrate itself induces a shape change in the active site of the enzyme, which results in a highly specific binding interaction ("induced-fit model"), a good example of the dependence of function on structure at the protein level (**Figure 3.33**).

A typical cell expresses several thousand different enzymes, each capable of catalyzing a different chemical reaction. Enzymes are generally named by adding the suffix *-ase* to the name of either the substrate or the type of reaction the enzyme catalyzes. For example, the reaction in which carbonic acid is broken down into carbon dioxide and water is catalyzed by the enzyme **carbonic anhydrase.**

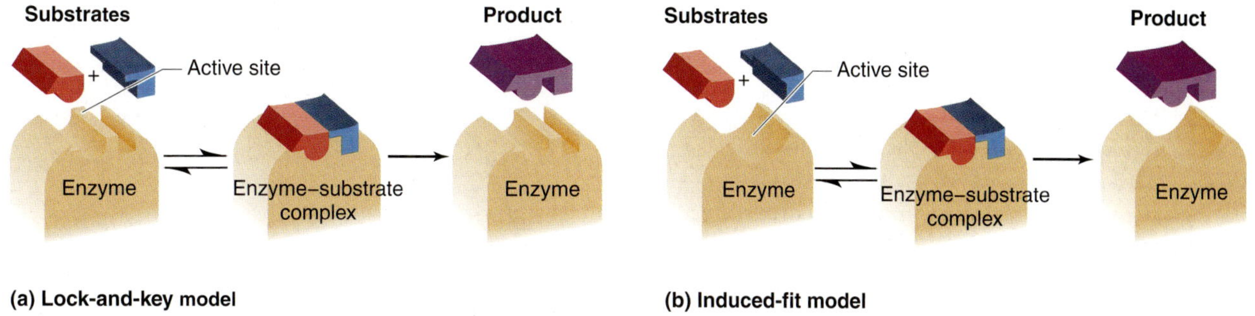

Figure 3.33 AP|R Binding of substrate to the active site of an enzyme catalyzes the formation of products. From M. S. Silberberg, *Chemistry: The Molecular Nature of Matter and Change*, 3rd ed., p. 701. The McGraw-Hill Companies, Inc., New York.

The catalytic activity of an enzyme can be extremely large. For example, one molecule of carbonic anhydrase can catalyze the conversion of about 100,000 substrate molecules to products in one second! The major characteristics of enzymes are listed in **Table 3.7**.

Cofactors

Many enzymes are inactive without small amounts of other substances known as **cofactors.** In some cases, the cofactor is a trace metal, such as magnesium, iron, zinc, or copper. Binding of one of the metals to an enzyme alters the enzyme's conformation so that it can interact with the substrate; this is a form of allosteric modulation. Because only a few enzyme molecules need be present to catalyze the conversion of large amounts of substrate to product, very small quantities of these trace metals are sufficient to maintain enzyme activity.

In other cases, the cofactor is an organic molecule that directly participates as one of the substrates in the reaction, in which case the cofactor is termed a **coenzyme.** Enzymes that require coenzymes catalyze reactions in which a few atoms (for example, hydrogen, acetyl, or methyl groups) are either removed from or added to a substrate. For example,

$$\text{R—2H} + \text{Coenzyme} \xrightarrow{\text{Enzyme}} \text{R} + \text{Coenzyme—2H}$$

What distinguishes a coenzyme from an ordinary substrate is the fate of the coenzyme. In our example, the two hydrogen atoms that transfer to the coenzyme can then be transferred from the coenzyme to another substrate with the aid of a second enzyme. This second reaction converts the coenzyme back to its original form so that it becomes available to accept two more hydrogen atoms. A single coenzyme molecule can act over and over again to transfer molecular fragments from one reaction to another. Therefore, as with metallic cofactors, only small quantities of coenzymes are necessary to maintain the enzymatic reactions in which they participate.

Coenzymes are derived from several members of a special class of nutrients known as **vitamins.** For example, the coenzymes **NAD$^+$** (nicotinamide adenine dinucleotide) and **FAD** (flavin adenine dinucleotide) are derived from the B vitamins niacin and riboflavin, respectively. As we will see, they play major roles in energy metabolism by transferring hydrogen from one substrate to another.

TABLE 3.7 Characteristics of Enzymes
An enzyme undergoes no net chemical change as a consequence of the reaction it catalyzes.
The binding of substrate to an enzyme's active site has all the characteristics—chemical specificity, affinity, competition, and saturation—of a ligand binding to a protein.
An enzyme increases the rate of a chemical reaction but does not cause a reaction to occur that would not occur in its absence.
Some enzymes increase both the forward and reverse rates of a chemical reaction and thus do not change the chemical equilibrium finally reached. They only increase the rate at which equilibrium is achieved.
An enzyme lowers the activation energy of a reaction but does not alter the net amount of energy that is added to or released by the reactants in the course of the reaction.

3.12 Regulation of Enzyme-Mediated Reactions

The rate of an enzyme-mediated reaction depends on substrate concentration and on the concentration and activity (defined later in this section) of the enzyme that catalyzes the reaction. Body temperature is normally nearly constant, so changes in temperature do not directly alter the rates of metabolic reactions. Increases in body temperature can occur during a fever, however, and around muscle tissue during exercise; such increases in temperature increase the rates of all metabolic reactions, including enzyme-catalyzed ones, in the affected tissues.

Substrate Concentration

Substrate concentration may be altered as a result of factors that alter the supply of a substrate from outside a cell. For example, there may be changes in its blood concentration due to changes in diet or the rate of substrate absorption from the intestinal tract. Intracellular substrate concentration can also be altered by cellular reactions that either utilize the substrate, and thus decrease its concentration, or synthesize the substrate, and thereby increase its concentration.

The rate of an enzyme-mediated reaction increases as the substrate concentration increases, as illustrated in **Figure 3.34**, until it reaches a maximal rate, which remains constant despite further increases in substrate concentration. The maximal rate is reached when the enzyme becomes saturated with substrate—that is, when the active binding site of every enzyme molecule is occupied by a substrate molecule.

Enzyme Concentration

At any substrate concentration, including saturating concentrations, the rate of an enzyme-mediated reaction can be increased by increasing the enzyme concentration. In most metabolic reactions, the substrate concentration is much greater than the concentration of enzyme available to catalyze the reaction. Therefore, if the number of enzyme molecules is doubled,

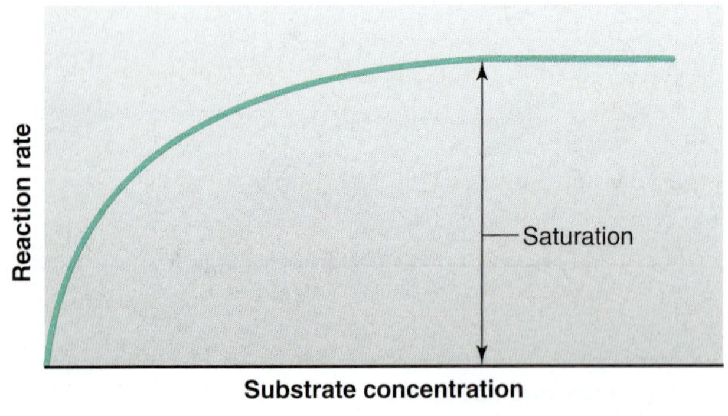

Figure 3.34 Rate of an enzyme-catalyzed reaction as a function of substrate concentration.

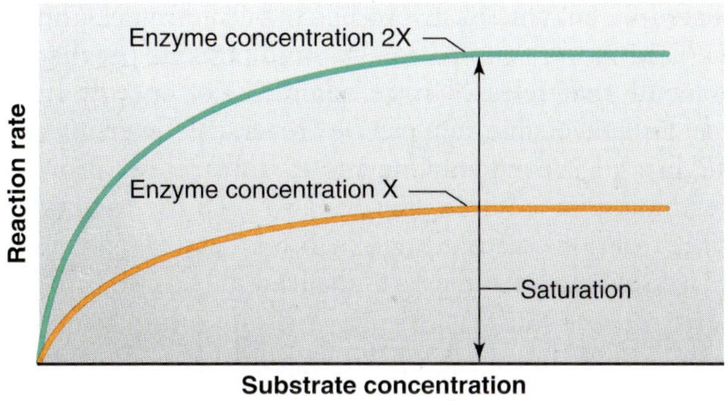

Figure 3.35 Rate of an enzyme-catalyzed reaction as a function of substrate concentration at two enzyme concentrations, X and 2X. Enzyme concentration 2X is twice the enzyme concentration of X, resulting in a reaction that proceeds twice as fast at any substrate concentration.

twice as many active sites will be available to bind substrate and twice as many substrate molecules will be converted to product (**Figure 3.35**). Certain reactions proceed faster in some cells than in others because more enzyme molecules are present.

To change the concentration of an enzyme, either the rate of enzyme synthesis or the rate of enzyme breakdown must be altered. Because enzymes are proteins, this involves changing the rates of protein synthesis or breakdown.

Enzyme Activity

In addition to changing the rate of enzyme-mediated reactions by changing the *concentration* of either substrate or enzyme, the rate can be altered by changing **enzyme activity.** A change in enzyme activity occurs when either allosteric or covalent modulation alters the properties (for example, the structure) of the enzyme's active site. Such modulation alters the rate at which the binding site converts substrate to product, the affinity of the binding site for substrate, or both.

Figure 3.36 illustrates the effect of increasing the affinity of an enzyme's active site without changing the substrate or enzyme concentration. If the substrate concentration is less than the saturating concentration, the increased affinity of the enzyme's binding site results in an increased number of active sites bound to substrate and, consequently, an increase in the reaction rate.

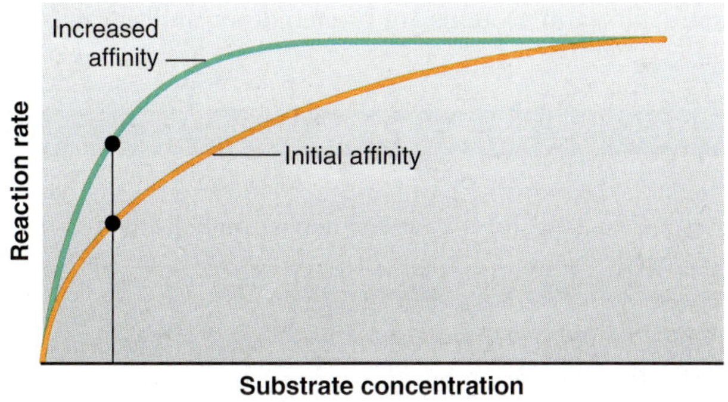

Figure 3.36 At a constant substrate concentration, increasing the affinity of an enzyme for its substrate by allosteric or covalent modulation increases the rate of the enzyme-mediated reaction. Note that increasing the enzyme's affinity does not increase the *maximal* rate of the enzyme-mediated reaction.

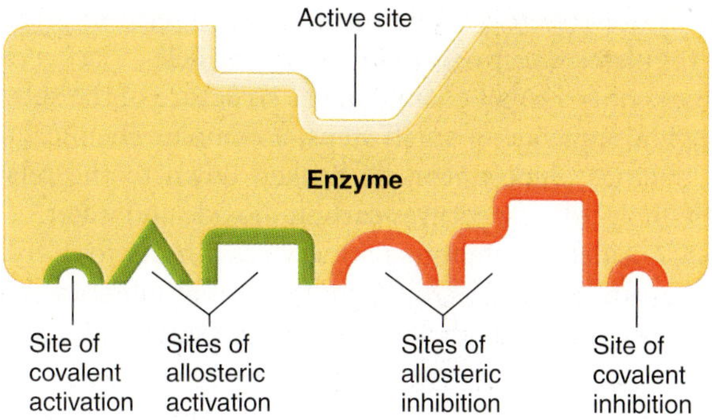

Figure 3.37 APR On a single enzyme, multiple sites can modulate enzyme activity, and therefore the reaction rate, by allosteric and covalent activation or inhibition.

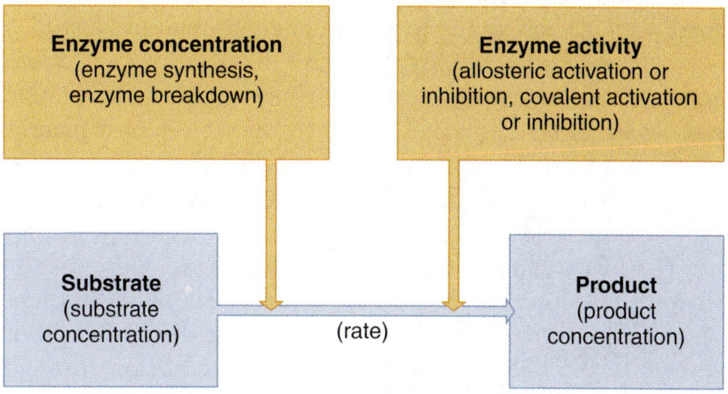

Figure 3.38 Factors that affect the rate of enzyme-mediated reactions.

PHYSIOLOGICAL INQUIRY

- What would happen in an enzyme-mediated reaction if the product formed was immediately used up or converted to another product by the cell?

Answer can be found at end of chapter.

The regulation of metabolism through the control of enzyme activity is an extremely complex process because, in many cases, more than one agent can alter the activity of an enzyme (**Figure 3.37**). The modulator molecules that allosterically alter enzyme activities may be product molecules of other cellular reactions. The result is that the overall rates of metabolism can adjust to meet various metabolic demands. In contrast, covalent modulation of enzyme activity is mediated by protein kinase enzymes that are themselves activated by various chemical signals the cell receives from, for example, a hormone.

Figure 3.38 summarizes the factors that regulate the rate of an enzyme-mediated reaction.

3.13 Multienzyme Reactions

The sequence of enzyme-mediated reactions leading to the formation of a particular product is known as a **metabolic pathway.** For example, the 19 reactions that break glucose down to carbon dioxide and water constitute the metabolic pathway for glucose catabolism, a key homeostatic process that regulates energy availability in all cells. Each reaction produces only a small change in the structure of the substrate. By such a sequence of small steps, a complex chemical structure, such as glucose, can be broken down to the relatively simple molecular structures carbon dioxide and water.

Consider a metabolic pathway containing four enzymes (e_1, e_2, e_3, and e_4) and leading from an initial substrate A to the end-product E, through a series of intermediates B, C, and D:

$$A \overset{e_1}{\rightleftharpoons} B \overset{e_2}{\rightleftharpoons} C \overset{e_3}{\rightleftharpoons} D \overset{e_4}{\longrightarrow} E$$

The irreversibility of the last reaction is of no consequence for the moment. By mass action, increasing the concentration of A will lead to an increase in the concentration of B (provided e_1 is not already saturated with substrate), and so on until eventually there is an increase in the concentration of the end-product E.

Because different enzymes have different concentrations and activities, it would be extremely unlikely that the reaction rates of all these steps would be exactly the same. Consequently, one step is likely to be slower than all the others. This step is known as the **rate-limiting reaction** in a metabolic pathway. None of the reactions that occur later in the sequence, including the formation of end product, can proceed more rapidly than the rate-limiting reaction because their substrates are supplied by the previous steps. By regulating the concentration or activity of the rate-limiting enzyme, the rate of flow through the whole pathway can be increased or decreased. Thus, it is not necessary to alter all the enzymes in a metabolic pathway to control the rate at which the end product is produced.

Rate-limiting enzymes are often the sites of allosteric or covalent regulation. For example, if enzyme e_2 is rate-limiting in the pathway just described, and if the end-product E inhibits the activity of e_2, **end-product inhibition** occurs (**Figure 3.39**). As the concentration of the product increases, the inhibition of further product formation increases. Such inhibition, which is a form of negative feedback (Chapter 1), frequently occurs in synthetic pathways in which the formation of end product is effectively shut down when it is not being utilized. This prevents unnecessary excessive accumulation of the end product and contributes to the homeostatic balance of the product.

Control of enzyme activity also can be critical for *reversing* a metabolic pathway. Consider the pathway we have been discussing, ignoring the presence of end-product inhibition of enzyme e_2. The pathway consists of three reversible reactions mediated by e_1, e_2, and e_3, followed by an irreversible reaction mediated by enzyme e_4. E can be converted into D, however, if the reaction is coupled to the simultaneous breakdown of a molecule that releases large quantities of energy. In other words, an irreversible step can be "reversed" by an alternative route, using a second enzyme and its substrate to provide the large amount of required energy. Two such high-energy irreversible reactions are indicated by bowed arrows to emphasize that two separate enzymes are involved in the two directions:

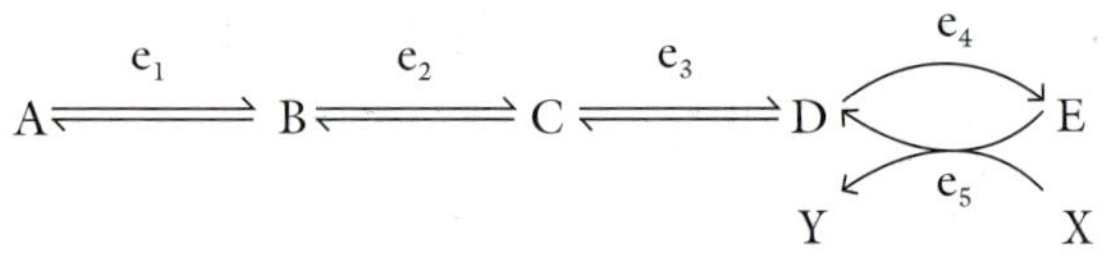

The direction of flow through the pathway can be regulated by controlling the concentration and/or activities of e_4 and e_5. If e_4 is activated and e_5 inhibited, the flow will proceed from A to E; whereas inhibition of e_4 and activation of e_5 will produce flow from E to A.

Another situation involving the differential control of several enzymes arises when there is a branch in a metabolic pathway. A single metabolite C may be the substrate for more than one enzyme, as illustrated by the pathway:

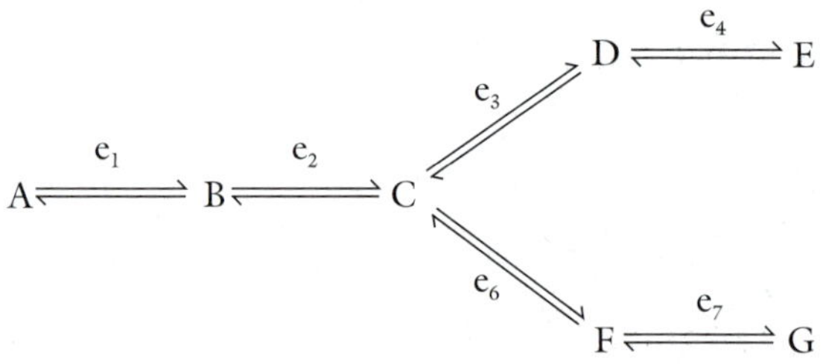

Altering the concentration and/or activities of e_3 and e_6 regulates the flow of metabolite C through the two branches of the pathway.

Considering the thousands of reactions that occur in the body and the permutations and combinations of possible control points, the overall result is staggering. The details of regulating the many metabolic pathways at the enzymatic level are beyond the scope of this book. In the remainder of this chapter, we consider only (1) the overall characteristics of the pathways by which cells obtain energy; and (2) the major pathways by which carbohydrates, fats, and proteins are broken down and synthesized.

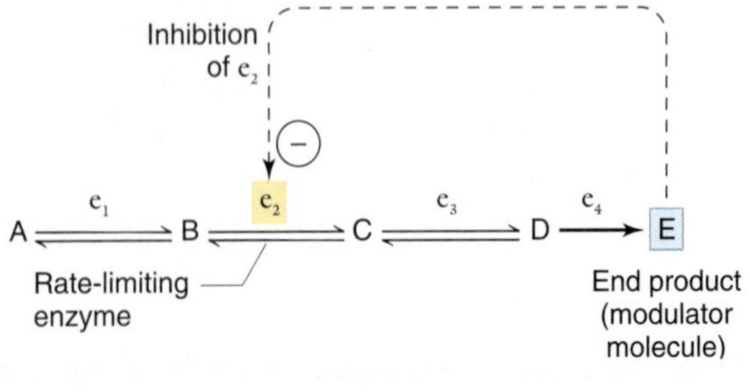

Figure 3.39 End-product inhibition of the rate-limiting enzyme in a metabolic pathway. The end-product E becomes the modulator molecule that produces inhibition of enzyme e_2.

SECTION D SUMMARY

In adults, the rates at which organic molecules are continuously synthesized (anabolism) and broken down (catabolism) are approximately equal.

Chemical Reactions

I. The difference in the energy content of reactants and products is the amount of energy (measured in calories) released or added during a reaction.

II. The energy released during a chemical reaction is either released as heat or transferred to other molecules.

III. The four factors that can alter the rate of a chemical reaction are listed in Table 3.5.

IV. The activation energy required to initiate the breaking of chemical bonds in a reaction is usually acquired through collisions between molecules.
V. Catalysts increase the rate of a reaction by lowering the activation energy.
VI. The characteristics of reversible and irreversible reactions are listed in Table 3.6.
VII. The net direction in which a reaction proceeds can be altered, according to the law of mass action, by increases or decreases in the concentrations of reactants or products.

Enzymes

I. Nearly all chemical reactions in the body are catalyzed by enzymes, the characteristics of which are summarized in Table 3.7.
II. Some enzymes require small concentrations of cofactors for activity.
  a. The binding of trace metal cofactors maintains the conformation of the enzyme's binding site so that it is able to bind substrate.
  b. Coenzymes, derived from vitamins, transfer small groups of atoms from one substrate to another. The coenzyme is regenerated in the course of these reactions and can do its work over and over again.

Regulation of Enzyme-Mediated Reactions

I. The rates of enzyme-mediated reactions can be altered by changes in temperature, substrate concentration, enzyme concentration, and enzyme activity. Enzyme activity is altered by allosteric or covalent modulation.

Multienzyme Reactions

I. The rate of product formation in a metabolic pathway can be controlled by allosteric or covalent modulation of the enzyme mediating the rate-limiting reaction in the pathway. The end product often acts as a modulator molecule, inhibiting the rate-limiting enzyme's activity.
II. An "irreversible" step in a metabolic pathway can be reversed by the use of two enzymes, one for the forward reaction and one for the reverse direction via another, energy-yielding reaction.

SECTION D REVIEW QUESTIONS

1. How do molecules acquire the activation energy required for a chemical reaction?
2. List the four factors that influence the rate of a chemical reaction and state whether increasing the factor will increase or decrease the rate of the reaction.
3. What characteristics of a chemical reaction make it reversible or irreversible?
4. List five characteristics of enzymes.
5. What is the difference between a cofactor and a coenzyme?
6. From what class of nutrients are coenzymes derived?
7. Why are small concentrations of coenzymes sufficient to maintain enzyme activity?
8. List three ways to alter the rate of an enzyme-mediated reaction.
9. How can an "irreversible step" in a metabolic pathway be reversed?

SECTION D KEY TERMS

activation energy 74
active site 75
anabolism 73
calorie 73
carbonic anhydrase 75
catabolism 73
catalyst 74
chemical equilibrium 74
coenzyme 76
cofactor 76
end-product inhibition 78
enzyme 75
enzyme activity 77
FAD 76
irreversible reaction 74
kilocalorie 73
law of mass action 75
metabolic pathway 77
metabolism 73
NAD^+ 76
rate-limiting reaction 78
reversible reaction 74
substrate 75
vitamin 76

SECTION E Metabolic Pathways

Enzymes are involved in many important physiological reactions that together promote a homeostatic state. For example, enzymes are vital for the regulated production of cellular energy (ATP), which, in turn, is needed for such widespread events as muscle contraction, nerve cell function, and chemical signal transduction.

Cells use three distinct but linked metabolic pathways to transfer the energy released from the breakdown of nutrient molecules to ATP. They are known as (1) glycolysis, (2) the Krebs cycle, and (3) oxidative phosphorylation (**Figure 3.40**). In the following section, we will describe the major characteristics of these three pathways, including the location of the pathway enzymes in a cell, the relative contribution of each pathway to ATP production, the sites of carbon dioxide formation and oxygen utilization, and the key molecules that enter and leave each pathway. Later, in Chapter 16, we will refer to these pathways when we describe the physiology of energy balance in the human body.

Several facts should be noted in Figure 3.40. First, glycolysis operates only on carbohydrates. Second, all the categories of macromolecular nutrients—carbohydrates, fats, and proteins—contribute to ATP production via the Krebs cycle and oxidative phosphorylation. Third, mitochondria are the sites of the Krebs cycle and oxidative phosphorylation. Finally, one important generalization to keep in mind is that glycolysis can occur in either the presence or absence of oxygen, whereas both the Krebs cycle and oxidative phosphorylation require oxygen.

3.14 Cellular Energy Transfer

Glycolysis

Glycolysis (from the Greek *glycos*, "sugar," and *lysis*, "breakdown") is a pathway that partially catabolizes carbohydrates, primarily glucose. It consists of 10 enzymatic reactions that convert a six-carbon molecule of glucose into two three-carbon

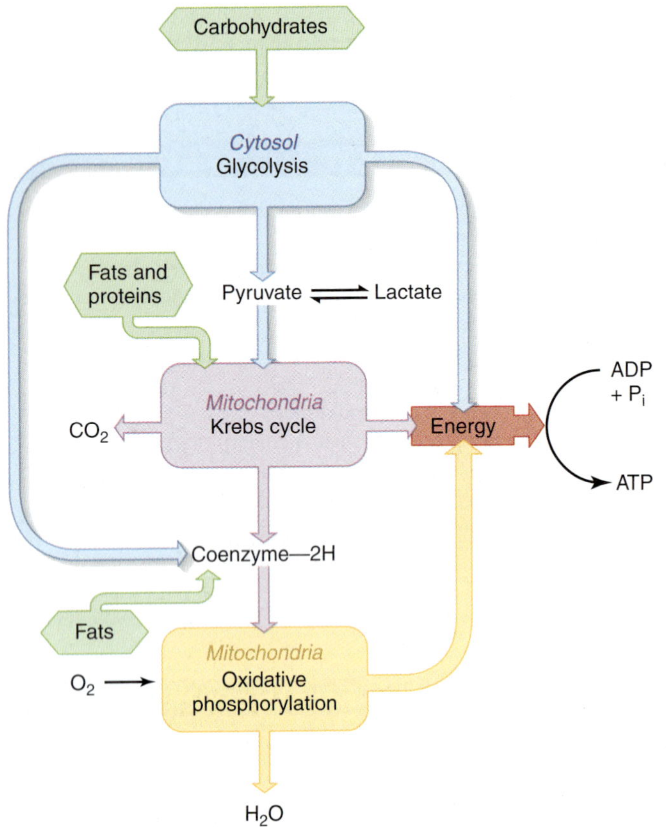

Figure 3.40 AP|R Pathways linking the energy released from the catabolism of nutrient molecules to the formation of ATP.

molecules of **pyruvate,** the ionized form of pyruvic acid (**Figure 3.41**). The reactions produce a net gain of two molecules of ATP and four atoms of hydrogen, two transferred to NAD^+ and two released as hydrogen ions:

$$\text{Glucose} + 2\ \text{ADP} + 2\ P_i + 2\ NAD^+ \longrightarrow 2\ \text{Pyruvate} + 2\ \text{ATP} + 2\ \text{NADH} + 2\ H^+ + 2\ H_2O$$

These 10 reactions, *none of which utilizes molecular oxygen,* take place in the cytosol. Note (see Figure 3.41) that all the intermediates between glucose and the end product pyruvate contain one or more ionized phosphate groups. Plasma membranes are impermeable to such highly ionized molecules; therefore, these molecules remain trapped within the cell.

The early steps in glycolysis (reactions 1 and 3) each *use*, rather than produce, one molecule of ATP to form phosphorylated intermediates. In addition, note that reaction 4 splits a six-carbon intermediate into two three-carbon molecules and reaction 5 converts one of these three-carbon molecules into the other. Thus, at the end of reaction 5, we have two molecules of 3-phosphoglyceraldehyde derived from one molecule of glucose. Keep in mind, then, that from this point on, *two* molecules of each intermediate are involved.

The first formation of ATP in glycolysis occurs during reaction 7, in which a phosphate group is transferred to ADP to form ATP. Because two intermediates exist at this point, reaction 7 produces two molecules of ATP, one from each intermediate. In this reaction, the mechanism of forming ATP is known as **substrate-level phosphorylation** because the phosphate group is transferred from a substrate molecule to ADP.

A similar substrate-level phosphorylation of ADP occurs during reaction 10, in which again two molecules of ATP are formed. Thus, reactions 7 and 10 generate a total of four molecules of ATP for every molecule of glucose entering the pathway. There is a net gain, however, of only two molecules of ATP during glycolysis because two molecules of ATP are used in reactions 1 and 3.

The end product of glycolysis, pyruvate, can proceed in one of two directions. If oxygen is present—that is, if **aerobic** conditions exist—much of the pyruvate can enter the Krebs cycle and be broken down into carbon dioxide, as described in the next section. Pyruvate is also converted to **lactate** (the ionized form of lactic acid) by a single enzyme-mediated reaction. In this reaction (**Figure 3.42**), two hydrogen atoms derived from $NADH^+ + H^+$ are transferred to each molecule of pyruvate to form lactate, and NAD^+ is regenerated. These hydrogens were originally transferred to NAD^+ during reaction 6 of glycolysis, so the coenzyme NAD^+ shuttles hydrogen between the two reactions during glycolysis. The overall reaction for the breakdown of glucose to lactate is

$$\text{Glucose} + 2\ \text{ADP} + 2\ P_i \longrightarrow 2\ \text{Lactate} + 2\ \text{ATP} + 2\ H_2O$$

As stated in the previous paragraph, under aerobic conditions, some of the pyruvate is not converted to lactate but instead enters the Krebs cycle. Therefore, the mechanism just described for regenerating NAD^+ from $NADH^+ + H^+$ by forming lactate does not occur to as great a degree. The hydrogens of NADH are transferred to oxygen during oxidative phosphorylation, regenerating NAD^+ and producing H_2O, as described in detail in the discussion that follows.

In most cells, the amount of ATP produced by glycolysis from one molecule of glucose is much smaller than the amount formed under aerobic conditions by the other two ATP-generating pathways—the Krebs cycle and oxidative phosphorylation. In special cases, however, glycolysis supplies most—or even all—of a cell's ATP. For example, erythrocytes contain the enzymes for glycolysis but have no mitochondria, which are required for the other pathways. All of their ATP production occurs, therefore, by glycolysis. Also, certain types of skeletal muscles contain considerable amounts of glycolytic enzymes but few mitochondria. During intense muscle activity, glycolysis provides most of the ATP in these cells and is associated with the production of large amounts of lactate. Despite these exceptions, most cells do not have sufficient concentrations of glycolytic enzymes or enough glucose to provide by glycolysis alone the high rates of ATP production necessary to meet their energy requirements.

What happens to the lactate that is formed during glycolysis? Some of it is released into the blood and taken up by the heart, brain, and other tissues where it is converted back to pyruvate and used as an energy source. Another portion of the secreted lactate is taken up by the liver where it is used as a precursor for the formation of glucose, which is then released into the blood where it becomes available as an energy source for all cells. The latter reaction is particularly important

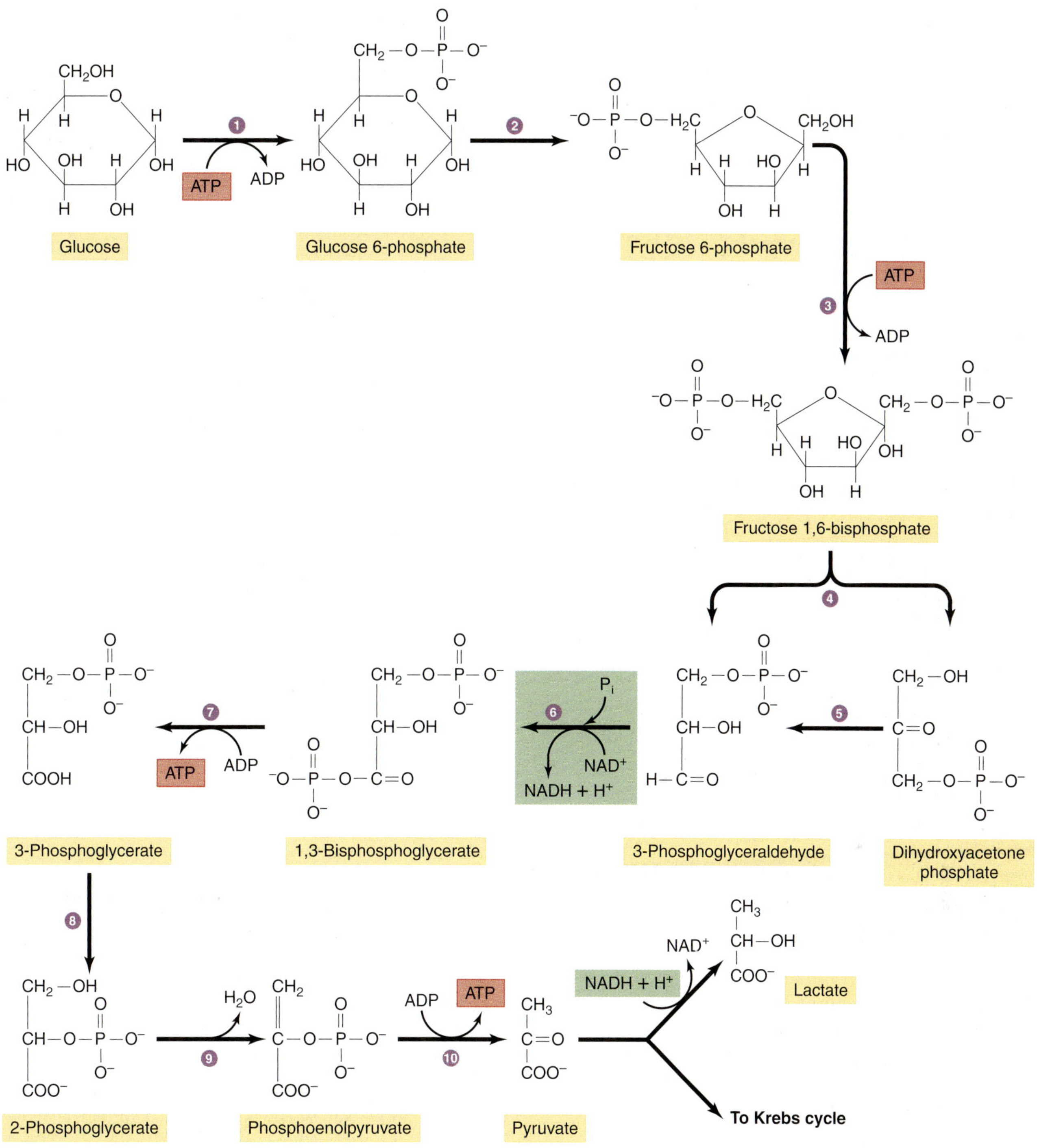

Figure 3.41 APIR Glycolytic pathway. During glycolysis, every molecule of glucose that enters the pathway produces a net synthesis of two molecules of ATP. Note that at the pH existing in the body, the products produced by the various glycolytic steps exist in the ionized, anionic form (pyruvate, for example). They are actually produced as acids (pyruvic acid, for example) that then ionize. Pyruvate is converted to lactate or enters the Krebs cycle; production of lactate is increased when the ATP demand of cells increases, as during exercise. *Note:* Beginning with step 5, two molecules of each intermediate are present even though only one is shown for clarity.

during periods in which energy demands are high, such as during exercise.

Our discussion of glycolysis has focused upon glucose as the major carbohydrate entering the glycolytic pathway. However, other carbohydrates such as fructose, derived from the disaccharide sucrose (table sugar), and galactose, from the disaccharide lactose (milk sugar), can also be catabolized by glycolysis because these carbohydrates are converted into several of the intermediates that participate in the early portion of the glycolytic pathway.

Krebs Cycle

The **Krebs cycle,** named in honor of Hans Krebs, who worked out the intermediate steps in this pathway (also known as the **citric acid cycle** or **tricarboxylic acid cycle**), is the second of the three pathways involved in nutrient catabolism

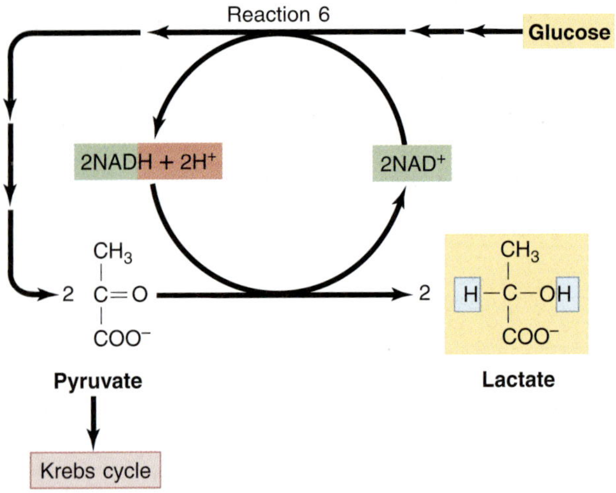

Figure 3.42 APR The coenzyme NAD$^+$ utilized in the glycolytic reaction 6 (see Figure 3.41) is regenerated when it transfers its hydrogen atoms to pyruvate during the formation of lactate. These reactions are increased in times of energy demand.

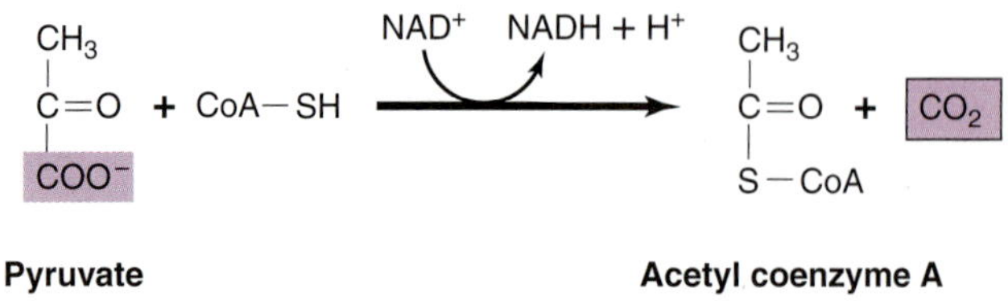

Figure 3.43 APR Formation of acetyl coenzyme A from pyruvate with the formation of a molecule of carbon dioxide.

and ATP production. It utilizes molecular fragments formed during carbohydrate, protein, and fat breakdown; it produces carbon dioxide, hydrogen atoms (half of which are bound to coenzymes), and small amounts of ATP. The enzymes for this pathway are located in the inner mitochondrial compartment, the matrix.

The primary molecule entering at the beginning of the Krebs cycle is **acetyl coenzyme A (acetyl CoA)**:

$$CH_3{-}\overset{\overset{\displaystyle O}{\|}}{C}{-}S{-}CoA$$

Coenzyme A (CoA) is derived from the B vitamin pantothenic acid and functions primarily to transfer acetyl groups, which contain two carbons, from one molecule to another. These acetyl groups come either from pyruvate—the end product of aerobic glycolysis—or from the breakdown of fatty acids and some amino acids.

Pyruvate, upon entering mitochondria from the cytosol, is converted to acetyl CoA and CO_2 (**Figure 3.43**). Note that this reaction produces the first molecule of CO_2 formed thus far in the pathways of nutrient catabolism, and that the reaction also transfers hydrogen atoms to NAD$^+$.

The Krebs cycle begins with the transfer of the acetyl group of acetyl CoA to the four-carbon molecule oxaloacetate to form the six-carbon molecule citrate (**Figure 3.44**). At the third step in the cycle, a molecule of CO_2 is produced—and again at the fourth step. Therefore, two carbon atoms entered the cycle as part of the acetyl group attached to CoA, and two carbons (although not the same ones) have left in the form of CO_2. Note also that the oxygen that appears in the CO_2 is derived not from molecular oxygen but from the carboxyl groups of Krebs-cycle intermediates.

In the remainder of the cycle, the four-carbon molecule formed in reaction 4 is modified through a series of reactions to produce the four-carbon molecule oxaloacetate, which becomes available to accept another acetyl group and repeat the cycle.

Now we come to a crucial fact: In addition to producing carbon dioxide, intermediates in the Krebs cycle generate hydrogen atoms, most of which are transferred to the coenzymes NAD$^+$ and FAD to form NADH and $FADH_2$. This hydrogen transfer to NAD$^+$ occurs in each of steps 3, 4, and 8, and to FAD in reaction 6. These hydrogens will be transferred from the coenzymes, along with the free H$^+$, to oxygen in the next stage of nutrient metabolism—oxidative phosphorylation. Because oxidative phosphorylation is necessary for regeneration of the hydrogen-free form of these coenzymes, *the Krebs cycle can operate only under aerobic conditions.* There is no pathway in the mitochondria that can remove the hydrogen from these coenzymes under anaerobic conditions.

So far, we have said nothing of how the Krebs cycle contributes to the formation of ATP. In fact, the Krebs cycle *directly* produces only one high-energy nucleotide triphosphate. This occurs during reaction 5 in which inorganic phosphate is transferred to guanosine diphosphate (GDP) to form guanosine triphosphate (GTP). The hydrolysis of GTP, like that of ATP, can provide energy for some energy-requiring reactions. In addition, the energy in GTP can be transferred to ATP by the reaction

$$GTP + ADP \rightleftharpoons GDP + ATP$$

The formation of ATP from GTP is the only mechanism by which ATP is formed within the Krebs cycle. Why, then, is the Krebs cycle so important? The reason is that the hydrogen atoms transferred to coenzymes during the cycle (plus the free hydrogen ions generated) are used in the next pathway, oxidative phosphorylation, to form large amounts of ATP.

The net result of the catabolism of one acetyl group from acetyl CoA by way of the Krebs cycle can be written

$$\text{Acetyl CoA} + 3\ NAD^+ + FAD + GDP + P_i + 2\ H_2O \longrightarrow 2\ CO_2 + CoA + 3\ NADH + 3\ H^+ + FADH_2 + GTP$$

Table 3.8 summarizes the characteristics of the Krebs-cycle reactions.

Oxidative Phosphorylation

Oxidative phosphorylation provides the third, and quantitatively most important, mechanism by which energy derived from nutrient molecules can be transferred to ATP. The basic principle behind this pathway is simple: The energy transferred to ATP is derived from the energy released when hydrogen ions combine with molecular oxygen to form water. The hydrogen comes from the NADH + H$^+$ and $FADH_2$ coenzymes generated by the Krebs cycle, by the metabolism

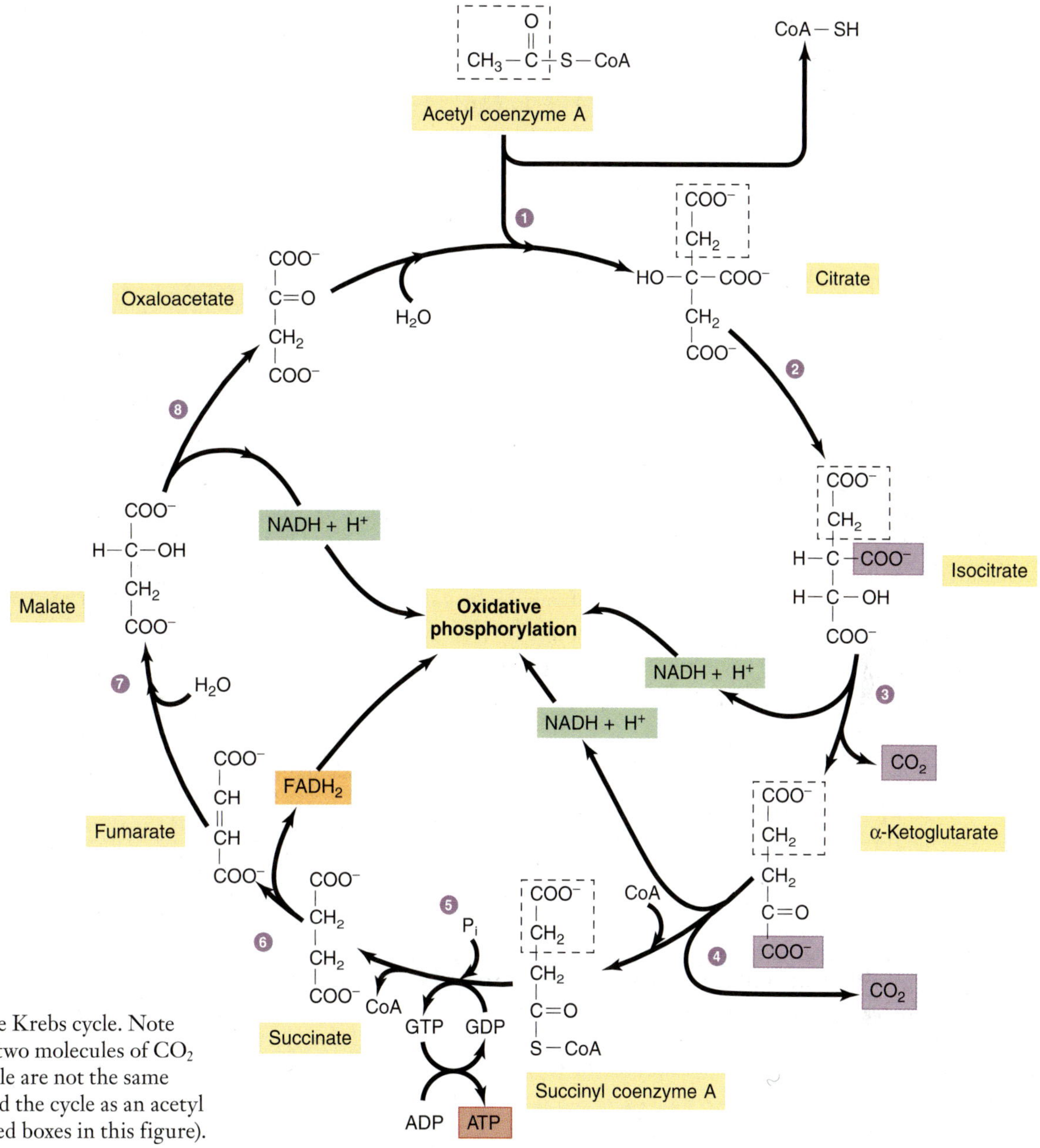

Figure 3.44 AP|R The Krebs cycle. Note that the carbon atoms in the two molecules of CO_2 produced by a turn of the cycle are not the same two carbon atoms that entered the cycle as an acetyl group (identified by the dashed boxes in this figure).

TABLE 3.8	Characteristics of the Krebs Cycle
Entering substrate	Acetyl coenzyme A—acetyl groups derived from pyruvate, fatty acids, and amino acids Some intermediates derived from amino acids
Enzyme location	Inner compartment of mitochondria (the mitochondrial matrix)
ATP production	1 GTP formed directly, which can be converted into ATP Operates only under aerobic conditions even though molecular oxygen is not used directly in this pathway
Coenzyme production	3 NADH + 3 H^+ and 2 $FADH_2$
Final products	2 CO_2 for each molecule of acetyl coenzyme A entering pathway Some intermediates used to synthesize amino acids and other organic molecules required for special cell functions
Net reaction	Acetyl CoA + 3 NAD^+ + FAD + GDP + P_i + 2 $H_2O \longrightarrow$ 2 CO_2 + CoA + 3 NADH + 3 H^+ + $FADH_2$ + GTP

of fatty acids (see the discussion that follows), and—to a much lesser extent—during glycolysis. The net reaction is

$$\frac{1}{2} O_2 + NADH + H^+ \longrightarrow H_2O + NAD^+ + \text{Energy}$$

Unlike the enzymes of the Krebs cycle, which are soluble enzymes in the mitochondrial matrix, the proteins that mediate oxidative phosphorylation are embedded in the inner mitochondrial membrane. The proteins for oxidative phosphorylation can be divided into two groups: (1) those that mediate the series of reactions that cause the transfer of hydrogen ions to molecular oxygen, and (2) those that couple the energy released by these reactions to the synthesis of ATP.

Some of the first group of proteins contain iron and copper cofactors and are known as **cytochromes** (because in pure form they are brightly colored). Their structure resembles the red iron–containing hemoglobin molecule, which binds oxygen in red blood cells. The cytochromes and associated proteins form the components of the **electron-transport chain,** in which two electrons from hydrogen atoms are initially transferred either from NADH + H^+ or $FADH_2$ to one of the elements in this chain. These electrons are then successively transferred to other compounds in the chain, often to or from an iron or copper ion, until the electrons are finally transferred to molecular oxygen, which then combines with hydrogen ions (protons) to form water. These hydrogen ions, like the electrons, come from free hydrogen ions and the hydrogen-bearing coenzymes, having been released early in the transport chain when the electrons from the hydrogen atoms were transferred to the cytochromes.

Importantly, in addition to transferring the coenzyme hydrogens to water, this process regenerates the hydrogen-free form of the coenzymes, which then become available to accept two more hydrogens from intermediates in the Krebs cycle, glycolysis, or fatty acid pathway (as described in the discussion that follows). Therefore, the electron-transport chain provides the *aerobic* mechanism for regenerating the hydrogen-free form of the coenzymes, whereas, as described earlier, the *anaerobic* mechanism, which applies only to glycolysis, is coupled to the formation of lactate.

At certain steps along the electron-transport chain, small amounts of energy are released. As electrons are transferred from one protein to another along the electron-transport chain, some of the energy released is used by the cytochromes to pump hydrogen ions from the matrix into the intermembrane space—the compartment between the inner and outer mitochondrial membranes (**Figure 3.45**). This creates a source of potential energy in the form of a hydrogen-ion-concentration gradient across the membrane. As you will learn in Chapter 4, solutes such as hydrogen ions move—or diffuse—along concentration gradients, but the presence of a lipid bilayer blocks the diffusion of most water-soluble molecules and ions. Embedded in the inner mitochondrial membrane, however, is an enzyme called **ATP synthase.** This enzyme forms a channel in the inner mitochondrial membrane, allowing the hydrogen ions to flow back to the matrix side, a process that is known as **chemiosmosis.** In the process, the energy of the concentration gradient is converted into chemical bond energy by ATP synthase, which catalyzes the formation of ATP from ADP and P_i.

$FADH_2$ enters the electron-transport chain at a point beyond that of NADH and therefore does not contribute quite as much to chemiosmosis. The processes associated with chemiosmosis are not perfectly stoichiometric, however, because some of the NADH that is produced in glycolysis and the Krebs cycle is used for other cellular activities, such as the synthesis of certain organic molecules. Also, some of the hydrogen ions in the mitochondria are used for other activities besides the generation of ATP. Therefore, the transfer of electrons to oxygen typically produces on average approximately 2.5 and 1.5 molecules of ATP for each molecule of NADH + H^+ and $FADH_2$, respectively.

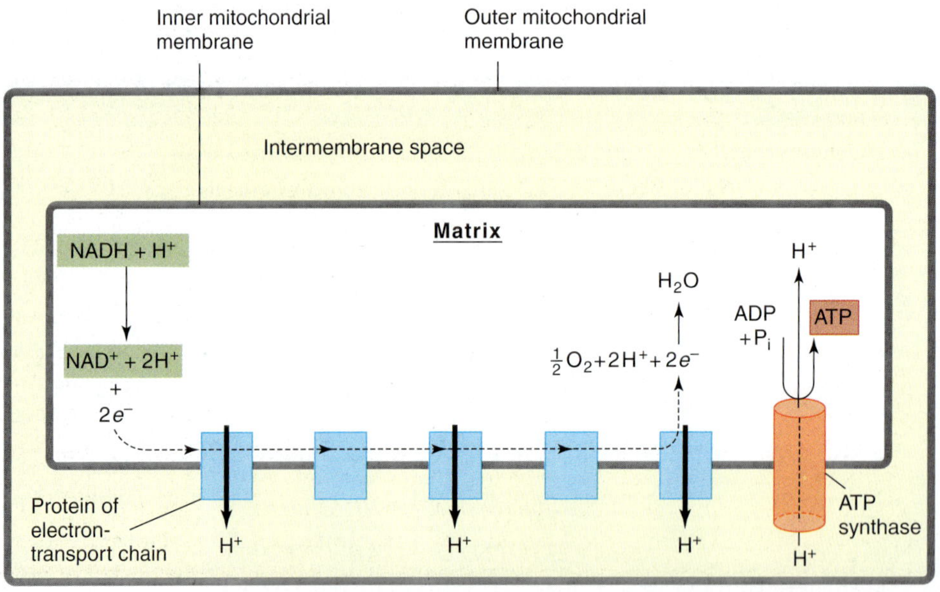

Figure 3.45 APR ATP is formed during oxidative phosphorylation by the flow of electrons along a series of proteins shown here as blue rectangles on the inner mitochondrial membrane. Each time an electron hops from one site to another along the transport chain, it releases energy, which is used by three of the transport proteins to pump hydrogen ions into the intermembrane space of the mitochondria. The hydrogen ions then flow down their concentration gradient across the inner mitochondrial membrane through a channel created by ATP synthase, shown here in red. The energy derived from this concentration gradient and flow of hydrogen ions is used by ATP synthase to synthesize ATP from ADP + P_i. A maximum of two to three molecules of ATP can be produced per pair of electrons donated, depending on the point at which a particular coenzyme enters the electron-transport chain. For simplicity, only the coenzyme NADH is shown.

TABLE 3.9	Characteristics of Oxidative Phosphorylation
Entering substrates	Hydrogen atoms obtained from $NADH + H^+$ and $FADH_2$ formed (1) during glycolysis, (2) by the Krebs cycle during the breakdown of pyruvate and amino acids, and (3) during the breakdown of fatty acids Molecular oxygen
Enzyme location	Inner mitochondrial membrane
ATP production	2–3 ATP formed from each $NADH + H^+$ 1–2 ATP formed from each $FADH_2$
Final products	H_2O—one molecule for each pair of hydrogens entering pathway
Net reaction	$\frac{1}{2}O_2 + NADH + H^+ + 3\ ADP + 3\ P_i \longrightarrow H_2O + NAD^+ + 3\ ATP$

In summary, most ATP formed in the body is produced during oxidative phosphorylation as a result of processing hydrogen atoms that originated largely from the Krebs cycle during the breakdown of carbohydrates, fats, and proteins. The mitochondria, where the oxidative phosphorylation and the Krebs-cycle reactions occur, are thus considered the powerhouses of the cell. In addition, most of the oxygen we breathe is consumed within these organelles, and most of the carbon dioxide we exhale is produced within them as well.

Table 3.9 summarizes the key features of oxidative phosphorylation.

3.15 Carbohydrate, Fat, and Protein Metabolism

Now that we have described the three pathways by which energy is transferred to ATP, let's consider how each of the three classes of energy-yielding nutrient molecules—carbohydrates, fats, and proteins—enters the ATP-generating pathways. We will also consider the synthesis of these molecules and the pathways and restrictions governing their conversion from one class to another. These anabolic pathways are also used to synthesize molecules that have functions other than the storage and release of energy. For example, with the addition of a few enzymes, the pathway for fat synthesis is also used for synthesis of the phospholipids found in membranes.

The material presented in this section should serve as a foundation for understanding how the body copes with changes in nutrient availability. The physiological mechanisms that regulate appetite, digestion, and absorption of food; transport of energy sources in the blood and across plasma membranes; and the body's responses to fasting and starvation are covered in Chapter 16.

Carbohydrate Metabolism

Carbohydrate Catabolism

In the previous sections, we described the major pathways of carbohydrate catabolism: the breakdown of glucose to pyruvate or lactate by way of the glycolytic pathway, and the metabolism of pyruvate to carbon dioxide and water by way of the Krebs cycle and oxidative phosphorylation.

The amount of energy released during the catabolism of glucose to carbon dioxide and water is 686 kcal/mol of glucose:

$$C_6H_{12}O_6 + 6\ O_2 \longrightarrow 6\ H_2O + 6\ CO_2 + 686\ \text{kcal/mol}$$

About 40% of this energy is transferred to ATP. **Figure 3.46** summarizes the points at which ATP forms during glucose catabolism. A net gain of two ATP molecules occurs by substrate-level phosphorylation during glycolysis, and two more are formed during the Krebs cycle from GTP, one from each of the two molecules of pyruvate entering the cycle. The majority of ATP molecules glucose catabolism produces—up to 34 ATP per molecule—form during oxidative phosphorylation from the hydrogens generated at various steps during glucose breakdown.

Because in the absence of oxygen only two molecules of ATP can form from the breakdown of glucose to lactate, the evolution of aerobic metabolic pathways greatly increases the amount of energy available to a cell from glucose catabolism. For example, if a muscle consumed 38 molecules of ATP during a contraction, this amount of ATP could be supplied by the breakdown of one molecule of glucose in the presence of oxygen or 19 molecules of glucose under anaerobic conditions.

However, although only two molecules of ATP are formed per molecule of glucose under anaerobic conditions, large amounts of ATP can still be supplied by the glycolytic pathway if large amounts of glucose are broken down to lactate. This is not an efficient utilization of nutrients, but it does permit continued ATP production under anaerobic conditions, such as occur during intense exercise.

Glycogen Storage

A small amount of glucose can be stored in the body to provide a reserve supply for use when glucose is not being absorbed into the blood from the small intestine. Recall from Chapter 2 that it is stored as the polysaccharide **glycogen,** mostly in skeletal muscles and the liver.

Glycogen is synthesized from glucose by the pathway illustrated in **Figure 3.47**. The enzymes for both glycogen synthesis and glycogen breakdown are located in the cytosol. The first step in glycogen synthesis, the transfer of phosphate from a molecule of ATP to glucose, forming glucose 6-phosphate, is the same as the first step in glycolysis. Thus, glucose 6-phosphate can either be broken down to pyruvate or used to form glycogen.

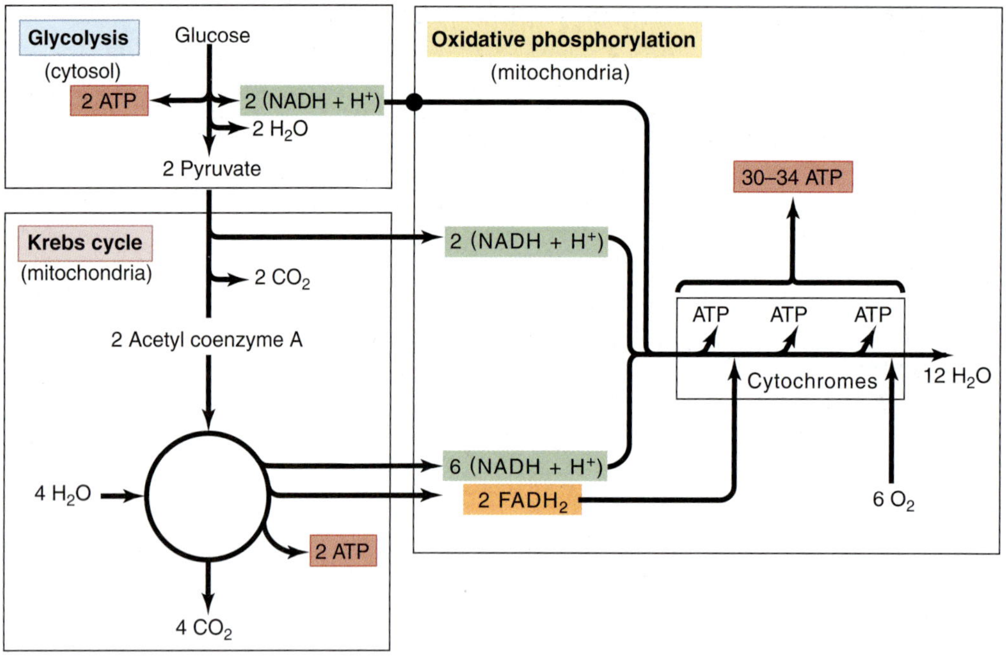

$$C_6H_{12}O_6 + 6\ O_2 + 38\ ADP + 38\ P_i \longrightarrow 6\ CO_2 + 6\ H_2O + 34\text{–}38\ ATP$$

Figure 3.46 APR Pathways of glycolysis and aerobic glucose catabolism and their linkage to ATP formation. The value of 38 ATP molecules is a theoretical maximum assuming that all molecules of NADH produced in glycolysis and the Krebs cycle enter into the oxidative phosphorylation pathway, and all of the free hydrogen ions are used in chemiosmosis for ATP synthesis.

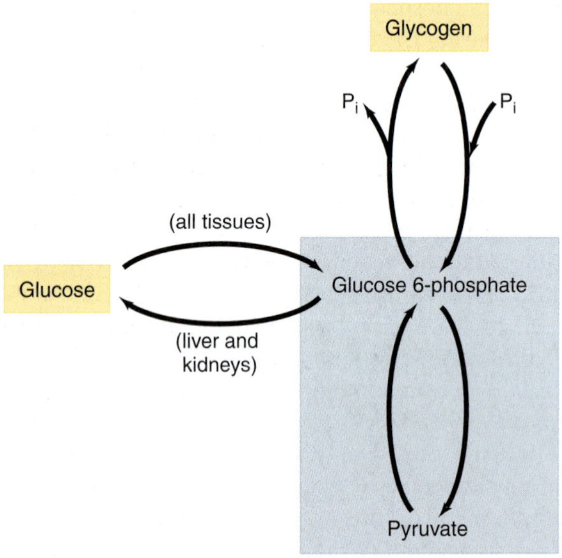

Figure 3.47 Pathways for glycogen synthesis and breakdown. Each bowed arrow indicates one or more irreversible reactions that require different enzymes to catalyze the reaction in the forward and reverse directions.

As indicated in Figure 3.47, different enzymes synthesize and break down glycogen. The existence of two pathways containing enzymes that are subject to both covalent and allosteric modulation provides a mechanism for regulating the flow between glucose and glycogen. When an excess of glucose is available to a liver or muscle cell, the enzymes in the glycogen-synthesis pathway are activated and the enzyme that breaks down glycogen is simultaneously inhibited. This combination leads to the net storage of glucose in the form of glycogen.

When less glucose is available, the reverse combination of enzyme stimulation and inhibition occurs, and net breakdown of glycogen to glucose 6-phosphate (known as **glycogenolysis**) ensues. Two paths are available to this glucose 6-phosphate: (1) in most cells, including skeletal muscle, it enters the glycolytic pathway where it is catabolized to provide the energy for ATP formation; (2) in liver and kidney cells, glucose 6-phosphate can be converted to free glucose by removal of the phosphate group, and the glucose is then able to pass out of the cell into the blood to provide energy for other cells.

Glucose Synthesis

In addition to being formed in the liver from the breakdown of glycogen, glucose can be synthesized in the liver and kidneys from intermediates derived from the catabolism of glycerol (a sugar alcohol) and some amino acids. This process of generating new molecules of glucose from noncarbohydrate precursors is known as **gluconeogenesis.** The major substrate in gluconeogenesis is pyruvate, formed from lactate as described earlier, and from several amino acids during protein breakdown. In addition, glycerol derived from the hydrolysis of triglycerides can be converted into glucose via a pathway that does not involve pyruvate.

The pathway for gluconeogenesis in the liver and kidneys (**Figure 3.48**) makes use of many but not all of the enzymes used in glycolysis because most of these reactions are reversible. However, reactions 1, 3, and 10 (see Figure 3.41) are irreversible, and additional enzymes are required, therefore, to form glucose from pyruvate. Pyruvate is converted to phosphoenolpyruvate by a series of mitochondrial reactions in which CO_2 is added to pyruvate to form the four-carbon Krebs-cycle intermediate oxaloacetate. An additional series of reactions leads to the transfer of a four-carbon intermediate derived from oxaloacetate out of the mitochondria and its conversion to phosphoenolpyruvate in the cytosol. Phosphoenolpyruvate then reverses the steps of glycolysis back to the level of reaction 3, in which a different enzyme from that used in glycolysis is required to convert fructose 1,6-bisphosphate to fructose 6-phosphate. From this point on, the reactions are again reversible, leading to glucose

6-phosphate, which can be converted to glucose in the liver and kidneys or stored as glycogen. Because energy in the form of heat and ATP generation is released during the glycolytic breakdown of glucose to pyruvate, energy must be added to reverse this pathway. A total of six ATP are consumed in the reactions of gluconeogenesis per molecule of glucose formed.

Many of the same enzymes are used in glycolysis and gluconeogenesis, so the questions arise: What controls the direction of the reactions in these pathways? What conditions determine whether glucose is broken down to pyruvate or whether pyruvate is converted into glucose? The answers lie in the concentrations of glucose or pyruvate in a cell and in the control the enzymes exert in the irreversible steps in the pathway. This control is carried out via various hormones that alter the concentrations and activities of these key enzymes. For example, if blood glucose concentrations fall below normal, certain hormones are secreted into the blood and act on the liver. There, the hormones preferentially induce the expression of the gluconeogenic enzymes, thereby favoring the formation of glucose.

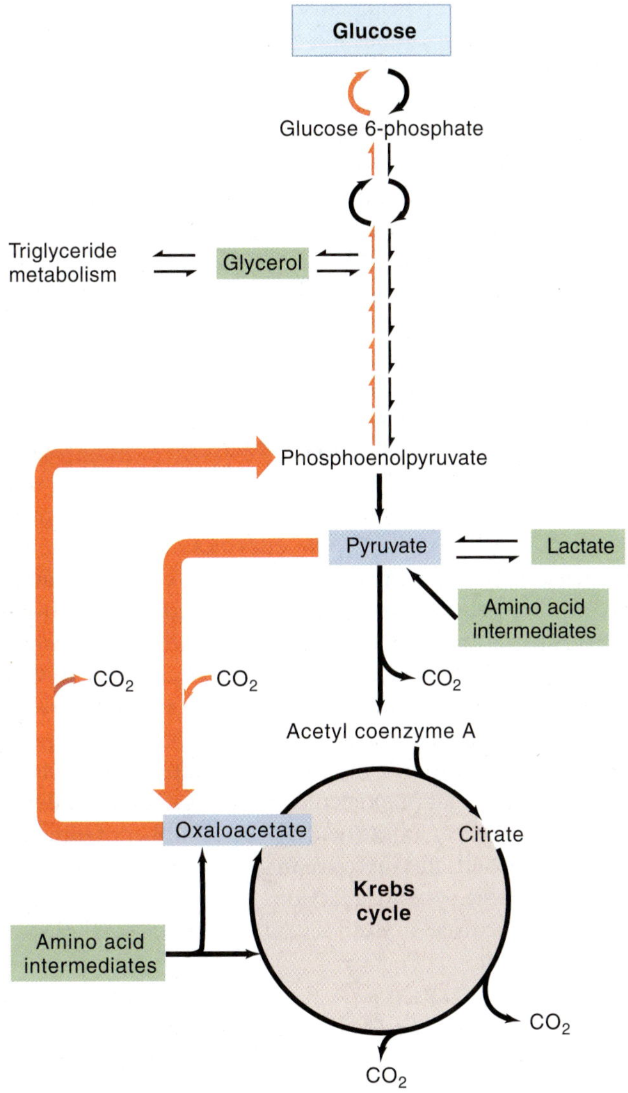

Figure 3.48 Gluconeogenic pathway by which pyruvate, lactate, glycerol, and various amino acid intermediates can be converted into glucose in the liver (and kidneys). Note the points at which each of these precursors, supplied by the blood, enters the pathway.

Fat Metabolism

Fat Catabolism

Triglyceride (fat) consists of three fatty acids bound to glycerol (Chapter 2). Fat typically accounts for approximately 80% of the energy stored in the body (**Table 3.10**). Under resting conditions, approximately half the energy used by muscle, liver, and the kidneys is derived from the catabolism of fatty acids.

Although most cells store small amounts of fat, most of the body's fat is stored in specialized cells known as **adipocytes.** Almost the entire cytoplasm of each of these cells is filled with a single, large fat droplet. Clusters of adipocytes form **adipose tissue,** most of which is in deposits underlying the skin or surrounding internal organs. The function of adipocytes is to synthesize and store triglycerides during periods of food uptake and then, when food is not being absorbed from the small intestine, to release fatty acids and glycerol into the blood for uptake and use by other cells to provide the energy needed for ATP formation. The factors controlling fat storage and release from adipocytes during different physiological states will be described in Chapter 16. Here, we will emphasize the pathway by which most cells catabolize fatty acids to provide the energy for ATP synthesis, and the pathway by which other molecules are used to synthesize fatty acids.

Figure 3.49 shows the pathway for fatty acid catabolism, which is achieved by enzymes present in the mitochondrial matrix. The breakdown of a fatty acid is initiated by linking a molecule of coenzyme A to the carboxyl end of the fatty acid. This initial step is accompanied by the breakdown of ATP to AMP and two P_i.

The coenzyme-A derivative of the fatty acid then proceeds through a series of reactions, collectively known as **beta oxidation,** which splits off a molecule of acetyl coenzyme A from the end of the fatty acid and transfers two pairs of hydrogen atoms to coenzymes (one pair to FAD and the other to NAD^+). The hydrogen atoms from the coenzymes then enter the oxidative-phosphorylation pathway to form ATP.

When an acetyl coenzyme A is split from the end of a fatty acid, another coenzyme A is added (ATP is not required for this step), and the sequence is repeated. Each passage through this sequence shortens the fatty acid chain by two carbon atoms until all the carbon atoms have transferred to coenzyme-A molecules. As we saw, these molecules then lead to production of CO_2 and ATP via the Krebs cycle and oxidative phosphorylation.

How much ATP is formed as a result of the total catabolism of a fatty acid? Most fatty acids in the body contain 14 to

TABLE 3.10 Energy Content of a 70 kg Person

	Total-Body Content (kg)	Energy Content (kcal/g)	Total-Body Energy Content (kcal)	%
Triglycerides	15.6	9	140,000	78
Proteins	9.5	4	38,000	21
Carbohydrates	0.5	4	2000	1

22 carbons, 16 and 18 being most common. The catabolism of one 18-carbon saturated fatty acid yields 146 ATP molecules. In contrast, as we have seen, the catabolism of one glucose molecule yields a maximum of 38 ATP molecules. Thus, taking into account the difference in molecular weight of the fatty acid and glucose, the amount of ATP formed from the catabolism of a gram of fat is about 2½ times greater than the amount of ATP produced by catabolizing 1 gram of carbohydrate. If an average person stored most of his or her energy as carbohydrate rather than fat, body weight would have to be approximately 30% greater in order to store the same amount of usable energy, and the person would consume more energy moving this extra weight around. Thus, a major step in energy economy occurred when animals evolved the ability to store energy as fat.

Fat Synthesis

The synthesis of fatty acids occurs by reactions that are almost the reverse of those that degrade them. However, the enzymes in the synthetic pathway are in the cytosol, whereas (as we have just seen) the enzymes catalyzing fatty acid breakdown are in the mitochondria. Fatty acid synthesis begins with cytoplasmic acetyl coenzyme A, which transfers its acetyl group to another molecule of acetyl coenzyme A to form a four-carbon chain. By repetition of this process, long-chain fatty acids are built up two carbons at a time. This accounts for the fact that all the fatty acids synthesized in the body contain an even number of carbon atoms.

Once the fatty acids are formed, triglycerides can be synthesized by linking fatty acids to each of the three hydroxyl groups in glycerol, more specifically, to a phosphorylated form of glycerol called **α-glycerol phosphate.** The synthesis of triglyceride is carried out by enzymes associated with the membranes of the smooth endoplasmic reticulum.

Compare the molecules produced by glucose catabolism with those required for synthesis of both fatty acids and α-glycerol phosphate. First, acetyl coenzyme A, the starting material for fatty acid synthesis, can be formed from pyruvate, the end product of glycolysis. Second, the other ingredients required for fatty acid synthesis—hydrogen-bound coenzymes and ATP—are produced during carbohydrate catabolism. Third, α-glycerol phosphate can be formed from a glucose intermediate. It should not be surprising, therefore, that much of the carbohydrate in food is converted into fat and stored in adipose tissue shortly after its absorption from the gastrointestinal tract.

Importantly, fatty acids—or, more specifically, the acetyl coenzyme A derived from fatty acid breakdown—cannot be used to synthesize *new* molecules of glucose. We can see the reasons for this by examining the pathways for glucose synthesis (see Figure 3.48). First, because the reaction in which pyruvate is broken down to acetyl coenzyme A and carbon dioxide is irreversible, acetyl coenzyme A cannot be converted into pyruvate, a molecule that could lead to the production of glucose. Second, the equivalents of the two carbon atoms in acetyl coenzyme A are converted into two molecules of carbon dioxide during their passage through the Krebs cycle before reaching oxaloacetate, another takeoff point for glucose synthesis; therefore, they cannot be used to synthesize *net* amounts of oxaloacetate.

Therefore, *glucose can readily be converted into fat, but the fatty acid portion of fat cannot be converted to glucose.*

Protein and Amino Acid Metabolism

In contrast to the complexities of protein synthesis, protein catabolism requires only a few enzymes, collectively called **proteases,** to break the peptide bonds between amino acids (a process called **proteolysis**). Some of these enzymes remove one amino acid at a time from the ends of the protein chain, whereas others break peptide bonds between specific amino acids within the chain, forming peptides rather than free amino acids.

Amino acids can be catabolized to provide energy for ATP synthesis, and they can also provide intermediates for the synthesis of a number of molecules other than proteins. Because there are 20 different amino acids, a large number of intermediates can be formed, and there are many pathways for processing them. A few basic types of reactions common to most of these pathways can provide an overview of amino acid catabolism.

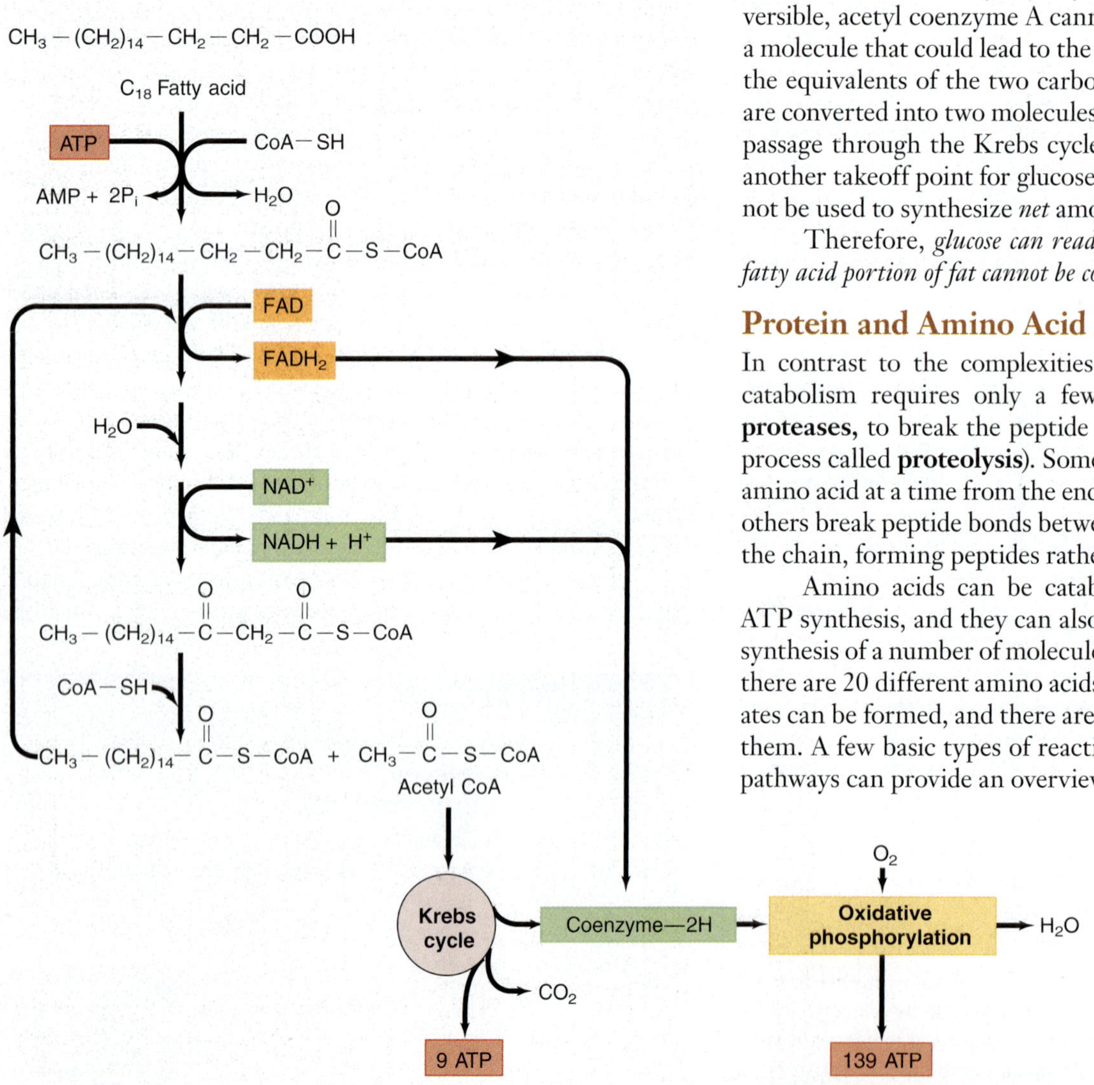

Figure 3.49 Pathway of fatty acid catabolism in mitochondria. The energy equivalent of two ATP is consumed at the start of the pathway, for a *net* gain of 146 ATP for this C18 fatty acid.

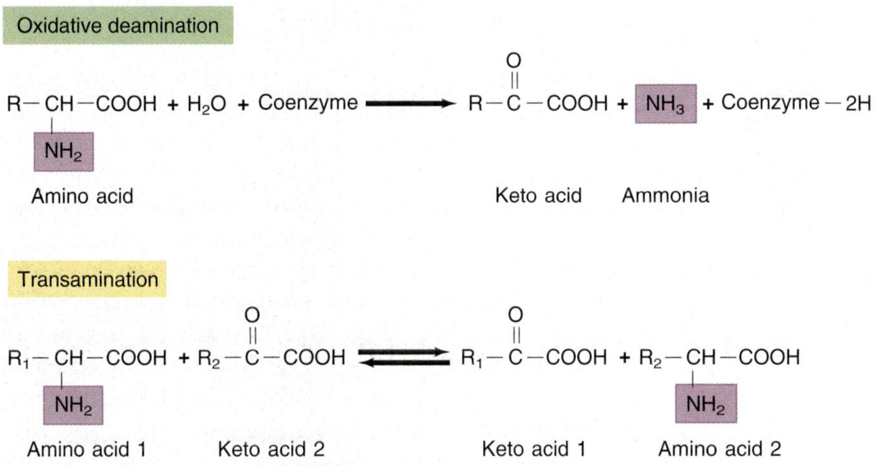

Figure 3.50 Oxidative deamination and transamination of amino acids.

Unlike most carbohydrates and fats, amino acids contain nitrogen atoms (in their amino groups) in addition to carbon, hydrogen, and oxygen atoms. Once the nitrogen-containing amino group is removed, the remainder of most amino acids can be metabolized to intermediates capable of entering either the glycolytic pathway or the Krebs cycle.

Figure 3.50 illustrates the two types of reactions by which the amino group is removed. In the first reaction, **oxidative deamination,** the amino group gives rise to a molecule of ammonia (NH_3) and is replaced by an oxygen atom derived from water to form a **keto acid,** a categorical name rather than the name of a specific molecule. The second means of removing an amino group is known as **transamination** and involves transfer of the amino group from an amino acid to a keto acid. Note that the keto acid to which the amino group is transferred becomes an amino acid. Cells can also use the nitrogen derived from amino groups to synthesize other important nitrogen-containing molecules, such as the purine and pyrimidine bases found in nucleic acids.

Figure 3.51 illustrates the oxidative deamination of the amino acid glutamic acid and the transamination of the amino acid alanine. Note that the keto acids formed are intermediates either in the Krebs cycle (α-ketoglutaric acid) or glycolytic pathway (pyruvic acid). Once formed, these keto acids can be metabolized to produce carbon dioxide and form ATP, or they can be used as intermediates in the synthetic pathway leading to the formation of glucose. As a third alternative, they can be used to synthesize fatty acids after their conversion to acetyl coenzyme A by way of pyruvic acid. Therefore, amino acids can be used as a source of energy, and some can be converted into carbohydrate and fat.

The ammonia that oxidative deamination produces is highly toxic to cells if allowed to accumulate. Fortunately, it passes through plasma membranes and enters the blood, which carries it to the liver. The liver contains enzymes that can combine two molecules of ammonia with carbon dioxide to form **urea,** which is relatively nontoxic and is the major nitrogenous waste product of protein catabolism. It enters the blood from the liver and is excreted by the kidneys into the urine.

Thus far, we have discussed mainly amino acid catabolism; now we turn to amino acid synthesis. The keto acids pyruvic acid and α-ketoglutaric acid can be derived from the breakdown of glucose; they can then be transaminated, as described previously, to form the amino acids glutamate and alanine. Therefore, glucose can be used to produce certain amino acids, provided other amino acids are available in the diet to supply amino groups for transamination. However, only 11 of the 20 amino acids can be formed by this process because nine of the specific keto acids cannot be synthesized from other intermediates. We have to obtain the nine amino acids corresponding to these keto acids from the food we eat; consequently, they are known as **essential amino acids.**

Figure 3.52 provides a summary of the multiple routes by which the body handles amino acids. The amino acid pools, which consist of the body's total free amino acids, are derived from (1) ingested protein, which is degraded to amino acids during digestion in the small intestine; (2) the synthesis of nonessential amino acids from the keto acids derived from carbohydrates and fat; and (3) the continuous breakdown of body proteins. These pools are the source of amino acids for the resynthesis of body protein and a host of specialized amino acid derivatives, as well as for conversion to carbohydrate and fat. A very small quantity of amino acids and protein is lost from the body via the urine; skin; hair; fingernails; and, in women, the menstrual fluid. The major route for the loss of amino acids is not their excretion but rather their deamination, with the eventual excretion of the nitrogen atoms as urea in the urine. The terms **negative nitrogen balance** and **positive nitrogen balance** refer to whether there is a net loss or gain, respectively, of amino acids in the body over any period of time.

If any of the essential amino acids are missing from the diet, a negative nitrogen balance—that is, loss greater than gain—always

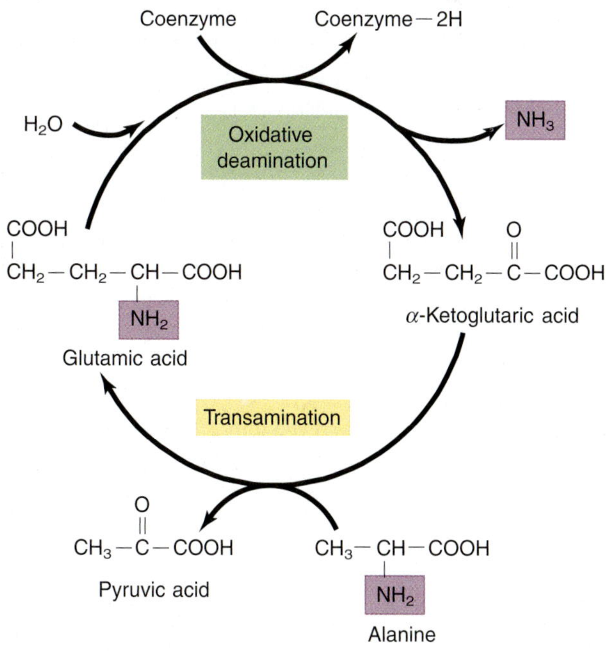

Figure 3.51 Oxidative deamination and transamination of the amino acids glutamic acid and alanine produce keto acids that can enter the carbohydrate pathways.

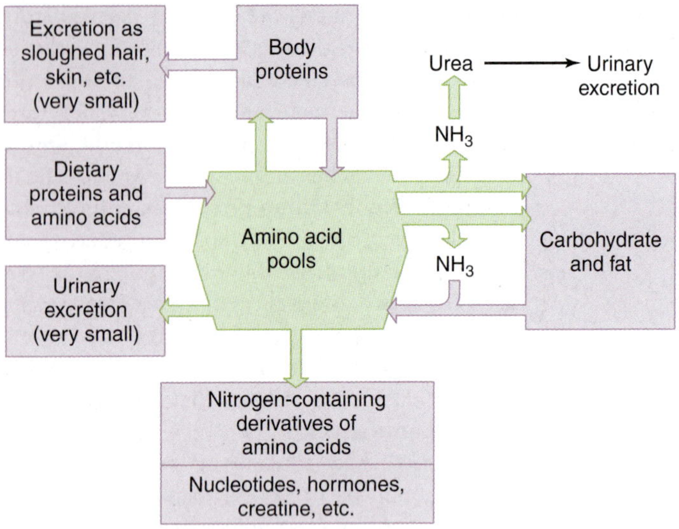

Figure 3.52 Pathways of amino acid metabolism.

results. The proteins that require a missing essential amino acid cannot be synthesized, and the other amino acids that would have been incorporated into these proteins are metabolized. This explains why a dietary requirement for protein cannot be specified without regard to the amino acid composition of that protein. Protein is graded in terms of how closely its relative proportions of essential amino acids approximate those in the average body protein. The highest-quality proteins are found in animal products, whereas the quality of most plant proteins is lower. Nevertheless, it is quite possible to obtain adequate quantities of all essential amino acids from a mixture of plant proteins alone.

Metabolism Summary

Having discussed the metabolism of the three major classes of organic molecules, we can now briefly review how each class is related to the others and to the process of synthesizing ATP. **Figure 3.53** illustrates the major pathways we have discussed and the relationships between the common intermediates. All three classes of molecules can enter the Krebs cycle through some intermediate; therefore, all three can be used as a source of energy for the synthesis of ATP. Glucose can be converted into fat or into some amino acids by way of common intermediates such as pyruvate, oxaloacetate, and acetyl coenzyme A. Similarly, some amino acids can be converted into glucose and fat. Fatty acids cannot be converted into glucose because of the irreversibility of the reaction converting pyruvate to acetyl coenzyme A, but the glycerol portion of triglycerides can be converted into glucose. Fatty acids can be used to synthesize portions of the keto acids used to form some amino acids. Metabolism is therefore a highly integrated process in which all classes of nutrient macromolecules can be used to provide energy and in which each class of molecule can be used to synthesize most but not all members of other classes.

3.16 Essential Nutrients

About 50 substances required for normal or optimal body function cannot be synthesized by the body or are synthesized in amounts inadequate to keep pace with the rates at which they are broken down or excreted. Such substances are known as **essential nutrients** (**Table 3.11**). Because they are all removed from the body at some finite rate, they must be continually supplied in the foods we eat.

The term *essential nutrient* is reserved for substances that fulfill two criteria: (1) they must be essential for health, and (2) they must not be synthesized by the body in adequate amounts. Therefore, glucose, although "essential" for normal metabolism, is not classified as an essential nutrient because the body normally can synthesize all it requires, from amino acids, for example. Furthermore, the quantity of an essential nutrient that must be present in the diet to maintain health is not a criterion for determining whether the substance is essential. Approximately 1500 g of water, 2 g of the amino acid methionine, and only about 1 mg of the vitamin thiamine are required per day.

Water is an essential nutrient because the body loses far more water in the urine and from the skin and respiratory tract than it can synthesize. (Recall that water forms as an end product of oxidative phosphorylation as well as from several other metabolic reactions.) Therefore, to maintain water balance, water intake is essential.

The mineral elements are examples of substances the body cannot synthesize or break down but that the body continually loses in the urine, feces, and various secretions. The major

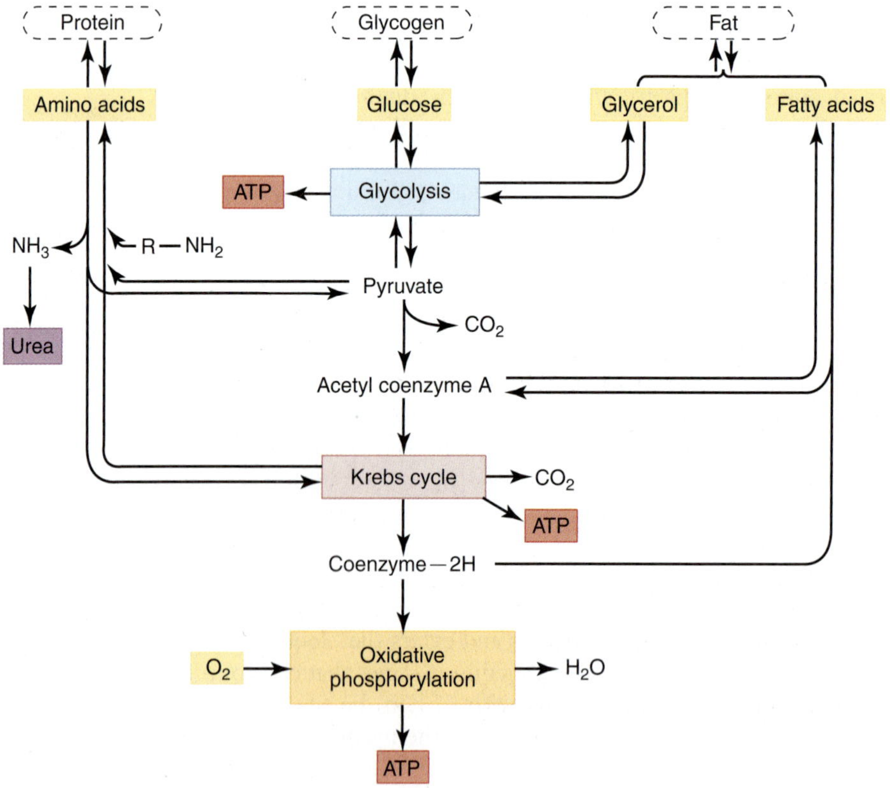

Figure 3.53 The relationships between the pathways for the metabolism of protein, carbohydrate (glycogen), and fat (triglyceride).

TABLE 3.11 Essential Nutrients	
Water	
Mineral Elements	
7 major mineral elements (see Table 2.1)	
13 trace elements (see Table 2.1)	
Essential Amino Acids	
Histidine	
Isoleucine	
Leucine	
Lysine	
Methionine	
Phenylalanine	
Threonine	
Tryptophan	
Valine	
Essential Fatty Acids	
Linoleic acid	
Linolenic acid	
Vitamins	
Water-soluble vitamins	
B_1: thiamine	Vitamin B complex
B_2: riboflavin	Vitamin B complex
B_6: pyridoxine	Vitamin B complex
B_{12}: cobalamine	Vitamin B complex
Niacin	Vitamin B complex
Pantothenic acid	Vitamin B complex
Folic acid	Vitamin B complex
Biotin	Vitamin B complex
Lipoic acid	
Vitamin C	
Fat-soluble vitamins	
Vitamin A	
Vitamin D	
Vitamin E	
Vitamin K	
Other Essential Nutrients	
Inositol	
Choline	
Carnitine	

minerals must be supplied in fairly large amounts, whereas only small quantities of the trace elements are required.

We have already noted that nine of the 20 amino acids are essential. Two fatty acids, linoleic and linolenic acid, which contain a number of double bonds and serve important roles in chemical messenger systems, are also essential nutrients. Three additional essential nutrients—inositol, choline, and carnitine—have functions that will be described in later chapters but do not fall into any common category other than being essential nutrients. Finally, the class of essential nutrients known as vitamins deserves special attention.

Vitamins

Vitamins are a group of 14 organic essential nutrients required in very small amounts in the diet. The exact chemical structures of the first vitamins to be discovered were unknown, and they were simply identified by letters of the alphabet. Vitamin B turned out to be composed of eight substances now known as the vitamin B complex. Plants and bacteria have the enzymes necessary for vitamin synthesis, and we get our vitamins by eating either plants or meat from animals that have eaten plants.

The vitamins as a class have no particular chemical structure in common, but they can be divided into the **water-soluble vitamins** and the **fat-soluble vitamins.** The water-soluble vitamins form portions of coenzymes such as NAD^+, FAD, and coenzyme A. The fat-soluble vitamins (A, D, E, and K) in general do not function as coenzymes. For example, vitamin A (retinol) is used to form the light-sensitive pigment in the eye, and lack of this vitamin leads to night blindness. The specific functions of each of the fat-soluble vitamins will be described in later chapters.

The catabolism of vitamins does not provide chemical energy, although some vitamins participate as coenzymes in chemical reactions that release energy from other molecules. Increasing the amount of a vitamin in the diet beyond a certain minimum does not necessarily increase the activity of those enzymes for which the vitamin functions as a coenzyme. Only very small quantities of coenzymes participate in the chemical reactions that require them, and increasing the concentration above this level does not increase the reaction rate.

The fate of large quantities of ingested vitamins varies depending upon whether the vitamin is water-soluble or fat-soluble. As the amount of water-soluble vitamins in the diet is increased, so is the amount excreted in the urine; therefore, the accumulation of these vitamins in the body is limited. On the other hand, fat-soluble vitamins can accumulate in the body because they are poorly excreted by the kidneys and because they dissolve in the fat stores in adipose tissue. The intake of very large quantities of fat-soluble vitamins can produce toxic effects.

SECTION E SUMMARY

Cellular Energy Transfer

I. The end products of glycolysis under aerobic conditions are ATP and pyruvate; the end products under anaerobic conditions are ATP and lactate.
   a. Carbohydrates are the only major nutrient molecules that can enter the glycolytic pathway, and the enzymes that facilitate this pathway are located in the cytosol.
   b. Hydrogen atoms generated by glycolysis are transferred either to NAD^+, which then transfers them to pyruvate to form lactate, thereby regenerating the original coenzyme molecule; or to the oxidative-phosphorylation pathway.
   c. The formation of ATP in glycolysis occurs by substrate-level phosphorylation, a process in which a phosphate group is transferred from a phosphorylated metabolic intermediate directly to ADP.

II. The Krebs cycle catabolizes molecular fragments derived from nutrient molecules and produces carbon dioxide, hydrogen atoms, and ATP. The enzymes that mediate the cycle are located in the mitochondrial matrix.
   a. Acetyl coenzyme A, the acetyl portion of which is derived from all three types of nutrient macromolecules, is the major substrate entering the Krebs cycle. Amino acids can also enter at several places in the cycle by being converted to cycle intermediates.

b. During one rotation of the Krebs cycle, two molecules of carbon dioxide are produced, and four pairs of hydrogen atoms are transferred to coenzymes. Substrate-level phosphorylation produces one molecule of GTP, which can be converted to ATP.

III. Oxidative phosphorylation forms ATP from ADP and P_i, using the energy released when molecular oxygen ultimately combines with hydrogen atoms to form water.

a. The enzymes for oxidative phosphorylation are located on the inner membranes of mitochondria.

b. Hydrogen atoms derived from glycolysis, the Krebs cycle, and the breakdown of fatty acids are delivered, most bound to coenzymes, to the electron-transport chain. The electron-transport chain then regenerates the hydrogen-free forms of the coenzymes NAD^+ and FAD by transferring the hydrogens to molecular oxygen to form water.

c. The reactions of the electron-transport chain produce a hydrogen ion gradient across the inner mitochondrial membrane. The flow of hydrogen ions back across the membrane provides the energy for ATP synthesis.

Carbohydrate, Fat, and Protein Metabolism

I. The aerobic catabolism of carbohydrates proceeds through the glycolytic pathway to pyruvate. Pyruvate enters the Krebs cycle and is broken down to carbon dioxide and hydrogens, which are then transferred to coenzymes.

a. About 40% of the chemical energy in glucose can be transferred to ATP under aerobic conditions; the rest is released as heat.

b. Under aerobic conditions, a maximum of 38 molecules of ATP can form from one molecule of glucose: up to 34 from oxidative phosphorylation, two from glycolysis, and two from the Krebs cycle.

c. Under anaerobic conditions, two molecules of ATP can form from one molecule of glucose during glycolysis.

II. Carbohydrates are stored as glycogen, primarily in the liver and skeletal muscles.

a. Different enzymes synthesize and break down glycogen. The control of these enzymes regulates the flow of glucose to and from glycogen.

b. In most cells, glucose 6-phosphate is formed by glycogen breakdown and is catabolized to produce ATP. In liver and kidney cells, glucose can be derived from glycogen and released from the cells into the blood.

III. New glucose can be synthesized (gluconeogenesis) from some amino acids, lactate, and glycerol via the enzymes that catalyze reversible reactions in the glycolytic pathway. Fatty acids cannot be used to synthesize new glucose.

IV. Fat, stored primarily in adipose tissue, provides about 80% of the stored energy in the body.

a. Fatty acids are broken down, two carbon atoms at a time, in the mitochondrial matrix by beta oxidation to form acetyl coenzyme A and hydrogen atoms, which combine with coenzymes.

b. The acetyl portion of acetyl coenzyme A is catabolized to carbon dioxide in the Krebs cycle, and the hydrogen atoms generated there, plus those generated during beta oxidation, enter the oxidative-phosphorylation pathway to form ATP.

c. The amount of ATP formed by the catabolism of 1 g of fat is about 2½ times greater than the amount formed from 1 g of carbohydrate.

d. Fatty acids are synthesized from acetyl coenzyme A by enzymes in the cytosol and are linked to α-glycerol phosphate, produced from carbohydrates, to form triglycerides by enzymes in the smooth endoplasmic reticulum.

V. Proteins are broken down to free amino acids by proteases.

a. The removal of amino groups from amino acids leaves keto acids, which can be either catabolized via the Krebs cycle to provide energy for the synthesis of ATP or converted into glucose and fatty acids.

b. Amino groups are removed by (i) oxidative deamination, which gives rise to ammonia; or by (ii) transamination, in which the amino group is transferred to a keto acid to form a new amino acid.

c. The ammonia formed from the oxidative deamination of amino acids is converted to urea by enzymes in the liver and then excreted in the urine by the kidneys.

VI. Some amino acids can be synthesized from keto acids derived from glucose, whereas others cannot be synthesized by the body and must be provided in the diet.

Essential Nutrients

I. Approximately 50 essential nutrients are necessary for health but cannot be synthesized in adequate amounts by the body and must therefore be provided in the diet.

II. A large intake of water-soluble vitamins leads to their rapid excretion in the urine, whereas a large intake of fat-soluble vitamins leads to their accumulation in adipose tissue and may produce toxic effects.

SECTION E REVIEW QUESTIONS

1. What are the end products of glycolysis under aerobic and anaerobic conditions?
2. What are the major substrates entering the Krebs cycle, and what are the products formed?
3. Why does the Krebs cycle operate only under aerobic conditions even though it does not use molecular oxygen in any of its reactions?
4. Identify the molecules that enter the oxidative-phosphorylation pathway and the products that form.
5. Where are the enzymes for the Krebs cycle located? The enzymes for oxidative phosphorylation? The enzymes for glycolysis?
6. How many molecules of ATP can form from the breakdown of one molecule of glucose under aerobic conditions? Under anaerobic conditions?
7. What molecules can be used to synthesize glucose?
8. Why can't fatty acids be used to synthesize glucose?
9. Describe the pathways used to catabolize fatty acids to carbon dioxide.
10. Why is it more efficient to store energy as fat than as glycogen?
11. Describe the pathway by which glucose is converted into fat.
12. Describe the two processes by which amino groups are removed from amino acids.
13. What can keto acids be converted into?
14. What is the source of the nitrogen atoms in urea, and in what organ is urea synthesized?
15. Why is water considered an essential nutrient whereas glucose is not?
16. What is the consequence of ingesting large quantities of water-soluble vitamins? Fat-soluble vitamins?

SECTION E KEY TERMS

acetyl coenzyme A (acetyl CoA) 82
adipocyte 87
adipose tissue 87
aerobic 80
α-glycerol phosphate 88
ATP synthase 84
beta oxidation 87
chemiosmosis 84
citric acid cycle 81
cytochrome 84
electron-transport chain 84
essential amino acid 89
essential nutrient 90
fat-soluble vitamin 91
gluconeogenesis 87
glycogen 86
glycogenolysis 86
glycolysis 79
keto acid 89
Krebs cycle 81
lactate 80
negative nitrogen balance 89
oxidative deamination 89
oxidative phosphorylation 82
positive nitrogen balance 89
protease 88
proteolysis 88
pyruvate 80
substrate-level phosphorylation 80
transamination 89
tricarboxylic acid cycle 81
urea 89
water-soluble vitamin 91

CHAPTER 3

Clinical Case Study: An Elderly Man Develops Muscle Damage After Changing His Diet

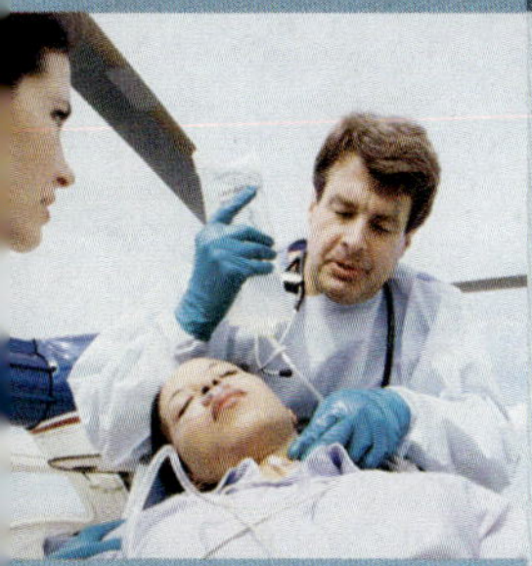

An elderly man and his wife moved from New Jersey to Florida to begin their retirement. The husband had recently been told by his physician in New Jersey that he needed to lose weight and start exercising or he ran the risk of developing type 2 diabetes mellitus. As part of his effort to become healthier, the man began walking daily and adding more fruits and vegetables to his diet in place of red meats and other fatty foods. About 2 weeks after making these changes, he began to feel weakness, tenderness, and cramps in his legs and arms. Eventually, the cramps developed into severe pain, and he also noticed a second alarming change, that his urine had become reddish brown in color. He was admitted into the hospital, where it was determined that he had widespread damage to his skeletal muscles. The dying muscle cells were releasing their intracellular contents into the man's blood; as these substances were filtered by the man's kidneys, they entered the urine and turned the urine a dark color.

After questioning the man, his Florida physician determined that the only change in the man's life and routine—apart from his move to Florida—were the changes in his diet and exercise level. Partly because the exercise (slow walks around the block) was deemed to be very mild, it was ruled out as a contributor to the muscle damage. His medical history revealed that the man had been taking a medication called a "statin" every day for 15 years to decrease his concentration of blood cholesterol. (You will learn more about cholesterol and statins in Chapters 12 and 16.) A rare side effect of statins is damage to skeletal muscle; however, why should this side effect appear suddenly after 15 years, and how could it be linked with this man's change in diet?

Further questioning revealed that the man and his wife had moved to a town that happened to have a large grapefruit orchard in which local residents typically picked their own grapefruits. This seemed like a fortuitous way to supplement his diet with a healthy and fresh citrus fruit, and consequently the man had been drinking up to five large glasses a day of freshly squeezed grapefruit juice since his arrival in town. This information solved the puzzle of what had happened to this man. Grapefruit juice contains a number of compounds called furanocoumarins. These compounds are inhibitors of a very important enzyme located in the small intestine and liver, called cytochrome P450 3A4 (or CYP3A4). The function of CYP3A4 is to metabolize substances in the body that are potentially toxic, including compounds ingested in the diet. Many oral medications are metabolized by this enzyme; you can think of this as the body's way of rejecting ingested compounds that it does not recognize. Recall from Figures 3.37 and 3.38 that one of the key features of enzymes is that their activity can be regulated in several ways. Furanocoumarins inhibit CYP3A4 by covalent inhibition.

Some of the statins, including the one our patient was taking, are metabolized by CYP3A4 in the small intestine. This must be factored into the amount, or dose, of the drug that is given to patients, so that enough of the drug gets into the bloodstream to exert its beneficial effect on decreasing cholesterol concentrations. When the man began drinking grapefruit juice, however, the furanocoumarins inhibited his CYP3A4. Therefore, when he took his usual dose of statin, the amount of the drug entering the blood was greater than normal, and this continued each day as he continued taking his medication. Eventually, the blood concentrations of the statin became very high, and he started to experience muscle damage and other side effects. Once this was determined, the man was advised to substitute other citrus drinks (most of which do not contain furanocoumarins) for grapefruit juice and to stop taking his cholesterol medication until his blood concentrations returned to normal. Additional treatments were initiated to treat his muscle damage.

This case is a fascinating study of how enzymes are regulated and what may happen when an enzyme that should be active instead is inhibited. It also points out the importance of reading the labels on all medications about possibly harmful drug and food interactions.

See Chapter 19 for complete, integrative case studies.

CHAPTER 3 TEST QUESTIONS

Answers found in Appendix A.

1. Which cell structure contains the enzymes required for oxidative phosphorylation?
   a. inner membrane of mitochondria
   b. smooth endoplasmic reticulum
   c. rough endoplasmic reticulum
   d. outer membrane of mitochondria
   e. matrix of mitochondria
2. Which sequence regarding protein synthesis is correct?
   a. translation ⟶ transcription ⟶ mRNA synthesis
   b. transcription ⟶ splicing of primary RNA transcript ⟶ translocation of mRNA ⟶ translation
   c. splicing of introns ⟶ transcription ⟶ mRNA synthesis translation
   d. transcription ⟶ translation ⟶ mRNA production
   e. tRNA enters nucleus ⟶ transcription begins ⟶ mRNA moves to cytoplasm ⟶ protein synthesis begins
3. Which is *incorrect* regarding ligand–protein binding reactions?
   a. Allosteric modulation of the protein's binding site occurs directly at the binding site itself.
   b. Allosteric modulation can alter the affinity of the protein for the ligand.
   c. Phosphorylation of the protein is an example of covalent modulation.
   d. If two ligands can bind to the binding site of the protein, competition for binding will occur.
   e. Binding reactions are either electrical or hydrophobic in nature.
4. According to the law of mass action, in the following reaction,

   $$CO_2 + H_2O \rightleftharpoons H_2CO_3$$

   a. Increasing the concentration of carbon dioxide will slow down the forward (left-to-right) reaction.
   b. Increasing the concentration of carbonic acid will accelerate the rate of the reverse (right-to-left) reaction.
   c. Increasing the concentration of carbon dioxide will speed up the reverse reaction.
   d. Decreasing the concentration of carbonic acid will slow down the forward reaction.
   e. No enzyme is required for either the forward or reverse reaction.
5. Which of the following can be converted to glucose by gluconeogenesis in the liver?
   a. fatty acid
   b. triglyceride
   c. glycerol
   e. glycogen
   d. ATP
6. Which of the following is true?
   a. Triglycerides have the least energy content per gram of the three major energy sources in the body.
   b. Fat catabolism generates new triglycerides for storage in adipose tissue.
   c. By mass, the total-body content of carbohydrates exceeds that of total triglycerides.
   d. Catabolism of fatty acids occurs in two-carbon steps.
   e. Triglycerides are the major lipids found in plasma membranes.

CHAPTER 3 GENERAL PRINCIPLES ASSESSMENT

Answers found in Appendix A.

1. How does the general principle that *structure is a determinant of—and has coevolved with—function* pertain to cells or cellular organelles? For example, what might be the significance of the extensive folds of the inner mitochondrial membranes shown in Figure 3.13? (See Figure 3.45 for a hint.) How do the illustrations in Figures 3.28 and 3.32b apply to the relationship between structure and function at the molecular (protein) level?
2. *Physiological processes are dictated by the laws of chemistry and physics.* Referring back to Figure 3.27, explain how this principle applies to the interaction between proteins and ligands.
3. *Physiological processes require the transfer and balance of matter and energy.* How is this general principle illustrated in Figure 3.53, and how does this relate to another key physiological principle that *homeostasis is essential for health and survival?* (You may want to refer back to Figure 1.6 and imagine that the box labeled "Active product" is "ATP.")

CHAPTER 3 QUANTITATIVE AND THOUGHT QUESTIONS

Answers found at www.mhhe.com/widmaier13.

1. A base sequence in a portion of one strand of DNA is A—G—T—G—C—A—A—G—T—C—T. Predict
   a. the base sequence in the complementary strand of DNA.
   b. the base sequence in RNA transcribed from the sequence shown.
2. The triplet code in DNA for the amino acid histidine is G—T—A. Predict the mRNA codon for this amino acid and the tRNA anticodon.
3. If a protein contains 100 amino acids, how many nucleotides will be present in the gene that codes for this protein?

4. A variety of chemical messengers that normally regulate acid secretion in the stomach bind to proteins in the plasma membranes of the acid-secreting cells. Some of these binding reactions lead to increased acid secretion, others to decreased secretion. In what ways might a drug that causes decreased acid secretion be acting on these cells?
5. In one type of diabetes, the plasma concentration of the hormone insulin is normal but the response of the cells that insulin usually binds to is markedly decreased. Suggest a reason for this in terms of the properties of protein-binding sites.
6. The following graph shows the relation between the amount of acid secreted and the concentration of compound X, which stimulates acid secretion in the stomach by binding to a membrane protein. At a plasma concentration of 2 pM, compound X produces an acid secretion of 20 mmol/h.

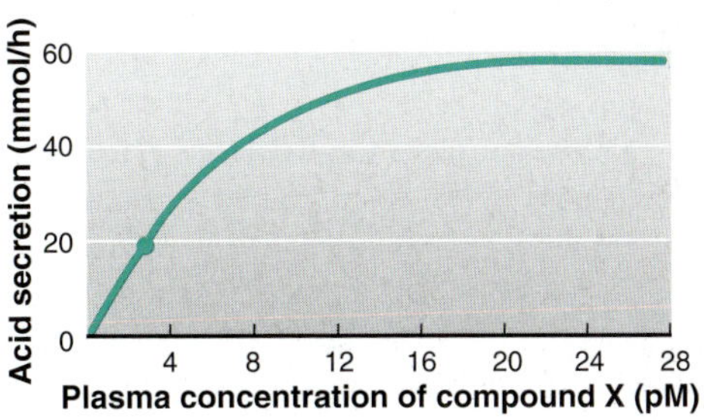

   a. Specify two ways in which acid secretion by compound X could be increased to 40 mmol/h.
   b. Why will increasing the concentration of compound X to 28 pM fail to produce more acid secretion than increasing the concentration of X to 20 pM?
7. In the following metabolic pathway, what is the rate of formation of the end-product E if substrate A is present at a saturating concentration? The maximal rates (products formed per second) of the individual steps are indicated.

$$A \xrightarrow{30} B \xrightarrow{5} C \xrightarrow{20} D \xrightarrow{40} E$$

8. If the concentration of oxygen in the blood delivered to a muscle is increased, what effect will it have on the muscle's rate of ATP production?
9. During prolonged starvation, when glucose is not being absorbed from the gastrointestinal tract, what molecules can be used to synthesize new glucose?
10. How might certain forms of liver disease produce an increase in the blood concentrations of ammonia?

CHAPTER 3 ANSWERS TO PHYSIOLOGICAL INQUIRIES

Figure 3.4 The intracellular fluid compartment includes all of the water in the cytoplasm plus the water in the nucleus. See Chapter 1 for a discussion of the different water compartments in the body.

Figure 3.9 Because tight junctions form a barrier to the transport of most substances across an epithelium, the food you consume remains in the intestine until it is digested into usable components. Thereafter, the digested products can be absorbed across the epithelium in a controlled manner.

Figure 3.19 An example of an alternatively spliced mRNA might appear as follows, where exon number 2 is missing from the mRNA.

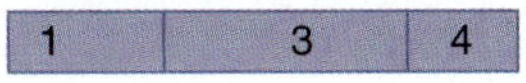

Figure 3.28 It would be easier to design drugs to interact with protein X because it has less chemical specificity. Any of a number of similar-shaped ligands (drugs) could theoretically interact with the protein.

Figure 3.31 Unless the dose of the ligand was sufficiently high to fully saturate both proteins X and Y, the effect of the ligand would probably be to increase blood pressure because at any given ligand concentration, protein Y would have a higher percent saturation than protein X. However, because protein X also binds the ligand to some extent, it would counteract some of the effects of protein Y.

Figure 3.38 If the product were rapidly removed or converted to another product, then the rate of conversion of the substrate into product would increase according to the law of mass action. This is actually typical of what happens in cells.

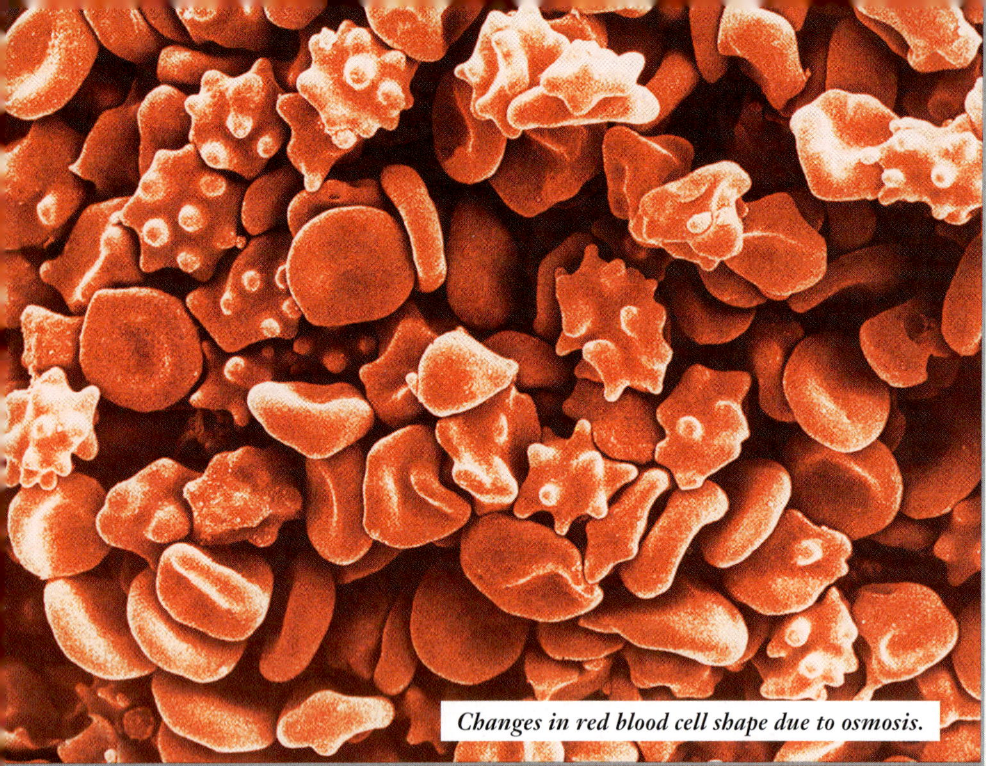

Changes in red blood cell shape due to osmosis.

4 Movement of Molecules Across Cell Membranes

You learned in Chapter 3 that the contents of a cell are separated from the surrounding extracellular fluid by a thin bilayer of lipids and protein, which forms the plasma membrane. You also learned that membranes associated with mitochondria, endoplasmic reticulum, lysosomes, the Golgi apparatus, and the nucleus divide the intracellular fluid into several membrane-bound compartments. The movements of molecules and ions between the various cell organelles and the cytosol, and between the cytosol and the extracellular fluid, depend on the properties of these membranes. The rates at which different substances move through membranes vary considerably and in some cases can be controlled—increased or decreased—in response to various signals. This chapter focuses upon the transport functions of membranes, with emphasis on the plasma membrane. The controlled movement of solutes such as ions, glucose, and gases, as well as the movement of water across membranes, is of profound importance in physiology. As just a few examples, such transport mechanisms are essential for cells to maintain their size and shape, energy balance, and their ability to send and respond to electrical or chemical signals from other cells.

As you read the first section, think how diffusion is a good example of the general principle introduced in Chapter 1 that physiological processes are dictated by the laws of chemistry and physics. In the subsequent sections, consider how the principles of homeostasis and of controlled exchange of materials apply.

4.1 Diffusion

One of the fundamental physical features of molecules of any substance, whether solid, liquid, or gas, is that they are in a continuous state of movement or vibration. The energy for this movement comes from heat; the warmer a substance is, the faster its molecules move. In solutions, such rapidly moving molecules cannot travel very far before colliding with other molecules, undergoing millions of collisions every second. Each collision alters the direction of the molecule's movement, so that the path of any one molecule becomes unpredictable. Because a molecule may at any instant be moving in any direction, such movement is random, with no preferred direction of movement.

The random thermal motion of molecules in a liquid or gas will eventually distribute them uniformly throughout a container. Thus, if we start with a solution in which a solute is more concentrated in one region than another (**Figure 4.1a**), random thermal motion will redistribute the solute from regions of higher concentration to regions of lower concentration until the solute reaches a uniform concentration throughout the solution (**Figure 4.1b**). This movement of molecules from one location to another solely as a result of their random thermal motion is known as **simple diffusion.**

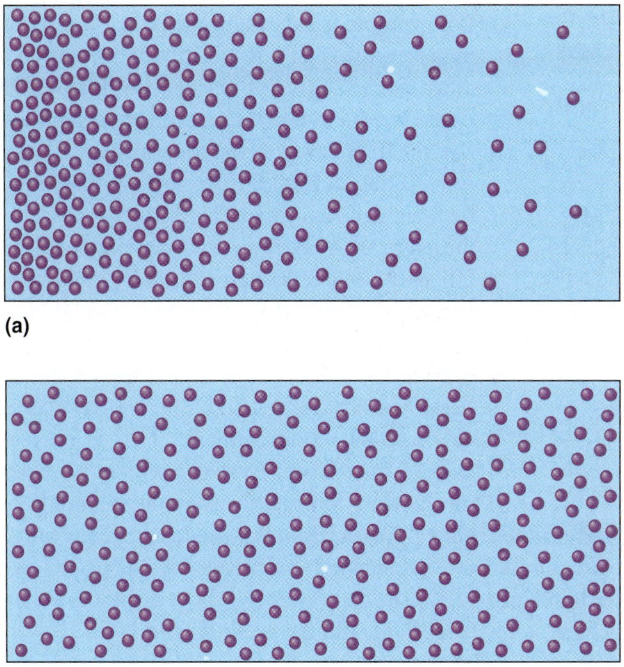

(a)

(b)

Figure 4.1 AP|R Simple diffusion. (a) Molecules initially concentrated in one region of a solution will, due to their random thermal motion, undergo a net diffusion from the region of higher concentration to the region of lower concentration. (b) With time, the molecules will become uniformly distributed throughout the solution.

Many processes in living organisms are closely associated with simple diffusion. For example, oxygen, nutrients, and other molecules enter and leave the smallest blood vessels (capillaries) by simple diffusion, and the movement of many substances across plasma membranes and organelle membranes occurs by simple diffusion. In this way, simple diffusion is one of the key mechanisms by which cells maintain homeostasis. For the remainder of the text, we will often follow convention and refer only to "diffusion" when describing simple diffusion. You will learn later about another type of diffusion called facilitated diffusion.

Magnitude and Direction of Diffusion

Figure 4.2 illustrates the diffusion of glucose between two compartments of equal volume separated by a permeable barrier. Initially, glucose is present in compartment 1 at a concentration of 20 mmol/L, and there is no glucose in compartment 2. The random movements of the glucose molecules in compartment 1 move some of them into compartment 2. The amount of material crossing a surface in a unit of time is known as a **flux.** This one-way flux of glucose from compartment 1 to compartment 2 depends on the concentration of glucose in compartment 1. If the number of molecules in a unit of volume is doubled, the flux of molecules across the surface of the unit will also be doubled because twice as many molecules will be moving in any direction at a given time.

After a short time, some of the glucose molecules that have entered compartment 2 will randomly move back into compartment 1 (see Figure 4.2, time B). The magnitude of the glucose flux from compartment 2 to compartment 1 depends upon the concentration of glucose in compartment 2 at any time.

The **net flux** of glucose between the two compartments at any instant is the difference between the two one-way fluxes. The net flux determines the net gain of molecules in compartment 2 per unit time and the net loss from compartment 1 per unit time.

Eventually, the concentrations of glucose in the two compartments become equal at 10 mmol/L. Glucose molecules continue to move randomly, and some will find their way from one compartment to the other. However, the two one-way fluxes are now equal in magnitude but opposite in direction; therefore, the *net* flux of glucose is zero (see Figure 4.2, time C). The system has now reached **diffusion equilibrium.** No further change in the glucose concentrations of the two compartments will occur because of the equal rates of diffusion of glucose molecules in both directions between the two compartments.

Several important properties of diffusion can be emphasized using this example. Three fluxes can be identified—the difference determines both the direction and the magnitude of the net flux.

At any concentration difference, however, the magnitude of the net flux depends on several additional factors: (1) temperature—the more elevated the temperature, the greater the speed of molecular movement and the faster the net flux; (2) mass of the molecule—large molecules such as proteins have a greater mass and lower speed than smaller molecules such as glucose and, consequently, have a slower net flux; (3) surface area—the greater the surface area between two regions, the greater the space available for diffusion and, therefore, the faster the net flux; and (4) the medium through which the molecules are moving—molecules diffuse more rapidly in air than in water. This is because collisions are less frequent in a gas phase, and, as we will see, when a membrane is involved, its chemical composition influences diffusion rates.

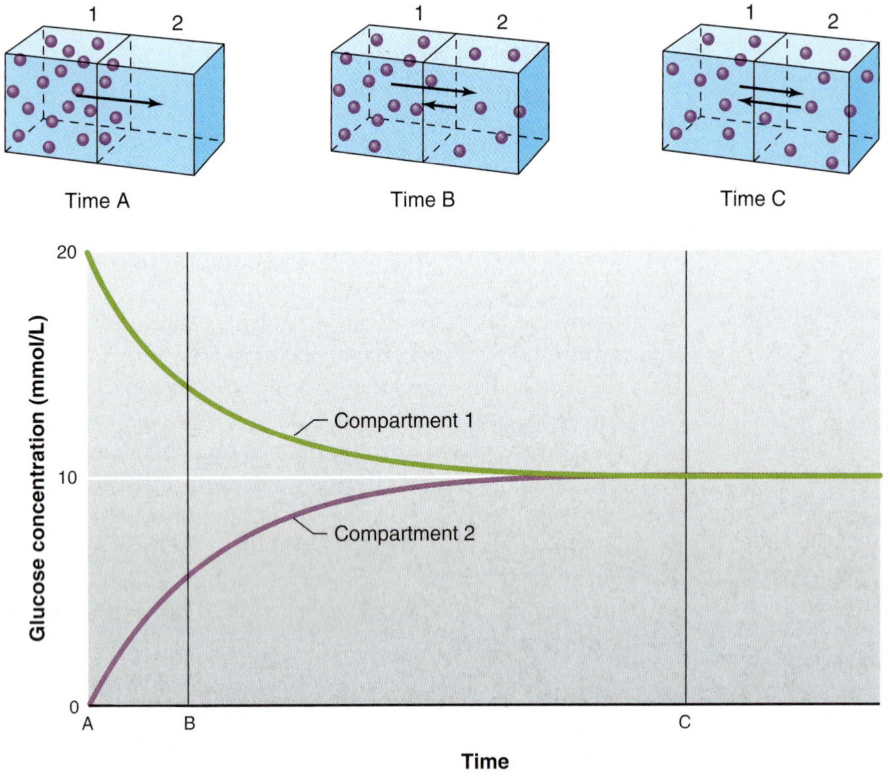

Figure 4.2 AP|R Diffusion of glucose between two compartments of equal volume separated by a barrier permeable to glucose. Initially, time A, compartment 1 contains glucose at a concentration of 20 mmol/L, and no glucose is present in compartment 2. At time B, some glucose molecules have moved into compartment 2, and some of these are moving back into compartment 1. The length of the arrows represents the magnitudes of the one-way movements. At time C, diffusion equilibrium has been reached, the concentrations of glucose are equal in the two compartments (10 mmol/L), and the *net* movement is zero. In the graph at the bottom of the figure, the green line represents the concentration in compartment 1, and the purple line represents the concentration in compartment 2. Note that at time C, glucose concentration is 10 mmol/L in both compartments. At that time, diffusion equilibrium has been reached.

PHYSIOLOGICAL INQUIRY

- If at time C, additional glucose could be added to compartment 1 such that its concentration was instantly increased to 15 mmol/L, what would the graph look like following time C? Draw the new graph on the figure and indicate the glucose concentrations in compartments 1 and 2 at diffusion equilibrium. (*Note:* It is not actually possible to instantly change the concentration of a substance in this way because it will immediately begin diffusing to the other compartment as it is added.)

Answer can be found at end of chapter.

two one-way fluxes occurring in opposite directions from one compartment to the other, and the net flux, which is the difference between them (**Figure 4.3**). The net flux is the most important component in diffusion because it is the net rate of material transfer from one location to another. Although the movement of individual molecules is random, *the net flux is always greater from regions of higher concentration to regions of lower concentration.* For this reason, we often say that substances move "downhill" by diffusion. The greater the difference in concentration between any two regions, the greater the magnitude of the net flux. Therefore, the concentration

Diffusion Rate Versus Distance

The distance over which molecules diffuse is an important factor in determining the rate at which they can reach a cell from the blood or move throughout the interior of a cell after crossing the plasma membrane. Although individual molecules travel at high speeds, the number of collisions they undergo prevents them from traveling very far in a straight line. Diffusion times increase in proportion to the *square* of the distance over which the molecules diffuse. For example, it takes glucose only a few seconds to reach diffusion equilibrium at a point 10 μm away from a source of glucose, but it would take over 11 years to reach the same concentration at a point 10 cm away from the source.

Thus, although diffusion equilibrium can be reached rapidly over distances of cellular dimensions, it takes a very long time when distances of a few centimeters or more are involved. For an organism as large as a human being, the diffusion of oxygen and nutrients from the body surface to tissues located only a few centimeters below the surface would be far too slow to provide adequate nourishment. This is overcome by the circulatory system, which provides a mechanism for rapidly moving materials over large distances using a pressure source (the heart). This process, known as bulk flow, is described in Chapter 12. Diffusion, on the other hand, provides movement over the short distances between the blood, interstitial fluid, and intracellular fluid.

Diffusion Through Membranes

The rate at which a substance diffuses across a plasma membrane can be measured by monitoring the rate at which its intracellular concentration approaches diffusion equilibrium with its concentration in the extracellular fluid. For simplicity's sake, assume that because the volume of extracellular fluid

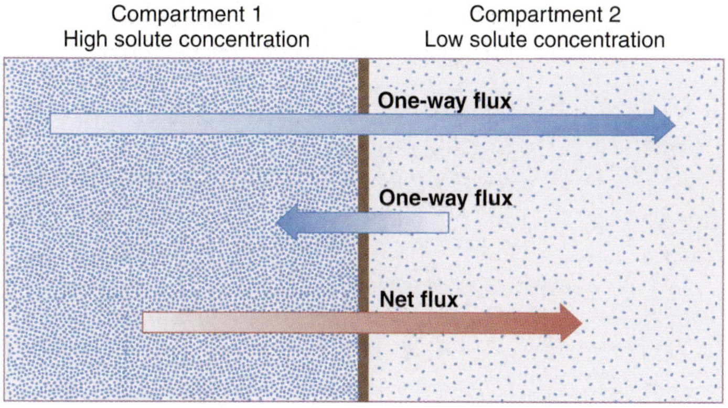

Figure 4.3 AP|R The two one-way fluxes occurring during the simple diffusion of solute across a boundary and the net flux, which is the difference between the two one-way fluxes. The net flux always occurs in the direction from higher to lower concentration. The length of the arrows indicates the magnitude of the flux.

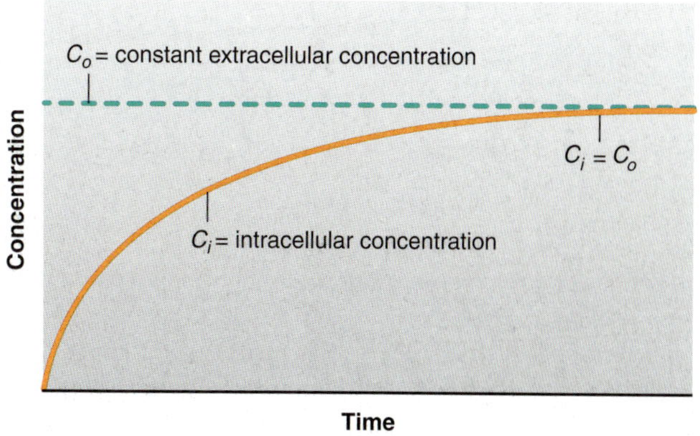

Figure 4.4 The increase in intracellular concentration as a solute diffuses from a constant extracellular concentration until diffusion equilibrium ($C_i = C_o$) is reached across the plasma membrane of a cell.

is large, its solute concentration will remain essentially constant as the substance diffuses into the intracellular volume (**Figure 4.4**). As with all diffusion processes, the net flux J of material across the membrane is from the region of greater concentration (the extracellular solution in this case) to the region of less concentration (the intracellular fluid). The magnitude of the net flux is directly proportional to the difference in concentration across the membrane ($C_o - C_i$, where o and i stand for concentrations outside and inside the cell), the surface area of the membrane A, and the membrane permeability coefficient P as described by the Fick diffusion equation:

$$J = PA(C_o - C_i)$$

The numerical value of the permeability coefficient P is an experimentally determined number for a particular type of molecule at a given temperature; it reflects the ease with which the molecule is able to move through a given membrane. In other words, the greater the permeability coefficient, the faster the net flux across the membrane for any given concentration difference and membrane surface area. Due to the magnitude of their permeability coefficients, molecules typically diffuse a thousand to a million times slower through membranes than through a water layer of equal thickness. Membranes, therefore, act as barriers that considerably slow the diffusion of molecules across their surfaces. The major factor limiting diffusion across a membrane is its chemical composition, namely the hydrophobic interior of its lipid bilayer, as described next.

Diffusion Through the Lipid Bilayer

When the permeability coefficients of different organic molecules are examined in relation to their molecular structures, a correlation emerges. Whereas most polar molecules diffuse into cells very slowly or not at all, nonpolar molecules diffuse much more rapidly across plasma membranes—that is, they have large permeability constants. The reason is that nonpolar molecules can dissolve in the nonpolar regions of the membrane occupied by the fatty acid chains of the membrane phospholipids. In contrast, polar molecules have a much lower solubility in the membrane lipids. Increasing the lipid solubility of a substance by decreasing the number of polar or ionized groups it contains will increase the number of molecules dissolved in the membrane lipids. This will increase the flux of the substance across the membrane. Oxygen, carbon dioxide, fatty acids, and steroid hormones are examples of nonpolar molecules that diffuse rapidly through the lipid portions of membranes. Most of the organic molecules that make up the intermediate stages of the various metabolic pathways (Chapter 3) are ionized or polar molecules, often containing an ionized phosphate group; therefore, they have a low solubility in the lipid bilayer. Most of these substances are retained within cells and organelles because they cannot diffuse across the lipid bilayer of membranes, unless the membrane contains special proteins such as channels, as we see next. This is an excellent example of the general principle that physiological processes are dictated by the laws of chemistry and physics.

Diffusion of Ions Through Protein Channels

Ions such as Na^+, K^+, Cl^-, and Ca^{2+} diffuse across plasma membranes at much faster rates than would be predicted from their very low solubility in membrane lipids. Also, different cells have quite different permeabilities to these ions, whereas nonpolar substances have similar permeabilities in nearly all cells. Moreover, artificial lipid bilayers containing no protein are practically impermeable to these ions; this indicates that the protein component of the membrane is responsible for these permeability differences.

As we have seen (Chapter 3), integral membrane proteins can span the lipid bilayer. Some of these proteins form **ion channels** that allow ions to diffuse across the membrane. A single protein may have a conformation resembling that of a doughnut, with the hole in the middle providing the channel for ion movement. More often, several proteins aggregate, each forming a subunit of the walls of a channel (**Figure 4.5**). The diameters of ion channels are very small, only slightly larger than those of the ions that pass through them. The small size of the channels prevents larger molecules from entering or leaving.

An important characteristic of ion channels is that they can show selectivity for the type of ion or ions that can diffuse through them. This selectivity is based on the channel diameter, the charged and polar surfaces of the protein subunits

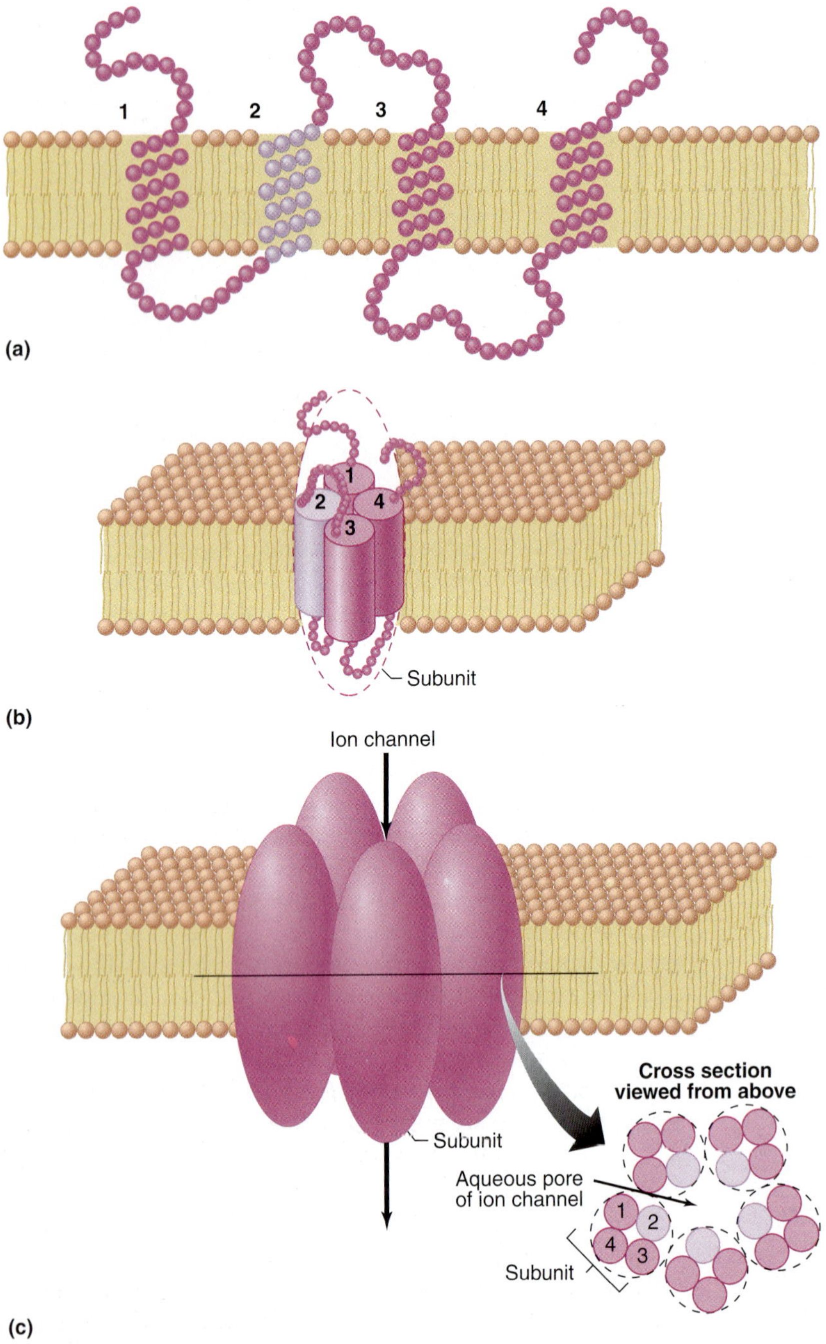

Figure 4.5 Model of an ion channel composed of five polypeptide subunits. Individual amino acids are represented as beads. (a) A channel subunit consisting of an integral membrane protein containing four transmembrane segments (1, 2, 3, and 4), each of which has an alpha-helical configuration within the membrane. Although this model has only four transmembrane segments, some channel proteins have as many as 12. (b) The same subunit as in (a) shown in three dimensions within the membrane, with the four transmembrane helices aggregated together and shown as cylinders. (c) The ion channel consists of five of the subunits illustrated in (b), which form the sides of the channel. As shown in cross section, the helical transmembrane segment 2 (light purple) of each subunit forms each side of the channel opening. The presence of ionized amino acid side chains along this region determines the selectivity of the channel to ions. Although this model shows the five subunits as identical, many ion channels are formed from the aggregation of several different types of subunit polypeptides.

PHYSIOLOGICAL INQUIRY

- In Chapter 2, you learned that proteins have several levels of structure. Which levels of structures are evident in the drawing of the ion channel in this figure?

Answer can be found at end of chapter.

that form the channel walls and electrically attract or repel the ions, and on the number of water molecules associated with the ions (so-called waters of hydration). For example, some channels (K^+ channels) allow only potassium ions to pass, whereas others are specific for Na^+ (Na^+ channels). Still others allow diffusion of both Na^+ and K^+ but not other ions. For this reason, two membranes that have the same permeability to K^+ because they have the same number of K^+ channels may have quite different permeabilities to Na^+ if they contain different numbers of Na^+ channels.

Role of Electrical Forces on Ion Movement

Thus far, we have described the direction and magnitude of solute diffusion across a membrane in terms of the solute's concentration difference across the membrane, its solubility in the membrane lipids, the presence of membrane ion channels, and the area of the membrane. When describing the diffusion of ions, because they are charged, one additional factor must be considered: the presence of electrical forces acting upon the ions.

A separation of electrical charge exists across plasma membranes of all cells. This is known as a **membrane potential** (**Figure 4.6**), the magnitude of which is measured in units of millivolts. (The origin of a membrane potential will be described in Chapter 6 in the context of neuronal function.) The membrane potential provides an electrical force that influences the movement of ions across the membrane. A simple principle of physics is that like charges repel each other, whereas opposite charges attract. For example, if the inside of a cell has a net negative charge with respect to the outside, as

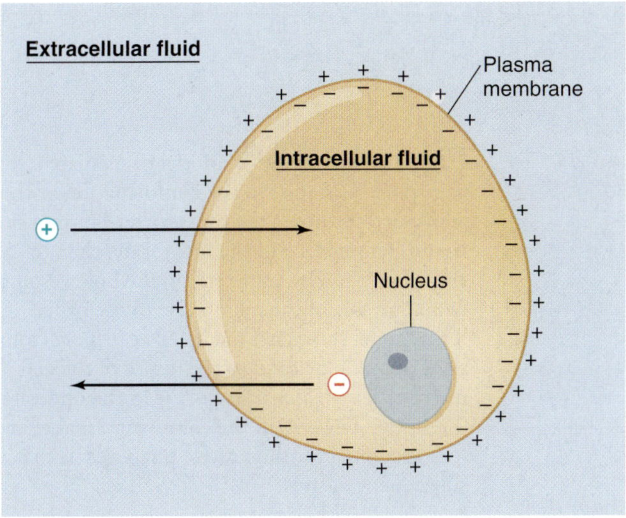

Figure 4.6 The separation of electrical charge across a plasma membrane (the membrane potential) provides the electrical force that drives positive ions (+) into a cell and negative ions (−) out.

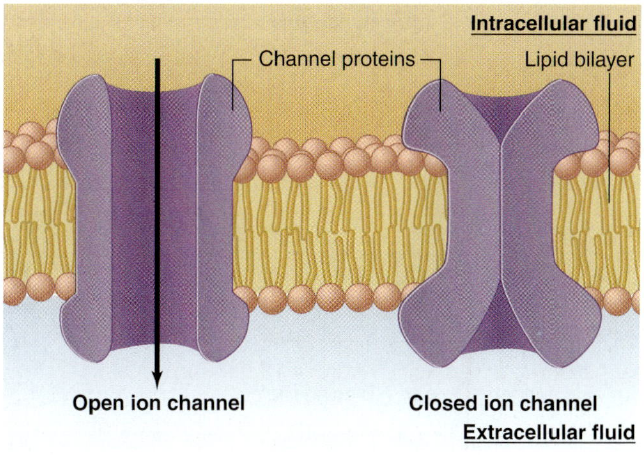

Figure 4.7 As a result of conformational changes in the proteins forming an ion channel, the channel may be open, allowing ions to diffuse across the membrane, or may be closed. The conformational change is grossly exaggerated for illustrative purposes. The actual conformational change is more likely to be just sufficient to allow or prevent an ion to fit through.

is generally true, there will be an electrical force attracting positive ions into the cell and repelling negative ions. Even if no difference in ion concentration existed across the membrane, there would still be a net movement of positive ions into and negative ions out of the cell because of the membrane potential. Consequently, the direction and magnitude of ion fluxes across membranes depend on both the concentration difference *and* the electrical difference (the membrane potential). These two driving forces are collectively known as the **electrochemical gradient** across a membrane.

The two forces that make up the electrochemical gradient may in some cases oppose each other. For example, the membrane potential may be driving potassium ions in one direction across the membrane while the concentration difference for K^+ is driving these ions in the opposite direction. The net movement of K^+ in this case would be determined by the relative magnitudes of the two opposing forces—that is, by the electrochemical gradient across the membrane.

Regulation of Diffusion Through Ion Channels

Ion channels can exist in an open or closed state (**Figure 4.7**), and changes in a membrane's permeability to ions can occur rapidly as these channels open or close. The process of opening and closing ion channels is known as **channel gating,** like the opening and closing of a gate in a fence. A single ion channel may open and close many times each second, suggesting that the channel protein fluctuates between these conformations. Over an extended period of time, at any given electrochemical gradient, the total number of ions that pass through a channel depends on how often the channel opens and how long it stays open.

Three factors can alter the channel protein conformations, producing changes in how long or how often a channel opens. First, the binding of specific molecules to channel proteins may directly or indirectly produce either an allosteric or covalent change in the shape of the channel protein. Such channels are termed **ligand-gated channels,** and the ligands that influence them are often chemical messengers. Second, changes in the membrane potential can cause movement of certain charged regions on a channel protein, altering its shape—these are **voltage-gated channels.** Third, physically deforming (stretching) the membrane may affect the conformation of some channel proteins—these are **mechanically gated channels.**

A single type of ion may pass through several different types of channels. For example, a membrane may contain ligand-gated K^+ channels, voltage-gated K^+ channels, and mechanically gated K^+ channels. Moreover, the same membrane may have several types of voltage-gated K^+ channels, each responding to a different range of membrane voltage, or several types of ligand-gated K^+ channels, each responding to a different chemical messenger. The roles of these gated channels in cell communication and electrical activity will be discussed in Chapters 5 through 7.

4.2 Mediated-Transport Systems

As stated in Chapter 1, a general principle of physiology is that controlled exchange of materials occurs between compartments and across cellular membranes. Although diffusion through gated channels accounts for some of the controlled transmembrane movement of ions, it does not account for all of it. Moreover, a number of other molecules, including amino acids and glucose, are able to cross membranes yet are too polar to diffuse through the lipid bilayer and too large to diffuse through channels. The passage of these molecules and the nondiffusional movements of ions are mediated by integral membrane proteins known as **transporters** (or carriers). The movement of substances through a membrane by these mechanisms is called **mediated transport,** which depends on conformational changes in these transporters.

The transported solute must first bind to a specific site on a transporter, a site exposed to the solute on one surface of the membrane (**Figure 4.8**). A portion of the transporter then undergoes a change in shape, exposing this same binding site to the solution on the opposite side of the membrane.

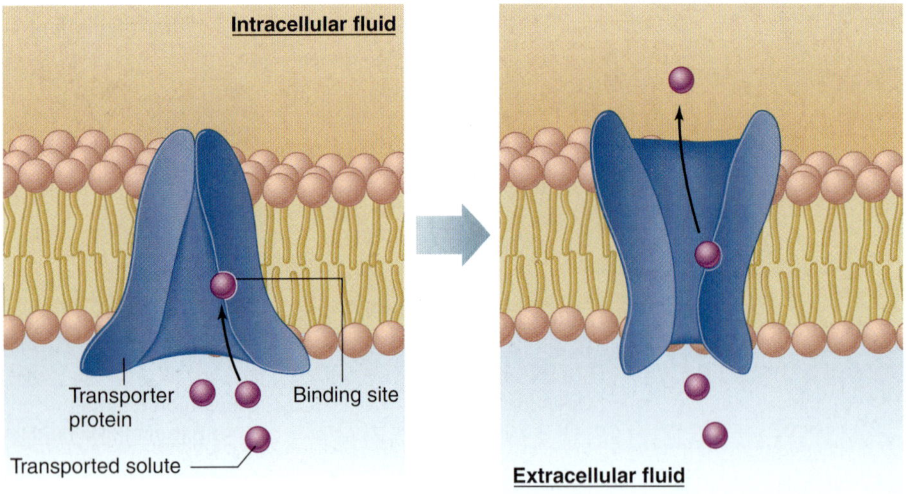

Figure 4.8 APIR Model of mediated transport. A change in the conformation of the transporter exposes the transporter binding site first to one surface of the membrane then to the other, thereby transferring the bound solute from one side of the membrane to the other. This model shows net mediated transport from the extracellular fluid to the inside of the cell. In many cases, the net transport is in the opposite direction. The size of the conformational change is exaggerated for illustrative purposes in this and subsequent figures.

The dissociation of the substance from the transporter binding site completes the process of moving the material through the membrane. Using this mechanism, molecules can move in either direction, getting on the transporter on one side and off at the other. The diagram of the transporter in Figure 4.8 is only a model, because the specific conformational changes of any transport protein are still uncertain.

Many of the characteristics of transporters and ion channels are similar. Both involve membrane proteins and show chemical specificity. They do, however, differ in the number of molecules or ions crossing the membrane by way of these membrane proteins. Ion channels typically move several thousand times more ions per unit time than do transporters. In part, this is because a transporter must change its shape for each molecule transported across the membrane, whereas an open ion channel can support a continuous flow of ions without a change in conformation. Imagine, for example, how many more cars can move over a bridge than can be shuttled back and forth by a ferry boat.

Many types of transporters are present in membranes, each type having binding sites that are specific for a particular substance or a specific class of related substances. For example, although both amino acids and sugars undergo mediated transport, a protein that transports amino acids does not transport sugars, and vice versa. Just as with ion channels, the plasma membranes of different cells contain different types and numbers of transporters; consequently, they exhibit differences in the types of substances transported and in their rates of transport.

Three factors determine the magnitude of solute flux through a mediated-transport system. The first of these is the extent to which the transporter binding sites are saturated, which depends on both the solute concentration and the affinity of the transporters for the solute. Second, the number of transporters in the membrane determines the flux at any level of saturation. The third factor is the rate at which the conformational change in the transport protein occurs. The flux through a mediated-transport system can be altered by changing any of these three factors.

For any transported solute, a finite number of specific transporters reside in a given membrane at any particular moment. As with any binding site, as the concentration of the solute to be transported is increased, the number of occupied binding sites increases until the transporters become saturated—that is, until all the binding sites are occupied. When the transporter binding sites are saturated, the maximal flux across the membrane has been reached and no further increase in solute flux will occur with increases in solute concentration. Contrast the solute flux resulting from mediated transport with the flux produced by diffusion through the lipid portion of a membrane (**Figure 4.9**). The flux due to diffusion increases in direct proportion to the increase in extracellular concentration, and there is no limit because diffusion does not involve binding to a fixed number of sites. (At very high ion concentrations, however, diffusion through ion channels may approach a limiting value because of the fixed number of channels available, just as an upper limit determines the rate at which cars can move over a bridge.)

When transporters are saturated, however, the maximal transport flux depends upon the rate at which the conformational changes in the transporters can transfer their binding sites from one surface to the other. This rate is much slower than the rate of ion diffusion through ion channels.

Thus far, we have described mediated transport as though all transporters had similar properties. In fact, two types of mediated transport exist—facilitated diffusion and active transport.

Facilitated Diffusion

As in simple diffusion, in **facilitated diffusion** the net flux of a molecule across a membrane always proceeds from higher to lower concentration, or "downhill" across a membrane; the key difference between these processes is that facilitated diffusion uses a transporter to move solute, as in Figure 4.8. Net facilitated diffusion continues until the concentrations of the solute on the two sides of the membrane become equal. At this point, equal numbers of molecules are binding to the transporter at the outer surface of the cell and moving into the cell as are binding at the inner surface and moving out. Neither simple diffusion nor facilitated diffusion is directly coupled to energy (ATP) derived from metabolism. For this reason, they are incapable of producing a net flux of solute from a lower to a higher concentration across a membrane.

Among the most important facilitated-diffusion systems in the body are those that mediate the transport of glucose across plasma membranes. Without such glucose transporters, or GLUTs as they are abbreviated, cells would be virtually

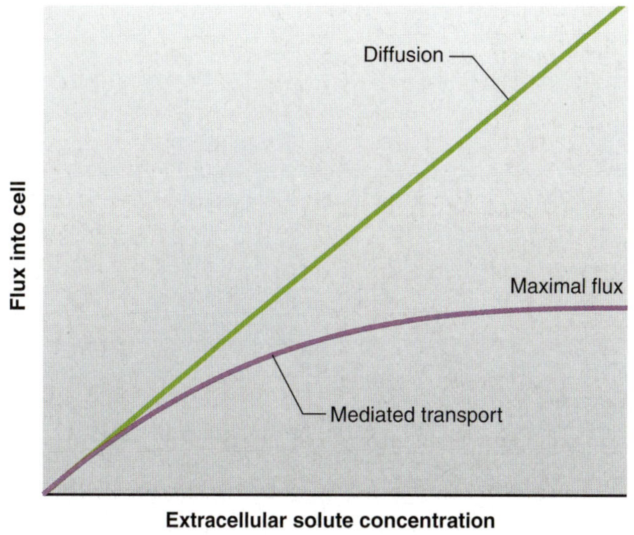

Figure 4.9 The flux of molecules diffusing into a cell across the lipid bilayer of a plasma membrane (green line) increases continuously in proportion to the extracellular concentration, whereas the flux of molecules through a mediated-transport system (purple line) reaches a maximal value.

PHYSIOLOGICAL INQUIRY

- What might determine the value for maximal flux of a mediated-transport system as shown here?

Answer can be found at end of chapter.

impermeable to glucose, which is a polar molecule. It might be expected that as a result of facilitated diffusion the glucose concentration inside cells would become equal to the extracellular concentration. This does not occur in most cells, however, because glucose is metabolized in the cytosol to glucose 6-phosphate almost as quickly as it enters (refer back to Figure 3.41). Consequently, the intracellular glucose concentration remains lower than the extracellular concentration, and there is a continuous net flux of glucose into cells.

Several distinct GLUTs are known to mediate the facilitated diffusion of glucose across cell membranes. Each GLUT is coded for by a different gene, and these genes are expressed in different types of cells. The transporters differ in the affinity of their binding sites for glucose; their maximal rates of transport when saturated; and the modulation of their transport activity by various chemical signals, such as the hormone insulin. As you will learn in Chapter 16, although glucose enters all cells by means of GLUTs, insulin primarily affects the type of transporter expressed in skeletal and cardiac muscle and adipose tissue. Insulin increases the recruitment of these glucose transporters from intracellular vesicles to the plasma membrane. The insertion of the GLUTs into the plasma membrane increases the rate of glucose movement into those cells. When insulin is not available, as in the disease ***type 1 diabetes mellitus,*** muscle and adipose cells cannot efficiently transport glucose into their cells because fewer GLUTs exist in the plasma membranes of those cells. This contributes to the accumulation of glucose in the extracellular fluid, which is a hallmark of the disease (described in detail in Chapter 16).

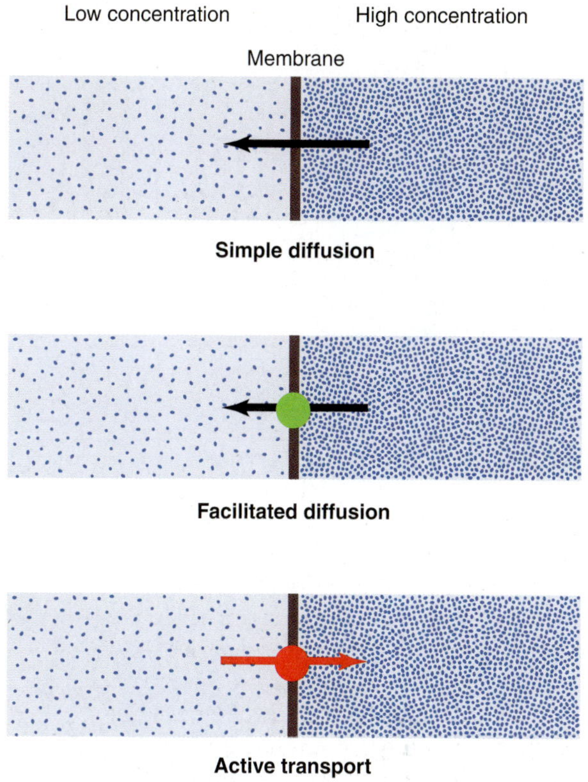

Figure 4.10 Direction of net solute flux crossing a membrane by simple diffusion (high to low concentration), facilitated diffusion (high to low concentration), and active transport (low to high concentration). The colored circles represent transporter molecules.

Active Transport

Active transport differs from facilitated diffusion in that it uses energy to move a substance *uphill* across a membrane—that is, against the substance's concentration gradient (**Figure 4.10**). As with facilitated diffusion, active transport requires a substance to bind to the transporter in the membrane. Because these transporters move the substance *uphill,* they are often referred to as pumps. As with facilitated-diffusion transporters, active-transport transporters exhibit specificity and saturation—that is, the flux via the transporter is maximal when all transporter binding sites are occupied.

The net movement from lower to higher concentrations and the maintenance of a higher steady-state concentration on one side of a membrane can be achieved only by the continuous input of energy into the active-transport process. Two means of coupling energy to transporters are known: (1) the direct use of ATP in **primary active transport,** and (2) the use of an electrochemical gradient across a membrane to drive the process in **secondary active transport.**

Primary Active Transport

The hydrolysis of ATP by a transporter provides the energy for primary active transport. The transporter itself is an enzyme called *ATPase* that catalyzes the breakdown of ATP and, in the process, phosphorylates itself. Phosphorylation of the transporter protein is a type of covalent modulation that changes the conformation of the transporter and the affinity of the transporter's solute binding site.

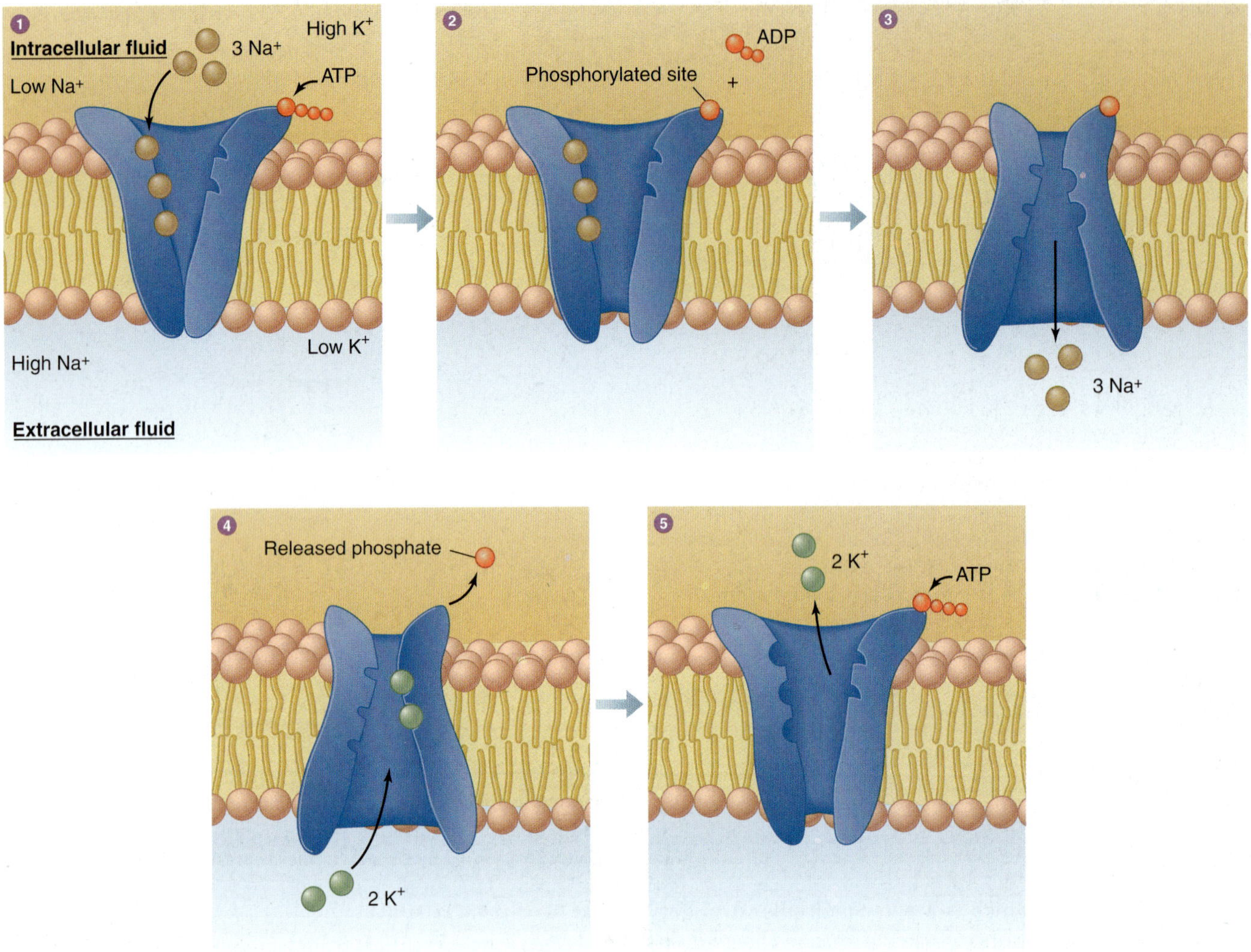

Figure 4.11 AP|R Active transport of Na^+ and K^+ mediated by the Na^+/K^+-ATPase pump. See text for the numbered sequence of events occurring during transport.

One of the best-studied examples of primary active transport is the movement of sodium and potassium ions across plasma membranes by the Na^+/K^+-ATPase pump. This transporter, which is present in all cells, moves sodium ions from intracellular to extracellular fluid, and potassium ions in the opposite direction. In both cases, the movements of the ions are against their respective concentration gradients. **Figure 4.11** illustrates the sequence the Na^+/K^+-ATPase pump is believed to use to transport these two ions in opposite directions. (1) Initially, the transporter, with an associated molecule of ATP, binds three sodium ions at high-affinity sites on the intracellular surface of the protein. Two binding sites also exist for K^+, but at this stage they are in a low-affinity state and therefore do not bind intracellular K^+. (2) Binding of Na^+ results in activation of an inherent ATPase activity of the transporter protein, causing phosphorylation of the cytosolic surface of the transporter and releasing a molecule of ADP. (3) Phosphorylation results in a conformational change of the transporter, exposing the bound sodium ions to the extracellular fluid and, at the same time, reducing the affinity of the binding sites for Na^+. The sodium ions are released from their binding sites. (4) The new conformation of the transporter results in an increased affinity of the two binding sites for K^+, allowing two molecules of K^+ to bind to the transporter on the extracellular surface. (5) Binding of K^+ results in dephosphorylation of the transporter. This returns the transporter to its original conformation, resulting in reduced affinity of the K^+ binding sites and increased affinity of the Na^+ binding sites. K^+ is therefore released into the intracellular fluid, allowing new molecules of Na^+ (and ATP) to be bound at the intracellular surface.

The pumping activity of the Na^+/K^+-ATPase primary active transporter establishes and maintains the characteristic distribution of high intracellular K^+ and low intracellular Na^+ relative to their respective extracellular concentrations (**Figure 4.12**). For each molecule of ATP hydrolyzed, this transporter moves three sodium ions out of a cell and two potassium ions into a cell. This results in a net transfer of positive charge to the outside of the cell; therefore, this transport process is not electrically neutral, a point that will be described in detail in Chapter 6 when we consider the electrical charge across plasma membranes of neurons. The Na^+/K^+-ATPase primary active transporter is found in every cell and helps establish and maintain the membrane potential of the cell.

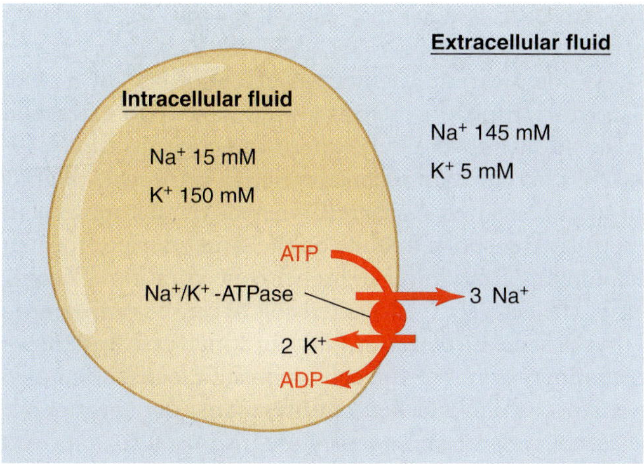

Figure 4.12 APIR The primary active transport of sodium and potassium ions in opposite directions by the Na^+/K^+-ATPase in plasma membranes is responsible for the low Na^+ and high K^+ intracellular concentrations. For each ATP hydrolyzed, three sodium ions move out of a cell and two potassium ions move in.

In addition to the Na^+/K^+-ATPase transporter, the major primary active-transport proteins found in most cells are (1) Ca^{2+}-ATPase; (2) H^+-ATPase; and (3) H^+/K^+-ATPase. Together, the activities of these and other active-transport systems account for a significant share of the total energy usage of the human body. Ca^{2+}-ATPase is found in the plasma membrane and several organelle membranes, including the membranes of the endoplasmic reticulum. In the plasma membrane, the direction of active calcium transport is from cytosol to extracellular fluid. In organelle membranes, it is from cytosol into the organelle lumen. Thus, active transport of Ca^{2+} out of the cytosol, via Ca^{2+}-ATPase, is one reason that the cytosol of most cells has a very low Ca^{2+} concentration, about 10^{-7} mol/L, compared with an extracellular Ca^{2+} concentration of 10^{-3} mol/L, 10,000 times greater. These transport mechanisms help ensure intracellular calcium ion homeostasis, an important function because of the many physiological activities in cells that are regulated by changes in calcium ion concentration (for example, release of cell secretions from storage vesicles into the extracellular fluid).

H^+-ATPase is in the plasma membrane and several organelle membranes, including the inner mitochondrial and lysosomal membranes. In the plasma membrane, the H^+-ATPase moves hydrogen ions out of cells and in this way helps maintain cellular pH. All enzymes in the body require a narrow range of pH for optimal activity; consequently, this active-transport process is vital for cell metabolism and survival.

H^+/K^+-ATPase is in the plasma membranes of the acid-secreting cells in the stomach and kidneys, where it pumps one hydrogen ion out of the cell and moves one K^+ in for each molecule of ATP hydrolyzed. The hydrogen ions enter the stomach lumen where they play an important role in the digestion of proteins.

Secondary Active Transport

In secondary active transport, the movement of an ion down its electrochemical gradient is coupled to the transport of another molecule, such as a nutrient like glucose or an amino acid. Thus, transporters that mediate secondary active transport have two binding sites, one for an ion—typically but not always Na^+—and another for the cotransported molecule. An example of such transport is shown in **Figure 4.13**. In this example, the electrochemical gradient for Na^+ is directed into the cell because of the higher concentration of Na^+ in the extracellular fluid and the excess negative charges inside the cell. The other solute to be transported, however, must move *against* its concentration gradient, uphill into the cell. High-affinity binding sites for Na^+ exist on the extracellular surface of the transporter. Binding of Na^+ increases the affinity of the binding site for the transported solute. The transporter then undergoes a conformational change, which exposes both binding sites to the intracellular side of the membrane. When the transporter

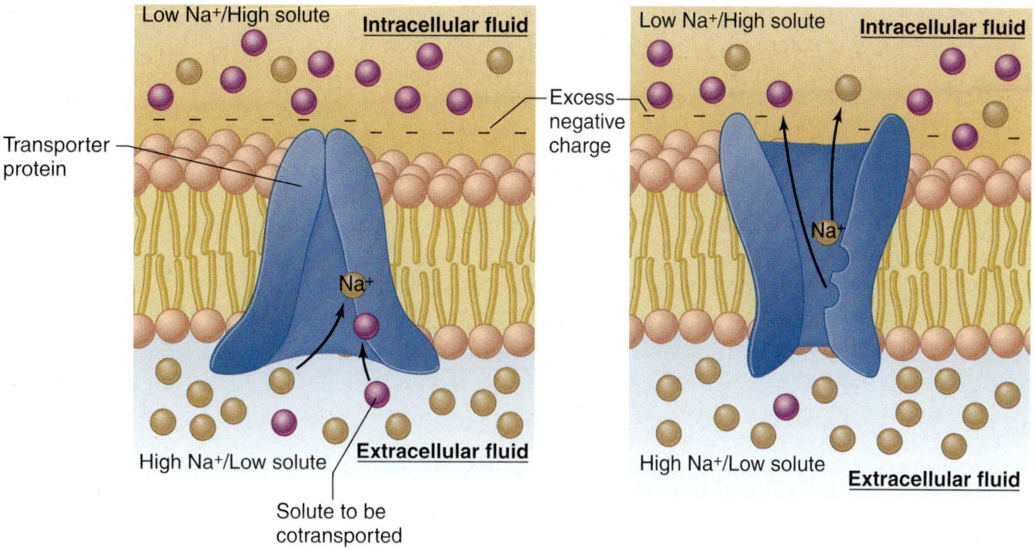

Figure 4.13 APIR Secondary active-transport model. In this example, the binding of a sodium ion to the transporter produces an allosteric increase in the affinity of the solute binding site at the extracellular surface of the membrane. Binding of Na^+ and solute causes a conformational change in the transporter that exposes the binding sites to the intracellular fluid. Na^+ diffuses down its electrochemical gradient into the cell, which returns the solute binding site to a low-affinity state.

PHYSIOLOGICAL INQUIRY

- Is ATP hydrolyzed in the process of transporting solutes with secondary active transport?

Answer can be found at end of chapter.

changes conformation, Na^+ moves into the intracellular fluid by simple diffusion down its electrochemical gradient. At the same time, the affinity of the solute binding site decreases, which releases the solute into the intracellular fluid. The solute can be thought of as entering the cell by "piggyback" with the sodium ion. Once the transporter releases both molecules, the protein assumes its original conformation. The most important distinction, therefore, between primary and secondary active transport is that secondary active transport uses the stored energy of an electrochemical gradient to move both an ion and a second solute across a plasma membrane. The creation and maintenance of the electrochemical gradient, however, depend on the action of primary active transporters.

The creation of a Na^+ concentration gradient across the plasma membrane by the primary active transport of Na^+ is a means of indirectly "storing" energy that can then be used to drive secondary active-transport pumps linked to Na^+. Ultimately, however, the energy for secondary active transport is derived from metabolism in the form of the ATP that is used by the Na^+/K^+-ATPase to create the Na^+ concentration gradient. If the production of ATP were inhibited, the primary active transport of Na^+ would cease and the cell would no longer be able to maintain an Na^+ concentration gradient across the membrane. This, in turn, would lead to a failure of the secondary active-transport systems that depend on the Na^+ gradient for their source of energy.

As noted earlier, the net movement of Na^+ by a secondary active-transport protein is always from high extracellular concentration into the cell, where the concentration of Na^+ is lower. Therefore, in secondary active transport, the movement of Na^+ is always *downhill*, whereas the net movement of the actively transported solute on the same transport protein is *uphill*, moving from lower to higher concentration. The movement of the actively transported solute can be either into the cell (in the same direction as Na^+), in which case it is known as **cotransport**, or out of the cell (opposite the direction of Na^+ movement), which is called **countertransport** (**Figure 4.14**). The terms *symport* and *antiport* are also used to refer to the processes of cotransport and countertransport, respectively.

In summary, the distribution of substances between the intracellular and extracellular fluid is often unequal (**Table 4.1**) due to the presence in the plasma membrane of primary and secondary active transporters, ion channels, and the membrane potential. **Table 4.2** provides a summary of the major characteristics of the different pathways by which substances move through cell membranes, whereas **Figure 4.15** illustrates the variety of commonly encountered channels and transporters associated with the movement of substances across a typical plasma membrane.

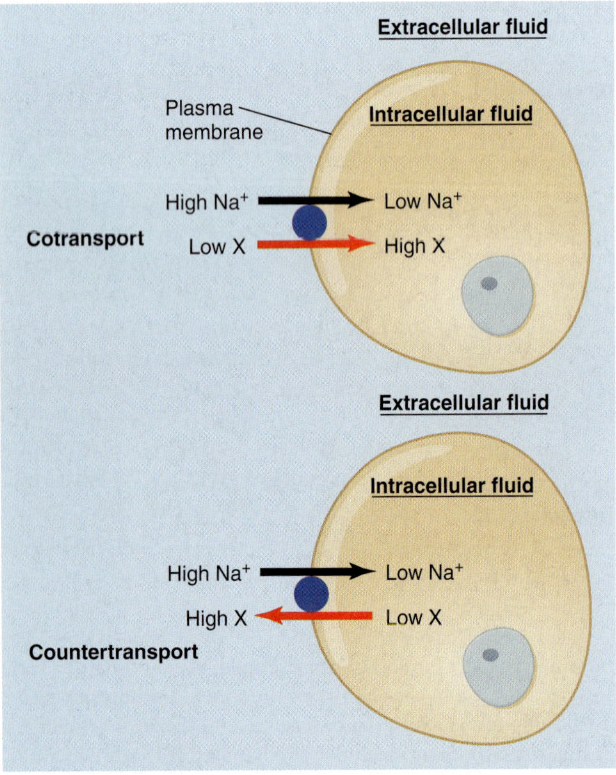

Figure 4.14 APIR Cotransport and countertransport during secondary active transport driven by Na^+. Sodium ions always move *down* their concentration gradient into a cell, and the transported solute always moves *up* its gradient. Both Na^+ and the transported solute X move in the same direction during cotransport, but in opposite directions during countertransport.

TABLE 4.1 Composition of Extracellular and Intracellular Fluids

	Extracellular Concentration (mM)	Intracellular Concentration (mM)*
Na^+	145	15
K^+	5	150
Ca^{2+}	1	0.0001
Mg^{2+}	1.5	12
Cl^-	100	7
HCO_3^-	24	10
P_i	2	40
Amino acids	2	8
Glucose	5.6	1
ATP	0	4
Protein	0.2	4

*The intracellular concentrations differ slightly from one tissue to another, depending on the expression of plasma membrane ion channels and transporters. The intracellular concentrations shown in the table are typical of most cells. For Ca^{2+}, values represent free concentrations. Total calcium levels, including the portion sequestered by proteins or in organelles, approach 2.5 mM (extracellular) and 1.5 mM (intracellular).

TABLE 4.2 Major Characteristics of Pathways by Which Substances Cross Membranes

	Diffusion		*Mediated Transport*		
	Through Lipid Bilayer	**Through Protein Channel**	**Facilitated Diffusion**	**Primary Active Transport**	**Secondary Active Transport**
Direction of net flux	High to low concentration	High to low concentration	High to low concentration	Low to high concentration	Low to high concentration
Equilibrium or steady state	$C_o = C_i$	$C_o = C_i$*	$C_o = C_i$	$C_o \neq C_i$	$C_o \neq C_i$
Use of integral membrane protein	No	Yes	Yes	Yes	Yes
Maximal flux at high concentration (saturation)	No	No	Yes	Yes	Yes
Chemical specificity	No	Yes	Yes	Yes	Yes
Use of energy and source	No	No	No	Yes: ATP	Yes: ion gradient (often Na^+)
Typical molecules using pathway	Nonpolar: O_2, CO_2, fatty acids	Ions: Na^+, K^+, Ca^{2+}	Polar: glucose	Ions: Na^+, K^+, Ca^{2+}, H^+	Polar: amino acids, glucose, some ions

*In the presence of a membrane potential, the intracellular and extracellular ion concentrations will not be equal at equilibrium.

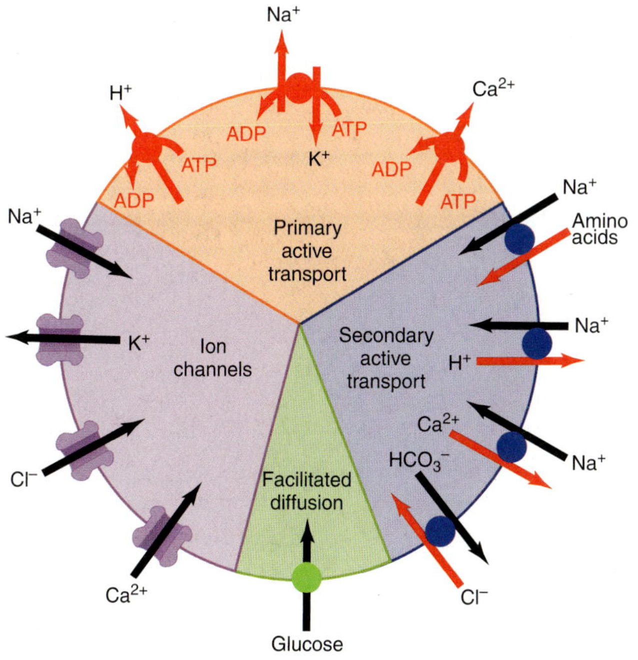

Figure 4.15 Movement of solutes across a typical plasma membrane involving membrane proteins. A specialized cell may contain additional transporters and channels not shown in this figure. Many of these membrane proteins can be modulated by various signals, leading to a controlled increase or decrease in specific solute fluxes across the membrane. The stoichiometry of cotransporters is not shown.

Not included in Table 4.2 is the mechanism by which water moves across membranes. The special case whereby this polar molecule moves between body fluid compartments is covered next.

4.3 Osmosis

Water is a polar molecule and yet it diffuses across the plasma membranes of most cells very rapidly. This process is mediated by a family of membrane proteins known as **aquaporins** that form channels through which water can diffuse. The type and number of these water channels differ in different membranes. Consequently, some cells are more permeable to water than others. In some cells, the number of aquaporin channels—and, therefore, the permeability of the membrane to water—can be altered in response to various signals. This is especially important in the epithelial cells that line certain ducts in the kidneys. As you will learn in Chapter 14, one of the major functions of the kidneys is to regulate the amount of water that gets excreted in the urine; this helps keep the total amount of water in the body fluid compartments homeostatic. The epithelial cells of the kidney ducts contain numerous aquaporins that can be increased or decreased in number depending on the water balance of the body at any time. For example, in an individual who is dehydrated, the numbers of aquaporins in the kidney epithelial cells will increase; this will permit additional water to move from the urine that is being formed in the renal ducts back into the blood. That is why the volume of urine decreases whenever an individual becomes dehydrated.

The net diffusion of water across a membrane is called **osmosis.** As with any diffusion process, a concentration difference must be present in order to produce a net flux. How can a difference in water concentration be established across a membrane?

The addition of a solute to water decreases the concentration of water in the solution compared to the concentration of pure water. For example, if a solute such as glucose is dissolved in water, the concentration of water in the resulting solution is less than that of pure water. A given volume of a glucose solution contains fewer water molecules than an equal volume of pure water because each glucose molecule occupies space formerly occupied by a water molecule (**Figure 4.16**). In quantitative terms, a liter of pure water weighs about 1000 g, and the molecular weight of water is 18. Thus, the concentration of water in pure water is 1000/18 = 55.5 M. The decrease in water concentration in a solution is approximately equal to the concentration of added solute. In other words, one solute molecule will displace one water molecule. The water concentration in a 1 M glucose solution is therefore approximately 54.5 M rather than 55.5 M. Just as adding water to a solution will dilute the solute, adding solute to water will "dilute" the water. The greater the solute concentration, the lower the water concentration.

The degree to which the water concentration is decreased by the addition of solute depends upon the *number* of particles (molecules or ions) of solute in solution (the solute concentration) and not upon the *chemical nature* of the solute. For example, 1 mol of glucose in 1 L of solution decreases the water concentration to the same extent as does 1 mol of an amino acid, or 1 mol of urea, or 1 mol of any other molecule that exists as a single particle in solution. On the other hand, a molecule that ionizes in solution decreases the water concentration in proportion to the number of ions formed. For example, many simple salts dissociate nearly completely in water. For simplicity's sake, we will assume the dissociation is 100% at body temperature and at concentrations found in the blood. Therefore, 1 mol of sodium chloride in solution gives rise to 1 mol of sodium ions and 1 mol of chloride ions, producing 2 mol of solute particles. This lowers the water concentration twice as much as 1 mol of glucose. By the same reasoning, if a 1 M $MgCl_2$ solution were to dissociate completely, it would lower the water concentration three times as much as would a 1 M glucose solution.

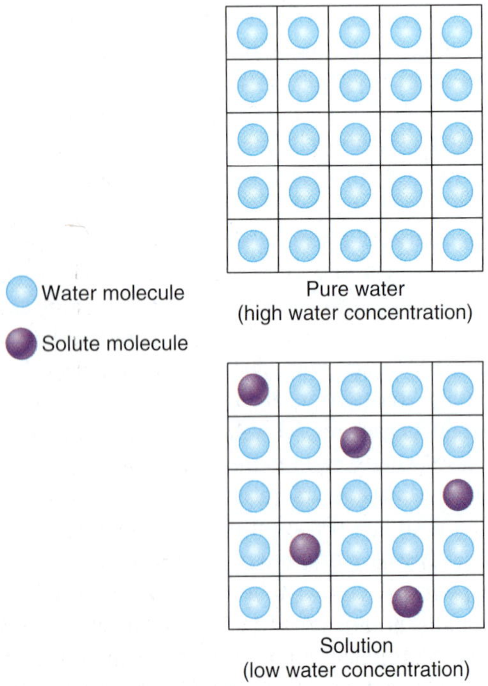

Figure 4.16 The addition of solute molecules to pure water lowers the water concentration in the solution.

Because the water concentration in a solution depends upon the number of solute particles, it is useful to have a concentration term that refers to the total concentration of solute particles in a solution, regardless of their chemical composition. The total solute concentration of a solution is known as its **osmolarity.** One **osmol** is equal to 1 mol of solute particles. Therefore, a 1 M solution of glucose has a concentration of 1 Osm (1 osmol per liter), whereas a 1 M solution of sodium chloride contains 2 osmol of solute per liter of solution. A liter of solution containing 1 mol of glucose and 1 mol of sodium chloride has an osmolarity of 3 Osm. A solution with an osmolarity of 3 Osm may contain 1 mol of glucose and 1 mol of sodium chloride, or 3 mol of glucose, or 1.5 mol of sodium chloride, or any other combination of solutes as long as the total solute concentration is equal to 3 Osm.

Although *osmolarity* refers to the concentration of solute particles, it also determines the water concentration in the solution because the higher the osmolarity, the lower the water concentration. The concentration of water in any two solutions having the same osmolarity is the same because the total number of solute particles per unit volume is the same.

Let us now apply these principles governing water concentration to osmosis of water across membranes. **Figure 4.17** shows two 1 L compartments separated by a membrane permeable to *both* solute and water. Initially, the concentration of solute is 2 Osm in compartment 1 and 4 Osm in compartment 2. This difference in solute concentration means there is also a difference in water concentration across the membrane: 53.5 M

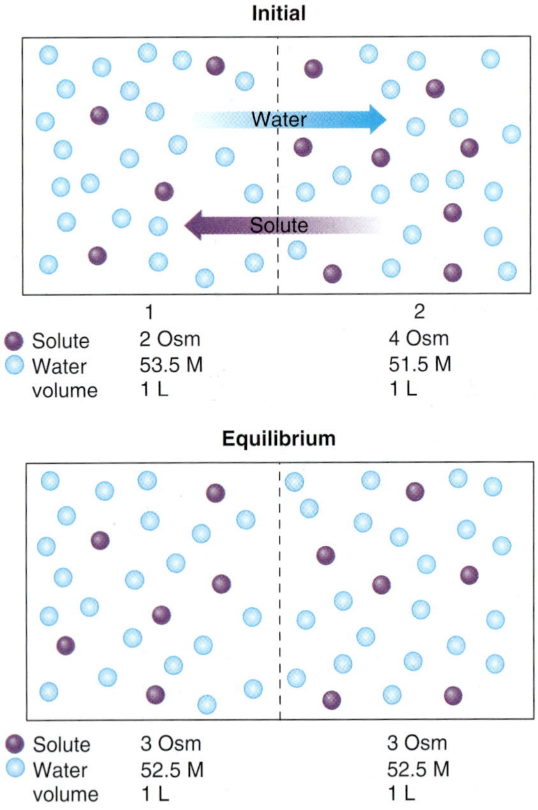

Figure 4.17 AP|R Between two compartments of equal volume, the net diffusion of water and solute across a membrane permeable to both leads to diffusion equilibrium of both, with no change in the volume of either compartment. (For clarity's sake, not all water molecules are shown in this figure or in Figure 4.18.)

in compartment 1 and 51.5 M in compartment 2. Therefore, a net diffusion of water from the higher concentration in compartment 1 to the lower concentration in compartment 2 will take place, and a net diffusion of solute in the opposite direction, from 2 to 1. When diffusion equilibrium is reached, the two compartments will have identical solute and water concentrations, 3 Osm and 52.5 M, respectively. One mol of water will have diffused from compartment 1 to compartment 2, and 1 mol of solute will have diffused from 2 to 1. Because 1 mol of solute has replaced 1 mol of water in compartment 1, and vice versa in compartment 2, no change in the volume occurs for either compartment.

If the membrane is now replaced by one *permeable to water but impermeable to solute* (**Figure 4.18**), the same *concentrations* of water and solute will be reached at equilibrium as before, but a change in the *volumes* of the compartments will also occur. Water will diffuse from 1 to 2, but there will be no solute diffusion in the opposite direction because the membrane is impermeable to solute. Water will continue to diffuse into compartment 2, therefore, until the water concentrations on the two sides become equal. The solute concentration in compartment 2 decreases as it is diluted by the incoming water, and the solute in compartment 1 becomes more concentrated as water moves out. When the water reaches diffusion equilibrium, the osmolarities of the compartments will be equal; therefore, the solute concentrations must also be equal. To reach this state of

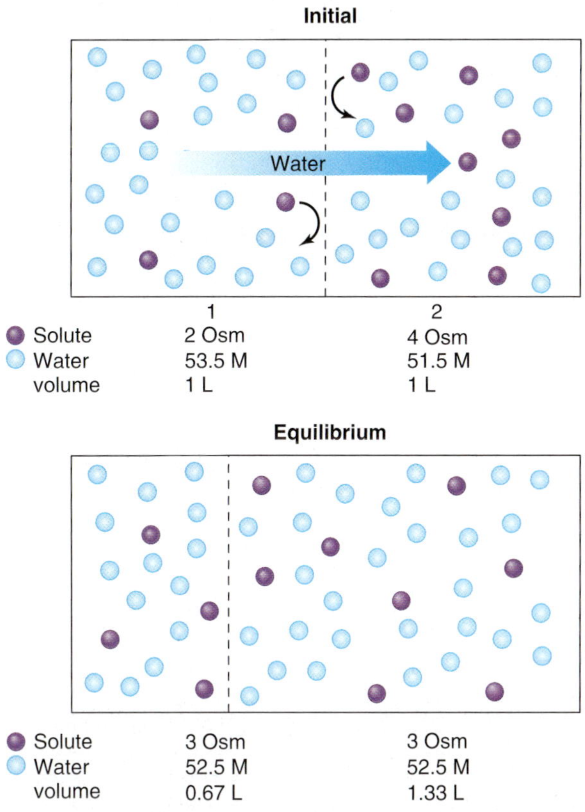

Figure 4.18 AP|R The movement of water across a membrane that is permeable to water but not to solute leads to an equilibrium state involving a change in the volumes of the two compartments. In this case, a net diffusion of water (0.33 L) occurs from compartment 1 to 2. (We will assume that the membrane in this example stretches as the volume of compartment 2 increases so that no significant change in compartment pressure occurs.)

equilibrium, enough water must pass from compartment 1 to 2 to increase the volume of compartment 2 by one-third and decrease the volume of compartment 1 by an equal amount. Note that it is the presence of a membrane impermeable to solute that leads to the volume changes associated with osmosis.

The two compartments in our example were treated as if they were infinitely expandable, so the net transfer of water did not create a pressure difference across the membrane. In contrast, if the walls of compartment 2 in Figure 4.18 had only a limited capacity to expand, as occurs across plasma membranes, the movement of water into compartment 2 would raise the pressure in compartment 2, which would oppose further net water entry. Thus, the movement of water into compartment 2 can be prevented by the application of pressure to compartment 2. This leads to an important definition. When a solution containing solutes is separated from pure water by a **semipermeable membrane** (a membrane permeable to water but not to solutes), the pressure that must be applied to the solution to prevent the net flow of water into it is known as the **osmotic pressure** of the solution. The greater the osmolarity of a solution, the greater the osmotic pressure. It is important to recognize that osmotic pressure does not push water molecules into a solution. Rather, it represents the amount of pressure that would have to be applied to a solution to *prevent* the net flow of water into the solution. Like osmolarity, the osmotic pressure associated with a solution is a measure of the solution's water concentration—the lower the water concentration, the higher the osmotic pressure.

Extracellular Osmolarity and Cell Volume

We can now apply the principles learned about osmosis to cells, which meet all the criteria necessary to produce an osmotic flow of water across a membrane. Both the intracellular and extracellular fluids contain water, and cells are surrounded by a membrane that is very permeable to water but impermeable to many substances. Substances that cannot cross the plasma membrane are called **nonpenetrating solutes;** that is, they do not penetrate through the lipid bilayer.

Most of the extracellular solute particles are sodium and chloride ions, which can diffuse into the cell through ion channels in the plasma membrane or enter the cell during secondary active transport. As we have seen, however, the plasma membrane contains Na^+/K^+-ATPase pumps that actively move sodium ions out of the cell. Therefore, Na^+ moves into cells and is pumped back out, behaving as if it never entered in the first place. For this reason, extracellular Na^+ behaves as a nonpenetrating solute. Any chloride ions that enter cells are also removed as quickly as they enter, due to the electrical repulsion generated by the membrane potential and the action of secondary transporters. Like Na^+, therefore, extracellular chloride ions behave as if they were nonpenetrating solutes.

Inside the cell, the major solute particles are potassium ions and a number of organic solutes. Most of the latter are large polar molecules unable to diffuse through the plasma membrane. Although potassium ions can diffuse out of a cell through K^+ channels, they are actively transported back by the Na^+/K^+-ATPase pump. The net effect, as with extracellular Na^+ and Cl^-, is that K^+ behaves as if it were a nonpenetrating solute, but in this case one confined to the intracellular fluid.

Therefore, Na^+ and Cl^- outside the cell and K^+ and organic solutes inside the cell behave as nonpenetrating solutes on the two sides of the plasma membrane.

The osmolarity of the extracellular fluid is normally in the range of 285–300 mOsm (we will round off to a value of 300 for the rest of this text unless otherwise noted). Because water can diffuse across plasma membranes, water in the intracellular and extracellular fluids will come to diffusion equilibrium. At equilibrium, therefore, the osmolarities of the intracellular and extracellular fluids are the same—approximately 300 mOsm. Changes in extracellular osmolarity can cause cells, such as the red blood cells shown in the chapter-opening photo, to shrink or swell as water molecules move across the plasma membrane.

If cells with an intracellular osmolarity of 300 mOsm are placed in a solution of nonpenetrating solutes having an osmolarity of 300 mOsm, they will neither swell nor shrink because the water concentrations in the intracellular and extracellular fluids are the same, and the solutes cannot leave or enter. Such solutions are said to be **isotonic** (**Figure 4.19**), meaning any solution that does not cause a change in cell size. Isotonic solutions have the same concentration of *nonpenetrating* solutes as normal extracellular fluid. By contrast, **hypotonic** solutions have a nonpenetrating solute concentration lower than that found in cells; therefore, water moves by osmosis into the cells, causing them to swell. Similarly, solutions containing greater than 300 mOsm of nonpenetrating solutes (**hypertonic** solutions) cause cells to shrink as water diffuses out of the cell into the fluid with the lower water concentration. The concentration of *nonpenetrating* solutes in a solution, not the total osmolarity, determines its tonicity—isotonic, hypotonic, or hypertonic. Penetrating solutes do not contribute to the tonicity of a solution.

Another set of terms—**isoosmotic, hypoosmotic,** and **hyperosmotic**—denotes the osmolarity of a solution relative to that of normal extracellular fluid without regard to whether the solute is penetrating or nonpenetrating. The two sets of terms are therefore not synonymous. For example, a 1 L solution containing 150 mOsm each of nonpenetrating Na^+ and Cl^- and 100 mOsm of urea, which can rapidly cross plasma membranes, would have a total osmolarity of 400 mOsm and would be hyperosmotic. It would, however, also be an isotonic solution, producing no change in the equilibrium volume of cells immersed in it. *Initially*, cells placed in this solution would shrink as water moved into the extracellular fluid. However, urea would quickly diffuse into the cells and reach the same concentration as the urea in the extracellular solution; consequently, both the intracellular and extracellular solutions would soon reach the same osmolarity. Therefore, at equilibrium, there would be no difference in the water concentration across the membrane and thus no change in final cell volume; this would be the case even though the extracellular fluid would remain hyperosmotic relative to the normal value of 300 mOsm. **Table 4.3** provides a comparison of the various terms used to describe the osmolarity and tonicity of solutions.

4.4 Endocytosis and Exocytosis

In addition to diffusion and mediated transport, there is another pathway by which substances can enter or leave cells, one that does not require the molecules to pass through the structural matrix of the plasma membrane. When sections of cells are observed under an electron microscope, regions of the plasma membrane can often be seen to have folded into the cell, forming small pockets that pinch off to produce intracellular, membrane-bound vesicles that enclose a small volume of extracellular fluid. This process is known as **endocytosis** (**Figure 4.20**). A similar process in the reverse direction, **exocytosis,** occurs when membrane-bound vesicles in the cytoplasm fuse with the plasma membrane and release their contents to the outside of the cell (see Figure 4.20).

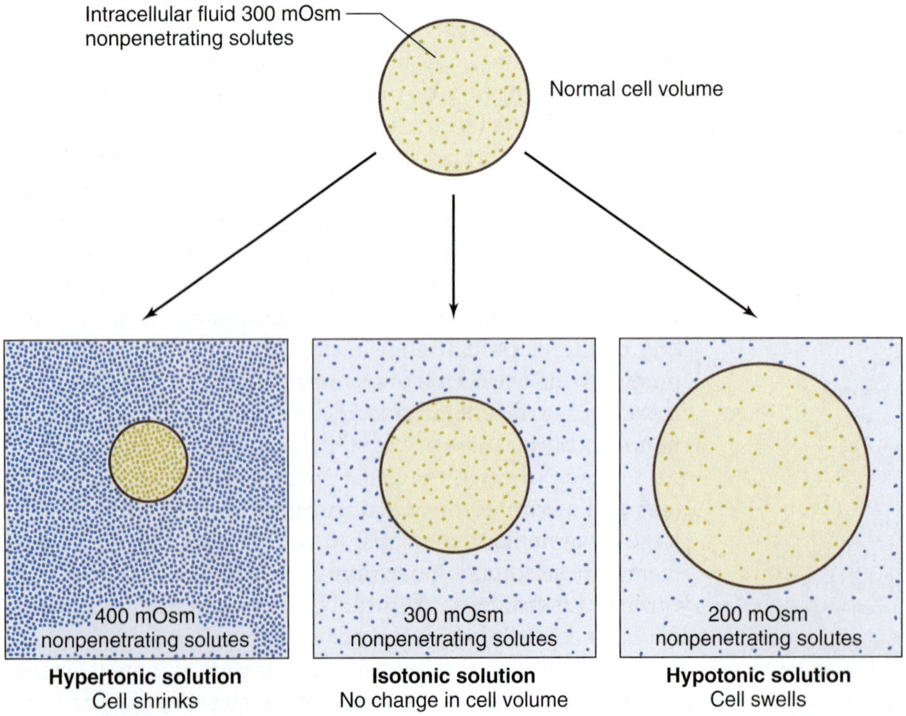

Figure 4.19 APIR Changes in cell volume produced by hypertonic, isotonic, and hypotonic solutions.

PHYSIOLOGICAL INQUIRY

- Blood volume must be restored in a person who has lost large amounts of blood due to serious injury. This is often accomplished by infusing isotonic NaCl solution into the blood. Why is this better than infusing an isoosmotic solution of a penetrating solute, such as urea?

Answer can be found at end of chapter.

TABLE 4.3	Terms Referring to the Osmolarity and Tonicity of Solutions*
Isotonic	A solution that does not cause a change in cell volume; one that contains 300 mOsmol/L of nonpenetrating solutes, regardless of the concentration of membrane-penetrating solutes present
Hypertonic	A solution that causes cells to shrink; one that contains greater than 300 mOsmol/L of nonpenetrating solutes, regardless of the concentration of membrane-penetrating solutes present
Hypotonic	A solution that causes cells to swell; one that contains less than 300 mOsmol/L of nonpenetrating solutes, regardless of the concentration of membrane-penetrating solutes present
Isoosmotic	A solution containing 300 mOsmol/L of solute, regardless of its composition of membrane-penetrating and nonpenetrating solutes
Hyperosmotic	A solution containing greater than 300 mOsmol/L of solutes, regardless of its composition of membrane-penetrating and nonpenetrating solutes
Hypoosmotic	A solution containing less than 300 mOsmol/L of solutes, regardless of its composition of membrane-penetrating and nonpenetrating solutes

*These terms are defined using an intracellular osmolarity of 300 mOsm, which is within the range for human cells but not an absolute fixed number.

Endocytosis

Three general types of endocytosis may occur in a cell. These are pinocytosis ("cell drinking"), phagocytosis ("cell eating"), and receptor-mediated endocytosis (**Figure 4.21**).

In **pinocytosis,** also known as **fluid endocytosis,** an endocytotic vesicle encloses a small volume of extracellular fluid. This process is nonspecific because the vesicle simply engulfs the water in the extracellular fluid along with whatever solutes are present. These solutes may include ions, nutrients, or any other small extracellular molecule. Large macromolecules, other cells, and cell debris do not normally enter a cell via this process.

In **phagocytosis,** cells engulf bacteria or large particles such as cell debris from damaged tissues. In this form of endocytosis, extensions of the plasma membrane called pseudopodia fold around the surface of the particle, engulfing it entirely. The pseudopodia, with their engulfed contents, then fuse into large vesicles called **phagosomes** that are internalized into the cell. Phagosomes migrate to and fuse with lysosomes in the cytoplasm, and the contents of the phagosomes are then destroyed by lysosomal enzymes and other molecules. Whereas most cells undergo pinocytosis, only a few special types of cells, such as those of the immune system (Chapter 18), carry out phagocytosis.

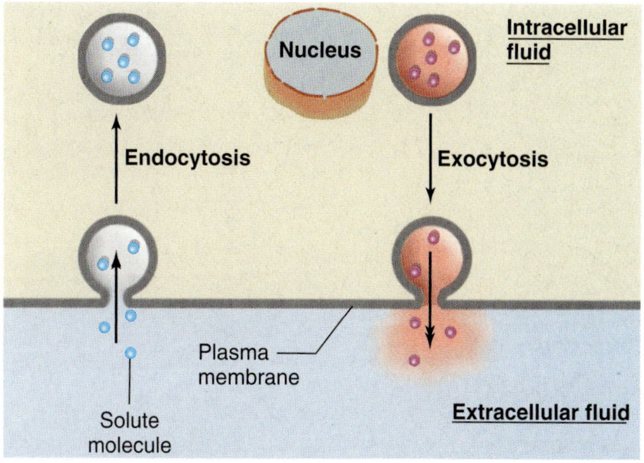

Figure 4.20 APIR Endocytosis and exocytosis.

In contrast to pinocytosis and phagocytosis, most cells have the capacity to *specifically* take up molecules that are important for cellular function or structure. In **receptor-mediated endocytosis,** certain molecules in the extracellular fluid bind to specific proteins on the outer surface of the plasma membrane. These proteins are called **receptors,** and each one recognizes one ligand with high affinity (see Section C of Chapter 3 for a discussion of ligand–protein interactions). In one form of receptor-mediated endocytosis, the receptor undergoes a conformational change when it binds a ligand. Through a series of steps, a cytosolic protein called **clathrin** is recruited to the plasma membrane. A class of proteins called adaptor proteins links the ligand-receptor complex to clathrin. The entire complex then forms a cagelike structure that leads to the aggregation of ligand-bound receptors into a localized region of membrane, forming a depression, or **clathrin-coated pit,** which then invaginates and pinches off to form a clathrin-coated vesicle. By localizing ligand-receptor complexes to discrete patches of plasma membrane prior to endocytosis, cells may obtain concentrated amounts of ligands without having to engulf large amounts of extracellular fluid from many different sites along the membrane. Receptor-mediated endocytosis, therefore, leads to a selective concentration in the endocytotic vesicle of a specific ligand bound to one type of receptor.

Cholesterol is one example of a ligand that enters cells via clathrin-dependent, receptor-mediated endocytosis. Cholesterol is an important building block for plasma and intracellular membranes, and most cells require a steady supply of this molecule. Cholesterol circulates in the blood, bound with proteins in particles called lipoproteins. The protein components of lipoproteins are recognized by plasma membrane receptors. When the receptors bind the lipoproteins, endocytosis ensues and the cholesterol is delivered to the intracellular fluid. The rate at which this occurs can be regulated. For example, if a cell has sufficient supplies of cholesterol, the rate at which it replenishes its supply of lipoprotein receptors may decrease. Conversely, receptor production increases when cholesterol supplies are low. This is a type of negative feedback that acts to maintain the cholesterol content of the cell within a homeostatic range.

Once an endocytotic vesicle pinches off from the plasma membrane in receptor-mediated endocytosis, the clathrin coat

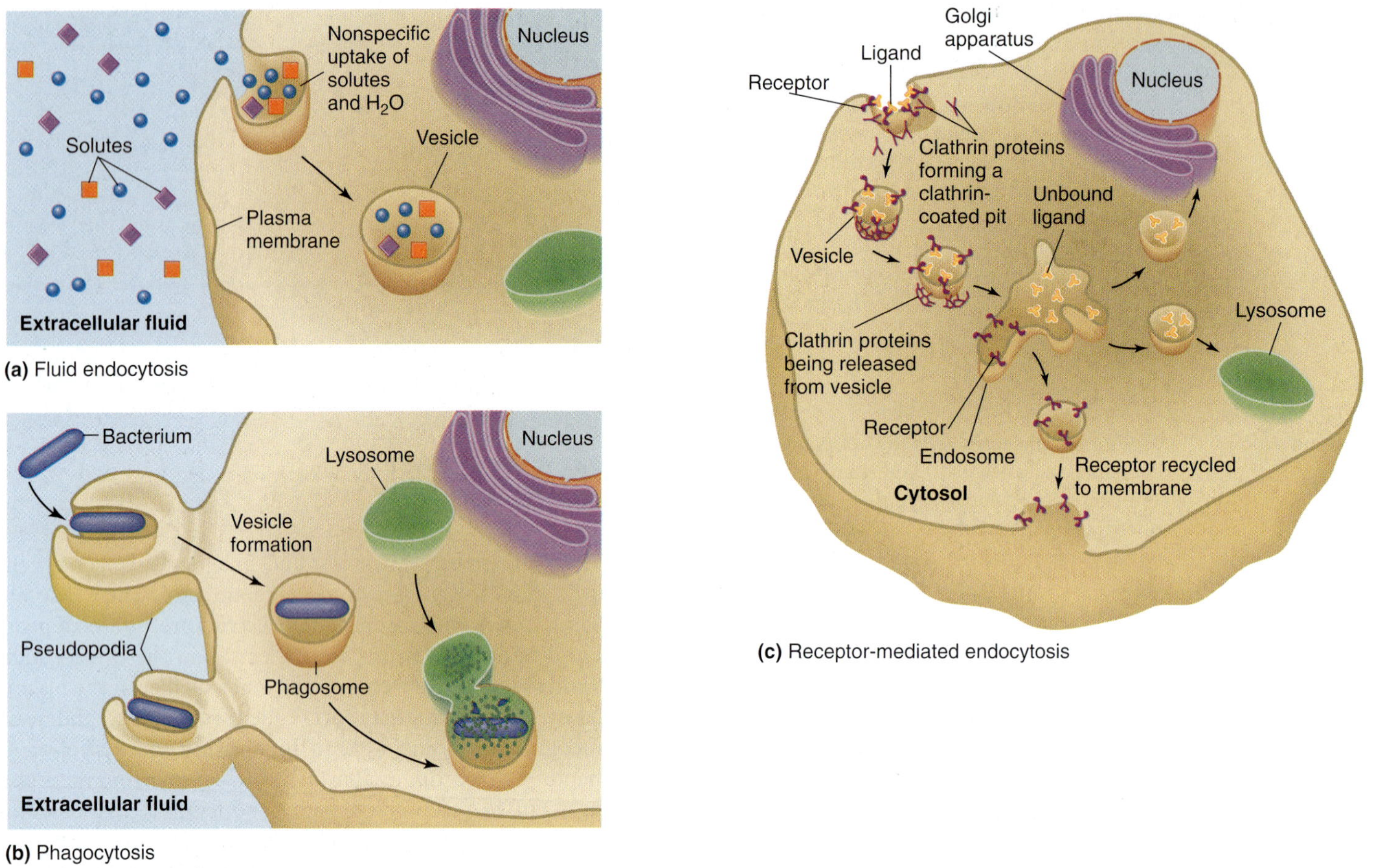

Figure 4.21 APIR Pinocytosis, phagocytosis, and receptor-mediated endocytosis. (a) In pinocytosis, solutes and water are nonspecifically brought into the cell from the extracellular fluid via endocytotic vesicles. (b) In phagocytosis, specialized cells form extensions of the plasma membrane called pseudopodia, which engulf bacteria or other large objects such as cell debris. The vesicles that form fuse with lysosomes, which contain enzymes and other molecules that destroy the vesicle contents. (c) In receptor-mediated endocytosis, a cell recognizes a specific extracellular ligand that binds to a plasma membrane receptor. The binding triggers endocytosis. In the example shown here, the ligand-receptor complexes are internalized via clathrin-coated vesicles, which merge with endosomes (for simplicity, adapter proteins are not shown). Ligands may be routed to the Golgi apparatus for further processing, or to lysosomes. The receptors are typically recycled to the plasma membrane.

is removed and clathrin proteins are recycled back to the membrane. The vesicles then have several possible fates, depending upon the cell type and the ligand that was engulfed. Some vesicles fuse with the membrane of an intracellular organelle, adding the contents of the vesicle to the lumen of that organelle. Other endocytotic vesicles pass through the cytoplasm and fuse with the plasma membrane on the opposite side of the cell, releasing their contents to the extracellular space. This provides a pathway for the transfer of large molecules, such as proteins, across the layers of cells that separate two fluid compartments in the body (for example, the blood and interstitial fluid). A similar process allows small amounts of macromolecules to move across the intestinal epithelium.

Most endocytotic vesicles fuse with a series of intracellular vesicles and tubular elements known as endosomes (Chapter 3), which lie between the plasma membrane and the Golgi apparatus. Like the Golgi apparatus, the endosomes perform a sorting function, distributing the contents of the vesicle and its membrane to various locations. Some of the contents of endocytotic vesicles are passed from the endosomes to the Golgi apparatus, where the ligands are modified and processed. Other vesicles fuse with lysosomes, organelles that contain digestive enzymes that break down large molecules such as proteins, polysaccharides, and nucleic acids. The fusion of endosomal vesicles with the lysosomal membrane exposes the contents of the vesicle to these digestive enzymes. Finally, in many cases, the receptors that were internalized with the vesicle get recycled back to the plasma membrane.

Another fate of endocytotic vesicles is seen in a special type of receptor-mediated endocytosis called potocytosis. **Potocytosis** is similar to other types of receptor-mediated endocytosis in that an extracellular ligand typically binds to a plasma membrane receptor, initiating formation of an intracellular vesicle. In potocytosis, however, the ligands appear to be primarily restricted to low-molecular-weight molecules such as certain vitamins, but have also been found to include the lipoprotein complexes just described. Potocytosis differs from clathrin-dependent, receptor-mediated endocytosis in the fate of the endocytotic vesicle. In potocytosis, tiny vesicles called **caveolae** (singular: *caveolus,* "little cave") pinch off from the plasma membrane and deliver their contents directly to the cell cytosol rather than merging with lysosomes or other organelles. The small molecules within the caveolae may diffuse into the cytosol via channels or be transported by carriers. Although their functions are still being actively investigated, caveolae have been implicated in a variety of important cellular functions, including cell signaling, transcellular transport, and cholesterol homeostasis.

Each episode of endocytosis removes a small portion of the membrane from the cell surface. In cells that have a great deal of endocytotic activity, more than 100% of the plasma membrane may be internalized in an hour, yet the membrane surface area remains constant. This is because the membrane is replaced at about the same rate by vesicle membrane that fuses with the plasma membrane during *exocytosis.* Some of the plasma membrane proteins taken into the cell during endocytosis are stored in the membranes of endosomes and, upon receiving the appropriate signal, can be returned to fuse with the plasma membrane during exocytosis.

Exocytosis

Exocytosis performs two functions for cells: (1) it provides a way to replace portions of the plasma membrane that endocytosis has removed and, in the process, a way to add new membrane components as well; and (2) it provides a route by which membrane-impermeable molecules (such as protein hormones) that the cell synthesizes can be secreted into the extracellular fluid.

How does the cell package substances that are to be secreted by exocytosis into vesicles? Chapter 3 described the entry of newly formed proteins into the lumen of the endoplasmic reticulum and the protein's processing through the Golgi apparatus. From the Golgi apparatus, the proteins to be secreted travel to the plasma membrane in vesicles from which they can be released into the extracellular fluid by exocytosis. In some cases, substances enter vesicles via mediated transporters in the vesicle membrane.

The secretion of substances by exocytosis is triggered in most cells by stimuli that lead to an increase in cytosolic calcium concentration in the cell. As will be described in Chapters 5 and 6, these stimuli open calcium channels in the plasma membrane and/or the membranes of intracellular organelles. The resulting increase in cytosolic calcium concentration activates proteins required for the vesicle membrane to fuse with the plasma membrane and release the vesicle contents into the extracellular fluid. Material stored in secretory vesicles is available for rapid secretion in response to a stimulus, without delays that might occur if the material had to be synthesized after the stimulus arrived. Exocytosis is the mechanism by which most neurons communicate with each other through the release of neurotransmitters stored in secretory vesicles that merge with the plasma membrane. It is also a major way in which many types of hormones are released from endocrine cells into the extracellular fluid.

Cells that actively undergo exocytosis recover bits of membrane via a process called compensatory endocytosis. This process, the mechanisms of which are still uncertain but that may involve both clathrin- and non-clathrin-mediated events, restores membrane material to the cytoplasm that can be made available for the formation of new secretory vesicles. It also helps prevent the plasma membrane's unchecked expansion.

4.5 Epithelial Transport

As described in Chapter 1, epithelial cells line hollow organs or tubes and regulate the absorption or secretion of substances across these surfaces. One surface of an epithelial cell generally faces a hollow or fluid-filled chamber, and the plasma membrane on this side is referred to as the **apical membrane** (also known as the luminal or mucosal membrane) of the epithelium (refer back to Figures 1.2 and 3.9). The plasma membrane on the opposite surface, which is usually adjacent to a network of blood vessels, is referred to as the **basolateral membrane** (also known as the serosal membrane).

The two pathways by which a substance can cross a layer of epithelial cells are (1) the **paracellular pathway,** in which diffusion occurs *between* the adjacent cells of the epithelium; and (2) the **transcellular pathway,** in which a substance moves *into* an epithelial cell across either the apical or basolateral membrane, diffuses through the cytosol, and exits across the opposite membrane. Diffusion through the paracellular pathway is limited by the presence of tight junctions between adjacent cells, because these junctions form a seal around the apical end of the epithelial cells (Chapter 3). Although small ions and water can diffuse to some degree through tight junctions, the amount of paracellular diffusion is limited by the tightness of the junctional seal and the relatively small area available for diffusion.

During transcellular transport, the movement of molecules through the plasma membranes of epithelial cells occurs via the pathways (diffusion and mediated transport) already described for movement across membranes. However, the transport and permeability characteristics of the apical and basolateral membranes are not the same. These two membranes often contain different ion channels and different transporters for mediated transport. As a result of these differences, substances can undergo a net movement from a low concentration on one side of an epithelium to a higher concentration on the other side. Examples include the absorption of material from the gastrointestinal tract into the blood, the movement of substances between the kidney tubules and the blood during urine formation, and the secretion of salts and water by glands such as sweat glands.

Figure 4.22 and **Figure 4.23** illustrate two examples of active transport across an epithelium. Na^+ is actively transported across most epithelia from lumen to blood side in absorptive processes, and from blood side to lumen during secretion. In our example, the movement of Na^+ from the lumen into the epithelial cell occurs by diffusion through Na^+ channels in the apical membrane (see Figure 4.22). Na^+ diffuses into the cell because the intracellular concentration of Na^+ is kept low by the active transport of Na^+ back out of the cell across the basolateral membrane on the opposite side, where all of the Na^+/K^+-ATPase pumps are located. In other words, Na^+ moves downhill into the cell and then uphill out of it. The net result is that Na^+ can be moved from lower to higher concentration across the epithelium.

Figure 4.23 illustrates the active absorption of organic molecules across an epithelium. In this case, the entry of an organic molecule X across the luminal plasma membrane occurs via a secondary active transporter linked to the downhill movement of Na^+ into the cell. In the process, X moves from a lower concentration in the luminal fluid to a higher concentration in the cell. The substance exits across the basolateral membrane by facilitated diffusion, which moves the material from its higher concentration in the cell to a lower concentration in the extracellular fluid on the blood side. The

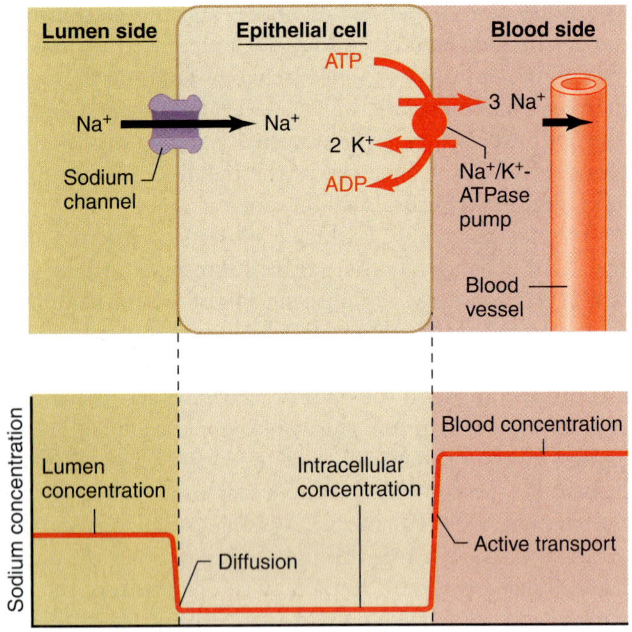

Figure 4.22 Active transport of Na^+ across an epithelial cell. The transepithelial transport of Na^+ always involves primary active transport out of the cell across one of the plasma membranes, typically via an Na^+/K^+-ATPase pump as shown here. The movement of Na^+ into the cell across the plasma membrane on the opposite side is always downhill. Sometimes, as in this example, it is by diffusion through Na^+ channels, whereas in other epithelia this downhill movement occurs through a secondary active transporter. Shown below the cell is the concentration profile of the transported solute across the epithelium.

PHYSIOLOGICAL INQUIRY

- What would happen in this situation if the cell's ATP supply decreased significantly?

Answer can be found at end of chapter.

concentration of the substance may be considerably higher on the blood side than in the lumen because the blood-side concentration can approach equilibrium with the high intracellular concentration created by the apical membrane entry step.

Although water is not actively transported across cell membranes, net movement of water across an epithelium can occur by osmosis as a result of the active transport of solutes, notably Na^+, across the epithelium. The active transport of Na^+, as previously described, results in a decrease in the Na^+ concentration on one side of an epithelial layer (the luminal side in our example) and an increase on the other. These changes in solute concentration are accompanied by changes in the water concentration on the two sides because a change in solute concentration, as we have seen, produces a change in water concentration. The water concentration difference will cause water to move by osmosis from the low-Na^+ side to the high-Na^+ side of the epithelium (**Figure 4.24**). Therefore, net movement of solute across an epithelium is accompanied by a flow of water in the same direction. If the epithelial cells are highly permeable to water, large net movements of water can occur with very small differences in osmolarity. As you will learn in Chapter 14, this is a major way in which epithelial cells of the kidney absorb water from the urine back into the blood. It is also the major way in which water is absorbed from the intestines into the blood (Chapter 15).

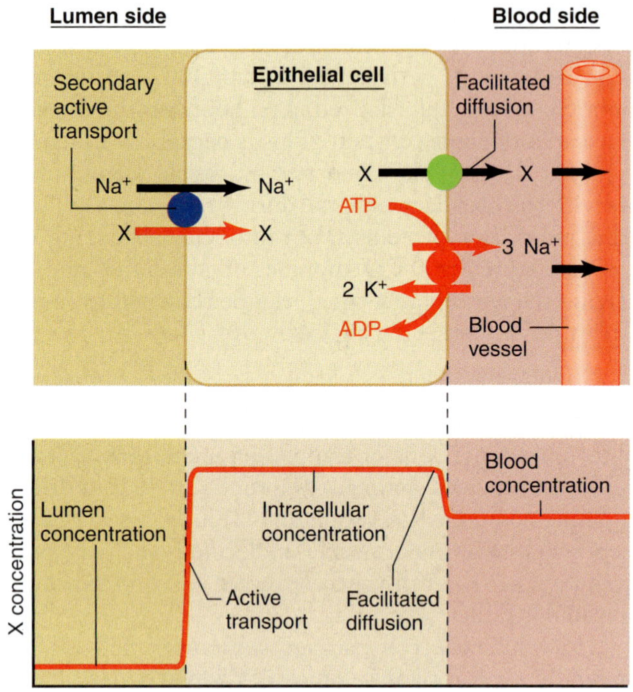

Figure 4.23 The transepithelial transport of most organic solutes (X) involves their movement into a cell through a secondary active transport driven by the downhill flow of Na^+. The organic substance then moves out of the cell at the blood side down a concentration gradient by means of facilitated diffusion. Shown below the cell is the concentration profile of the transported solute across the epithelium.

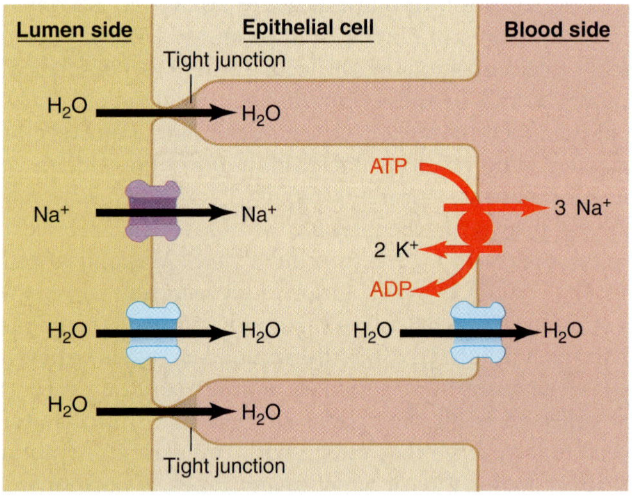

Figure 4.24 Net movements of water across an epithelium are dependent on net solute movements. The active transport of Na^+ across the cells and into the surrounding interstitial spaces produces an elevated osmolarity in this region and a decreased osmolarity in the lumen. This leads to the osmotic flow of water across the epithelium in the same direction as the net solute movement. The water diffuses through water channels in the membrane and across the tight junctions between the epithelial cells.

SUMMARY

Diffusion

I. Simple diffusion is the movement of molecules from one location to another by random thermal motion.
   a. The net flux between two compartments always proceeds from higher to lower concentrations.
   b. Diffusion equilibrium is reached when the concentrations of the diffusing substance in the two compartments become equal.

II. The magnitude of the net flux J across a membrane is directly proportional to the concentration difference across the membrane $C_o - C_i$, the surface area of the membrane A, and the membrane permeability coefficient P.

III. Nonpolar molecules diffuse through the hydrophobic portions of membranes much more rapidly than do polar or ionized molecules because nonpolar molecules can dissolve in the fatty acyl tails in the lipid bilayer.

IV. Ions diffuse across membranes by passing through ion channels formed by integral membrane proteins.
   a. The diffusion of ions across a membrane depends on both the concentration gradient and the membrane potential.
   b. The flux of ions across a membrane can be altered by opening or closing ion channels.

Mediated-Transport Systems

I. The mediated transport of molecules or ions across a membrane involves binding the transported solute to a transporter protein in the membrane. Changes in the conformation of the transporter move the binding site to the opposite side of the membrane, where the solute dissociates from the protein.
   a. The binding sites on transporters exhibit chemical specificity, affinity, and saturation.
   b. The magnitude of the flux through a mediated-transport system depends on the degree of transporter saturation, the number of transporters in the membrane, and the rate at which the conformational change in the transporter occurs.

II. Facilitated diffusion is a mediated-transport process that moves molecules from higher to lower concentrations across a membrane by means of a transporter until the two concentrations become equal. Metabolic energy is not required for this process.

III. Active transport is a mediated-transport process that moves molecules against an electrochemical gradient across a membrane by means of a transporter and an input of energy.
   a. Primary active transport uses the phosphorylation of the transporter by ATP to drive the transport process.
   b. Secondary active transport uses the binding of ions (often Na^+) to the transporter to drive the secondary-transport process.
   c. In secondary active transport, the downhill flow of an ion is linked to the uphill movement of a second solute either in the same direction as the ion (cotransport) or in the opposite direction of the ion (countertransport).

Osmosis

I. Water crosses membranes by (a) diffusing through the lipid bilayer, and (b) diffusing through protein channels in the membrane.

II. Osmosis is the diffusion of water across a membrane from a region of higher water concentration to a region of lower water concentration. The osmolarity—total solute concentration in a solution—determines the water concentration: the higher the osmolarity of a solution, the lower the water concentration.

III. Osmosis across a membrane that is permeable to water but impermeable to solute leads to an increase in the volume of the compartment on the side that initially had the higher osmolarity, and a decrease in the volume on the side that initially had the lower osmolarity.

IV. Application of sufficient pressure to a solution will prevent the osmotic flow of water into the solution from a compartment of pure water. This pressure is called the osmotic pressure. The greater the osmolarity of a solution, the greater its osmotic pressure. Net water movement occurs from a region of lower osmotic pressure to one of higher osmotic pressure.

V. The osmolarity of the extracellular fluid is about 300 mOsm. Because water comes to diffusion equilibrium across cell membranes, the intracellular fluid has an osmolarity equal to that of the extracellular fluid.
   a. Na^+ and Cl^- ions are the major effectively nonpenetrating solutes in the extracellular fluid; potassium ions and various organic solutes are the major effectively nonpenetrating solutes in the intracellular fluid.
   b. Table 4.3 lists the terms used to describe the osmolarity and tonicity of solutions containing different compositions of penetrating and nonpenetrating solutes.

Endocytosis and Exocytosis

I. During endocytosis, regions of the plasma membrane invaginate and pinch off to form vesicles that enclose a small volume of extracellular material.
   a. The three classes of endocytosis are (i) fluid endocytosis, (ii) phagocytosis, and (iii) receptor-mediated endocytosis.
   b. Most endocytotic vesicles fuse with endosomes, which in turn transfer the vesicle contents to lysosomes for digestion by lysosomal enzymes.
   c. Potocytosis is a special type of receptor-mediated endocytosis in which vesicles called caveolae deliver their contents directly to the cytosol.

II. Exocytosis, which occurs when intracellular vesicles fuse with the plasma membrane, provides a means of adding components to the plasma membrane and a route by which membrane-impermeable molecules, such as proteins the cell synthesizes, can be released into the extracellular fluid.

Epithelial Transport

I. Molecules can cross an epithelial layer of cells by two pathways: (a) through the extracellular spaces between the cells—the paracellular pathway; and (b) through the cell, across both the luminal and basolateral membranes as well as the cell's cytoplasm—the transcellular pathway.

II. In epithelial cells, the permeability and transport characteristics of the apical and basolateral plasma membranes differ, resulting in the ability of cells to actively transport a substance between the fluid on one side of the cell and the fluid on the opposite side.

III. The active transport of Na^+ through an epithelium increases the osmolarity on one side of the cell and decreases it on the other, causing water to move by osmosis in the same direction as the transported Na^+.

REVIEW QUESTIONS

1. What determines the direction in which net diffusion of a nonpolar molecule will occur?
2. In what ways can the net solute flux between two compartments separated by a permeable membrane be increased?
3. Why are membranes more permeable to nonpolar molecules than to most polar and ionized molecules?
4. Ions diffuse across cell membranes by what pathway?
5. When considering the diffusion of ions across a membrane, what driving force, in addition to the ion concentration gradient, must be considered?
6. Describe the mechanism by which a transporter of a mediated-transport system moves a solute from one side of a membrane to the other.
7. What determines the magnitude of flux across a membrane in a mediated-transport system?
8. What characteristics distinguish simple diffusion from facilitated diffusion?
9. What characteristics distinguish facilitated diffusion from active transport?
10. Describe the direction in which sodium ions and a solute transported by secondary active transport move during cotransport and countertransport.
11. How can the concentration of water in a solution be decreased?
12. If two solutions with different osmolarities are separated by a water-permeable membrane, why will a change occur in the volumes of the two compartments if the membrane is impermeable to the solutes but no change in volume will occur if the membrane is permeable to solutes?
13. Why do sodium and chloride ions in the extracellular fluid and potassium ions in the intracellular fluid behave as though they were nonpenetrating solutes?
14. What is the approximate osmolarity of the extracellular fluid? Of the intracellular fluid?
15. What change in cell volume will occur when a cell is placed in a hypotonic solution? In a hypertonic solution?
16. Under what conditions will a hyperosmotic solution be isotonic?
17. How do the mechanisms for actively transporting glucose and Na^+ across an epithelium differ?
18. By what mechanism does the active transport of Na^+ lead to the osmotic flow of water across an epithelium?

KEY TERMS

active transport 103
apical membrane 113
aquaporin 107
basolateral membrane 113
caveolus 112
channel gating 101
clathrin 111
clathrin-coated pit 111
cotransport 106
countertransport 106
diffusion equilibrium 97
electrochemical gradient 101
endocytosis 110
exocytosis 110
facilitated diffusion 102
fluid endocytosis 111
flux 97
hyperosmotic 110
hypertonic 110
hypoosmotic 110
hypotonic 110
ion channel 99
isoosmotic 110
isotonic 110
ligand-gated channel 101
mechanically gated channel 101
mediated transport 101
membrane potential 100
net flux 97
nonpenetrating solute 109
osmol 108
osmolarity 108
osmosis 107
osmotic pressure 109
paracellular pathway 113
phagocytosis 111
phagosome 111
pinocytosis 111
potocytosis 112
primary active transport 103
receptor 111
receptor-mediated endocytosis 111
secondary active transport 103
semipermeable membrane 109
simple diffusion 97
transcellular pathway 113
transporter 101
voltage-gated channel 101

CLINICAL TERMS

exercise-associated hyponatremia 115
type 1 diabetes mellitus 103

CHAPTER 4

Clinical Case Study: A Novice Marathoner Collapses After a Race

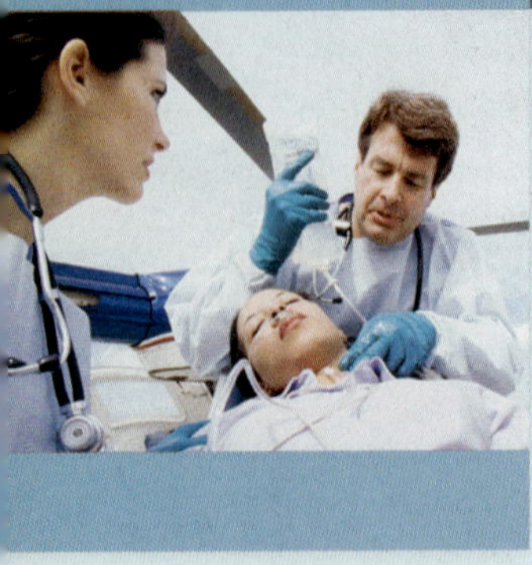

A 22-year-old, 102-pound (46.4 kg) woman who had occasionally competed in short-distance races, decided to compete in her first marathon. She was in good health but was completely inexperienced in long-distance runs. During the hour before the race, she drank two 20-ounce bottles of water (about 1.2 liters) in anticipation of the water loss she expected to occur due to perspiration over the next few hours. The race took place on an unseasonably cool day in April. As she ran, she was careful to drink a cup of water (5–10 ounces) at each water station, roughly each mile along the course. Being a newcomer to competing in marathons, she had already been running for 3 hours at the 20-mile mark and was beginning to feel extremely fatigued. Soon after, her leg muscles began cramping and she felt slightly sick to her stomach. Thinking she was losing too much fluid, she stopped for a moment at a water station and drank several cups of water, then continued on. After another 2 miles, she became nauseated and consumed a full 20-ounce bottle of water; a mile later, she began to feel confused and disoriented and developed a headache. At that point, she became panicked that she would not finish the race; even though she did not feel thirsty, she finished yet another bottle of water. Twenty minutes later, she collapsed, lost consciousness, and was taken by ambulance to a local hospital. She was diagnosed with ***exercise-associated hyponatremia*** (EAH), a condition in which the concentration of Na^+ in the blood decreases to dangerously low levels (in her case, to 115 mM; see Table 4.1 for comparison).

(continued)

(continued)

It was clear to her physicians what caused the EAH. When we exercise, perspiration helps cool us down. Perspiration is a dilute solution of several ions, particularly Na^+ (the other major ones being Cl^- and K^+). The result of excessive sweating is that the total amount of water and Na^+ in the body becomes depleted. Our patient was exercising very hard and for a very long time but was not losing as much fluid as she had anticipated because of the cold weather. She was wise to be aware of the potential for fluid loss, but she was not aware that drinking pure water in such quantities could significantly dilute her body fluids. As the concentration of Na^+ in her extracellular fluid decreased, the electrochemical gradient for Na^+ across her cells—including her muscle and brain cells—also decreased as a consequence. As noted in this chapter and described in detail in Chapters 6 and 9, the electrochemical gradient for Na^+ is part of what regulates the function of skeletal muscle and brain cells. As a result of disrupting this gradient, our patient's muscles and neurons began to malfunction, accounting in part for the cramps and mental confusion.

In addition, however, recall from Figure 4.19 what happens to cells when the concentrations of nonpenetrating solutes across the cell membrane are changed. As our patient's extracellular fluid became more dilute than her intracellular fluid, water moved by osmosis into her cells. Many types of cells, including those of the brain, are seriously damaged when they swell due to water influx. It is even worse in the brain than elsewhere because there is no room for the brain to expand within the skull. As brain cells swell, the fluid pressure in the brain increases, compressing blood vessels and restricting blood flow. When blood flow is reduced, oxygen and nutrient levels decrease and metabolic waste products build up, further contributing to brain cell malfunction. Thus, the combination of water influx, increased pressure, and changes in the electrochemical gradient for Na^+ all contributed to the mental disturbances and subsequent loss of consciousness in our patient.

Interestingly, the nausea triggered by the EAH probably is responsible in part for activating the release of a hormone called antidiuretic hormone (ADH) from the pituitary gland. You will learn about this hormone and gland in Chapters 11, 12, and 14, but for now it is worth noting that the primary function of ADH is to stimulate the kidneys to retain water in the body by producing less urine. This might happen, for example, when someone is dehydrated, as was described earlier in this chapter. In the case of our subject, however, this hormone was counterproductive, because she was already overhydrated. The decrease in urine production caused by nausea-induced increases in antidiuretic hormone only made things worse.

What do you think would be an appropriate way to treat EAH? Remember, the patient is not dehydrated. In fact, one of the best predictors of EAH in patients like ours is weight *gain* during a marathon; such individuals actually weigh more at the end of a race than at the beginning because of all the water they drink! The treatment is an intravenous infusion of an isotonic solution of NaCl to bring the total levels of Na^+ in the body fluids back toward normal. At the same time, however, the extracellular fluid volume is reduced with a diuretic (a medication that increases urine production). In addition, patients may also receive medications to prevent or stop seizures. As you will learn in Chapters 6 and 8, a seizure is uncontrolled, unregulated activity of the neurons in the brain; one potential cause of a seizure is a large imbalance in extracellular ion concentrations in the brain. In our patient, gradual restoration of Na^+ levels and treatment for the nausea and headache were sufficient to save her life, but careful monitoring of her progress over the course of a 24-hour hospital stay was required.

Clinical term: exercise-associated hyponatremia (EAH)

See Chapter 19 for complete, integrative case studies.

CHAPTER 4 TEST QUESTIONS

Answers found in Appendix A.

1. Which properties are characteristic of ion channels?
   a. They are usually lipids.
   b. They exist on one side of the plasma membrane, usually the intracellular side.
   c. They can open and close depending on the presence of any of three types of "gates."
   d. They permit movement of ions against concentration gradients.
   e. They mediate facilitated diffusion.
2. Which of the following does *not* directly or indirectly require an energy source?
   a. primary active transport
   b. operation of the Na^+/K^+-ATPase pump
   c. the mechanism used by cells to produce a calcium ion gradient across the plasma membrane
   d. facilitated transport of glucose across a plasma membrane
   e. secondary active transport
3. If a small amount of urea were added to an isoosmotic saline solution containing cells, what would be the result?
   a. The cells would shrink and remain that way.
   b. The cells would first shrink but then be restored to normal volume after a brief period of time.
   c. The cells would swell and remain that way.
   d. The cells would first swell but then be restored to normal volume after a brief period of time.
   e. The urea would have no effect, even transiently.
4. Which is/are true of epithelial cells?
   a. They can only move uncharged molecules across their surfaces.
   b. They may have segregated functions on apical (luminal) and basolateral surfaces.
   c. They cannot form tight junctions.
   d. They depend upon the activity of Na^+/K^+-ATPase pumps for much of their transport functions.
   e. Both b and d are correct.
5. Which is *incorrect?*
   a. Diffusion of a solute through a membrane is considerably quicker than diffusion of the same solute through a water layer of equal thickness.
   b. A single ion, such as K^+, can diffuse through more than one type of channel.
   c. Lipid-soluble solutes diffuse more readily through the phospholipid bilayer of a plasma membrane than do water-soluble ones.

d. The rate of facilitated diffusion of a solute is limited by the number of transporters in the membrane at any given time.
e. A common example of cotransport is that of an ion and an organic molecule.

6. In considering diffusion of ions through an ion channel, which driving force/forces must be considered?
a. the ion concentration gradient
b. the electrical gradient
c. osmosis
d. facilitated diffusion
e. both a and b

CHAPTER 4 GENERAL PRINCIPLES ASSESSMENT *Answers found in Appendix A.*

1. How does the information presented in Figures 4.8–4.10 and 4.17 illustrate the general principle that *homeostasis is essential for health and survival?*
2. Give two examples from this chapter that illustrate the general principle that *controlled exchange of materials occurs between compartments and across cellular membranes.*
3. Another general physiological principle states that *physiological processes are dictated by the laws of chemistry and physics.* How does this relate to the movement of solutes through lipid bilayers and its dependence on electrochemical gradients? How is heat related to solute movement?

CHAPTER 4 QUANTITATIVE AND THOUGHT QUESTIONS *Answers found at www.mhhe.com/widmaier13.*

1. In two cases (A and B), the concentrations of solute X in two 1 L compartments separated by a membrane through which X can diffuse are

	Concentration of X (mM)	
Case	Compartment 1	Compartment 2
A	3	5
B	32	30

a. In what direction will the net flux of X take place in case A and in case B?
b. When diffusion equilibrium is reached, what will the concentration of solute in each compartment be in case A and in case B?
c. Will A reach diffusion equilibrium faster, slower, or at the same rate as B?

2. When the extracellular concentration of the amino acid alanine is increased, the net flux of the amino acid leucine into a cell is decreased. How might this observation be explained?
3. If a transporter that mediates active transport of a substance has a lower affinity for the transported substance on the extracellular surface of the plasma membrane than on the intracellular surface, in what direction will there be a net transport of the substance across the membrane? (Assume that the rate of transporter conformational change is the same in both directions.)
4. Why will inhibition of ATP synthesis by a cell lead eventually to a decrease and, ultimately, cessation in secondary active transport?
5. Given the following solutions, which has the lowest water concentration? Which two have the same osmolarity?

	Concentration (mM)			
Solution	Glucose	Urea	NaCl	$CaCl_2$
A	20	30	150	10
B	10	100	20	50
C	100	200	10	20
D	30	10	60	100

6. Assume that a membrane separating two compartments is permeable to urea but not permeable to NaCl. If compartment 1 contains 200 mmol/L of NaCl and 100 mmol/L of urea, and compartment 2 contains 100 mmol/L of NaCl and 300 mmol/L of urea, which compartment will have increased in volume when osmotic equilibrium is reached?
7. What will happen to cell volume if a cell is placed in each of the following solutions?

	Concentration of X, mM	
Solution	NaCl (Nonpenetrating)	Urea (Penetrating)
A	150	100
B	100	150
C	200	100
D	100	50

8. Characterize each of the solutions in question 7 as isotonic, hypotonic, hypertonic, isoosmotic, hypoosmotic, or hyperosmotic.
9. By what mechanism might an increase in intracellular Na^+ concentration lead to an increase in exocytosis?

CHAPTER 4 ANSWERS TO PHYSIOLOGICAL INQUIRIES

Figure 4.2 As shown in the accompanying graph, there would be a net flux of glucose from compartment 1 to compartment 2, with diffusion equilibrium occurring at 12.5 mmol/L.

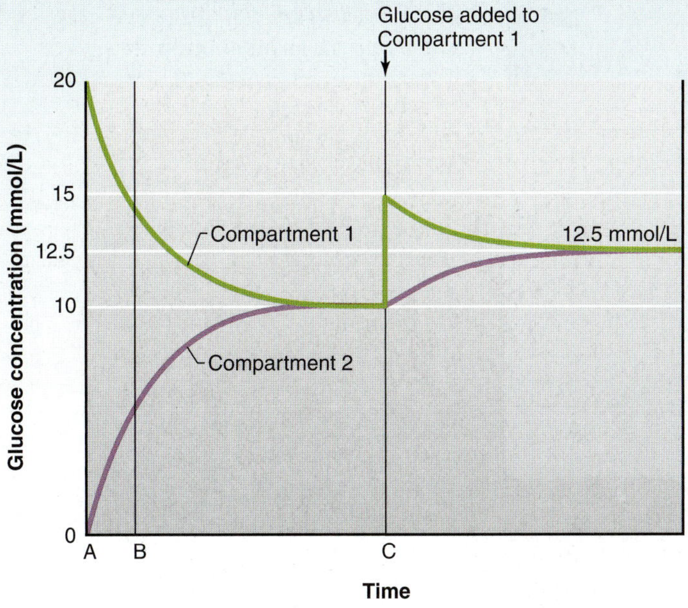

Figure 4.5 The primary structure of the protein is represented by the beads—the amino acid sequence shown in (a). The secondary structure includes all the helical regions in the lipid bilayer, shown in (a) and (b). The tertiary structure is the folded conformation shown in (b). The quaternary structure is the association of the five subunit polypeptides into one protein, shown in (c).

Figure 4.9 Maximal flux depends on the number of transporter molecules in the membrane and their inherent rate of conformational change when binding solute. If we assume that the rate of conformational change stays constant, then the greater the number of transporters, the greater the maximal flux that can occur.

Figure 4.13 ATP is not hydrolyzed when a solute moves across a membrane by secondary active transport. However, ATP *is* hydrolyzed by an ion pump (typically the Na^+/K^+-ATPase primary active transporter) to establish the ion concentration gradient that is used during secondary active transport. Therefore, secondary active transport *indirectly* requires ATP.

Figure 4.19 Because it is a nonpenetrating solute, infusion of isotonic NaCl restores blood volume without causing a redistribution of water between body fluid compartments due to osmosis. An isoosmotic solution of a penetrating solute, however, would only partially restore blood volume because some water would enter the intracellular fluid by osmosis as the solute enters cells. This could also result in damage to cells as their volume expands beyond normal.

Figure 4.22 Active transport of Na^+ across the basolateral (blood side) membrane would decrease, resulting in an increased intracellular concentration of Na^+. This would reduce the rate of Na^+ diffusion into the cell through the Na^+ channel on the lumen side because the diffusion gradient would be smaller.

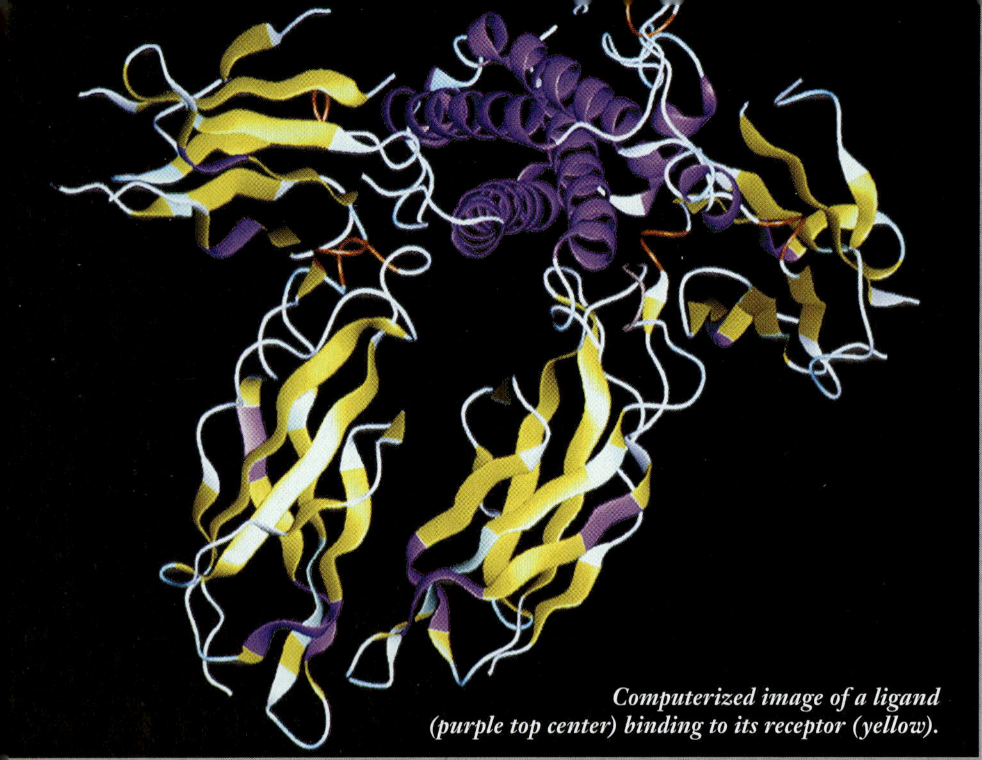

Computerized image of a ligand (purple top center) binding to its receptor (yellow).

5 Control of Cells by Chemical Messengers

You learned in Chapter 1 how homeostatic control systems help maintain a normal balance of the body's internal environment. The operation of control systems requires that cells be able to communicate with each other, often over long distances. Much of this intercellular communication is mediated by chemical messengers. This chapter describes how these messengers interact with their target cells and how these interactions trigger intracellular signals that lead to the cell's response. Throughout this chapter, you should carefully distinguish *inter*cellular (between cells) and *intra*cellular (within a cell) chemical messengers and communication. The material in this chapter will provide a foundation for understanding how the nervous, endocrine, and other organ systems function. Before starting, you should review the material covered in Section C of Chapter 3 for background on ligand–protein interactions.

The material in this chapter illustrates the general physiological principle that information flow between cells, tissues, and organs is an essential feature of homeostasis and allows for integration of physiological processes. These many and varied processes will be covered in detail beginning in Chapter 6 and will continue throughout the book, but the mechanisms of information flow that link different structures and processes share many common features, as described here.

5.1 Receptors

In Chapter 1, you learned that several classes of chemical messengers can communicate a signal from one cell to another. These messengers include molecules such as neurotransmitters, whose signals are mediated rapidly and over a short distance. Other messengers, such as hormones, communicate more slowly and over greater distances. Whatever the chemical messenger, however, the cell receiving the signal must have a way to detect the signal's presence. Once a cell detects a signal, a mechanism is required to transduce that signal into a biologically meaningful response, such as the cell-division response to the delivery of growth-promoting signals.

The first step in the action of any intercellular chemical messenger is the binding of the messenger to specific target-cell proteins known as **receptors** or **receptor proteins.** In the general language of Chapter 3, a chemical messenger is a ligand, and the receptor has a binding site for that ligand. The binding of a messenger to a receptor activates the receptor; this initiates a sequence of events in the cell leading to the cell's response to that messenger, a process called **signal transduction.** In this section, we consider some general features common to many receptors, describe the interactions between receptors and their ligands, and give some examples of how receptors are regulated.

Receptors and Their Interactions with Ligands

What is the nature of the receptors that bind intercellular chemical messengers? They are proteins or glycoproteins located either in the cell's plasma membrane or inside the cell, either in the cytosol or the nucleus. The plasma membrane is the much more common location, because a very large number of messengers are water-soluble and therefore cannot diffuse across the lipid-rich (hydrophobic) plasma membrane. In contrast, a much smaller number of lipid-soluble messengers pass through membranes (mainly by diffusion but in some cases assisted by mediated transport) to bind to their receptors located inside the cell.

Plasma membrane receptors are transmembrane proteins; that is, they span the entire membrane thickness. A typical plasma membrane receptor is illustrated in **Figure 5.1**. Like other transmembrane proteins, a plasma membrane receptor has hydrophobic segments within the membrane, one or more hydrophilic segments extending out from the membrane into the extracellular fluid, and other hydrophilic segments extending into the intracellular fluid. Arriving chemical messengers bind to the extracellular parts of the receptor.

Specificity

The binding of a chemical messenger to its receptor initiates the events leading to the cell's response. The existence of receptors explains a very important characteristic of intercellular communication—**specificity** (see **Table 5.1** for a glossary of terms concerning receptors). Although a given chemical messenger may come into contact with many different cells, it influences certain cell types and not others. This is because cells differ in the types of receptors they possess. Only certain cell types—sometimes just one—express the specific receptor required to bind a given chemical messenger (**Figure 5.2**). In many cases, the receptor proteins for a group of messengers are structurally related. For example, there are "superfamilies" of hormone receptors such as the steroid hormone receptors.

Even though different cell types may possess the receptors for the same messenger, the responses of the various cell types to that messenger may differ from each other.

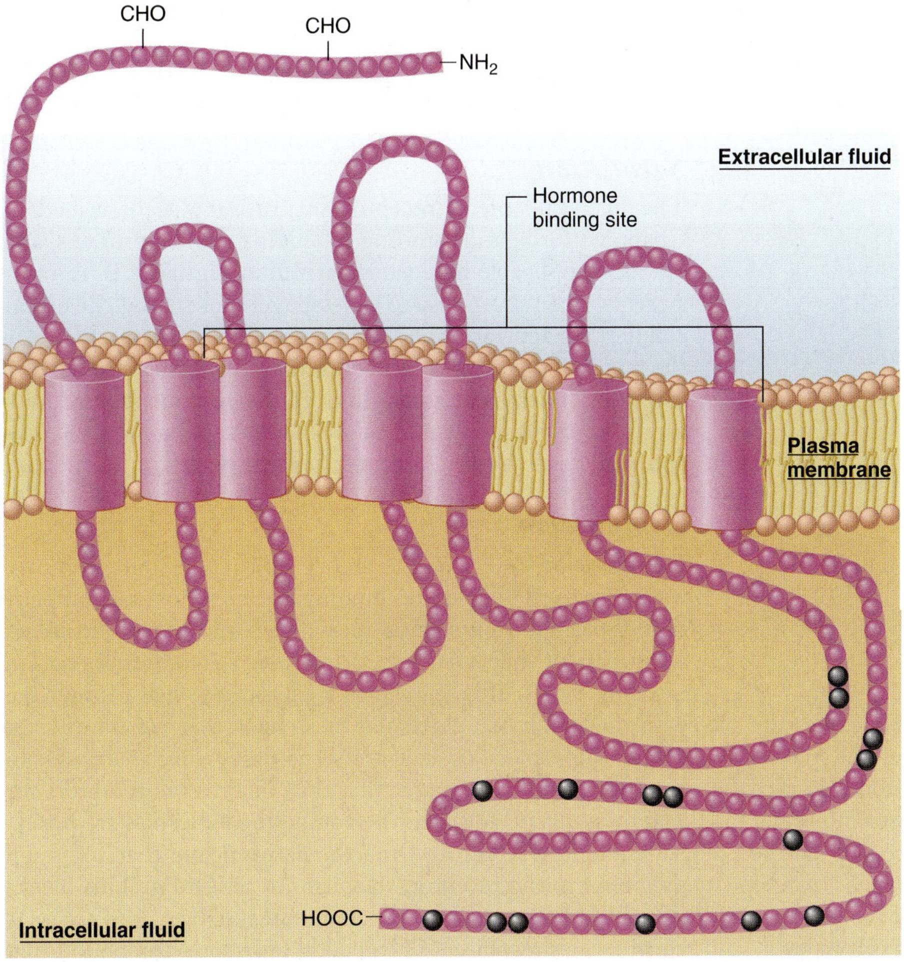

Figure 5.1 Structure of a receptor that binds the hormone epinephrine. The seven clusters of amino acids embedded in the phospholipid bilayer represent hydrophobic portions of the protein's alpha helix (shown here as cylinders). Note that the binding site for the hormone includes several of the segments that extend into the extracellular fluid. Portions of the extracellular segments can be linked to carbohydrates (CHO). The amino acids denoted by black circles represent some of the sites at which intracellular enzymes can phosphorylate, and thereby regulate, the receptor.

TABLE 5.1	A Glossary of Terms Concerning Receptors
Receptor (receptor protein)	A specific protein in either the plasma membrane or the interior of a target cell that a chemical messenger binds with, thereby invoking a biologically relevant response in that cell.
Specificity	The ability of a receptor to bind only one type or a limited number of structurally related types of chemical messengers.
Saturation	The degree to which receptors are occupied by messengers. If all are occupied, the receptors are fully saturated; if half are occupied, the saturation is 50%, and so on.
Affinity	The strength with which a chemical messenger binds to its receptor.
Competition	The ability of different molecules to compete with a ligand for binding to its receptor. Competitors generally are similar in structure to the natural ligand.
Antagonist	A molecule that competes with a ligand for binding to its receptor but does not activate signaling normally associated with the natural ligand. Therefore, an antagonist prevents the actions of the natural ligand. Antihistamines are examples of antagonists.
Agonist	A chemical messenger that binds to a receptor and triggers the cell's response; often refers to a drug that mimics a normal messenger's action. Decongestants are examples of agonists.
Down-regulation	A decrease in the total number of target-cell receptors for a given messenger; may occur in response to chronic high extracellular concentration of the messenger.
Up-regulation	An increase in the total number of target-cell receptors for a given messenger; may occur in response to a chronic low extracellular concentration of the messenger.
Increased sensitivity	The increased responsiveness of a target cell to a given messenger; may result from up-regulation of receptors.

For example, the neurotransmitter norepinephrine causes the smooth muscle of certain blood vessels to contract but, via the same type of receptor, inhibits insulin secretion from the pancreas. In essence, then, the receptor functions as a molecular switch that elicits the cell's response when "switched on" by the messenger binding to it. Just as identical types of switches can be used to turn on a light or a radio, a single type of receptor can be used to produce different responses in different cell types.

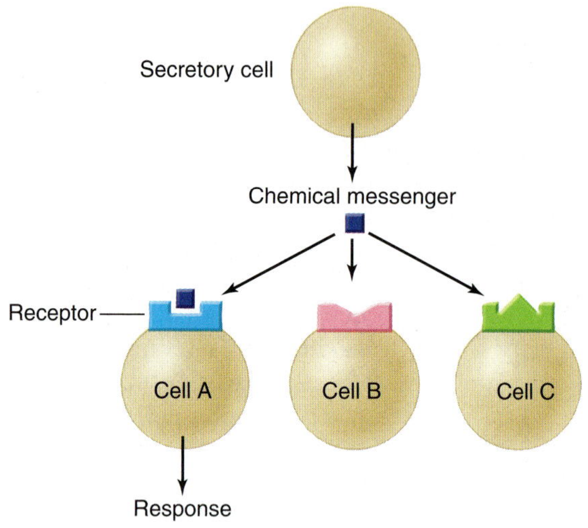

Figure 5.2 Specificity of receptors for chemical messengers. Only cell A has the appropriate receptor for this chemical messenger; therefore, it is the only one among the group that is a target cell for the messenger.

Affinity

The degree to which a particular messenger binds to its receptor is determined by the **affinity** of the receptor for the messenger. A receptor with high affinity will bind at lower concentrations of a messenger than will a receptor of low affinity (refer back to Figure 3.36). Differences in affinity of receptors for their ligands have important implications for the use of therapeutic drugs in treating illness; receptors with high affinity for a ligand require much less of the ligand (that is, a lower dose) to become activated.

Saturation

The phenomenon of receptor **saturation** was described in Chapter 3 for ligands binding to binding sites on proteins, and are fully applicable here (summarized in **Figure 5.3**). In most systems, a cell's response to a messenger increases as the extracellular concentration of the messenger increases, because the number of receptors occupied by messenger molecules increases. There is an upper limit to this responsiveness, however, because only a finite number of receptors are available, and they become fully saturated at some point.

Competition

Competition refers to the ability of a molecule to compete with a natural ligand for binding to its receptor. Competition typically occurs with messengers that have a similarity in part of their structures, and it also underlies the action of many drugs. If researchers or physicians wish to interfere with the action of a particular messenger, they can administer competing molecules that are structurally similar enough to the endogenous messenger that they bind to the receptors for that messenger. However, the competing molecules are different enough in structure from the native ligand that, although they bind to the receptor, they cannot activate it. This blocks the endogenous messenger from binding and yet does not trigger the cell's response. The general term for a compound that

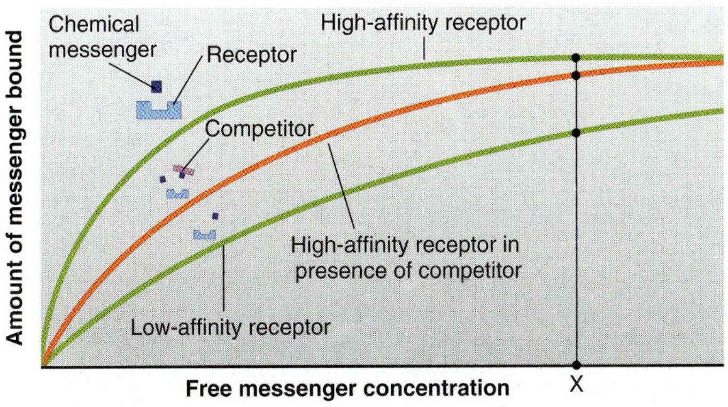

Figure 5.3 Characteristics of receptors binding to messengers. The receptors with high affinity will have more bound messenger at a given messenger concentration (e.g., concentration X). The presence of a competitor will reduce the amount of messenger bound, until at very high concentrations the receptors become saturated with messenger. Note in the illustration that the low-affinity receptor in this case has a slightly different shape in its ligand-binding region compared to the high-affinity receptor. Also note the similarity in parts of the shapes of the natural messenger and its competitor.

blocks the action of a chemical messenger is **antagonist;** when an antagonist works by competing with a chemical messenger for its binding site, it is known as a competitive antagonist. One example is a type of drug called a beta-blocker, which is sometimes used in the treatment of high blood pressure and other diseases. Beta-blockers antagonize the ability of epinephrine and norepinephrine to bind to one of their receptors—the beta-adrenergic receptor. Because epinephrine and norepinephrine normally act to increase blood pressure (Chapter 12), beta-blockers tend to decrease blood pressure by acting as antagonists. Antihistamines are another example and are useful in treating allergic symptoms brought on due to excess histamine secretion from cells known as mast cells (Chapter 18). Antihistamines are antagonists that block histamine from binding to its receptors on cells and triggering an allergic response.

On the other hand, some drugs that compete with natural ligands for a particular receptor type do trigger the cell's response exactly as if the true (endogenous) chemical messenger had combined with the receptor. Such drugs, known as **agonists,** are used therapeutically to mimic the messenger's action. For example, the common decongestant drugs ***phenylephrine*** and ***oxymetazoline,*** found in many types of nasal sprays, mimic the action of epinephrine on a different class of receptors, called alpha-adrenergic receptors, in blood vessels. When alpha-adrenergic receptors are activated, the smooth muscles of inflamed, dilated blood vessels in the nose contract, resulting in constriction of those vessels in the nasal passages and fewer sniffles.

Regulation of Receptors

Receptors are themselves subject to physiological regulation. The number of receptors a cell has, or the affinity of the receptors for their specific messenger, can be increased or decreased in certain systems. An important example is the phenomenon of **down-regulation.** When a high extracellular concentration of a messenger is maintained for some time, the total number of the target cell's receptors for that messenger may decrease—that is, down-regulate. Down-regulation has the effect of reducing the target cells' responsiveness to frequent or intense stimulation by a messenger—that is, desensitizing them—and thus represents a local negative feedback mechanism.

Change in the opposite direction, called **up-regulation,** also occurs. Cells exposed for a prolonged period to very low concentrations of a messenger may come to have many more receptors for that messenger, thereby developing increased sensitivity to it. The greater the number of receptors available to bind a ligand, the greater the likelihood that such binding will occur. For example, when the nerves to a muscle are damaged, the delivery of neurotransmitters from those nerves to the muscle is decreased or eliminated. With time, under these conditions, the muscle will contract in response to a much smaller amount of neurotransmitter than normal. This happens because the receptors for the neurotransmitter have been up-regulated, resulting in increased sensitivity.

Up-regulation and down-regulation are possible because there is a continuous synthesis and degradation of receptors. The main cause of down-regulation of plasma membrane receptors is **internalization.** The binding of a messenger to its receptor can stimulate the internalization of the complex; that is, the messenger-receptor complex is taken into the cell by receptor-mediated endocytosis (see Chapter 4). This increases the rate of receptor degradation inside the cell. Consequently, at elevated hormone concentrations, the number of plasma membrane receptors of that type gradually decreases during down-regulation.

The opposite events also occur and contribute to up-regulation. The cell may contain stores of receptors in the membranes of intracellular vesicles. These are then inserted into the plasma membrane during up-regulation. Receptor regulation is an excellent example of the general physiological principle of homeostasis, because it acts to return signal strength toward normal when the concentration of messenger molecules varies above or below normal.

5.2 Signal Transduction Pathways

What are the sequences of events by which the binding of a chemical messenger to a receptor causes the cell to respond in a specific way?

The combination of messenger with receptor causes a change in the conformation (three-dimensional shape) of the receptor. This event, known as **receptor activation,** is the initial step leading to the cell's responses to the messenger. These cellular responses can take the form of changes in (1) the permeability, transport properties, or electrical state of the plasma membrane; (2) metabolism; (3) secretory activity; (4) rate of proliferation and differentiation; or (5) contractile or other activities.

Despite the seeming variety of responses, there is a common denominator: they are all directly due to alterations of particular cell proteins. Let us examine a few examples of messenger-induced responses, all of which are described more fully in subsequent chapters. The neurotransmitter-induced generation of electrical signals in neurons reflects the altered conformation of membrane proteins (ion channels) through which ions can diffuse between extracellular and intracellular fluid. Similarly, changes in the rate of glucose secretion by the liver induced by the hormone epinephrine reflect the altered activity and concentration of enzymes in the metabolic pathways for glucose synthesis. Finally, muscle contraction induced by the neurotransmitter acetylcholine results from the altered conformation of contractile proteins.

Thus, receptor activation by a messenger is only the first step leading to the cell's ultimate response (contraction, secretion, and so on). The diverse sequences of events that link receptor activation to cellular responses are termed **signal transduction pathways.** The "signal" is the receptor activation, and "transduction" denotes the process by which a stimulus is transformed into a response.

Signal transduction pathways differ between lipid-soluble and water-soluble messengers. As described earlier, the receptors for these two broad chemical classes of messenger are in different locations—the former inside the cell and the latter in the plasma membrane of the cell. The rest of this chapter describes the major features of the signal transduction pathways that these two broad categories of receptors initiate.

Pathways Initiated by Lipid-Soluble Messengers

Lipid-soluble messengers usually act on cells by binding to intracellular receptor proteins. Lipid-soluble messengers include all steroid hormones and the thyroid hormones. Chemically, these hormones are all hydrophobic, and the steroid receptors constitute the **steroid-hormone-receptor superfamily.** Although plasma membrane receptors for a few of these messengers have been identified, most of the receptors in this superfamily are intracellular. When not bound to a messenger, the receptors are inactive. In a few cases, the inactive receptors are located in the cytosol and move into the nucleus after binding their hormone. Most of the inactive receptors, however, already reside in the cell nucleus, where they bind to and are activated by their respective ligands. In both cases, receptor activation leads to altered rates of the transcription of one or more genes in a particular cell.

The messenger diffuses out of capillaries from plasma to the interstitial fluid. From there, the messenger diffuses across the plasma membrane and nuclear envelope to enter the nucleus and bind to the receptor there (**Figure 5.4**). The activated receptor complex then functions in the nucleus as a transcription factor, defined as a regulatory protein that directly influences gene transcription. The hormone–receptor complex binds to DNA at a regulatory region of a gene, an event that typically increases the rate of that gene's transcription into mRNA. The mRNA molecules move out of the nucleus to direct the synthesis, on ribosomes, of the protein the gene encodes. The result is an increase in the cellular concentration of the protein and/or its rate of secretion, accounting for the cell's ultimate response to the messenger. For example, if the protein encoded by the gene is an enzyme, the cell's response is an increase in the rate of the reaction catalyzed by that enzyme.

Two other points are important. First, more than one gene may be subject to control by a single receptor type. For

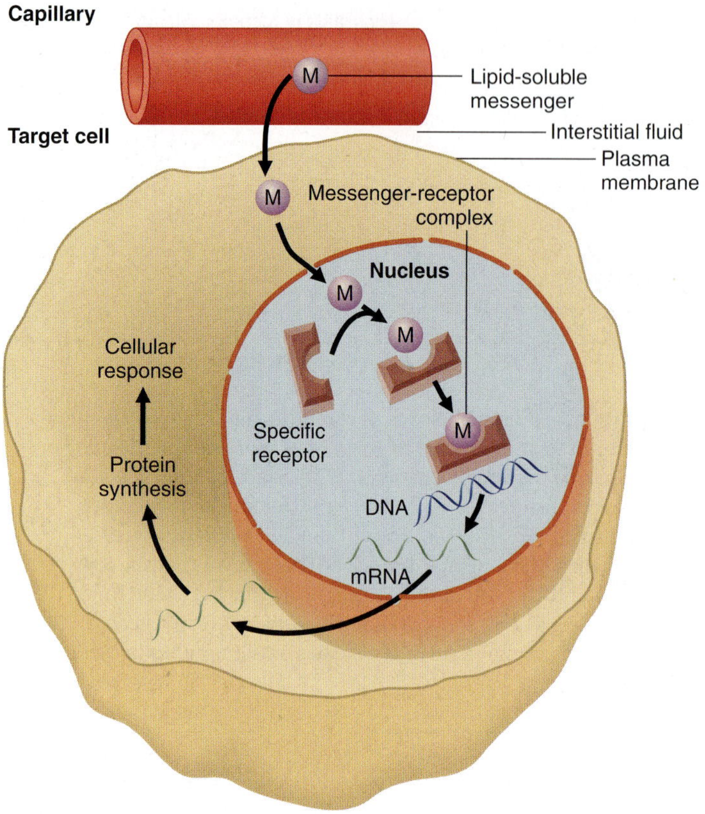

Figure 5.4 APIR Mechanism of action of lipid-soluble messengers. This figure shows the receptor for these messengers in the nucleus. In some cases, the unbound receptor is in the cytosol rather than the nucleus, in which case the binding occurs there, and the messenger-receptor complex moves into the nucleus. For simplicity, a single messenger is shown binding to a single receptor. In many cases, however, two messenger-receptor complexes must bind together in order to activate a gene.

example, the glucocorticoid hormone cortisol acts via its intracellular receptor to activate numerous genes involved in the coordinated control of cellular metabolism and energy balance. Second, in some cases, the transcription of a gene or genes may be *decreased* rather than increased by the activated receptor. Cortisol, for example, inhibits transcription of several genes whose protein products mediate inflammatory responses that occur following injury or infection; for this reason, cortisol has important anti-inflammatory effects.

Pathways Initiated by Water-Soluble Messengers

Water-soluble messengers cannot readily enter cells by diffusion through the lipid bilayer of the plasma membrane. Instead, they exert their actions on cells by binding to the extracellular portion of receptor proteins embedded in the plasma membrane. Water-soluble messengers include most peptide and protein hormones, neurotransmitters, and paracrine–autocrine compounds. On the basis of the signal transduction pathways they initiate, plasma membrane receptors can be classified into the types listed in **Table 5.2** and illustrated in **Figure 5.5**.

Some notes on general terminology are essential for this discussion. First, the extracellular chemical messengers that reach the cell and bind to their specific plasma membrane

TABLE 5.2	Classification of Receptors Based on Their Locations and the Signal Transduction Pathways They Use

I. Intracellular receptors (Figure 5.4) (for lipid-soluble messengers): Function in the nucleus as transcription factors or suppressors to alter the rate of transcription of particular genes

II. Plasma membrane receptors (Figure 5.5) (for water-soluble messengers)
  A. Receptors that are ligand-gated ion channels
  B. Receptors that themselves function as enzymes, such as receptor tyrosine kinases
  C. Receptors that are bound to and activate cytoplasmic janus kinases
  D. G-protein-coupled receptors that activate G proteins, which in turn act upon effector proteins—either ion channels or enzymes—in the plasma membrane

receptors are often referred to as **first messengers. Second messengers,** then, are substances that enter or are generated in the cytoplasm as a result of receptor activation by the first messenger. The second messengers diffuse throughout the cell to serve as chemical relays from the plasma membrane to the biochemical machinery inside the cell. The third essential general term is **protein kinase,** which is the name for an enzyme that phosphorylates other proteins by transferring a phosphate group to them from ATP. Phosphorylation of a protein changes its three-dimensional conformation and, consequently, alters the protein's activity. There are many different protein kinases, and each type is able to phosphorylate only specific proteins. The important point is that a variety of protein kinases are involved in signal transduction pathways. These pathways may involve a series of reactions in which a particular inactive protein kinase is activated by phosphorylation and then catalyzes the phosphorylation of another inactive protein kinase, and so on. At the ends of these sequences, the ultimate phosphorylation of key proteins, such as transporters, metabolic enzymes, ion channels, and contractile proteins, underlies the cell's biochemical response to the first messenger. Different proteins respond differently to phosphorylation; some are activated and some are inactivated (inhibited).

As described in Chapter 3, other enzymes do the reverse of protein kinases; that is, they dephosphorylate proteins. These enzymes, termed protein phosphatases, also participate in signal transduction pathways, but their roles are less understood than those of the protein kinases and will not be described further in this chapter.

Receptors That Are Ligand-Gated Ion Channels

In the first type of plasma membrane receptor listed in Table 5.2, the protein that acts as the receptor is also an ion channel. Activation of the receptor by a first messenger (the ligand) results in a conformational change of the receptor such that it forms an open channel through the plasma membrane (**Figure 5.5a**). Because the opening of ion channels has been compared to the opening of a gate in a fence, these types of channels are known as **ligand-gated ion channels.** They are particularly prevalent in the plasma membranes of neurons, as you will learn in Chapter 6.

The opening of ligand-gated ion channels in response to binding of a first messenger results in an increase in the net diffusion across the plasma membrane of one or more types of ions specific to that channel. As you will see in Chapter 6, such a change in ion diffusion results in a change in the electrical charge, or membrane potential, of a cell. This change in membrane potential constitutes the cell's response to the messenger. In addition, when the channel is a Ca^{2+} channel, its opening results in an increase by diffusion in cytosolic Ca^{2+} concentration. Increasing cytosolic Ca^{2+} is another essential event in the transduction pathway for many signaling systems.

Receptors That Function as Enzymes

The receptors in the second category of plasma membrane receptors listed in Table 5.2 have intrinsic enzyme activity. With one major exception (discussed later), the many receptors that possess intrinsic enzyme activity are all protein kinases (**Figure 5.5b**). Of these, the great majority specifically phosphorylate tyrosine residues. Consequently, these receptors are known as **receptor tyrosine kinases.**

The typical sequence of events for receptors with intrinsic tyrosine kinase activity is as follows. The binding of a specific messenger to the receptor changes the conformation of the receptor so that its enzymatic portion, located on the cytoplasmic side of the plasma membrane, is activated. This results in autophosphorylation of the receptor; that is, the receptor phosphorylates some of its own tyrosine residues. The newly created phosphotyrosines on the cytoplasmic portion of the receptor then serve as docking sites for cytoplasmic proteins. The bound docking proteins then bind and activate other proteins, which in turn activate one or more signaling pathways within the cell. The common denominator of these pathways is that they all involve activation of cytoplasmic proteins by phosphorylation. Most of the receptors with intrinsic tyrosine kinase activity bind first messengers that typically influence cell proliferation and differentiation, and are often called growth factors.

There is one physiologically important exception to the generalization that plasma membrane receptors with inherent enzyme activity function as protein kinases. In this exception, the receptor functions both as a receptor and as a **guanylyl cyclase** to catalyze the formation, in the cytoplasm, of a molecule known as **cyclic GMP (cGMP).** In turn, cGMP functions as a second messenger to activate a protein kinase called **cGMP-dependent protein kinase.** This kinase phosphorylates specific proteins that then mediate the cell's response to the original messenger. As described in Chapter 7, receptors that function both as ligand-binding molecules and as guanylyl cyclases are abundantly expressed in the retina of the eye, where they are important for processing visual inputs. This

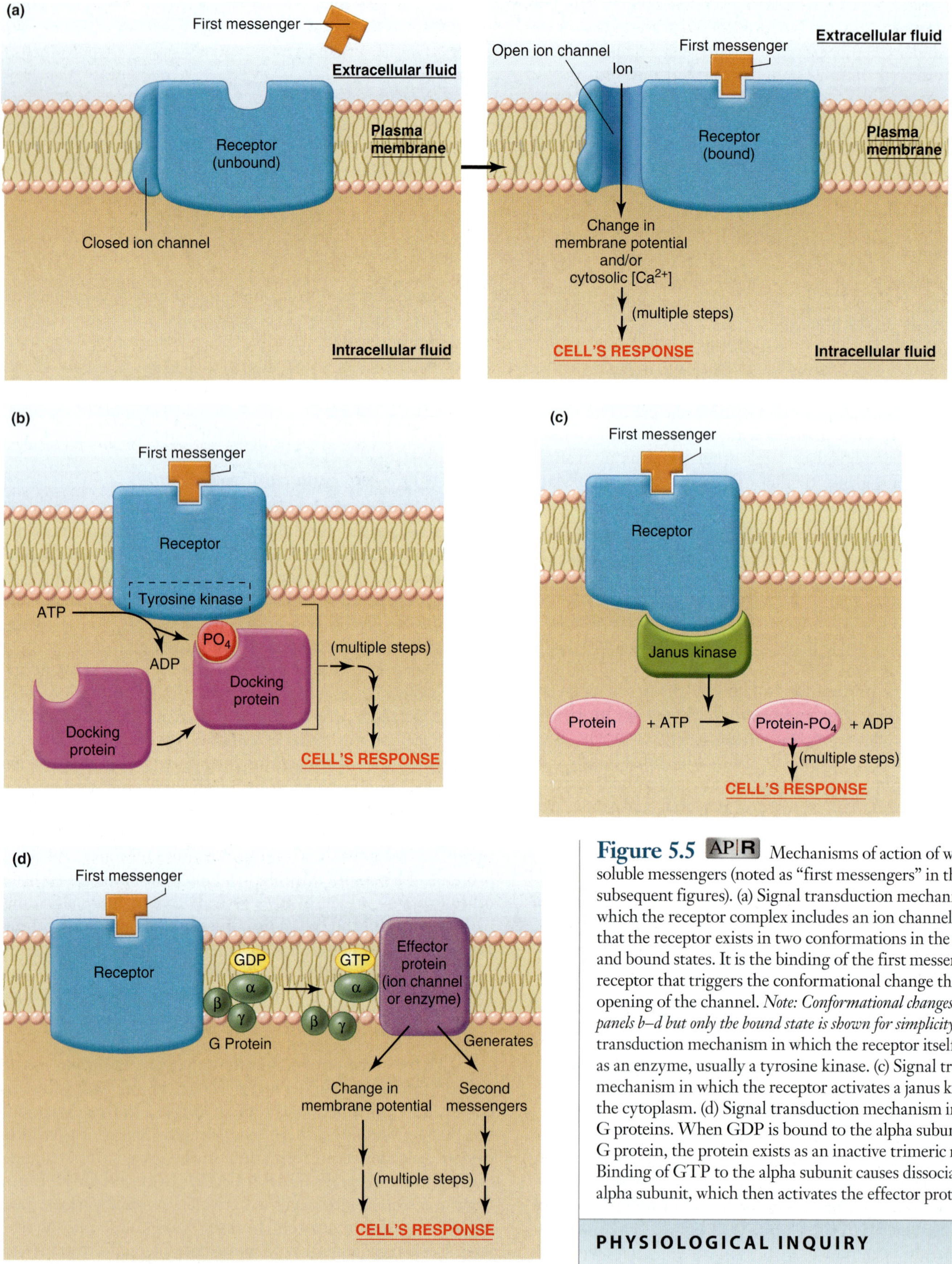

Figure 5.5 AP|R Mechanisms of action of water-soluble messengers (noted as "first messengers" in this and subsequent figures). (a) Signal transduction mechanism in which the receptor complex includes an ion channel. Note that the receptor exists in two conformations in the unbound and bound states. It is the binding of the first messenger to its receptor that triggers the conformational change that leads to opening of the channel. *Note: Conformational changes also occur in panels b–d but only the bound state is shown for simplicity.* (b) Signal transduction mechanism in which the receptor itself functions as an enzyme, usually a tyrosine kinase. (c) Signal transduction mechanism in which the receptor activates a janus kinase in the cytoplasm. (d) Signal transduction mechanism involving G proteins. When GDP is bound to the alpha subunit of the G protein, the protein exists as an inactive trimeric molecule. Binding of GTP to the alpha subunit causes dissociation of the alpha subunit, which then activates the effector protein.

PHYSIOLOGICAL INQUIRY

- Many cells express more than one of the four types of receptors depicted in this figure. Why might this be?

Answer can be found at end of chapter.

signal transduction pathway is used by only a small number of messengers and should not be confused with the much more prevalent cAMP system to be described in a later section. Also, in certain cells, guanylyl cyclase enzymes are present in the cytoplasm. In these cases, a first messenger—the gas nitric oxide (NO)—diffuses into the cytosol of the cell and combines with the guanylyl cyclase to trigger the formation of cGMP. Nitric oxide is a lipid-soluble gas produced from the amino acid arginine by the action of an enzyme called nitric oxide synthase, which is present in numerous cell types including the cells that line the interior of blood vessels. When released from such cells, NO acts locally in a paracrine fashion to relax the smooth muscle component of certain blood vessels, which allows the blood vessel to dilate, or open, more. As you will learn in Chapter 12, the ability of certain blood vessels to dilate is an important part of the homeostatic control of the circulation of blood and of blood pressure.

Receptors That Interact with Cytoplasmic Janus Kinases

Recall that in the previous category, the receptor itself has intrinsic enzyme activity. In the next category of receptors (see Table 5.2 and **Figure 5.5c**), the enzymatic activity—again, tyrosine kinase activity—resides not in the receptor but in a family of separate cytoplasmic kinases, called **janus kinases (JAKs)**, which are associated with the receptor. In these cases, the receptor and its associated janus kinase function as a unit. The binding of a first messenger to the receptor causes a conformational change in the receptor that leads to activation of the janus kinase. Different receptors associate with different members of the janus kinase family, and the different janus kinases phosphorylate different target proteins, many of which act as transcription factors. The result of these pathways is the synthesis of new proteins, which mediate the cell's response to the first messenger. One significant example of signals mediated primarily via receptors linked to janus kinases are those of the cytokines—proteins secreted by cells of the immune system that play a critical role in immune defenses (Chapter 18).

G-Protein-Coupled Receptors

The fourth category of plasma membrane receptors in Table 5.2 is by far the largest, including hundreds of distinct receptors (**Figure 5.5d**). Bound to the inactive receptor is a protein complex located on the cytosolic surface of the plasma membrane and belonging to the family of proteins known as **G proteins.** G proteins contain three subunits, called the alpha, beta, and gamma subunits. The alpha subunit can bind GDP and GTP. The beta and gamma subunits help anchor the alpha subunit in the membrane. The binding of a first messenger to the receptor changes the conformation of the receptor. This activated receptor increases the affinity of the alpha subunit of the G protein for GTP. When bound to GTP, the alpha subunit dissociates from the beta and gamma subunits of the trimeric G protein. This dissociation allows the activated alpha subunit to link up with still another plasma membrane protein, either an ion channel or an enzyme. These ion channels and enzymes are effector proteins that mediate the next steps in the sequence of events leading to the cell's response.

In essence, then, a G protein serves as a switch to couple a receptor to an ion channel or to an enzyme in the plasma membrane. Consequently, these receptors are known as **G-protein-coupled receptors.** The G protein may cause the ion channel to open, with a resulting change in electrical signals or, in the case of Ca^{2+} channels, changes in the cytosolic Ca^{2+} concentration. Alternatively, the G protein may activate or inhibit the membrane enzyme with which it interacts. Such enzymes, when activated, cause the generation of second messengers inside the cell.

Once the alpha subunit of the G protein activates its effector protein, a GTPase activity inherent in the alpha subunit cleaves the GTP into GDP and P_i. This cleavage renders the alpha subunit inactive, allowing it to recombine with its beta and gamma subunits.

There are several subfamilies of plasma membrane G proteins, each with multiple distinct members, and a single receptor may be associated with more than one type of G protein. Moreover, some G proteins may couple to more than one type of plasma membrane effector protein. In this way, a first-messenger-activated receptor, via its G-protein couplings, can call into action a variety of plasma membrane proteins such as ion channels and enzymes. These molecules can, in turn, induce a variety of cellular events.

To illustrate some of the major points concerning G proteins, plasma membrane effector proteins, second messengers, and protein kinases, the next two sections describe the two most common effector protein enzymes regulated by G proteins—adenylyl cyclase and phospholipase C. In addition, the subsequent portions of the signal transduction pathways in which they participate are described.

Adenylyl Cyclase and Cyclic AMP

In this pathway (**Figure 5.6**), activation of the receptor by the binding of the first messenger (for example, the hormone epinephrine) allows the receptor to activate its associated G protein, in this example known as G_s (the subscript *s* denotes "stimulatory"). This causes G_s to activate its effector protein, the membrane enzyme called **adenylyl cyclase** (also known as adenylate cyclase). The activated adenylyl cyclase, with its catalytic site located on the cytosolic surface of the plasma membrane, catalyzes the conversion of cytosolic ATP to cyclic 3′,5′-adenosine monophosphate, or **cyclic AMP (cAMP)** (**Figure 5.7**). Cyclic AMP then acts as a second messenger (see Figure 5.6). It diffuses throughout the cell to trigger the sequence of events leading to the cell's ultimate response to the first messenger. The action of cAMP eventually terminates when it is broken down to AMP, a reaction catalyzed by the enzyme **cAMP phosphodiesterase** (see Figure 5.7). This enzyme is also subject to physiological control. Thus, the cellular concentration of cAMP can be changed either by altering the rate of its messenger-mediated synthesis or the rate of its phosphodiesterase-mediated breakdown. Caffeine and theophylline, the active ingredients of coffee and tea, are widely consumed stimulants that work partly by inhibiting phosphodiesterase activity, thereby prolonging the actions of cAMP within cells.

What does cAMP actually do inside the cell? It binds to and activates an enzyme known as **cAMP-dependent protein kinase,** also called protein kinase A (see Figure 5.6). Recall that

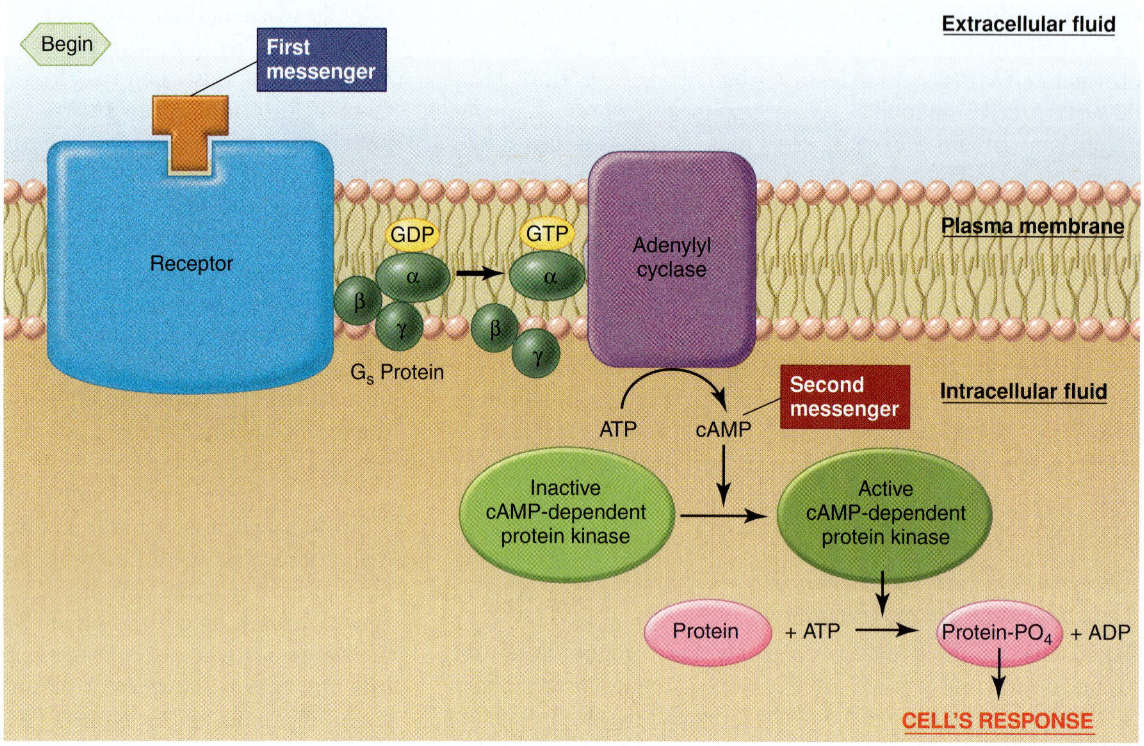

Figure 5.6 APIR Cyclic AMP second-messenger system. Not shown in the figure is the existence of another regulatory protein, G_i, which certain receptors can react with to cause inhibition of adenylyl cyclase.

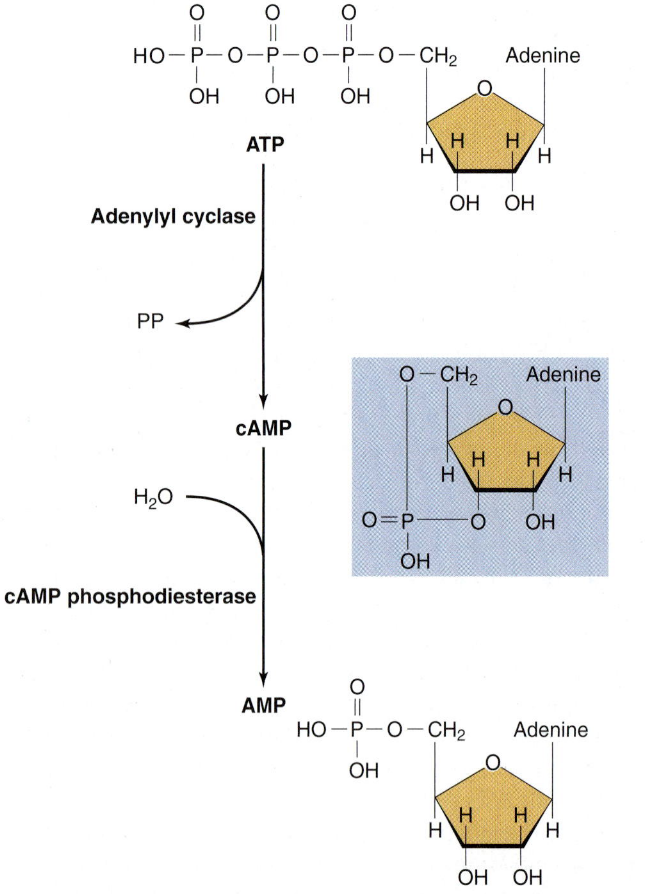

Figure 5.7 Structure of ATP, cAMP, and AMP. ATP is converted to cAMP by the action of the plasma membrane enzyme adenylyl cyclase. cAMP is inactivated by the cytosolic enzyme cAMP phosphodiesterase, which converts cAMP into the noncyclized form AMP.

protein kinases phosphorylate other proteins—often enzymes—by transferring a phosphate group to them. The changes in the activity of proteins phosphorylated by cAMP-dependent protein kinase bring about the cell's response (secretion, contraction, and so on). Again, recall that each of the various protein kinases that participate in the multiple signal transduction pathways described in this chapter has its own specific substrates.

In essence, then, the activation of adenylyl cyclase by a G protein initiates an "amplification cascade" of events that converts proteins in sequence from inactive to active forms. **Figure 5.8** illustrates the benefit of such a cascade. While it is active, a single enzyme molecule is capable of transforming into product not one but many substrate molecules, let us say 100. Therefore, one active molecule of adenylyl cyclase may catalyze the generation of 100 cAMP molecules. At each of the two subsequent enzyme-activation steps in our example, another 100-fold amplification occurs. Therefore, the end result is that a single molecule of the first messenger could, in this example, cause the generation of 1 million product molecules. This helps to explain how hormones and other messengers can be effective at extremely low extracellular concentrations. To take an actual example, one molecule of the hormone epinephrine can cause the liver to generate and release 10^8 molecules of glucose.

In addition, activated cAMP-dependent protein kinase can diffuse into the cell nucleus, where it can phosphorylate a protein that then binds to specific regulatory regions of certain genes. Such genes are said to be cAMP-responsive. Therefore, the effects of cAMP can be rapid and independent of changes in gene activity, as in the example of epinephrine and glucose production, or slower and dependent upon the formation of new gene products.

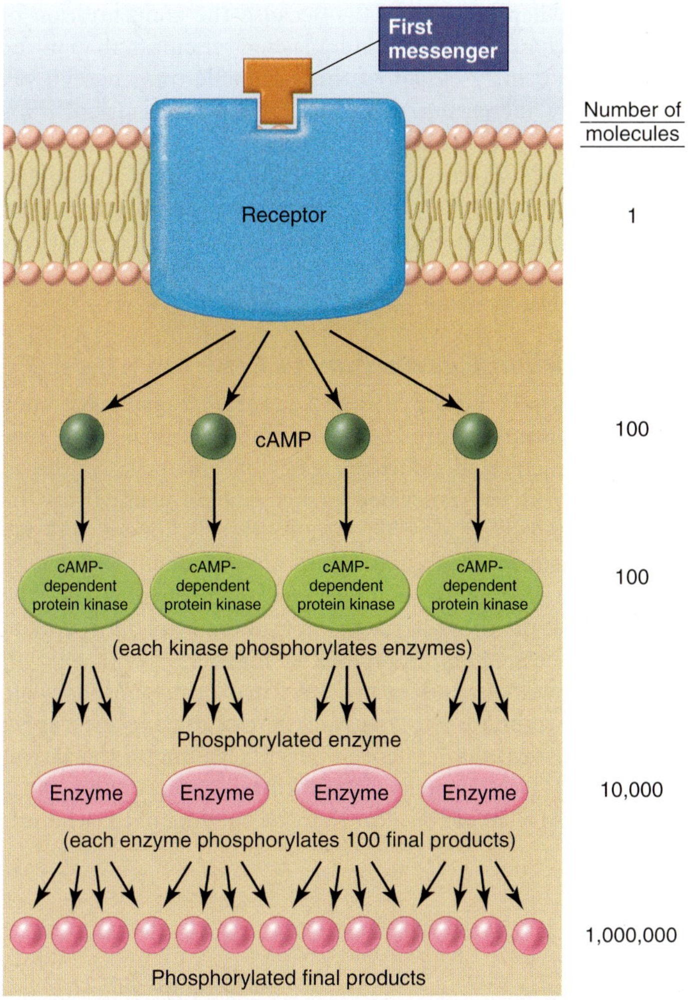

Figure 5.8 APIR Example of signal amplification. In this example, a single molecule of a first messenger results in 1 million final products. Other second-messenger pathways have similar amplification processes. The steps between receptor activation and cAMP generation are omitted for simplicity.

PHYSIOLOGICAL INQUIRY

- What are the advantages of having an enzyme like adenylyl cyclase involved in the initial response to receptor activation by a first messenger?

Answer can be found at end of chapter.

How can cAMP's activation of a single molecule, cAMP-dependent protein kinase, be common to the great variety of biochemical sequences and cell responses initiated by cAMP-generating first messengers? The answer is that cAMP-dependent protein kinase can phosphorylate a large number of different proteins (**Figure 5.9**). In this way, activated cAMP-dependent protein kinase can exert multiple actions within a single cell and different actions in different cells. For example, epinephrine acts via the cAMP pathway on fat cells to stimulate the breakdown of triglyceride, a process that is mediated by one particular phosphorylated enzyme that is chiefly expressed in adipose cells. In the liver, epinephrine acts via cAMP to stimulate both glycogenolysis and gluconeogenesis, processes that are mediated by phosphorylated enzymes that differ from those in fat cells.

Whereas phosphorylation mediated by cAMP- dependent protein kinase activates certain enzymes, it inhibits others. For example, the enzyme catalyzing the rate-limiting step in glycogen synthesis is inhibited by phosphorylation. This explains how epinephrine inhibits glycogen synthesis at the same time it stimulates glycogen breakdown by activating the enzyme that catalyzes the latter response.

Not mentioned thus far is the fact that receptors for some first messengers, upon activation by their messengers, *inhibit* adenylyl cyclase. This inhibition results in less, rather than more, generation of cAMP. This occurs because these receptors are associated with a different G protein known as G_i

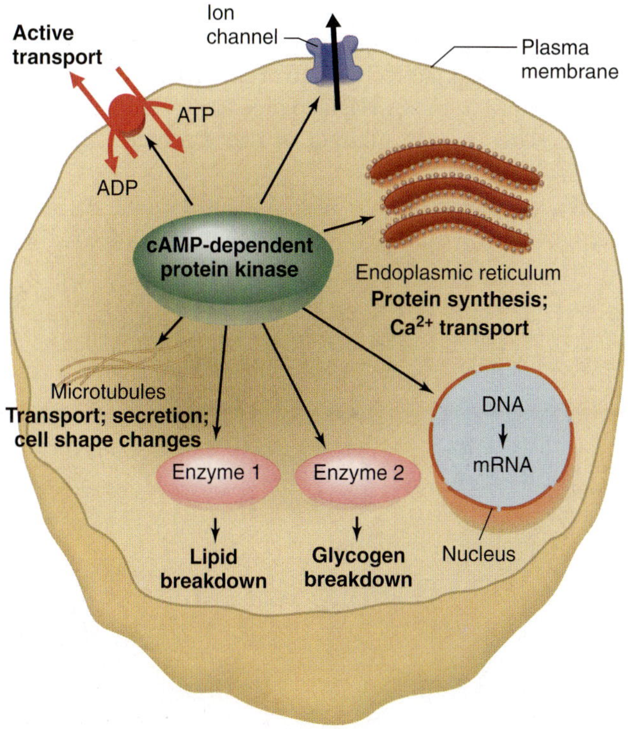

Figure 5.9 APIR The variety of cellular responses induced by cAMP is due mainly to the fact that activated cAMP-dependent protein kinase can phosphorylate many different proteins, activating or inhibiting them. In this figure, the protein kinase is shown phosphorylating seven different proteins—a microtubular protein, an ATPase, an ion channel, a protein in the endoplasmic reticulum, a protein involved in stimulating the transcription of a gene into mRNA, and two enzymes.

PHYSIOLOGICAL INQUIRY

- Does a given protein kinase, such as cAMP-dependent protein kinase, phosphorylate the same proteins in all cells in which the kinase is present?

Answer can be found at end of chapter.

(the subscript *i* denotes "inhibitory"). Activation of G_i causes the inhibition of adenylyl cyclase. The result is to decrease the concentration of cAMP in the cell and thereby the phosphorylation of key proteins inside the cell. Many cells express both stimulatory and inhibitory G proteins in their membranes, providing a means of tightly regulating intracellular cAMP concentrations. This common cellular feature highlights the general principle that most physiological functions are controlled by multiple regulatory systems, often working in opposition.

Phospholipase C, Diacylglycerol, and Inositol Trisphosphate

In this system, a G protein called G_q is activated by a receptor bound to a first messenger. Activated G_q then activates a plasma membrane effector enzyme called **phospholipase C.** This enzyme catalyzes the breakdown of a plasma membrane phospholipid known as phosphatidylinositol bisphosphate, abbreviated PIP_2, to **diacylglycerol** (**DAG**) and **inositol trisphosphate** (**IP_3**) (**Figure 5.10**). Both DAG and IP_3 then function as second messengers but in very different ways.

DAG activates members of a family of related protein kinases known collectively as **protein kinase C,** which, in a fashion similar to cAMP-dependent protein kinase, then phosphorylates a large number of other proteins, leading to the cell's response.

IP_3, in contrast to DAG, does not exert its second-messenger role by directly activating a protein kinase. Rather, cytosolic IP_3 binds to receptors located on the endoplasmic reticulum. These receptors are ligand-gated Ca^{2+} channels that open when bound to IP_3. Because the concentration of Ca^{2+} is much greater in the endoplasmic reticulum than in the cytosol, Ca^{2+} diffuses out of this organelle into the cytosol, significantly increasing cytosolic Ca^{2+} concentration. This increased Ca^{2+} concentration then continues the sequence of events leading to the cell's response to the first messenger. We will pick up this thread in more detail in a later section. However, it is worth noting that one of the actions of Ca^{2+} is to help activate some forms of protein kinase C (which is how this kinase got its name—*C* for "calcium").

Control of Ion Channels by G Proteins

A comparison of Figure 5.5d and Figure 5.9 emphasizes one more important feature of G-protein function—the ability to both directly and indirectly gate ion channels. As shown in Figure 5.5d and described earlier, an ion channel can be the effector protein for a G protein. This is known as direct G-protein gating of plasma membrane ion channels because the G protein interacts directly with the channel. All the events occur in the plasma membrane and are independent of second messengers. Now look at Figure 5.9, and you will see that cAMP-dependent protein kinase can phosphorylate a plasma membrane ion channel, thereby causing it to open. As we have seen, the sequence of events leading to the activation of cAMP-dependent protein kinase proceeds through a G protein, so it should be clear that the opening of this channel

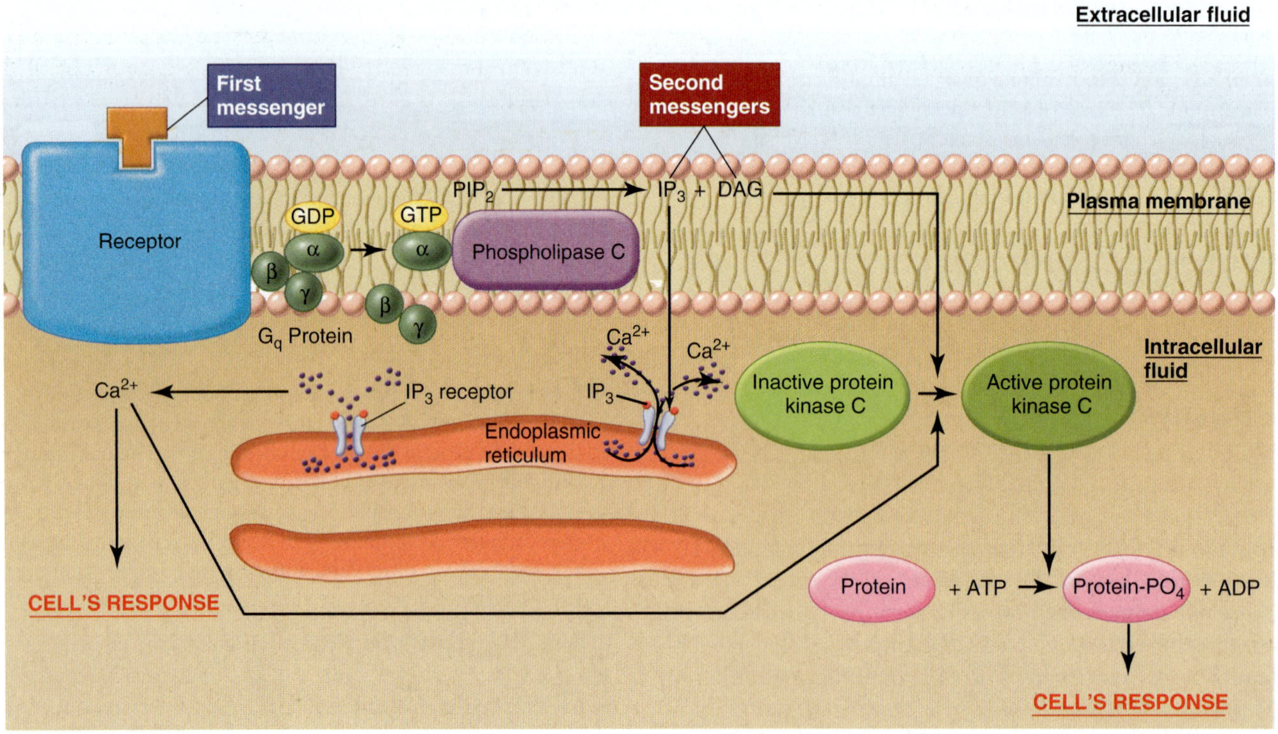

Figure 5.10 APR Mechanism by which an activated receptor stimulates the enzymatically mediated breakdown of PIP_2 to yield IP_3 and DAG. IP_3 then binds to a receptor on the endoplasmic receptor. This receptor is a ligand-gated ion channel that, when opened, allows the release of calcium ions from the endoplasmic reticulum into the cytosol. Together with DAG, Ca^{2+} activates protein kinase C.

TABLE 5.3	Summary of Mechanisms by Which Receptor Activation Influences Ion Channels
The ion channel is part of the receptor.	
A G protein directly gates the channel.	
A G protein gates the channel indirectly via a second messenger.	

TABLE 5.4 Ca^{2+} as a Second Messenger
Common Mechanisms by Which Stimulation of a Cell Leads to an Increase in Cytosolic Ca^{2+} Concentration
I. Receptor activation
A. Plasma-membrane Ca^{2+} channels open in response to a first messenger; the receptor itself may contain the channel, or the receptor may activate a G protein that opens the channel via a second messenger.
B. Ca^{2+} is released from the endoplasmic reticulum; this is typically mediated by IP_3.
C. Active Ca^{2+} transport out of the cell is inhibited by a second messenger.
II. Opening of voltage-gated Ca^{2+} channels
Major Mechanisms by Which an Increase in Cytosolic Ca^{2+} Concentration Induces the Cell's Responses
I. Ca^{2+} binds to calmodulin. On binding Ca^{2+}, the calmodulin changes shape, which allows it to activate or inhibit a large variety of enzymes and other proteins. Many of these enzymes are protein kinases.
II. Ca^{2+} combines with Ca^{2+}-binding intermediary proteins other than calmodulin. These proteins then act in a manner analogous to calmodulin.
III. Ca^{2+} combines with and alters response proteins directly, without the intermediation of any specific Ca^{2+}-binding protein.

is indirectly dependent on that G protein. To generalize, the *indirect G-protein gating* of ion channels utilizes a second-messenger pathway for the opening or closing of the channel. Not just cAMP-dependent protein kinase but protein kinases involved in other signal transduction pathways can participate in reactions leading to such indirect gating. **Table 5.3** summarizes the three ways by which receptor activation by a first messenger leads to opening or closing of ion channels, causing a change in membrane potential.

Ca^{2+} as a Second Messenger

The calcium ion (Ca^{2+}) functions as a second messenger in a great variety of cellular responses to stimuli, both chemical and electrical. The physiology of Ca^{2+} as a second messenger requires an analysis of two broad questions: (1) How do stimuli cause the cytosolic Ca^{2+} concentration to increase? (2) How does the increased Ca^{2+} concentration elicit the cells' responses? Note that, for simplicity, our two questions are phrased in terms of an *increase* in cytosolic concentration. There are, in fact, first messengers that elicit a *decrease* in cytosolic Ca^{2+} concentration and therefore a decrease in calcium's second-messenger effects. Now for the answer to the first question.

By means of active-transport systems in the plasma membrane and cell organelles, Ca^{2+} is maintained at an extremely low concentration in the cytosol. Consequently, there is always a large electrochemical gradient favoring diffusion of Ca^{2+} into the cytosol via Ca^{2+} channels found in both the plasma membrane and the endoplasmic reticulum. A stimulus to the cell can alter this steady state by influencing the active-transport systems and/or the ion channels, resulting in a change in cytosolic Ca^{2+} concentration. The most common ways that receptor activation by a first messenger increases the cytosolic Ca^{2+} concentration have already been presented in this chapter and are summarized in the top part of **Table 5.4**.

Now we turn to the question of how the increased cytosolic Ca^{2+} concentration elicits the cells' responses (see bottom of Table 5.4). The common denominator of Ca^{2+} actions is its ability to bind to various cytosolic proteins, altering their conformation and thereby activating their function. One of the most important of these is a protein found in most cells known as **calmodulin** (**Figure 5.11**). On binding with Ca^{2+}, calmodulin changes shape, and this allows calcium–calmodulin to activate or inhibit a large variety of enzymes and other proteins, many of them protein kinases. Activation or inhibition of **calmodulin-dependent protein kinases** leads, via phosphorylation, to activation or inhibition of proteins involved in the cell's ultimate responses to the first messenger.

Calmodulin is not, however, the only intracellular protein influenced by Ca^{2+} binding. For example, you will learn in Chapter 9 how Ca^{2+} binds to a protein called troponin in certain types of muscle to initiate contraction.

As a final note, it was described earlier in this chapter that the receptors for lipid-soluble messengers, once activated by hormone binding, act in the nucleus as transcription factors to increase or decrease the rate of gene transcription. There are many other transcription factors inside cells, however, and the signal transduction pathways initiated by plasma membrane receptors often activate these transcription factors, typically by phosphorylation. Therefore, many first messengers that bind to plasma membrane receptors can also alter gene transcription via second messengers. For example, several of the proteins that cAMP-dependent protein kinase phosphorylates function as transcription factors.

Other Messengers

In a few places in this text, you will learn about messengers that are not as readily classified as those just described. Among these are the eicosanoids. The **eicosanoids** are a family of molecules produced from the polyunsaturated fatty acid **arachidonic acid,** which is present in plasma membrane phospholipids. The eicosanoids include the **cyclic endoperoxides,** the **prostaglandins,** the **thromboxanes,** and the **leukotrienes** (**Figure 5.12**). They are generated in many

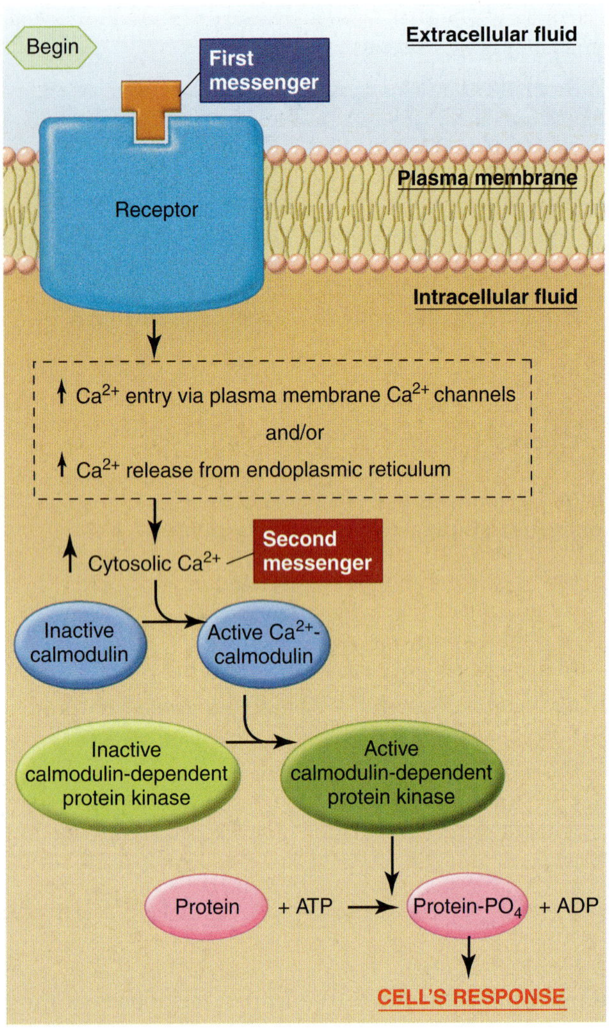

Figure 5.11 Ca^{2+}, calmodulin, and the calmodulin-dependent protein kinase system. (There are multiple calmodulin-dependent protein kinases.) Table 5.4 summarizes the mechanisms for increasing cytosolic Ca^{2+} concentration.

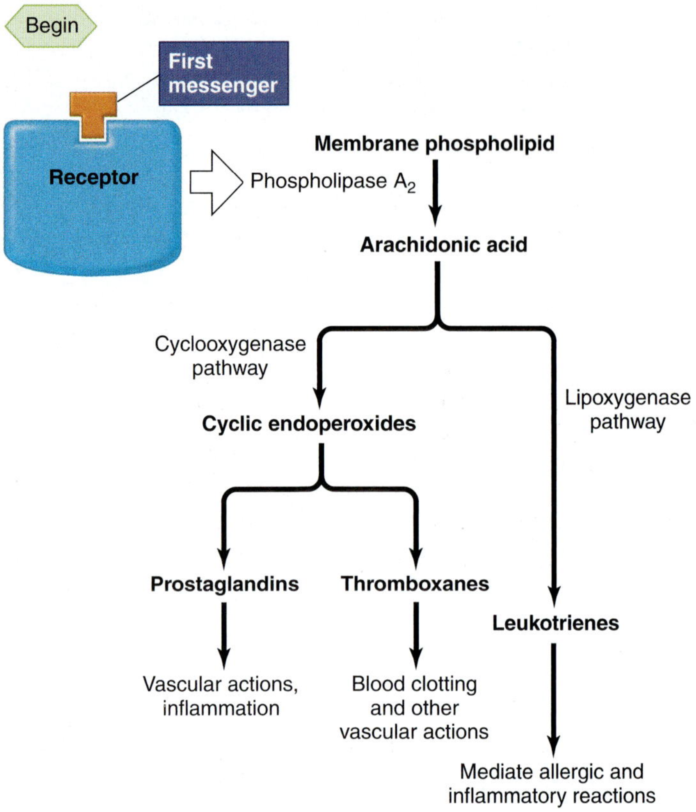

Figure 5.12 Pathways for eicosanoid synthesis and some of their major functions. Phospholipase A_2 is the one enzyme common to the formation of all the eicosanoids; it is the site at which stimuli act. Anti-inflammatory steroids inhibit phospholipase A_2. The step mediated by cyclooxygenase is inhibited by aspirin and other nonsteroidal anti-inflammatory drugs (NSAIDs). There are also drugs available that inhibit the lipoxygenase enzyme, thereby blocking the formation of leukotrienes. These drugs may be helpful in controlling asthma, in which excess leukotrienes have been implicated in the allergic and inflammatory components of the disease.

PHYSIOLOGICAL INQUIRY

- Based on the pathways shown in this figure, why are people advised to avoid taking aspirin or other NSAIDs prior to a surgical procedure?

Answer can be found at end of chapter.

kinds of cells in response to different types of extracellular signals; these include a variety of growth factors, immune defense molecules, and even other eicosanoids. Thus, eicosanoids may act as both extracellular and intracellular messengers, depending on the cell type.

The synthesis of eicosanoids begins when an appropriate stimulus—hormone, neurotransmitter, paracrine substance, drug, or toxic agent—binds its receptor and activates **phospholipase A_2**, an enzyme localized to the plasma membrane of the stimulated cell. As shown in Figure 5.12, this enzyme splits off arachidonic acid from the membrane phospholipids, and the arachidonic acid can then be metabolized by two pathways. One pathway is initiated by an enzyme called **cyclooxygenase (COX)** and leads ultimately to formation of the cyclic endoperoxides, prostaglandins, and thromboxanes. The other pathway is initiated by the enzyme **lipoxygenase** and leads to formation of the leukotrienes. Within both of these pathways, synthesis of the various specific eicosanoids is enzyme-mediated. Thus, beyond phospholipase A_2, the eicosanoid-pathway enzymes expressed in a particular cell determine which eicosanoids the cell synthesizes in response to a stimulus.

Each of the major eicosanoid subdivisions contains more than one member, as indicated by the use of the plural in referring to them (*prostaglandins*, for example). On the basis of structural differences, the different molecules within each subdivision are designated by a letter—for example, PGA and PGE for prostaglandins of the A and E types, which then may be further subdivided—for example, PGE_2.

Once they have been synthesized in response to a stimulus, the eicosanoids may in some cases act as intracellular messengers, but more often they are released immediately and act locally. For this reason, the eicosanoids are usually categorized as paracrine and autocrine substances. After they act, they are quickly metabolized by local enzymes to inactive forms. The eicosanoids exert a wide array of effects, particularly on blood vessels and in inflammation. Many of these will be described in future chapters.

Certain drugs influence the eicosanoid pathway and are among the most commonly used in the world today. ***Aspirin***, for example, inhibits cyclooxygenase and, therefore, blocks the synthesis of the endoperoxides, prostaglandins, and thromboxanes. It and other drugs that also block cyclooxygenase are collectively termed ***nonsteroidal anti-inflammatory drugs (NSAIDs)***. Their major uses are to reduce pain, fever, and inflammation. The term *nonsteroidal* distinguishes them from synthetic glucocorticoids (analogs of steroid hormones made by the adrenal glands) that are used in large doses as anti-inflammatory drugs; these steroids inhibit phospholipase A_2 and therefore block the production of all eicosanoids.

Cessation of Activity in Signal Transduction Pathways

Once initiated, signal transduction pathways are eventually shut off, preventing chronic overstimulation of a cell, which can be detrimental. The key event is usually the cessation of receptor activation. Responses to messengers are transient events that persist only briefly and subside when the receptor is no longer bound to the first messenger. A major way that receptor activation ceases is by a decrease in the concentration of first-messenger molecules in the region of the receptor. This occurs as enzymes in the vicinity metabolize the first messenger, as the first messenger is taken up by adjacent cells, or as it simply diffuses away.

In addition, receptors can be inactivated in at least three other ways: (1) the receptor becomes chemically altered (usually by phosphorylation), which may reduce its affinity for a first messenger, and so the messenger is released; (2) phosphorylation of the receptor may prevent further G-protein binding to the receptor; and (3) plasma membrane receptors may be removed when the combination of first messenger and receptor is taken into the cell by endocytosis. The processes described here are physiologically controlled. For example, in many cases the inhibitory phosphorylation of a receptor is mediated by a protein kinase that was initially activated in response to the first messenger. This receptor inactivation constitutes negative feedback.

This concludes our description of the basic principles of signal transduction pathways. It is essential to recognize that the pathways do not exist in isolation but may be active simultaneously in a single cell, undergoing complex interactions. This is possible because a single first messenger may trigger changes in the activity of more than one pathway and, much more importantly, because many different first messengers—often dozens—may simultaneously influence a cell. Moreover, a great deal of "cross talk" can occur at one or more levels among the various signal transduction pathways. For example, active molecules generated in the cAMP pathway can alter the activity of receptors and signaling molecules generated by other pathways.

Finally, for reference purposes, **Table 5.5** summarizes the biochemistry of the second messengers described in this chapter.

TABLE 5.5 Reference Table of Important Second Messengers

Substance	Source	Effects
Ca^{2+}	Enters cell through plasma membrane ion channels or is released from endoplasmic reticulum.	Activates calmodulin and other Ca^{2+}-binding proteins; calcium–calmodulin activates calmodulin-dependent protein kinases. Also activates protein kinase C.
Cyclic AMP (cAMP)	A G protein activates plasma membrane adenylyl cyclase, which catalyzes the formation of cAMP from ATP.	Activates cAMP-dependent protein kinase (protein kinase A).
Cyclic GMP (cGMP)	Generated from guanosine triphosphate in a reaction catalyzed by a plasma membrane receptor with guanylyl cyclase activity.	Activates cGMP-dependent protein kinase (protein kinase G).
Diacylglycerol (DAG)	A G protein activates plasma membrane phospholipase C, which catalyzes the generation of DAG and IP_3 from plasma membrane phosphatidylinositol bisphosphate (PIP_2).	Activates protein kinase C.
Inositol trisphosphate (IP_3)	See DAG above.	Releases Ca^{2+} from endoplasmic reticulum.

SUMMARY

Receptors

I. Receptors for chemical messengers are proteins or glycoproteins located either inside the cell or, much more commonly, in the plasma membrane. The binding of a messenger by a receptor manifests specificity, saturation, and competition.

II. Receptors are subject to physiological regulation by their own messengers. This includes down- and up-regulation.

III. Different cell types express different types of receptors; even a single cell may express multiple receptor types.

Signal Transduction Pathways

I. Binding a chemical messenger activates a receptor, and this initiates one or more signal transduction pathways leading to the cell's response.

II. Lipid-soluble messengers bind to receptors inside the target cell. The activated receptor acts in the nucleus as a transcription factor to alter the rate of transcription of specific genes, resulting in a change in the concentration or secretion of the proteins the genes encode.

III. Water-soluble messengers bind to receptors on the plasma membrane. The pathways induced by activation of the receptor often involve second messengers and protein kinases.

a. The receptor may be a ligand-gated ion channel. The channel opens, resulting in an electrical signal in the membrane and, when Ca^{2+} channels are involved, an increase in the cytosolic Ca^{2+} concentration.

b. The receptor may itself be an enzyme. With one exception, the enzyme activity is that of a protein kinase, usually a tyrosine kinase. The exception is the receptor that functions as a guanylyl cyclase to generate cyclic GMP.

c. The receptor may activate a cytosolic janus kinase associated with it.

d. The receptor may interact with an associated plasma membrane G protein, which in turn interacts with plasma membrane effector proteins—ion channels or enzymes.

e. Very commonly, the receptor may stimulate, via a G_s protein, or inhibit, via a G_i protein, the membrane effector enzyme adenylyl cyclase, which catalyzes the conversion of cytosolic ATP to cyclic AMP. Cyclic AMP acts as a second messenger to activate intracellular cAMP-dependent protein kinase, which phosphorylates proteins that mediate the cell's ultimate responses to the first messenger.

f. The receptor may activate, via a G_q protein, the plasma membrane enzyme phospholipase C, which catalyzes the formation of diacylglycerol (DAG) and inositol trisphosphate (IP_3). DAG activates protein kinase C, and IP_3 acts as a second messenger to release Ca^{2+} from the endoplasmic reticulum.

IV. The receptor, via a G protein, may directly open or close (gate) an adjacent ion channel. This differs from indirect G-protein gating of channels, in which a second messenger acts upon the channel.

V. The calcium ion is one of the most widespread second messengers.

a. An activated receptor can increase cytosolic Ca^{2+} concentration by causing certain Ca^{2+} channels in the plasma membrane and/or endoplasmic reticulum to open.

b. Ca^{2+} binds to one of several intracellular proteins, most often calmodulin. Calcium-activated calmodulin activates or inhibits many proteins, including calmodulin-dependent protein kinases.

VI. Eicosanoids are derived from arachidonic acid, which is released from phospholipids in the plasma membrane. They exert widespread intracellular and extracellular effects on cell activity.

VII. The signal transduction pathways triggered by activated plasma membrane receptors may influence genetic expression by activating transcription factors.

VIII. Cessation of receptor activity occurs when the first-messenger molecule concentration decreases or when the receptor is chemically altered or internalized, in the case of plasma membrane receptors.

REVIEW QUESTIONS

1. What is the chemical nature of receptors? Where are they located?
2. Explain why different types of cells may respond differently to the same chemical messenger.
3. Describe how the metabolism of receptors can lead to down-regulation or up-regulation.
4. What is the first step in the action of a messenger on a cell?
5. Describe the signal transduction pathway that lipid-soluble messengers use.
6. Classify plasma membrane receptors according to the signal transduction pathways they initiate.
7. What is the result of opening a membrane ion channel?
8. Contrast receptors that have intrinsic enzyme activity with those associated with cytoplasmic janus kinases.
9. Describe the role of plasma membrane G proteins.
10. Draw a diagram describing the adenylyl cyclase–cAMP system.
11. Draw a diagram illustrating the phospholipase C/DAG/IP_3 system.
12. How does the calcium–calmodulin system function?

KEY TERMS

CLINICAL TERMS

Clinical Case Study: A Child with Unexplained Weight Gain and Calcium Imbalance

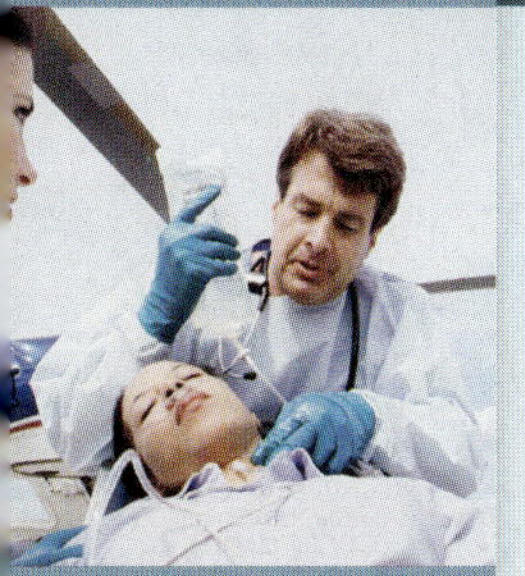

A 3-year-old girl was seen by her pediatrician to determine the cause of a recent increase in the rate of her weight gain. Her height was normal (95 cm/37.4 inches) but she weighed 16.5 kg (36.3 pounds), which is in the 92nd percentile for her age. The girl's mother—who was very short and overweight—stated that the child seemed listless at times and was rarely very active. She was also prone to muscle cramps and complained to her mother that her fingers and toes "felt funny," which the pediatrician was able to interpret as tingling sensations. She had a good appetite but not one that appeared unusual or extreme. The doctor suspected that the child had developed a deficiency in the amount of thyroid hormone in her blood. This hormone is produced by the thyroid gland in the neck (see Chapter 11) and is responsible in part for normal metabolism, that is, the rate at which calories are expended. Too little thyroid hormone typically results in weight gain and may also cause fatigue or lack of energy. A blood test was performed, and indeed the girl's thyroid hormone concentration was low. Because there are several conditions that may result in a deficiency of thyroid hormone, an additional exam was performed. During that exam, the physician noticed that the fourth metacarpals on each of the girl's hands were shorter than normal, and he could feel hard bumps (nodules) just beneath the girl's skin at various sites on her body. He ordered a blood test for Ca^{2+} and another hormone called parathyroid hormone (PTH).

PTH gets its name because the glands that produce it lie adjacent (*para*) to the thyroid gland. PTH normally acts on the kidneys and bones to maintain calcium ion homeostasis in the blood. For example, should Ca^{2+} concentrations in the blood decrease for any reason, PTH secretion will increase and stimulate the release of Ca^{2+} from bones into the blood. It also stimulates the retention of Ca^{2+} by the kidneys, such that less Ca^{2+} is lost in the urine. These two factors help to restore blood Ca^{2+} concentrations—a classic example of homeostasis through negative feedback. The doctor suspected that the nodules he felt were Ca^{2+} deposits and that the shortened fingers were the result of improper bone formation during development due to a Ca^{2+} imbalance. Abnormally low blood Ca^{2+} concentrations would also explain the cramps and tingling sensations. This is because extracellular Ca^{2+} concentration is critical for normal function of muscles and nerves, as well as for healthy bones and growth. The results of the blood test confirmed that Ca^{2+} concentrations were lower than normal. A logical explanation for why Ca^{2+} levels were low would be because PTH concentrations were low. Paradoxically, however, PTH concentrations were increased in the girl's blood. This means that PTH was present but was unable to act on its targets—the bones and kidneys—to maintain Ca^{2+} balance in the blood. What could prevent PTH from doing its job? How might this be related to the thyroid hormone imbalance that was responsible for the weight gain?

A genetic condition in which PTH concentrations in the blood are high but Ca^{2+} concentrations are low is ***pseudohypoparathyroidism.*** The prefix *hypo* in this context refers to "less than normal amounts of" PTH in the blood. This girl's condition seemed to fit a diagnosis of hypoparathyroidism, because her Ca^{2+} concentrations were low and she consequently demonstrated several symptoms characteristic of low Ca^{2+}. However, because her PTH concentrations were *not* low—in fact, they were higher than normal—the condition is called *pseudo,* or "false," hypoparathyroidism. A blood sample was taken from the girl and the white blood cells were subjected to DNA analysis. That analysis revealed that the girl was heterozygous for a mutation in the *GNAS1* gene, which encodes the alpha subunit of the stimulatory G protein (G_s alpha). Recall from Figure 5.6 that G_s couples certain plasma membrane receptor proteins to adenylyl cyclase and the production of cAMP, an important second messenger in many cells. PTH is known to act by binding to a cell surface receptor and activating adenylyl cyclase via this pathway. Because the girl had reduced expression of normal G_s alpha, her cells were unable to respond adequately to PTH, and consequently her blood concentrations of Ca^{2+} could not be maintained within the normal range.

PTH, however, is not the only signaling molecule in the body that acts through a G_s-coupled receptor; as you have learned in this chapter, there are many other such molecules. One of them is a hormone from the pituitary gland that stimulates thyroid hormone production by the thyroid gland. This explains why our patient had low thyroid hormone concentrations in addition to her PTH/Ca^{2+} imbalance.

Pseudohypoparathyroidism is a rare disorder, but it illustrates a larger and extremely important medical concern called target-organ resistance. Such diseases are characterized by normal or even elevated blood concentrations of signaling molecules such as PTH but insensitivity (that is, resistance) of a target organ (or organs) to the molecule. In our patient, the cause of the resistance was insufficient G_s-alpha action due to an inherited mutation; in other cases (such as type 2 diabetes mellitus, described in Chapter 16), it may result from defects in other aspects of cell signaling pathways. It is likely that the girl inherited the mutation from her mother, who showed some similar symptoms.

The girl was treated with a thyroid hormone pill each day, calcium tablets twice per day, and a derivative of vitamin D (which helps the intestines absorb Ca^{2+}) twice per day. She will need to remain on this treatment plan for the rest of her life. In addition, it will be important for her physician to monitor other physiological functions mediated by other hormones that are known to act via G_s alpha.

Clinical term: pseudohypoparathyroidism

See Chapter 19 for complete, integrative case studies.

CHAPTER 5 TEST QUESTIONS *Answers found in Appendix A.*

1–3: Match a receptor feature (a–e) with each choice.

1. Defines the situation when all receptor binding sites are occupied by a messenger
2. Defines the strength of receptor binding to a messenger
3. Reflects the fact that a receptor normally binds only to a single messenger

Receptor feature:

a. affinity
b. saturation
c. competition
d. down-regulation
e. specificity

4. Which of the following intracellular or plasma membrane proteins require/requires Ca^{2+} for full activity?
   a. calmodulin
   b. janus kinase (JAK)
   c. cAMP-dependent protein kinase
   d. guanylyl cyclase
   e. all of the above
5. Which is correct?
   a. cAMP-dependent protein kinase phosphorylates tyrosine residues.
   b. Protein kinase C is activated by cAMP.
   c. The subunit of G_s proteins that activates adenylyl cyclase is the beta subunit.
   d. Lipid-soluble messengers typically act on receptors in the cell cytosol or nucleus.
   e. The binding site of a typical plasma membrane receptor for its messenger is located on the cytosolic surface of the receptor.
6. Inhibition of which enzyme/enzymes would inhibit the conversion of arachidonic acid to leukotrienes?
   a. cyclooxygenase
   b. lipoxygenase
   c. phospholipase A_2
   d. adenylyl cyclase
   e. both b and c

7–10: Match each type of molecule with the correct choice (a–e); a given choice may be used once, more than once, or not at all.

Molecule:

7. second messenger
8. example of a first messenger
9. part of a trimeric protein in membranes
10. enzyme

Choices:

a. neurotransmitter or hormone
b. cAMP-dependent protein kinase
c. calmodulin
d. Ca^{2+}
e. alpha subunit of G proteins

CHAPTER 5 GENERAL PRINCIPLES ASSESSMENT *Answers found in Appendix A.*

1. What examples from this chapter demonstrate the general physiological principle that *controlled exchange of materials occurs between compartments and across cell membranes?* Specifically, how is this related to another general principle, namely, *information flow between cells, tissues, and organs is an essential feature of homeostasis and allows for integration of physiological processes?*
2. Another principle states that *physiological processes require the transfer and balance of matter and energy.* How is energy balance related to intracellular signaling?

CHAPTER 5 QUANTITATIVE AND THOUGHT QUESTIONS *Answers found at www.mhhe.com/widmaier13.*

1. Patient A is given a drug that blocks the synthesis of all eicosanoids, whereas patient B is given a drug that blocks the synthesis of leukotrienes but none of the other eicosanoids. What enzymes do these drugs most likely block?
2. Certain nerves to the heart release the neurotransmitter norepinephrine. If these nerves are removed in experimental animals, the heart becomes extremely sensitive to the administration of a drug that is an agonist of norepinephrine. Explain why this may happen, in terms of receptor physiology.
3. A particular hormone is known to elicit—completely by way of the cyclic AMP system—six different responses in its target cell. A drug is found that eliminates one of these responses but not the other five. Which of the following, if any, could the drug be blocking: the hormone's receptors, G_s protein, adenylyl cyclase, or cyclic AMP?
4. If a drug were found that blocked all Ca^{2+} channels directly linked to G proteins, would this eliminate the role of Ca^{2+} as a second messenger? Why or why not?
5. Explain why the effects of a first messenger do not immediately cease upon removal of the messenger.

CHAPTER 5 ANSWERS TO PHYSIOLOGICAL INQUIRIES

Figure 5.5 Expressing more than one type of receptor allows a cell to respond to more than one type of first messenger. For example, one first messenger might activate a particular biochemical pathway in a cell by activating one type of receptor and signaling pathway. By contrast, another first messenger acting on a different receptor and activating a different signaling pathway might inhibit the same biochemical process. In this way, the biochemical process can be tightly regulated.

Figure 5.8 Enzymes can generate large amounts of product without being consumed. This is an extremely efficient way to generate a second messenger like cAMP. Enzymes have many other advantages (see Table 3.7), including the ability to have their activities fine-tuned by other inputs (see Figures 3.36 to 3.38). This enables the cell to adjust its response to a first messenger depending on the other conditions present.

Figure 5.9 Not necessarily. In some cases, a kinase may phosphorylate the same protein in many different types of cells. However, many cells also express certain cell-specific proteins that are not found in all tissues, and some of these proteins may be substrates for cAMP-dependent protein kinase. Thus, the proteins that are phosphorylated by a given kinase depend upon the cell type, which makes the cellular response tissue-specific. As an example, in the kidneys, cAMP-dependent protein kinase phosphorylates proteins that insert water channels in cell membranes and thereby reduce urine volume, whereas in heart muscle the same kinase phosphorylates Ca^{2+} channels that increase the strength of muscle contraction.

Figure 5.12 Aspirin and NSAIDs block the cyclooxygenase pathway. This includes the pathway to the production of thromboxanes, which as shown in the figure are important for blood clotting. Because of the risk of bleeding that occurs with any type of surgery, the use of such drugs prior to the surgery may increase the likelihood of excessive bleeding.

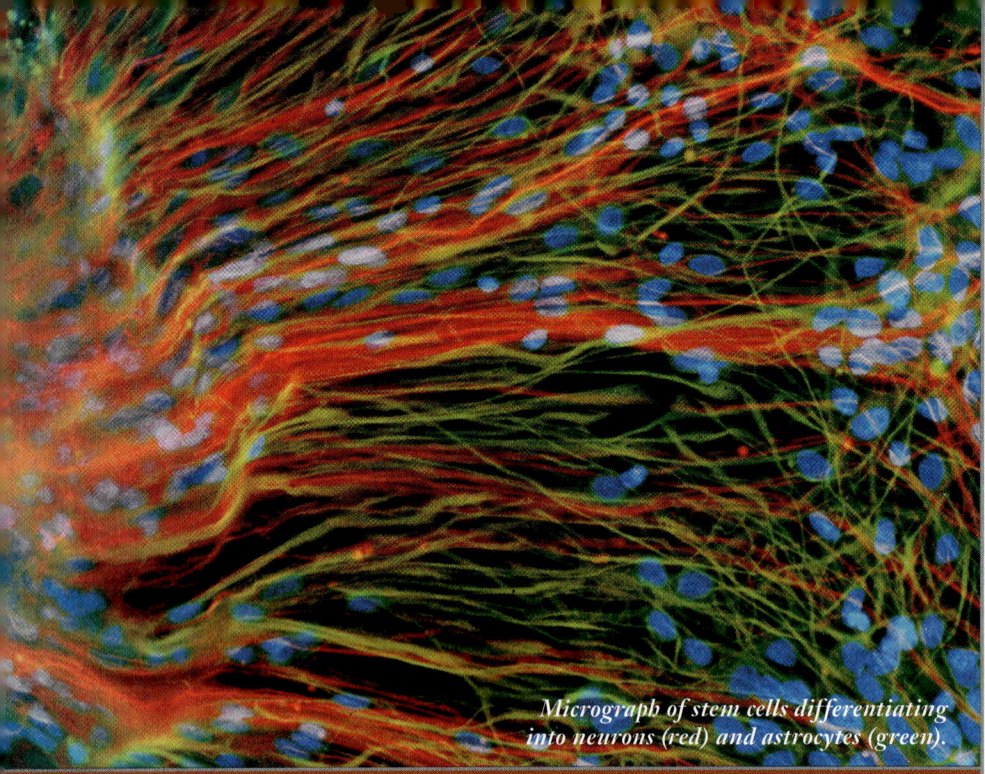

Micrograph of stem cells differentiating into neurons (red) and astrocytes (green).

6 Neuronal Signaling and the Structure of the Nervous System

Chapters 1–5 examined the principle of homeostasis, the basic chemistry of the body, and the general structure and function of all body cells. Now we turn our attention to the structure and function of a specific organ system and its cells—the nervous system. The nervous system is composed of trillions of cells distributed in a network throughout the brain, spinal cord, and periphery. It plays a key role in the maintenance of homeostasis. It does this by mediating information flow that coordinates the activity of widely dispersed cells, tissues, and organs, both internally and with the external environment. Among its many functions are activation of muscle contraction (Chapters 9 and 10), integration of blood oxygen, carbon dioxide, and pH levels with respiratory system activity (Chapter 13), regulation of volumes and pressures in the circulation by acting on the cardiovascular system (Chapter 12) and urinary system (Chapter 14), and modulating digestive system motility and secretion (Chapter 15). The nervous system is one of the two major control systems of the body; the other is the endocrine system (Chapter 11). Unlike the relatively slow, long-lasting signals of the endocrine system, the nervous system sends rapid electrical signals along nerve cell membranes.

As you read about the structure and function of neurons and the nervous system in this chapter, you will encounter numerous examples of the general principles of physiology that were outlined in Chapter 1. Section A highlights how the structure of neurons contributes to their specialized functions in mediating the information flow between organs and integration of homeostatic processes. In Section B, controlled exchange of materials (ions) across cellular membranes and the laws of chemistry and physics will be key principles underlying the electrical properties of neurons. Information flow that allows for integration of physiological processes between cells of the nervous system is the theme of Section C; and in Section D, you will see how the nervous system illustrates the general principle of physiology that most physiological functions are controlled by multiple regulatory systems, often working in opposition.

SECTION A

Neural Tissue

The various structures of the nervous system are intimately interconnected, but for convenience we divide them into two parts: (1) the **central nervous system** (**CNS**), composed of the brain and spinal cord; and (2) the **peripheral nervous system** (**PNS**), consisting of the nerves that connect the brain and spinal cord with the body's muscles, glands, sense organs, and other tissues.

The basic unit of the nervous system is the individual nerve cell, or **neuron.** Neurons operate by generating electrical signals that move from one part of the cell to another part of the same cell or to neighboring cells. In most neurons, the electrical signal causes the release of chemical messengers—**neurotransmitters**—to communicate with other cells. Most neurons serve as integrators because their output reflects the balance of inputs they receive from up to hundreds of thousands of other neurons.

6.1 Structure and Maintenance of Neurons

Neurons occur in a wide variety of sizes and shapes, but all share features that allow cell-to-cell communication. Long extensions, or **processes,** connect neurons to each other and perform the neurons' input and output functions. As shown in **Figure 6.1**, most neurons contain a cell body and two types of processes—dendrites and axons.

As in other types of cells, a neuron's **cell body** (or **soma**) contains the nucleus and ribosomes and thus has the genetic information and machinery necessary for protein synthesis. The **dendrites** are a series of highly branched outgrowths of the cell body. In the PNS, dendrites receive incoming sensory information and transfer it to integrating regions of sensory neurons. In the CNS, dendrites and the cell body receive most of the inputs from other neurons, with the dendrites generally taking a more important role. Branching dendrites increase a cell's surface area—some neurons may have as many as 400,000 dendrites. Knoblike outgrowths called **dendritic spines** increase the surface area of dendrites still further, and there are often ribosomes present. The presence of protein-synthesis machinery allows dendritic spines to remodel their shape in response to variation in synaptic activity, which may play a key role in complex processes like learning and memory. Thus, the structure of dendrites in the CNS increases a cell's capacity to receive signals from many other neurons.

The **axon,** sometimes also called a **nerve fiber,** is a long process that extends from the cell body and carries outgoing signals to its target cells. In humans, axons range in length from a few microns to over a meter. The region of the axon that arises from the cell body is known as the **initial segment** (or **axon hillock**). The initial segment is the "trigger zone" where, in most neurons, propagated electrical signals are generated. These signals then propagate away from the cell body along the axon or, sometimes, back along the dendrites. The axon may have branches, called **collaterals.** Near their ends, both the axon and its collaterals undergo further branching (see Figure 6.1). The greater the degree of branching of the axon and axon collaterals, the greater the cell's sphere of influence.

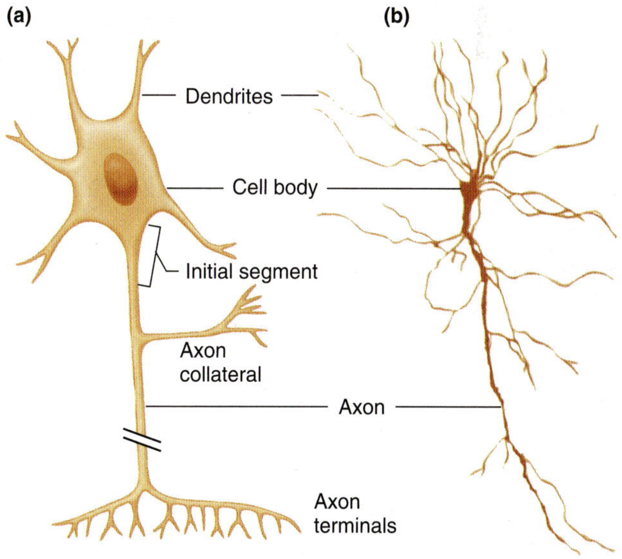

Figure 6.1 APIR (a) Diagrammatic representation of one type of neuron. The break in the axon indicates that axons may extend for long distances; in fact, they may be 5000 to 10,000 times longer than the cell body is wide. This neuron is a common type, but there is a wide variety of neuronal morphologies, some of which have no axons. (b) A neuron as observed through a microscope. The axon terminals cannot be seen at this magnification.

Each branch ends in an **axon terminal,** which is responsible for releasing neurotransmitters from the axon. These chemical messengers diffuse across an extracellular gap to the cell opposite the terminal. Alternatively, some neurons release their chemical messengers from a series of bulging areas along the axon known as **varicosities.**

The axons of many neurons are covered by sheaths of **myelin** (**Figure 6.2**), which usually consists of 20 to 200 layers of highly modified plasma membrane wrapped around the axon by a nearby supporting cell. In the brain and spinal cord, these myelin-forming cells are the **oligodendrocytes.** Each oligodendrocyte may branch to form myelin on as many as 40 axons. In the PNS, cells called **Schwann cells** form individual myelin sheaths surrounding 1- to 1.5-mm-long segments at regular intervals along some axons. The spaces between adjacent sections of myelin where the axon's plasma membrane is exposed to extracellular fluid are called the **nodes of Ranvier.** As we will see, the myelin sheath speeds up conduction of the electrical signals along the axon and conserves energy.

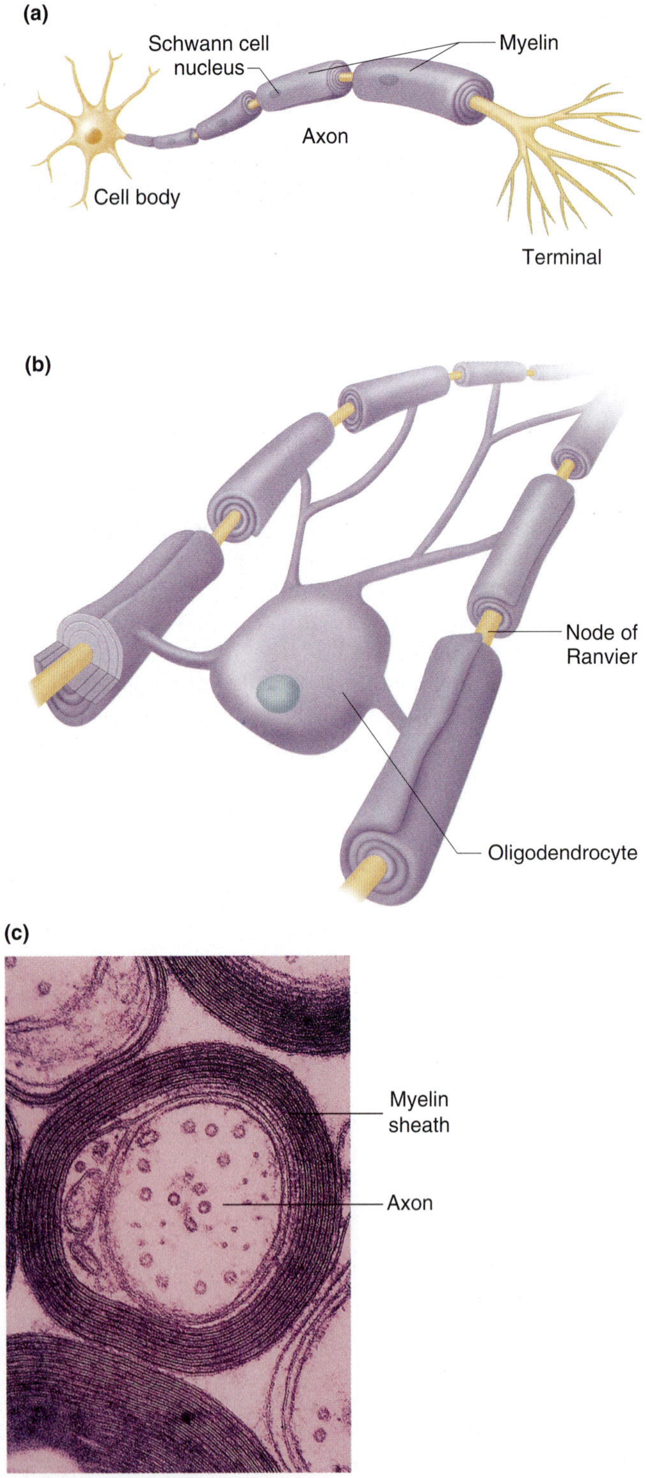

Figure 6.2 AP|R (a) Myelin formed by Schwann cells, and (b) oligodendrocytes on axons. (c) Electron micrograph of transverse sections of myelinated axons in brain.

To maintain the structure and function of the cell axon, various organelles and other materials must move as far as 1 meter between the cell body and the axon terminals. This movement, termed **axonal transport,** depends on a scaffolding of microtubule "rails" running the length of the axon and specialized types of motor proteins known as **kinesins** and **dyneins** (**Figure 6.3**). At one end, these double-headed motor proteins bind to their cellular cargo, and the other end uses energy derived from the hydrolysis of ATP to "walk" along the microtubules. Kinesin transport mainly occurs from the cell body toward the axon terminals (**anterograde**) and is important in moving nutrient molecules, enzymes, mitochondria, neurotransmitter-filled vesicles, and other organelles. Dynein movement is in the other direction (**retrograde**), carrying recycled membrane vesicles, growth factors, and other chemical signals that can affect the neuron's morphology, biochemistry, and connectivity. Retrograde transport is also the route by which some harmful agents invade the CNS, including tetanus toxin and the herpes simplex, rabies, and polio viruses.

6.2 Functional Classes of Neurons

Neurons can be divided into three functional classes: afferent neurons, efferent neurons, and interneurons (**Figure 6.4**). **Afferent neurons** convey information from the tissues and organs of the body *toward* the CNS. **Efferent neurons** convey information *away from* the CNS to effector cells like muscle, gland, or other cell types. **Interneurons** connect neurons *within* the CNS. As a rough estimate, for each afferent neuron entering the CNS, there are 10 efferent neurons and 200,000 interneurons. Thus, the great majority of neurons are interneurons.

At their peripheral ends (the ends farthest from the CNS), afferent neurons have **sensory receptors,** which respond to various physical or chemical changes in their environment by generating electrical signals in the neuron. The receptor region may be a specialized portion of the plasma membrane or a separate cell closely associated with the neuron ending. (Recall from Chapter 5 that the term *receptor* has two distinct meanings, the one defined here and the other referring to the specific proteins a chemical messenger combines with to exert its effects on a target cell.) Afferent neurons propagate electrical signals from their receptors into the brain or spinal cord.

Afferent neurons have a shape that is distinct from that diagrammed in Figure 6.1, because they have only a single process associated with the cell body, usually considered an axon. Shortly after leaving the cell body, the axon divides. One branch, the peripheral process, begins where the dendritic branches converge from the receptor endings. The other branch, the

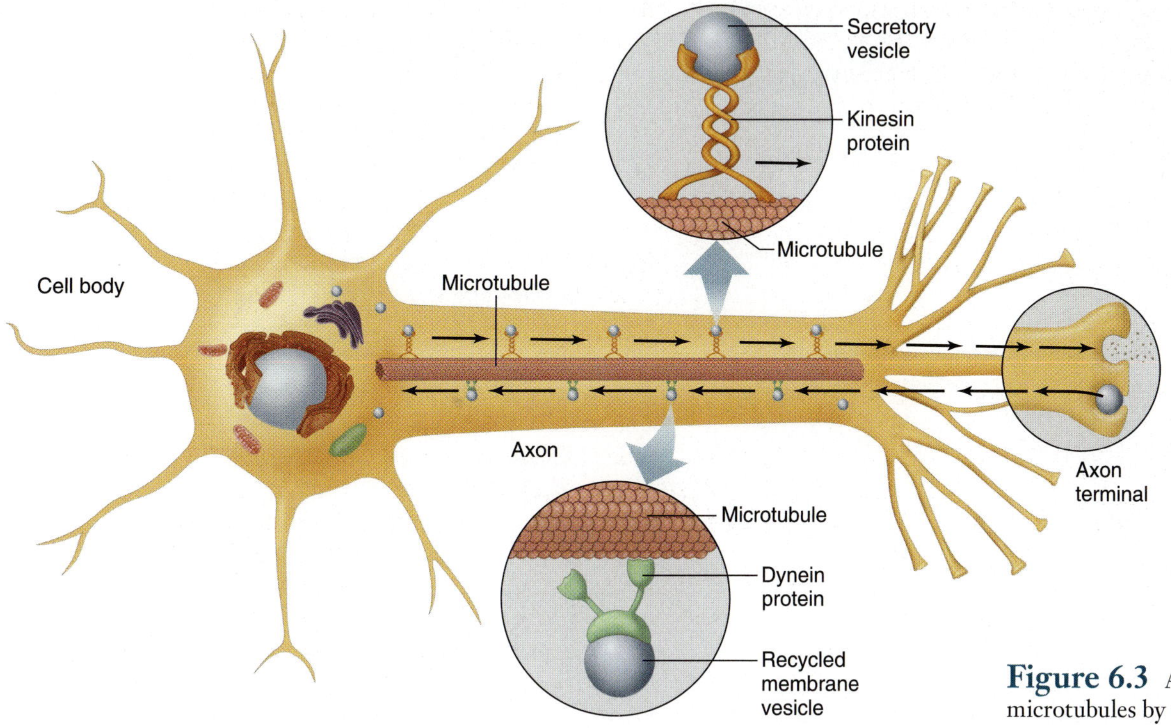

Figure 6.3 Axonal transport along microtubules by dynein and kinesin.

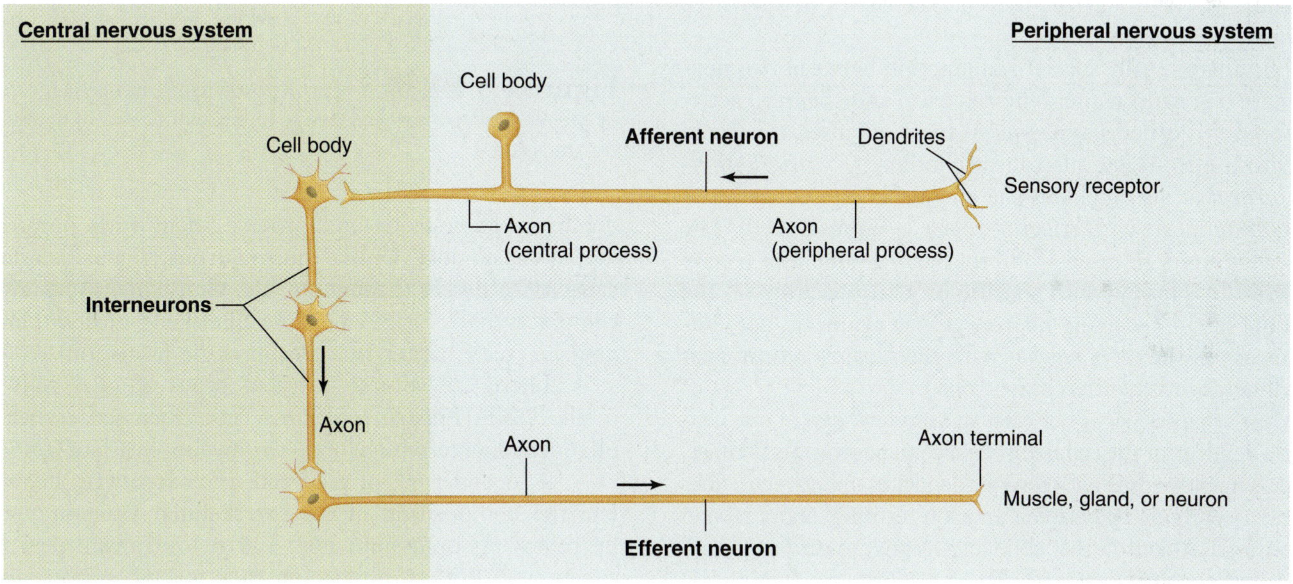

Figure 6.4 AP|R Three classes of neurons. The arrows indicate the direction of transmission of neural activity. Afferent neurons in the PNS generally receive input at sensory receptors. Efferent components of the PNS may terminate on muscle, gland, neuron, or other effector cells. Both afferent and efferent components may consist of two neurons, not one as shown here.

central process, enters the CNS to form junctions with other neurons. Note in Figure 6.4 that for afferent neurons, both the cell body and the long axon are outside the CNS and only a part of the central process enters the brain or spinal cord.

Efferent neurons have a shape like that shown in Figure 6.1. Generally, their cell bodies and dendrites are within the CNS, and the axons extend out to the periphery. There are exceptions, however, such as in the enteric nervous system of the gastrointestinal tract described in Chapter 15. Groups of afferent and efferent neuron axons, together with connective tissue and blood vessels, form the **nerves** of the PNS. Note that *nerve fiber* is a term sometimes used to refer to a single axon, whereas a *nerve* is a bundle of axons (fibers) bound together by connective tissue.

Interneurons lie entirely within the CNS. They account for over 99% of all neurons and have a wide range of physiological properties, shapes, and functions. The number of interneurons interposed between specific afferent and efferent neurons varies according to the complexity of the action they control. The knee-jerk reflex elicited by tapping below the kneecap activates thigh muscles without interneurons—the afferent neurons interact directly with efferent neurons. In contrast, when you

TABLE 6.1 Characteristics of Three Classes of Neurons

I. Afferent neurons	
	A. Transmit information into the CNS from receptors at their peripheral endings
	B. Single process from the cell body splits into a long peripheral process (axon) that is in the PNS and a short central process (axon) that enters the CNS
II. Efferent neurons	
	A. Transmit information out of the CNS to effector cells, particularly muscles, glands, neurons, and other cells
	B. Cell body with multiple dendrites and a small segment of the axon are in the CNS; most of the axon is in the PNS
III. Interneurons	
	A. Function as integrators and signal changers
	B. Integrate groups of afferent and efferent neurons into reflex circuits
	C. Lie entirely within the CNS
	D. Account for > 99% of all neurons

hear a song or smell a certain perfume that evokes memories of someone you know, millions of interneurons may be involved.

Table 6.1 summarizes the characteristics of the three functional classes of neurons.

The anatomically specialized junction between two neurons where one neuron alters the electrical and chemical activity of another is called a **synapse.** At most synapses, the signal is transmitted from one neuron to another by *neurotransmitters*, a term that also includes the chemicals efferent neurons use to communicate with effector cells (e.g., a muscle cell). The neurotransmitters released from one neuron alter the receiving neuron by binding with specific protein receptors on the membrane of the receiving neuron. (Once again, do not confuse this use of the term *receptor* with the sensory receptors at the peripheral ends of afferent neurons.)

Most synapses occur between an axon terminal of one neuron and a dendrite or the cell body of a second neuron. Sometimes, however, synapses occur between two dendrites or between a dendrite and a cell body or between an axon terminal and a second axon terminal. A neuron that conducts a signal toward a synapse is called a **presynaptic neuron,** whereas a neuron conducting signals away from a synapse is a **postsynaptic neuron. Figure 6.5** shows how, in a multineuronal pathway, a single neuron can be postsynaptic to one cell and presynaptic to another. A postsynaptic neuron may have thousands of synaptic junctions on the surface of its dendrites and cell body, so that signals from many presynaptic neurons can affect it. Interconnected in this way, the many millions of neurons in the nervous system exemplify the general principle of physiology that information flow between cells, tissues, and organs is an essential feature of homeostasis and allows for complex integration of physiological processes.

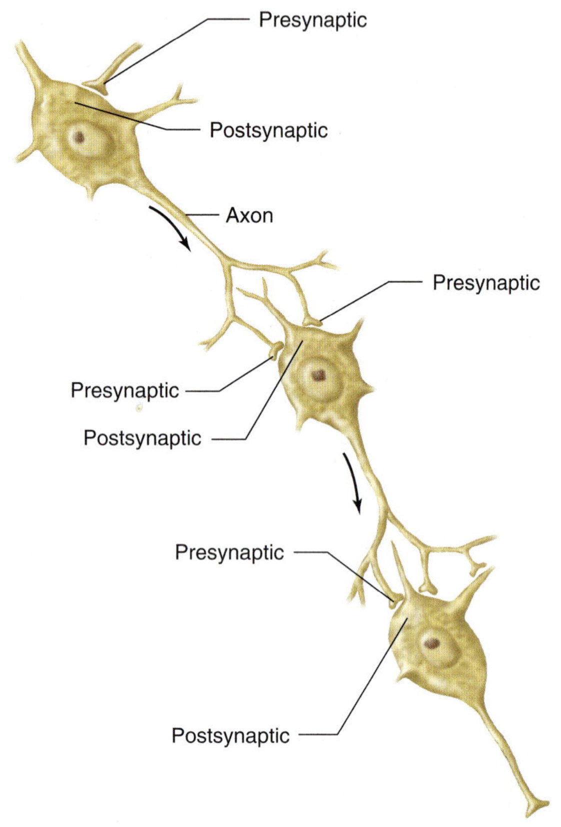

Figure 6.5 APIR A neuron postsynaptic to one cell can be presynaptic to another. Arrows indicate direction of neural transmission.

6.3 Glial Cells

According to recent analyses, neurons account for only about half of the cells in the human CNS. The remainder are **glial cells** (*glia*, "glue"). Glial cells surround the soma, axon, and dendrites of neurons and provide them with physical and metabolic support. Unlike most neurons, glial cells retain the capacity to divide throughout life. Consequently, many CNS tumors actually originate from glial cells rather than from neurons (see Chapter 19 for a thorough discussion).

There are several different types of glial cells found in the CNS (**Figure 6.6**). One type discussed earlier is the oligodendrocyte, which forms the myelin sheath of CNS axons.

A second type of glial cell, the **astrocyte,** helps regulate the composition of the extracellular fluid in the CNS by removing potassium ions and neurotransmitters around synapses. Another important function of astrocytes is to stimulate the formation of tight junctions (review Figure 3.9) between the cells that make up the walls of capillaries found in the CNS. This forms the **blood–brain barrier,** which is a much more selective filter for exchanged substances than is present between the blood and most other tissues. Astrocytes also sustain the neurons metabolically—for example, by providing glucose and removing ammonia. In developing embryos, astrocytes guide neurons as they migrate to their ultimate destination, and they stimulate neuronal growth by secreting growth factors. In addition, astrocytes have many neuronlike characteristics. For example, they have ion channels, receptors for certain neurotransmitters and the enzymes for processing them, and the capability of generating weak electrical responses. Thus, in addition to all their other roles, it is speculated that astrocytes may take part in information signaling in the brain.

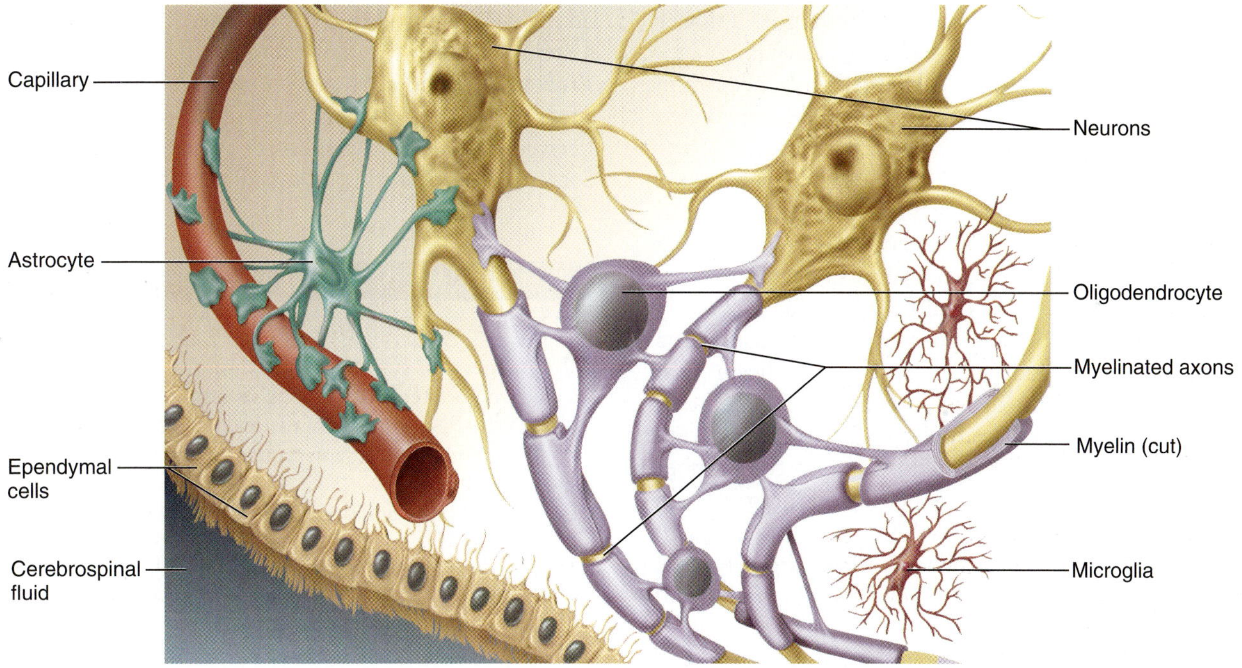

Figure 6.6 APIR Glial cells of the central nervous system.

The **microglia,** a third type of glial cell, are specialized, macrophage-like cells (Chapter 18) that perform immune functions in the CNS, and may also contribute to synapse remodeling and plasticity. Lastly, **ependymal cells** line the fluid-filled cavities within the brain and spinal cord and regulate the production and flow of cerebrospinal fluid, which will be described later.

Schwann cells, the glial cells of the PNS, have most of the properties of the CNS glia. As mentioned earlier, Schwann cells produce the myelin sheath of the axons of the peripheral neurons.

6.4 Neural Growth and Regeneration

The elaborate networks of neuronal processes that characterize the nervous system are remarkably similar in all human beings and depend upon the outgrowth of specific axons to specific targets.

Development of the nervous system in the embryo begins with a series of divisions of undifferentiated precursor cells (**stem cells**) that can develop into neurons or glia. After the last cell division, each neuronal daughter cell differentiates, migrates to its final location, and sends out processes that will become its axon and dendrites. A specialized enlargement, the **growth cone,** forms the tip of each extending axon and is involved in finding the correct route and final target for the process.

As the axon grows, it is guided along the surfaces of other cells, most commonly glial cells. Which route the axon follows depends largely on attracting, supporting, deflecting, or inhibiting influences exerted by several types of molecules. Some of these molecules, such as cell adhesion molecules, reside on the membranes of the glia and embryonic neurons. Others are soluble **neurotrophic factors** (growth factors for neural tissue) in the extracellular fluid surrounding the growth cone or its distant target.

Once the target of the advancing growth cone is reached, synapses form. The synapses are active, however, before their final maturation. This early activity, in part, determines their final function. During these early stages of neural development, which occur during all trimesters of pregnancy and into infancy, alcohol and other drugs, radiation, malnutrition, and viruses can exert effects that cause permanent damage to the developing fetal nervous system.

A surprising aspect of development of the nervous system occurs after growth and projection of the axons. Many of the newly formed neurons and synapses degenerate. In fact, as many as 50% to 70% of neurons undergo a programmed self-destruction called **apoptosis** in the developing CNS. Exactly why this seemingly wasteful process occurs is unknown, although neuroscientists speculate that this refines or fine-tunes connectivity in the nervous system.

Throughout the life span, our brain has an amazing ability to modify its structure and function in response to stimulation or injury, a characteristic known as **plasticity.** This involves both the generation of new neurons and remodeling of synaptic connections, and is stimulated by exercise and by engaging in cognitively challenging activities.

The degree of neural plasticity varies with age. For example, an infant suffering from seizures (uncontrolled excessive neural activity) can have nearly half of the brain removed, and because of extensive remodeling the brain can recover full functionality into adulthood. If the same procedure were performed on an adult, it would result in permanent deficits in the functions served by the excised brain regions. For many neural systems, the critical time window for development occurs at a fairly young age. In visual pathways, for example, regions of the brain involved in processing visual stimuli are permanently impaired if no visual stimulation is received during a critical time, which peaks between 1 and 2 years of age.

By contrast, the ability to learn a language undergoes a slower and more subtle change in plasticity—humans learn languages relatively easily and quickly until adolescence, but learning becomes slower and more difficult as we proceed from adolescence through adulthood.

The basic shapes and locations of major neuronal circuits in the mature CNS do not change once formed. However, the creation and removal of synaptic contacts begun during fetal development continue throughout life as part of normal growth, learning, and aging. Also, although it was previously thought that production of new neurons ceased around the time of birth, a growing body of evidence now indicates that the ability to produce new neurons is retained in some brain regions throughout life. For example, cognitive stimulation and exercise have both been shown to increase the number of neurons in brain regions associated with learning even in adults. In addition, the effectiveness of some antidepressant medications has been shown to depend upon the production of new neurons in limbic system regions involved in emotion and motivation (Chapter 8).

If axons are severed, they can repair themselves and restore significant function provided that the damage occurs outside the CNS and does not affect the neuron's cell body. After such an injury, the axon segment that is separated from the cell body degenerates. The part of the axon still attached to the cell body then gives rise to a growth cone, which grows out to the effector organ so that function can be restored. Return of function following a peripheral nerve injury is delayed because axon regrowth proceeds at a rate of only 1 mm per day. So, for example, if afferent neurons from your thumb were damaged by an injury in the area of your shoulder, it might take 2 years for sensation in your thumb to be restored.

Spinal injuries typically crush rather than cut the tissue, leaving the axons intact. In this case, a primary problem is self-destruction (apoptosis) of the nearby oligodendrocytes. When these cells die and their associated axons lose their myelin sheath, the axons cannot transmit information effectively. Severed axons within the CNS may grow small new extensions, but no significant regeneration of the axon occurs across the damaged site, and there are no well-documented reports of significant return of function. Functional regeneration is prevented either by some basic difference of CNS neurons or some property of their environment, such as inhibitory factors associated with nearby glia.

Researchers are trying a variety of ways to provide an environment that will support axonal regeneration in the CNS. They are creating tubes to support regrowth of the severed axons, redirecting the axons to regions of the spinal cord that lack growth-inhibiting factors, preventing apoptosis of the oligodendrocytes so myelin can be maintained, and supplying neurotrophic factors that support recovery of the damaged tissue.

Medical researchers are also attempting to restore function to damaged or diseased spinal cords and brains by implanting undifferentiated stem cells that will develop into new neurons and replace missing neurotransmitters or neurotrophic factors. Initial stem cell research focused on the use of embryonic and fetal stem cells which, while yielding promising results, raises ethical concerns. Recently, however, researchers have developed promising techniques using stem cells isolated from adults, and using adult cells that have been induced to revert to a stem-cell-like state. For example, in patients with ***Parkinson disease***, a degenerative nervous system disease resulting in progressive loss of movement, the implantation of neural stem cells derived from healthy regions of a patient's own brain has been somewhat successful in restoring motor function.

SECTION A SUMMARY

Structure and Maintenance of Neurons

I. The nervous system is divided into two parts. The central nervous system (CNS) consists of the brain and spinal cord, and the PNS consists of nerves outside of the CNS.

II. The basic unit of the nervous system is the nerve cell, or neuron.

III. The cell body and dendrites receive information from other neurons.

IV. The axon (nerve fiber), which may be covered with sections of myelin separated by nodes of Ranvier, transmits information to other neurons or effector cells.

Functional Classes of Neurons

I. Neurons are classified in three ways:
   a. *Afferent neurons* transmit information into the CNS from receptors at their peripheral endings.
   b. *Efferent neurons* transmit information out of the CNS to effector cells.
   c. *Interneurons* lie entirely within the CNS and form circuits with other interneurons or connect afferent and efferent neurons.

II. Neurotransmitters, which are released by a presynaptic neuron and combine with protein receptors on a postsynaptic neuron, transmit information across a synapse.

Glial Cells

I. The CNS also contains glial cells, which help regulate the extracellular fluid composition, sustain the neurons metabolically, form myelin and the blood–brain barrier, serve as guides for developing neurons, provide immune functions, and regulate cerebrospinal fluid.

Neural Growth and Regeneration

I. Neurons develop from stem cells, migrate to their final locations, and send out processes to their target cells.

II. Cell division to form new neurons and the plasticity to remodel after injury markedly decrease between birth and adulthood.

III. After degeneration of a severed axon, damaged peripheral neurons may regrow the axon to their target organ. Functional regeneration of severed CNS axons does not usually occur.

SECTION A REVIEW QUESTIONS

1. Describe the direction of information flow through a neuron in response to input from another neuron. What is the relationship between the presynaptic neuron and the postsynaptic neuron?
2. Contrast the two uses of the word *receptor*.
3. Where are afferent neurons, efferent neurons, and interneurons located in the nervous system? Are there places where all three could be found?

SECTION A KEY TERMS

SECTION A CLINICAL TERMS

SECTION B

Membrane Potentials

6.5 Basic Principles of Electricity

This section provides an excellent demonstration of the general principle of physiology that physiological processes are dictated by the laws of chemistry and physics, notably those that determine the net flux of charged molecules. As discussed in Chapter 4, the predominant solutes in the extracellular fluid are sodium and chloride ions. The intracellular fluid contains high concentrations of potassium ions and ionized nonpenetrating molecules, particularly phosphate compounds and proteins with negatively charged side chains. Electrical phenomena resulting from the distribution of these charged particles occur at the cell's plasma membrane and play a significant role in signal integration and cell-to-cell communication, the two major functions of the neuron.

A fundamental physical principle is that charges of the same type repel each other—positive charge repels positive charge, and negative charge repels negative charge. In contrast, oppositely charged substances attract each other and will move toward each other if not separated by some barrier (**Figure 6.7**).

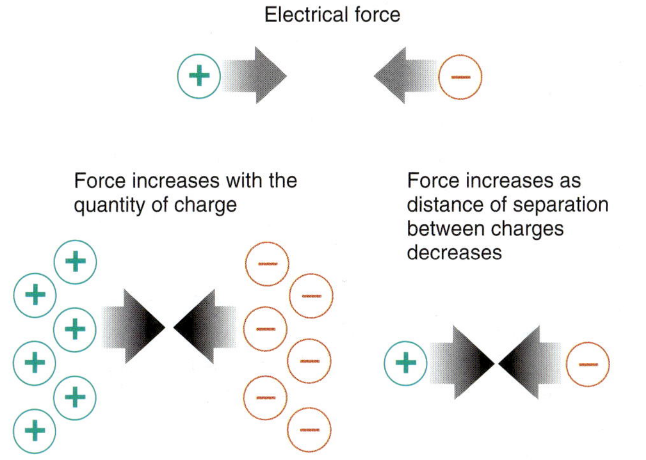

Figure 6.7 The electrical force of attraction between positive and negative charges increases with the quantity of charge and with decreasing distance between charges.

Separated electrical charges of opposite sign have the potential to do work if they are allowed to come together. This potential is called an **electrical potential** or, because it is determined by the difference in the amount of charge between two points, a **potential difference.** The electrical potential difference is often referred to simply as the **potential.** The units of electrical potential are volts. The total charge that can be separated in most biological systems is very small, so the potential differences are small and are measured in millivolts (1 mV = 0.001 V).

The movement of electrical charge is called a **current.** The electrical potential between charges tends to make them flow, producing a current. If the charges are opposite, the current brings them toward each other; if the charges are alike, the current increases the separation between them. The amount of charge that moves—in other words, the current—depends on the potential difference between the charges and on the nature of the material or structure through which they are moving. The hindrance to electrical charge movement is known as **resistance.** If resistance is high, the current flow will be low. The effect of voltage V and resistance R on current I is expressed in **Ohm's law:**

$$I = \frac{V}{R}$$

Materials that have a high electrical resistance reduce current flow and are known as insulators. Materials that have a low resistance allow rapid current flow and are called conductors.

Water that contains dissolved ions is a relatively good conductor of electricity because the ions can carry the current. As we have seen, the intracellular and extracellular fluids contain many ions and can therefore carry current. Lipids, however, contain very few charged groups and cannot carry current. Therefore, the lipid layers of the plasma membrane are regions of high electrical resistance separating the intracellular fluid and the extracellular fluid, two low-resistance aqueous compartments.

6.6 The Resting Membrane Potential

All cells under resting conditions have a potential difference across their plasma membranes, with the inside of the cell negatively charged with respect to the outside (**Figure 6.8**). This potential is the **resting membrane potential.**

By convention, extracellular fluid is designated as the voltage reference point, and the polarity (positive or negative) of the membrane potential is stated in terms of the sign of the excess charge on the inside of the cell by comparison. For example, if the intracellular fluid has an excess of negative charge and the potential difference across the membrane has a magnitude of 70 mV, we say that the membrane potential is −70 mV (inside relative to outside).

The magnitude of the resting membrane potential varies from about −5 to −100 mV, depending upon the type of cell. In neurons, it is generally in the range of −40 to −90 mV. The resting membrane potential holds steady unless changes in electrical current alter the potential.

The resting membrane potential exists because of a tiny excess of negative ions inside the cell and an excess of positive ions outside. The excess negative charges inside are electrically attracted to the excess positive charges outside the cell, and vice versa. Thus, the excess charges (ions) collect in a thin shell tight against the inner and outer surfaces of the plasma membrane (**Figure 6.9**), whereas the bulk of the intracellular and extracellular fluid remains electrically neutral. Unlike the diagrammatic representation in Figure 6.9, the number of positive and negative charges that have to be separated across a membrane to account for the potential is actually an infinitesimal fraction of the total number of charges in the two compartments.

Table 6.2 lists the concentrations of sodium, potassium, and chloride ions in the extracellular fluid and in the intracellular fluid of a representative neuron. Each of these ions has a 10- to 30-fold difference in concentration between the inside and the outside of the cell. Although this table appears to contradict our earlier assertion that the bulk of the intracellular and extracellular fluid is electrically neutral, there are many other ions not listed, including Mg^{2+}, Ca^{2+}, H^+, HCO_3^-, HPO_4^{2-}, SO_4^{2-}, amino acids, and proteins. When all ions are accounted for, each solution is indeed electrically neutral. Of the ions that can flow across the membrane and affect its electrical potential, Na^+, K^+, and Cl^- are present in the highest concentrations, and the membrane permeability to each is independently determined. Na^+ and K^+ generally play the most important roles in generating the resting membrane potential, but in some cells Cl^- is also a factor. Notice that the Na^+ and Cl^- concentrations are lower inside the cell than outside, and that the K^+ concentration is greater inside the cell. The concentration differences for Na^+ and K^+ are established by the action of the sodium–potassium ion pump (Na^+/K^+-ATPase, Chapter 4) that pumps Na^+ out of the cell and K^+ into it. The reason for the Cl^- distribution varies between cell types, as will be described later.

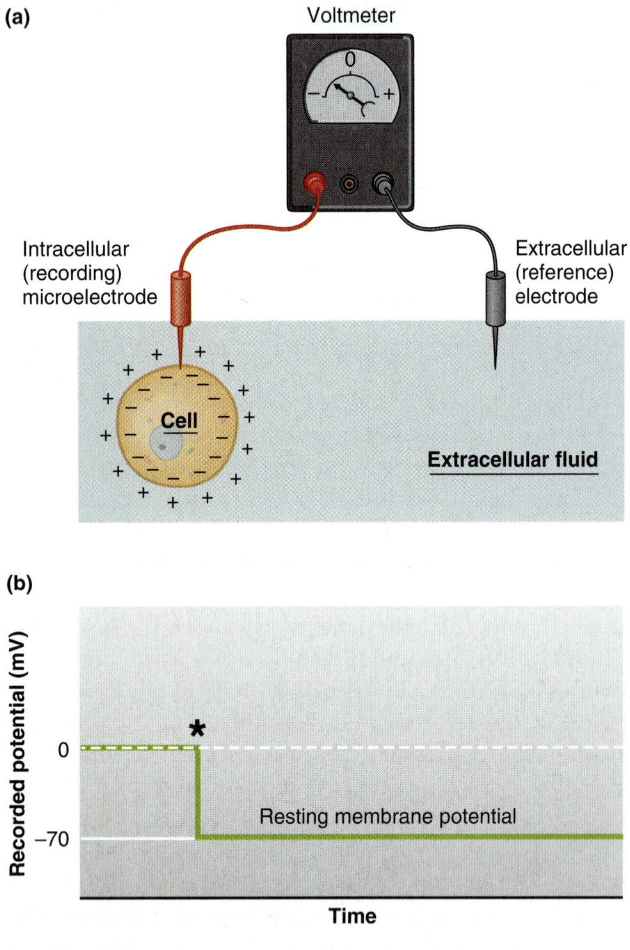

Figure 6.8 (a) Apparatus for measuring membrane potentials. The voltmeter records the difference between the intracellular and extracellular electrodes. (b) The potential difference across a plasma membrane as measured by an intracellular microelectrode. The asterisk indicates the moment the electrode entered the cell.

PHYSIOLOGICAL INQUIRY

- If you reversed the position of these two electrodes, would the graph in part (b) look different?

Answer can be found at end of chapter.

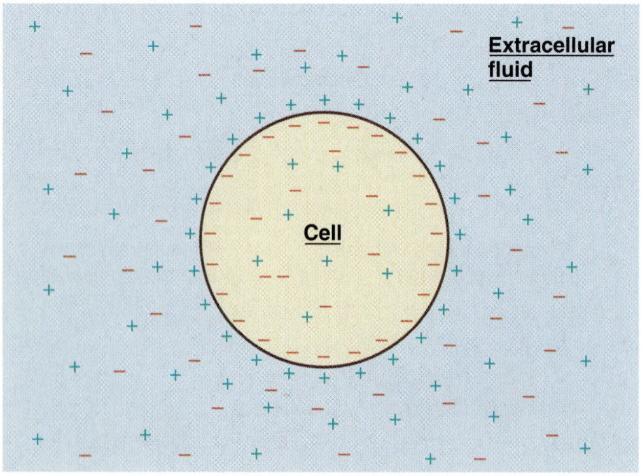

Figure 6.9 The excess positive charges outside the cell and the excess negative charges inside collect in a tight shell against the plasma membrane. In reality, these excess charges are only an extremely small fraction of the total number of ions inside and outside the cell.

TABLE 6.2 Distribution of Major Mobile Ions Across the Plasma Membrane of a Typical Nerve Cell

	Concentration (mmol/L)	
Ion	**Extracellular**	**Intracellular**
Na^+	145	15
Cl^-	100	7*
K^+	5	150

A more accurate measure of electrical driving force can be obtained using mEq/L, which factors in ion valence. Because all the ions in this table have a valence of 1, the mEq/L is the same as the mmol/L concentration.

*Intracellular Cl^- concentration varies significantly between neurons due to differences in expression of membrane transporters and channels.

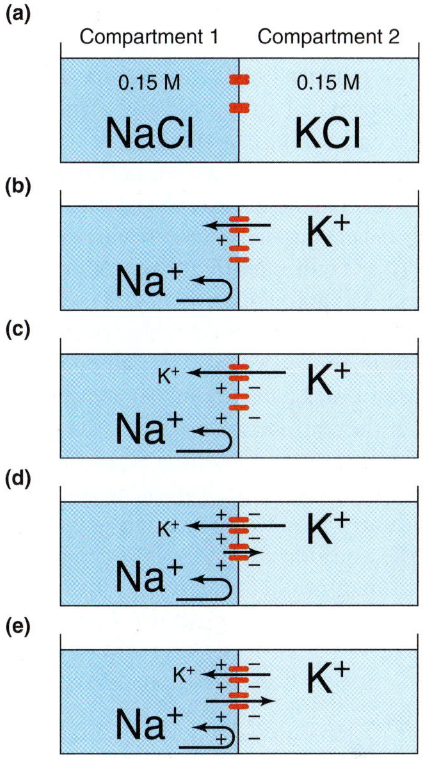

Figure 6.10 Generation of a potential across a membrane due to diffusion of K^+ through K^+ channels (red). Arrows represent ion movements; as in Figure 4.3, arrow length represents the magnitude of the flux. So few K^+ ions cross the membrane that ion concentrations do not change significantly on either side of the membrane from step (a) to step (e). See the text for a complete explanation of the steps a–e.

PHYSIOLOGICAL INQUIRY

- In setting up this experiment, 0.15 mole of NaCl was placed in compartment 1, 0.15 mole of KCl was placed in compartment 2, and each compartment has a volume of 1 liter. What is the approximate total solute concentration in each compartment at equilibrium?

Answer can be found at end of chapter.

The magnitude of the resting membrane potential depends mainly on two factors: (1) differences in specific ion concentrations in the intracellular and extracellular fluids; and (2) differences in membrane permeabilities to the different ions, which reflect the number of open channels for the different ions in the plasma membrane.

To understand how concentration differences for Na^+ and K^+ create membrane potentials, first consider what happens when the membrane is permeable (has open channels) to only one ion (**Figure 6.10**). In this hypothetical situation, it is assumed that the membrane contains K^+ channels but no Na^+ or Cl^- channels. Initially, compartment 1 contains 0.15 M NaCl, compartment 2 contains 0.15 M KCl, and no ion movement occurs because the channels are closed (**Figure 6.10a**). There is no potential difference across the membrane because the two compartments contain equal numbers of positive and negative ions. The positive ions are different—Na^+ versus K^+, but the *total* numbers of positive ions in the two compartments are the same, and each positive ion balances a chloride ion.

However, if these K^+ channels are opened, K^+ will diffuse down its concentration gradient from compartment 2 into compartment 1 (**Figure 6.10b**). Sodium ions will not be able to move across the membrane. After a few potassium ions have moved into compartment 1, that compartment will have an excess of positive charge, leaving behind an excess of negative charge in compartment 2 (**Figure 6.10c**). Thus, a potential difference has been created across the membrane.

This introduces another major factor that can cause net movement of ions across a membrane: an electrical potential. As compartment 1 becomes increasingly positive and compartment 2 increasingly negative, the membrane potential difference begins to influence the movement of the potassium ions. The negative charge of compartment 2 tends to attract them back into their original compartment, and the positive charge of compartment 1 tends to repulse them (**Figure 6.10d**).

As long as the flux or movement of ions due to the K^+ concentration gradient is greater than the flux due to the membrane potential, net movement of K^+ will occur from compartment 2 to compartment 1 (see Figure 6.10d) and the membrane potential will progressively increase. However, eventually, the membrane potential will become negative enough to produce a flux equal but opposite to the flux produced by the concentration gradient (**Figure 6.10e**). The membrane potential at which these two fluxes become equal in magnitude but opposite in direction is called the **equilibrium potential** for that ion—in this case, K^+. At the equilibrium potential for an ion, there is no *net* movement of the ion because the opposing fluxes are equal, and the potential will undergo no further change. It is worth emphasizing once again that the number of ions crossing the membrane to establish this equilibrium potential is insignificant compared to the number originally present in compartment 2, so there is no significant change in the K^+ concentration in either compartment between step (a) and step (e).

The magnitude of the equilibrium potential (in mV) for any type of ion depends on the concentration gradient for that ion across the membrane. If the concentrations on the two sides were equal, the flux due to the concentration gradient would be zero and the equilibrium potential would also be zero. The larger the concentration gradient, the larger the equilibrium potential because a larger, electrically driven movement of ions will be required to balance the movement due to the concentration difference.

Now consider the situation in which the membrane separating the two compartments is replaced with one that contains only Na^+ channels. A parallel situation will occur (**Figure 6.11**). Sodium ions (Na^+) will initially move from compartment 1 to compartment 2. When compartment 2 is positive with respect to compartment 1, the difference in electrical charge across the membrane will begin to drive Na^+ from compartment 2 back to compartment 1 and, eventually, net movement of Na^+ will cease. Again, at the equilibrium potential, the movement of ions due to the concentration gradient is equal but opposite to the movement due to the electrical gradient, and an insignificant number of sodium ions actually move in achieving this state.

Thus, the equilibrium potential for one ion species can be different in magnitude *and* direction from those for other ion species, depending on the concentration gradients between

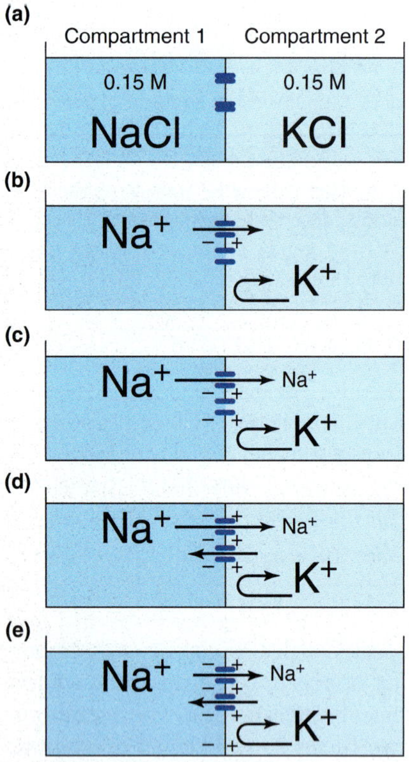

Figure 6.11 Generation of a potential across a membrane due to diffusion of Na^+ through Na^+ channels (blue). Arrows represent ion movements; as in Figure 4.3, arrow length indicates the magnitude of the flux. So few Na^+ ions cross the membrane that ion concentrations do not change significantly from step (a) to step (e). See the text for a more complete explanation.

PHYSIOLOGICAL INQUIRY

- In this hypothetical system, what equilibrium state would result if open channels for both Na^+ and K^+ were present?

Answer can be found at end of chapter.

the intracellular and extracellular compartments for each ion. If the concentration gradient for any ion is known, the equilibrium potential for that ion can be calculated by means of the Nernst equation.

The **Nernst equation** describes the equilibrium potential for any ion species—that is, the electrical potential necessary to balance a given ionic concentration gradient across a membrane so that the net flux of the ion is zero. The Nernst equation is

$$E_{\text{ion}} = \frac{61}{Z}\log\left(\frac{C_{\text{out}}}{C_{\text{in}}}\right)$$

where

E_{ion} = equilibrium potential for a particular ion, in mV
C_{in} = intracellular concentration of the ion
C_{out} = extracellular concentration of the ion
Z = the valence of the ion

61 = a constant value that takes into account the universal gas constant, the temperature (37°C), and the Faraday electrical constant

Using the concentration gradients from Table 6.2, the equilibrium potentials for Na^+ (E_{Na}) and K^+ (E_K) are

$$E_{Na} = \frac{61}{+1}\log\left(\frac{145}{15}\right) = +60\text{ mV}$$

$$E_K = \frac{61}{+1}\log\left(\frac{5}{150}\right) = -90\text{ mV}$$

Thus, at these typical concentrations, Na^+ flux through open channels will tend to bring the membrane potential toward +60 mV, whereas K^+ flux will bring it toward −90 mV. If the concentration gradients change, the equilibrium potentials will change.

The hypothetical situations presented in Figures 6.10 and 6.11 are useful for understanding how individual permeating ions like Na^+ and K^+ influence membrane potential, but keep in mind that real cells are far more complicated. Many charged molecules contribute to the overall electrical properties of cell membranes. For example, most of the negative charge inside neurons is accounted for not by chloride ions but by impermeable organic anions—in particular, proteins and phosphate compounds. Thus, when there is a net flux of K^+ out of a cell, these are the main ion species contributing to the negative charge on the inside of the membrane. Another complication in real cells is that they are rarely permeable to only a single ion at a time.

When channels for more than one ion species are open in the membrane at the same time, the permeabilities and concentration gradients for all the ions must be considered when accounting for the membrane potential. For a given concentration gradient, the greater the membrane permeability to an ion species, the greater the contribution that ion species will make to the membrane potential. Given the concentration gradients and relative membrane permeabilities (P_{ion}) for Na^+, K^+, and Cl^-, the potential of a membrane (V_m) can be calculated using the **Goldman-Hodgkin-Katz (GHK) equation:**

$$V_m = 61\log\frac{P_K[K_{\text{out}}] + P_{Na}[Na_{\text{out}}] + P_{Cl}[Cl_{\text{in}}]}{P_K[K_{\text{in}}] + P_{Na}[Na_{\text{in}}] + P_{Cl}[Cl_{\text{out}}]}$$

The GHK equation is essentially an expanded version of the Nernst equation that takes into account individual ion permeabilities. In fact, setting the permeabilities of any two ions to zero gives the equilibrium potential for the remaining ion. Note that the Cl^- concentrations are reversed as compared to Na^+ and K^+ (the inside concentration is in the numerator and the outside in the denominator), because Cl^- is an anion and its movement has the opposite effect on the membrane potential. Ion gradients and permeabilities vary widely in different excitable cells of the human body and in other animals, and yet the GHK equation can be used to determine the resting membrane potential of any cell if the conditions are known. For example, if the relative permeability values of a cell were $P_K = 1$, $P_{Na} = 0.04$, and $P_{Cl} = 0.45$ and the ion concentrations were equal to those listed in Table 6.2, the resting membrane potential would be

$$V_m = 61 \log \frac{(1)(5) + (.04)(145) + (.45)(7)}{(1)(150) + (.04)(15) + (.45)(100)} = -70 \text{ mV}$$

The contributions of Na^+, K^+ and Cl^- to the overall membrane potential are thus a function of their concentration gradients and relative permeabilities. The concentration gradients determine their equilibrium potentials, and the relative permeability determines how strongly the resting membrane potential is influenced toward those potentials. In mammalian neurons, the K^+ permeability may be as much as 100 times greater than that for Na^+ and Cl^-, so neuronal resting membrane potentials are typically fairly close to the equilibrium potential for K^+ (**Figure 6.12**). The value of the Cl^- equilibrium potential is also near the resting membrane potential in many neurons, but for reasons we will return to shortly, Cl^- actually has minimal importance in determining neuronal resting membrane potentials compared to K^+ and Na^+.

In summary, the resting potential is generated across the plasma membrane largely because of the movement of K^+ out of the cell down its concentration gradient through open K^+ channels (called **leak K^+ channels**). This makes the inside of the cell negative with respect to the outside. Even though K^+ flux has more impact on the resting membrane potential than does Na^+ flux, the resting membrane potential is not *equal* to the K^+ equilibrium potential, because having a small number of open Na^+ channels does pull the membrane potential slightly toward the Na^+ equilibrium potential. Thus, at the resting membrane potential, ion channels allow net movement both of Na^+ into the cell and K^+ out of the cell.

Over time, the concentrations of intracellular sodium and potassium ions do not change, however, because of the action of the Na^+/K^+-ATPase pump. In a resting cell, the number of ions the pump moves equals the number of ions that leak down their concentration and/or electrical gradients (described collectively in Chapter 4 as the *electrochemical gradient*). As long as the concentration gradients remain stable and the ion permeabilities of the plasma membrane do not change, the electrical potential across the resting membrane will also remain constant.

Thus far, we have described the membrane potential as due purely and directly to the passive movement of ions down their electrochemical gradients, with the concentration gradients maintained by membrane pumps. However, the Na^+/K^+-ATPase pump not only maintains the concentration gradients for these ions but also helps to establish the membrane potential more directly. The Na^+/K^+-ATPase pumps actually move three sodium ions out of the cell for every two potassium ions that they bring in. This unequal transport of positive ions makes the inside of the cell more negative than it would be from ion diffusion alone. When a pump moves net charge across the membrane and contributes directly to the membrane potential, it is known as an **electrogenic pump.**

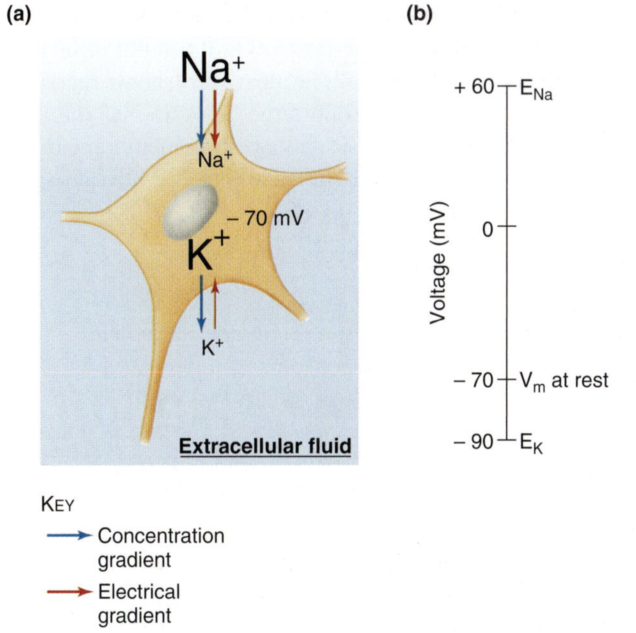

Figure 6.12 Forces influencing sodium and potassium ions at the resting membrane potential. (a) At a resting membrane potential of −70 mV, both the concentration and electrical gradients favor inward movement of Na^+, whereas the K^+ concentration and electrical gradients are in opposite directions. (b) The greater permeability and movement of K^+ maintain the resting membrane potential at a value near E_K.

PHYSIOLOGICAL INQUIRY

- Would decreasing a neuron's intracellular fluid $[K^+]$ by 1 mM have the same effect on resting membrane potential as raising the extracellular fluid $[K^+]$ by 1 mM?

Answer can be found at end of chapter.

In most cells, the electrogenic contribution to the membrane potential is quite small. Even though the electrogenic contribution of the Na^+/K^+-ATPase pump is small, the pump always makes an essential *indirect* contribution to the membrane potential because it maintains the concentration gradients that result in ion diffusion and charge separation.

Figure 6.13 summarizes the development of a resting membrane potential in three conceptual steps. First, the action of the Na^+/K^+-ATPase pump sets up the concentration gradients for Na^+ and K^+ (**Figure 6.13a**). These concentration gradients determine the equilibrium potentials for the two ions—that is, the value to which each ion would bring the membrane potential if it were the only permeating ion. Simultaneously, the pump has a small electrogenic effect on the membrane due to the fact that three sodium ions are pumped out for every two potassium ions pumped in. The next step shows that initially there is a greater flux of K^+ out of the cell than Na^+ into the cell (**Figure 6.13b**). This is because in a resting membrane there is a greater permeability to K^+ than there is to Na^+. Because there is greater net efflux than influx of positive ions during this step, a significant negative membrane potential develops, with the value approaching that of the K^+ equilibrium potential. In the steady-state resting neuron, the flux of ions across the membrane reaches a dynamic balance (**Figure 6.13c**). Because the membrane potential is not equal to the equilibrium potential for either ion, there is a small but steady leak of Na^+ into the cell and K^+ out of the cell. The concentration gradients do not dissipate over time, however, because ion movement by the Na^+/K^+-ATPase pump exactly balances the rate at which the ions leak in the opposite direction.

Now let's return to the behavior of chloride ions in excitable cells. The plasma membranes of many cells also have Cl^- channels but do not contain chloride ion pumps. Therefore, in these cells, Cl^- concentrations simply shift until the equilibrium potential for Cl^- is equal to the resting membrane potential. In other words, the negative membrane potential determined by Na^+ and K^+ moves Cl^- out of the cell, and the Cl^- concentration inside the cell becomes lower than that outside. This concentration gradient produces a diffusion of Cl^- back into the cell that exactly opposes the movement out because of the electrical potential.

In contrast, some cells have a nonelectrogenic active-transport system that moves Cl^- out of the cell, generating a strong concentration gradient. In these cells, the Cl^- equilibrium potential is negative to the resting membrane potential, and net Cl^- diffusion into the cell contributes to the excess negative charge inside the cell; that is, net Cl^- diffusion makes the membrane potential more negative than it would be if only Na^+ and K^+ were involved.

6.7 Graded Potentials and Action Potentials

You have just learned that all cells have a resting membrane potential due to the presence of ion pumps and leak channels in the cell membrane. In addition, however, some cells have another group of ion channels that can be gated (opened or closed) under certain conditions. Such channels give a cell the ability to produce electrical signals that can transmit information between different regions of the membrane. This property is known as **excitability,** and such membranes are called **excitable membranes.** Cells of this type include all neurons and muscle cells, as well as some endocrine, immune, and reproductive cells. The electrical signals occur in two forms: graded potentials and action potentials. Graded potentials are important in signaling over short distances, whereas action potentials are long-distance signals that are particularly important in neuronal and muscle cell membranes.

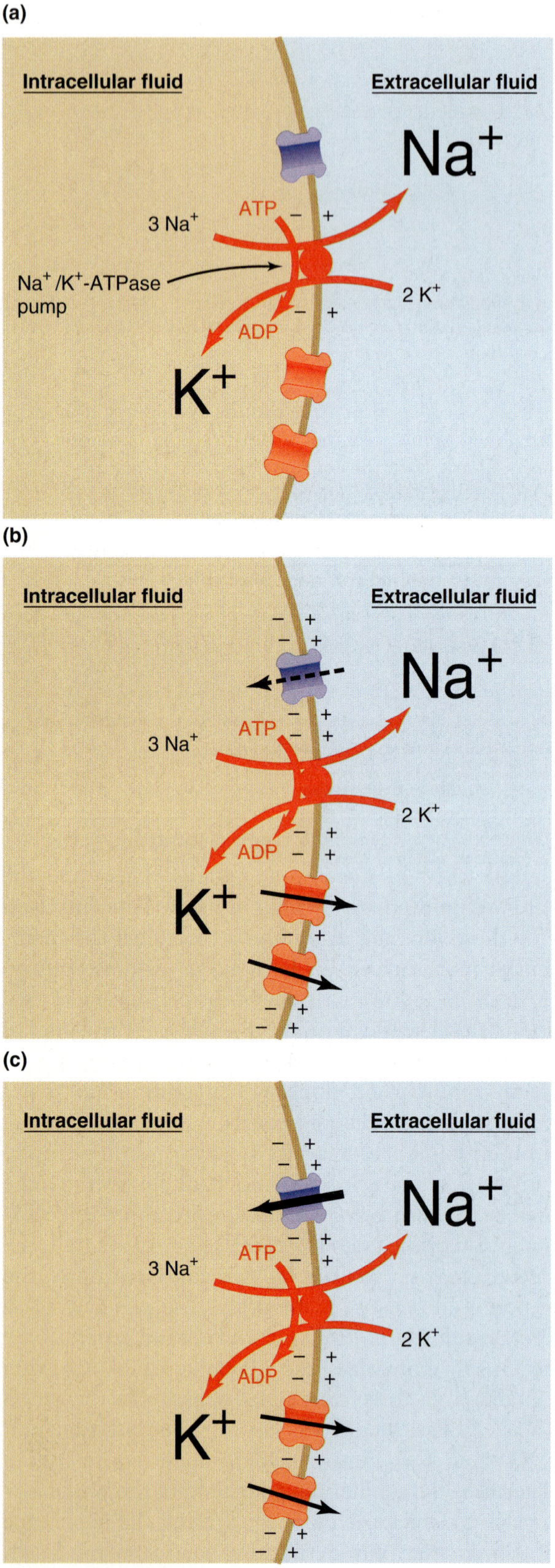

Figure 6.13 AP|R Summary of steps establishing the resting membrane potential. (a) An Na^+/K^+-ATPase pump establishes concentration gradients and generates a small negative potential. (b) Greater net movement of K^+ than Na^+ makes the membrane potential more negative on the inside. (c) At a steady negative resting membrane potential, ion fluxes through the channels and pump balance each other. The K^+ permeability (shown in red) is mainly due to K^+ leak channels, while Na^+ permeability (purple) is due mainly to other transport processes (see Figure 4.15).

The terms *depolarize*, *repolarize*, and *hyperpolarize* are used to describe the direction of changes in the membrane potential relative to the resting potential (**Figure 6.14**). The resting membrane potential is "polarized," simply meaning that the outside and inside of a cell have a different net charge. The membrane is **depolarized** when its potential becomes less negative (closer to zero) than the resting level. **Overshoot** refers to a reversal of the membrane potential polarity—that is, when the inside of a cell becomes positive relative to the outside. When a membrane potential that has been depolarized is returning toward the resting value, it is **repolarizing.** The membrane is **hyperpolarized** when the potential is more negative than the resting level.

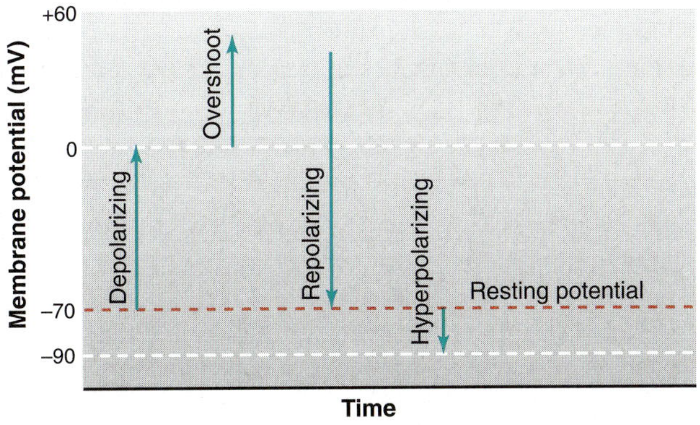

Figure 6.14 Depolarizing, repolarizing, hyperpolarizing, and overshoot changes in membrane potential relative to the resting potential.

The changes in membrane potential that the neuron uses as signals occur because of changes in the permeability of the cell membrane to ions. Recall from Chapter 4 that gated channels in a membrane may be opened or closed by mechanical, electrical, or chemical stimuli. When a neuron receives a chemical signal from a neighboring neuron, for instance, some gated channels will open, allowing greater ionic current across the membrane. The greater movement of ions down their electrochemical gradient alters the membrane potential so that it is either depolarized or hyperpolarized relative to the resting state. We will see that particular characteristics of these gated channels play a role in determining the nature of the electrical signal generated.

Graded Potentials

Graded potentials are changes in membrane potential that are confined to a relatively small region of the plasma membrane. They are usually produced when some specific change in the cell's environment acts on a specialized region of the membrane. They are called graded potentials simply because the magnitude of the potential change can vary (is "graded"). Graded potentials are given various names related to the location of the potential or the function they perform—for instance, receptor potential, synaptic potential, and pacemaker potential are all different types of graded potentials (**Table 6.3**).

Whenever a graded potential occurs, charge flows between the place of origin of this potential and adjacent regions of the plasma membrane, which are still at the resting potential. In **Figure 6.15a**, a small region of a membrane

TABLE 6.3 A Miniglossary of Terms Describing the Membrane Potential

Potential or potential difference	The voltage difference between two points
Membrane potential or transmembrane potential	The voltage difference between the inside and outside of a cell
Equilibrium potential	The voltage difference across a membrane that produces a flux of a given ion species that is equal but opposite to the flux due to the concentration gradient of that same ion species
Resting membrane potential or resting potential	The steady transmembrane potential of a cell that is not producing an electrical signal
Graded potential	A potential change of variable amplitude and duration that is conducted decrementally; has no threshold or refractory period
Action potential	A brief all-or-none depolarization of the membrane, which reverses polarity in neurons; has a threshold and refractory period and is conducted without decrement
Synaptic potential	A graded potential change produced in the postsynaptic neuron in response to the release of a neurotransmitter by a presynaptic terminal; may be depolarizing (an excitatory postsynaptic potential or EPSP) or hyperpolarizing (an inhibitory postsynaptic potential or IPSP)
Receptor potential	A graded potential produced at the peripheral endings of afferent neurons (or in separate receptor cells) in response to a stimulus
Pacemaker potential	A spontaneously occurring graded potential change that occurs in certain specialized cells
Threshold potential	The membrane potential at which an action potential is initiated

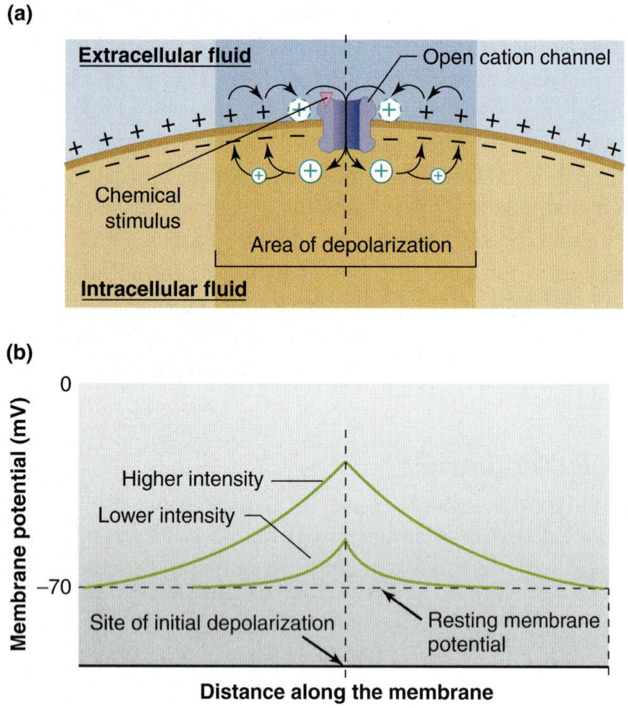

Figure 6.15 Depolarization and graded potential caused by a chemical stimulus. (a) Inward positive current through ligand-gated cation channels depolarizes a region of the membrane, and local currents spread the depolarization to adjacent regions. (b) The intensity of the initial stimulus determines the magnitude of membrane depolarization, and at increasing distances from the initial site the amount of depolarization is less.

PHYSIOLOGICAL INQUIRY

- If the ligand-gated ion channel allowed only the outward flow of K^+ from the cell, how would this figure and graph be different?

Answer can be found at end of chapter.

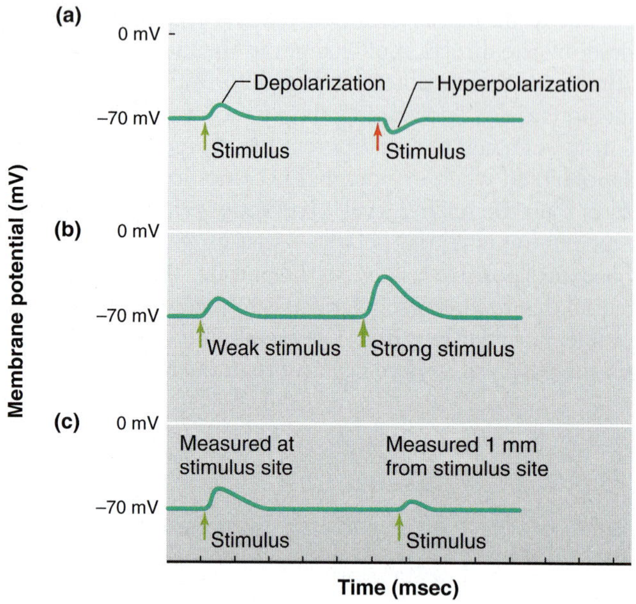

Figure 6.16 Graded potentials can be recorded under experimental conditions in which the stimulus strength can vary. Such experiments show that graded potentials (a) can be depolarizing or hyperpolarizing, (b) can vary in size, (c) are conducted decrementally. The resting membrane potential is −70 mV.

has been depolarized by transient application of a chemical signal, briefly opening membrane cation channels and producing a potential less negative than that of adjacent areas. Positive charges inside the cell (mainly K^+ ions) will move through the intracellular fluid away from the depolarized region and toward the more negative, resting regions of the membrane. Simultaneously, outside the cell, positive charge will move from the more positive region of the resting membrane toward the less positive regions the depolarization just created. Note that this local current moves positive charges toward the depolarization site along the outside of the membrane and away from the depolarization site along the inside of the membrane. Thus, it produces a decrease in the amount of charge separation in the membrane regions surrounding the open ion channel. In other words, depolarization spreads to adjacent areas along the membrane.

Depending upon the initiating event, graded potentials can occur in either a depolarizing or a hyperpolarizing direction (**Figure 6.16a**), and their magnitude is related to the magnitude of the initiating event (**Figure 6.15b**, **Figure 6.16b**).

In addition to the movement of ions on the inside and the outside of the cell, charge is lost across the membrane because the membrane is permeable to ions through open membrane channels. The result is that the change in membrane potential decreases as the distance increases from the initial site of the potential change (Figure 6.15b, **Figure 6.16c**). Current flows much like water flows through a leaky hose, decreasing just as water flow decreases the farther along the hose you are from the faucet. In fact, plasma membranes are so leaky to ions that these currents die out almost completely within a few millimeters of their point of origin. Because of this, local current is **decremental;** that is, the flow of charge decreases as the distance from the site of origin of the graded potential increases (**Figure 6.17**).

Because the electrical signal decreases with distance, graded potentials (and the local current they generate) can function as signals only over very short distances (a few millimeters). However, if additional stimuli occur before the graded potential has died away, these can add to the depolarization from the first stimulus. This process, termed **summation,** is particularly important for sensation, as Chapter 7 will discuss. Graded potentials are the only means of communication used by some neurons, whereas in other neurons, graded potentials initiate signals that travel longer distances, as described next.

Action Potentials

Action potentials are very different from graded potentials. They are large alterations in the membrane potential; the membrane potential may change by as much as 100 mV. For example, a cell might depolarize from −70 to +30 mV, and then repolarize to its resting potential. Action potentials are generally very rapid (as brief as 1–4 milliseconds) and may

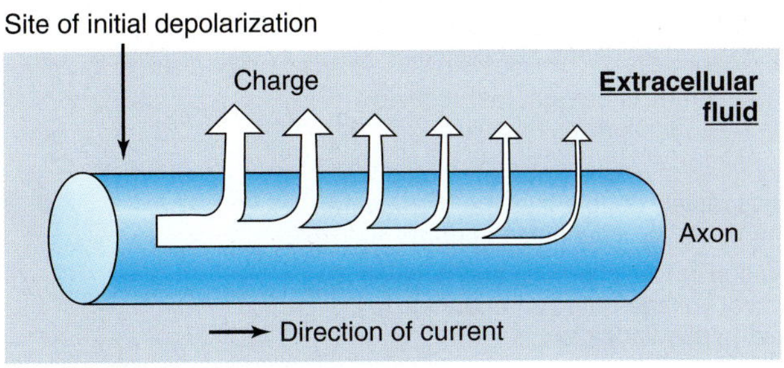

Figure 6.17 Leakage of charge (predominately potassium ions) across the plasma membrane reduces the local current at sites farther along the membrane from the site of initial depolarization.

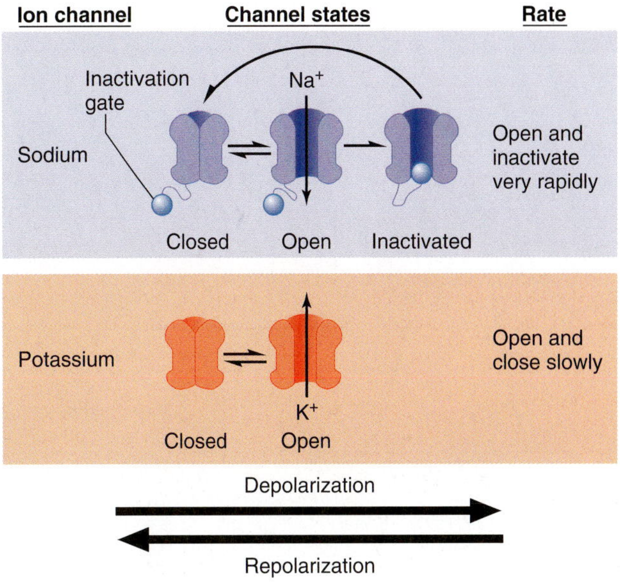

Figure 6.18 AP|R Behavior of voltage-gated Na^+ and K^+ channels. Depolarization of the membrane causes Na^+ channels to rapidly open, then undergo inactivation followed by the opening of K^+ channels. When the membrane repolarizes to negative voltages, both channels return to the closed state.

repeat at frequencies of several hundred per second. The propagation of action potentials down the axon is the mechanism the nervous system uses to communicate over long distances.

What properties of ion channels allow them to generate these large, rapid changes in membrane potential, and how are action potentials propagated along an excitable membrane? These questions are addressed in the following sections.

Voltage-Gated Ion Channels

As described in Chapter 4, there are many types of ion channels and several different mechanisms that regulate the opening of the different types. **Ligand-gated channels** open in response to the binding of signaling molecules (as shown in Figure 6.15), and **mechanically gated channels** open in response to physical deformation (stretching) of the plasma membranes. Whereas these types of channels often cause graded potentials that can serve as the initiating stimulus for an action potential, it is **voltage-gated channels** that give a membrane the ability to undergo action potentials. There are dozens of different types of voltage-gated ion channels, varying by which ion they conduct (for example, Na^+, K^+, Ca^{2+}, or Cl^-) and in how they behave as the membrane voltage changes. For now, we will focus on the particular types of Na^+ and K^+ channels that mediate most neuronal action potentials.

Figure 6.18 summarizes the relevant characteristics of these channels. Na^+ and K^+ channels are similar in having sequences of charged amino acid residues in their structure that make the channels reversibly change shape in response to changes in membrane potential. When the membrane is at a negative potential (for example, at the resting membrane potential), both types of channels tend to close, whereas membrane depolarization tends to open them. Two key differences, however, allow these channels to play different roles in the production of action potentials. First, Na^+ channels respond much faster to changes in membrane voltage. When an area of a membrane is suddenly depolarized, local Na^+ channels open before the K^+ channels do, and if the membrane is then repolarized to negative voltages, the K^+ channels are also slower to close. The second key difference is that Na^+ channels have an extra feature in their structure known as an **inactivation gate.** This structure, sometimes visualized as a "ball and chain," limits the flux of sodium ions by blocking the channel shortly after depolarization opens it. When the membrane repolarizes, the channel closes, forcing the inactivation gate back out of the pore and allowing the channel to return to the closed state. Integrating these channel properties with the basic principles governing membrane potentials, we can now explain how action potentials occur.

Action Potential Mechanism

In our previous coverage of resting membrane potential and graded potentials, we saw that the membrane potential depends upon the concentration gradients and membrane permeabilities of different ions, particularly Na^+ and K^+. This is true of the action potential as well. During an action potential, transient changes in membrane permeability allow sodium and potassium ions to move down their electrochemical gradients. **Figure 6.19** illustrates the steps that occur during an action potential.

In step 1 of the figure, the resting membrane potential is close to the K^+ equilibrium potential because there are more open K^+ channels than Na^+ channels. Note that these leak channels are distinct from the voltage-gated channels just described. An action potential begins with a depolarizing stimulus—for example, when a neurotransmitter binds to a specific ligand-gated ion channel and allows Na^+ to enter the cell (review Figure 6.15). This initial depolarization stimulates the opening of some voltage-gated Na^+ channels, and further entry of Na^+ through those channels adds to the local membrane depolarization. When the membrane reaches a critical **threshold potential** (step 2), depolarization becomes a **positive feedback** loop. Na^+ entry causes depolarization, which opens more voltage-gated Na^+ channels, which causes more depolarization, and so on. This process is represented as a rapid depolarization of the membrane potential (step 3), and it overshoots so that the membrane actually becomes positive

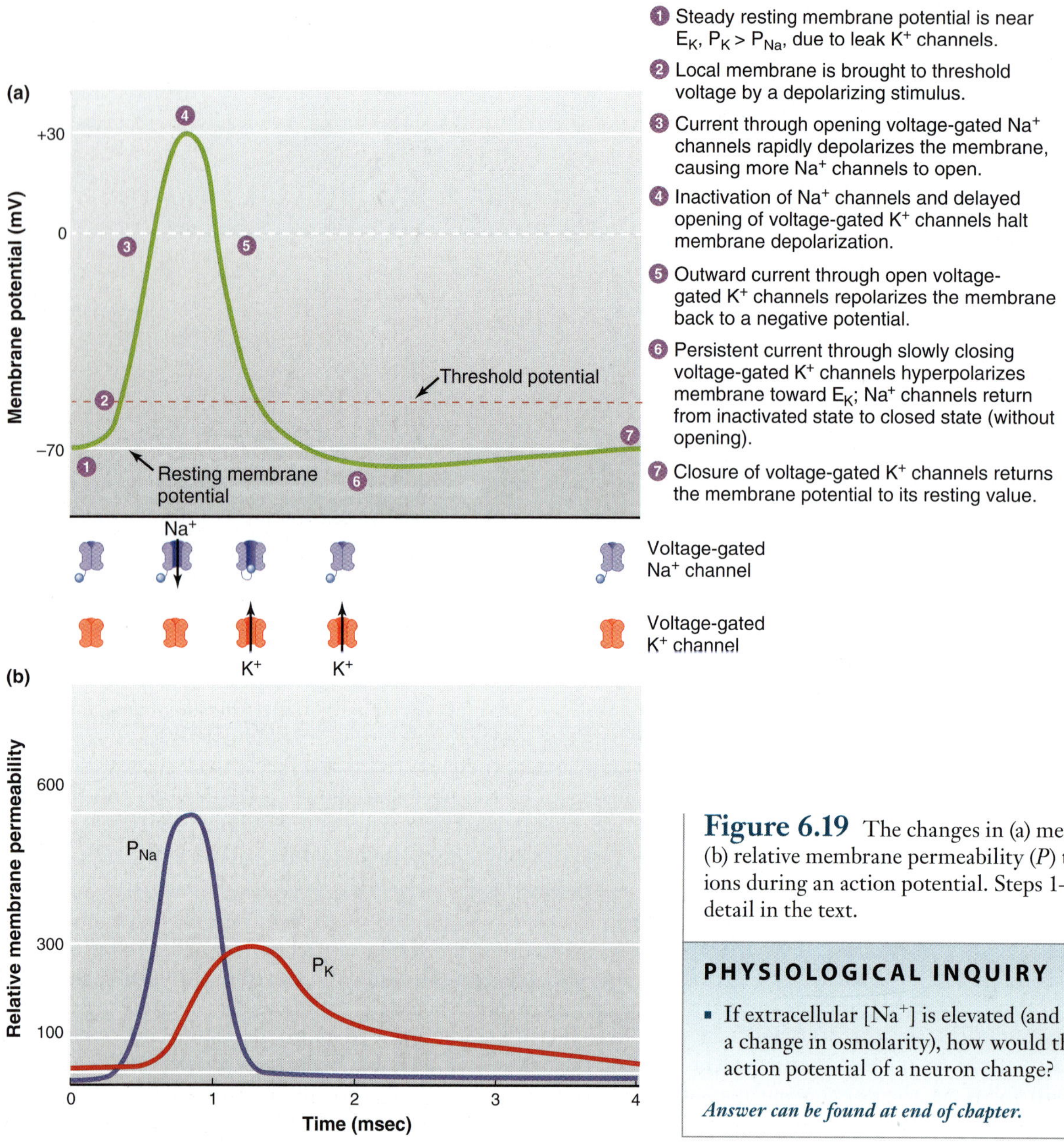

Figure 6.19 The changes in (a) membrane potential (mV) and (b) relative membrane permeability (*P*) to sodium and potassium ions during an action potential. Steps 1–7 are described in more detail in the text.

PHYSIOLOGICAL INQUIRY

- If extracellular $[Na^+]$ is elevated (and you ignore any effects of a change in osmolarity), how would the resting potential and action potential of a neuron change?

Answer can be found at end of chapter.

on the inside and negative on the outside. In this phase, the membrane approaches but does not quite reach the Na^+ equilibrium potential (+60 mV).

As the membrane potential approaches its peak value (step 4), the Na^+ permeability abruptly declines as inactivation gates break the cycle of positive feedback by blocking the open Na^+ channels. Meanwhile, the depolarized state of the membrane has begun to open the relatively sluggish voltage-gated K^+ channels, and the resulting elevated K^+ flux out of the cell rapidly repolarizes the membrane toward its resting value (step 5). The return of the membrane to a negative potential causes voltage-gated Na^+ channels to go from their inactivated state back to the closed state (without opening, as described earlier) and K^+ channels to also return to the closed state. Because voltage-gated K^+ channels close relatively slowly, immediately after an action potential there is a period when K^+ permeability remains above resting levels and the membrane is transiently hyperpolarized toward the K^+ equilibrium potential (step 6). This portion of the action potential is known as the **afterhyperpolarization.** Once the voltage-gated K^+ channels finally close, however, the resting membrane potential is restored (step 7). Whereas voltage-gated Na^+ channels operate in a positive feedback mode at the beginning of an action potential, voltage-gated K^+ channels bring the action potential to an end and induce their own closing through a **negative feedback** process (**Figure 6.20**).

You may think that large movements of ions across the membrane are required to produce such large changes in membrane potential. Actually, the number of ions that cross the membrane during an action potential is extremely small compared to the total number of ions in the cell, producing only infinitesimal changes in the intracellular ion concentrations. Yet, if this tiny number of additional ions crossing the membrane with repeated action potentials were not eventually moved back across the membrane, the concentration gradients of Na^+ and K^+ would gradually dissipate and action potentials

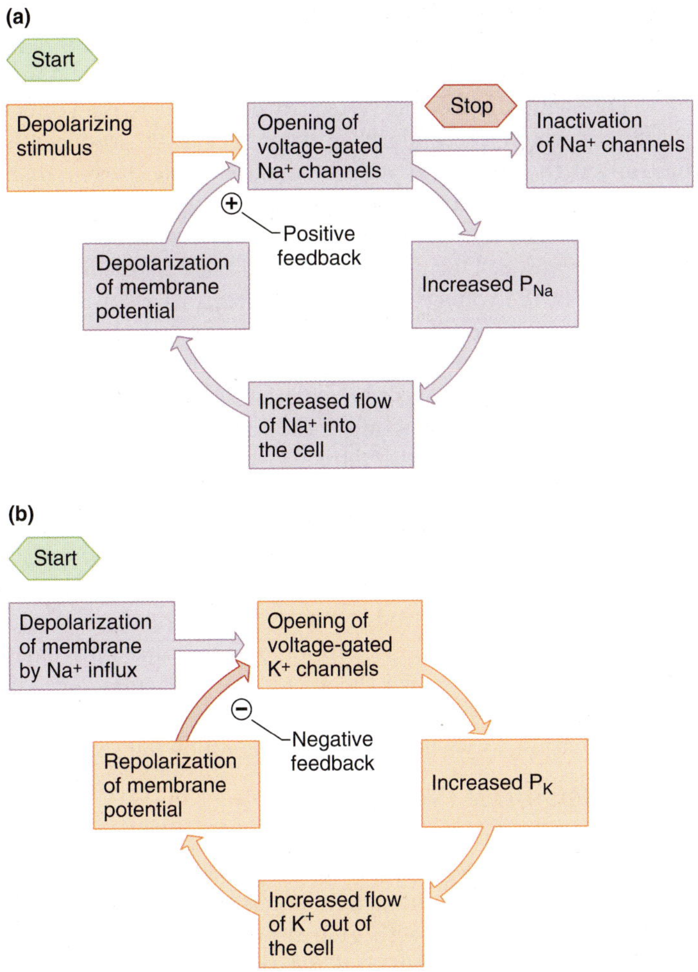

Figure 6.20 Feedback control in voltage-gated ion channels. (a) Na^+ channels exert positive feedback on membrane potential. (b) K^+ channels exert negative feedback.

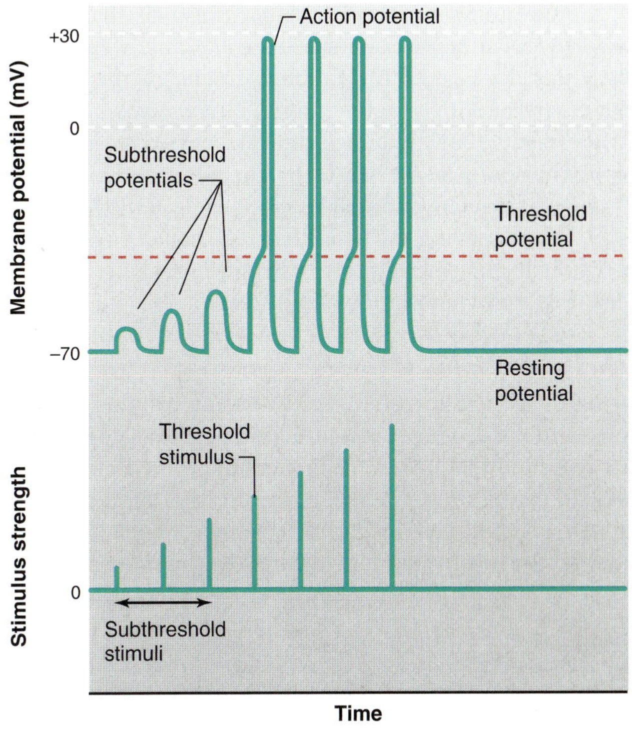

Figure 6.21 Changes in the membrane potential with increasing strength of excitatory stimuli. When the membrane potential reaches threshold, action potentials are generated. Increasing the stimulus strength above threshold level does not cause larger action potentials. (The afterhyperpolarization has been omitted from this figure for clarity, and the absolute value of threshold is not indicated because it varies from cell to cell.)

could no longer be generated. As may be expected, cellular accumulation of Na^+ and loss of K^+ are prevented by the continuous action of the membrane Na^+/K^+-ATPase pumps.

As explained previously, not all membrane depolarizations in excitable cells trigger the positive feedback process that leads to an action potential. Action potentials occur only when the initial stimulus plus the current through the Na^+ channels it opens are sufficient to elevate the membrane potential beyond the threshold potential. Stimuli that are just strong enough to depolarize the membrane to this level are **threshold stimuli** (**Figure 6.21**). The threshold of most excitable membranes is about 15 mV less negative than the resting membrane potential. Thus, if the resting potential of a neuron is −70 mV, the threshold potential may be −55 mV. At depolarizations less than threshold, the positive feedback cycle cannot get started. In such cases, the membrane will return to its resting level as soon as the stimulus is removed and no action potential will be generated. These weak depolarizations are called **subthreshold potentials,** and the stimuli that cause them are **subthreshold stimuli.**

Stimuli stronger than those required to reach threshold elicit action potentials, but as can be seen in Figure 6.21, the action potentials resulting from such stimuli have exactly the same amplitude as those caused by threshold stimuli. This is because once threshold is reached, membrane events are no longer dependent upon stimulus strength. Rather, the depolarization generates an action potential because the positive feedback cycle is operating. Action potentials either occur maximally or they do not occur at all. Another way of saying this is that action potentials are **all-or-none.**

The firing of a gun is a mechanical analogy that shows the principle of all-or-none behavior. The magnitude of the explosion and the velocity at which the bullet leaves the gun do not depend on how hard the trigger is squeezed. Either the trigger is pulled hard enough to fire the gun, or it is not; the gun cannot be fired halfway.

Because the amplitude of a single action potential does not vary in proportion to the amplitude of the stimulus, an action potential cannot convey information about the magnitude of the stimulus that initiated it. How then do you distinguish between a loud noise and a whisper, a light touch and a pinch? This information, as we will discuss later, depends upon the number and patterns of action potentials transmitted per unit of time (i.e., their frequency) and not upon their magnitude.

The generation of action potentials is prevented by ***local anesthetics*** such as ***procaine*** (***Novocaine***) and ***lidocaine*** (***Xylocaine***) because these drugs block voltage-gated Na^+ channels, preventing them from opening in response to depolarization. Without action potentials, graded signals generated in sensory neurons—in response to injury, for example—cannot reach the brain and give rise to the sensation of pain.

Some animals produce toxins (poisons) that work by interfering with nerve conduction in the same way that local anesthetics do. For example, some organs of the pufferfish produce an extremely potent toxin, ***tetrodotoxin,*** that binds to voltage-gated Na^+ channels and prevents the Na^+ component of the action potential. In Japan, chefs who prepare this delicacy are specially trained to completely remove the toxic organs before serving the pufferfish dish called fugu. Individuals who eat improperly prepared fugu may die, even if they ingest only a tiny quantity of tetrodotoxin.

Refractory Periods

During the action potential, a second stimulus, no matter how strong, will not produce a second action potential (**Figure 6.22**). That region of the membrane is then said to be in its **absolute refractory period.** This occurs during the period when the voltage-gated Na^+ channels are either already open or have proceeded to the inactivated state during the first action potential.

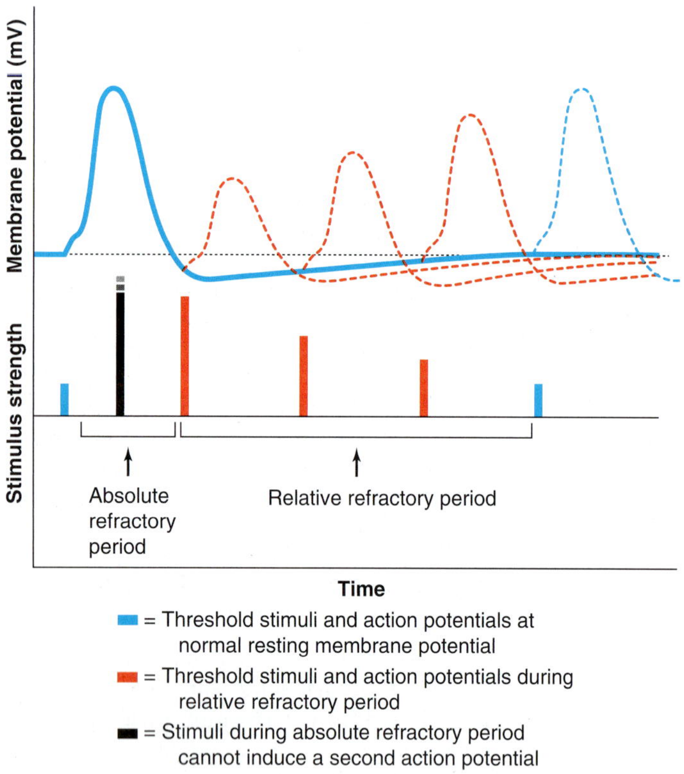

Figure 6.22 Absolute and relative refractory periods of the action potential determined by a paired-pulse protocol. After a threshold stimulus that results in an action potential (first stimulus and solid voltage trace), a second stimulus given at various times after the first can be used to determine refractory periods. All stimuli shown are of the minimum size needed to stimulate an action potential. During the absolute refractory period, a second stimulus (black), no matter how strong, will not produce a second action potential. In the relative refractory period (stimuli and action potentials shown in red), a second action potential can be triggered, but a larger stimulus is required to reach threshold, mainly because K^+ permeability is still above resting levels. Action potentials are reduced in size during the relative refractory period, due both to the inactivation of some Na^+ channels and the persistence of some open K^+ channels.

The inactivation gate that has blocked these channels must be removed by repolarizing the membrane and closing the pore before the channels can reopen to the second stimulus.

Following the absolute refractory period, there is an interval during which a second action potential can be produced—but only if the stimulus strength is considerably greater than usual. This is the **relative refractory period,** which can last 1 to 15 msec or longer and coincides roughly with the period of afterhyperpolarization. During the relative refractory period, some but not all of the voltage-gated Na^+ channels have returned to a resting state and some of the K^+ channels that repolarized the membrane are still open. From this relative refractory state, it is possible for a new stimulus to depolarize the membrane above the threshold potential, but only if the stimulus is large in magnitude or outlasts the relative refractory period.

The refractory periods limit the number of action potentials an excitable membrane can produce in a given period of time. Most neurons respond at frequencies of up to 100 action potentials per second, and some may produce much higher frequencies for brief periods. Refractory periods contribute to the separation of these action potentials so that individual electrical signals pass down the axon. The refractory periods also are the key in determining the direction of action potential propagation, as we will discuss in the following section.

Action Potential Propagation

The action potential can only travel the length of a neuron if each point along the membrane is depolarized to its threshold potential as the action potential moves down the axon (**Figure 6.23**). As with graded potentials (refer back to Figure 6.15a), the membrane is depolarized at each point along the way with respect to the adjacent portions of the membrane, which are still at the resting membrane potential. The difference between the potentials causes current to flow, and this local current depolarizes the adjacent membrane where it causes the voltage-gated Na^+ channels located there to open. The current entering during an action potential is sufficient to easily depolarize the adjacent membrane to the threshold potential.

The new action potential produces local currents of its own that depolarize the region adjacent to it (Figure 6.23b), producing yet another action potential at the next site, and so on, to cause **action potential propagation** along the length of the membrane. Thus, there is a sequential opening and closing of Na^+ and K^+ channels along the membrane. It is like lighting a trail of gunpowder—the action potential does not move, but it "sets off" a new action potential in the region of the axon just ahead of it. Because each regeneration of the action potential depends on the positive feedback cycle of a new group of Na^+ channels where the action potential is occurring, the action potential arriving at the end of the membrane is virtually identical in form to the initial one. Thus, action potentials do not decrease in magnitude with distance like graded potentials.

Because a membrane area that has just undergone an action potential is refractory and cannot immediately undergo another, the only direction of action potential propagation is away from a region of membrane that has recently been active. This is again similar to a burning trail of gunpowder—the fire can only spread in the forward direction where the gunpowder is fresh, and not backward where the gunpowder has already burned.

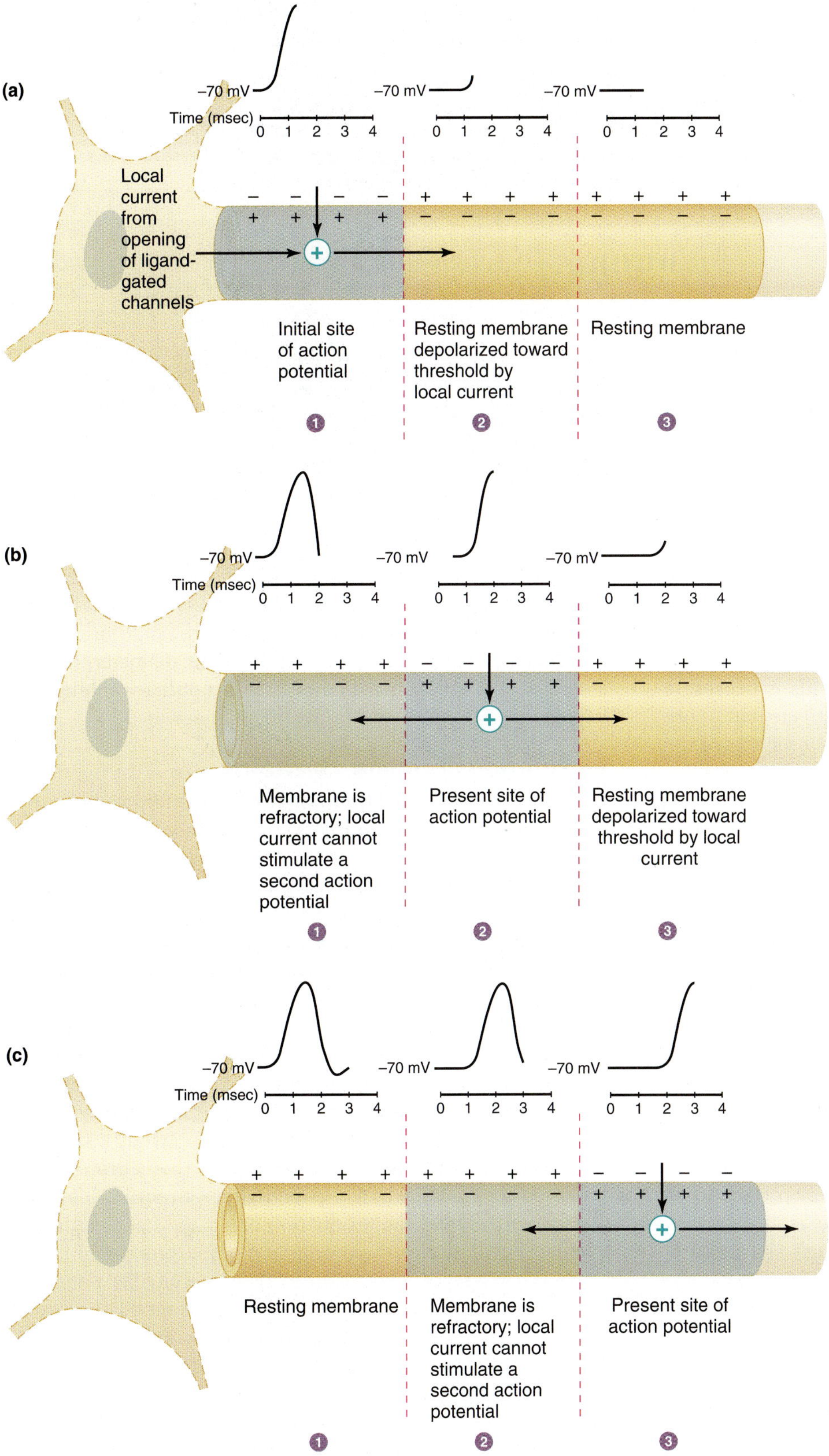

Figure 6.23 APIR One-way propagation of an action potential. For simplicity, potentials are shown only on the upper membrane, local currents are shown only on the inside of the membrane, and repolarizing currents are not shown. (a) Local current from the opening of ligand-gated ion channels in the cell body and dendrites causes an action potential to be initiated in region 1, and local current depolarizes region 2. (b) Action potential in region 2 generates local currents; region 3 is depolarized toward threshold, but region 1 is refractory. (c) Action potential in region 3 generates local currents, but region 2 is refractory.

PHYSIOLOGICAL INQUIRY

- Striking the ulnar nerve in your elbow against a hard surface (sometimes called "hitting your funny bone") initiates action potentials near the midpoint of sensory and motor axons traveling in that nerve. In which direction will those action potentials propagate?

Answer can be found at end of chapter.

If the membrane through which the action potential must travel is not refractory, excitable membranes can conduct action potentials in either direction, with the direction of propagation determined by the stimulus location. For example, the action potentials in skeletal muscle cells are initiated near the middle of the cells and propagate toward the two ends. In most neurons, however, action potentials are initiated at one end of the cell and propagate toward the other end, as shown in Figure 6.23. The propagation ceases when the action potential reaches the end of an axon.

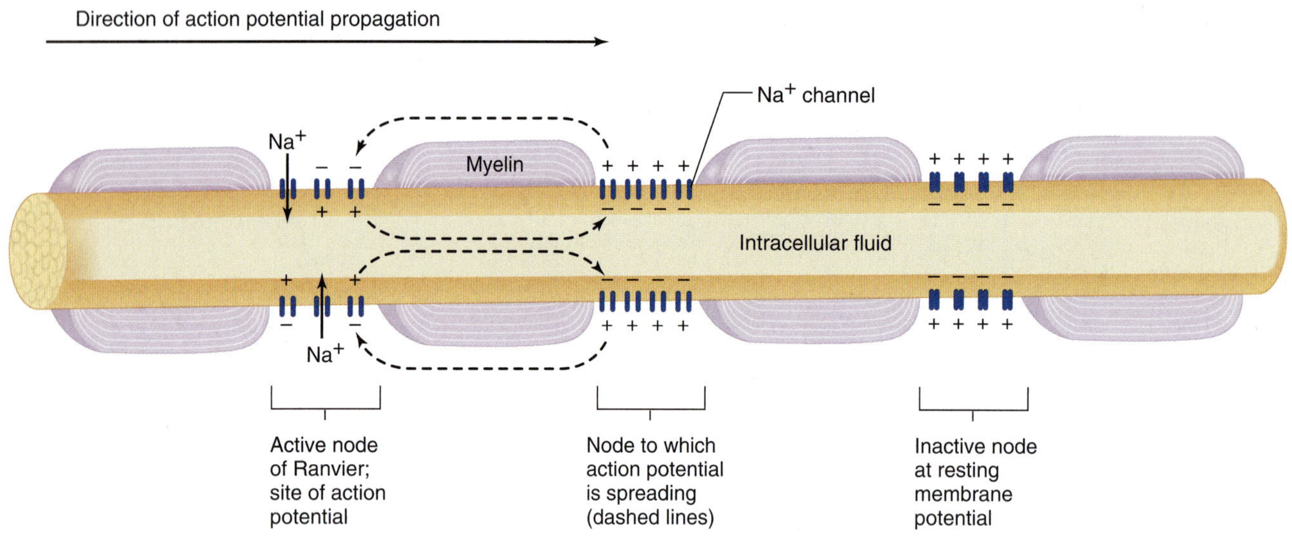

Figure 6.24 Myelinization and saltatory conduction of action potentials. K^+ channels are not depicted.

The velocity with which an action potential propagates along a membrane depends upon fiber diameter and whether or not the fiber is myelinated. The larger the fiber diameter, the faster the action potential propagates. This is because a large fiber offers less internal resistance to local current; more ions will flow in a given time, bringing adjacent regions of the membrane to threshold faster.

Myelin is an insulator that makes it more difficult for charge to flow between intracellular and extracellular fluid compartments. Because there is less "leakage" of charge across the myelin, a local current can spread farther along an axon. Moreover, the concentration of voltage-gated Na^+ channels in the myelinated region of axons is low. Therefore, action potentials occur only at the nodes of Ranvier, where the myelin coating is interrupted and the concentration of voltage-gated Na^+ channels is high (**Figure 6.24**). Action potentials appear to jump from one node to the next as they propagate along a myelinated fiber; for this reason, such propagation is called **saltatory conduction** (Latin, *saltare*, "to leap"). However, it is important to understand that an action potential does not, in fact, jump from region to region but rather is regenerated at each node.

Propagation via saltatory conduction is faster than propagation in nonmyelinated fibers of the same axon diameter. This is because less charge leaks out through the myelin-covered sections of the membrane, more charge arrives at the node adjacent to the active node, and an action potential is generated there sooner than if the myelin were not present. Moreover, because ions cross the membrane only at the nodes of Ranvier, the membrane pumps need to restore fewer ions. Myelinated axons are therefore metabolically more efficient than unmyelinated ones. Thus, myelin adds speed, reduces metabolic cost, and saves room in the nervous system because the axons can be thinner.

Conduction velocities range from about 0.5 m/sec (1 mi/h) for small-diameter, unmyelinated fibers to about 100 m/sec (225 mi/h) for large-diameter, myelinated fibers. At 0.5 m/sec, an action potential would travel the distance from the toe to the brain of an average-sized person in about 4 sec; at a velocity of 100 m/sec, it only takes about 0.02 sec. Perhaps you've dropped a heavy object on your toe and noticed that an immediate, sharp pain (carried by large-diameter, myelinated neurons) occurs before the onset of a dull, throbbing ache (transmitted along small, unmyelinated neurons).

Generation of Action Potentials

In our description of action potentials thus far, we have spoken of "stimuli" as the initiators of action potentials. These stimuli bring the membrane to the threshold potential, and voltage-gated Na^+ channels initiate the action potential. How is the threshold potential attained, and how do various types of neurons actually generate action potentials?

In afferent neurons, the initial depolarization to threshold is achieved by a graded potential—here called a **receptor potential.** Receptor potentials are generated in the sensory receptors at the peripheral ends of the neurons, which are at the ends farthest from the CNS. In all other neurons, the depolarization to threshold is due either to a graded potential generated by synaptic input to the neuron, known as a **synaptic potential,** or to a spontaneous change in the neuron's membrane potential, known as a **pacemaker potential.** The next section will address the production of synaptic potentials, and Chapter 7 will discuss the production of receptor potentials.

Triggering of action potentials by pacemaker potentials is an inherent property of certain neurons (and other excitable cells, including certain smooth muscle and cardiac muscle cells). In these cells, the activity of different types of ion channels in the plasma membrane causes a graded depolarization of the membrane—the pacemaker potential. If threshold is reached, an action potential occurs; the membrane then repolarizes and again begins to depolarize. There is no stable, resting membrane potential in such cells because of the continuous change in membrane permeability. The rate at which the membrane depolarizes to threshold determines the action potential frequency. Pacemaker potentials are implicated in many rhythmic behaviors, such as breathing, the heartbeat, and movements within the walls of the stomach and intestines.

TABLE 6.4 Differences Between Graded Potentials and Action Potentials

Graded Potential	Action Potential
Amplitude varies with size of the initiating event.	All-or-none. Once membrane is depolarized to threshold, amplitude is independent of the size of the initiating event.
Can be summed.	Cannot be summed.
Has no threshold.	Has a threshold that is usually about 15 mV depolarized relative to the resting potential.
Has no refractory period.	Has a refractory period.
Amplitude decreases with distance.	Is conducted without decrement; the depolarization is amplified to a constant value at each point along the membrane.
Duration varies with initiating conditions.	Duration is constant for a given cell type under constant conditions.
Can be a depolarization or a hyperpolarization.	Is only a depolarization.
Initiated by environmental stimulus (receptor), by neurotransmitter (synapse), or spontaneously.	Initiated by a graded potential.
Mechanism depends on ligand-gated channels or other chemical or physical changes.	Mechanism depends on voltage-gated channels.

Because of the effects of graded changes in membrane potential on action potential generation, a review of graded and action potentials is recommended. The differences between graded potentials and action potentials are listed in **Table 6.4**.

SECTION B SUMMARY

Basic Principles of Electricity

I. Separated electrical charges create the potential to do work, as occurs when charged particles produce an electrical current as they flow down a potential gradient. The lipid barrier of the plasma membrane is a high-resistance insulator that keeps charged ions separated, whereas ionic current flows readily in the aqueous intracellular and extracellular fluids.

The Resting Membrane Potential

I. Membrane potentials are generated mainly by the diffusion of ions and are determined by both the ionic concentration differences across the membrane and the membrane's relative permeability to different ions.
   a. Plasma membrane Na^+/K^+-ATPase pumps maintain low intracellular Na^+ concentration and high intracellular K^+ concentration.
   b. In almost all resting cells, the plasma membrane is much more permeable to K^+ than to Na^+, so the membrane potential is close to the K^+ equilibrium potential—that is, the inside is negative relative to the outside.
   c. The Na^+/K^+-ATPase pumps directly contribute a small component of the potential because they are electrogenic.

Graded Potentials and Action Potentials

I. Neurons signal information by graded potentials and action potentials (APs).

II. Graded potentials are local potentials whose magnitude can vary and that die out within 1 or 2 mm of their site of origin.

III. An AP is a rapid change in the membrane potential during which the membrane rapidly depolarizes and repolarizes. At the peak, the potential reverses and the membrane becomes positive inside. APs provide long-distance transmission of information through the nervous system.
   a. APs occur in excitable membranes because these membranes contain many voltage-gated Na^+ channels. These channels open as the membrane depolarizes, causing a positive feedback opening of more voltage-gated Na^+ channels and moving the membrane potential toward the Na^+ equilibrium potential.
   b. The AP ends as the Na^+ channels inactivate and K^+ channels open, restoring resting conditions.
   c. Depolarization of excitable membranes triggers an AP only when the membrane potential exceeds a threshold potential.
   d. Regardless of the size of the stimulus, if the membrane reaches threshold, the AP generated is the same size.
   e. A membrane is refractory for a brief time following an AP.
   f. APs are propagated without any change in size from one site to another along a membrane.
   g. In myelinated nerve fibers, APs are regenerated at the nodes of Ranvier in saltatory conduction.
   h. APs can be triggered by depolarizing graded potentials in sensory neurons, at synapses, or in some cells by pacemaker potentials.

SECTION B REVIEW QUESTIONS

1. Describe how negative and positive charges interact.
2. Contrast the abilities of intracellular and extracellular fluids and membrane lipids to conduct electrical current.
3. Draw a simple cell; indicate where the concentrations of Na^+, K^+, and Cl^- are high and low and the electrical potential difference across the membrane when the cell is at rest.
4. Explain the conditions that give rise to the resting membrane potential. What effect does membrane permeability have on this potential? What role do Na^+/K^+-ATPase membrane pumps play in the membrane potential? Is this role direct or indirect?
5. Which two factors involving ion diffusion determine the magnitude of the resting membrane potential?
6. Explain why the resting membrane potential is not equal to the K^+ equilibrium potential.
7. Draw a graded potential and an action potential on a graph of membrane potential versus time. Indicate zero membrane potential, resting membrane potential, and threshold potential; indicate when the membrane is depolarized, repolarizing, and hyperpolarized.
8. List the differences between graded potentials and action potentials.
9. Describe how ion movement generates the action potential.
10. What determines the activity of the voltage-gated Na^+ channel?
11. Explain threshold and the relative and absolute refractory periods in terms of the ionic basis of the action potential.
12. Describe the propagation of an action potential. Contrast this event in myelinated and unmyelinated axons.
13. List three ways in which action potentials can be initiated in neurons.

SECTION B KEY TERMS

absolute refractory period 156
action potential 152
action potential propagation 156
afterhyperpolarization 154
all-or-none 155
current 145
decremental 152
depolarized 151
electrical potential 145
electrogenic pump 149
equilibrium potential 147
excitability 150
excitable membrane 150
Goldman-Hodgkin-Katz (GHK) equation 148
graded potential 151
hyperpolarized 151
inactivation gate 153
leak K^+ channels 149
ligand-gated channels 153
mechanically gated channels 153
negative feedback 154
Nernst equation 148
Ohm's law 145
overshoot 151
pacemaker potential 158
positive feedback 153
potential 145
potential difference 145
receptor potential 158
relative refractory period 156
repolarizing 151
resistance 145
resting membrane potential 146
saltatory conduction 158
subthreshold potential 155
subthreshold stimulus 155
summation 152
synaptic potential 158
threshold potential 153
threshold stimulus 155
voltage-gated channels 153

SECTION B CLINICAL TERMS

lidocaine (Xylocaine) 155
local anesthetics 155
procaine (Novocaine) 155
tetrodotoxin 156

SECTION C

Synapses

As defined earlier, a synapse is an anatomically specialized junction between two neurons, at which the electrical activity in a presynaptic neuron influences the electrical activity of a postsynaptic neuron. Anatomically, synapses include parts of the presynaptic and postsynaptic neurons and the extracellular space between these two cells. According to recent estimates, there are more than 10^{14} (100 trillion!) synapses in the CNS.

Activity at synapses can increase or decrease the likelihood that the postsynaptic neuron will fire action potentials by producing a brief, graded potential in the postsynaptic membrane. The membrane potential of a postsynaptic neuron is brought closer to threshold (depolarized) at an **excitatory synapse,** and it is either driven farther from threshold (hyperpolarized) or stabilized at its resting potential at an **inhibitory synapse.**

Hundreds or thousands of synapses from many different presynaptic cells can affect a single postsynaptic cell (**convergence**), and a single presynaptic cell can send branches to affect many other postsynaptic cells (**divergence, Figure 6.25**). Convergence allows information from many sources to influence a cell's activity; divergence allows one cell to affect multiple pathways.

The level of excitability of a postsynaptic cell at any moment (i.e., how close its membrane potential is to threshold) depends on the number of synapses active at any one time and the number that are excitatory or inhibitory. If the membrane of the postsynaptic neuron reaches threshold, it will generate action potentials that are propagated along its axon to the terminal branches, which in turn influence the excitability of other cells.

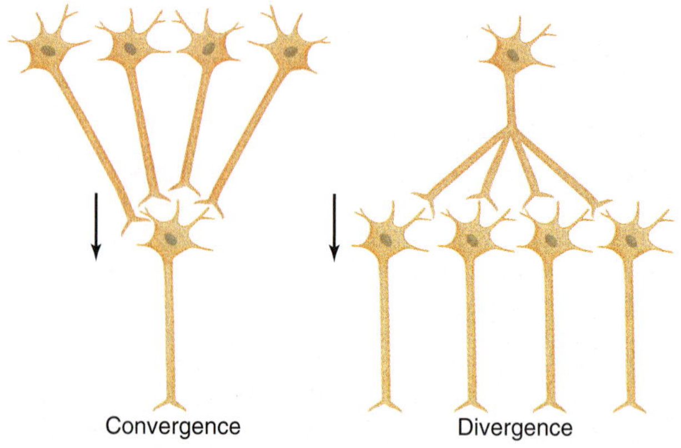

Figure 6.25 Convergence of neural input from many neurons onto a single neuron, and divergence of output from a single neuron onto many others. Arrows indicate the direction of transmission of neural activity.

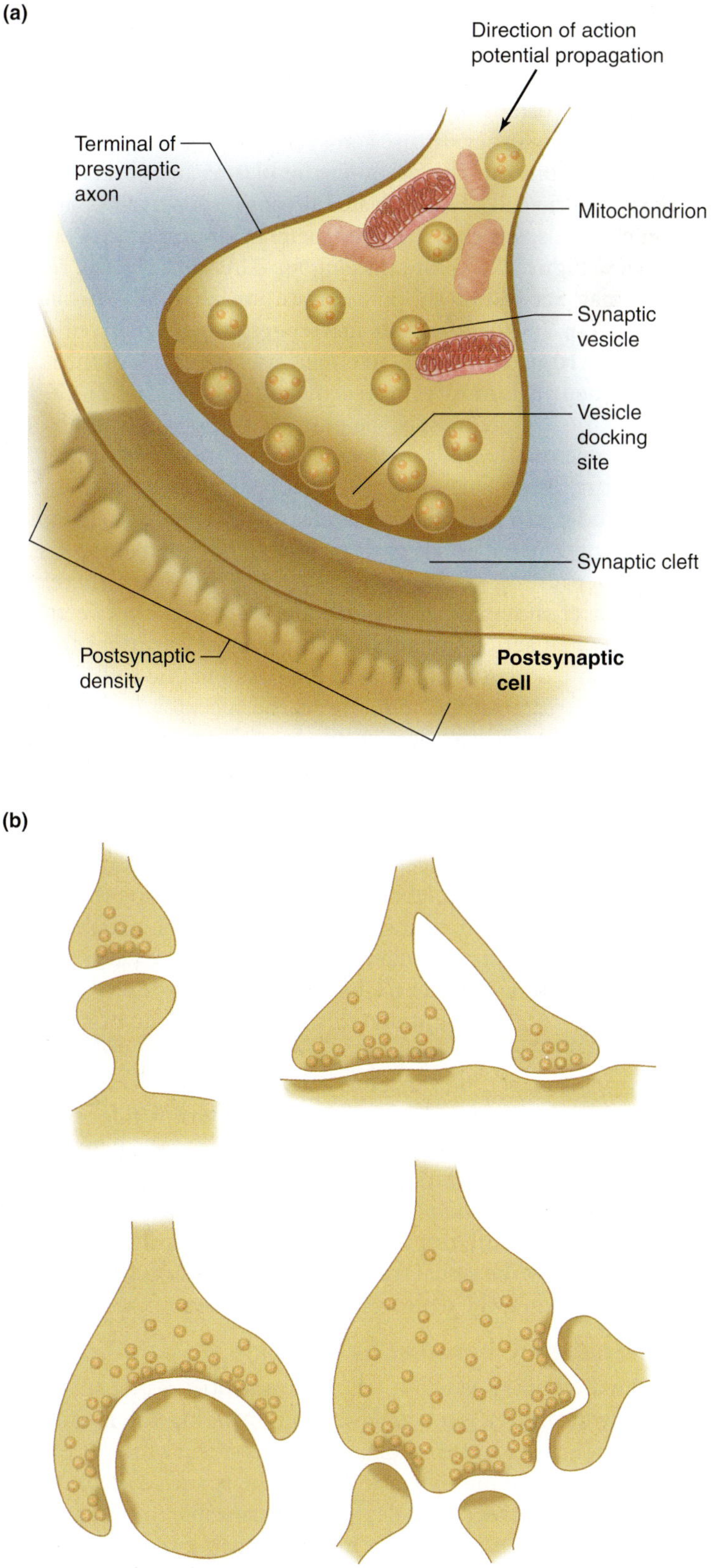

Figure 6.26 APIR (a) Diagram of a chemical synapse. Some vesicles are docked at the presynaptic membrane, ready for release. The postsynaptic membrane is distinguished microscopically by the postsynaptic density, which contains proteins associated with the receptors. (b) Synapses appear in many forms, as demonstrated here. The presynaptic terminals all contain synaptic vesicles. Redrawn from Walmsley et al.

6.8 Functional Anatomy of Synapses

There are two types of synapses: electrical and chemical. At **electrical synapses,** the plasma membranes of the presynaptic and postsynaptic cells are joined by gap junctions (Chapter 3). These allow the local currents resulting from arriving action potentials to flow directly across the junction through the connecting channels from one neuron to the other. This depolarizes the membrane of the second neuron to threshold, continuing the propagation of the action potential. Communication between cells via electrical synapses is extremely rapid. Until recently, it was thought that electrical synapses were rare in the adult mammalian nervous system. However, they have now been described in widespread locations, and neuroscientists suspect they may play important roles. Among the possible functions are synchronization of electrical activity of neurons clustered in local CNS networks and communication between glial cells and neurons. Multiple isoforms of gap-junction proteins have been described, and the conductance of some of these is modulated by factors such as membrane voltage, intracellular pH, and Ca^{2+} concentration. More research will be required to gain a complete understanding of this modulation and all of the complex roles of electrical synapses in the nervous system. Their function is better understood in cardiac and smooth muscle tissues, where they are also numerous (see Chapter 9).

Figure 6.26a shows the basic structure of a typical **chemical synapse.** The axon of the presynaptic neuron ends in a slight swelling, the axon terminal, which holds the **synaptic vesicles** that contain neurotransmitter molecules. The postsynaptic membrane adjacent to the axon terminal has a high density of membrane proteins that make up a specialized area called the **postsynaptic density.** Note that in actuality the size and shape of the presynaptic and postsynaptic elements can vary greatly (**Figure 6.26b**). A 10 to 20 nm extracellular space, the **synaptic cleft,** separates the presynaptic and postsynaptic neurons and prevents *direct* propagation of the current from the presynaptic neuron to the postsynaptic cell. Instead, signals are transmitted across the synaptic cleft by means of a chemical messenger—a neurotransmitter—released from the presynaptic axon terminal. Sometimes more than one neurotransmitter may be simultaneously released from an axon, in which case the additional neurotransmitter is called a **cotransmitter.** These neurotransmitters have different receptors on the postsynaptic cell.

6.9 Mechanisms of Neurotransmitter Release

As indicated in **Figure 6.27,** neurotransmitters are stored in small vesicles with lipid bilayer membranes. Prior to activation, many vesicles are docked on the presynaptic membrane at release regions known as **active zones,** whereas others are dispersed within the terminal. Neurotransmitter release is initiated when an action potential reaches the presynaptic terminal membrane. A key feature of neuron terminals is that in addition to the Na^+ and K^+ channels found elsewhere in the neuron, they also possess voltage-gated Ca^{2+} channels. Depolarization during the action potential opens these Ca^{2+} channels, and because the electrochemical gradient favors Ca^{2+} influx, Ca^{2+} flows into the axon terminal.

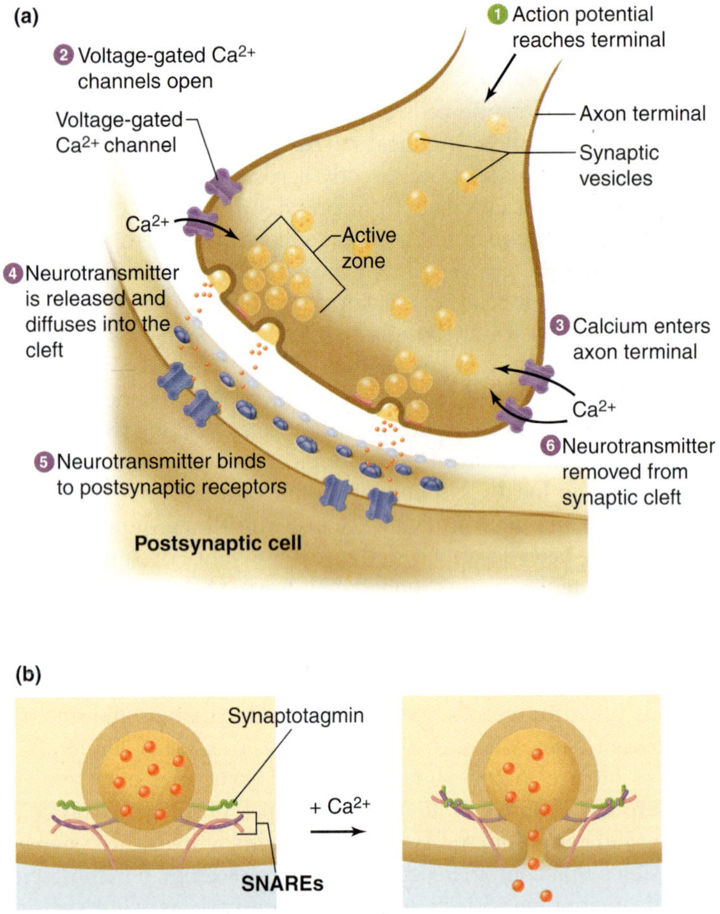

Figure 6.27 APR (a) Mechanisms of signaling at a chemical synapse. (b) Magnified view showing details of neurotransmitter release. Calcium ions trigger synaptotagmin and SNARE proteins to induce membrane fusion and neurotransmitter release. (SNARE = Soluble *N*-ethylmaleimide-sensitive factor attachment protein receptor)

Calcium ions activate processes that lead to the fusion of docked vesicles with the synaptic terminal membrane (**Figure 6.27b**). Prior to the arrival of an action potential, vesicles are loosely docked in the active zones by the interaction of a group of proteins, some of which are anchored in the vesicle membrane and others that are found in the membrane of the terminal. These are collectively known as **SNARE proteins** (soluble *N*-ethylmaleimide-sensitive factor attachment protein receptors). Calcium ions entering during depolarization bind to a separate family of proteins associated with the vesicle, **synaptotagmins,** triggering a conformational change in the SNARE complex that leads to membrane fusion and neurotransmitter release. After fusion, vesicles can undergo at least two possible fates. At some synapses, vesicles completely fuse with the membrane and are later recycled by endocytosis from the membrane at sites outside the active zone (see Figure 4.21). At other synapses, especially those at which action potential firing frequencies are high, vesicles may fuse only briefly while they release their contents and then reseal the pore and withdraw back into the nerve terminal (a mechanism called "kiss-and-run fusion").

6.10 Activation of the Postsynaptic Cell

Once neurotransmitters are released from the presynaptic axon terminal, they diffuse across the cleft. A fraction of these molecules bind to receptors on the plasma membrane of the postsynaptic cell. The activated receptors themselves may be ion channels, which designates them as **ionotropic receptors** (review Figure 6.15a for an example). Alternatively, the receptors may act indirectly on separate ion channels through a G protein and/or a second messenger, a type referred to as **metabotropic receptors.** In either case, the result of the binding of neurotransmitter to receptor is the opening or closing of specific ion channels in the postsynaptic plasma membrane, which eventually leads to changes in the membrane potential in that neuron. These channels belong, therefore, to the class of ligand-gated channels controlled by receptors, as discussed in Chapter 5, and are distinct from voltage-gated channels.

Because of the sequence of events involved, there is a very brief **synaptic delay**—about 0.2 msec—between the arrival of an action potential at a presynaptic terminal and the membrane potential changes in the postsynaptic cell.

Neurotransmitter binding to the receptor is a transient and reversible, noncovalent event. As with any binding site, the bound ligand—in this case, the neurotransmitter—is in equilibrium with the unbound form. Thus, if the concentration of unbound neurotransmitter in the synaptic cleft decreases, the number of occupied receptors will decrease. The ion channels in the postsynaptic membrane return to their resting state when the neurotransmitters are no longer bound. Unbound neurotransmitters are removed from the synaptic cleft when they (1) are actively transported back into the presynaptic axon terminal (in a process called **reuptake**) or, in some cases, into nearby glial cells; (2) diffuse away from the receptor site; or (3) are enzymatically transformed into inactive substances, some of which are transported back into the presynaptic axon terminal for reuse.

The two kinds of chemical synapses—excitatory and inhibitory—are differentiated by the effects of the neurotransmitter on the postsynaptic cell. Whether the effect is excitatory or inhibitory depends on the type of ion channel influenced by the signal transduction mechanism brought into operation when the neurotransmitter binds to its receptor.

Excitatory Chemical Synapses

At an excitatory synapse, the postsynaptic response to the neurotransmitter is a depolarization, bringing the membrane potential closer to threshold. The usual effect of the activated receptor on the postsynaptic membrane at such synapses is to open nonselective channels that are permeable to Na^+ and K^+. These ions then are free to move according to the electrical and chemical gradients across the membrane.

Both electrical and concentration gradients drive Na^+ into the cell, whereas for K^+, the electrical gradient opposes the concentration gradient (review Figure 6.12). Opening channels that are permeable to both ions therefore results in the simultaneous movement of a relatively small number of potassium ions out of the cell and a larger number of sodium ions into the cell. Thus, the *net* movement of positive ions is into the postsynaptic cell, causing a slight depolarization. This membrane potential

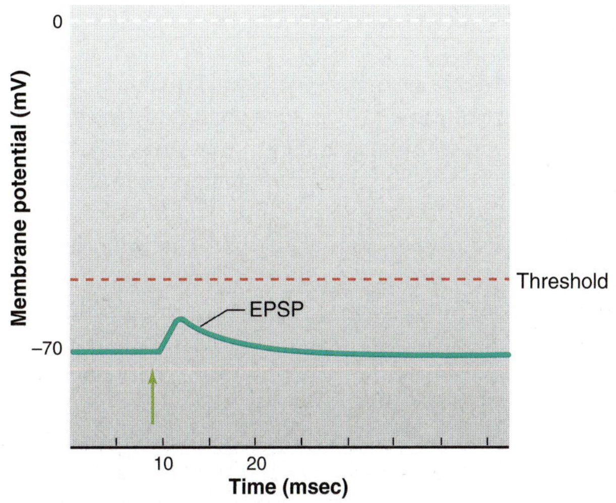

Figure 6.28 Excitatory postsynaptic potential (EPSP). Stimulation of the presynaptic neuron is marked by the green arrow. (Drawn larger than normal; typical EPSP = 0.5 mV)

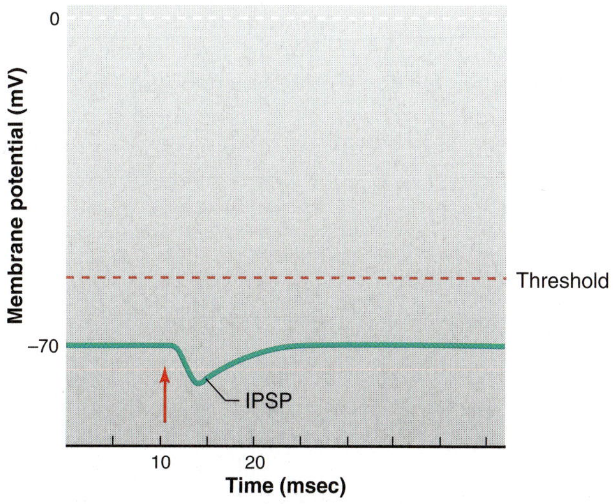

Figure 6.29 Inhibitory postsynaptic potential (IPSP). Stimulation of the presynaptic neuron is marked by the red arrow. (This hyperpolarization is drawn larger than a typical IPSP.)

change is called an **excitatory postsynaptic potential (EPSP, Figure 6.28)**. The EPSP is a graded potential that decreases in magnitude as it spreads away from the synapse by local current. Its only function is to bring the membrane potential of the postsynaptic neuron closer to threshold.

Inhibitory Chemical Synapses

At inhibitory synapses, the potential change in the postsynaptic neuron is generally a hyperpolarizing graded potential called an **inhibitory postsynaptic potential (IPSP, Figure 6.29)**. Alternatively, there may be no IPSP but rather *stabilization* of the membrane potential at its existing value. In either case, activation of an inhibitory synapse lessens the likelihood that the postsynaptic cell will depolarize to threshold and generate an action potential.

At an inhibitory synapse, the activated receptors on the postsynaptic membrane open Cl^- or K^+ channels; Na^+ permeability is not affected. In those cells that actively regulate intracellular Cl^- concentrations via active transport out of the cell, the Cl^- equilibrium potential is more negative than the resting potential. Therefore, as Cl^- channels open, Cl^- enters the cell, producing a hyperpolarization—that is, an IPSP. In cells that do not actively transport Cl^-, the equilibrium potential for Cl^- is equal to the resting membrane potential. Therefore, an increase in Cl^- permeability does not change the membrane potential but is able to increase chloride's influence on the membrane potential. This makes it more difficult for excitatory inputs from other synapses to change the potential when these chloride channels are simultaneously open (**Figure 6.30**). Increased K^+ permeability, when it occurs in the postsynaptic cell, also produces an IPSP. Earlier, we noted that if a cell membrane were permeable only to potassium ions, the resting membrane potential would equal the K^+ equilibrium potential; that is, the resting membrane potential would be about −90 mV instead of −70 mV. Thus, with increased K^+ permeability, more potassium ions leave the cell and the membrane moves closer to the K^+ equilibrium potential, causing a hyperpolarization.

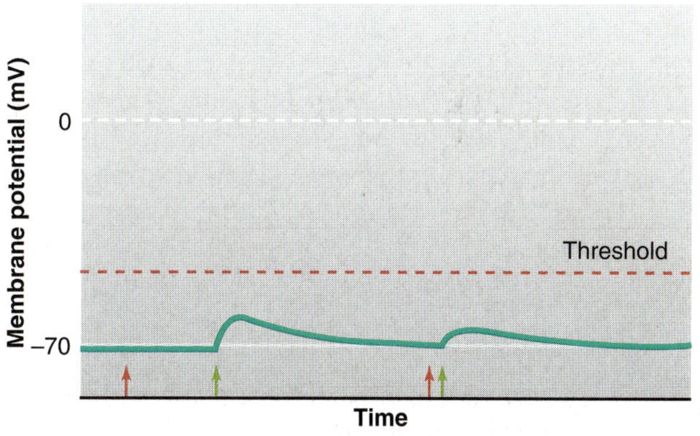

Figure 6.30 Synaptic inhibition of postsynaptic cells where E_{Cl} is equal to the resting membrane potential. Stimulation of a presynaptic neuron releasing a neurotransmitter that opens chloride channels (red arrows) has no direct effect on the postsynaptic membrane potential. However, when an excitatory synapse is simultaneously activated (green arrows), chloride movement into the cell diminishes the EPSP.

6.11 Synaptic Integration

In most neurons, one excitatory synaptic event by itself is not enough to reach threshold in the postsynaptic neuron. For example, a single EPSP may be only 0.5 mV, whereas changes of about 15 mV are necessary to depolarize the neuron's membrane to threshold. This being the case, an action potential can be initiated only by the combined effects of many excitatory synapses.

Of the thousands of synapses on any one neuron, probably hundreds are active simultaneously or close enough in time that the effects can add together. The membrane potential of the postsynaptic neuron at any moment is, therefore, the result of all the synaptic activity affecting it at that moment. A depolarization of the membrane toward threshold occurs when excitatory synaptic input predominates, and either a hyperpolarization or stabilization occurs when inhibitory input predominates.

A simple experiment can demonstrate how EPSPs and IPSPs interact, as shown in **Figure 6.31**. Assume there are three synaptic inputs to the postsynaptic cell. The synapses from axons A and B are excitatory, and the synapse from axon C is inhibitory. There are laboratory stimulators on axons A, B, and C so that each can be activated individually. An electrode is placed in the cell body of the postsynaptic neuron that will record the membrane potential. In part 1 of the experiment, we will test the interaction of two EPSPs by stimulating axon A and then, after a short time, stimulating it again. Part 1 of Figure 6.31 shows that no interaction occurs between the two EPSPs. The reason is that the change in membrane potential associated with an EPSP is fairly short-lived. Within a few milliseconds (by the time we stimulate axon A for the second time), the postsynaptic cell has returned to its resting condition.

In part 2, we stimulate axon A for the second time before the first EPSP has died away; the second synaptic potential adds to the previous one and creates a greater depolarization than from one input alone. This is called **temporal summation** because the input signals arrive from the same presynaptic cell at different *times*. The potentials summate because there are a greater number of open ion channels and, therefore, a greater flow of positive ions into the cell. In part 3 of Figure 6.31, axon B is first stimulated alone to determine its response, and then axons A and B are stimulated simultaneously. The EPSPs resulting from input from the two separate neurons also summate in the postsynaptic neuron, resulting in a greater degree of depolarization. Although it clearly is necessary that stimulation of A and B occur closely in time for summation to occur, this is called **spatial summation** because the two inputs occurred at different *locations* on the cell. The interaction of multiple EPSPs through spatial and temporal summation can increase the inward flow of positive ions and bring the postsynaptic membrane to threshold so that action potentials are initiated (see part 4 of Figure 6.31).

So far, we have tested only the patterns of interaction of excitatory synapses. Because EPSPs and IPSPs are due to oppositely directed local currents, they tend to cancel each other, and there is little or no net change in membrane potential when both A and C are stimulated (see Figure 6.31, part 5). Inhibitory potentials can also show spatial and temporal summation.

Depending on the postsynaptic membrane's resistance and on the amount of charge moving through the ligand-gated channels, the synaptic potential will spread to a greater or lesser degree across the plasma membrane of the cell. The membrane of a large area of the cell becomes slightly depolarized during activation of an excitatory synapse and slightly hyperpolarized or stabilized during activation of an inhibitory synapse, although these graded potentials will decrease with distance from the synaptic junction (**Figure 6.32**). Inputs from more than one synapse can result in summation of the synaptic potentials, which may then trigger an action potential.

In the previous examples, we referred to the threshold of the postsynaptic neuron as though it were the same for all parts of the cell. However, different parts of the neuron have different thresholds. In general, the initial segment has a more negative threshold (i.e., much closer to the resting potential) than the membrane of the cell body and dendrites. This is due to a higher density of voltage-gated Na^+ channels in this area of the membrane. Therefore, the initial segment is most responsive to small changes in the membrane potential that occur in response to synaptic potentials on the cell body and dendrites. The initial segment reaches threshold whenever enough EPSPs summate. The resulting action potential is then propagated from this point down the axon.

The fact that the initial segment usually has the lowest threshold explains why the locations of individual synapses on the postsynaptic cell are important. A synapse located near the initial segment will produce a greater voltage change in the initial segment than will a synapse on the outermost branch of a

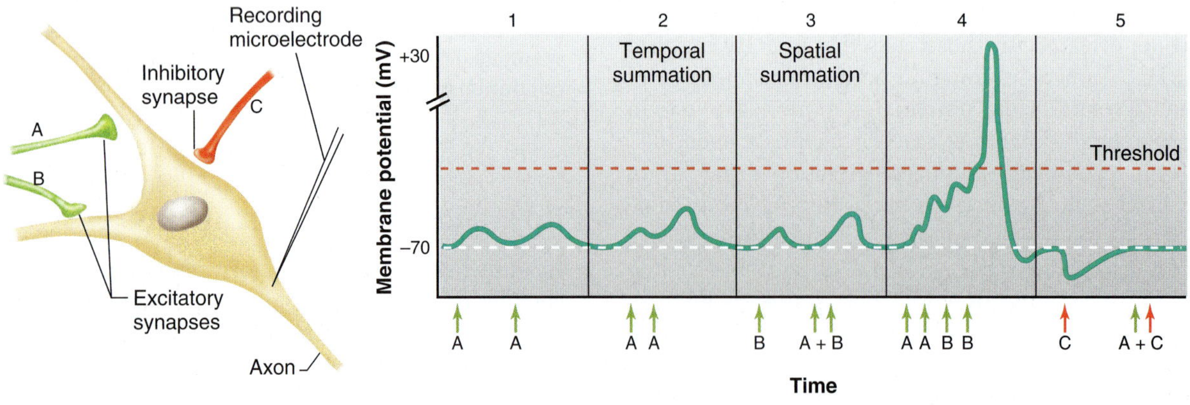

Figure 6.31 Interaction of EPSPs and IPSPs at the postsynaptic neuron. Presynaptic neurons (A–C) were stimulated at times indicated by the arrows, and the resulting membrane potential was recorded in the postsynaptic cell by a recording microelectrode.

PHYSIOLOGICAL INQUIRY

- How might the traces in panel 5 be different if the excitatory synapse (A) was much closer to the initial segment than the inhibitory synapse (C)?

Answer can be found at end of chapter.

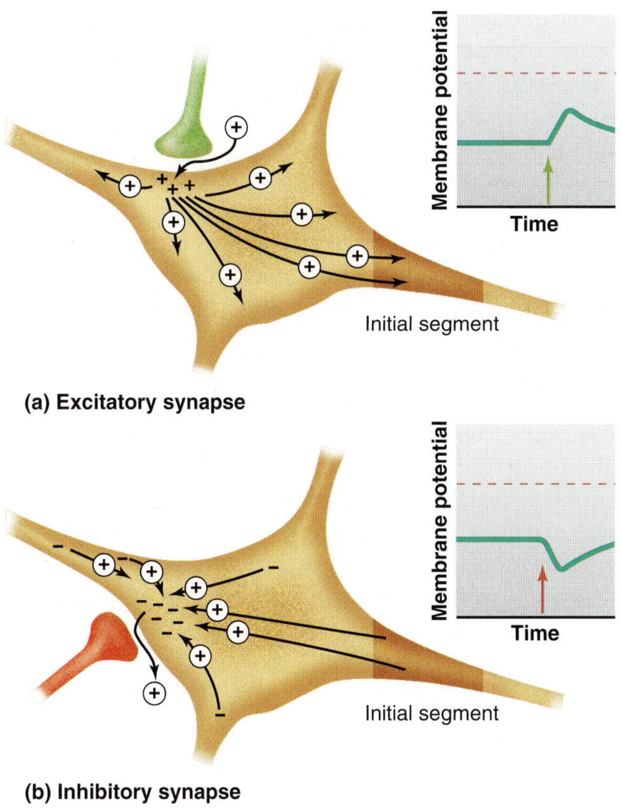

Figure 6.32 Comparison of excitatory and inhibitory synapses, showing current direction through the postsynaptic cell following synaptic activation. (a) Current through the postsynaptic cell is away from the excitatory synapse and may depolarize the initial segment. (b) Current through the postsynaptic cell is toward the inhibitory synapse and may hyperpolarize the initial segment. The arrow on the graph indicates moment of stimulus.

dendrite because it will expose the initial segment to a larger local current. In some neurons, however, signals from dendrites distant from the initial segment may be boosted by the presence of some voltage-gated Na^+ channels in parts of those dendrites.

Postsynaptic potentials last much longer than action potentials. In the event that cumulative EPSPs cause the initial segment to still be depolarized to threshold after an action potential has been fired and the refractory period is over, a second action potential will occur. In fact, as long as the membrane is depolarized to threshold, action potentials will continue to arise. Neuronal responses almost always occur in bursts of action potentials rather than as single, isolated events.

6.12 Synaptic Strength

Individual synaptic events—whether excitatory or inhibitory—have been presented as though their effects are constant and reproducible. Actually, enormous variability occurs in the postsynaptic potentials that follow a presynaptic input. The effectiveness or strength of a given synapse is influenced by both presynaptic and postsynaptic mechanisms.

A presynaptic terminal does not release a constant amount of neurotransmitter every time it is activated. One reason for this variation involves Ca^{2+} concentration. Calcium ions that have entered the terminal during previous action potentials are pumped out of the cell or (temporarily) into intracellular organelles. If Ca^{2+} removal does not keep up with entry, as can occur during high-frequency stimulation, Ca^{2+} concentration in the terminal, and consequently the amount of neurotransmitter released upon subsequent stimulation, will be greater than usual. The greater the amount of neurotransmitter released, the greater the number of ion channels opened in the postsynaptic membrane and the larger the amplitude of the EPSP or IPSP in the postsynaptic cell.

The neurotransmitter output of some presynaptic terminals is also altered by activation of membrane receptors on the terminals themselves. Activation of these presynaptic receptors influences Ca^{2+} influx into the terminal and thus the number of neurotransmitter vesicles that release neurotransmitter into the synaptic cleft. These presynaptic receptors may be associated with a second synaptic ending known as an **axo–axonic synapse,** in which an axon terminal of one neuron ends on an axon terminal of another. For example, in **Figure 6.33,** the neurotransmitter released by A binds with receptors on B, resulting in a change in the amount of neurotransmitter released from B in response to action potentials. Thus, neuron A has no direct effect on neuron C, but it has an important influence on the ability of B to influence C. Neuron A is thus exerting a presynaptic effect on the synapse between B and C. Depending upon the type of presynaptic receptors activated by the neurotransmitter from neuron A, the presynaptic effect may decrease the amount of neurotransmitter released from B (**presynaptic inhibition**) or increase it (**presynaptic facilitation**).

Axo–axonic synapses such as A in Figure 6.33 can alter the Ca^{2+} concentration in axon terminal B or even affect neurotransmitter synthesis there. The mechanisms bringing about these effects vary from synapse to synapse. The receptors on the

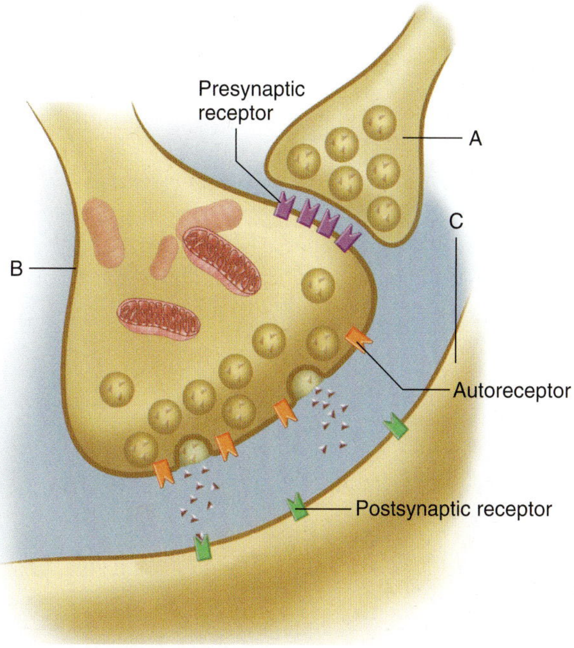

Figure 6.33 APR A presynaptic (axo–axonic) synapse between axon terminal A and axon terminal B. Cell C is postsynaptic to cell B.

axon terminal of neuron B could be ionotropic, in which case the membrane potential of the terminal is rapidly and directly affected by neurotransmitter from A; or they might be metabotropic, in which case the alteration of synaptic machinery by second messengers is generally slower in onset and longer in duration. In either case, if the Ca^{2+} concentration in axon terminal B increases, the number of vesicles releasing neurotransmitter from B increases. Decreased Ca^{2+} reduces the number of vesicles releasing transmitter. Axo–axonic synapses are important because they selectively control one specific input to the postsynaptic neuron C. This type of synapse is particularly common in the modulation of sensory input, for example, in the modulation of pain pathways (discussed in the next chapter, see Figure 7.16).

Some receptors on the presynaptic terminal are not associated with axo–axonic synapses. Instead, they are activated by neurotransmitters or other chemical messengers released by nearby neurons or glia or even by the axon terminal itself. In the last case, the receptors are called **autoreceptors** (see Figure 6.33) and provide an important feedback mechanism that the neuron can use to regulate its own neurotransmitter output. In most cases, the released neurotransmitter acts on autoreceptors to decrease its own release, thereby providing negative feedback control.

Postsynaptic mechanisms for varying synaptic strength also exist. For example, as described in Chapter 5, many types and subtypes of receptors exist for each kind of neurotransmitter. The different receptor types operate by different signal transduction mechanisms and can have different—sometimes even opposite—effects on the postsynaptic mechanisms they influence. A given signal transduction mechanism may be regulated by multiple neurotransmitters, and the various second-messenger systems affecting a channel may interact with each other.

Recall, too, from Chapter 5 that the number of receptors is not constant, varying with up- and down-regulation, for example. Also, the ability of a given receptor to respond to its neurotransmitter can change. Thus, in some systems, a receptor responds normally when first exposed to a neurotransmitter but then eventually fails to respond despite the continued presence of the receptor's neurotransmitter, a phenomenon known as **receptor desensitization.** This is part of the reason that drug abusers sometimes develop a tolerance to drugs that elevate certain brain neurotransmitters, forcing them to take increasing amounts of the drug to get the desired effect (see Chapter 8).

Imagine the complexity when a cotransmitter (or several cotransmitters) is released with the neurotransmitter to act upon postsynaptic receptors and maybe upon presynaptic receptors as well! Clearly, the possible variations in transmission are great at even a single synapse, and these provide mechanisms by which synaptic strength can be altered in response to changing conditions, part of the phenomenon of *plasticity* described at the beginning of this chapter.

Modification of Synaptic Transmission by Drugs and Disease

The great majority of therapeutic, illicit, and so-called "recreational" drugs that act on the nervous system do so by altering synaptic mechanisms and thus synaptic strength. Drugs act by interfering with or stimulating normal processes in the neuron involved in neurotransmitter synthesis, storage, and release, and in receptor activation. The synaptic mechanisms labeled in **Figure 6.34** are important to synaptic function and are vulnerable to the effects of drugs.

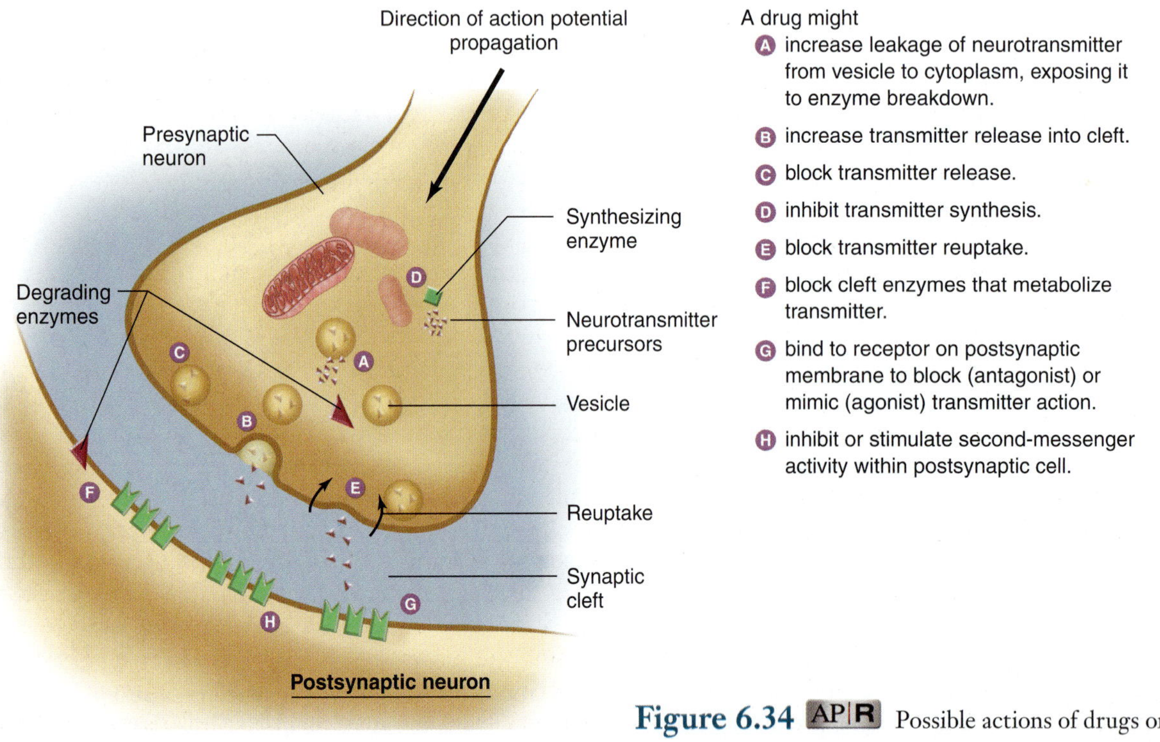

Figure 6.34 AP|R Possible actions of drugs on a synapse.

The long-term effects of drugs are sometimes difficult to predict because the imbalances the initial drug action produces are soon counteracted by feedback mechanisms that normally regulate the processes. For example, if a drug interferes with the action of a neurotransmitter by inhibiting the rate-limiting enzyme in its synthetic pathway, the neurons may respond by increasing the rate of precursor transport into the axon terminals to maximize the use of any available enzyme.

Recall from Chapter 5 that drugs that bind to a receptor and produce a response similar to the normal activation of that receptor are called **agonists,** and drugs that bind to the receptor but are unable to activate it are **antagonists.** By occupying the receptors, antagonists prevent binding of the normal neurotransmitter at the synapse. Specific agonists and antagonists can affect receptors on both presynaptic and postsynaptic membranes.

Diseases can also affect synaptic mechanisms. For example, the neurological disorder tetanus is caused by the bacillus *Clostridium tetani*, which produces a toxin (***tetanus toxin***). This toxin is a protease that destroys SNARE proteins in the presynaptic terminal so that fusion of vesicles with the membrane is prevented, inhibiting neurotransmitter release. Tetanus toxin specifically affects inhibitory neurons in the CNS that normally are important in suppressing the neurons that lead to skeletal muscle activation. Therefore, tetanus toxin results in an increase in muscle contraction and a rigid, or spastic paralysis. Toxins of the *Clostridium botulinum* bacilli, which cause ***botulism,*** also block neurotransmitter release from synaptic vesicles by destroying SNARE proteins. However, they target the excitatory synapses that activate skeletal muscles; consequently, botulism is characterized by reduced muscle contraction, or a flaccid paralysis. Low doses of one type of botulinum toxin (***Botox***) are injected therapeutically to treat a number of conditions, including facial wrinkles, severe sweating, uncontrollable blinking, misalignment of the eyes, and others.

Table 6.5 summarizes the factors that determine synaptic strength.

TABLE 6.5 Factors That Determine Synaptic Strength

I. Presynaptic factors
- A. Availability of neurotransmitter
  - 1. Availability of precursor molecules
  - 2. Amount (or activity) of the rate-limiting enzyme in the pathway for neurotransmitter synthesis
- B. Axon terminal membrane potential
- C. Axon terminal Ca^{2+}
- D. Activation of membrane receptors on presynaptic terminal
  - 1. Axo–axonic synapses
  - 2. Autoreceptors
  - 3. Other receptors
- E. Certain drugs and diseases, which act via the above mechanisms A–D

II. Postsynaptic factors
- A. Immediate past history of electrical state of postsynaptic membrane (e.g., excitation or inhibition from temporal or spatial summation)
- B. Effects of other neurotransmitters or neuromodulators acting on postsynaptic neuron
- C. Up- or down-regulation and desensitization of receptors
- D. Certain drugs and diseases

III. General factors
- A. Area of synaptic contact
- B. Enzymatic destruction of neurotransmitter
- C. Geometry of diffusion path
- D. Neurotransmitter reuptake

6.13 Neurotransmitters and Neuromodulators

We have emphasized the role of neurotransmitters in eliciting EPSPs and IPSPs. However, certain chemical messengers elicit complex responses that cannot be described as simply EPSPs or IPSPs. The word *modulation* is used for these complex responses, and the messengers that cause them are called **neuromodulators.** The distinctions between neuromodulators and neurotransmitters are not always clear. In fact, certain neuromodulators are often synthesized by the presynaptic cell and coreleased with the neurotransmitter. To add to the complexity, many hormones, paracrine factors, and messengers used by the immune system serve as neuromodulators.

Neuromodulators often modify the postsynaptic cell's response to specific neurotransmitters, amplifying or dampening the effectiveness of ongoing synaptic activity. Alternatively, they may change the presynaptic cell's synthesis, release, reuptake, or metabolism of a transmitter. In other words, they alter the effectiveness of the synapse.

In general, the receptors for neurotransmitters influence ion channels that directly affect excitation or inhibition of the postsynaptic cell. These mechanisms operate within milliseconds. Receptors for neuromodulators, on the other hand, more often bring about changes in metabolic processes in neurons, often via G proteins coupled to second-messenger systems. Such changes, which can occur over minutes, hours, or even days, include alterations in enzyme activity or, through influences on DNA transcription, in protein synthesis. Thus, neurotransmitters are involved in rapid communication, whereas neuromodulators tend to be associated with slower events such as learning, development, motivational states, and some types of sensory or motor activities.

The number of substances known to act as neurotransmitters or neuromodulators is large and still growing. Table 6.6 provides a framework for categorizing that list. A huge amount of information has accumulated concerning the synthesis, metabolism, and mechanisms of action of these messengers—material well beyond the scope of this book. The following sections will therefore present only some basic generalizations about some of the neurotransmitters that are deemed most important. For simplicity's sake, we use the term *neurotransmitter* in a general sense, realizing that sometimes the messenger may be described more appropriately as a neuromodulator. A note on terminology should also be included here. Neurons are often referred to using the suffix *-ergic;* the missing prefix is the type of neurotransmitter the neuron releases. For example, *dopaminergic* applies to neurons that release the neurotransmitter dopamine.

TABLE 6.6 Classes of Some of the Chemicals Known or Presumed to Be Neurotransmitters or Neuromodulators

I. Acetylcholine (ACh)
II. Biogenic amines A. Catecholamines 1. Dopamine (DA) 2. Norepinephrine (NE) 3. Epinephrine (Epi) B. Serotonin (5-hydroxytryptamine, 5-HT) C. Histamine
III. Amino acids A. Excitatory amino acids; for example, glutamate B. Inhibitory amino acids; for example, gamma-aminobutyric acid (GABA) and glycine
VI. Neuropeptides For example, endogenous opioids, oxytocin, tachykinins
V. Gases For example, nitric oxide, carbon monoxide, hydrogen sulfide
VI. Purines For example, adenosine and ATP

Acetylcholine

Acetylcholine (ACh) is a major neurotransmitter in the PNS at the neuromuscular junction (Chapter 9) and in the brain. Neurons that release ACh are called **cholinergic** neurons. The cell bodies of the brain's cholinergic neurons are concentrated in relatively few areas, but their axons are widely distributed.

Acetylcholine is synthesized from choline (a common nutrient found in many foods) and acetyl coenzyme A in the cytoplasm of synaptic terminals and stored in synaptic vesicles. After it is released and activates receptors on the postsynaptic membrane, the concentration of ACh at the postsynaptic membrane decreases (thereby stopping receptor activation) due to the action of the enzyme **acetylcholinesterase.** This enzyme is located on the presynaptic and postsynaptic membranes and rapidly destroys ACh, releasing choline and acetate. The choline is then transported back into the presynaptic axon terminals where it is reused in the synthesis of new ACh. The ACh concentration at the receptors is also reduced by simple diffusion away from the synapse and eventual breakdown of the molecule by an enzyme in the blood. Some chemical weapons, such as the nerve gas ***Sarin,*** inhibit acetylcholinesterase, causing a buildup of ACh in the synaptic cleft. This results in overstimulation of postsynaptic ACh receptors, initially causing uncontrolled muscle contractions but ultimately leading to receptor desensitization and paralysis.

There are two general types of ACh receptors, and they are distinguished by their responsiveness to two different chemicals. Recall that although a receptor is considered specific for a given ligand, such as ACh, most receptors will recognize natural or synthetic compounds that exhibit some degree of chemical similarity to that ligand. Some ACh receptors respond not only to acetylcholine but to the drug nicotine and have therefore come to be known as **nicotinic receptors.** ***Nicotine*** is a plant alkaloid compound that constitutes 1% to 2% of tobacco products. It is also contained in treatments for smoking cessation, such as nasal sprays, chewing gums, and transdermal patches. Nicotine's hydrophobic structure allows rapid absorption through lung capillaries, mucous membranes, skin, and the blood–brain barrier. The nicotinic acetylcholine receptor is an excellent example of a receptor that contains an ion channel (i.e., a ligand-gated channel). In this case, the channel is permeable to both sodium and potassium ions, but because Na^+ has the larger electrochemical driving force, the net effect of opening these channels is depolarization. Nicotinic receptors are present at the neuromuscular junction and, as Chapter 9 will explain, several nicotinic receptor antagonists are toxins that induce paralysis. Nicotinic receptors in the brain are important in cognitive functions and behavior. For example, one cholinergic system that employs nicotinic receptors plays a major role in attention, learning, and memory by reinforcing the ability to detect and respond to meaningful stimuli. The presence of nicotinic receptors on presynaptic terminals in reward pathways of the brain explains why tobacco products are among the most highly addictive substances known.

The other general type of cholinergic receptor is stimulated not only by acetylcholine but by the mushroom poison muscarine; therefore, these are called **muscarinic receptors.** These receptors couple with G proteins, which then alter the activity of a number of different enzymes and ion channels. They are prevalent at some cholinergic synapses in the brain and at junctions where a major division of the PNS innervates peripheral glands and organs, like salivary glands and the heart. ***Atropine*** is an antagonist of muscarinic receptors with many clinical uses, such as in eyedrops that relax the muscles of the iris, thereby dilating the pupils for an eye exam.

Neurons associated with the ACh system degenerate in people with ***Alzheimer disease*** (also called *Alzheimer's disease*), a brain disease that is usually age related and is the most common cause of declining intellectual function in late life. Alzheimer disease affects 10% to 15% of people over age 65, and 50% of people over age 85. Because of the degeneration of cholinergic neurons, this disease is associated with a decreased amount of ACh in certain areas of the brain and even the loss of the postsynaptic neurons that would have responded to it. These defects and those in other neurotransmitter systems that are affected in this disease are related to the declining language and perceptual abilities, confusion, and memory loss that characterize Alzheimer disease sufferers. Several genetic mechanisms have been identified as potential contributors to increased risk of developing Alzheimer disease. One example is a gene on chromosome 19 that codes for a protein involved in carrying cholesterol in the bloodstream. Mutations of genes on chromosomes 1, 14, and 21 are associated with abnormally increased concentrations of ***beta-amyloid protein,*** which is associated with neuronal cell death in a severe form of the disease that can begin as early as 30 years of age. This emerging picture of genetic risk factors is complex, and in some cases it appears that multiple genes are simultaneously involved. Some research also suggests that lifestyle factors like diet, exercise, social engagement, and mental stimulation may play a role in determining whether cholinergic neurons are lost and Alzheimer disease develops.

Biogenic Amines

The **biogenic amines** are small, charged molecules that are synthesized from amino acids and contain an amino group (R—NH_2). The most common biogenic amines are dopamine, norepinephrine, serotonin, and histamine. Epinephrine, another biogenic amine, is not a common neurotransmitter in the CNS but is the major *hormone* secreted by the adrenal medulla. Norepinephrine is an important neurotransmitter in both the central and peripheral components of the nervous system.

Catecholamines

Dopamine, norepinephrine (NE), and **epinephrine** all contain a catechol ring (a six-carbon ring with two adjacent hydroxyl groups) and an amine group, which is why they are called **catecholamines.** The catecholamines are formed from the amino acid tyrosine and share the same two initial steps in their synthetic pathway (**Figure 6.35**). Synthesis of catecholamines begins with the uptake of tyrosine by the axon terminals and its conversion to another precursor, L-dihydroxy-phenylalanine (**L-dopa**) by the rate-limiting enzyme in the pathway, tyrosine hydroxylase. Depending on the enzymes present in the terminals, any one of the three catecholamines may ultimately be released. Autoreceptors on the presynaptic terminals strongly modulate synthesis and release of the catecholamines.

After activation of the receptors on the postsynaptic cell, the catecholamine concentration in the synaptic cleft declines, mainly because a membrane transporter protein actively transports the catecholamine back into the axon terminal. The catecholamine neurotransmitters are also broken down in both the extracellular fluid and the axon terminal by enzymes such as **monoamine oxidase (MAO).** Drugs known as MAO inhibitors increase the amount of norepinephrine and dopamine in a synapse by slowing their metabolic degradation. They are used in the treatment of mood disorders such as some types of depression.

Within the CNS, the cell bodies of the catecholamine-releasing neurons lie in parts of the brain called the brainstem and hypothalamus. Although these neurons are relatively few in number, their axons branch greatly and go to virtually all parts of the brain and spinal cord. These neurotransmitters play essential roles in states of consciousness, mood, motivation, directed attention, movement, blood pressure regulation, and hormone release, functions that will be covered in more detail in Chapters 8, 10, 11, and 12.

For historical reasons having to do with nineteenth-century British physiologists referring to secretions of the adrenal gland as "adrenaline," the adjective **"adrenergic"** is commonly used to describe neurons that release norepinephrine or epinephrine and also to describe the receptors to which those chemicals bind. There are two major classes of receptors for norepinephrine and epinephrine: **alpha-adrenergic receptors** and **beta-adrenergic receptors** (also called alpha-adrenoceptors and beta-adrenoceptors). All catecholamine receptors are metabotropic, and thus use second messengers to transfer a signal from the surface of the cell to the cytoplasm. Beta-adrenoceptors act via stimulatory G proteins to increase cAMP in the postsynaptic cell. There are three subclasses of beta-receptors, β_1, β_2, and β_3, which function in different ways in different tissues (as will be described in Section D and Table 6.11). Alpha-adrenoceptors exist in two subclasses, α_1 and α_2. They act presynaptically to inhibit norepinephrine release (α_2) or postsynaptically to either stimulate or inhibit the activity of different types of K^+ channels (α_1). The subclasses of alpha- and beta-receptors are distinguished by the drugs that influence them and their second-messenger systems.

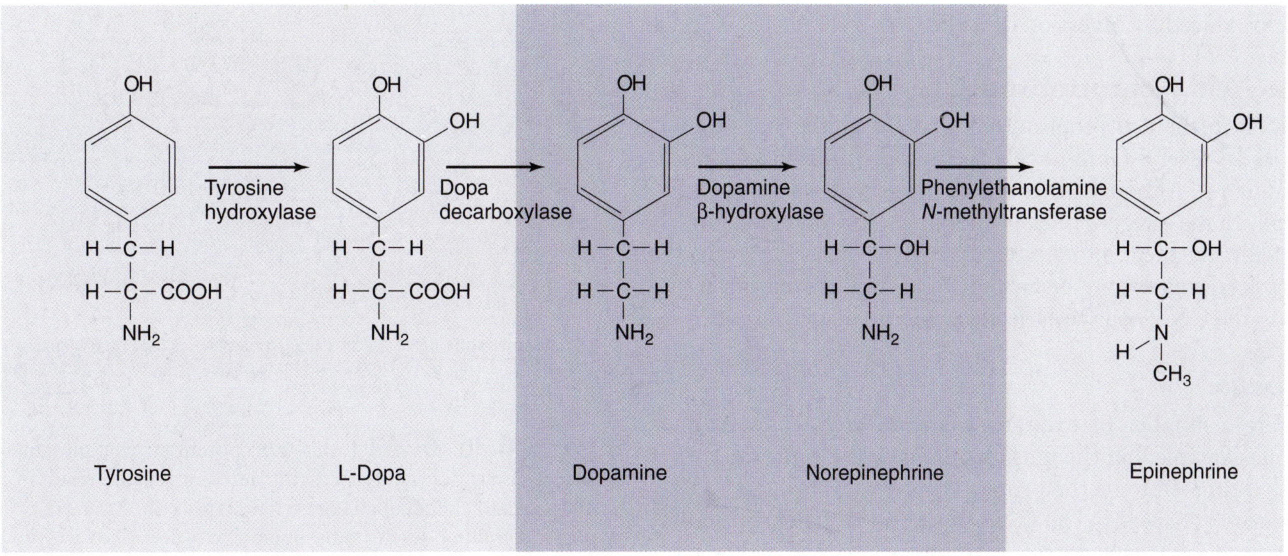

Figure 6.35 Catecholamine biosynthetic pathway. Tyrosine hydroxylase is the rate-limiting enzyme, but which neurotransmitter is ultimately released from a neuron depends on which of the other three enzymes are present in that cell. The dark-colored box indicates the more common CNS catecholamine neurotransmitters.

Serotonin

Though not a catecholamine, **serotonin** (5-hydroxytryptamine, or 5-HT) is an important biogenic amine. It is produced from tryptophan, an essential amino acid. Its effects generally have a slow onset, indicating that it works as a neuromodulator. Serotonergic neurons innervate virtually every structure in the brain and spinal cord and operate via at least 16 different receptor types.

In general, serotonin has an excitatory effect on pathways that are involved in the control of muscles, and an inhibitory effect on pathways that mediate sensations. The activity of serotonergic neurons is lowest or absent during sleep and highest during states of alert wakefulness. In addition to their contributions to motor activity and sleep, serotonergic pathways also function in the regulation of food intake, bone remodeling, reproductive behavior, and emotional states such as mood and anxiety.

Selective serotonin reuptake inhibitors such as ***paroxetine*** (***Paxil***) are thought to aid in the treatment of depression by inactivating the 5-HT transporter and increasing the synaptic concentration of the neurotransmitter. Interestingly, such drugs are often associated with decreased appetite but paradoxically cause weight gain due to disruption of enzymatic pathways that regulate fuel metabolism. Recent reports also suggest that bone density may be reduced in people taking this class of drugs. This is one example of how the use of reuptake inhibitors for a specific neurotransmitter—one with widespread actions—can cause unwanted side effects. Serotonin is found in both neural and nonneural cells, with the majority located outside of the CNS. In fact, approximately 90% of the body's total serotonin is found in the digestive system, 8% is in blood platelets and immune cells, and only 1% to 2% is found in the brain.

The drug lysergic acid diethylamide (***LSD***) stimulates the 5-HT_{2A} subtype of serotonin receptor and alters its interaction with glutamate receptors in the brain. Though the mechanism is not completely understood, alteration of this receptor complex produces the intense visual hallucinations that are produced by ingestion of LSD.

Amino Acid Neurotransmitters

In addition to the neurotransmitters that are synthesized from amino acids, several amino acids themselves function as neurotransmitters. Although the amino acid neurotransmitters chemically fit the category of biogenic amines, neurophysiologists traditionally put them into a category of their own. The amino acid neurotransmitters are by far the most prevalent neurotransmitters in the CNS, and they affect virtually all neurons there.

Glutamate

There are a number of **excitatory amino acids, aspartate** being one example, but the most common by far is **glutamate,** which is estimated to be the primary neurotransmitter at 50% of excitatory synapses in the CNS. As with other neurotransmitter systems, pharmacological manipulation of the receptors for glutamate has permitted identification of specific receptor subtypes by their ability to bind natural and synthetic ligands. Although metabotropic glutamate receptors do exist, the vast majority are ionotropic, with two important subtypes being found in postsynaptic membranes. They are designated as **AMPA receptors** (identified by their binding to α-amino-3 hydroxy-5 methyl-4 isoxazole propionic acid) and **NMDA receptors** (which bind *N*-methyl-D-aspartate).

Cooperative activity of AMPA and NMDA receptors has been implicated in one type of a phenomenon called **long-term potentiation (LTP)**. This mechanism couples frequent activity across a synapse with lasting changes in the strength of signaling across that synapse, and is thus thought to be one of the major cellular processes involved in learning and memory. **Figure 6.36** outlines the mechanism in stepwise fashion. When a presynaptic neuron fires action potentials (step 1), glutamate is released from presynaptic terminals (step 2) and binds to both AMPA and NMDA receptors on postsynaptic membranes (step 3). AMPA receptors function just like the excitatory postsynaptic receptors discussed earlier—when glutamate binds, the channel becomes permeable to both Na^+ and K^+, but the larger entry of Na^+ creates a depolarizing EPSP of the postsynaptic cell (step 4). By contrast, NMDA-receptor channels also mediate a substantial Ca^{2+} flux, but opening them requires more than just glutamate binding. A magnesium ion blocks NMDA channels when the membrane voltage is near the negative resting potential, and to drive it out of the way the membrane must be significantly depolarized by the current through AMPA channels (step 5). This explains why it requires a high frequency of presynaptic action potentials to complete

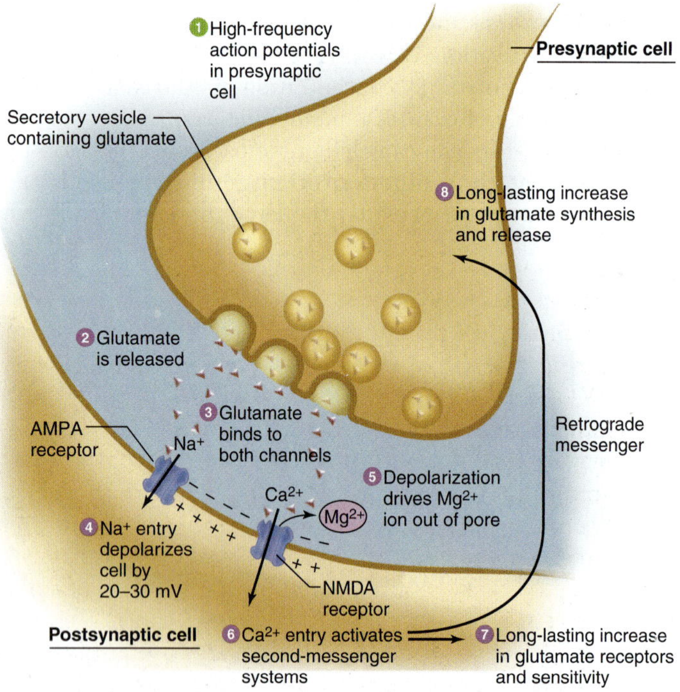

Figure 6.36 APIR Long-term potentiation at glutamatergic synapses. Episodes of intense firing across a synapse result in structural and chemical changes that amplify the strength of synaptic signaling during subsequent activation. See text for description of each step; details of the mechanism linking steps 1 and 2 were described in Figure 6.27. Note that both AMPA and NMDA receptors are nonspecific cation channels that also allow K^+ flux, but the net Na^+ and Ca^{2+} fluxes indicated are most relevant to the LTP mechanism, as described in the text.

the long-term potentiation mechanism. At low frequencies, there is insufficient temporal summation of AMPA-receptor EPSPs to provide the 20–30 mV of depolarization needed to move the magnesium ion, and so the NMDA receptors do not open. When the depolarization is sufficient, however, NMDA receptors do open, allowing Ca^{2+} to enter the postsynaptic cell (step 6). Calcium ions then activate a second-messenger cascade in the postsynaptic cell that includes persistent activation of multiple different protein kinases, stimulation of gene expression and protein synthesis, and ultimately a long-lasting increase in the sensitivity of the postsynaptic neuron to glutamate (step 7). This second-messenger system can also activate long-term enhancement of presynaptic glutamate release via retrograde signals that have not yet been identified (step 8). Each subsequent action potential arriving along this presynaptic cell will cause a greater depolarization of the postsynaptic membrane. Thus, repeatedly and intensely activating a particular pattern of synaptic firing (as you might when studying for an exam) causes chemical and structural changes that facilitate future activity along those same pathways (as might occur when recalling what you learned).

NMDA receptors have also been implicated in mediating **excitotoxicity.** This is a phenomenon in which the injury or death of some brain cells (due, for example, to blocked or ruptured blood vessels) rapidly spreads to adjacent regions. When glutamate-containing cells die and their membranes rupture, the flood of glutamate excessively stimulates AMPA and NMDA receptors on nearby neurons. The excessive stimulation of those neurons causes the accumulation of toxic concentrations of intracellular Ca^{2+}, which in turn kills those neurons and causes *them* to rupture, and the wave of damage progressively spreads. Recent experiments and clinical trials suggest that administering NMDA receptor antagonists may help minimize the spread of cell death following injuries to the brain.

GABA

GABA (gamma-aminobutyric acid) is the major inhibitory neurotransmitter in the brain. Although it is not one of the 20 amino acids used to build proteins, it is classified with the amino acid neurotransmitters because it is a modified form of glutamate. With few exceptions, GABA neurons in the brain are small interneurons that dampen activity within neural circuits. Postsynaptically, GABA may bind to ionotropic or metabotropic receptors. The ionotropic receptor increases Cl^- flux into the cell, resulting in hyperpolarization of the postsynaptic membrane. In addition to the GABA binding site, this receptor has several additional binding sites for other compounds, including steroids, barbiturates, and benzodiazepines. Benzodiazepine drugs such as ***alprazolam*** **(*Xanax*)** and ***diazepam*** **(*Valium*)** reduce anxiety, guard against seizures, and induce sleep by increasing Cl^- flux through the GABA receptor.

Synapses that use GABA are also among the many targets of the ethanol (ethyl alcohol) found in alcoholic beverages. Ethanol stimulates GABA synapses and simultaneously inhibits excitatory glutamate synapses, with the overall effect being global depression of the electrical activity of the brain. Thus, as a person's blood alcohol content increases, there is a progressive reduction in overall cognitive ability, along with sensory perception inhibition (hearing and balance, in particular), loss of motor coordination, impaired judgment, memory loss, and unconsciousness. Very high doses of ethanol are sometimes fatal, due to suppression of brainstem centers responsible for regulating the cardiovascular and respiratory systems. Dopaminergic and endogenous opioid signaling pathways (discussed in the next section) are also affected by ethanol, which results in short-term mood elevation or euphoria. The involvement of these pathways underlies the development of long-term alcohol dependence in some people.

Glycine

Glycine is the major neurotransmitter released from inhibitory interneurons in the spinal cord and brainstem. It binds to ionotropic receptors on postsynaptic cells that allow Cl^- to enter, thus preventing them from approaching the threshold for firing action potentials. Normal function of glycinergic neurons is essential for maintaining a balance of excitatory and inhibitory activity in spinal cord integrating centers that regulate skeletal muscle contraction. This becomes apparent in cases of poisoning with the neurotoxin ***strychnine***, an antagonist of glycine receptors sometimes used to kill rodents. Victims experience hyperexcitability throughout the nervous system, which leads to convulsions, spastic contraction of skeletal muscles, and ultimately death due to impairment of the muscles of respiration.

Neuropeptides

The **neuropeptides** are composed of two or more amino acids linked together by peptide bonds. About 100 neuropeptides have been identified, but their physiological roles are not all known. It seems that evolution has selected the same chemical messengers for use in widely differing circumstances, and many of the neuropeptides have been previously identified in nonneural tissue where they function as hormones or paracrine substances. They generally retain the name they were given when first discovered in the nonneural tissue.

The neuropeptides are formed differently than other neurotransmitters, which are synthesized in the axon terminals by very few enzyme-mediated steps. The neuropeptides, in contrast, are derived from large precursor proteins, which in themselves have little, if any, inherent biological activity. The synthesis of these precursors, directed by mRNA, occurs on ribosomes, which exist only in the cell body and large dendrites of the neuron, often a considerable distance from axon terminals or varicosities where the peptides are released.

In the cell body, the precursor protein is packaged into vesicles, which are then moved by axonal transport into the terminals or varicosities (review Figure 6.3), where the protein is cleaved by specific peptidases. Many of the precursor proteins contain multiple peptides, which may be different or be copies of one peptide. Neurons that release one or more of the peptide neurotransmitters are collectively called **peptidergic.** In many cases, neuropeptides are cosecreted with another type of neurotransmitter and act as neuromodulators.

The amount of peptide released from vesicles at synapses is significantly lower than the amount of nonpeptidergic neurotransmitters such as catecholamines. In addition, neuropeptides can diffuse away from the synapse and affect other neurons at some distance, in which case they are referred to as neuromodulators. The actions of these neuromodulators are longer lasting (on the order of several hundred milliseconds) than when peptides or other molecules act as neurotransmitters. After release, peptides can interact with either ionotropic or metabotropic receptors. They are eventually broken down by peptidases located in neuronal membranes.

Endogenous opioids—a group of neuropeptides that includes **beta-endorphin,** the **dynorphins,** and the **enkephalins**—have attracted much interest because their receptors are the sites of action of opiate drugs such as ***morphine*** and ***codeine.*** The opiate drugs are powerful ***analgesics*** (that is, they relieve pain without loss of consciousness), and the endogenous opioids undoubtedly play a role in regulating pain. The opioids have been implicated as a possible contributor to a runner's "second wind," when the athlete feels a boost of energy and a decrease in pain and effort, and in the general feeling of well-being experienced after a bout of strenuous exercise, the so-called "runner's high." There is also evidence that the opioids play a role in eating and drinking behavior, in regulation of the cardiovascular system, and in mood and emotion.

Substance P, another of the neuropeptides, is a transmitter released by afferent neurons that relay sensory information into the CNS. It is known to be involved in pain sensation.

Gases

Surprisingly, certain very short-lived gases also serve as neurotransmitters. **Nitric oxide** is the best understood, but recent research indicates that **carbon monoxide** and **hydrogen sulfide** are also emitted by neurons as signals. Gases are not released by exocytosis of presynaptic vesicles, nor do they bind to postsynaptic plasma membrane receptors. They are produced by enzymes in axon terminals (in response to Ca^{2+} entry) and simply diffuse from their sites of origin in one cell into the intracellular fluid of other neurons or effector cells, where they bind to and activate proteins. For example, nitric oxide released from neurons activates guanylyl cyclase in recipient cells, which increases the concentration of the second-messenger cyclic GMP.

Nitric oxide plays a role in a bewildering array of neurally mediated events—learning, development, drug tolerance, penile and clitoral erection, and sensory and motor modulation, to name a few. Paradoxically, it is also implicated in neural damage that results, for example, from the stoppage of blood flow to the brain or from a head injury. In later chapters, we will see that nitric oxide is produced not only in the central and peripheral nervous systems but also by a variety of nonneural cells; it also plays an important paracrine role in the cardiovascular and immune systems, among others.

Purines

Other nontraditional neurotransmitters include the purines, **ATP** and **adenosine,** which act principally as neuromodulators. ATP is present in all presynaptic vesicles and is coreleased with one or more other neurotransmitters in response to Ca^{2+} influx into the terminal. Adenosine is derived from ATP via enzyme activity occurring in the extracellular compartment. Both presynaptic and postsynaptic receptors have been described for adenosine, and the roles these substances play in the nervous system and other tissues are active areas of research.

6.14 Neuroeffector Communication

Thus far, we have described the effects of neurotransmitters released at synapses between neurons. Many neurons of the PNS end, however, not at synapses on other neurons but at neuroeffector junctions on muscle, gland, and other cells. The neurotransmitters released by these efferent neurons' terminals or varicosities provide the link by which electrical activity of the nervous system regulates effector cell activity.

The events that occur at neuroeffector junctions are similar to those at synapses between neurons. The neurotransmitter is released from the efferent neuron upon the arrival of an action potential at the neuron's axon terminals or varicosities. The neurotransmitter then diffuses to the surface of the effector cell, where it binds to receptors on that cell's plasma membrane. The receptors may be directly under the axon terminal or varicosity, or they may be some distance away so that the diffusion path the neurotransmitter follows is long. The receptors on the effector cell may be either ionotropic or metabotropic. The response (such as altered muscle contraction or glandular secretion) of the effector cell will be described in later chapters. As we will see in the next section, the major neurotransmitters released at neuroeffector junctions are acetylcholine and norepinephrine.

SECTION C SUMMARY

I. An excitatory synapse brings the membrane of the postsynaptic cell closer to threshold. An inhibitory synapse prevents the postsynaptic cell from approaching threshold by hyperpolarizing or stabilizing the membrane potential.

II. Whether a postsynaptic cell fires action potentials depends on the number of synapses that are active and whether they are excitatory or inhibitory.

III. Neurotransmitters are chemical messengers that pass from one neuron to another and modify the electrical or metabolic function of the recipient cell.

Functional Anatomy of Synapses

I. Electrical synapses consist of gap junctions that allow current to flow between adjacent cells.

II. In chemical synapses, neurotransmitter molecules are stored in synaptic vesicles in the presynaptic axon terminal, and when released transmit the signal from a presynaptic to a postsynaptic neuron.

Mechanisms of Neurotransmitter Release

I. Depolarization of the axon terminal increases the Ca^{2+} concentration within the terminal, which causes the release of neurotransmitter into the synaptic cleft.

II. The neurotransmitter diffuses across the synaptic cleft and binds to receptors on the postsynaptic cell; the activated receptors usually open ion channels.

Activation of the Postsynaptic Cell

I. At an excitatory synapse, the electrical response in the postsynaptic cell is called an excitatory postsynaptic potential (EPSP). At inhibitory synapses, it is either an inhibitory postsynaptic potential (IPSP) or a stabilization of the membrane potential near resting levels.

II. Usually at an excitatory synapse, channels in the postsynaptic cell that are permeable to Na^+, K^+, and other small positive ions open, but Na^+ flux dominates, because it has the largest electrochemical gradient. At inhibitory synapses, channels to Cl^- or K^+ open.

Synaptic Integration

I. The postsynaptic cell's membrane potential is the result of temporal and spatial summation of the EPSPs and IPSPs at the many active excitatory and inhibitory synapses on the cell.
II. Action potentials are generally initiated by the temporal and spatial summation of many EPSPs.

Synaptic Strength

I. Synaptic strength is modified by presynaptic and postsynaptic events, drugs, and diseases (see Table 6.5).

Neurotransmitters and Neuromodulators

I. In general, neurotransmitters cause EPSPs and IPSPs, and neuromodulators cause, via second messengers, more complex metabolic effects in the postsynaptic cell.
II. The actions of neurotransmitters are usually faster than those of neuromodulators.
III. A substance can act as a neurotransmitter at one type of receptor and as a neuromodulator at another.
IV. The major classes of known or suspected neurotransmitters and neuromodulators are listed in Table 6.6.

Neuroeffector Communication

I. The synapse between a neuron and an effector cell is called a neuroeffector junction.
II. The events at a neuroeffector junction (release of neurotransmitter into an extracellular space, diffusion of neurotransmitter to the effector cell, and binding with a receptor on the effector cell) are similar to those at synapses between neurons.

SECTION C REVIEW QUESTIONS

1. Describe the structure of presynaptic axon terminals, and the mechanism of neurotransmitter release.
2. Contrast the postsynaptic mechanisms of excitatory and inhibitory synapses.
3. Explain how synapses allow neurons to act as integrators; include the concepts of facilitation, temporal and spatial summation, and convergence in your explanation.
4. List at least eight ways in which the effectiveness of synapses may be altered.
5. Discuss differences between neurotransmitters and neuromodulators.
6. List the major classes of neurotransmitters, and give examples of each.
7. Detail the mechanism of long-term potentiation, and explain what role it might play in learning and memory.

SECTION C KEY TERMS

SECTION C CLINICAL TERMS

SECTION **D**

Structure of the Nervous System

We now survey the anatomy and broad functions of the major structures of the central and peripheral nervous systems. **Figure 6.37** provides a conceptual overview of the organization of the nervous system for you to refer to as we discuss the various subdivisions in this section and in later chapters.

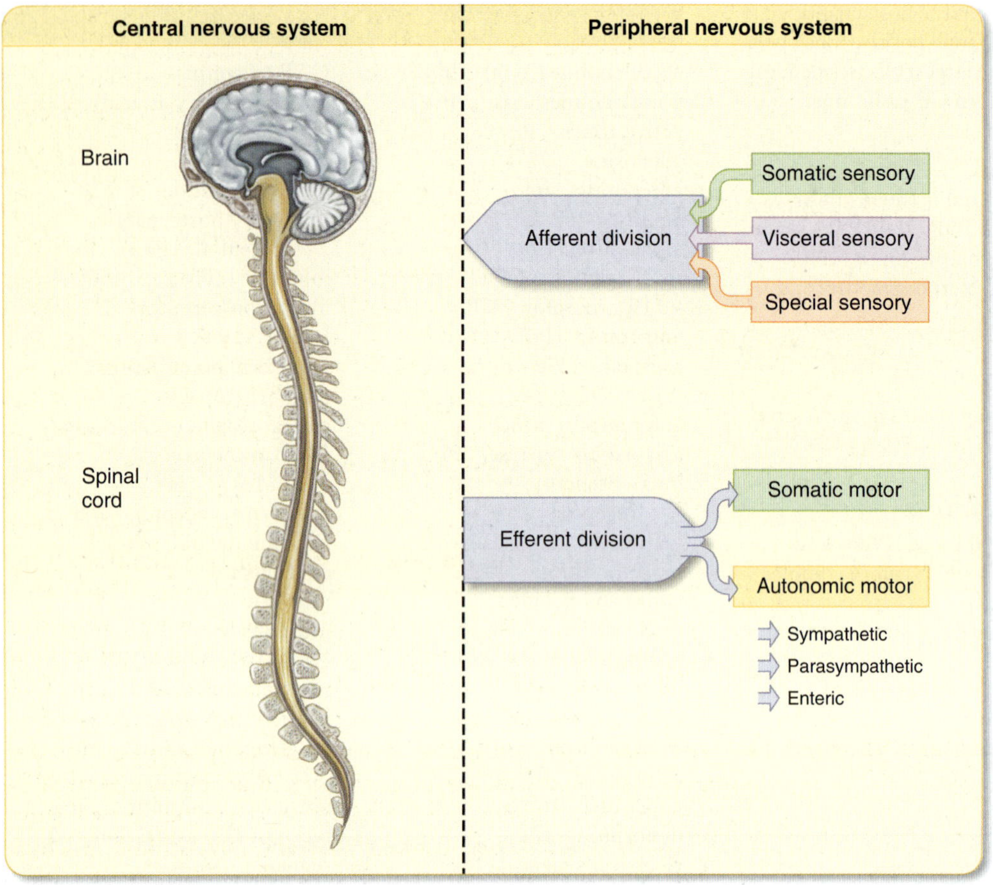

Figure 6.37 Overview of the structural and functional organization of the nervous system.

First, we must introduce some important terminology. Recall that a long extension from a single neuron is called an axon or a nerve fiber and that the term *nerve* refers to a group of many axons that are traveling together to and from the same general location in the PNS. There are no nerves in the CNS. Rather, a group of axons traveling together in the CNS is called a **pathway,** a **tract,** or, when it links the right and left halves of the CNS, a **commissure.** Two general types of pathways occur in the CNS. The first are sometimes referred to as *long neural pathways* and consist of neurons with relatively long axons that carry information directly between the brain and spinal cord or between large regions of the brain. The second type are *multisynaptic pathways* and include many neurons with branching axons and many synaptic connections. Because synapses are the sites where new information can be integrated into neural messages, these pathways perform complex neural processing, while long neural pathways transmit signals with relatively less alteration. The cell bodies of neurons with similar functions are often clustered together. Groups of neuron cell bodies in the PNS are called ganglia (singular, **ganglion**). In the CNS, they are called nuclei (singular, **nucleus**), not to be confused with cell nuclei.

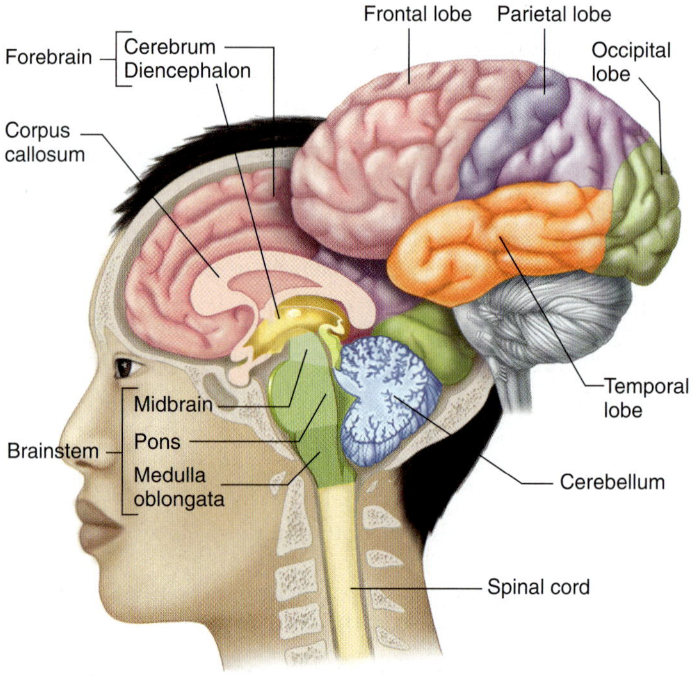

Figure 6.38 AP|R The surface of the cerebral cortex and the divisions of the brain shown in sagittal section. The outer surface of the cerebrum (cortex) is divided into four lobes as shown.

6.15 Central Nervous System: Brain

During development, the CNS forms from a long tube. As the anterior part of the tube, which becomes the brain, folds during its continuing formation, four different regions become apparent. These regions become the four subdivisions of the brain: the **cerebrum, diencephalon, brainstem,** and **cerebellum** (**Figure 6.38**). The cerebrum and diencephalon together constitute the **forebrain.** The brainstem consists of the **midbrain, pons,** and **medulla oblongata.** The brain also

TABLE 6.7 Summary of Functions of the Major Parts of the Brain

I. Forebrain
- A. Cerebral hemispheres
  1. Contain the cerebral cortex, which participates in perception (Chapter 7); the generation of skilled movements (Chapter 10); reasoning, learning, and memory (Chapter 8)
  2. Contain subcortical nuclei, including those that participate in coordination of skeletal muscle activity (Chapter 10)
  3. Contain interconnecting fiber pathways
- B. Thalamus
  1. Acts as a synaptic relay station for sensory pathways on their way to the cerebral cortex (Chapter 7)
  2. Participates in control of skeletal muscle coordination (Chapter 10)
  3. Plays a key role in awareness (Chapter 8)
- C. Hypothalamus
  1. Regulates anterior pituitary gland function (Chapter 11)
  2. Regulates water balance (Chapter 14)
  3. Participates in regulation of autonomic nervous system (Chapters 6 and 16)
  4. Regulates eating and drinking behavior (Chapter 16)
  5. Regulates reproductive system (Chapters 11 and 17)
  6. Reinforces certain behaviors (Chapter 8)
  7. Generates and regulates circadian rhythms (Chapters 1, 7, and 16)
  8. Regulates body temperature (Chapter 16)
  9. Participates in generation of emotional behavior (Chapter 8)
- D. Limbic system
  1. Participates in generation of emotions and emotional behavior (Chapter 8)
  2. Plays essential role in most kinds of learning (Chapter 8)

II. Cerebellum
- A. Coordinates movements, including those for posture and balance (Chapter 10)
- B. Participates in some forms of learning (Chapter 8)

III. Brainstem
- A. Contains all the fibers passing between the spinal cord, forebrain, and cerebellum
- B. Contains the reticular formation and its various integrating centers, including those for cardiovascular and respiratory activity (Chapters 12 and 13)
- C. Contains nuclei for cranial nerves III through XII

contains four interconnected cavities, the **cerebral ventricles,** which are filled with fluid.

Overviews of the brain subdivisions are included here and in Table 6.7, but details of their functions are given more fully in Chapters 7, 8, and 10.

Forebrain

The larger component of the forebrain, the cerebrum, consists of the right and left **cerebral hemispheres** as well as some associated structures on the underside of the brain. The central core of the forebrain is formed by the diencephalon.

The cerebral hemispheres (**Figure 6.39**) consist of the **cerebral cortex**—an outer shell of **gray matter** composed primarily of cell bodies that give the area a gray appearance—and an inner layer of **white matter,** composed primarily of myelinated fiber tracts. This in turn overlies cell clusters, which are also gray matter and are collectively termed the **subcortical nuclei.** The fiber tracts consist of the many nerve fibers that bring information into the cerebrum, carry information out, and connect different areas within a hemisphere. The cortex layers of the left and right cerebral hemispheres, although largely separated by a deep longitudinal division, are connected by a massive bundle of nerve fibers known as the **corpus callosum.**

The cortex of each cerebral hemisphere is divided into four lobes, named after the overlying skull bones covering the brain: the **frontal, parietal, occipital,** and **temporal lobes.** Although it averages only 3 mm in thickness, the cortex is highly folded. This results in an area containing cortical neurons that is four times larger than it would be if unfolded, yet does not appreciably increase the volume of the brain. Such elaboration of structural surface area to enhance function in organs throughout the body affirms the general principle of physiology that structure and function are related. This folding also results in the characteristic external appearance of the human cerebrum, with its sinuous ridges called gyri (singular, **gyrus**) separated by grooves called sulci (singular, **sulcus**). The cells of the human cerebral cortex are organized in six distinct layers, composed of varying sizes and numbers of two basic types: pyramidal cells (named for the shape of their cell bodies) and nonpyramidal cells. The **pyramidal cells** form the major output cells of the cortex, sending their axons to other parts of the cortex and to other parts of the CNS. Nonpyramidal cells are mostly involved in receiving inputs into the cortex and in local processing of information. This elaboration of the human cerebral cortex into multiple cell layers, like its highly folded structure, allows for an increase in the number and integration of neurons for signal processing. This is supported by the fact that an increase in the number of cell layers in the cerebral cortex has paralleled the increase in behavioral and cognitive complexity in vertebrate evolution. For example, reptiles have just three layers in the cortex, and dolphins have five. Some regions of the human brain with ancient evolutionary origins, such as the olfactory cortex, persist in having only three cell layers.

The cerebral cortex is one of the most complex integrating areas of the nervous system. In the cerebral cortex, basic afferent information is collected and processed into meaningful perceptual images, and control over the systems that govern the movement of the skeletal muscles is refined. Nerve fibers enter the cortex predominantly from the diencephalon, specifically from a region known as the thalamus as well as from other regions of the cortex and areas of the brainstem. Some of the input fibers convey information about specific events in the environment, whereas others control levels of cortical excitability, determine states of arousal, and direct attention to specific stimuli.

The subcortical nuclei are heterogeneous groups of gray matter that lie deep within the cerebral hemispheres. Predominant among them are the **basal nuclei** (often, but less correctly referred to as **basal ganglia**), which play an important role in controlling movement and posture and in more complex aspects of behavior.

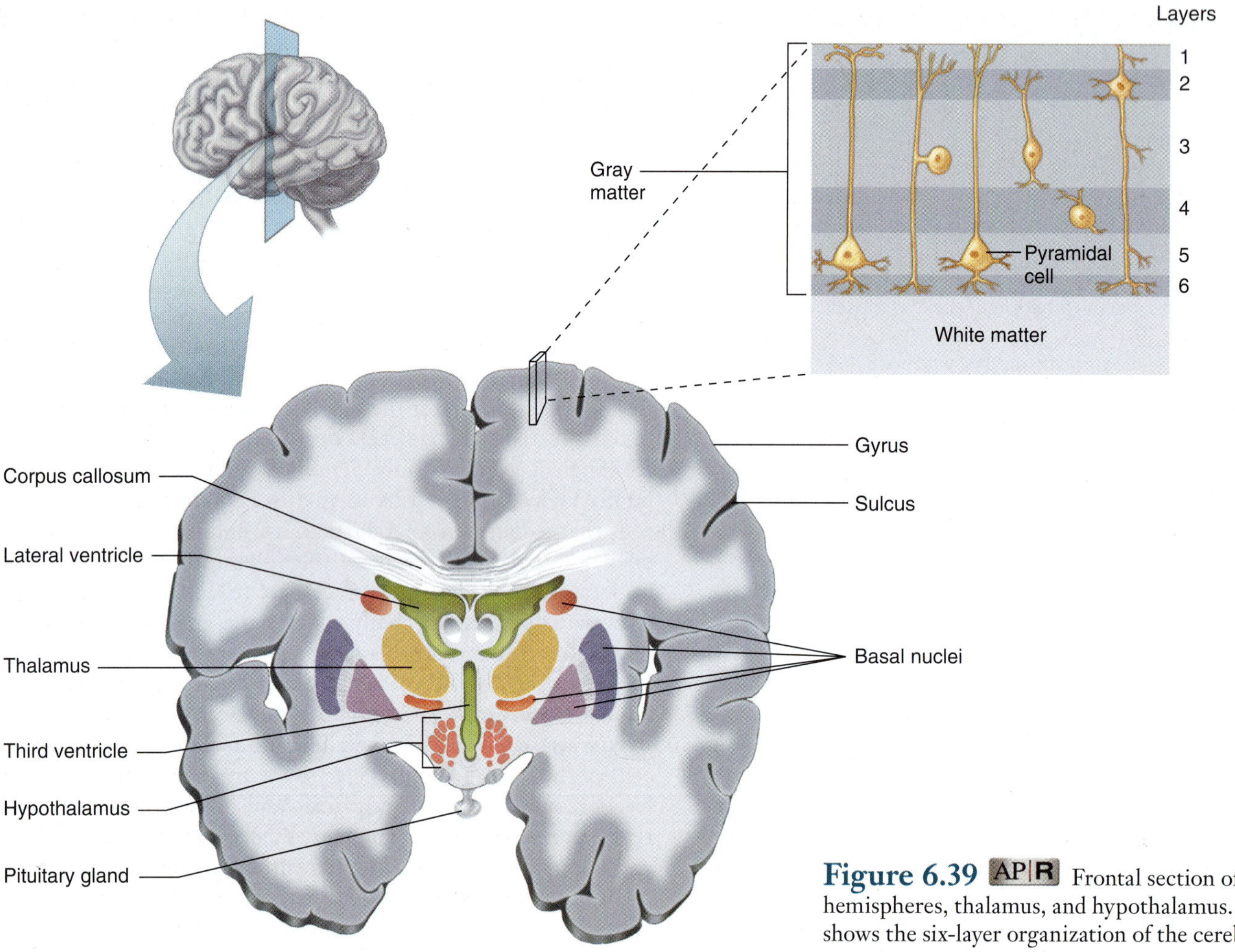

Figure 6.39 AP|R Frontal section of the cerebral hemispheres, thalamus, and hypothalamus. The inset shows the six-layer organization of the cerebral cortex.

The diencephalon, which is divided in two by the narrow third cerebral ventricle, is the second component of the forebrain. It contains the thalamus, hypothalamus, and epithalamus. The **thalamus** is a collection of several large nuclei that serve as synaptic relay stations and important integrating centers for most inputs to the cortex, and it plays a key role in general arousal. The thalamus also is involved in focusing attention. For example, it is responsible for filtering out extraneous sensory information such as might occur when you try to concentrate on a private conversation at a loud, crowded party.

The **hypothalamus** lies below the thalamus and is on the undersurface of the brain. Although it is a tiny region that accounts for less than 1% of the brain's weight, it contains different cell groups and pathways that form the master command center for neural and endocrine coordination. Indeed, the hypothalamus is the single most important control area for homeostatic regulation of the internal environment. Behaviors having to do with preservation of the individual (for example, eating and drinking) and preservation of the species (reproduction) are among the many functions of the hypothalamus. The hypothalamus lies directly above and is connected by a stalk to the **pituitary gland,** an important endocrine structure that the hypothalamus regulates (Chapter 11).

The **epithalamus** is a small mass of tissue that includes the **pineal gland,** which has a role in regulating circadian rhythms through release of the hormone melatonin.

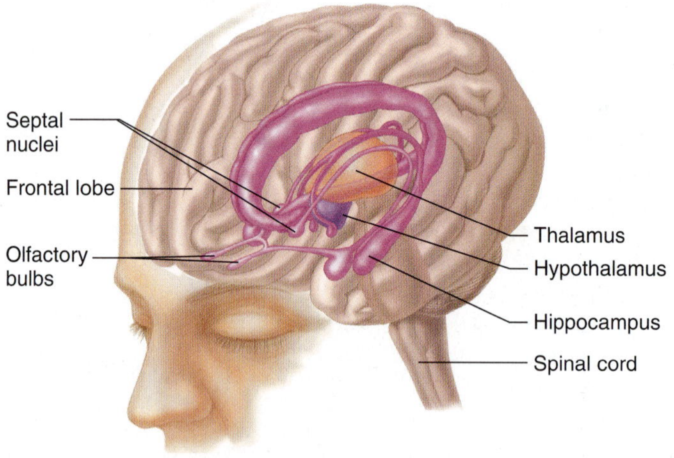

Figure 6.40 AP|R Structures of the limbic system (violet) and their anatomical relation to the hypothalamus (purple) are shown in this partially transparent view of the brain.

Thus far, we have described discrete anatomical areas of the forebrain. Some of these forebrain areas, consisting of both gray and white matter, are also classified together in a functional system called the **limbic system.** This interconnected group of brain structures includes portions of frontal-lobe cortex, temporal lobe, thalamus, and hypothalamus, as well as the fiber pathways that connect them (**Figure 6.40**).

Besides being connected with each other, the parts of the limbic system connect with many other parts of the CNS. Structures within the limbic system are associated with learning, emotional experience and behavior, and a wide variety of visceral and endocrine functions (see Chapter 8). In fact, the hypothalamus coordinates much of the output of the limbic system into behavioral and endocrine responses.

Cerebellum

The cerebellum consists of an outer layer of cells, the cerebellar cortex (do not confuse this with the cerebral cortex), and several deeper cell clusters. Although the cerebellum does not initiate voluntary movements, it is an important center for coordinating movements and for controlling posture and balance. To carry out these functions, the cerebellum receives information from the muscles and joints, skin, eyes, vestibular apparatus, viscera, and the parts of the brain involved in control of movement. Although the cerebellum's function is almost exclusively motor, it also may be involved in some forms of learning.

Brainstem

All the nerve fibers that relay signals between the forebrain, cerebellum, and spinal cord pass through the brainstem. Running through the core of the brainstem and consisting of loosely arranged neuron cell bodies intermingled with bundles of axons is the **reticular formation,** the one part of the brain absolutely essential for life. It receives and integrates input from all regions of the CNS and processes a great deal of neural information. The reticular formation is involved in motor functions, cardiovascular and respiratory control, and the mechanisms that regulate sleep and wakefulness and that focus attention. Most of the biogenic amine neurotransmitters are released from the axons of cells in the reticular formation and, because of the far-reaching projections of these cells, these neurotransmitters affect all levels of the nervous system.

Some reticular formation neurons send axons for considerable distances up or down the brainstem and beyond to most regions of the brain and spinal cord. This pattern explains the very large scope of influence that the reticular formation has over other parts of the CNS and explains the widespread effects of the biogenic amines.

The pathways that convey information from the reticular formation to the upper portions of the brain stimulate arousal and wakefulness. They also direct attention to specific events by selectively stimulating neurons in some areas of the brain while inhibiting others. The fibers that descend from the reticular formation to the spinal cord influence activity in both efferent and afferent neurons. Considerable interaction takes place between the reticular pathways that go up to the forebrain, down to the spinal cord, and to the cerebellum. For example, all three components function in controlling muscle activity.

The reticular formation encompasses a large portion of the brainstem, and many areas within the reticular formation serve distinct functions. For example, some reticular formation neurons are clustered together, forming brainstem nuclei and integrating centers. These include the cardiovascular, respiratory, swallowing, and vomiting centers, all of which we will discuss in later chapters. The reticular formation also has nuclei important in eye-movement control and the reflexive orientation of the body in space.

In addition, the brainstem contains nuclei involved in processing information for 10 of the 12 pairs of **cranial nerves.** These are the peripheral nerves that connect directly with the brain and innervate the muscles, glands, and sensory receptors of the head, as well as many organs in the thoracic and abdominal cavities.

6.16 Central Nervous System: Spinal Cord

The spinal cord lies within the bony vertebral column (**Figure 6.41**). It is a slender cylinder of soft tissue about as big around as your little finger. The central butterfly-shaped area (in cross section) of gray matter is composed of interneurons, the cell bodies and dendrites of efferent neurons, the entering axons of afferent neurons, and glial cells. The regions of gray matter projecting toward the back of the body are called the **dorsal horns,** whereas those oriented toward the front are the **ventral horns.**

The gray matter is surrounded by white matter, which consists of groups of myelinated axons. These groups of fiber tracts run longitudinally through the cord, some descending to relay information *from* the brain to the spinal cord, others ascending to transmit information *to* the brain. Pathways also transmit information between different levels of the spinal cord.

Groups of afferent fibers that enter the spinal cord from the peripheral nerves enter on the dorsal side of the cord via the **dorsal roots.** Small bumps on the dorsal roots, the

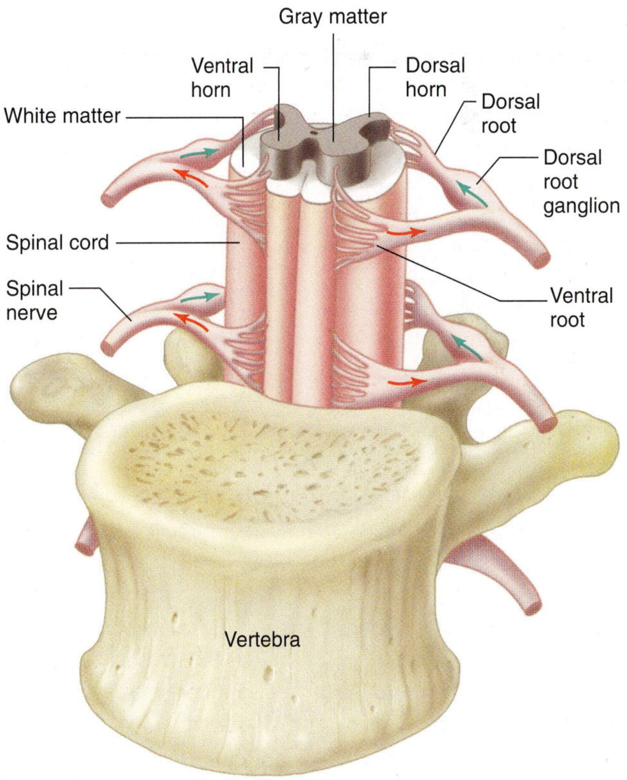

Figure 6.41 AP|R Section of the spinal cord, ventral view. The arrows indicate the direction of transmission of neural activity.

dorsal root ganglia, contain the cell bodies of these afferent neurons. The axons of efferent neurons leave the spinal cord on the ventral side via the **ventral roots.** A short distance from the cord, the dorsal and ventral roots from the same level combine to form a **spinal nerve,** one on each side of the spinal cord.

6.17 Peripheral Nervous System

Neurons in the PNS transmit signals between the CNS and receptors and effectors in all other parts of the body. As noted earlier, the axons are grouped into bundles called nerves. The PNS has 43 pairs of nerves: 12 pairs of cranial nerves and 31 pairs of spinal nerves that connect with the spinal cord. **Table 6.8** lists the cranial nerves and summarizes the information they transmit. The 31 pairs of spinal nerves are designated by the vertebral levels from which they exit: cervical, thoracic, lumbar, sacral, and coccygeal (**Figure 6.42**). Neurons in the spinal nerves at each level generally communicate with nearby structures, controlling muscles and glands as well as receiving sensory input. The eight pairs of cervical nerves innervate the neck, shoulders, arms, and hands. The 12 pairs of thoracic nerves are associated with the chest and upper abdomen. The five pairs of lumbar nerves are associated with the lower abdomen, hips, and legs; the five pairs of sacral nerves are associated with the genitals and lower digestive tract. A single pair of coccygeal nerves associated with the tailbone brings the total to 31 pairs.

These peripheral nerves can contain nerve fibers that are the axons of efferent neurons, afferent neurons, or both. Therefore, fibers in a nerve may be classified as belonging to the **efferent** or the **afferent division** of the PNS (refer back to Figure 6.37). All the spinal nerves contain both afferent and efferent fibers, whereas some of the cranial nerves contain only afferent fibers (the optic nerves from the eyes, for example) or only efferent fibers (the hypoglossal nerve to muscles of the tongue, for example).

As noted earlier, afferent neurons convey information from sensory receptors at their peripheral endings to the CNS. The long part of their axon is outside the CNS and is part of the PNS. Afferent neurons are sometimes called primary afferents or first-order neurons because they are the first cells entering the CNS in the synaptically linked chains of neurons that handle incoming information.

TABLE 6.8 The Cranial Nerves

Name	Fibers	Comments
I. Olfactory	Afferent	Carries input from receptors in olfactory (smell) neuroepithelium*
II. Optic	Afferent	Carries input from receptors in eye*
III. Oculomotor	Efferent	Innervates skeletal muscles that move eyeball up, down, and medially, and raise upper eyelid; innervates smooth muscles that constrict pupil and alter lens shape for near and far vision
	Afferent	Transmits information from receptors in muscles
IV. Trochlear	Efferent	Innervates skeletal muscles that move eyeball downward and laterally
	Afferent	Transmits information from receptors in muscles
V. Trigeminal	Efferent	Innervates skeletal chewing muscles
	Afferent	Transmits information from receptors in skin; skeletal muscles of face, nose, and mouth; and teeth sockets
VI. Abducens	Efferent	Innervates skeletal muscles that move eyeball laterally
	Afferent	Transmits information from receptors in muscles
VII. Facial	Efferent	Innervates skeletal muscles of facial expression and swallowing; innervates nose, palate, and lacrimal and salivary glands
	Afferent	Transmits information from taste buds in front of tongue and mouth
VIII. Vestibulocochlear	Afferent	Transmits information from receptors in inner ear
IX. Glossopharyngeal	Efferent	Innervates skeletal muscles involved in swallowing and parotid salivary gland
	Afferent	Transmits information from taste buds at back of tongue and receptors in auditory-tube skin
X. Vagus	Efferent	Innervates skeletal muscles of pharynx and larynx and smooth muscle and glands of thorax and abdomen
	Afferent	Transmits information from receptors in thorax and abdomen
XI. Accessory	Efferent	Innervates sternocleidomastoid and trapezius muscles in the neck
XII. Hypoglossal	Efferent	Innervates skeletal muscles of tongue

*The olfactory and optic pathways are CNS structures so are not technically "nerves."

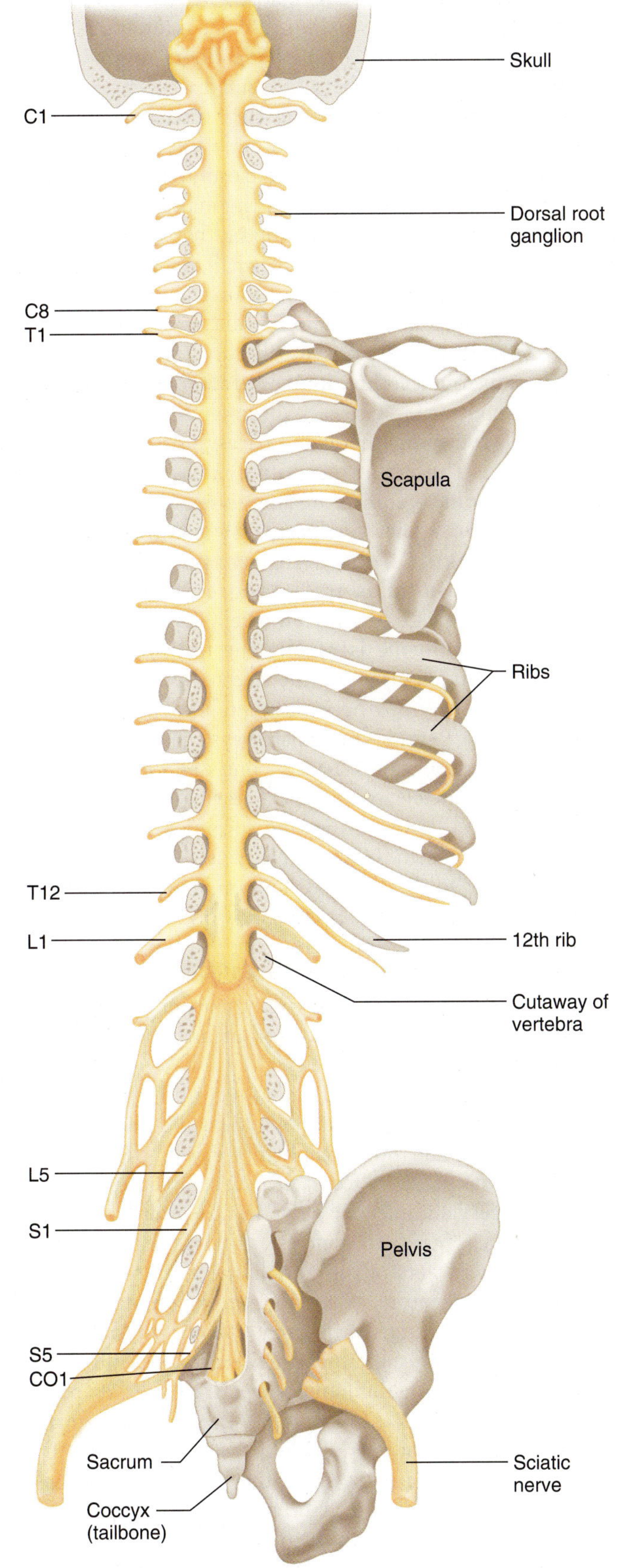

Efferent neurons carry signals out from the CNS to muscles, glands, and other tissues. The efferent division of the PNS is more complicated than the afferent, being subdivided into a **somatic nervous system** and an **autonomic nervous system.** These terms are somewhat misleading because they suggest the presence of additional nervous systems distinct from the central and peripheral systems. Keep in mind that these terms together make up the efferent division of the PNS.

The simplest distinction between the somatic and autonomic systems is that the neurons of the somatic division innervate skeletal muscle, whereas the autonomic neurons innervate smooth and cardiac muscle, glands, neurons in the gastrointestinal tract, and other tissues. Other differences are listed in **Table 6.9**.

The somatic portion of the efferent division of the PNS is made up of all the nerve fibers going from the CNS to skeletal muscle cells. The cell bodies of these neurons are located in groups in the brainstem or the ventral horn of the spinal cord. Their large-diameter, myelinated axons leave the CNS and pass without any synapses to skeletal muscle cells. The neurotransmitter these neurons release is acetylcholine. Because activity in the somatic neurons leads to contraction of the innervated skeletal muscle cells, these neurons are called **motor neurons.** Excitation of motor neurons leads only to the *contraction* of skeletal muscle cells; there are no somatic neurons that inhibit skeletal muscles. Muscle relaxation involves the inhibition of the motor neurons in the spinal cord.

TABLE 6.9 Peripheral Nervous System: Somatic and Autonomic Divisions

Somatic
Consists of a single neuron between CNS and skeletal muscle cells
Innervates skeletal muscle cells
Can lead only to muscle cell excitation
Autonomic
Has two-neuron chain (connected by a synapse) between CNS and effector organ
Innervates smooth and cardiac muscle, glands, GI neurons, but not skeletal muscle cells
Can be either excitatory or inhibitory

Figure 6.42 APIR Dorsal view of the spinal cord and spinal nerves. Parts of the skull and vertebrae have been cut away; the ventral roots of the spinal nerves are not visible. In general, the eight cervical nerves (C) control the muscles and glands and receive sensory input from the neck, shoulders, arms, and hands. The 12 thoracic nerves (T) are associated with the shoulders, chest, and upper abdomen. The five lumbar nerves (L) are associated with the lower abdomen, hips, and legs; and the five sacral nerves (S) are associated with the genitals and lower digestive tract. Redrawn from *Fundamental Neuroanatomy* by Walle J. H. Nauta and Michael Fiertag. Copyright © 1986 by W. H. Freeman and Company. Reprinted by permission.

6.18 Autonomic Nervous System

The efferent innervation of tissues other than skeletal muscle is by way of the autonomic nervous system. A special case occurs in the gastrointestinal tract, where autonomic neurons innervate a nerve network in the wall of the intestinal tract. This network is called the **enteric nervous system,** and although often classified as a subdivision of the autonomic efferent nervous system, it also includes sensory neurons and interneurons. Chapter 15 will describe this network in more detail.

In contrast to the somatic nervous system, the autonomic nervous system is made up of two neurons in series that connect the CNS and the effector cells (**Figure 6.43**). The first neuron has its cell body in the CNS. The synapse between the two neurons is outside the CNS in a cell cluster called an **autonomic ganglion.** The neurons passing between the CNS and the ganglia are called **preganglionic neurons;** those passing between the ganglia and the effector cells are **postganglionic neurons.**

Anatomical and physiological differences within the autonomic nervous system are the basis for its further subdivision into **sympathetic** and **parasympathetic divisions** (review Figure 6.37). The neurons of the sympathetic and parasympathetic divisions leave the CNS at different levels—the sympathetic fibers from the thoracic (chest) and lumbar regions of the spinal cord, and the parasympathetic fibers from the brainstem and the sacral portion of the spinal cord (**Figure 6.44**). Therefore, the sympathetic division is also called the thoracolumbar division, and the parasympathetic division is called the craniosacral division.

The two divisions also differ in the location of ganglia. Most of the sympathetic ganglia lie close to the spinal cord and form the two chains of ganglia—one on each side of the cord—known as the **sympathetic trunks** (see Figure 6.44 and **Figure 6.45**). Other sympathetic ganglia, called collateral ganglia—the celiac, superior mesenteric, and inferior mesenteric ganglia—are in the abdominal cavity, closer to the innervated organ (see Figure 6.44). In contrast, the parasympathetic ganglia lie within, or very close to, the organs that the postganglionic neurons innervate.

Preganglionic sympathetic neurons leave the spinal cord only between the first thoracic and second lumbar segments, whereas sympathetic *trunks* extend the entire length of the cord, from the cervical levels high in the neck down to the sacral levels. The gangliain the extra lengths of sympathetic trunks receive preganglionic neurons from the thoracolumbar regions because some of the preganglionic neurons, once in the sympathetic trunks, turn to travel upward or downward for several segments before forming synapses with postganglionic neurons (see Figure 6.45, numbers 1 and 4). Other possible paths the sympathetic fibers might take are shown in Figure 6.45, numbers 2, 3, and 5.

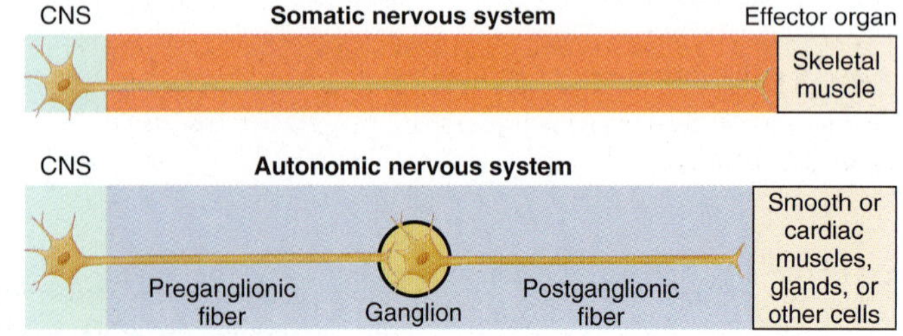

Figure 6.43 Efferent division of the PNS, including an overall plan of the somatic and autonomic nervous systems.

Due in part to differences in their anatomy, the overall activation pattern within the sympathetic and parasympathetic systems tends to be different. The close anatomical association of the sympathetic ganglia and the marked divergence of presynaptic sympathetic neurons make that division tend to respond as a single unit. Although small segments are occasionally activated independently, it is more typical for increased sympathetic activity to occur body-wide when circumstances warrant activation. The parasympathetic system, in contrast, exhibits less divergence; thus, it tends to activate specific organs in a pattern finely tailored to each given physiological situation.

In both the sympathetic and parasympathetic divisions, acetylcholine is the neurotransmitter released between pre- and postganglionic neurons in autonomic ganglia, and the postganglionic cells have predominantly nicotinic acetylcholine receptors (**Figure 6.46**). In the parasympathetic division, acetylcholine is also the neurotransmitter between the postganglionic neuron and the effector cell. In the sympathetic division, norepinephrine is usually the transmitter between the postganglionic neuron and the effector cell. We say "usually" because a few sympathetic postganglionic endings release acetylcholine (e.g., sympathetic pathways that regulate sweating). At many autonomic synapses, one or more cotransmitters are stored and released with the major neurotransmitter. These include ATP, dopamine, and several of the neuropeptides, all of which seem to play a relatively small role.

In addition to the classical autonomic neurotransmitters just described, there is a widespread network of postganglionic neurons recognized as nonadrenergic and noncholinergic. These neurons use nitric oxide and other neurotransmitters to mediate some forms of blood vessel dilation and to regulate various gastrointestinal, respiratory, urinary, and reproductive functions.

Many of the drugs that stimulate or inhibit various components of the autonomic nervous system affect receptors for acetylcholine and norepinephrine. Recall that there are several types of receptors for each neurotransmitter. A great majority of acetylcholine receptors in the autonomic ganglia are nicotinic receptors. In contrast, the acetylcholine receptors on cellular targets of postganglionic autonomic neurons are muscarinic receptors. The cholinergic receptors on skeletal muscle fibers, innervated by the *somatic* motor neurons, not autonomic neurons, are nicotinic receptors (**Table 6.10**).

One set of postganglionic neurons in the sympathetic division never develops axons. Instead, these neurons form an endocrine gland, the adrenal medulla (see Figure 6.46). Upon activation by preganglionic sympathetic axons, cells of the **adrenal medulla** release a mixture of about 80% epinephrine and 20% norepinephrine into the blood (plus small amounts of other substances, including dopamine, ATP, and neuropeptides). These catecholamines, properly called *hormones* rather than *neurotransmitters* in this circumstance, are transported via the blood to effector cells having receptors sensitive to them. The receptors may be the same adrenergic receptors that are located near the release sites of sympathetic postganglionic neurons

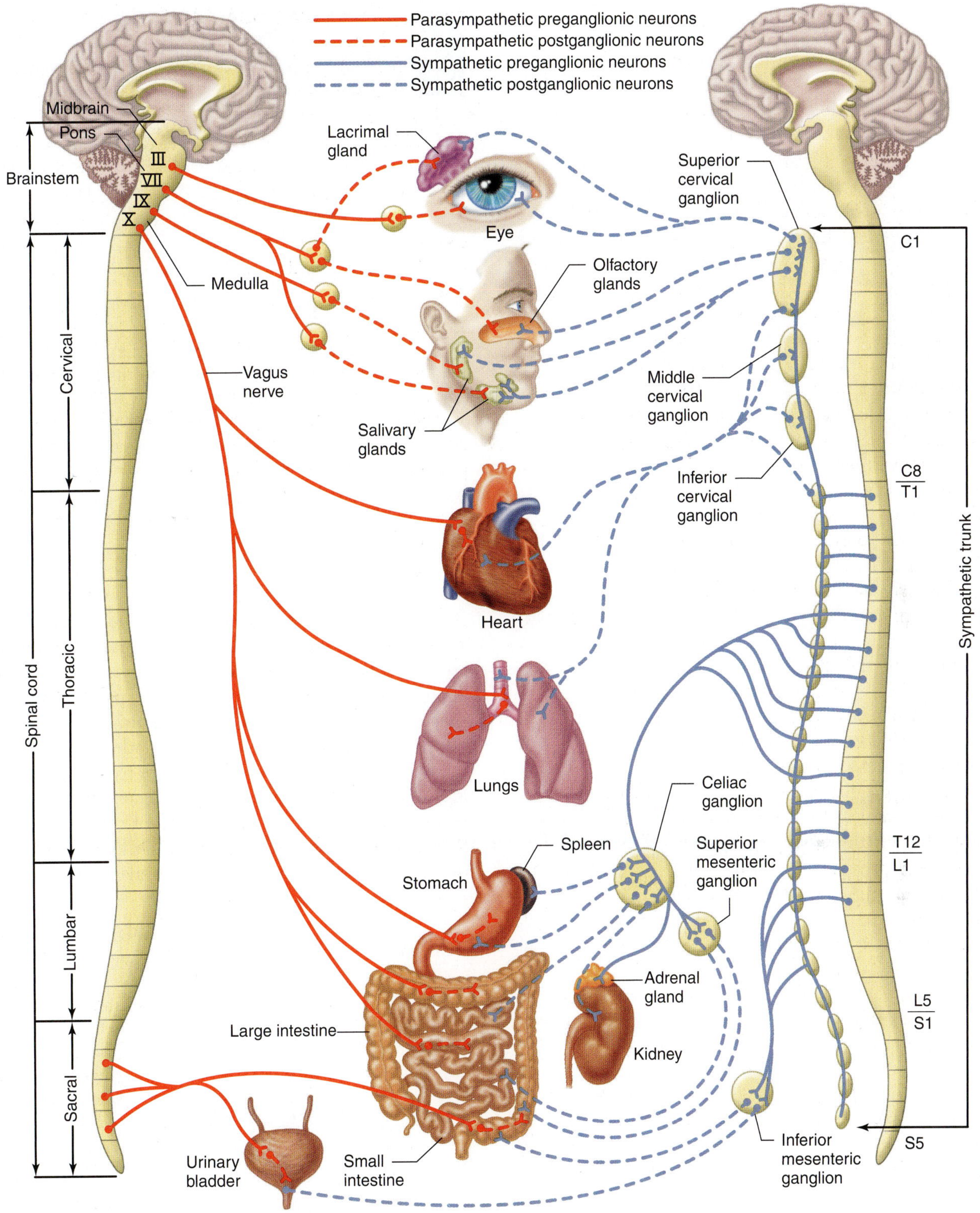

Figure 6.44 AP|R The parasympathetic (at left) and sympathetic (at right) divisions of the autonomic nervous system. Although single nerves are shown exiting the brainstem and spinal cord, all represent paired (left and right) nerves. Only one sympathetic trunk is indicated, although there are two, one on each side of the spinal cord. The celiac, superior mesenteric, and inferior mesenteric ganglia are collateral ganglia. Not shown are the fibers passing to the liver, blood vessels, genitalia, and skin glands.

and are normally activated by the norepinephrine released from these neurons. In other cases, the receptors may be located in places that are not near the neurons and are therefore activated only by the circulating epinephrine or norepinephrine. The overall effect of these catecholamines is slightly different due to the fact that some adrenergic receptor subtypes have a higher affinity for epinephrine (e.g., β_2), whereas others have a higher affinity for norepinephrine (e.g., α_1).

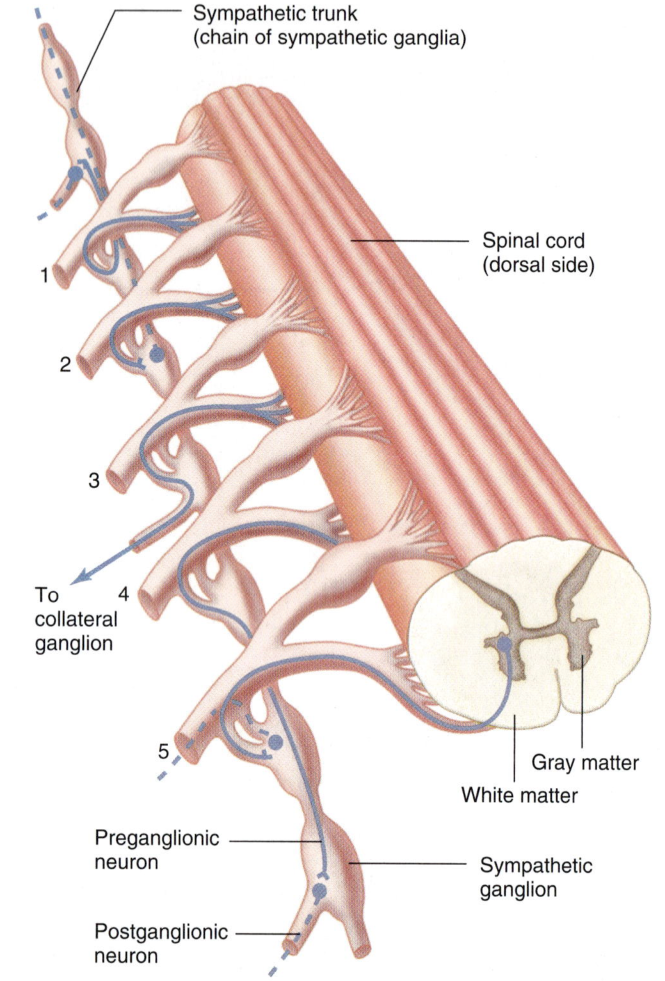

Figure 6.45 AP|R Relationship between a sympathetic trunk and spinal nerves (1 through 5) with the various courses that preganglionic sympathetic neurons (solid lines) take through the sympathetic trunk. Dashed lines represent postganglionic neurons. A mirror image of this exists on the opposite side of the spinal cord.

TABLE 6.10 Locations of Receptors for Acetylcholine, Norepinephrine, and Epinephrine

I. Receptors for acetylcholine
  A. Nicotinic receptors
    1. On postganglionic neurons in the autonomic ganglia
    2. At neuromuscular junctions of skeletal muscle
    3. On some CNS neurons
  B. Muscarinic receptors
    1. On smooth muscle
    2. On cardiac muscle
    3. On gland cells
    4. On some CNS neurons
    5. On some neurons of autonomic ganglia (although the great majority of receptors at this site are nicotinic)

II. Receptors for norepinephrine and epinephrine
  A. On smooth muscle
  B. On cardiac muscle
  C. On gland cells
  D. On other tissue cells (e.g., adipose, bone, renal tubules)
  E. On some CNS neurons

Table 6.11 is a reference list of the effects of autonomic nervous system activity, which will be described in later chapters. Note that the heart and many glands and smooth muscles are innervated by both sympathetic and parasympathetic fibers; that is, they receive **dual innervation.** Whatever effect one division has on the effector cells, the other division usually has the opposite effect. (Several exceptions to this rule are indicated in Table 6.11.) Moreover, the two divisions are usually activated reciprocally; that is, as the activity of one division increases, the activity of the other decreases. Think of this like a person driving a car with one foot on the brake and the other on the

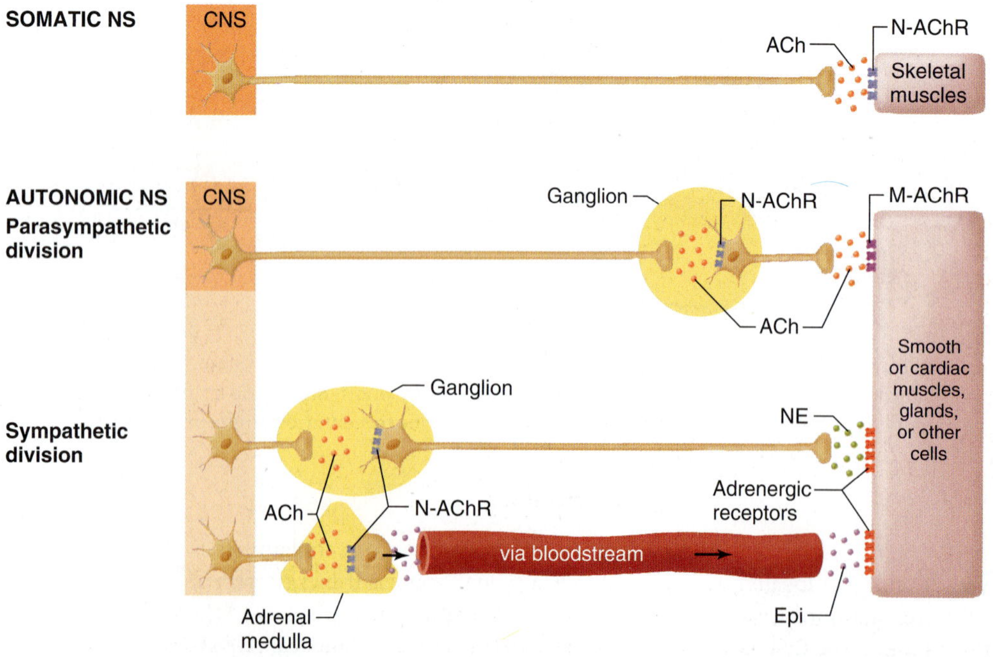

Figure 6.46 Transmitters used in the various components of the peripheral efferent nervous system. Notice that the first neuron exiting the CNS—whether in the somatic or the autonomic nervous system—releases acetylcholine. In a very few cases, postganglionic sympathetic neurons may release a transmitter other than norepinephrine. (ACh, acetylcholine; NE, norepinephrine; Epi, epinephrine; N-AChR, nicotinic acetylcholine receptor; M-AChR, muscarinic acetylcholine receptor)

PHYSIOLOGICAL INQUIRY

- How would the effects differ between a drug that blocks muscarinic acetylcholine receptors and one that blocks nicotinic acetylcholine receptors?

Answer can be found at end of chapter.

TABLE 6.11 Some Effects of Autonomic Nervous System Activity

Effector Organ	Sympathetic Nervous System Effect and Receptor Types*	Parasympathetic Nervous System Effect (All M-ACh Receptors)
Eyes		
Iris muscle	Contracts radial muscle (widens pupil), α_1	Contracts sphincter muscle (makes pupil smaller)
Ciliary muscle	Relaxes (flattens lens for far vision), β_2	Contracts (allows lens to become more convex for near vision)
Heart		
SA node	Increases heart rate, β_1	Decreases heart rate
Atria	Increases contractility, β_1, β_2	Decreases contractility
AV node	Increases conduction velocity, β_1, β_2	Decreases conduction velocity
Ventricles	Increases contractility, β_1, β_2	Decreases contractility slightly
Arterioles		
Coronary	Constricts, α_1, α_2 Dilates, β_2	—†
Skin	Constricts, α_1, α_2	—
Skeletal muscle	Constricts, α_1 Dilates, β_2	—
Abdominal viscera	Constricts, α_1	—
Kidneys	Constricts, α_1	—
Salivary glands	Constricts, α_1, α_2	Dilates
Veins	Constricts, α_1, α_2 Dilates, β_2	—
Lungs		
Bronchial muscle	Relaxes, β_2	Contracts
Salivary glands	Stimulates secretion, α_1 Stimulates enzyme secretion, β_1	Stimulates watery secretion
Stomach		
Motility, tone	Decreases, α_1, α_2, β_2	Increases
Sphincters	Contracts, α_1	Relaxes
Secretion	Inhibits (?)	Stimulates
Intestine		
Motility	Decreases, α_1, α_2, β_1, β_2	Increases
Sphincters	Contracts (usually), α_1	Relaxes (usually)
Secretion	Inhibits, $x\alpha_2$	Stimulates
Gallbladder	Relaxes, β_2	Contracts
Liver	Glycogenolysis and gluconeogenesis, α_1, β_2	—
Pancreas		
Exocrine glands	Inhibits secretion, α	Stimulates secretion
Endocrine glands	Inhibits secretion, α_2 Stimulates secretion, β_2	—
Fat cells	Increases fat breakdown, α_2, β_3	—
Kidneys	Increases renin secretion, β_1	—
Urinary bladder		
Bladder wall	Relaxes, β_2	Contracts
Sphincter	Contracts, α_1	Relaxes
Uterus	Contracts in pregnancy, α_1 Relaxes, β_2	Variable
Reproductive tract (male)	Ejaculation, α_1	Erection
Skin		
Muscles causing hair erection	Contracts, α_1	—
Sweat glands	Secretion from hands, feet, and armpits, α_1 Generalized abundant, dilute secretion, M-AChR	— —
Lacrimal glands	Minor secretion, α_1	Major secretion
Nasopharyngeal glands	—	Secretion

*Note that many effector organs contain both alpha-adrenergic and beta-adrenergic receptors. Activation of these receptors may produce either the same or opposing effects. For simplicity, except for the arterioles and a few other cases, only the dominant sympathetic effect is given when the two receptors oppose each other.

† A dash means these cells are not innervated by this branch of the autonomic nervous system or that these nerves do not play a significant physiological role.

Table adapted from Laurence L. Brunton, John S. Lazo, and Keither L. Parker, eds., *Goodman and Gilman's The Pharmacological Basis of Therapeutics*, 11th ed., McGraw-Hill, New York, 2006.

accelerator. Either depressing the brake (parasympathetic) or relaxing the accelerator (sympathetic) will slow the car. Dual innervation by neurons that cause opposite responses provides a very fine degree of control over the effector organ; this is perhaps one of the most obvious examples of the general principle of physiology that most physiological functions are controlled by multiple regulatory systems, often working in opposition.

A useful generalization is that the sympathetic system increases its activity under conditions of physical or psychological stress. Indeed, a generalized activation of the sympathetic system is called the **fight-or-flight response,** describing the situation of an animal forced to either challenge an attacker or run from it. All resources for physical exertion are activated: heart rate and blood pressure increase; blood flow increases to the skeletal muscles, heart, and brain; the liver releases glucose; and the pupils dilate. Simultaneously, the activity of the gastrointestinal tract and blood flow to it are inhibited by sympathetic firing. In contrast, when the parasympathetic system is activated, a person is in a **rest-or-digest state** in which homeostatic functions are predominant.

The two divisions of the autonomic nervous system rarely operate independently, and autonomic responses generally represent the regulated interplay of both divisions. Autonomic responses usually occur without conscious control or awareness, as though they were indeed autonomous (in fact, the autonomic nervous system has been called the "involuntary" nervous system). However, it is wrong to assume that this is always the case, for some visceral or glandular responses can be learned and thus, to an extent, voluntarily controlled.

A complex pattern of stimulation and desensitization of the nicotinic acetylcholine receptors at autonomic ganglia underlies many of the physiological effects of *nicotine.* At low doses, nicotine activates autonomic ganglia and stimulates the release of catecholamines from the adrenal medulla. The sympathetic components of these pathways dominate control of the cardiovascular system under these conditions, and so heart rate and blood pressure increase. Persistent high blood pressure and increased work on the heart are part of the reason that chronic nicotine use contributes to cardiovascular disease. In the gastrointestinal system, parasympathetic effects tend to dominate, leading to activation of intestinal smooth muscle motor activity. At higher doses of nicotine, brainstem control centers that regulate gastrointestinal functions can be overactivated and vomiting or diarrhea can sometimes occur, especially in individuals who have had little prior nicotine exposure. After initial activation, nicotinic acetylcholine receptors eventually become desensitized by high nicotine doses, which results in depression of all autonomic signaling pathways.

6.19 Blood Supply, Blood–Brain Barrier, and Cerebrospinal Fluid

As mentioned earlier, the brain lies within the skull, and the spinal cord lies within the vertebral column. Between the soft neural tissues and the bones that house them are three types of membranous coverings called **meninges:** the thick **dura mater** next to the bone, the **arachnoid mater** in the middle, and the thin **pia mater** next to the nervous tissue (**Figure 6.47**). The **subarachnoid space** between the arachnoid mater and pia mater is filled with **cerebrospinal fluid** (**CSF**). The meninges and their specialized parts protect and support the CNS, and they circulate and absorb the cerebrospinal fluid. ***Meningitis*** is an infection of the meninges that occurs in the CSF of the subarachnoid space and that can result in increased intracranial pressure, seizures, and loss of consciousness.

Ependymal cells make up a specialized epithelial structure called the **choroid plexus,** which produces CSF at a rate that completely replenishes it about three times per day. The black arrows in Figure 6.47 show the flow of CSF. It circulates through the interconnected ventricular system to the brainstem, where it passes through small openings out to the subarachnoid space surrounding the brain and spinal cord. Aided by circulatory, respiratory, and postural pressure changes, the fluid ultimately flows to the top of the outer surface of the brain, where most of it enters the bloodstream through one-way valves in large veins. CSF can provide important diagnostic information for diseases of the nervous system, such as meningitis. Fluid samples are generally obtained by inserting a large needle into the spinal canal below the level of the second lumbar vertebra, where the spinal cord ends (see Figure 6.42).

Thus, the CNS literally floats in a cushion of cerebrospinal fluid. Because the brain and spinal cord are soft, delicate tissues, they are somewhat protected by this shock-absorbing fluid from sudden and jarring movements. If the outflow is obstructed, cerebrospinal fluid accumulates, causing ***hydrocephalus*** ("water on the brain"). In severe, untreated cases, the resulting elevation of pressure in the ventricles causes compression of the brain's blood vessels, which may lead to inadequate blood flow to the neurons, neuronal damage, and cognitive dysfunction.

Under normal conditions, glucose is the only substrate metabolized by the brain to supply its energy requirements, and most of the energy from the oxidative breakdown of glucose is transferred to ATP. The brain's glycogen stores are negligible, so it depends upon a continuous blood supply of glucose and oxygen. In fact, the most common form of brain damage is caused by a decreased blood supply to a region of the brain. When neurons in the region are without a blood supply and deprived of nutrients and oxygen for even a few minutes, they cease to function and die. This neuronal death, when it results from vascular disease, is called a ***stroke.***

Although the adult brain makes up only 2% of the body weight, it receives 12% to 15% of the total blood supply, which supports its high oxygen utilization. If the blood flow to a region of the brain is reduced to 10% to 25% of its normal level, energy-dependent membrane ion pumps begin to fail, membrane ion gradients decrease, extracellular K^+ concentration increases, and membranes depolarize.

The exchange of substances between blood and extracellular fluid in the CNS is different from the more-or-less unrestricted diffusion of nonprotein substances from blood to extracellular fluid in the other organs of the body. A complex group of **blood–brain barrier** mechanisms closely control both the kinds of substances that enter the extracellular fluid of the brain and the rates at which they enter. These mechanisms minimize the ability of many harmful substances to reach the neurons, but they also reduce the access of some potentially helpful therapeutic drugs.

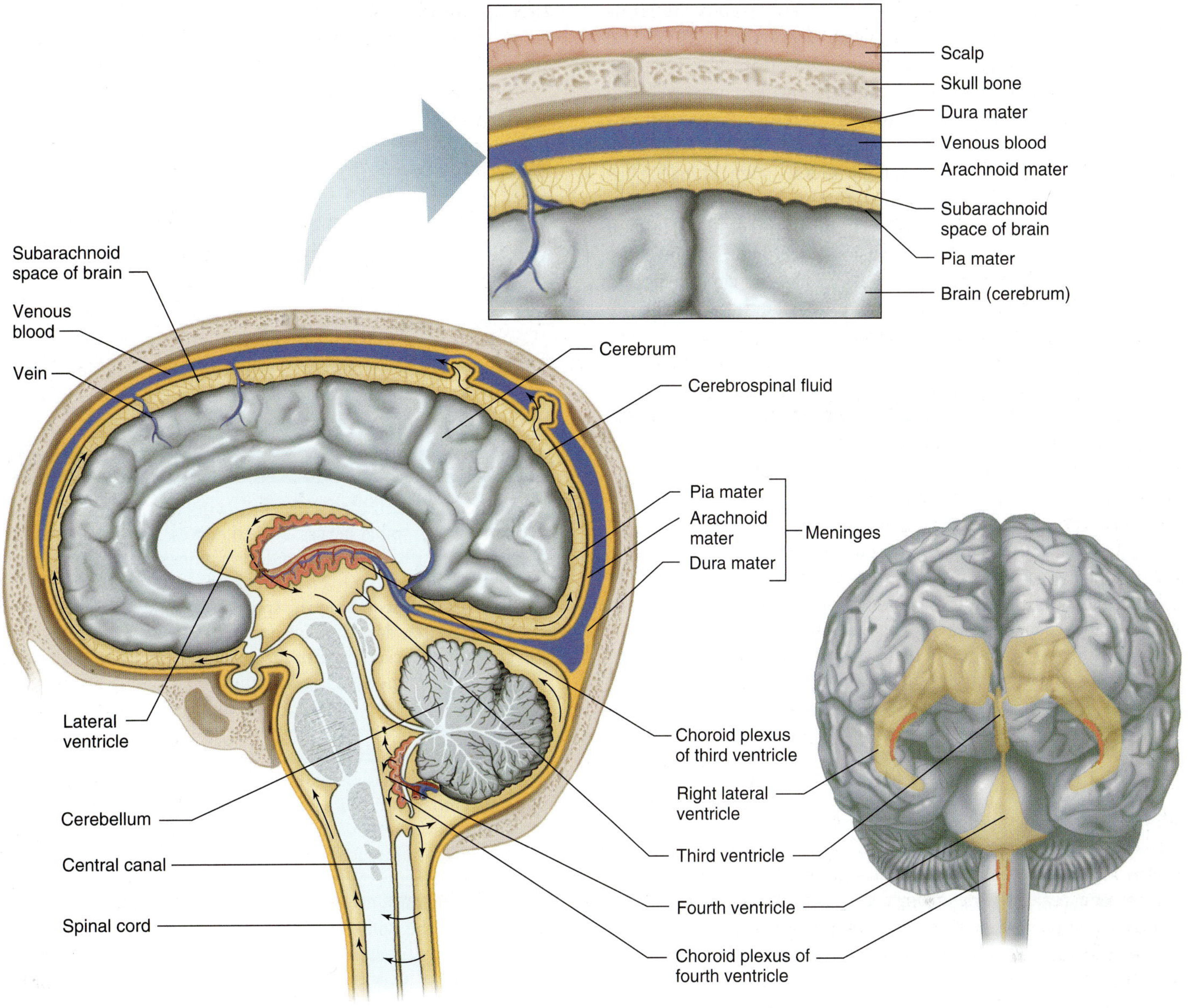

Figure 6.47 APR The four interconnected ventricles of the brain. The lateral ventricles form the first two. The choroid plexus forms the cerebrospinal fluid (CSF), which flows out of the ventricular system at the brainstem (arrows).

The blood–brain barrier is formed by the cells that line the smallest blood vessels in the brain. It has anatomical structures, such as tight junctions, and physiological transport systems that handle different classes of substances in different ways. Substances that dissolve readily in the lipid components of the plasma membranes enter the brain quickly. Therefore, the extracellular fluid of the brain and spinal cord is a product of—but chemically different from—the blood.

The blood–brain barrier accounts for some drug actions, too, as we can see from the following scenario. Morphine differs chemically from heroin only slightly: morphine has two hydroxyl groups, whereas heroin has two acetyl groups (—$COCH_3$). This small difference renders heroin more lipid-soluble and able to cross the blood–brain barrier more readily than morphine. As soon as heroin enters the brain, however, enzymes remove the acetyl groups from heroin and change it to morphine. The morphine, less soluble in lipid, is then effectively trapped in the brain, where it may have prolonged effects. Other drugs that have rapid effects in the CNS because of their high lipid solubility are barbiturates, nicotine, caffeine, and alcohol.

Many substances that do not dissolve readily in lipids, such as glucose and other important substrates of brain metabolism, nonetheless enter the brain quite rapidly by combining with membrane transport proteins in the cells that line the smallest brain blood vessels. Similar transport systems also move substances out of the brain and into the blood, preventing the buildup of molecules that could interfere with brain function.

A barrier is also present between the blood in the capillaries of the choroid plexuses and the cerebrospinal fluid, and cerebrospinal fluid is thus a selective secretion. For example, K^+ and Ca^{2+} concentrations are slightly lower in cerebrospinal fluid than in plasma, whereas the Na^+ and Cl^- concentrations are slightly higher. The choroid plexus vessel walls also have limited permeability to toxic heavy metals such as lead, thus affording a degree of protection to the brain.

The cerebrospinal fluid and the extracellular fluid of the CNS are, over time, in diffusion equilibrium. Thus, the restrictive, selective barrier mechanisms in the capillaries and choroid plexuses regulate the extracellular environment of the neurons of the brain and spinal cord.

SECTION D SUMMARY

Central Nervous System: Brain

I. The brain is divided into six regions: cerebrum, diencephalon, midbrain, pons, medulla oblongata, and cerebellum.

II. The cerebrum, made up of right and left cerebral hemispheres, and the diencephalon together form the forebrain. The cerebral cortex forms the outer shell of the cerebrum and is divided into the parietal, frontal, occipital, and temporal lobes.

III. The diencephalon contains the thalamus and hypothalamus.

IV. The limbic system is a set of deep forebrain structures associated with learning and emotion.

V. The cerebellum plays a role in posture, movement, and some kinds of memory.

VI. The midbrain, pons, and medulla oblongata form the brainstem, which contains the reticular formation.

Central Nervous System: Spinal Cord

I. The spinal cord is divided into two areas: central gray matter, which contains nerve cell bodies and dendrites; and white matter, which surrounds the gray matter and contains myelinated axons organized into ascending or descending tracts.

II. The axons of the afferent and efferent neurons form the spinal nerves.

Peripheral Nervous System

I. The PNS consists of 43 paired nerves—12 pairs of cranial nerves and 31 pairs of spinal nerves, as well as neurons found in the gastrointestinal tract wall. Most nerves contain the axons of both afferent and efferent neurons.

II. The efferent division of the PNS is divided into somatic and autonomic parts. The somatic fibers innervate skeletal muscle cells and release the neurotransmitter acetylcholine.

Autonomic Nervous System

I. The autonomic nervous system innervates cardiac and smooth muscle, glands, gastrointestinal tract neurons, and other tissue cells. Each autonomic pathway consists of a preganglionic neuron with its cell body in the CNS and a postganglionic neuron with its cell body in an autonomic ganglion outside the CNS.

II. The autonomic nervous system is divided into sympathetic and parasympathetic components. Enteric neurons within the walls of the GI tract are also sometimes considered as a separate subcategory of the autonomic system. Preganglionic neurons in both the sympathetic and parasympathetic divisions release acetylcholine; the postganglionic parasympathetic neurons release mainly acetylcholine; and the postganglionic sympathetic neurons release mainly norepinephrine.

III. The adrenal medulla is a hormone-secreting part of the sympathetic nervous system and secretes mainly epinephrine.

IV. Many effector organs that the autonomic nervous system innervates receive dual innervation from the sympathetic and parasympathetic division of the autonomic nervous system.

Blood Supply, Blood–Brain Barrier, and Cerebrospinal Fluid

I. Inside the skull and vertebral column, the brain and spinal cord are enclosed in and protected by the meninges.

II. Brain tissue depends on a continuous supply of glucose and oxygen for metabolism.

III. The brain ventricles and the space within the meninges are filled with cerebrospinal fluid, which is formed in the ventricles.

IV. The blood–brain barrier closely regulates the chemical composition of the extracellular fluid of the CNS.

SECTION D REVIEW QUESTIONS

1. Make an organizational chart showing the CNS, PNS, brain, spinal cord, spinal nerves, cranial nerves, forebrain, brainstem, cerebrum, diencephalon, midbrain, pons, medulla oblongata, and cerebellum.
2. Draw a cross section of the spinal cord showing the gray and white matter, dorsal and ventral roots, dorsal root ganglion, and spinal nerve. Indicate the general locations of pathways.
3. List two functions of the thalamus.
4. List the functions of the hypothalamus, and discuss how they relate to homeostatic control.
5. Make a PNS chart indicating the relationships among afferent and efferent divisions, somatic and autonomic nervous systems, and sympathetic and parasympathetic divisions.
6. Contrast the somatic and autonomic divisions of the efferent nervous system; mention at least three characteristics of each.
7. Name the neurotransmitter released at each synapse or neuroeffector junction in the somatic and autonomic systems.
8. Contrast the sympathetic and parasympathetic components of the autonomic nervous system; mention at least four characteristics of each.
9. Explain how the adrenal medulla can affect receptors on various effector organs despite the fact that its cells have no axons.
10. The chemical composition of the CNS extracellular fluid is different from that of blood. Explain how this difference is achieved.

SECTION D KEY TERMS

adrenal medulla 180
afferent division 178
arachnoid mater 184
autonomic ganglion 180
autonomic nervous system 179
basal ganglia 175
basal nuclei 175
blood–brain barrier 184
brainstem 174
cerebellum 174
cerebral cortex 175
cerebral hemisphere 175
cerebral ventricle 175
cerebrospinal fluid (CSF) 184
cerebrum 174
choroid plexus 184
commissure 174
corpus callosum 175
cranial nerve 177
diencephalon 174
dorsal horn 177
dorsal root 177
dorsal root ganglia 178
dual innervation 182
dura mater 184
efferent division 178
enteric nervous system 180
epithalamus 176
fight-or-flight response 184
forebrain 174
frontal lobe 175
ganglion 174

SECTION D CLINICAL TERMS

CHAPTER 6 Clinical Case Study: A Woman Develops Pain, Visual Problems, and Tingling in Her Legs

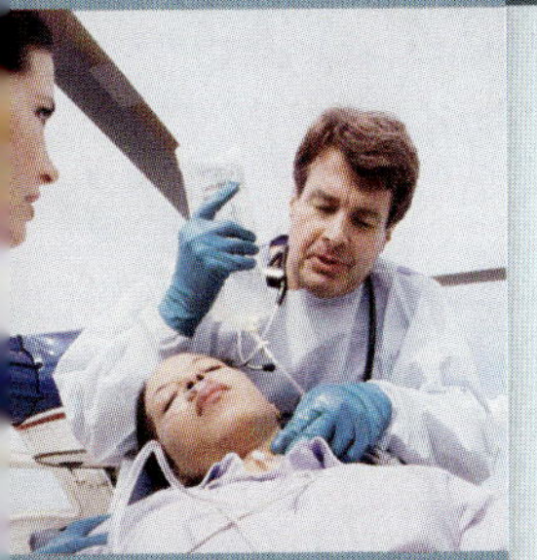

A 37-year-old female visits her doctor because of back pain and numbness and tingling in her legs. Sensory tests also show reduced ability to sense light touch and to feel a pinprick on both legs. X-rays show no abnormalities of the vertebrae or her spinal canal that might obstruct or damage nerve pathways. She is prescribed anti-inflammatory medications and sent home, and her symptoms gradually subside. Three months later, she comes back to the clinic because her symptoms have returned. In addition to back pain and sensory disturbances in her legs, however, she now also reports experiencing double vision when she looks to one side, and persistent dizziness. A sample of her cerebrospinal fluid obtained by lumbar puncture shows the presence of an abnormally high concentration of the disease-fighting proteins called antibodies (see Chapter 18), which suggests excess immune system activity within her CNS. Magnetic resonance imaging (MRI) is used to visualize her nervous system tissues, and several abnormal spots, or lesions, are noted in her mid-thoracic spinal cord, in her brainstem, and near the ventricles of her brain (see Figure 19.6 for an explanation of MRI). Her condition is tentatively diagnosed as multiple sclerosis, which is confirmed when a follow-up MRI performed 4 months later shows an increase in the number and size of lesions in her nervous system.

In the disease ***multiple sclerosis*** (***MS***), a loss of myelin occurs at one or several places in the nervous system. Multiple sclerosis ranks second only to trauma as a cause of neurological disability arising in young and middle-aged adults. It most commonly strikes between the ages of 20 and 50 and twice as often in females as in males. It currently affects approximately 400,000 Americans and as many as 3 million people worldwide. Multiple sclerosis is an autoimmune condition in which the myelin sheaths surrounding axons in the CNS are attacked and destroyed by antibodies and cells of the immune system. The loss of insulating myelin sheaths results in increased leak of K^+ through newly exposed channels. This results in hyperpolarization and failure of action potential conduction of neurons in the brain and spinal cord. Depending upon the location of the affected neurons, symptoms can include muscle weakness, fatigue, decreased motor coordination, slurred speech, blurred or hazy vision, bladder dysfunction, pain or other sensory disturbances, and cognitive dysfunction. In many patients, the symptoms are markedly worsened when body temperature is elevated, for example, by exercise, a hot shower, or hot weather.

The severity and rate of progression of MS vary enormously among individuals, ranging from isolated, episodic attacks with complete recovery in between to steadily progressing neurological disability. In the latter case, MS can ultimately be fatal as brainstem centers responsible for respiratory and cardiovascular function are destroyed. Because of the variability in presentation, diagnosing MS can be difficult. A person having several of these symptoms on two or more occasions separated by more than a month is a candidate for further testing. Nerve-conduction tests can detect slowed or failed action potential conduction in the motor, sensory, and visual systems. Cerebrospinal fluid analysis can reveal the presence of an abnormal immune reaction against myelin. The most definitive evidence, however, is usually the visualization by MRI of multiple, progressive, scarred (sclerotic) areas within the brain and spinal cord, from which this disease derives its name.

The cause of multiple sclerosis is not known, but it appears to result from a combination of genetic and environmental factors. It tends to run in families and is more common among Caucasians than in other racial groups. The involvement of environmental triggers is suggested by occasional clusters of disease outbreaks and also by the observation that the prevalence of MS in people of Japanese descent rises significantly when they move to the United States. Among the suspects for the environmental trigger is infection early in life with a virus, such as those that cause measles, cold sores, chicken pox, or influenza. There is presently no cure for multiple sclerosis, but anti-inflammatory agents and drugs that suppress the immune response have been proven to reduce the severity and slow the progression of the disease.

Clinical term: multiple sclerosis (MS)

See Chapter 19 for complete, integrative case studies.

CHAPTER 6 TEST QUESTIONS

Answers found in Appendix A.

1. Which best describes an afferent neuron?
   a. The cell body is in the CNS and the peripheral axon terminal is in the skin.
   b. The cell body is in the dorsal root ganglion and the central axon terminal is in the spinal cord.
   c. The cell body is in the ventral horn of the spinal cord and the axon ends on skeletal muscle.
   d. The dendrites are in the PNS and the axon terminal is in the dorsal root.
   e. All parts of the cell are within the CNS.

2. Which incorrectly pairs a glial cell type with an associated function?
   a. astrocytes; formation of the blood–brain barrier
   b. microglia; performance of immune function in the CNS
   c. oligodendrocytes; formation of myelin sheaths on axons in the PNS
   d. ependymal cells; regulation of production of cerebrospinal fluid
   e. astrocytes; removal of potassium ions and neurotransmitters from the brain's extracellular fluid

3. If the extracellular Cl^- concentration is 110 mmol/L and a particular neuron maintains an intracellular Cl^- concentration of 4 mmol/L, at what membrane potential would Cl^- be closest to electrochemical equilibrium in that cell?
   a. +80 mV
   b. +60 mV
   c. 0 mV
   d. −86 mV
   e. −100 mV

4. Consider the following five experiments in which the concentration gradient for Na^+ was varied. In which case(s) would Na^+ tend to leak out of the cell if the membrane potential was experimentally held at +42 mV?

Experiment	Extracellular Na^+ (mmol/L)	Intracellular Na^+ (mmol/L)
A	50	15
B	60	15
C	70	15
D	80	15
E	90	15

   a. A only
   b. B only
   c. C only
   d. A, B, and C
   e. D and E

5. Which is a true statement about the resting membrane potential in a typical neuron?
   a. The membrane potential is closer to the Na^+ equilibrium potential than to the K^+ equilibrium potential.
   b. The Cl^- permeability is higher than that for Na^+ or K^+.
   c. The membrane potential is at the equilibrium potential for K^+.
   d. There is no ion movement at the steady resting membrane potential.
   e. Ion movement by the Na^+/K^+-ATPase pump is equal and opposite to the leak of ions through Na^+ and K^+ channels.

6. If a ligand-gated channel permeable to both Na^+ and K^+ was briefly opened at a specific location on the membrane of a typical resting neuron, what would result?
   a. Local currents on the inside of the membrane would flow away from that region.
   b. Local currents on the outside of the membrane would flow away from that region.
   c. Local currents would travel without decrement all along the cell's length.
   d. A brief local hyperpolarization of the membrane would result.
   e. Fluxes of Na^+ and K^+ would be equal, so no local currents would flow.

7. Which ion channel state correctly describes the phase of the action potential it is associated with?
   a. Voltage-gated Na^+ channels are inactivated in a resting neuronal membrane.
   b. Open voltage-gated K^+ channels cause the depolarizing upstroke of the action potential.
   c. Open voltage-gated K^+ channels cause afterhyperpolarization.
   d. The sizable leak through voltage-gated K^+ channels determines the value of the resting membrane potential.
   e. Opening of voltage-gated Cl^- channels is the main factor causing rapid repolarization of the membrane at the end of an action potential.

8. Two neurons, A and B, synapse onto a third neuron, C. If neurotransmitter from A opens ligand-gated channels permeable to Na^+ and K^+ and neurotransmitter from B opens ligand-gated Cl^- channels, which of the following statements is true?
   a. An action potential in neuron A causes a depolarizing EPSP in neuron B.
   b. An action potential in neuron B causes a depolarizing EPSP in neuron C.
   c. Simultaneous action potentials in A and B will cause hyperpolarization of neuron C.
   d. Simultaneous action potentials in A and B will cause less depolarization of neuron C than if only neuron A fired an action potential.
   e. An action potential in neuron B will bring neuron C closer to its action potential threshold than would an action potential in neuron A.

9. Which correctly associates a neurotransmitter with one of its characteristics?
   a. Dopamine is a catecholamine synthesized from the amino acid tyrosine.
   b. Glutamate is released by most inhibitory interneurons in the spinal cord.
   c. Serotonin is an endogenous opioid associated with "runner's high."
   d. GABA is the neurotransmitter that mediates long-term potentiation.
   e. Neuropeptides are synthesized in the axon terminals of the neurons that release them.

10. Which of these synapses does not have acetylcholine as its primary neurotransmitter?
   a. synapse of a postganglionic parasympathetic neuron onto a heart cell
   b. synapse of a postganglionic sympathetic neuron onto a smooth muscle cell
   c. synapse of a preganglionic sympathetic neuron onto a postganglionic neuron
   d. synapse of a somatic efferent neuron onto a skeletal muscle cell
   e. synapse of a preganglionic sympathetic neuron onto adrenal medullary cells

CHAPTER 6 GENERAL PRINCIPLES ASSESSMENT

Answers found in Appendix A.

1. One of the general principles of physiology introduced in Chapter 1 is, *Most physiological functions are controlled by multiple regulatory systems, often working in opposition.* How do the structure and function of the autonomic nervous system demonstrate this principle?
2. What general principles of physiology are demonstrated by the mechanisms underlying neuronal resting membrane potentials?
3. Another general principle of physiology states, *Structure is a determinant of—and has coevolved with—function.* A common theme in humans and other organisms is elaboration of surface area of a structure to maximize its ability to perform some function. What structures of the human nervous system demonstrate this principle?

CHAPTER 6 QUANTITATIVE AND THOUGHT QUESTIONS

Answers found at www.mhhe.com/widmaier13.

1. Neurons are treated with a drug that instantly and permanently stops the Na^+/K^+-ATPase pumps. Assume for this question that the pumps are not electrogenic. What happens to the resting membrane potential immediately and over time?
2. Extracellular K^+ concentration in a person is increased with no change in intracellular K^+ concentration. What happens to the resting potential and the action potential?
3. A person has received a severe blow to the head but appears to be all right. Over the next week, however, he develops loss of appetite, thirst, and loss of sexual capacity but no loss in sensory or motor function. What part of the brain do you think may have been damaged?
4. A person is taking a drug that causes, among other things, dryness of the mouth and speeding of the heart rate but no impairment of the ability to use the skeletal muscles. What type of receptor does this drug probably block? (Table 6.11 will help you answer this.)
5. Some cells are treated with a drug that blocks Cl^- channels, and the membrane potential of these cells becomes slightly depolarized (less negative). From these facts, predict whether the plasma membrane of these cells actively transports Cl^- and, if so, in what direction.
6. If the enzyme acetylcholinesterase was blocked with a drug, what malfunctions would occur in the heart and skeletal muscle?
7. The compound tetraethylammonium (TEA) blocks the voltage-gated changes in K^+ permeability that occur during an action potential. After experimental treatment of neurons with TEA, what changes would you expect in the action potential? In the afterhyperpolarization?
8. A resting neuron has a membrane potential of −80 mV (determined by Na^+ and K^+ gradients), there are no Cl^- pumps, the cell is slightly permeable to Cl^-, and ECF $[Cl^-]$ is 100 mM. What is the intracellular $[Cl^-]$?

CHAPTER 6 ANSWERS TO PHYSIOLOGICAL INQUIRIES

Figure 6.8 If the electrodes were reversed, the graph would start at 0 mV as before, but when the electrode was inserted the potential difference recorded would jump to +70 mV rather than −70 mV.

Figure 6.10 NaCl and KCl ionize in solution virtually completely, so initially each compartment would have a total solute concentration of approximately 0.3 osmols per liter (see Chapter 4 to review the difference between moles and osmols). Because an insignificant number of potassium ions actually move in establishing the equilibrium potential, the final solute concentrations of the compartments would not be significantly different.

Figure 6.11 Na^+ and K^+ would move down their concentration gradients in opposite directions, each canceling charge carried by the other. Thus, at equilibrium, there would be no membrane potential and both compartments would have 0.15 M Cl^-, 0.075 M Na^+, and 0.075 M K^+.

Figure 6.12 No. Changing the ECF [K^+] has a greater effect on E_K (and thus the resting membrane potential). This is because the ratio of external to internal K^+ is changed more when ECF concentration goes from 5 to 6 mM (a 20% increase) than when ICF concentration is decreased from 150 to 149 mM (a 0.7% decrease). You can confirm this with the Nernst equation. Inserting typical values, when $[K_{out}] = 5$ mM and $[K_{in}] = 150$ mM, the calculated value of $E_K = -90.1$ mV. If you change $[K_{in}]$ to 149 mM, the calculated value of $E_K = -89.9$ mV, which is not very different. By comparison, changing $[K_{out}]$ to 6 mM causes a greater change, with the resulting $E_K = -85.3$ mV.

Figure 6.15 Because the exit of K^+ from the cell would make the inside of the cell more negative in the area of the channel, positive current would flow toward the channel's location on the inside of the cell and away from the channel on the outside. The graph would simply be inverted; there would be hyperpolarization at the initial site of the channel, which would be smaller in magnitude at increasing distances from the site.

Figure 6.19 The value of the resting potential would change very little because the permeability of resting membranes to Na^+ is very low. However, during an action potential, the membrane voltage would rise more steeply and reach a more positive value due to the larger electrochemical gradient for Na^+ entry through open voltage-gated channels.

Figure 6.23 In all of the neurons, action potentials will propagate in both directions from the elbow—up the arm toward the spinal cord and down the arm toward the hand. Action potentials traveling upward along afferent pathways will continue through synapses into the CNS to be perceived as pain, tingling, vibration, and other sensations of the lower arm. In contrast, action potential signals traveling backward up motor axons will die out once they reach the cell bodies because synapses found there are "one way" in the opposite direction.

Figure 6.31 The greater the distance between the synapse and the initial segment (the location of the electrode), the greater the decrement of a graded potential. Therefore, if synapse A were closer to the axon hillock than synapse C, summing the two would most likely result in a small depolarizing potential. The farther from the hillock synapse C is, the more closely the depolarization would come to resemble the trace occurring in response to synapse A firing alone.

Figure 6.46 The muscarinic receptor blocker would only inhibit parasympathetic pathways, where acetylcholine released from postganglionic neurons binds to muscarinic receptors on target organs. This would reduce the ability to stimulate "rest-or-digest" processes and leave the sympathetic "fight-or-flight" response intact. On the other hand, a nicotinic acetylcholine receptor blocker would inhibit all autonomic control of target organs because those receptors are found at the ganglion in both parasympathetic and sympathetic pathways.

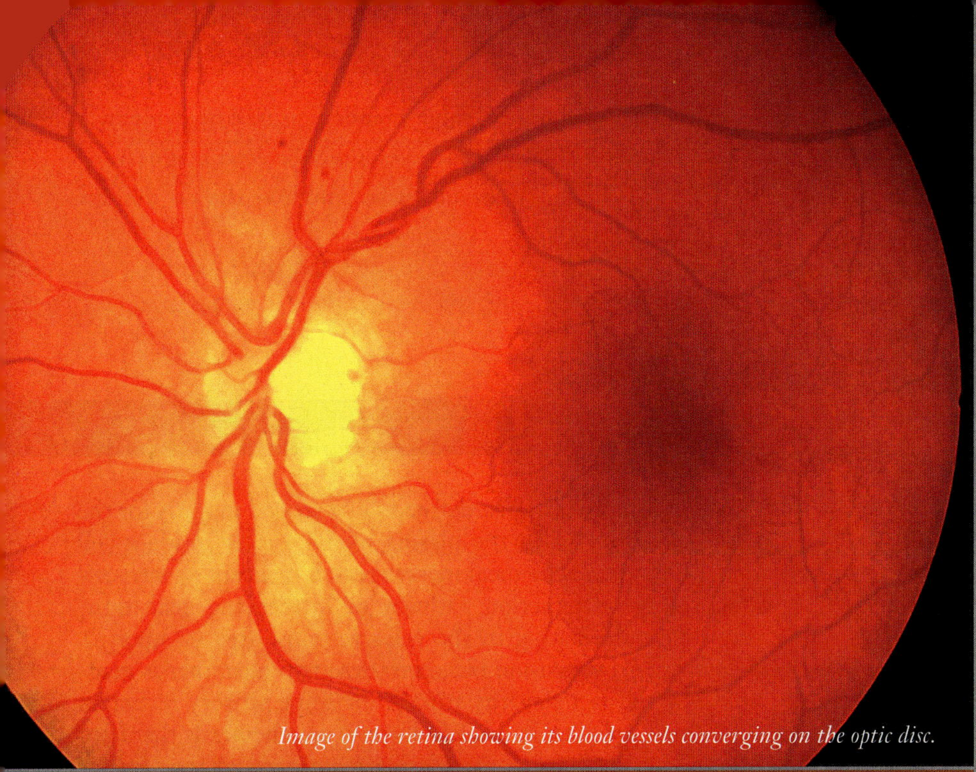

Image of the retina showing its blood vessels converging on the optic disc.

7 Sensory Physiology

Chapter 6 provided an overview of the structure and function of the nervous system, and explained in detail how electrical signals are generated and transmitted by excitable membranes. It also generally described two functional divisions of the nervous system: the afferent division, by which the CNS receives information, and the efferent division, which transmits outgoing commands. In this chapter, you will learn in more detail about the structure and function of sensory systems comprising the afferent division of the nervous system. In addition, you will learn how those systems help maintain homeostasis by providing the CNS with information about conditions in the external and internal environments. Such information is communicated to the CNS from the skin, muscles, and viscera as well as from the visual, auditory, vestibular, and chemical sensory systems.

A number of general principles of physiology will be evident in this discussion of sensory systems. One is that information flow between cells, tissues and organs is an essential feature of homeostasis that allows for integration of physiological processes. Sensory systems gather information in the form of various physical and chemical stimuli and convert those stimuli into action potentials that are conducted to integrating centers for processing. An amazing variety of examples of the relationship between structure and function will be apparent in the form of specialized receptors that allow the different sensory systems to detect specific types of stimuli, such as pressure, light, or airborne chemicals. An understanding of some simple laws of chemistry and physics is important for appreciating how some stimuli are detected and encoded, as will be evident in the discussions of how the eye detects electromagnetic radiation of particular wavelengths, and how the ear detects sound waves.

SECTION A

General Principles

A **sensory system** is a part of the nervous system that consists of sensory receptors that receive stimuli from the external or internal environment, the neural pathways that conduct information from the receptors to the brain or spinal cord, and those parts of the brain that deal primarily with processing the information. Information that a sensory system processes may or may not lead to conscious awareness of the stimulus. For example, whereas you would immediately notice a change when leaving an air-conditioned house on a hot summer day, your blood pressure can fluctuate significantly without your awareness. Regardless of whether the information reaches consciousness, it is called **sensory information.** If the information does reach consciousness, it can also be called a **sensation.** A person's awareness of the sensation (and, typically, understanding of its meaning) is called **perception.** For example, feeling pain is a sensation, but awareness that a tooth hurts is a perception. Sensations and perceptions occur after the CNS modifies or processes sensory information. This processing can accentuate, dampen, or otherwise filter sensory afferent information.

The initial step of sensory processing is the transduction of stimulus energy first into graded potentials—the receptor potentials—and then into action potentials in afferent neurons. The pattern of action potentials in particular neurons is a code that provides information about the stimulus such as its intensity, its location, and the specific type of input that is being sensed. Primary sensory areas of the central nervous system that receive this input then communicate with other regions of the brain or spinal cord in further processing of the information, which may include determination of reflexive efferent responses, perception, storage into memory, comparison with past memories, and assignment of emotional significance.

7.1 Sensory Receptors

Information about the external world and about the body's internal environment exists in different forms—pressure, temperature, light, odorants, sound waves, chemical concentrations, and so on. **Sensory receptors** at the peripheral ends of afferent neurons change this information into graded potentials that can initiate action potentials, which travel into the central nervous system. The receptors are either specialized endings of the primary afferent neurons themselves (**Figure 7.1a**) or separate receptor cells (some of which are actually specialized neurons) that signal the primary afferent neurons by releasing neurotransmitters (**Figure 7.1b**).

To avoid confusion, be aware that the term *receptor* has two completely different meanings. One meaning is that of "sensory receptor," as just defined. The second usage is for the individual proteins in the plasma membrane or inside a cell that bind specific chemical messengers, triggering an intracellular signal transduction pathway or influencing gene transcription, culminating in the cell's response (see Chapter 5). The potential confusion between these two meanings is magnified by the fact that the stimuli for some sensory receptors (e.g., those involved in taste and smell) are chemicals that bind to receptor proteins in the plasma membrane of the sensory receptor. If you are in doubt as to which meaning is intended, add the modifier "sensory" or "protein" to see which makes sense in the context.

The energy or chemical that impinges upon and activates a sensory receptor is known as a **stimulus.** There are many types of sensory receptors, each of which responds much more readily to one form of stimulus than to others. The type of stimulus to which a particular receptor responds in normal functioning is known as its **adequate stimulus.** In addition, within the general stimulus type that serves as a receptor's adequate stimulus, a particular receptor may respond best (i.e., at lowest threshold) to a limited subset of stimuli. For example, different individual receptors in the eye respond best to light (the adequate stimulus) of different wavelengths.

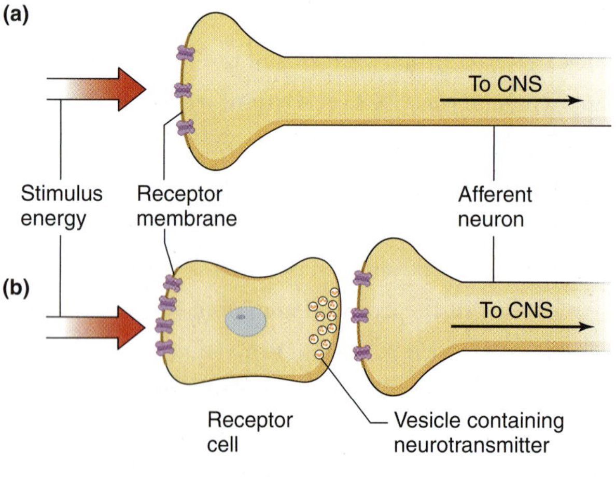

Figure 7.1 Schematic diagram of two types of sensory receptors. The sensitive membrane region that responds to a stimulus is either (a) an ending of an afferent neuron or (b) on a separate cell adjacent to an afferent neuron. Ion channels (shown in purple) on the receptor membrane alter ion flux and initiate stimulus transduction. Note that in some cases the stimulus (red arrows) does not act directly on ion channels but activates them indirectly through mechanisms specific to that sensory system.

Most sensory receptors are exquisitely sensitive to their specific adequate stimulus. For example, some olfactory receptors respond to as few as three or four odor molecules in the inspired air, and visual receptors can respond to a single photon, the smallest quantity of light.

Virtually all sensory receptors, however, can be activated by different types of stimuli if the intensity is sufficient. For example, the receptors of the eye normally respond to light, but they can be activated by an intense mechanical stimulus. For example, a poke in the eye can result in "seeing stars"—the sensation of *light* is still perceived even though the photoreceptors are stimulated by a mechanical stimulus. Regardless of how the receptor is stimulated, any given receptor gives rise to only one sensation.

Several general classes of receptors are characterized by the type of stimulus to which they are sensitive. As the name indicates, **mechanoreceptors** respond to mechanical stimuli, such as pressure or stretch, and are responsible for many types of sensory information, including touch, blood pressure, and muscle tension. These stimuli alter the permeability of ion channels on the receptor membrane, changing the membrane potential. **Thermoreceptors** detect sensations of cold or warmth, and **photoreceptors** respond to particular ranges of light wavelengths. **Chemoreceptors** respond to the binding of particular chemicals to the receptor membrane. This type of receptor provides the senses of smell and taste and detects blood pH and oxygen concentration. **Nociceptors** are a general category of detectors that sense pain due to actual or potential tissue damage. They can be activated by a variety of stimuli such as heat, mechanical stimuli like excess stretch, or chemical substances in the extracellular fluid of damaged tissues.

The Receptor Potential

Regardless of the original form of the signal that activates sensory receptors, the information must be translated into the language of graded potentials or action potentials. The process by which a stimulus—a photon of light, say, or the mechanical stretch of a tissue—is transformed into an electrical response is known as **sensory transduction.** The transduction process in all sensory receptors involves the opening or closing of ion channels that receive information about the internal and external world, either directly or through a second-messenger system. The ion channels are present in a specialized region of the receptor membrane located at the distal tip of the cell's single axon or on associated specialized sensory cells (see Figure 7.1). The gating of these ion channels allows a change in ion flux across the receptor membrane, which in turn produces a change in the membrane potential. This change is a graded potential called a **receptor potential.** (See Figure 6.16 to review the general properties of graded potentials.) The different mechanisms that affect ion channels in the various types of sensory receptors are described throughout this chapter.

In afferent neurons with specialized receptor tips, the receptor membrane region where the initial ion channel changes occur does not generate action potentials. Instead, local current flows a short distance along the axon to a region where the membrane has voltage-gated ion channels and can generate action potentials. In myelinated afferent neurons, this region is usually at the first node of Ranvier. The receptor potential, like the synaptic potential discussed in Chapter 6, is a graded response to different stimulus intensities (**Figure 7.2**) and diminishes as it travels along the membrane.

If the receptor membrane is on a separate cell, the receptor potential there alters the release of neurotransmitter from that cell. The neurotransmitter diffuses across the extracellular cleft between the receptor cell and the afferent neuron and binds to receptor proteins on the afferent neuron. Thus, this junction is a synapse. The combination of neurotransmitter with its binding sites generates a graded potential in the afferent neuron analogous to either an excitatory postsynaptic potential or, in some cases, an inhibitory postsynaptic potential.

As is true of all graded potentials, the magnitude of a receptor potential (or a graded potential in the axon adjacent to the receptor cell) decreases with distance from its origin. However, if the amount of depolarization at the first excitable patch of membrane in the afferent neuron (e.g., at the first node of Ranvier)

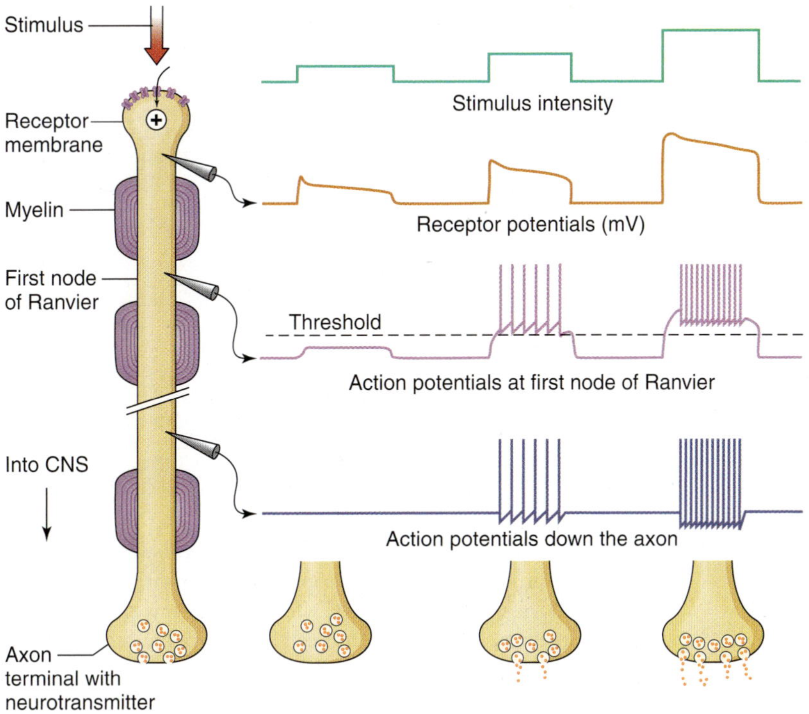

Figure 7.2 Stimulation of an afferent neuron with a receptor ending. Electrodes measure graded potentials and action potentials at various points in response to different stimulus intensities. Action potentials arise at the first node of Ranvier in response to a suprathreshold stimulus, and the action potential frequency and neurotransmitter release increase as the stimulus and receptor potential become larger.

PHYSIOLOGICAL INQUIRY

- How would this afferent pathway be affected by exposing this entire neuron to a drug that blocks voltage-gated Ca^{2+} channels?

Answer can be found at end of chapter.

is large enough to bring the membrane to threshold, action potentials are initiated, which then propagate along the afferent neuron (see Figure 7.2).

As long as the receptor potential keeps the afferent neuron depolarized to a level at or above threshold, action potentials continue to fire and propagate along the afferent neuron. Moreover, an increase in the graded potential magnitude causes an increase in the action potential frequency in the afferent neuron (up to the limit imposed by the neuron's refractory period) and an increase in neurotransmitter release at the afferent neuron's central axon terminal (see Figure 7.2). Although the magnitude of the receptor potential determines the *frequency* of the action potentials, it does not determine the *amplitude* of those action potentials. Factors that control the magnitude of the receptor potential include stimulus strength, rate of change of stimulus strength, temporal summation of successive receptor potentials (see Figure 6.31), and a process called adaptation.

Adaptation is a decrease in receptor sensitivity, which results in a decrease in action potential frequency in an afferent neuron despite the continuous presence of a stimulus. Degrees of adaptation vary widely among different types of sensory receptors (**Figure 7.3**). **Slowly adapting receptors** maintain a persistent or slowly decaying receptor potential during a constant stimulus, initiating action potentials in afferent neurons for the duration of the stimulus. These receptors are common in systems sensing parameters that need to be constantly monitored, such as joint and muscle receptors that participate in the maintenance of steady postures. Conversely, **rapidly adapting receptors** generate a receptor potential and action potentials at the onset of a stimulus but very quickly cease responding. Adaptation may be so rapid that only a single action potential is generated. Some rapidly adapting receptors only initiate action potentials at the onset of a stimulus—a so-called "on response"—whereas others respond with a burst at the beginning of the stimulus and again upon its removal—called "on–off responses." Rapidly adapting receptors are important for monitoring sensory stimuli that move or change quickly (like receptors in the skin that sense vibration) and those that persist but do not need to be monitored closely (like receptors that detect the pressure of a chair only when you first sit down).

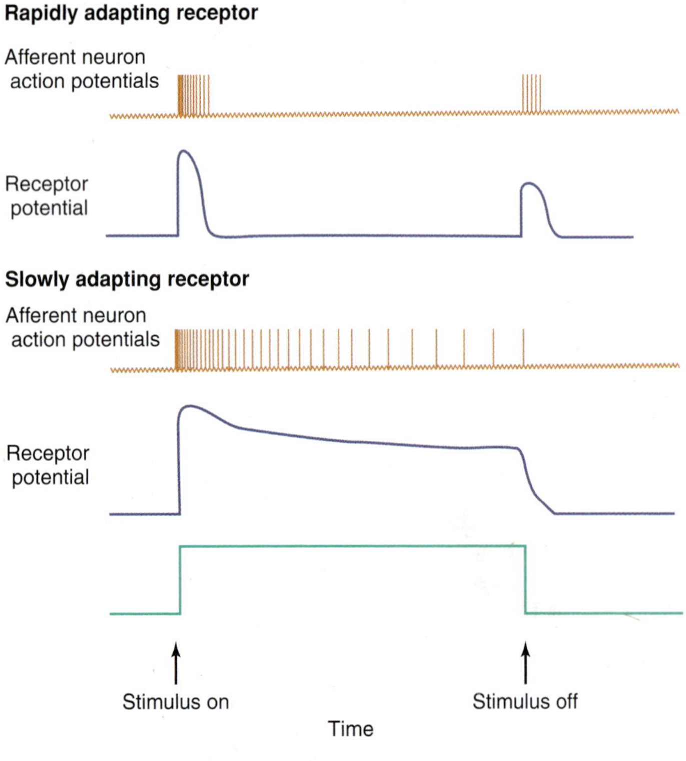

Figure 7.3 Responses of slowly adapting and rapidly adapting receptors to a prolonged, constant stimulus. Rapidly adapting receptors respond only briefly before adapting to a constant stimulus, whereas slowly adapting receptors have persistent receptor potentials and afferent neuronal action potentials. The rapidly adapting receptor shown has an "off response" at the end of the stimulus, which is not always the case.

7.2 Primary Sensory Coding

Coding is the conversion of stimulus energy into a signal that conveys the relevant sensory information to the central nervous system. Important characteristics of a stimulus include the type of input it represents, its intensity, and the location of the body it affects. Coding begins at the receptive neurons in the peripheral nervous system.

A single afferent neuron with all its receptor endings makes up a **sensory unit.** In a few cases, the afferent neuron has a single receptor, but generally the peripheral end of an afferent neuron divides into many fine branches, each terminating with a receptor.

The area of the body that leads to activity in a particular afferent neuron when stimulated is called the **receptive field** for that neuron (**Figure 7.4**). Receptive fields of neighboring afferent neurons usually overlap so that stimulation of a single point activates several sensory units. Thus, activation of

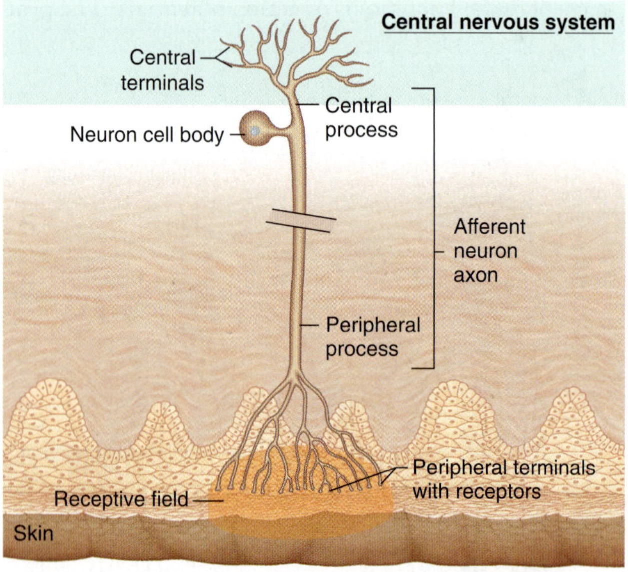

Figure 7.4 A sensory unit including the location of sensory receptors, the processes reaching peripherally and centrally from the cell body, and the terminals in the CNS. Also shown is the receptive field of this neuron. Afferent neuron cell bodies are located in dorsal root ganglia of the spinal cord for sensory inputs from the body and cranial nerve ganglia for sensory inputs from the head.

a single sensory unit almost never occurs. As we will see, the degree of overlap varies in different parts of the body.

Stimulus Type

Another term for stimulus type (heat, cold, sound, or pressure, for example) is stimulus **modality.** Modalities can be divided into submodalities. Cold and warm are submodalities of temperature, whereas salty, sweet, bitter, and sour are submodalities of taste. The type of sensory receptor a stimulus activates plays the primary role in coding the stimulus modality.

As mentioned earlier, a given receptor type is particularly sensitive to one stimulus modality—the adequate stimulus—because of the signal transduction mechanisms and ion channels incorporated in the receptor's plasma membrane. For example, receptors for vision contain pigment molecules whose shapes are transformed by light, which in turn alters the activity of membrane ion channels and generates a receptor potential. In contrast, receptors in the skin do not have light-sensitive pigment molecules, so they cannot respond to light.

All the receptors of a single afferent neuron are preferentially sensitive to the same type of stimulus; for example, they are all sensitive to cold or all to pressure. Adjacent sensory units, however, may be sensitive to different types of stimuli. Because the receptive fields for different modalities overlap, a single stimulus, such as an ice cube on the skin, can simultaneously give rise to the sensations of touch and temperature.

Stimulus Intensity

How do we distinguish a strong stimulus from a weak one when the information about both stimuli is relayed by action potentials that are all the same amplitude? The frequency of action potentials in a single afferent neuron is one way, because increased stimulus strength means a larger receptor potential, and this in turn leads to more frequent action potentials (review Figure 7.2).

As the strength of a local stimulus increases, receptors on adjacent branches of an afferent neuron are activated, resulting in a summation of their local currents. **Figure 7.5** shows an experiment in which increased stimulus intensity to the receptors of a sensory unit is reflected in increased action potential frequency in its afferent neuron.

In addition to increasing the firing frequency in a single afferent neuron, stronger stimuli usually affect a larger area and activate similar receptors on the endings of *other* afferent neurons. For example, when you touch a surface lightly with a finger, the area of skin in contact with the surface is small, and only the receptors in that skin area are stimulated. Pressing down firmly increases the area of skin stimulated. This "calling in" of receptors on additional afferent neurons is known as **recruitment.**

Stimulus Location

A third type of information to be signaled is the location of the stimulus—in other words, where the stimulus is being applied. It should be noted that in vision, hearing, and smell, stimulus location is interpreted as arising from the site from which the stimulus originated rather than the place on our body where the stimulus was actually applied. For example, we interpret the sight and sound of a barking dog as arising from the dog in the yard rather than in a specific region of our eyes and ears. We will have more to say about this later; we deal here with the senses in which the stimulus is localized to a site on the body.

Stimulus location is coded by the site of a stimulated receptor, as well as by the fact that action potentials from each

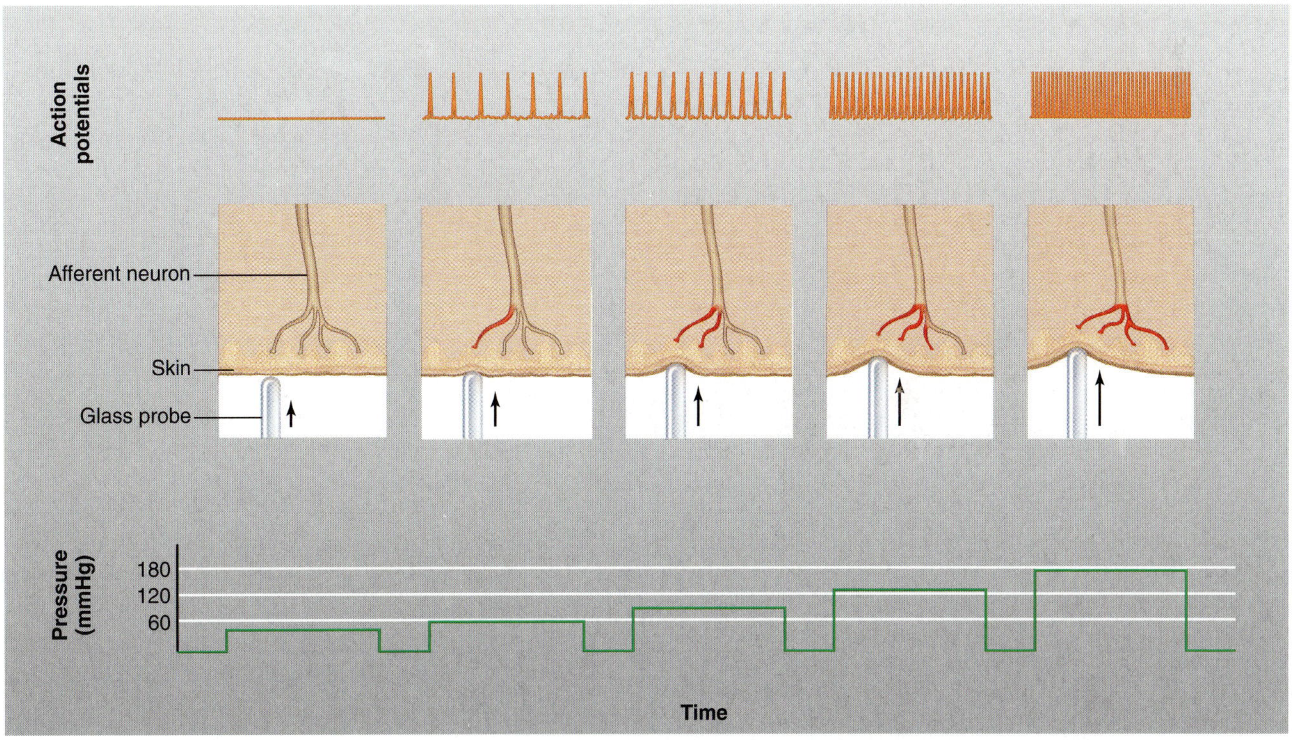

Figure 7.5 Action potentials in an afferent fiber leading from the pressure receptors of a slowly adapting, single sensory unit increase in frequency as more branches of the afferent neuron are stimulated by pressures of increasing magnitude.

receptor travel along unique pathways to a specific region of the CNS associated only with that particular modality and body location. These distinct anatomical pathways are sometimes referred to as **labeled lines.** The precision, or **acuity,** with which we can locate and discern one stimulus from an adjacent one depends upon the amount of convergence of neuronal input in the specific ascending pathways. The greater the convergence, the less the acuity. Other factors affecting acuity are the size of the receptive field covered by a single sensory unit (**Figure 7.6a**), the density of sensory units, and the amount of overlap in nearby receptive fields. For example, it is easy to discriminate between two adjacent stimuli (two-point discrimination) applied to the skin on your lips, where the sensory units are small and numerous, but it is harder to do so on the back, where the relatively few sensory units are large and widely spaced (**Figure 7.6b**). Locating sensations from internal organs is less precise than from the skin because there are fewer afferent neurons in the internal organs and each has a larger receptive field.

It is fairly easy to see why a stimulus to a neuron that has a small receptive field can be located more precisely than a stimulus to a neuron with a large receptive field (see Figure 7.6). However, more subtle mechanisms also exist that allow us to localize distinct stimuli within the receptive field of a single neuron. In some cases, receptive field overlap aids stimulus localization even though, intuitively, overlap would seem to "muddy" the image. In the next few paragraphs, we will examine how this works.

An afferent neuron responds most vigorously to stimuli applied at the center of its receptive field because the receptor density—that is, the number of its receptor endings in a given area—is greatest there. The response decreases as the stimulus is moved toward the receptive field periphery. Thus, a stimulus activates more receptors and generates more action potentials in its associated afferent neuron if it occurs at the center of the receptive field (point A in **Figure 7.7**). The firing frequency of the afferent neuron is also related to stimulus strength, however. Thus, a high frequency of impulses in the single afferent nerve fiber of Figure 7.7 could mean either that a moderately intense stimulus was applied to the center at point A or that a stronger stimulus was applied near the periphery at point B. Therefore, neither the intensity nor the location of the stimulus can be detected precisely with a single afferent neuron.

Because the receptor endings of different afferent neurons overlap, however, a stimulus will trigger activity in more than one sensory unit. In **Figure 7.8,** neurons A and C, stimulated near the edges of their receptive fields where the receptor density is low, fire action potentials less frequently than does neuron B, stimulated at the center of its receptive field. A high action potential frequency in neuron B occurring

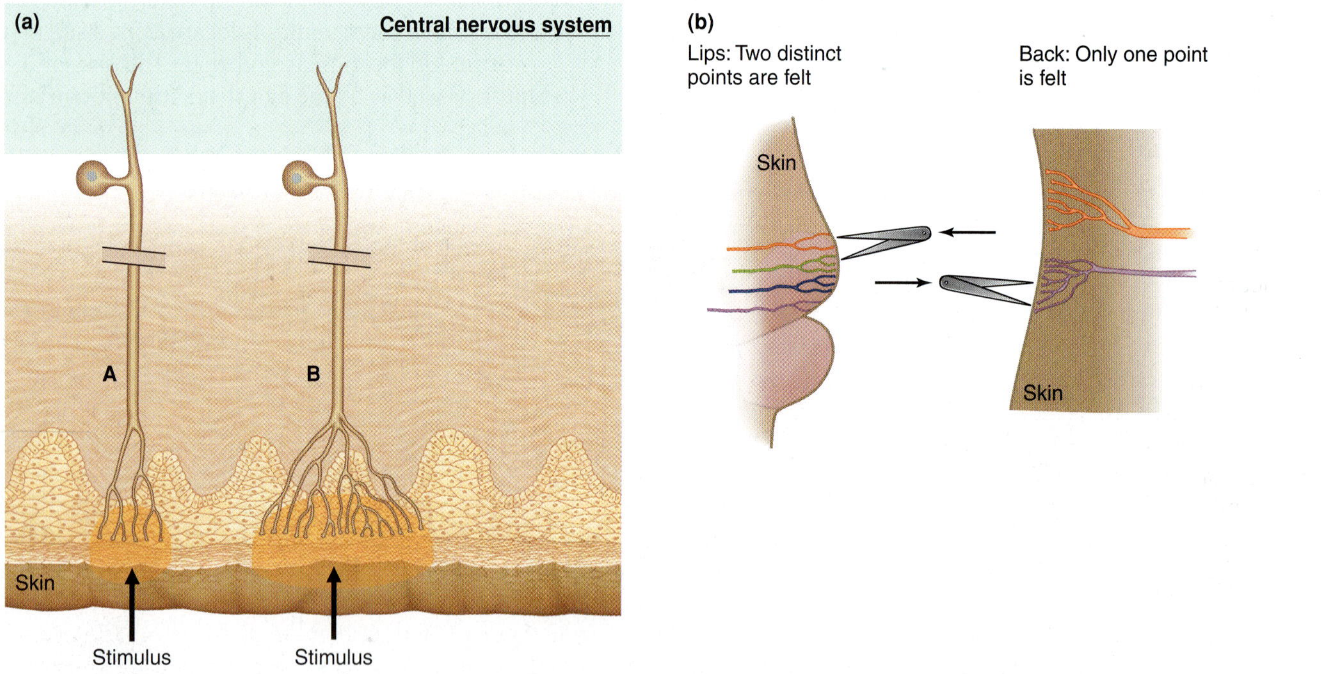

Figure 7.6 The influence of sensory unit size and density on acuity. (a) The information from neuron A indicates the stimulus location more precisely than does that from neuron B because A's receptive field is smaller. (b) Two-point discrimination is finer on the lips than on the back, due to the lips' numerous sensory units with small receptive fields.

PHYSIOLOGICAL INQUIRY

- Referring to part (b) of the figure, make a prediction about the relative size of the brain region devoted to processing lip sensations versus that for the brain region that processes sensations from the skin of your back.

Answer can be found at end of chapter.

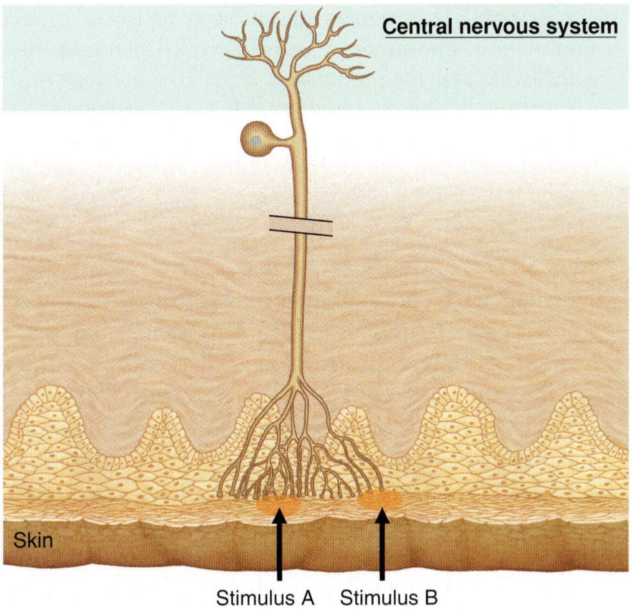

Figure 7.7 Two stimulus points, A and B, in the receptive field of a single afferent neuron. The density of receptor terminals around area A is greater than around B, so the frequency of action potentials in response to a stimulus in area A will be greater than the response to a similar stimulus in B.

simultaneously with lower frequencies in A and C provides the brain with a more accurate localization of the stimulus near the center of neuron B's receptive field. Once this location is known, the brain can interpret the firing frequency of neuron B to determine stimulus intensity.

Lateral Inhibition

The phenomenon of **lateral inhibition** is an important mechanism enabling the localization of a stimulus site for some sensory systems. In lateral inhibition, information from afferent neurons whose receptors are at the edge of a stimulus is strongly inhibited compared to information from the stimulus's center. **Figure 7.9** shows one neuronal arrangement that accomplishes lateral inhibition. The afferent neuron in the center (B) has a higher initial firing frequency than do the neurons on either side (A and C). The number of action potentials transmitted in the lateral pathways is further decreased by inhibitory inputs from inhibitory interneurons stimulated by the central neuron. Although the lateral afferent neurons (A and C) also exert inhibition on the central pathway, their lower initial firing frequency has a smaller inhibitory effect on the central pathway. Thus, lateral inhibition enhances the *contrast* between the center and periphery of a stimulated region, thereby increasing the brain's ability to localize a sensory input. Lateral inhibition can occur at different levels in the sensory pathways but typically happens at an early stage.

Lateral inhibition can be demonstrated by pressing the tip of a pencil against your finger. With your eyes closed, you can localize the pencil point precisely, even though the region around the pencil tip is also indented, activating mechanoreceptors within this region (**Figure 7.10**). Exact localization is possible because lateral inhibition removes the information from the peripheral regions.

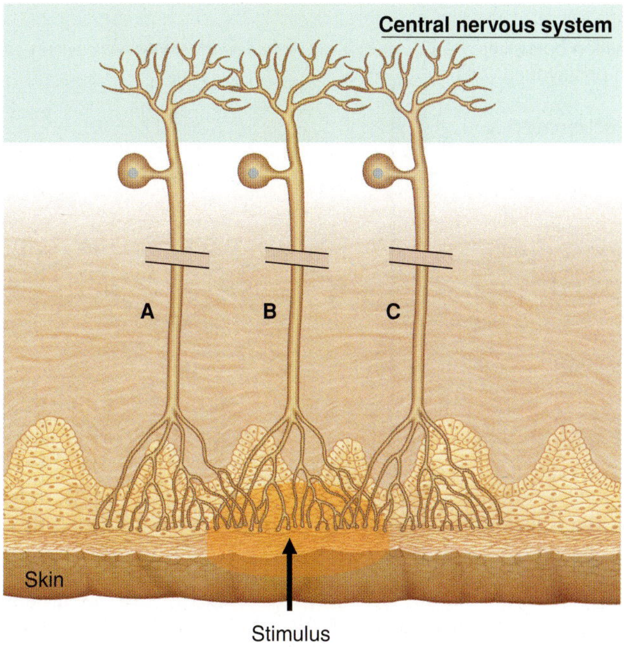

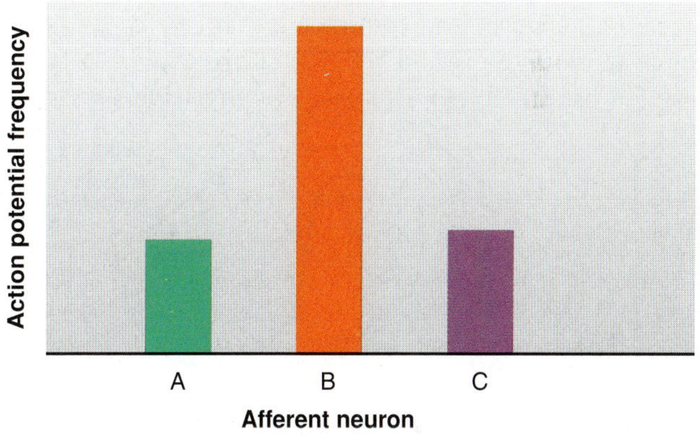

Figure 7.8 A stimulus point falls within the overlapping receptive fields of three afferent neurons. Note the difference in receptor response (i.e., the action potential frequency in the three neurons) due to the difference in receptor distribution under the stimulus (fewer receptor endings for A and C than for B).

Lateral inhibition is utilized to the greatest degree in the pathways providing the most accurate localization. For example, lateral inhibition within the retina of the eye creates amazingly sharp visual acuity, and skin hair movements are also well-localized due to lateral inhibition between parallel pathways ascending to the brain. On the other hand, neuronal pathways carrying temperature and pain information do not have significant lateral inhibition, so we locate these stimuli relatively poorly.

Central Control of Afferent Information

All sensory signals are subject to extensive modification at the various synapses along the sensory pathways before they reach higher levels of the central nervous system. Inhibition from collaterals from other ascending neurons (e.g., lateral inhibition) reduces or even abolishes much of the incoming information, as can inhibitory pathways descending from higher

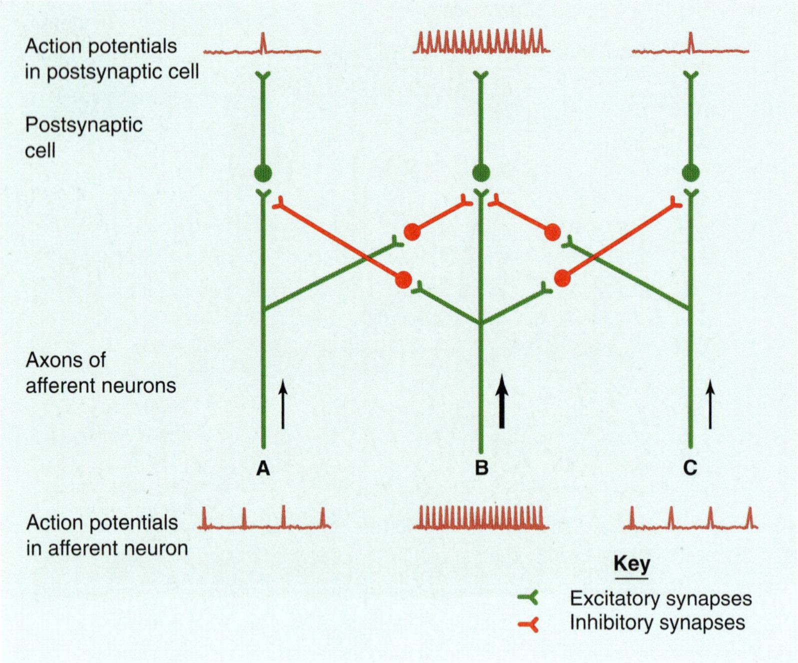

Figure 7.9 Afferent pathways showing lateral inhibition. Three sensory units have overlapping receptive fields. Because the central fiber B at the beginning of the pathway (bottom of figure) is firing at the highest frequency, it inhibits the lateral neurons (via inhibitory interneurons) to a greater extent than the lateral neurons inhibit the central pathway.

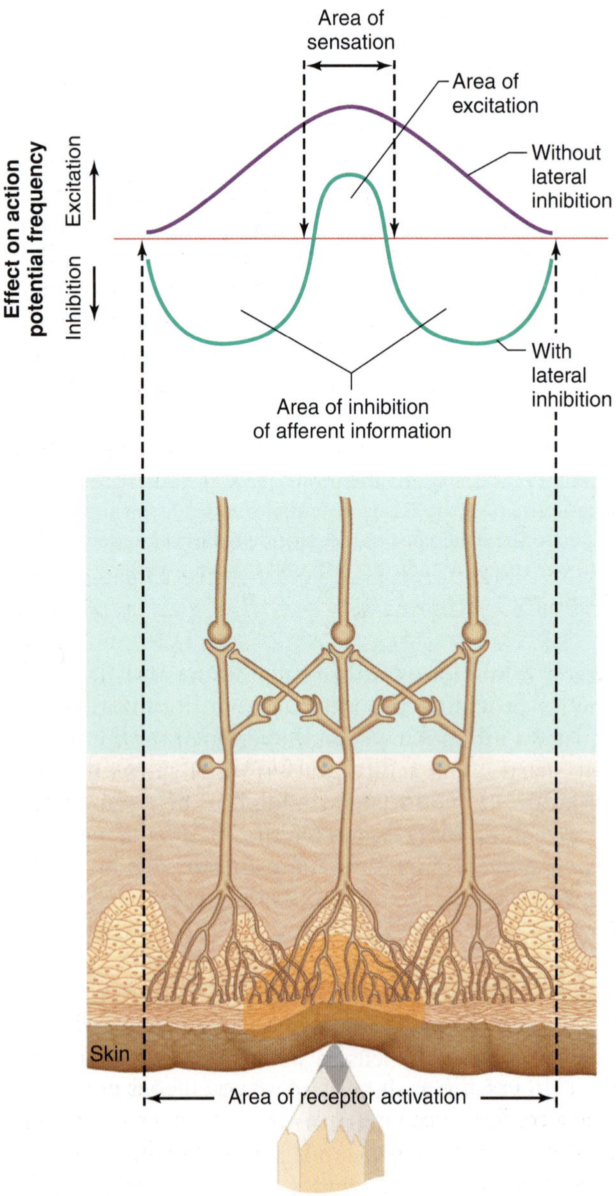

Figure 7.10 A pencil tip pressed against the skin activates receptors under the pencil tip and in the adjacent tissue. The sensory unit under the tip inhibits additional stimulated units at the edge of the stimulated area. Lateral inhibition produces a central area of excitation surrounded by an area in which the afferent information is inhibited. The sensation is localized to a more restricted region than that in which all three units are actually stimulated.

centers in the brain. The reticular formation and cerebral cortex (see Chapter 6), in particular, control the input of afferent information via descending pathways. The inhibitory controls may be exerted directly by synapses on the axon terminals of the primary afferent neurons (an example of presynaptic inhibition) or indirectly via interneurons that affect other neurons in the sensory pathways (**Figure 7.11**).

In some cases, for example, in the pain pathways, the afferent input is continuously inhibited to some degree. This provides the flexibility of either removing the inhibition, so as to allow a greater degree of signal transmission, or increasing the inhibition, so as to block the signal more completely.

Therefore, the sensory information that reaches the brain is significantly modified from the basic signal originally transduced into action potentials at the sensory receptors. The neuronal pathways within which these modifications take place are described next.

7.3 Ascending Neural Pathways in Sensory Systems

Afferent **sensory pathways** are generally formed by chains of three or more neurons connected by synapses. These chains of neurons travel in bundles of parallel pathways carrying information into the central nervous system. Some pathways terminate in parts of the cerebral cortex responsible for conscious recognition of the incoming information; others carry information not consciously perceived. Sensory pathways are also called **ascending pathways** because they project "up" to the brain.

The central processes of the afferent neurons enter the brain or spinal cord and synapse upon interneurons there. The central processes may diverge to terminate on several, or many, interneurons (**Figure 7.12a**) or converge so that the processes of many afferent neurons terminate upon a single interneuron (**Figure 7.12b**). The interneurons upon which the afferent neurons synapse are called second-order neurons, and these in turn synapse with third-order neurons, and so on, until the information (coded action potentials) reaches the cerebral cortex.

Most sensory pathways convey information about only a single type of sensory information. For example, one pathway conveys information only from mechanoreceptors, whereas another is influenced by information only from thermoreceptors. This allows the brain to distinguish the different types of sensory information even though all of it is being transmitted by essentially the same signal, the action potential. The ascending pathways in the spinal cord and brain that carry information about single types of stimuli are known as the **specific ascending pathways.** The specific ascending pathways pass to the brainstem and thalamus, and the final neurons in the pathways go from there to specific sensory areas of the cerebral cortex (**Figure 7.13**). (The olfactory pathways do not send pathways to the thalamus, instead sending some branches directly to the olfactory cortex and others to the limbic system.) For the most part, the specific pathways cross to the side of the central nervous system that is opposite to the location of their sensory receptors. Thus, information from receptors on the right side of the body is transmitted to the left cerebral hemisphere, and vice versa.

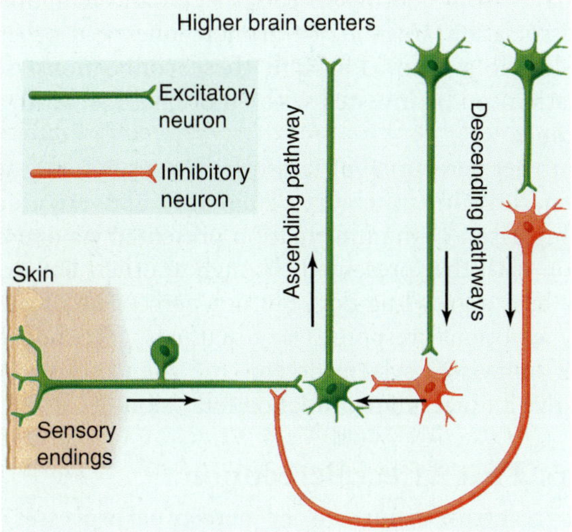

Figure 7.11 Descending pathways may influence sensory information by directly inhibiting the central terminals of the afferent neuron (an example of presynaptic inhibition) or via an interneuron that affects the ascending pathway by inhibitory synapses. Arrows indicate the direction of action potential transmission.

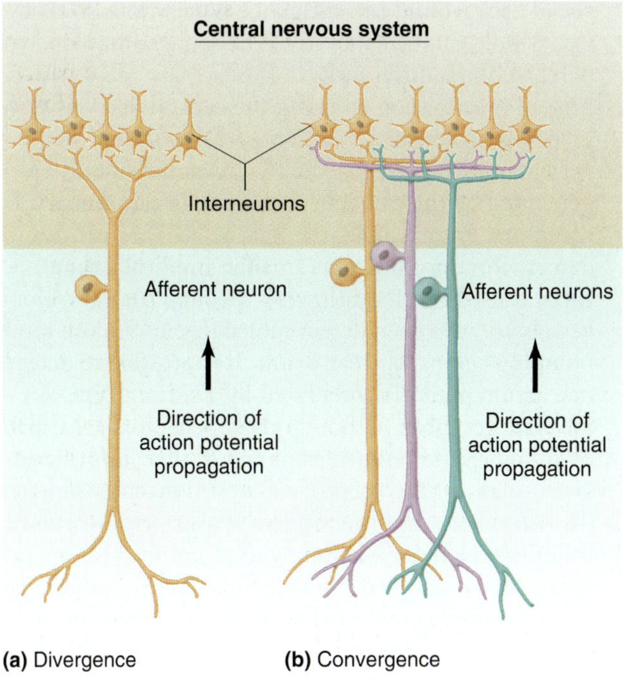

Figure 7.12 (a) Divergence of an afferent neuron onto many interneurons. (b) Convergence of input from several afferent neurons onto single interneurons.

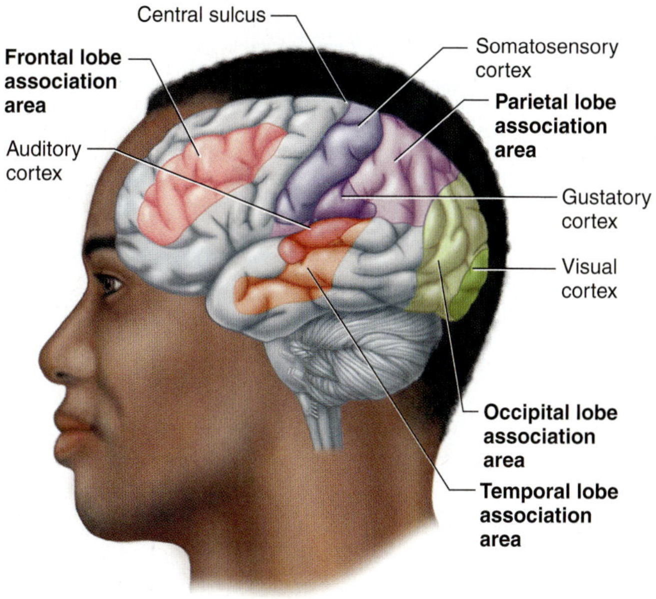

Figure 7.13 AP|R Primary sensory areas and areas of association cortex. The olfactory cortex is located toward the midline on the undersurface of the frontal lobes (not visible in this picture).

The specific ascending pathways that transmit information from somatic receptors project to the somatosensory cortex. **Somatic receptors** are those carrying information from the skin, skeletal muscle, bones, tendons, and joints. The **somatosensory cortex** is a strip of cortex that lies in the parietal lobe of the brain just posterior to the **central sulcus,** which separates the parietal and frontal lobes (see Figure 7.13). The specific ascending pathways from the eyes connect to a different primary cortical receiving area, the **visual cortex,** which is in the occipital lobe. The specific ascending pathways from the ears go to the **auditory cortex,** which is in the temporal lobe. Specific ascending pathways from the taste buds pass to the **gustatory cortex** adjacent to the region of the somatosensory cortex where information from the face is processed. The pathways serving olfaction project to portions of the limbic system and the **olfactory cortex,** which is located on the undersurface of the frontal and temporal lobes. Finally, the processing of afferent information does not end in the primary cortical receiving areas but continues from these areas to association areas in the cerebral cortex where complex integration occurs.

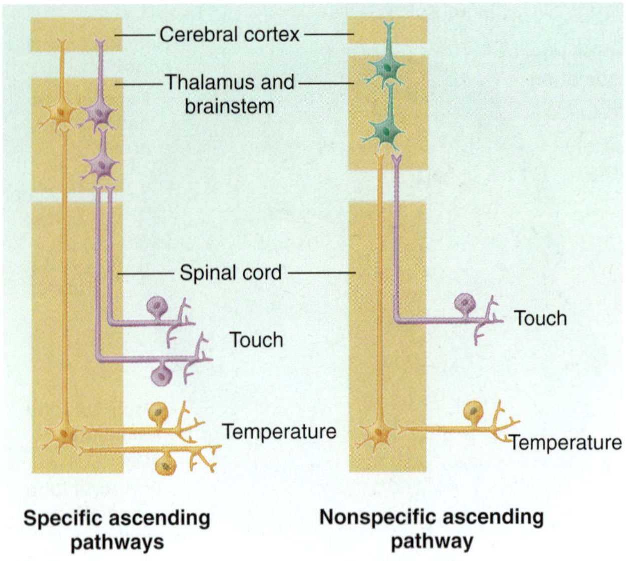

Figure 7.14 Diagrammatic representation of two specific ascending sensory pathways and a nonspecific ascending sensory pathway.

In contrast to the specific ascending pathways, neurons in the **nonspecific ascending pathways** are activated by sensory units of several different types and therefore signal general information (**Figure 7.14**). In other words, they indicate that *something* is happening, without specifying just what or where. A given ascending neuron in a nonspecific ascending pathway may respond, for example, to input from several afferent neurons, each activated by a different stimulus, such as maintained skin pressure, heating, and cooling. Such pathway neurons are called **polymodal neurons.** The nonspecific ascending pathways, as well as collaterals from the specific ascending pathways, end in the brainstem reticular formation and regions of the thalamus and cerebral cortex that are not highly discriminative but are important in controlling alertness and arousal.

7.4 Association Cortex and Perceptual Processing

The **cortical association areas** presented in Figure 7.13 lie outside the primary cortical sensory or motor areas but are adjacent to them. The cortical association areas are not considered part of the sensory pathways, but they play a role in the progressively more complex analysis of incoming information.

Although neurons in the earlier stages of the sensory pathways are necessary for perception, information from the primary sensory cortical areas undergoes further processing after it is relayed to a cortical association area. The region of association cortex closest to the primary sensory cortical area processes the information in fairly simple ways and serves basic sensory-related functions. Regions farther from the primary sensory areas process the information in more complicated ways. These include, for example, greater contributions from areas of the brain serving arousal, attention, memory, and language. Some of the neurons in these latter regions also integrate input concerning two or more types of sensory stimuli. Thus, an association area neuron receiving input from both the visual cortex and the "neck" region of the somatosensory cortex may integrate visual information with sensory information about head position. In this way, for example, a viewer understands a tree is vertical even if the viewer's head is tipped sideways.

Axons from neurons of the parietal and temporal lobes go to association areas in the frontal lobes and other parts of the limbic system. Through these connections, sensory information can be invested with emotional and motivational significance.

Further perceptual processing involves not only arousal, attention, learning, memory, language, and emotions but also comparison of the information presented via one type of sensation with that presented through another. For example, we may hear a growling dog, but our perception of the event and our emotional response vary markedly, depending upon whether our visual system detects the sound source to be a nearby live animal or an animal on television.

Factors That Affect Perception

We put great trust in our sensory–perceptual processes despite the inevitable modifications we know the nervous system makes. Several factors are known to affect our perceptions of the real world:

1. Sensory receptor mechanisms (e.g., adaptation) and processing of the information along afferent pathways can influence afferent information.
2. Factors such as emotions, personality, experience, and social background can influence perceptions so that two people can be exposed to the same stimuli and yet perceive them differently.
3. Not all information entering the central nervous system gives rise to conscious sensation. Actually, this is a very good thing because many unwanted signals are generated by the extreme sensitivity of our sensory receptors. For example, the hair cells of the ear can detect vibrations having a smaller amplitude than those caused by blood flowing through the ears' blood vessels and can even detect molecules in random motion bumping against the ear drum. It is possible to detect one action potential generated by a certain type of mechanoreceptor. Although these receptors are capable of giving rise to sensations, much of their information is canceled out by receptor or central mechanisms to be discussed later. In other afferent pathways, information is not canceled out—it simply does not feed into parts of the brain that give rise to a conscious sensation. To use an example cited earlier, stretch receptors in the walls of some of the largest blood vessels monitor blood pressure as part of reflex regulation of this pressure, but people usually do not have a conscious awareness of their blood pressure.

4. We lack suitable receptors for many types of potential stimuli. For example, we cannot directly detect ionizing radiation or radio waves.
5. Damaged neural networks may give faulty perceptions as in the phenomenon known as ***phantom limb***, in which a limb lost by accident or amputation is experienced as though it were still in place. The missing limb is perceived to be the site of tingling, touch, pressure, warmth, itch, wetness, pain, and even fatigue. It seems that the sensory neural networks in the central nervous system that are normally triggered by receptor activation are, instead, activated independently of peripheral input. The activated neural networks continue to generate the usual sensations, which the brain perceives as arising from the missing receptors.
6. Some drugs alter perceptions. In fact, the most dramatic examples of a clear difference between the real world and our perceptual world can be found in drug-induced hallucinations.
7. Various types of mental illness can alter perceptions of the world, like the hallucinations that can occur in the disease ***schizophrenia*** (discussed in detail in Chapter 8).

In summary, for perception to occur, there can be no separation of the three processes involved—transducing stimuli into action potentials by the receptor, transmitting information through the nervous system, and interpreting those inputs. Sensory information is processed at each synapse along the afferent pathways and at many levels of the central nervous system, with the more complex stages receiving input only after the more elementary systems have processed the information. This hierarchical processing of afferent information along individual pathways is an important organizational feature of sensory systems. As we will see, a second important feature is that information is processed by *parallel* pathways, each of which handles a limited aspect of the neural signals generated by the sensory transducers. A third feature is that information at each stage along the pathway is modified by "top-down" influences serving the emotions, attention, memory, and language. Every synapse along the afferent pathway adds an element of organization and contributes to the sensory experience so that what we perceive is not a simple—or even an absolutely accurate—image of the stimulus that originally activated our receptors.

We conclude our introduction to sensory system pathways and coding with a summary of the general principles of sensory stimulus processing (**Table 7.1**). In the next section, we will take a detailed look at mechanisms involved in specific sensory systems.

TABLE 7.1 Summary of General Principles of Sensory Stimulus Processing

Stimulus Feature	Stimulus Processing
Modality	The structure of specific sensory receptor types allows them to best detect certain modalities and submodalities. General classes of receptor types include mechanoreceptors, thermoreceptors, photoreceptors, and chemoreceptors. The type of stimulus that specifically activates a given receptor is called that receptor's adequate stimulus. Information in sensory pathways is organized such that initial cortical processing of the various modalities occurs in different parts of the brain.
Duration	Detecting stimulus duration occurs in two general ways, determined by a receptor property called adaptation. Some sensory receptors respond and generate receptor potentials the entire time that a stimulus is applied (slowly adapting, or tonic receptors), while others respond only briefly when a stimulus is first applied and sometimes again when the stimulus is removed (rapidly adapting, or phasic receptors).
Intensity	Sensory receptor potential amplitude tends to be graded according to the size of the stimulus applied, but action potential amplitude does not change with stimulus intensity. Rather, increasing stimulus intensity is encoded by the activation of increasing numbers of sensory neurons (recruitment) and by an increase in the frequency of action potentials propagated along sensory pathways.
Location	Stimuli of a given modality from a particular region of the body generally travel along dedicated, specific neural pathways to the brain, referred to as labeled lines. The acuity with which a stimulus can be localized depends on the size and density of receptive fields in each body region. A synaptic processing mechanism called lateral inhibition enhances localization as sensory signals travel through the CNS. Most specific ascending pathways synapse in the thalamus on the way to the cerebral cortex after crossing the midline, such that sensory information from the right side of the body is generally processed on the left side of the brain, and vice versa.
Sensation and perception	A consciously perceived stimulus is referred to as a sensation, and awareness of a stimulus combined with understanding of its meaning is called perception. This higher processing of sensory information occurs in association areas of the cerebral cortex.

SECTION A SUMMARY

I. Sensory processing begins with the transformation of stimulus energy into graded potentials and then into action potentials in neurons.

II. Information carried in a sensory system may or may not lead to a conscious awareness of the stimulus.

Sensory Receptors

I. Receptors translate information from the external and internal environments into graded potentials.
   a. Receptors may be either specialized endings of afferent neurons or separate cells that form synapses with the afferent neurons.
   b. Receptors respond best to one form of stimulus, but they may respond to other forms if the stimulus intensity is abnormally high.
   c. Regardless of how a specific receptor is stimulated, activation of that receptor can only lead to perception of one type of sensation. However, not all receptor activations lead to conscious sensations.

II. The transduction process in all sensory receptors involves—either directly or indirectly—the opening or closing of ion channels in the receptor. Ions then flow across the membrane, causing a receptor potential.
   a. Receptor potential magnitude and action potential frequency increase as stimulus strength increases.
   b. Receptor potential magnitude varies with stimulus strength, rate of change of stimulus application, temporal summation of successive receptor potentials, and adaptation.

Primary Sensory Coding

I. The type of stimulus perceived is determined in part by the type of receptor activated. All receptors of a given sensory unit respond to the same stimulus modality.

II. Stimulus intensity is coded by the rate of firing of individual sensory units and by the number of sensory units activated.

III. Localization of a stimulus depends on the size of the receptive field covered by a single sensory unit and on the overlap of nearby receptive fields. Lateral inhibition is a means by which ascending pathways increase sensory acuity.

IV. Information coming into the nervous system is subject to modification by both ascending and descending pathways.

Ascending Neural Pathways in Sensory Systems

I. A single afferent neuron with all its receptor endings is a sensory unit.
   a. Afferent neurons, which usually have more than one receptor of the same type, are the first neurons in sensory pathways.
   b. The receptive field for a neuron is the area of the body that causes activity in a sensory unit or other neuron in the ascending pathway of that unit.

II. Neurons in the specific ascending pathways convey information about only a single type of stimulus to specific primary receiving areas of the cerebral cortex.

III. Nonspecific ascending pathways convey information from more than one type of sensory unit to the brainstem reticular formation and regions of the thalamus that are not part of the specific ascending pathways.

Association Cortex and Perceptual Processing

I. Information from the primary sensory cortical areas is elaborated after it is relayed to a cortical association area.
   a. The primary sensory cortical area and the region of association cortex closest to it process the information in fairly simple ways and serve basic sensory-related functions.
   b. Regions of association cortex farther from the primary sensory areas process the sensory information in more complicated ways.
   c. Processing in the association cortex includes input from areas of the brain serving other sensory modalities, arousal, attention, memory, language, and emotions.

SECTION A REVIEW QUESTIONS

1. Distinguish between a sensation and a perception.
2. Define the term *adequate stimulus.*
3. Describe the general process of transduction in a receptor that is a cell separate from the afferent neuron. Include in your description the following terms: *specificity*, *stimulus*, *receptor potential*, *synapse*, *neurotransmitter*, *graded potential*, and *action potential.*
4. List several ways in which the magnitude of a receptor potential can vary.
5. Differentiate between the function of rapidly adapting and slowly adapting receptors.
6. Describe the relationship between sensory information processing in the primary cortical sensory areas and in the cortical association areas.
7. List several ways in which sensory information can be distorted.
8. How does the nervous system distinguish between stimuli of different types?
9. How does the nervous system code information about stimulus intensity?
10. Describe the general mechanism of lateral inhibition and explain its importance in sensory processing.
11. Make a diagram showing how a specific ascending pathway relays information from peripheral receptors to the cerebral cortex.

SECTION A KEY TERMS

acuity 196
adaptation 194
adequate stimulus 192
ascending pathway 198
auditory cortex 199
central sulcus 199
chemoreceptor 193
coding 194
cortical association area 200
gustatory cortex 199
labeled lines 196
lateral inhibition 197
mechanoreceptor 193
modality 195
nociceptor 193
nonspecific ascending pathway 200
olfactory cortex 199
perception 192
photoreceptor 193
polymodal neuron 200
rapidly adapting receptor 194
receptive field 194
receptor potential 193
recruitment 195
sensation 192
sensory information 192
sensory pathway 198
sensory receptor 192
sensory system 192
sensory transduction 193
sensory unit 194
slowly adapting receptor 194
somatic receptor 199
somatosensory cortex 199
specific ascending pathway 199
stimulus 192
thermoreceptor 193
visual cortex 199

SECTION A CLINICAL TERMS

phantom limb 201
schizophrenia 201

SECTION **B**

Specific Sensory Systems

7.5 Somatic Sensation

Sensation from the skin, skeletal muscles, bones, tendons, and joints—**somatic sensation**—is initiated by a variety of sensory receptors collectively called somatic receptors (**Figure 7.15**). Some of these receptors respond to mechanical stimulation of the skin, hairs, and underlying tissues, whereas others respond to temperature or chemical changes. Activation of somatic receptors gives rise to the sensations of touch, pressure, awareness of the position of the body parts and their movement, temperature, and pain. The receptors for visceral sensations, which arise in certain organs of the thoracic and abdominal cavities, are the same types as the receptors that give rise to somatic sensations. Some organs, such as the liver, have no sensory receptors at all. Each sensation is associated with a specific receptor type. In other words, distinct receptors exist for heat, cold, touch, pressure, limb position or movement, and pain.

Touch and Pressure

Stimulation of different types of mechanoreceptors in the skin (see Figure 7.15) leads to a wide range of touch and pressure experiences—hair bending, deep pressure, vibrations, and superficial touch, for example. These mechanoreceptors are highly specialized neuron endings encapsulated in elaborate cellular structures. The details of the mechanoreceptors vary, but, in general, the neuron endings are linked to networks of collagen fibers within a capsule that is often filled with fluid. These networks transmit the mechanical tension in the fluid-filled capsule to ion channels in the neuron endings and activate them.

The skin mechanoreceptors adapt at different rates. About half of them adapt rapidly, firing only when the stimulus is changing. Other types of mechanoreceptors adapt more slowly. Activation of rapidly adapting receptors gives rise to the sensations of touch, movement, and vibration, whereas slowly adapting receptors give rise to the sensation of pressure.

In both categories, some receptors have small, well-defined receptive fields and can provide precise information about the contours of objects indenting the skin. As might be expected, these receptors are concentrated at the fingertips. In contrast, other receptors have large receptive fields with obscure boundaries, sometimes covering a whole finger or a large part of the palm. These receptors are not involved in detailed spatial discrimination but signal information about skin stretch and joint movement.

Senses of Posture and Movement

The senses of posture and movement are complex. The major receptors responsible for these senses are the muscle-spindle stretch receptors and Golgi tendon organs. These mechanoreceptors occur in skeletal muscles and the fibrous tendons that connect them to bone. Muscle-spindle stretch receptors respond both to the absolute magnitude of muscle stretch and to the rate at which the stretch occurs, and Golgi tendon organs monitor muscle tension (both of these receptors are

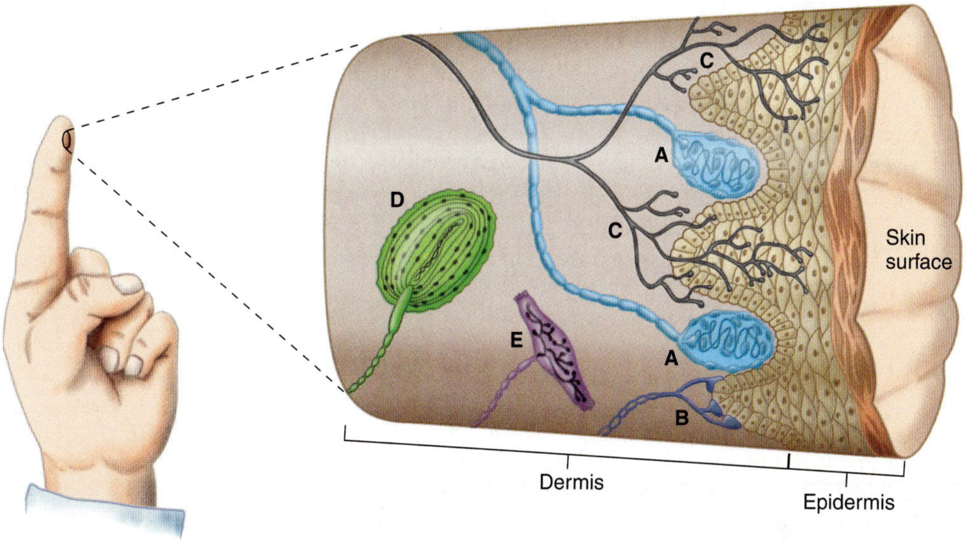

A. Meissner's corpuscle—rapidly adapting mechanoreceptor, touch and pressure
B. Merkel's corpuscle—slowly adapting mechanoreceptor, touch and pressure
C. Free neuron ending—slowly adapting, some are nociceptors, some are thermoreceptors, and some are mechanoreceptors
D. Pacinian corpuscles—rapidly adapting mechanoreceptor, vibration and deep pressure
E. Ruffini corpuscle—slowly adapting mechanoreceptor, skin stretch

Figure 7.15 APIR Skin receptors. Some nerve fibers have free endings not related to any apparent receptor structure. Thicker, myelinated axons, on the other hand, end in receptors that have a complex structure. Not drawn to scale; for example, Pacinian corpuscles are actually four to five times larger than Meissner's corpuscles. In skin with hair (like the back of the hand), there are receptors made up of free neuron endings wrapped around the hair follicles, and Meissner's corpuscles are absent.

PHYSIOLOGICAL INQUIRY

- Applying a pressure stimulus to the fluid-filled capsule of an isolated Pacinian corpuscle causes a brief burst of action potentials in the afferent neuron, which ceases until the pressure is removed, at which time another brief burst of action potentials occurs. If an experimenter removes the capsule and applies pressure directly to the afferent neuron ending, action potentials are continuously fired during the stimulus. Explain these results.

Answer can be found at end of chapter.

described in Chapter 10). Vision and the vestibular organs (the sense organs of balance) also support the senses of posture and movement. Mechanoreceptors in the joints, tendons, ligaments, and skin also play a role. The term **kinesthesia** refers to the sense of movement at a joint.

Temperature

Information about temperature is transmitted along small-diameter, afferent neurons with little or no myelination. These neurons originate in the tissues as free neuron endings—that is, they lack the elaborate capsular endings commonly seen in tactile receptors. The actual temperature sensors are ion channels in the plasma membranes of the axon terminals that belong to a family of proteins called **transient receptor potential (TRP) proteins.** Different isoforms of TRP channels have gates that open in different temperature ranges. When activated, all of these channel types allow flux of a nonspecific cation current that is dominated by a depolarizing inward flux of Na^+. The resulting receptor potential initiates action potentials in the afferent neuron, which travel along labeled lines to the brain where the temperature stimulus is perceived. The different channels have overlapping temperature ranges, which is somewhat analogous to the overlapping receptive fields of tactile receptors (review Figure 7.8). Interestingly, some of the TRP proteins can be opened by chemical ligands. This explains why capsaicin (a chemical found in chili peppers) and ethanol are perceived as being hot when ingested and menthol feels cool when applied to the skin. Some afferent neurons, especially those stimulated at the extremes of temperature, have proteins in their receptor endings that also respond to painful stimuli. These multipurpose neurons are therefore included among the polymodal neurons described earlier in relation to the nonspecific ascending pathways and are in part responsible for the perception of pain at extreme temperatures. These neurons represent only a subset of the pain receptors, which are described next.

Pain

Most stimuli that cause, or could potentially cause, tissue damage elicit a sensation of pain. Receptors for such stimuli are known as nociceptors. Nociceptors, like thermoreceptors, are free axon terminals of small-diameter afferent neurons with little or no myelination. They respond to intense mechanical deformation, extremes of temperature, and many chemicals. Examples of the latter include H^+, neuropeptide transmitters, bradykinin, histamine, cytokines, and prostaglandins, several of which are released by damaged cells. Some of these chemicals are secreted by cells of the immune system (described in Chapter 18) that have moved into the injured area. These substances act by binding to specific ligand-gated ion channels on the nociceptor plasma membrane.

The primary afferents having nociceptor endings synapse on ascending neurons after entering the central nervous system (**Figure 7.16a**). Glutamate and the neuropeptide

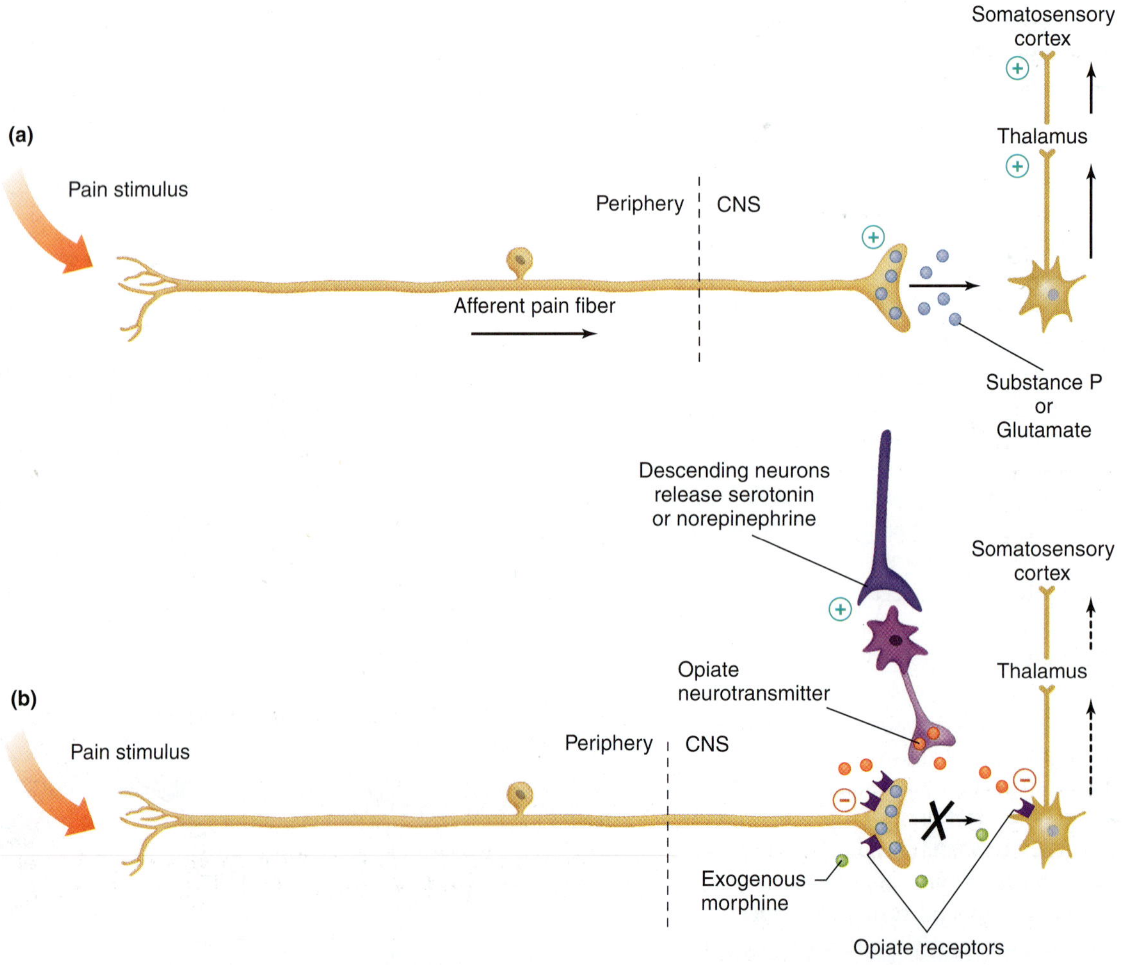

Figure 7.16 Cellular pathways of pain transmission and modulation. (a) Painful stimulation releases substance P or glutamate from afferent fibers in the dorsal horn of the spinal cord. (b) Descending inputs from the brainstem stimulate dorsal horn interneurons to release endogenous opiate neurotransmitters. Presynaptic opiate receptors inhibit neurotransmitter release from afferent pain fibers, and postsynaptic receptors inhibit ascending neurons. Morphine inhibits pain in a similar manner. In some cases, descending neurons may directly synapse onto and inhibit ascending neurons.

substance P are among the neurotransmitters released at these synapses.

When incoming nociceptive afferents activate interneurons, it may lead to the phenomenon of ***referred pain,*** in which the sensation of pain is experienced at a site other than the injured or diseased tissue. For example, during a heart attack, a person often experiences pain in the left arm. Referred pain occurs because both visceral and somatic afferents often converge on the same neurons in the spinal cord (**Figure 7.17**). Excitation of the somatic afferent fibers is the more usual source of afferent discharge, so we "refer" the location of receptor activation to the somatic source even though, in the case of visceral pain, the perception is incorrect. **Figure 7.18** shows the typical distribution of referred pain from visceral organs.

Pain differs significantly from the other somatosensory modalities. After transduction of a first noxious stimulus into action potentials in the afferent neuron, a series of changes can occur in components of the pain pathway—including the ion channels in the nociceptors themselves—that alters the way these components respond to subsequent stimuli. Both increased and decreased sensitivity to painful stimuli can occur. When these changes result in an increased sensitivity to painful stimuli, known as ***hyperalgesia,*** the pain can last for hours after the original stimulus is gone. Therefore, the pain experienced in response to stimuli that occur even a short time after the original stimulus (and the reactions to that pain) can be more intense than the initial pain. This type of pain response is common with severe burn injuries. Moreover, probably more than any other type of sensation, pain can be altered by past experiences, suggestion, emotions (particularly anxiety), and the simultaneous activation of other sensory

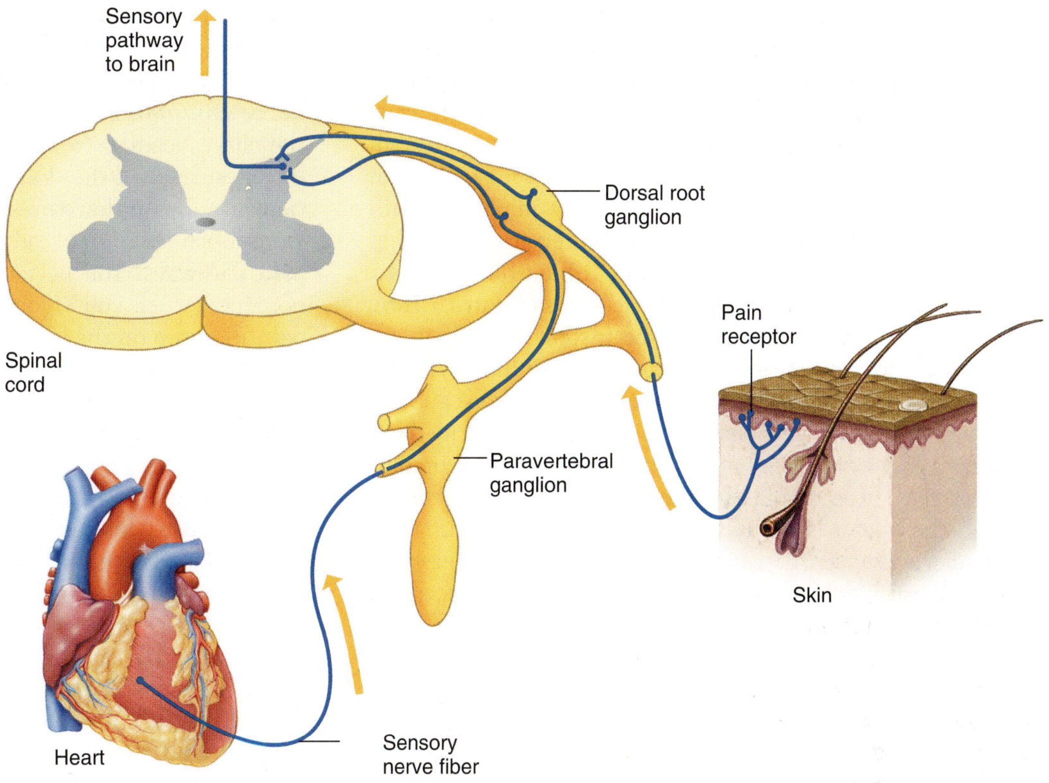

Figure 7.17 Convergence of visceral and somatic afferent neurons onto ascending pathways produces the phenomenon of referred pain.

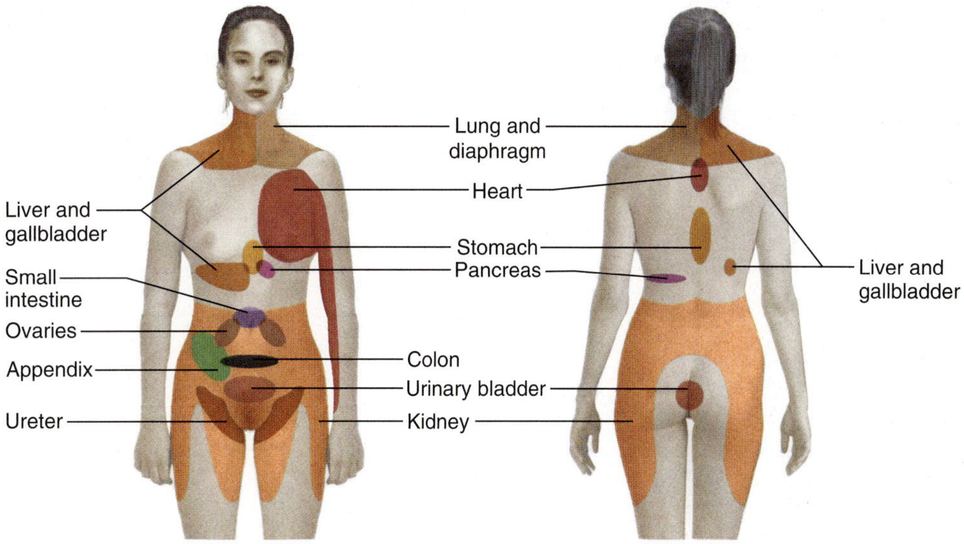

Figure 7.18 Regions of the body surface where we typically perceive referred pain from visceral organs.

PHYSIOLOGICAL INQUIRY

- A woman has had a sore neck for a few days. Why might a clinician listen carefully to her chest and upper back with a stethoscope during the examination?

Answer can be found at end of chapter.

modalities. Thus, the level of pain experienced is not solely a physical property of the stimulus.

Analgesia is the selective suppression of pain without effects on consciousness or other sensations. Electrical stimulation of specific areas of the central nervous system can produce a profound reduction in pain—a phenomenon called ***stimulation-produced analgesia***—by inhibiting pain pathways. This occurs because descending pathways that originate in these brain areas selectively inhibit the transmission of information originating in nociceptors (**Figure 7.16b**). The descending axons end at lower brainstem and spinal levels on interneurons in the pain pathways and inhibit synaptic transmission between the afferent nociceptor neurons and the secondary ascending neurons. Some of the neurons in these inhibitory pathways release morphinelike endogenous opioids (Chapter 6). These opioids inhibit the propagation of input through the higher levels of the pain system. Thus, treating a patient with morphine can provide relief in many cases of intractable pain by binding to and activating opioid receptors at the level of entry of the active nociceptor neurons. This is distinct from morphine's effect on the brain.

The endogenous-opioid systems also mediate other phenomena known to relieve pain. In clinical studies, 55% to 85% of patients experienced pain relief when treated with ***acupuncture***, an ancient Chinese therapy involving the insertion of needles into specific locations on the skin. This success rate was similar to that observed when patients were treated with morphine (70%). In studies comparing morphine to a ***placebo*** (injections of sugar that patients *thought* was the drug), as many as 35% of those receiving the placebo experienced pain relief. Acupuncture is thought to activate afferent neurons leading to spinal cord and midbrain centers that release endogenous opioids and other neurotransmitters implicated in pain relief. It seems likely that pathways descending from the cortex activate those same regions to exert the placebo effect. Thus, exploiting the body's built-in analgesia mechanisms can be an effective means of controlling pain.

Also of use for lessening pain is ***transcutaneous electrical nerve stimulation*** (***TENS***), in which the painful site itself or the nerves leading from it are stimulated by electrodes placed on the surface of the skin. TENS works because the stimulation of nonpain, low-threshold afferent fibers (e.g., the fibers from touch receptors) leads to the inhibition of neurons in the pain pathways. You perform a low-tech version of this phenomenon when you vigorously rub your scalp at the site of a painful bump on the head.

Neural Pathways of the Somatosensory System

After entering the central nervous system, the afferent nerve fibers from the somatic receptors synapse on neurons that form the specific ascending pathways projecting primarily to the somatosensory cortex via the brainstem and thalamus. They also synapse on interneurons that give rise to the nonspecific ascending pathways. There are two major types of somatosensory pathways from the body; these pathways are organized differently from each other in the spinal cord and brain (**Figure 7.19**). The ascending **anterolateral pathway,** also called the spinothalamic pathway, makes its first synapse between the sensory receptor neuron and a second neuron located in the gray matter of the spinal cord (**Figure 7.19a**). This second neuron immediately crosses to the opposite side of the spinal cord and then ascends through the anterolateral column of the cord to the thalamus, where it synapses on cortically projecting neurons. The anterolateral pathway processes pain and temperature information. The second major pathway for somatic sensation is the **dorsal column pathway** (**Figure 7.19b**). This, too, is named for the section of white matter (the dorsal columns of the spinal cord) through which the sensory receptor neurons project. In the dorsal column pathway, sensory neurons do not cross over or synapse immediately upon entering the spinal cord. Rather, they ascend on

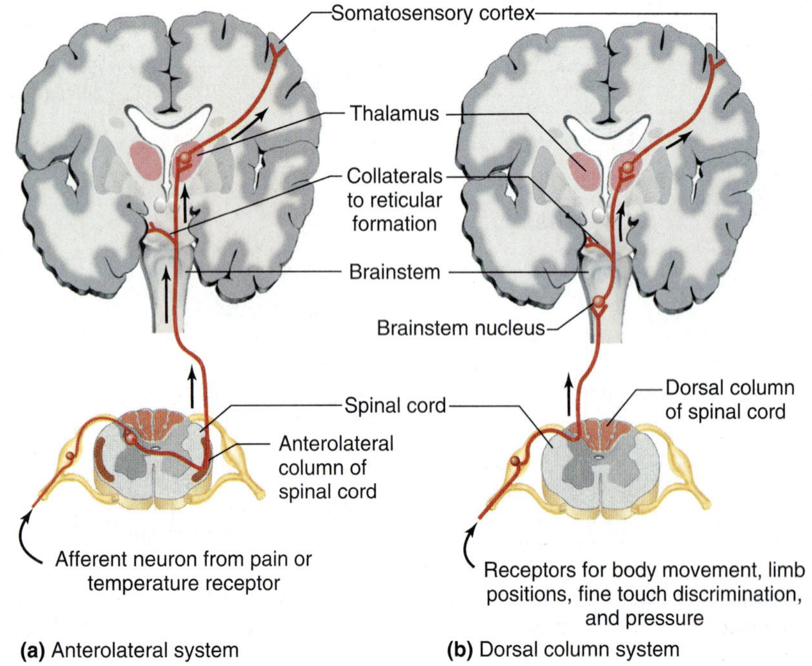

Figure 7.19 (a) The anterolateral system. (b) The dorsal column system. Information carried over collaterals to the reticular formation in (a) and (b) contribute to alertness and arousal mechanisms.

PHYSIOLOGICAL INQUIRY

- If an accident severed the left half of a person's spinal cord at the mid-thoracic level but the right half remained intact, what pattern of sensory deficits would occur?

Answer can be found at end of chapter.

the same side of the cord and make the first synapse in the brainstem. The secondary neuron then crosses in the brainstem as it ascends. As in the anterolateral pathway, the second synapse is in the thalamus, from which projections are sent to the somatosensory cortex.

Note that both pathways cross from the side where the afferent neurons enter the central nervous system to the opposite side either in the spinal cord (anterolateral system) or in the brainstem (dorsal column system). Consequently, sensory pathways from somatic receptors on the left side of the body terminate in the somatosensory cortex of the right cerebral hemisphere. Somatosensory information from the head and face does not travel to the brain within these two spinal cord pathways; it enters the brainstem directly via cranial nerves (review Table 6.8).

In the somatosensory cortex, the endings of the axons of the specific somatic pathways are grouped according to the peripheral location of the receptors that give input to the pathways (**Figure 7.20**). The parts of the body that are most densely innervated—fingers, thumb, and face—are represented by the largest areas of the somatosensory cortex. There are qualifications, however, to this seemingly precise picture. There is considerable overlap of the body part representations, and the sizes of the areas can change with sensory experience. The phantom limb phenomenon described in the first section of this chapter provides a good example of the dynamic nature of the somatosensory cortex. Studies of upper-limb amputees have shown that cortical areas formerly responsible for a missing arm and hand are commonly "rewired" to respond to sensory inputs originating in the face (note the proximity of the cortical regions representing these areas in Figure 7.20). As the somatosensory cortex undergoes this reorganization, a touch on a person's cheek might be perceived as a touch on his or her missing arm.

7.6 Vision

Vision is perhaps the most important sense for the day-to-day activities of humans. Perceiving a visual signal requires an organ—the eyes—capable of focusing and responding to light, and the appropriate neural pathways and structures to interpret the signal. We begin with an overview of light energy and eye structure.

Light

The receptors of the eye are sensitive only to that tiny portion of the vast spectrum of electromagnetic radiation that we call visible light (**Figure 7.21a**). Radiant energy is described in terms of wavelengths and frequencies. The **wavelength** is the distance between two successive wave peaks of the electromagnetic radiation (**Figure 7.21b**). Wavelengths vary from several kilometers at the long-wave radio end of the spectrum to trillionths of a meter at the gamma-ray end. The **frequency** (in hertz, the number of cycles per second) of the radiation wave varies inversely with wavelength. The wavelengths capable of stimulating the receptors of the eye—the **visible spectrum**—are between about 400 and 750 nm. Different wavelengths of light within this band are perceived as different colors.

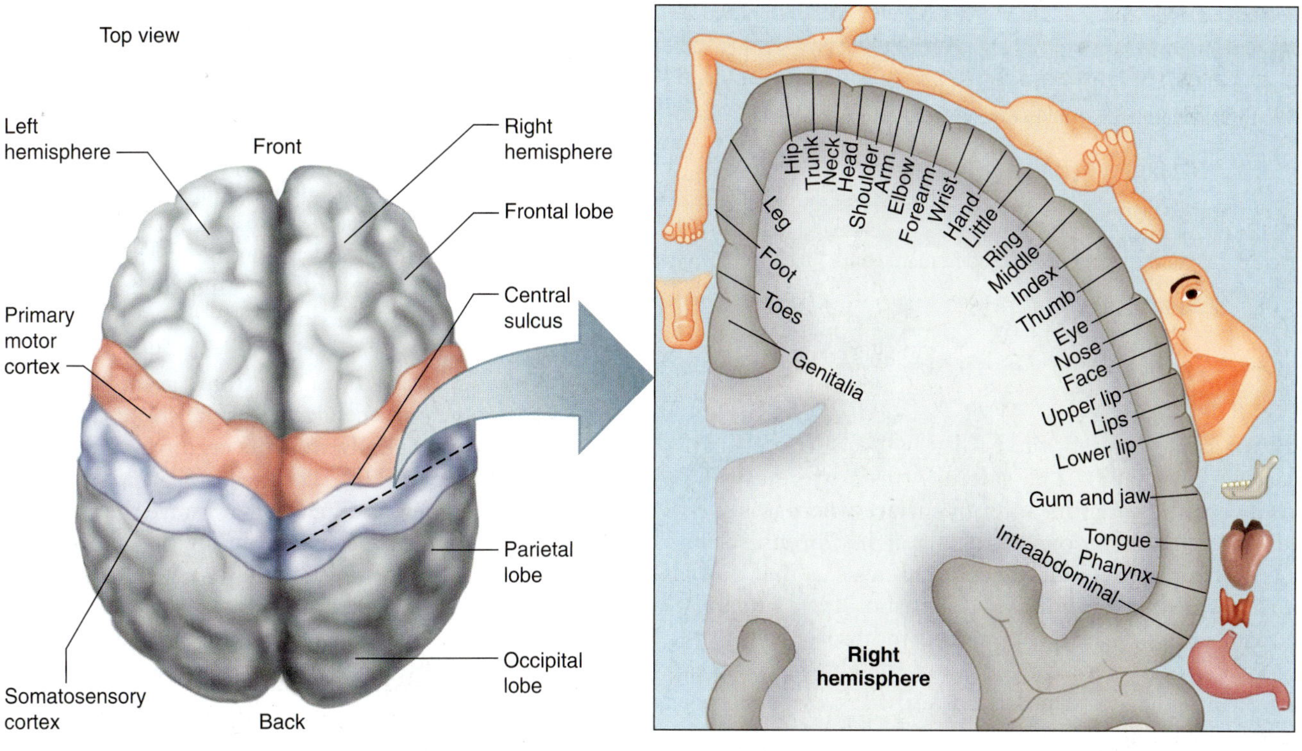

Figure 7.20 The location of pathway terminations for different parts of the body in somatosensory cortex, although there is actually much overlap between the cortical regions. The left half of the body is represented on the right hemisphere of the brain, and the right half of the body is represented on the left hemisphere, which is not shown here.

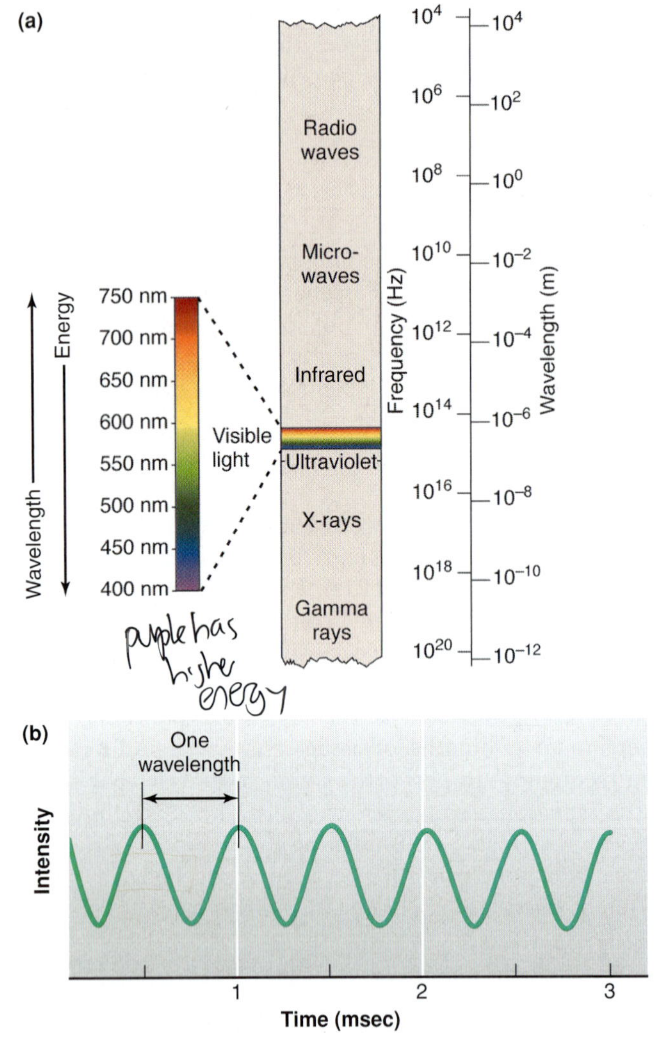

Figure 7.21 The electromagnetic spectrum. (a) Visible light ranges in wavelength from 400 to 750 nm (1 nm = 1 billionth of a meter). (b) Wavelength is the inverse of frequency.

PHYSIOLOGICAL INQUIRY

- What is the frequency of the electromagnetic wave shown in panel (b)? Would it be visible to the human eye?

Answer can be found at end of chapter.

Overview of Eye Anatomy

The eye is a three-layered, fluid-filled ball divided into two chambers (Figure 7.22). The **sclera** forms a white capsule around the eye, except at its anterior surface where it is specialized into the clear **cornea.** The tough, fibrous sclera serves as the insertion point for external muscles that move the eyeballs within their sockets. A portion of the underlying **choroid** layer is darkly pigmented to absorb light rays at the back of the eyeball. In the front, the choroid layer is specialized into the **iris** (the structure that gives your eyes their color), the **ciliary muscle,** and the **zonular fibers.** Circular and radial smooth muscle fibers of the iris determine the diameter of the **pupil,** the anterior opening that allows light into the eye. Activity of the ciliary muscle and the resulting tension on the zonular fibers determine the shape and consequently the focusing power of the crystalline **lens** just behind the iris.

The **retina** is formed from an extension of the developing brain in fetal life. It forms the inner, posterior surface of the eye, containing numerous types of neurons including the sensory cells of the eyes, called **photoreceptors.** Features of the retina can be viewed through the pupil with an ***ophthalmoscope,*** a handheld device that uses a light source and lenses to illuminate and magnify the image of the back of the eye. These features include

1. the **macula lutea** (Latin for "yellow spot"; often simply referred to as the macula): a small region at the center of the retina that is relatively free of blood vessels;
2. the **fovea centralis:** a central, shallow pit within the macula containing a high density of cones but relatively few light-obstructing retinal neurons—this region is specialized to deliver the highest visual acuity;
3. the **optic disc:** a distinct, circular region toward the nasal side of the retina where neurons carrying information from the photoreceptors exit the eye as the **optic nerve;** and
4. blood vessels: these enter the eye at the optic disc and branch extensively over the inner surface of the retina.

The eye is divided into two fluid-filled spaces. The anterior chamber of the eye, between the iris and the cornea, is filled with a clear fluid called **aqueous humor.** The posterior chamber of the eye, between the lens and the retina, is filled with a viscous, jellylike substance known as **vitreous humor.**

The Optics of Vision

A ray of light can be represented by a line drawn in the direction in which the wave is traveling. Light waves diverge in all directions from every point of a visible object. When a light wave crosses from air into a denser medium like glass or water, the wave changes direction at an angle that depends on the density of the medium and the angle at which it strikes the surface (Figure 7.23a). This bending of light waves, called **refraction,** is the mechanism allowing us to focus an accurate image of an object onto the retina.

When light waves diverging from a point on an object pass from air into the curved surfaces of the cornea and lens of the eye, they are refracted inward, converging back into a point on the retina (Figure 7.23b). The cornea plays a larger quantitative role than the lens in focusing light waves because the waves are refracted more in passing from air into the much denser environment of the cornea than they are when passing between fluid spaces of the eye and the lens, which are more similar in density. Objects in the center of the field of view are focused onto the fovea centralis, with the image formed upside down and reversed right to left relative to the original source. One of the fascinating features of the brain, however, is that it restores our perception of the image to its proper orientation.

Light waves from objects close to the eye strike the cornea at greater angles and must be refracted more in order to

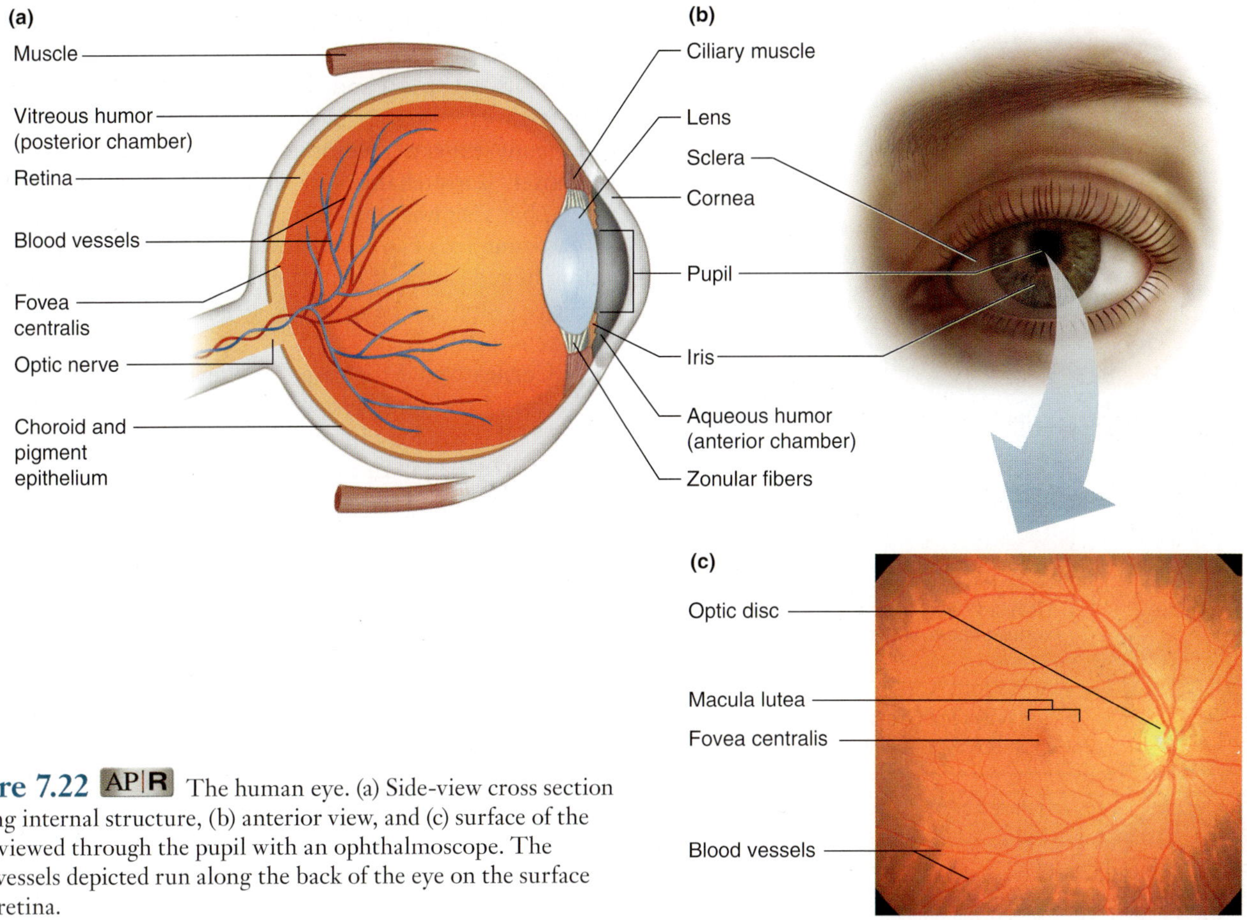

Figure 7.22 AP|R The human eye. (a) Side-view cross section showing internal structure, (b) anterior view, and (c) surface of the retina viewed through the pupil with an ophthalmoscope. The blood vessels depicted run along the back of the eye on the surface of the retina.

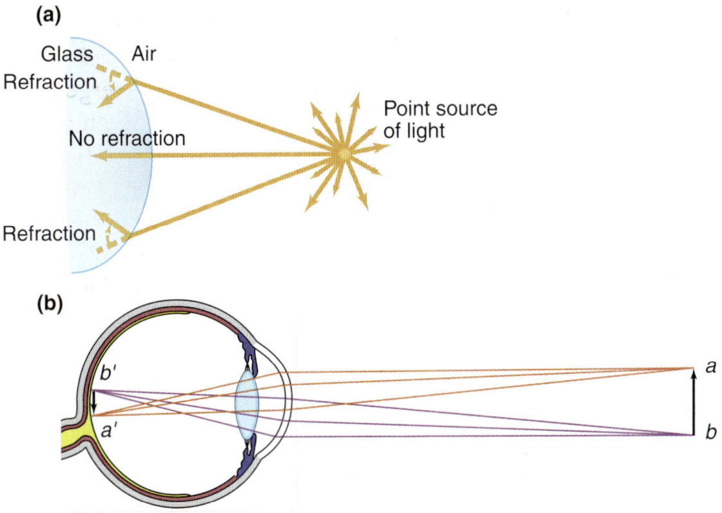

Figure 7.23 AP|R Focusing point sources of light. (a) When diverging light rays enter a dense medium at an angle to its convex surface, refraction bends them inward. (b) Refraction of light by the lens system of the eye. For simplicity, we show light refraction only at the surface of the cornea, where the greatest refraction occurs. Refraction also occurs in the lens and at other sites in the eye. Incoming light from *a* (above) and *b* (below) is bent in opposite directions, resulting in *b′* being above *a′* on the retina.

reconverge on the retina. Although, as previously noted, the cornea performs the greater part quantitatively of focusing the visual image on the retina, all *adjustments* for distance are made by changes in lens shape. Such changes are part of the process known as **accommodation.**

The shape of the lens is controlled by the ciliary muscle and the tension it applies to the zonular fibers, which attach the ciliary muscle to the lens (**Figure 7.24**). The ciliary muscle, which is stimulated by parasympathetic nerves, is circular, so that it draws nearer to the central lens as it contracts. As the muscle contracts, it lessens the tension on the zonular fibers. Conversely, when the ciliary muscle relaxes, the diameter of the ring of muscle increases and the tension on the zonular fibers also increases. Therefore, the shape of the lens is altered by contraction and relaxation of the ciliary muscle. To focus on distant objects, the ciliary muscle relaxes and the zonular fibers pull the lens into a flattened, oval shape. Contraction of the ciliary muscles focuses the eye on near objects by releasing the tension on the zonular fibers, which allows the natural elasticity of the lens to return it to a more spherical shape (**Figure 7.25**). The shape of the lens determines to what degree the light waves are refracted and how they project onto the retina. Constriction of the pupil also occurs when the ciliary muscle contracts, which helps sharpen the image further.

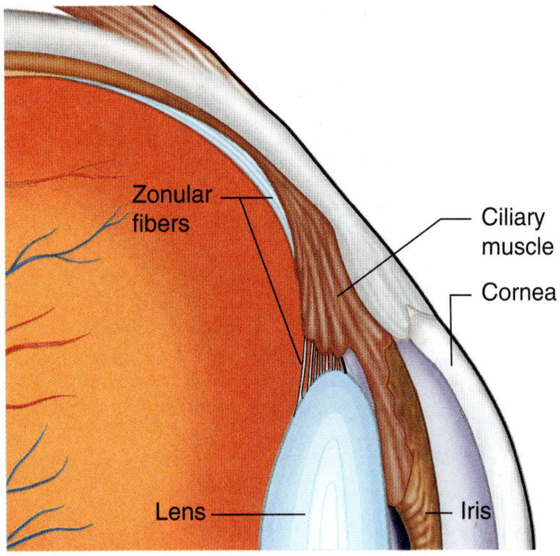

Figure 7.24 APIR Ciliary muscle, zonular fibers, and lens of the eye.

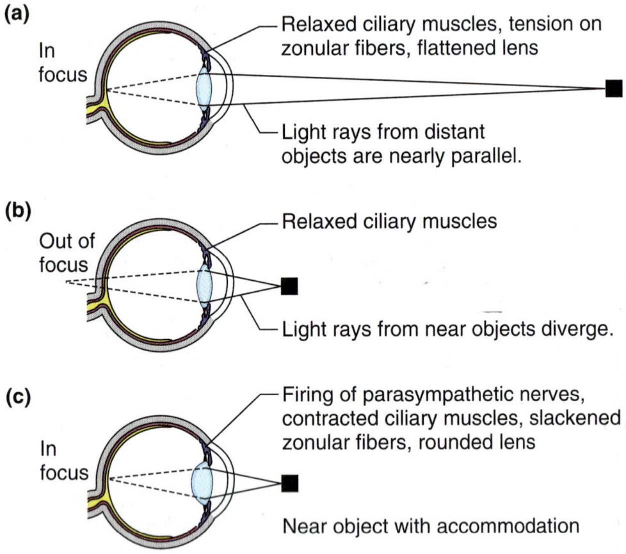

Figure 7.25 Accommodation for near vision. (a) Light rays from distant objects are more parallel, and they focus onto the retina when the lens is less curved. (b) Diverging light rays from near objects do not focus on the retina when the ciliary muscles are relaxed. (c) Accommodation increases the curvature of the lens, focusing the image of near objects onto the retina.

As people age, the lens tends to lose elasticity, reducing its ability to assume a spherical shape. The result is a progressive decline in the ability to accommodate for near vision. This condition, known as ***presbyopia,*** is a normal part of the aging process and is the reason that people around 45 years of age may have to begin wearing reading glasses or bifocals for close work.

The cells that make up most of the lens lose their internal membranous organelles early in life and are therefore transparent, but they lack the ability to replicate. The only lens cells that retain the capacity to divide are on the lens surface, and as new cells form, older cells come to lie deeper within the lens. With increasing age, the central part of the lens becomes denser and stiffer and may acquire a coloration that progresses from yellow to black.

Another change in lens color that sometimes occurs with aging is ***cataract,*** an opacity (clouding) of the lens that is one of the most common eye disorders. Cataracts are also associated with smoking and diseases such as diabetes. Because long-term exposure to ultraviolet radiation may also play a role, many experts recommend wearing sunglasses to delay the onset. Early changes in lens color do not interfere with vision, but vision is impaired as the process slowly continues. The opaque lens can be removed surgically. With the aid of an implanted artificial lens or compensating corrective lenses, effective vision can be restored, although the ability to accommodate is lost.

Cornea and lens shape and eyeball length determine the point where light rays converge. Defects in vision occur if the eyeball is too long in relation to the focusing power of the lens (**Figure 7.26a**). In this case, the images of faraway objects focus at a point in front of the retina. This ***nearsighted,*** or ***myopic,*** eye is unable to see distant objects clearly. Near objects are clear to a person with this condition but without the normal rounding of the lens that occurs via accommodation. In

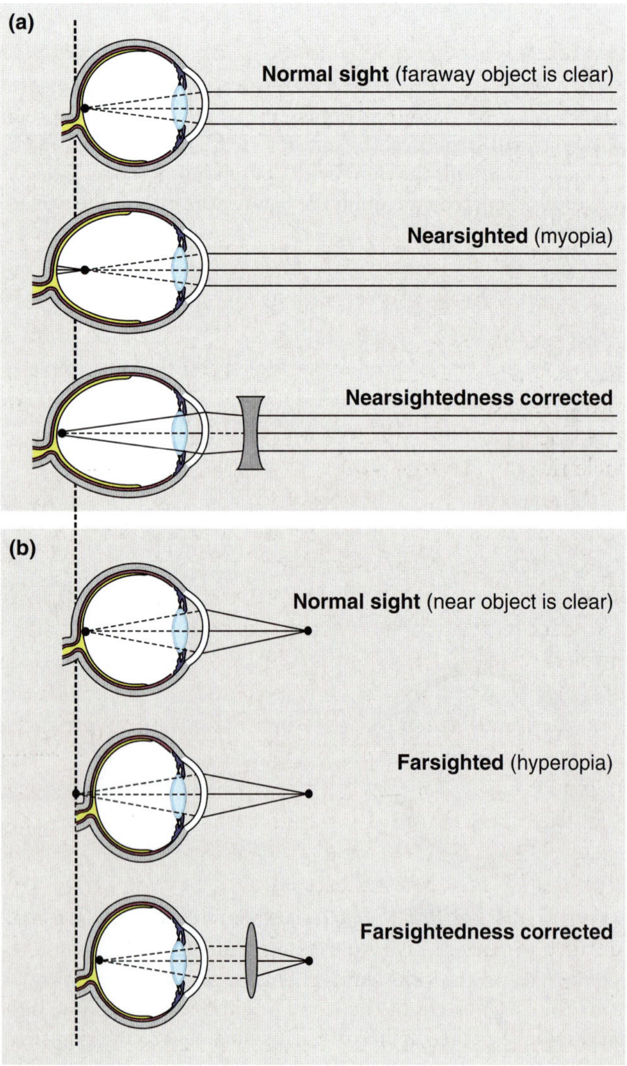

Figure 7.26 Correction of vision defects. (a) Nearsightedness (myopia). (b) Farsightedness (hyperopia).

contrast, if the eye is too short for the lens, images of near objects are focused behind the retina (**Figure 7.26b**). This eye is ***farsighted***, or ***hyperopic;*** though a person with this condition has poor near vision, distant objects can be seen if the accommodation reflex is activated to increase the curvature of the lens. These visual defects are easily correctable by manipulating the refraction of light entering the eye. The use of corrective lenses (such as glasses or contact lenses) for near- and farsighted vision is shown in Figure 7.26. In recent years, major advances in refractive surgery have involved reshaping the cornea with the use of lasers.

Defects in vision also occur when the lens or cornea does not have a smoothly spherical surface, a condition known as ***astigmatism***. Corrective lenses can usually compensate for these surface imperfections.

The size and shape of a person's eye over time depend in part on the volume of the aqueous humor and vitreous humor. These two fluids are colorless and permit the transmission of light from the front of the eye to the retina. The aqueous humor is constantly formed by special vascular tissue that overlies the ciliary muscle and drains away through a canal in front of the iris at the edge of the cornea. In some instances, the aqueous humor forms faster than it is removed, which results in increased pressure within the eye. ***Glaucoma***, a major cause of irreversible blindness, is a disease in which retinal cells are damaged as a result of increased pressure within the eye.

Just as the aperture of a camera can be varied to alter the amount of light that enters, the iris regulates the diameter of the pupil. The color of the iris is of no importance as long as the tissue is sufficiently opaque to prevent the passage of light. The iris is composed of two layers of smooth muscle that are innervated by autonomic nerves. Stimulation of sympathetic nerves to the iris enlarges the pupil by causing radially arranged muscle fibers to contract. Stimulation of parasympathetic fibers to the iris makes the pupil smaller by causing the muscle fibers that circle around the pupil to contract.

These neurally induced changes occur in response to light-sensitive reflexes integrated in the midbrain. Bright light causes a decrease in the diameter of the pupil, which reduces the amount of light entering the eye and restricts the light to the central part of the lens for more accurate vision. The constriction of the pupil also protects the retina from damage induced by very bright light, such as direct rays from the sun. Conversely, the pupil enlarges in dim light, when maximal light entry is needed. Changes also occur as a result of emotion or pain. For example, activation of the sympathetic nervous system dilates the pupils of a person who is angry (review Table 6.11). Abnormal or absent response of the pupil to changes in light can indicate damage to the midbrain from trauma or tumors or can also be a telltale sign when a person is under the influence of narcotics like heroin.

Photoreceptor Cells and Phototransduction

The retina, an extension of the central nervous system, contains photoreceptors and several other cell types that function in the transduction of light waves into visual information (**Figure 7.27**). The photoreceptor cells have a tip, or **outer segment,** composed of stacked layers of membrane called **discs.** The discs house the molecular machinery that responds to light. The photoreceptors also have an **inner segment,** which contains mitochondria and other organelles, and a synaptic terminal that connects the photoreceptor to other neurons in the retina. The two types of photoreceptors are called **rods** and **cones** because of the shapes of their light-sensitive outer segments. The rods are extremely sensitive and respond to very low levels of illumination, whereas the cones are considerably less sensitive and respond only when the light is bright. In cones, the light-sensitive discs are formed from in-foldings of the surface plasma membrane, whereas in rods, the disc membranes are intracellular structures.

Note that the light-sensitive portions of the photoreceptor cells face *away* from the incoming light, and the light must pass through all the cell layers of the retina before reaching and stimulating the photoreceptors. A remarkable specialization of the vertebrate retina prevents light rays from being blocked or scattered as they pass through these layers. Approximately 20% of the volume of the retina is taken up by a type of glial cells called **Müller cells** (not shown in Figure 7.27). These elongated, funnel-shaped cells span the distance from the inner surface of the retina directly to the photoreceptors, with an estimated abundance of 1:1 with cone cells and one per 10 rod cells. In addition to metabolically supporting retinal neurons and mediating neurotransmitter degradation, they appear to act like fiber-optic cables that deliver light rays through the retinal layers directly to the photoreceptor cells.

Two pigmented layers, the choroid and the **pigment epithelium** of the back of the retina, absorb light rays that bypass the photoreceptors. This prevents reflection and scattering of photons back through the rods and cones, which would cause the visual image to blur.

The photoreceptors contain molecules called **photopigments,** which absorb light. **Rhodopsin** is a unique photopigment in the retina for the rods, and there are also unique photopigments for each of three different types of cones. Photopigments consist of membrane-bound proteins called **opsins** bound to a **chromophore** molecule. The chromophore in all types of photopigments is **retinal** (reh-tin-AL), a derivative of vitamin A. This is the part of the photopigment that is light-sensitive. The opsin in each of the photopigments is different and binds to the chromophore in a different way. Because of this, each photopigment absorbs light most effectively at a specific part of the visible spectrum. For example, the photopigment found in one type of cone cell absorbs light most effectively at long wavelengths (designated as "red" cones), whereas another absorbs short wavelengths ("blue" cones).

The membranous discs of the outer segment are stacked perpendicular to the path of incoming light rays. This layered arrangement maximizes the membrane surface area, a relationship between structure and function that is a general principle of physiology observable in many body systems. In fact, each photoreceptor may contain over a billion molecules of photopigment, providing an extremely effective trap for light.

The photoreceptor is unique because it is the only type of sensory cell that is relatively depolarized (about −35 mV) when it is at rest (i.e., in the dark) and *hyperpolarized* (to about −70 mV) in response to its adequate stimulus. The mechanisms involved in mediating these membrane potential changes are shown in **Figure 7.28.** In the absence of light, action of the enzyme **guanylyl cyclase** converts GTP into a high intracellular concentration of the second-messenger molecule, cyclic GMP (cGMP). The cGMP maintains outer segment ligand-gated cation channels in an open state, and a persistent influx of Na^+ and Ca^{2+} results. Thus, in the dark, cGMP concentrations are high and the photoreceptor cell is maintained in a relatively depolarized state.

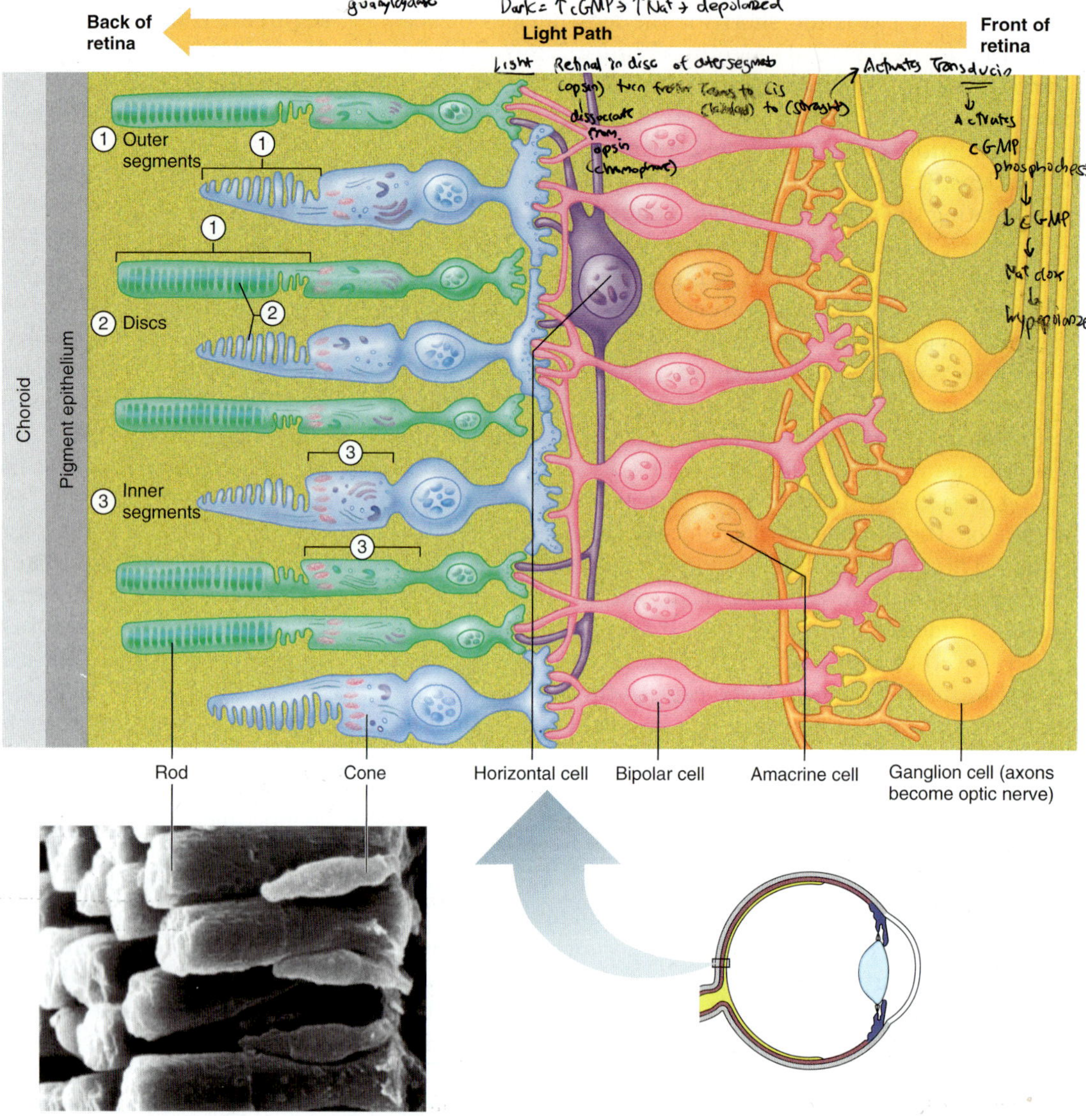

Figure 7.27 AP|R Organization of the retina. Light enters through the cornea and passes through the aqueous humor, pupil, vitreous humor, and the front surface of the retina before reaching the photoreceptor cells. The membranes that contain the light-sensitive proteins form discrete discs in the rods but are continuous with the plasma membrane in the cones, which accounts for the comblike appearance of these latter cells. Horizontal and amacrine cells, depicted here in purple and orange, provide lateral integration between neurons of the retina. Not shown are Müller cells, funnel-shaped glial cells that act as fiber-optic pathways for light from the front surface of the retina to the photoreceptors. At the lower left is a scanning electron micrograph of rods and cones. Redrawn from Dowling and Boycott.

When light of an appropriate wavelength shines on a photoreceptor cell, a cascade of events leads to hyperpolarization of the photoreceptor cell membrane. Molecules of retinal in the disc membrane assume a new conformation induced by the absorption of energy from photons and dissociate from the opsin. This, in turn, alters the shape of the opsin protein and promotes an interaction between the opsin and a protein called **transducin** that belongs to the G-protein family (see Chapter 5). Transducin activates the enzyme **cGMP-phosphodiesterase,** which rapidly degrades cGMP. The decrease in cytoplasmic cGMP concentration allows the cation channels to close, and the loss of depolarizing current allows the membrane potential to hyperpolarize. After its activation by light, retinal molecule changes back to its resting shape and is reassociated with the opsin by an enzyme-mediated mechanism.

If you move from a place of bright sunlight into a darkened room, a temporary "blindness" takes place until the photoreceptors can undergo **dark adaptation.** In the low levels of illumination of the darkened room, vision can only be supplied by the rods, which have greater sensitivity than the cones. During the exposure to bright light, however, the rhodopsin in the rods has been completely activated and retinal has dissociated from the opsin, making the rods insensitive to further stimulation by light. Rhodopsin cannot respond fully again until it is restored to its resting state by enzymatic reassociation of retinal with the opsin, a process requiring several minutes. Obtaining sufficient dietary vitamin A is essential for good night vision because it provides the chromophore retinal for rhodopsin.

Light adaptation occurs when you step from a dark place into a bright one. Initially, the eye is extremely sensitive to light as rods are overwhelmingly activated, and the visual image is too bright and has poor contrast. However, the rhodopsin is soon inactivated (sometimes said to be "bleached") as retinal dissociates from rhodopsin. As long as you remain

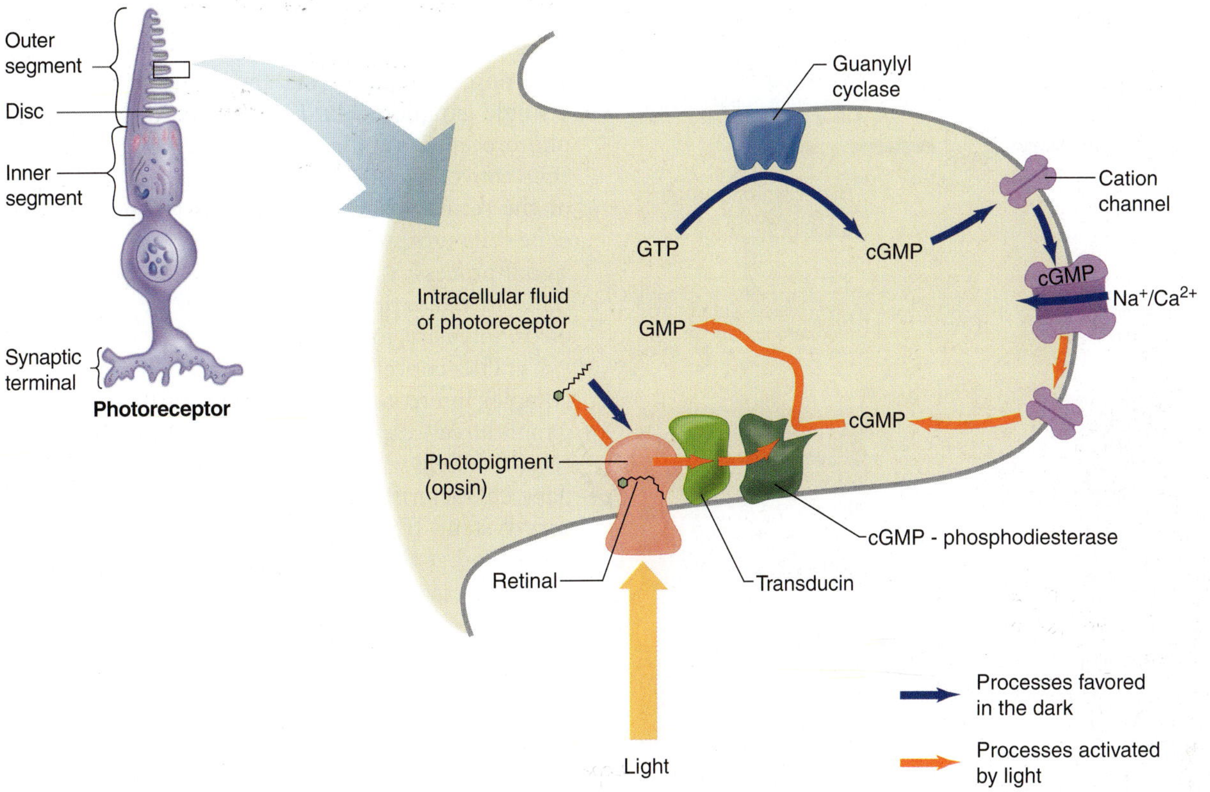

Figure 7.28 Phototransduction in a cone cell. In the absence of a light stimulus, cGMP binds to cation channels and opens them. When light strikes the chromophore (retinal) of the photopigment, it changes conformation and dissociates from the opsin. As a result, cGMP-phosphodiesterase in the membrane of the disc is stimulated, which decreases cGMP and thus closes the cation channels. For simplicity, the proteins are shown widely spaced in the membrane. In fact, all of these proteins are densely interspersed within the cone disc membrane. Phototransduction in rods is basically identical, except the membranous discs are contained completely within the cell's cytosol (see Figure 7.27), and the cGMP-gated ion channels are in the surface membrane rather than the disc membranes.

PHYSIOLOGICAL INQUIRY

- Explain why one early symptom of vitamin A deficiency is impaired vision at night (often called night blindness).

Answer can be found at end of chapter.

in bright light, the rods are unresponsive so that only the less-sensitive cones are operating, and the image is sharp and not overwhelmingly bright.

Neural Pathways of Vision

The distinct characteristics of the visual image are transmitted through the visual system along multiple, parallel pathways. The neural pathway of vision begins with the rods and cones. We just described in detail how the presence or absence of light influences photoreceptor cell membrane potential, and we will now consider how this information is encoded, processed, and transmitted to the brain.

Light signals are converted into action potentials through the interaction of photoreceptors with **bipolar cells** and **ganglion cells.** Photoreceptor and bipolar cells only undergo graded responses because they lack the voltage-gated channels that mediate action potentials in other types of neurons (review Figure 6.19). Ganglion cells have those channels and are therefore the first cells in the pathway where action potentials can be initiated. Photoreceptors interact with bipolar and ganglion cells in two distinct ways, designated as "ON-pathways" and "OFF-pathways." In both pathways, photoreceptors are depolarized in the absence of light, causing the neurotransmitter glutamate to be released onto bipolar cells. Light striking the photoreceptors of either pathway hyperpolarizes the photoreceptors, resulting in a decrease in glutamate release onto bipolar cells. Two key differences in the two pathways are that (1) bipolar cells of the ON-pathway spontaneously depolarize in the absence of input, whereas bipolar cells of the OFF-pathway hyperpolarize in the absence of input; and (2) glutamate receptors of ON-pathway bipolar cells are inhibitory, whereas glutamate receptors of OFF-pathway bipolar cells are excitatory. The net result is that the two pathways respond exactly the opposite in the presence and absence of light (**Figure 7.29**).

Glutamate released onto ON-pathway bipolar cells binds to metabotropic receptors that cause enzymatic breakdown of cGMP, which hyperpolarizes the bipolar cells by a mechanism

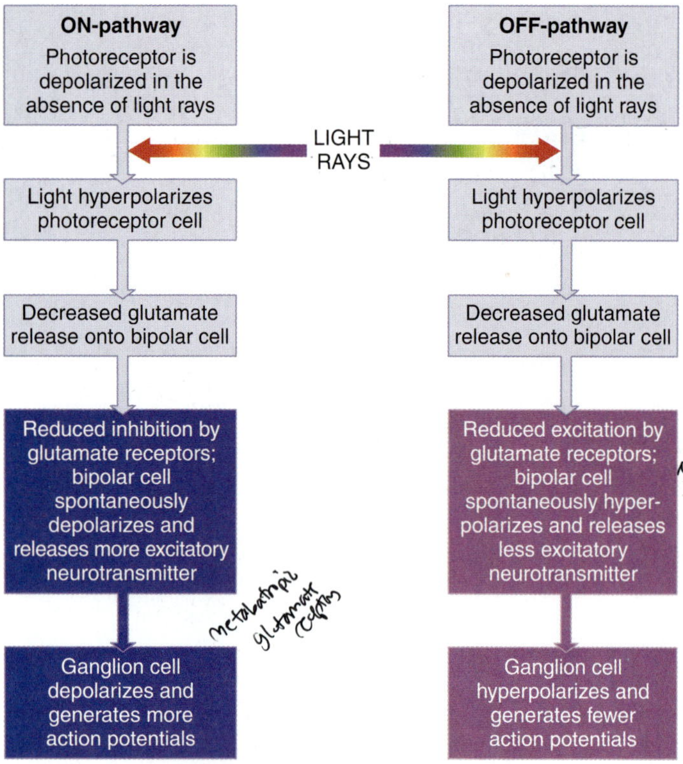

Figure 7.29 Effects of light on signaling in ON-pathway ganglion cells and OFF-pathway ganglion cells.

similar to that occurring when light strikes a photoreceptor cell. When the bipolar cells are hyperpolarized, they are prevented from releasing excitatory neurotransmitter onto their associated ganglion cells. Thus, in the absence of light, ganglion cells of the ON-pathway are not stimulated to fire action potentials. These processes reverse, however, when light strikes the photoreceptors: glutamate release from photoreceptors declines, ON-bipolar cells depolarize, excitatory neurotransmitter is released, the ganglion cells are depolarized, and an increased frequency of action potentials propagates to the brain.

OFF-pathway bipolar cells have ionotropic glutamate receptors that are nonselective cation channels, which depolarize the bipolar cells when glutamate binds. Depolarization of these bipolar cells stimulates them to release excitatory neurotransmitter onto their associated ganglion cells, stimulating them to fire action potentials. Thus, the OFF-pathway generates action potentials in the absence of light, and reversal of these processes inhibits action potentials when light does strike the photoreceptors. The coexistence of these ON- and OFF-pathways in each region of the retina greatly improves image resolution by increasing the brain's ability to perceive contrast at edges or borders.

Stimulation of ganglion cells is actually far more complex than just described—a significant amount of signal processing occurs within the retina before action potentials actually travel to the brain. Synapses between photoreceptors, bipolar cells, and ganglion cells are interconnected by a layer of **horizontal cells** and a layer of **amacrine cells,** which pass information between adjacent areas of the retina (review Figure 7.27). Furthermore, the retina is characterized by a large amount of convergence; many photoreceptors can synapse on each bipolar cell, and many bipolar cells synapse on a single ganglion cell. The amount of convergence varies by photoreceptor type and retinal region. As many as 100 rod cells converge onto a single bipolar cell in peripheral regions of the retina, whereas in the fovea region only one or a few cone cells synapse onto a bipolar cell. As a result of this retinal signal processing, individual ganglion cells respond differentially to the various characteristics of visual images, such as color, intensity, form, and movement.

The convergence of inputs from photoreceptors and complex interconnections of cells in the retina mean that each ganglion cell carries encoded information from a particular receptive field within the retina. Receptive fields in the retina have characteristics that differ from those in the somatosensory system. If you were to shine pinpoints of light onto the retina and at the same time record from a ganglion cell, you would discover that the receptive field for that cell is round. Furthermore, the response of the ganglion cell could demonstrate either an increased or decreased action potential frequency, depending on the location of the stimulus within that single field. Because of different inputs from bipolar cell pathways to the ganglion cell, each receptive field has an inner core ("center") that responds differently than the area around it (the "surround"). There can be "ON center/OFF surround" or "OFF center/ON surround" ganglion cells, so named because the responses are either depolarization (ON) or hyperpolarization (OFF) in the two areas of the field (**Figure 7.30**). The usefulness of this organization is that the existence of a clear edge between the "ON" and "OFF" areas of the receptive field increases the contrast between the area that is receiving light and the area around it, increasing visual acuity. As a result, a

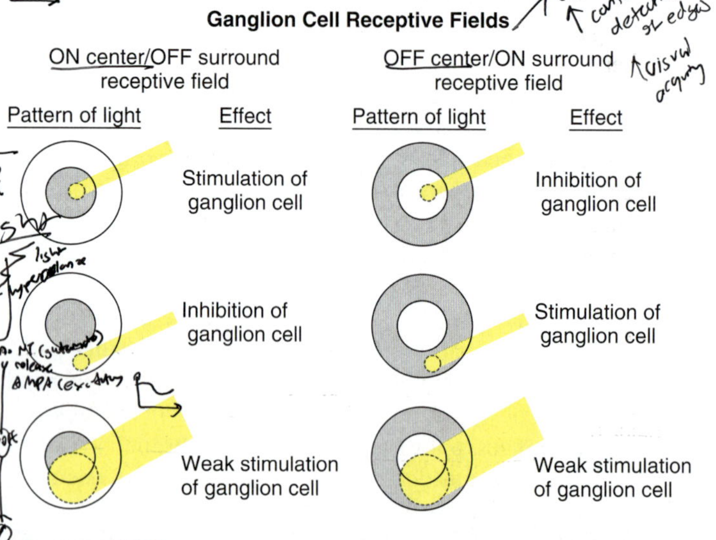

Figure 7.30 Types of ganglion cell receptive fields. ON center/OFF surround ganglion cells are stimulated when a pinpoint of light strikes the center of the receptive field and are inhibited when light strikes the surrounding area. The opposite occurs in OFF center/ON surround cells. In either case, light striking both regions results in intermediate activation due to offsetting influences. This is an example of lateral inhibition and enhances the detection of the edges of a visual stimulus, thus increasing visual acuity.

great deal of information processing takes place at this early stage of the sensory pathway.

The axons of the ganglion cells form the output from the retina—the optic nerve, which is cranial nerve II (**Figure 7.31a**). The two optic nerves meet at the base of the brain to form the **optic chiasm,** where some of the axons cross and travel within the **optic tracts** to the opposite side of the brain, providing both cerebral hemispheres with input from each eye. With both eyes open, the outer regions of our total visual field is perceived by only one eye (zones of **monocular vision**). In the central portion, the fields from the two eyes overlap (the zone of **binocular vision**) (**Figure 7.31b**). The ability to compare overlapping information from the two eyes in this central region allows for depth perception and improves our ability to judge distances.

Parallel processing of information continues all the way to and within the cerebral cortex to the highest stages of visual neural networks. Cells in this pathway respond to electrical signals that are generated initially by the photoreceptors' response to light. Optic nerve fibers project to several structures in the brain, the largest number passing to the thalamus (specifically to the lateral geniculate nucleus of the thalamus; see Figure 7.31), where the information (color, intensity, shape, movement, etc.) from the different ganglion cell types is kept distinct. In addition to the input from the retina, many neurons of the lateral geniculate nucleus also receive input from the brainstem reticular formation and input relayed back from the visual cortex, the primary visual area of the cerebral cortex. These nonretinal inputs can control the transmission of information from the retina to the visual cortex and may be involved in our ability to shift attention between vision and the other sensory modalities.

The lateral geniculate nucleus sends action potentials to the visual cortex (see Figures 7.13 and 7.31). Different aspects of visual information continue along in the parallel pathways coded by the ganglion cells, then are processed simultaneously in a number of independent ways in different parts of the cerebral cortex before they are reintegrated to produce the conscious sensation of sight and the perceptions associated with it. The cells of the visual pathways are organized to handle information about line, contrast, movement, and color. They do not, however, form a picture in the brain but only generate a spatial and temporal pattern of electrical activity that we *perceive* as a visual image.

We mentioned earlier that some neurons of the visual pathway project to regions of the brain other than the visual cortex. For example, a recently discovered class of ganglion cells containing an opsinlike pigment called **melanopsin** carries visual information to the **suprachiasmatic nucleus,** which lies just above the optic chiasm and functions as part of the "biological clock." It appears that information about the daily cycle of light intensity from these ganglion cells is used

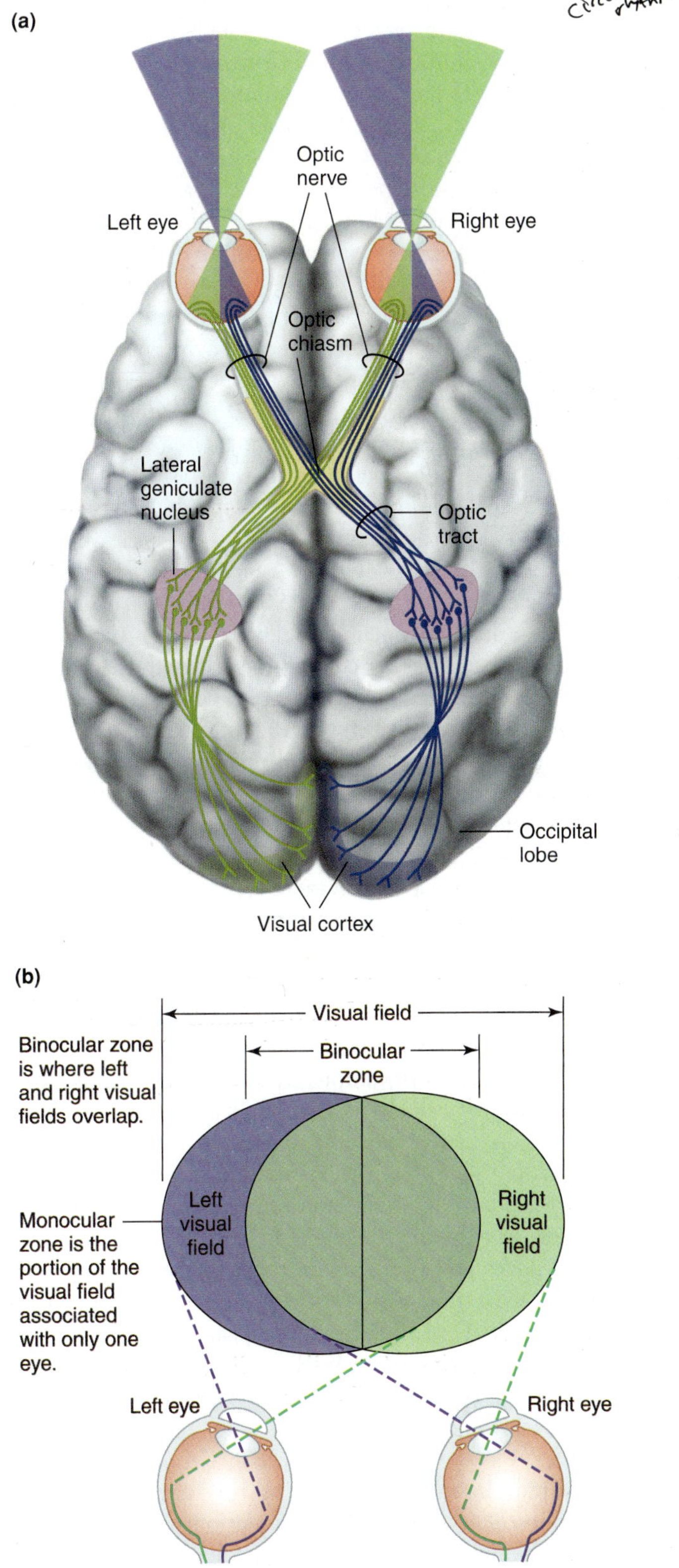

Figure 7.31 APR Visual pathways and fields. (a) Visual pathways viewed from above show how visual information from each eye field is distributed to the visual cortex of both occipital lobes. (b) Overlap of visual fields from the two eyes creates a binocular zone of vision, which allows for perception of depth and distance.

PHYSIOLOGICAL INQUIRY

- Three patients have suffered destruction of different portions of their visual pathway. Patient 1 has lost the right optic tract, patient 2 has lost the nerve fibers that cross at the optic chiasm, and patient 3 has lost the left occipital lobe. Draw a picture of what each person would perceive through each eye when looking at a white wall.

Answer can be found at end of chapter.

to entrain this neuronal clock to a 24-hour day—the circadian rhythm (review Figure 1.10). Other visual information passes to the brainstem and cerebellum, where it is used in the coordination of eye and head movements, fixation of gaze, and change in pupil size.

Color Vision

The colors we perceive are related to the wavelengths of light that the pigments in the objects of our visual world reflect, absorb, or transmit. For example, an object appears red because it absorbs shorter wavelengths, which would be perceived as blue, while simultaneously reflecting the longer wavelengths, perceived as red, to excite the photopigment of the retina most sensitive to red. Light perceived as white is a mixture of all wavelengths, and black is the absence of all light.

Color vision begins with activation of the photopigments in the cone photoreceptor cells. Human retinas have three kinds of cones—one responding optimally at long wavelengths ("L" or "red" cones), one at medium wavelengths ("M" or "green" cones), and the other stimulated best at short wavelengths ("S" or "blue" cones). Each type of cone is excited over a range of wavelengths, with the greatest response occurring near the center of that range. For any given wavelength of light, the three cone types are excited to different degrees (**Figure 7.32**). For example, in response to light of 531 nm wavelengths, the green cones respond maximally, the red cones less, and the blue not at all. Our sensation of the shade of green at this wavelength depends upon the relative outputs of these three types of cone cells and the comparison made by higher-order cells in the visual system.

The pathways for color vision follow those that Figure 7.31 describes. Ganglion cells of one type respond to a broad band of wavelengths. In other words, they receive input from all three types of cones, and they signal not a specific color but, rather, general brightness. Ganglion cells of a second type code for specific colors. These latter cells are also called **opponent color cells** because they have an excitatory input from one type of cone receptor and an inhibitory input from another. For example, the cell in **Figure 7.33** increases its rate of firing when viewing a blue light but decreases it when a yellow light replaces the blue. The cell gives a weak response when stimulated with a white light because the light contains both blue and yellow wavelengths. Other more complicated patterns also exist. The output from these cells is recorded by multiple, and as yet unclear, mechanisms in visual centers of the brain. Our ability to discriminate color also depends on the *intensity* of light striking the retina. In brightly lit conditions, the differential response of the cones allows for good color vision. In dim light, however, only the highly sensitive rods are able to respond. Though rods are activated over a range of wavelengths that overlap with those that activate the cones (see Figure 7.32), there is no mechanism for distinguishing between frequencies. Thus, objects that appear vividly colored in bright daylight are perceived in shades of gray as night falls and lighting becomes so dim that only rods can respond.

Color Blindness

At high light intensities, as in daylight vision, most people—92% of the male population and over 99% of the female population—have normal color vision. However, there are several types of defects in color vision that result from mutations in the cone pigments. The most common form of ***color blindness***, red–green color blindness, is present predominantly in men, affecting 1 out of 12. Color blindness in women is much rarer (1 out of 200). Men with red–green color blindness lack either the red or the green cone pigments entirely or have them in an abnormal form. Because of this, the discrimination between shades of these colors is poor.

Color blindness results from a recessive mutation in one or more genes encoding the cone pigments. Genes encoding the red and green cone pigments are located very close to each other on the X chromosome, whereas the gene encoding the blue chromophore is located on chromosome 7. Because of this close association of the red and green genes on the X chromosome, there is a greater likelihood that genetic recombination will occur during meiosis (see Chapter 17, Section A),

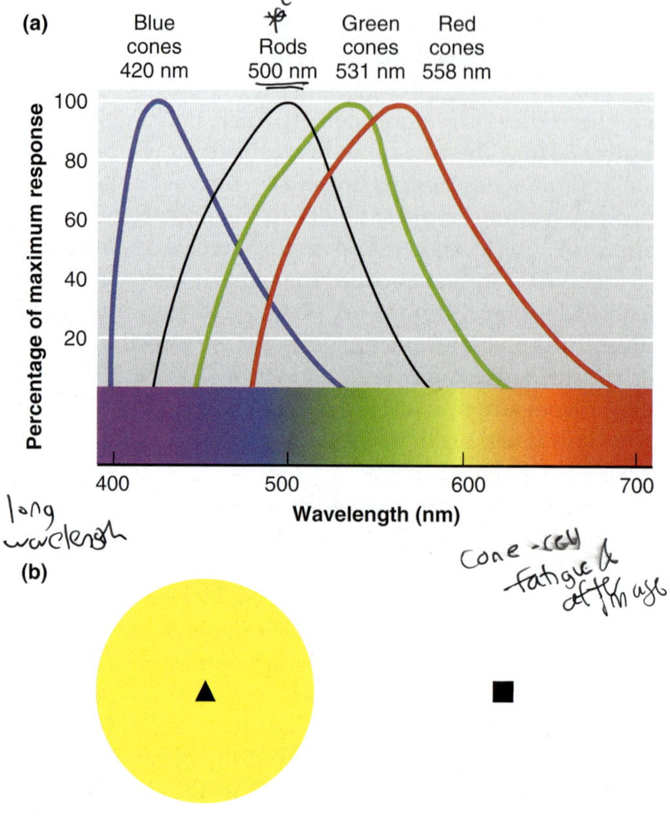

Figure 7.32 The sensitivities of the photopigments in the normal human retina. (a) The frequency of action potentials in the optic nerve is directly related to a photopigment's absorption of light. Under bright lighting conditions, the three types of cones respond over different frequency ranges. In dim light, only the rods respond. (b) Demonstration of cone cell fatigue and afterimage. Hold very still and stare at the triangle inside the yellow circle for 30 seconds. Then, shift your gaze to the square and wait for the image to appear around it.

PHYSIOLOGICAL INQUIRY

- What color was the image you saw while you stared at the square? Why did you perceive that particular color?

Answer can be found at end of chapter.

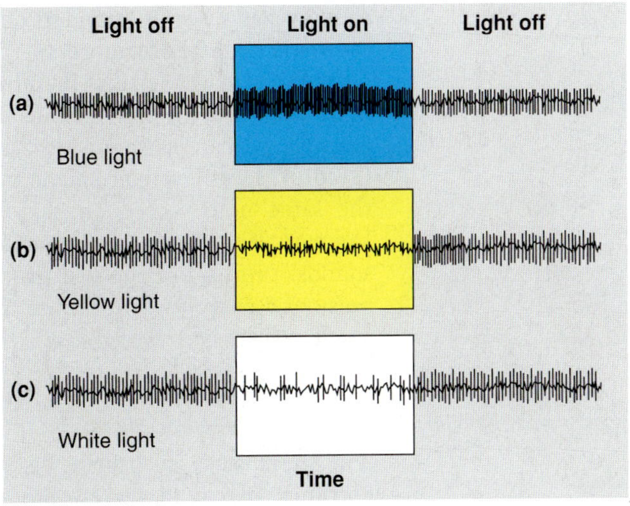

Figure 7.33 Response of a single opponent color ganglion cell to blue, yellow, and white lights. Redrawn from Hubel and Wiesel.

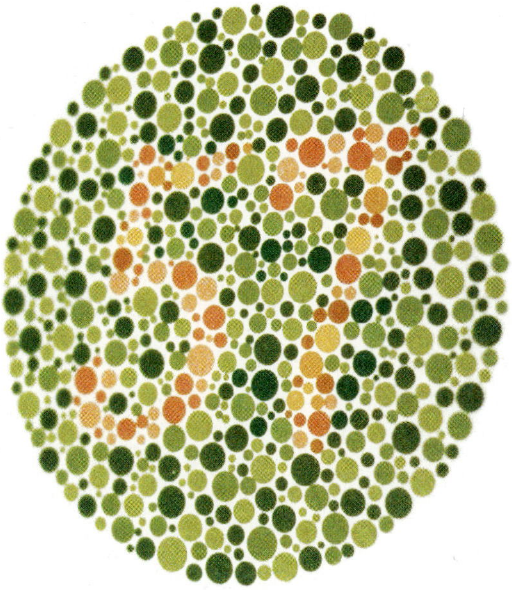

Figure 7.34 Image used for testing red–green color vision. With normal color vision, the number 57 is visible; no number is apparent to those with a red–green defect.

thus eliminating or changing the spectral characteristics of the red and green pigments produced. This, in part, accounts for the fact that red–green defects are not always complete and that some color-blind individuals under some conditions can distinguish shades of red or green. In males, the presence of only a single X chromosome means that a single recessive allele from the mother will result in color blindness, even though the mother herself may have normal color vision due to having one normal X chromosome. It also means that 50% of the male offspring of that mother will be expected to be color blind. Individuals who have red–green color blindness will not be able to see the number in **Figure 7.34.**

Eye Movement

The macula lutea region of the retina, within which the fovea centralis is located, is specialized in several ways to provide the highest visual acuity. It is comprised of densely packed cones with minimal convergence through the bipolar and ganglion cell layers. In addition, light rays are scattered less on the way to the outer segment of those cones than in other retinal regions, because the interneuron layers and the blood vessels are displaced to the edges. This central region becomes impaired in a condition known as ***macular degeneration,*** producing a defect characterized by loss of vision in the center of the visual field. The most common form of this disease increases with age, occurring in approximately 30% of individuals over the age of 75, and is therefore referred to as ***age-related macular degeneration (AMD).***

To focus the most important point in the visual image (the fixation point) on the fovea and keep it there, the eyeball must be able to move. Six skeletal muscles attached to the outside of each eyeball (identified in **Figure 7.35**) control its movement. These muscles perform two basic movements, fast and slow.

The fast movements, called **saccades,** are small, jerking movements that rapidly bring the eye from one fixation point to another to allow a search of the visual field. In addition, saccades move the visual image over the receptors, thereby preventing adaptation that would result from persistent photobleaching of photoreceptors in a given region of the retina. Saccades also occur during certain periods of sleep when dreaming occurs, though these movements are not thought to be involved in "watching" the visual imagery of dreams.

Slow eye movements are involved both in tracking visual objects as they move through the visual field and during compensation for movements of the head. The control centers for these compensating movements obtain their information about head movement from the vestibular system, which we will describe shortly. Control systems for the other slow movements of the eyes require the continuous feedback of visual information about the moving object.

7.7 Hearing

The sense of hearing (**audition**) is based on the physics of sound and the physiology of the external, middle, and inner ear. In addition, there is complex neural processing along pathways to the brain and within brain regions involved in sensing and perceiving acoustic information.

Sound

Sound energy is transmitted through a gaseous, liquid, or solid medium by setting up a vibration of the medium's molecules, air being the most common medium in which we hear sound energy. When there are no molecules, as in a vacuum, there can be no sound. Anything capable of disturbing molecules—for example, vibrating objects—can serve as a sound source. **Figure 7.36, a–d,** demonstrates the basic mechanism of sound production using a tuning fork as an example. When struck, the tuning fork vibrates, creating disturbances of air molecules that make up the sound wave. The sound wave consists of zones of compression, in which the molecules are close together and the pressure is increased, alternating with zones of rarefaction, in which the molecules are farther apart and the pressure is lower.

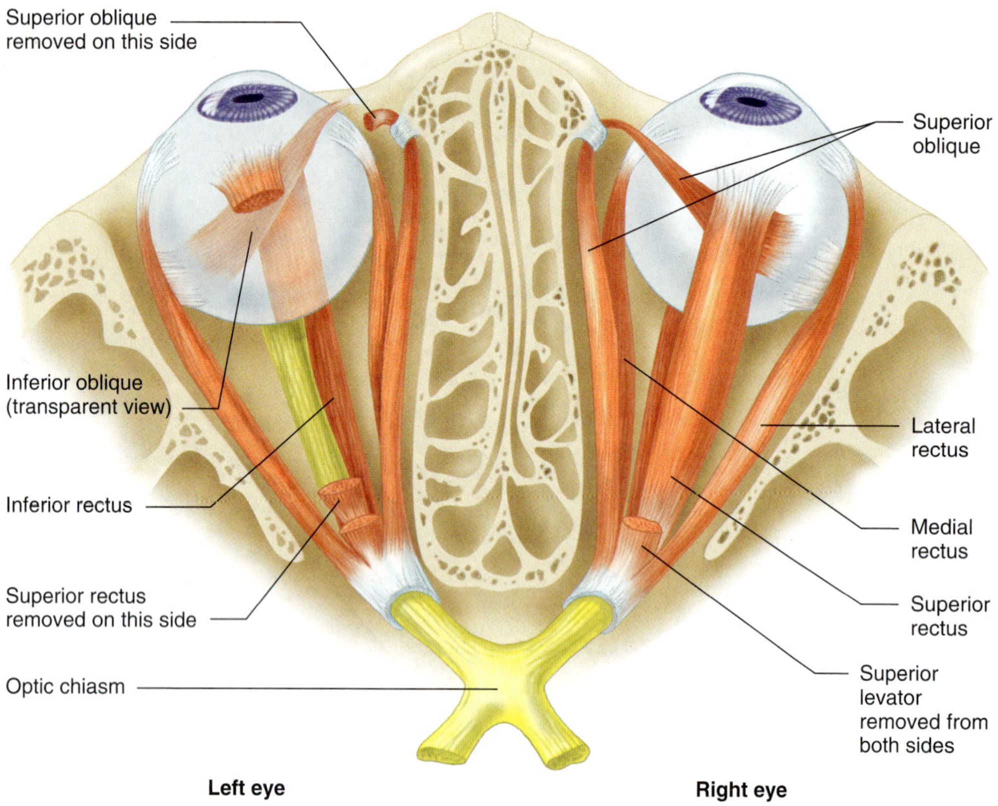

Figure 7.35 APIR A superior view of the muscles that move the eyes to direct the gaze and provide convergence.

As the air molecules bump against each other, the zones of compression and rarefaction ripple outward and the sound wave is transmitted over distance.

A sound wave measured over time (**Figure 7.36e**) consists of rapidly alternating pressures that vary continuously from a high during compression of molecules, to a low during rarefaction, and back again. The difference between the pressure of molecules in zones of compression and rarefaction determines the wave's amplitude, which is related to the loudness of the sound; the greater the amplitude, the louder the sound. The human ear can detect volume variations over an enormous range, from the sound of someone breathing in the room to a jet taking off on a nearby runway. Because of this incredible range, sound loudness is measured in decibels (dB), which are a logarithmic function of sound pressure. The threshold for human hearing is assigned a value of 0 dB, and an increase of 30 dB, for example, would represent a 1000-fold increase in sound intensity.

The frequency of vibration of the sound source (the number of zones of compression or rarefaction in a given time) determines the pitch we hear; the faster the vibration, the higher the pitch. The sounds heard most keenly by human ears are those from sources vibrating at frequencies between 1000 and 4000 Hz (hertz, or cycles per second), but the entire range of frequencies audible to human beings extends from 20 to 20,000 Hz. Most sounds are not pure tones but are mixtures of tones of a variety of frequencies. Sequences of pure tones of varying frequencies are generally perceived as musical. The addition of other frequencies, called overtones, to a pure tone's sound wave gives the sound its characteristic quality, or timbre.

We can distinguish hundreds of thousands of different sounds. For example, we can distinguish the note C (261.63 Hz) played on a piano from the same note played on a violin. We can also selectively *not* perceive sounds, tuning out the background noise of a party to concentrate on a single voice.

Sound Transmission in the Ear

The first step in hearing is the entrance of sound waves into the **external auditory canal** (**Figure 7.37**). The shapes of the outer ear (the pinna, or auricle) and the external auditory canal help to amplify and direct the sound. The sound waves reverberate from the sides and end of the external auditory canal, filling it with the continuous vibrations of pressure waves.

The **tympanic membrane** (eardrum) is stretched across the end of the external auditory canal, and as air molecules push against the membrane, they cause it to vibrate at the same frequency as the sound wave. Under higher pressure during a zone of compression, the tympanic membrane bows inward. The distance the membrane moves, although always very small, is a function of the force with which the air molecules hit it and is related to the sound pressure and therefore its loudness. During the subsequent zone of rarefaction, the membrane bows outward; when the sound ceases, it returns toward a midpoint. The exquisitely sensitive tympanic membrane responds to all the varying pressures of the sound waves, vibrating slowly in response to low-frequency sounds and rapidly in response to high-frequency sounds.

The tympanic membrane separates the external auditory canal from the **middle ear,** an air-filled cavity in the temporal bone of the skull. The pressures in the external auditory canal and middle ear cavity are normally equal to atmospheric pressure. The middle ear cavity is exposed to atmospheric pressure through the **eustachian tube,** which connects the middle ear to the pharynx. The slitlike ending of this tube in the pharynx is normally closed, but muscle movements open the tube during yawning, swallowing, or sneezing. A difference in pressure can be produced with sudden changes in altitude (as in an ascending or descending elevator or airplane). When the pressures outside the ear and in the ear canal change, the pressure in the middle ear initially remains constant because the eustachian tube is closed. This pressure difference can stretch the tympanic membrane and cause pain. This problem is relieved by voluntarily yawning or swallowing, which opens the eustachian tube and allows the pressure in the middle ear to equilibrate with the new atmospheric pressure.

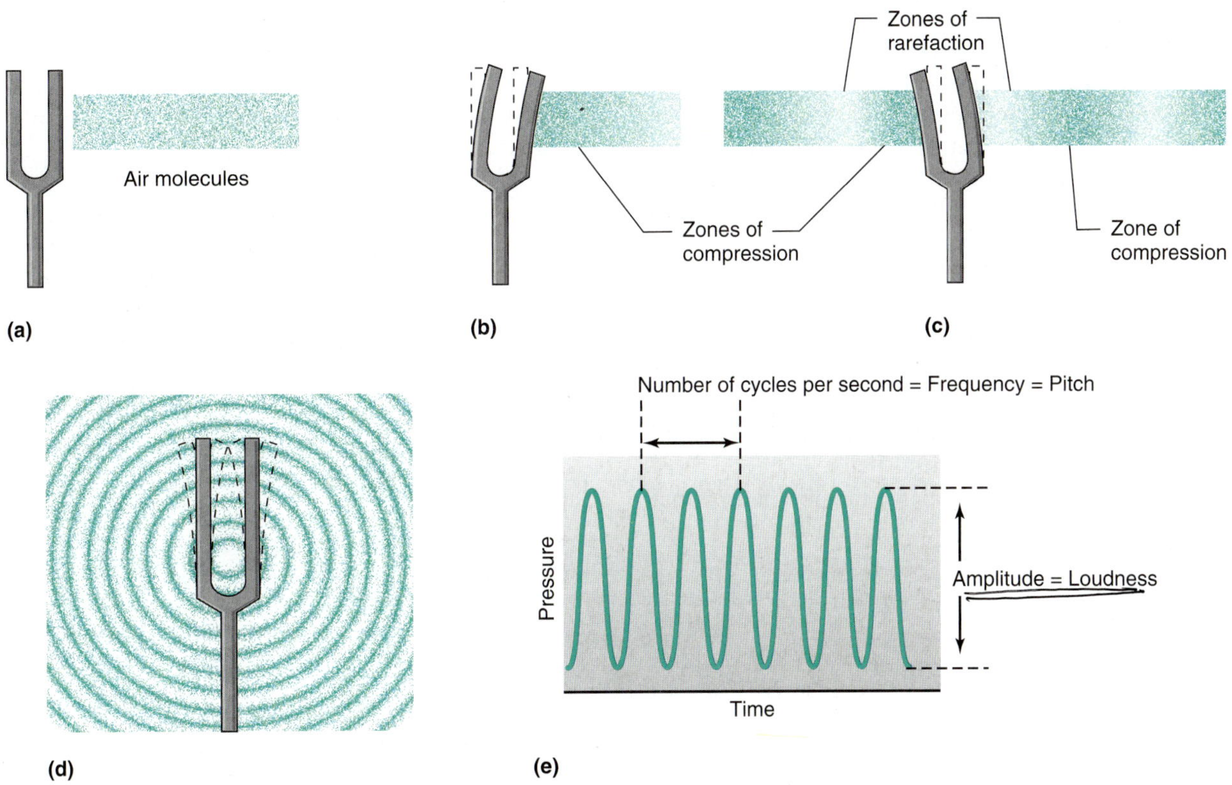

Figure 7.36 Formation of sound waves from a vibrating tuning fork.

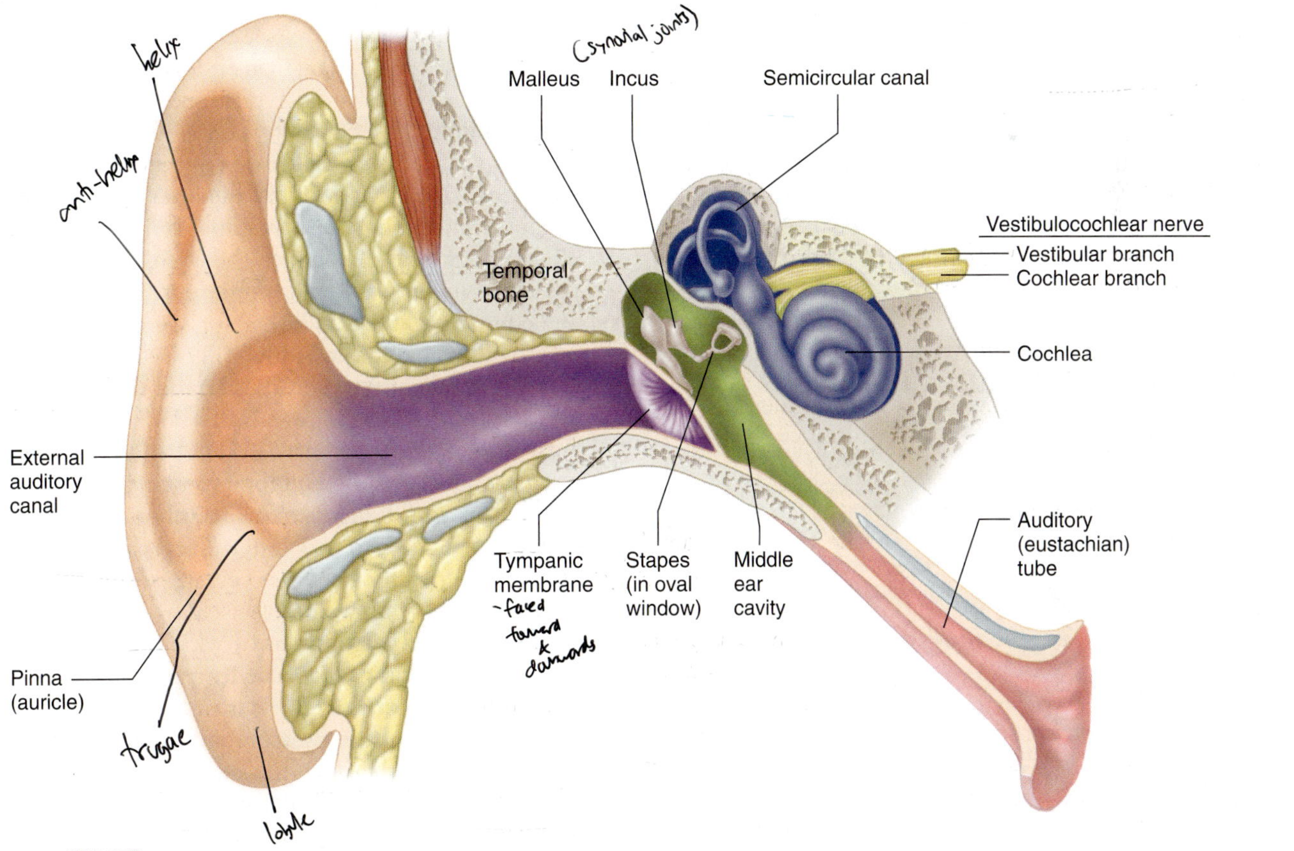

Figure 7.37 AP|R The human ear. In this and the following two figures, violet indicates the outer ear, green the middle ear, and blue the inner ear. The malleus, incus, and stapes are bones and components of the middle ear compartment. The eustachian tube is generally closed except during pharynx movements such as swallowing or yawning.

The second step in hearing is the transmission of sound energy from the tympanic membrane through the middle ear cavity to the **inner ear.** The inner ear, called the **cochlea,** is a spiral-shaped, fluid-filled space in the temporal bone. The temporal bone also houses other structures, including the semicircular canals, which contain the sensory organs for balance and movement. These fluid-filled passages are connected to the cochlea but will be discussed later.

Because liquid is more difficult to move than air, the sound pressure transmitted to the inner ear must be amplified. This is achieved by a movable chain of three small bones, the **malleus, incus,** and **stapes** (**Figure 7.38**). These bones act as a piston and couple the vibrations of the tympanic membrane to the **oval window,** a membrane-covered opening separating the middle and inner ears. The total force of a sound wave applied to the tympanic membrane is transferred to the oval window; however, because the oval window is much smaller than the tympanic membrane, the force per unit area (i.e., the pressure) is increased 15 to 20 times. Additional advantage is gained through the lever action of the middle ear bones. The amount of energy transmitted to the inner ear can be lessened by the contraction of two small skeletal muscles in the middle ear. The **tensor tympani muscle** attaches to the malleus, and contraction of the muscle dampens the bone's movement. The **stapedius** attaches to the stapes and similarly controls its mobility. These muscles contract reflexively to protect the delicate receptor apparatus of the inner ear from continuous, loud sounds. They cannot, however, protect against sudden, intermittent loud sounds, which is why it is crucial for people to wear ear protection in environments like a gun firing range. These muscles also contract reflexively when you vocalize to reduce the perception of loudness of your own voice, and optimize hearing over certain frequency ranges.

The entire system described thus far involves the transmission of sound energy into the cochlea. The cochlea is almost completely divided lengthwise by a membranous tube called the **cochlear duct,** which contains the sensory receptors of the auditory system (see Figure 7.38). The cochlear duct is filled with a fluid known as **endolymph,** a compartment of extracellular fluid that is atypical in that its K^+ concentration is high and its Na^+ concentration is low, like the intracellular fluid of most cells. On either side of the cochlear duct are compartments filled with a fluid called **perilymph,** which is similar in composition to cerebrospinal fluid (review Figure 6.47). The **scala vestibuli** is above the cochlear duct and begins at the oval window; the **scala tympani** is below the cochlear duct and connects to the middle ear at a second membrane-covered opening, the **round window.** The scala vestibuli and scala tympani are continuous at the far end of the cochlear duct at the **helicotrema** (see Figure 7.38).

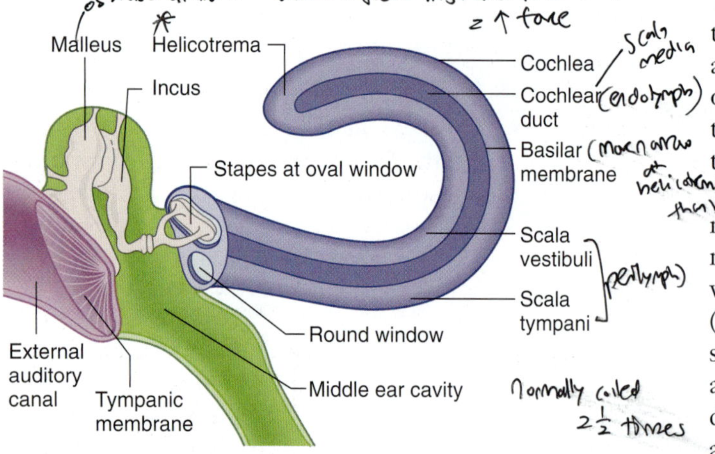

Figure 7.38 APR Relationship between the middle ear bones and the cochlea. The stapes attaches to the oval window, on the other side of which is the fluid-filled scala vestibuli. At the far end of this compartment is the helicotrema, an opening leading directly into the fluid-filled scala tympani. The membranous round window is between the scala tympani and middle ear. The cochlea is shown uncoiled for clarity. Redrawn from Kandel and Schwartz.

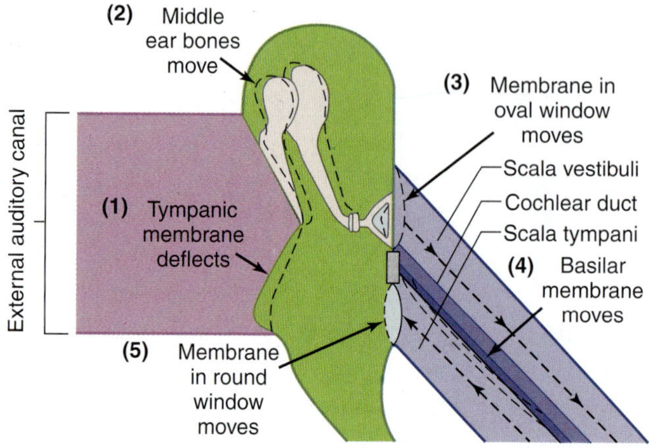

Figure 7.39 APR Transmission of sound vibrations through the middle and inner ear. (1) Sound waves coming through the external auditory canal move the tympanic membrane, which (2) moves the bones of the middle ear, (3) vibrates the membrane in the oval window, (4) causes oscillation of specific regions of the basilar membrane, and (5) causes pressure-relieving oscillations of the round window membrane. Redrawn from Davis and Silverman.

PHYSIOLOGICAL INQUIRY

- How might sounding an 80 dB warning tone just before the firing of an artillery gun (140 dB) reduce hearing damage?

Answer can be found at end of chapter.

Sound waves in the ear canal cause in-and-out movement of the tympanic membrane, which moves the chain of middle ear bones against the membrane covering the oval window, causing it to bow into the scala vestibuli and back out (**Figure 7.39**). This movement creates waves of pressure in the scala vestibuli. The wall of the scala vestibuli is largely bone, and there are only two paths by which the pressure waves can dissipate. One path is to the helicotrema, where the waves pass around the end of the cochlear duct into the scala tympani. However, most of the pressure is transmitted from the scala vestibuli across the cochlear duct. Pressure changes in the scala tympani are relieved by movements of the membrane within the round window.

The side of the cochlear duct nearest to the scala tympani is formed by the **basilar membrane** (**Figure 7.40**), upon which sits the **organ of Corti,** which contains the

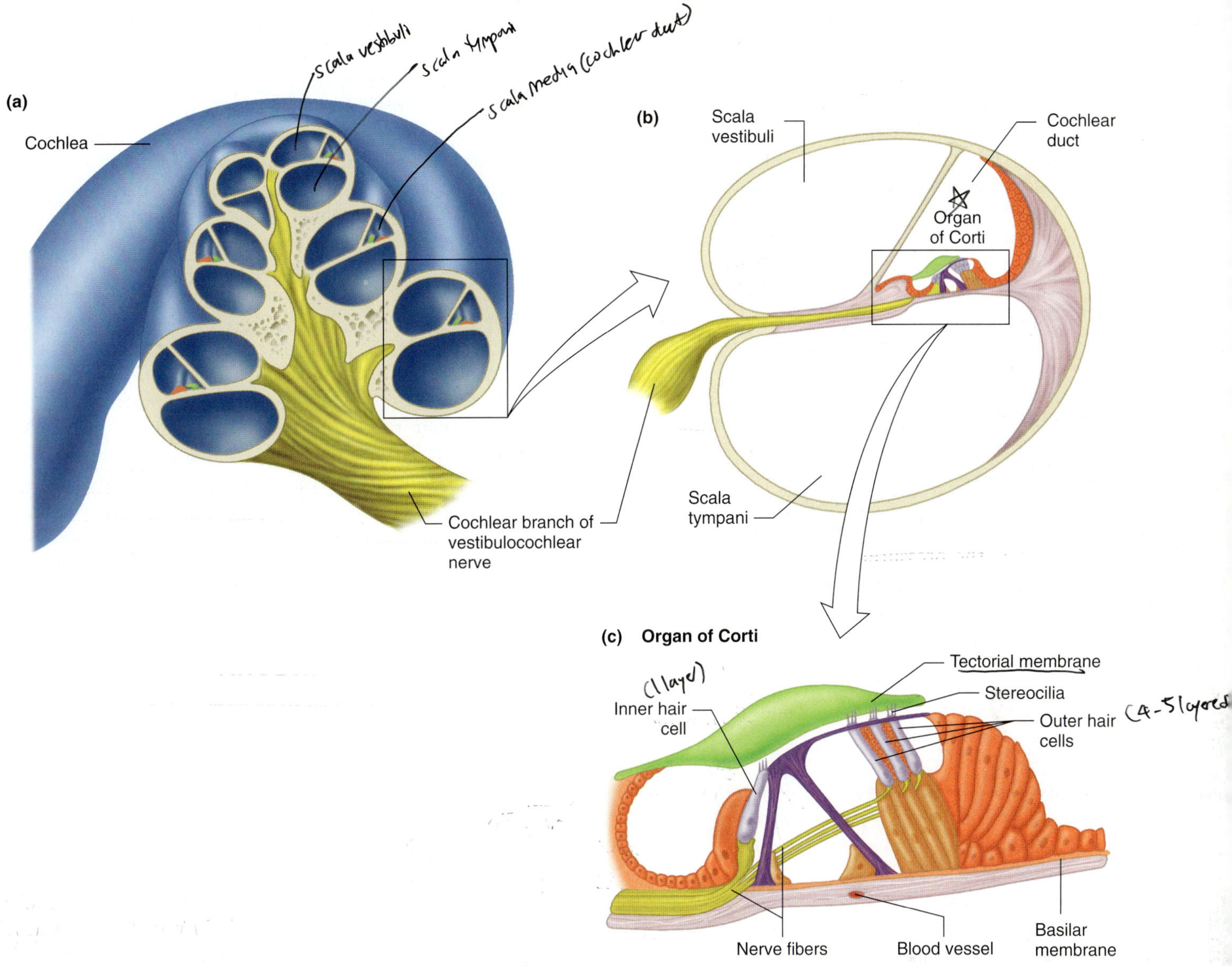

Figure 7.40 AP|R Cross section of the membranes and compartments of the inner ear with detailed view of the hair cells and other structures on the basilar membrane. Views (a), (b), and (c) show increasing magnification. Redrawn from Rasmussen.

ear's sensitive receptor cells. Pressure differences across the cochlear duct cause the basilar membrane to vibrate.

The region of maximal displacement of the vibrating basilar membrane varies with the frequency of the sound source. Nearest to the middle ear, the basilar membrane is relatively narrow and stiff, predisposing it to vibrate most easily—that is, it undergoes the greatest movement—in response to high-frequency (high-pitched) tones. The basilar membrane becomes progressively wider and less stiff toward the far end. Thus, as the frequency of received sound waves is lowered, the point of maximal vibrational movement occurs progressively farther along the membrane toward the helicotrema. The basilar membrane is thus a sort of frequency-analyzing map, with high pitches being detected nearest the middle ear and low pitches detected toward the far end.

Hair Cells of the Organ of Corti

The receptor cells of the organ of Corti are called **hair cells.** These cells are mechanoreceptors that have hairlike **stereocilia** protruding from one end (**Figure 7.41a**). There are two anatomically separate groups of hair cells, a single row of **inner hair cells** and three rows of **outer hair cells.** Stereocilia of inner hair cells extend into the endolymph fluid and actually transduce pressure waves caused by fluid movement in the cochlear duct into receptor potentials. The stereocilia of outer hair cells are embedded in an overlying **tectorial membrane** and mechanically alter its movement in a complex way that sharpens frequency tuning at each point along the basilar membrane.

The tectorial membrane overlies the organ of Corti. As pressure waves displace the basilar membrane, the hair cells move in relation to the stationary tectorial membrane, and, consequently, the stereocilia bend. When the stereocilia are bent toward the tallest member of a bundle, fibrous connections called **tip links** pull open mechanically gated cation channels, and the resulting charge influx from the K^+-rich endolymph fluid depolarizes the membrane (see Figure 7.41). This opens voltage-gated Ca^{2+} channels near the base of the cell, which triggers neurotransmitter release. Bending the hair cells in the opposite direction slackens the tip links, closing the channels and allowing the cell to rapidly repolarize. Thus, as sound waves vibrate the basilar membrane, the stereocilia are bent back and forth, the membrane potential of the hair cells rapidly oscillates, and bursts of neurotransmitter are released onto afferent neurons.

The neurotransmitter released from each hair cell is glutamate (just like in photoreceptor cells), which binds to and activates protein-binding sites on the terminals of 10 or so afferent neurons. This causes the generation of action potentials in the neurons, the axons of which join to form the cochlear branch of the **vestibulocochlear nerve** (cranial nerve VIII). The greater the energy (loudness) of the sound wave, the greater the frequency of action potentials generated in the afferent nerve fibers. Because of its position on the basilar membrane, each hair cell responds to a limited range of sound frequencies, with one particular frequency stimulating it most strongly.

In addition to the protective reflexes involving the tensor tympani and stapedius muscles, efferent nerve fibers from the brainstem regulate the activity of outer hair cells and dampen their response, which also protects them. Despite these protective mechanisms, the hair cells are easily damaged or even destroyed by exposure to high-intensity sounds such as those generated by rock concert speakers, jet plane engines, and construction equipment. Lesser noise levels also cause damage if exposure is chronic. The general mechanism of loud-sound-induced hair cell damage is thought to be due to breakage of the delicate tips of stereocilia caused by high-amplitude movements of the basilar membrane. Hearing impairment may be temporary at intermediate levels of exposure, because stereocilia tips can regenerate. However, if the sound is excessively loud or prolonged, the hair cells themselves die and are not replaced. In either temporary or permanent hearing loss, it is common for a person to experience ***tinnitis***, or "ringing in the ears," from persistent, inappropriate activation of afferent cochlear neurons following hair cell damage or loss. **Table 7.2** lists the volume level of common sounds and their effects on hearing.

Neural Pathways in Hearing

Cochlear nerve fibers enter the brainstem and synapse with interneurons there. Fibers from both ears often converge on the same neuron. Many of these interneurons are influenced by the different arrival times and intensities of the input from the two ears. The different arrival times of low-frequency sounds and the different intensities of high-frequency sounds are used to determine the direction of the sound source. If, for example, a sound is louder in the right ear or arrives sooner at the right ear than at the left, we assume that the sound source

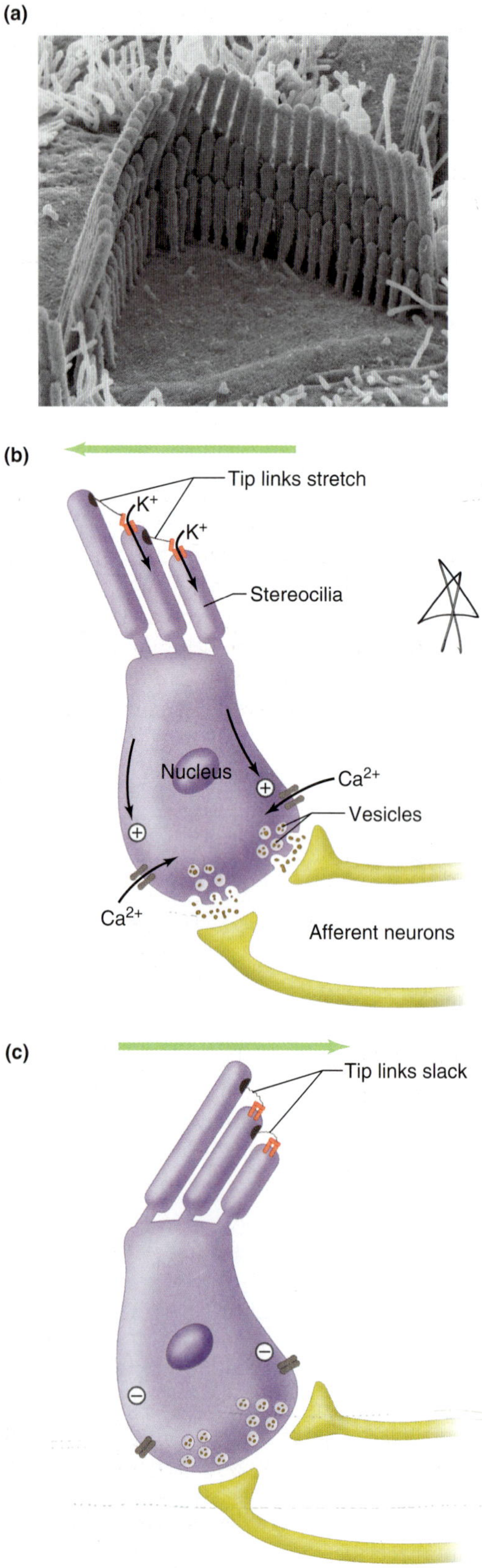

Figure 7.41 Mechanism for neurotransmitter release in a hair cell of the auditory system. (a) Scanning electron micrograph shows the size gradation in a bundle of outer hair cell stereocilia at the top of a single hair cell (tectorial membrane removed). (b) Bending stereocilia in one direction depolarizes the cell and stimulates neurotransmitter release. (c) Bending in the opposite direction repolarizes the cell and stops the release.

PHYSIOLOGICAL INQUIRY

- Furosemide is commonly used to treat high blood pressure because it increases the production of urine (it is a diuretic). It acts in the kidney by inhibiting a membrane protein responsible for pumping K^+, Na^+, and Cl^- across an epithelial membrane. Based on this information, propose a mechanism that might explain why one of the drug's side effects is hearing loss.

Answer can be found at end of chapter.

TABLE 7.2	Decibel Levels of Common Sounds and Their Effects	
Sound Source	**Decibel Level**	**Effects**
Breathing	10	Just audible
Rustling leaves	20	
Whisper	30	Very quiet
Refrigerator humming	40	
Quiet office conversation	50–60	Comfortable hearing level below 60 dB
Vacuum cleaner, hair dryer	70	Intrusive; interferes with telephone conversation
City traffic, garbage disposal	80	Annoying; constant exposure could damage hearing
Lawnmower, blender	90	Above 85 dB, 8 hours exposure causes hearing damage
Farm tractor	100	To prevent hearing loss, recommendation is for less than 15 minutes unprotected exposure
Chain saw	110	Regular exposure of more than 1 minute risks permanent hearing loss
Rock concert	110–140	Threshold of pain begins at around 125 dB
Shotgun blast, jet take-off (200-foot distance)	130	Some permanent hearing loss likely
Jet take-off (75-foot distance)	150	Tympanic membrane rupture, permanent damage

Adapted from National Institute on Deafness and Other Communication Disorders, National Institutes of Health, www.nidcd.nih.gov.

is on the right. The shape of the outer ear (the pinna; see Figure 7.37) and movements of the head are also important in localizing the sound source.

From the brainstem, the information is transmitted via a polysynaptic pathway to the thalamus and on to the auditory cortex in the temporal lobe (see Figure 7.13). The neurons responding to different pitches (frequencies) are mapped along the auditory cortex in a manner that corresponds to regions along the basilar membrane, much as stimuli from different regions of the body are represented at different sites in the somatosensory cortex. Different areas of the auditory system is further specialized; some neurons respond best to complex sounds such as those used in verbal communication. Others signal the location, movement, duration, or loudness of a sound. Descending influences on auditory nerve pathways modulate sound perception in complex ways, allowing us to selectively focus on particular sounds. For example, we can focus on a soloist's efforts above an orchestra's accompaniment and selectively suppress the echoes of a sound off of walls and floors when attempting to localize the sound's source.

Electronic devices can help compensate for damage to the intricate middle ear, cochlea, or neural structures. ***Hearing aids*** amplify incoming sounds, which then pass via the ear canal to the same cochlear mechanisms used for normal sound. When substantial damage has occurred, however, and hearing aids cannot correct the deafness, electronic devices known as ***cochlear implants*** may in some cases partially restore functional hearing. In response to sound, cochlear implants directly stimulate the cochlear nerve with tiny electrical currents so that sound signals are transmitted directly to the auditory pathways, bypassing the cochlea.

7.8 Vestibular System

Hair cells are also found in the **vestibular apparatus** of the inner ear. The vestibular apparatus is a connected series of endolymph-filled, membranous tubes that also connect with the cochlear duct (Figure 7.42). The hair cells detect changes in the motion and position of the head by a stereocilia transduction mechanism similar to that just discussed for cochlear hair cells. The vestibular apparatus consists of three membranous **semicircular canals** and two saclike swellings, the **utricle** and

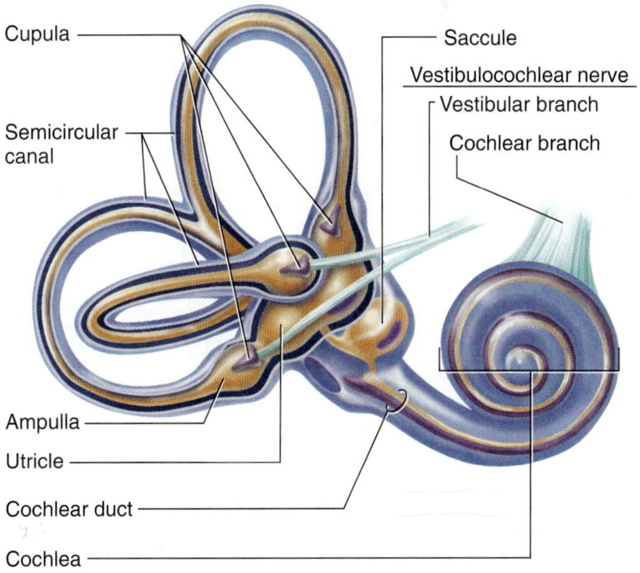

Figure 7.42 APIR A tunnel in the temporal bone contains a fluid-filled membranous duct system. The semicircular canals, utricle, and saccule make up the vestibular apparatus. This system is connected to the cochlear duct. The purple structures within the ampullae are the cupulae (singular, *cupula*), which contain the hair (receptor) cells. Redrawn from Hudspeth.

saccule, all of which lie in tunnels in the temporal bone on each side of the head. The bony tunnels of the inner ear, which house the vestibular apparatus and cochlea, have such a complicated shape that they are sometimes called the **labyrinth.**

The Semicircular Canals

The semicircular canals detect angular acceleration during *rotation* of the head along three perpendicular axes. The three axes of the semicircular canals are those activated while nodding the head up and down as in signifying "yes," shaking the head from side to side as in signifying "no," and tipping the head so the ear touches the shoulder (**Figure 7.43**).

Receptor cells of the semicircular canals, like those of the organ of Corti, contain stereocilia. These stereocilia are encapsulated within a gelatinous mass, the **cupula,** which extends across the lumen of each semicircular canal at the **ampulla,** a slight bulge in the wall of each duct (**Figure 7.44**). Whenever the head moves, the semicircular canal within its bony enclosure and the attached bodies of the hair cells all move with it. The fluid filling the duct, however, is not attached to the skull and, because of inertia, tends to retain its original position. Thus, the moving ampulla is pushed against the stationary fluid, which causes bending of the stereocilia and alteration in the rate of release of neurotransmitter from the hair cells. This neurotransmitter crosses the synapse and activates the neurons associated with the hair cells, initiating the propagation of action potentials toward the brain.

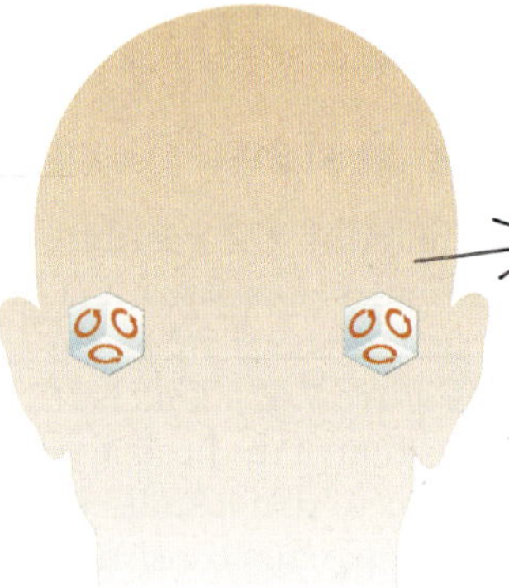

Figure 7.43 Orientation of the semicircular canals within the labyrinth. Each plane of orientation is perpendicular to the others. Together, they allow detection of movements in all directions.

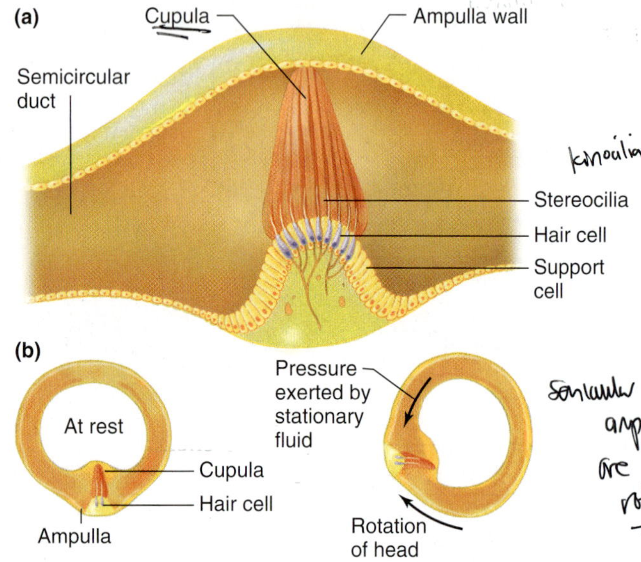

Figure 7.44 (a) Organization of a cupula and ampulla. (b) Relation of the cupula to the ampulla when the head is at rest and when it is accelerating.

The speed and magnitude of rotational head movements determine the direction in which the stereocilia are bent and which hair cells are stimulated. Movement of these mechanoreceptors causes changes in the membrane potential of the hair cell and neurotransmitter release by a mechanism similar to that in cochlear hair cells (review Figure 7.41). Neurotransmitter is released from the hair cells at rest, and the release increases or decreases from this resting rate according to the direction in which the hairs are bent. Each hair cell receptor has one direction of maximum neurotransmitter release; when its stereocilia are bent in this direction, the receptor cell depolarizes (**Figure 7.45**). When the stereocilia are bent in the opposite direction, the cell hyperpolarizes. The frequency of action potentials in the afferent nerve fibers that synapse with the hair cells is related to both the amount of force bending the stereocilia on the receptor cells and the direction in which this force is applied.

When the head continuously rotates at a steady velocity (like a figure skater's head during a spin), the duct fluid begins to move at the same rate as the rest of the head, and the stereocilia slowly return to their resting position. For this reason, the hair cells are stimulated only during acceleration or deceleration in the rate of rotation of the head.

The Utricle and Saccule

The utricle and saccule (see Figure 7.42) provide information about *linear* acceleration of the head, and about changes in head position relative to the forces of gravity. Here, too, the receptor cells are mechanoreceptors sensitive to the displacement of projecting hairs. The hair cells in the utricle point nearly

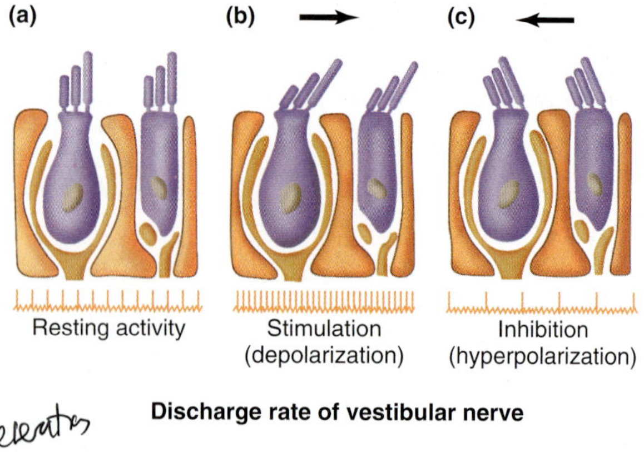

Figure 7.45 The relationship between the position of hairs in the ampulla and action potential firing in afferent neurons. (a) Resting activity. (b) Movement of hairs in one direction increases the action potential frequency in the afferent nerve activated by the hair cell. (c) Movement in the opposite direction decreases the rate relative to the resting state.

straight up when you stand, and they respond when you tip your head away from the horizontal plane, or to linear accelerations in the horizontal plane. In the saccule, hair cells project at right angles to those in the utricle, and they respond when you move from a lying to a standing position, or to vertical accelerations like those produced when you jump on a trampoline.

The utricle and saccule are slightly more complex than the ampullae. The stereocilia projecting from the hair cells are covered by a gelatinous substance in which tiny stones, or **otoliths**, are embedded. The otoliths, which are calcium carbonate crystals, make the gelatinous substance heavier than the surrounding fluid. In response to a change in position, the gelatinous otolithic material moves according to the forces of gravity and pulls against the hair cells so that the stereocilia on the hair cells bend and the receptor cells are stimulated. **Figure 7.46** demonstrates how otolith organs are stimulated by a change in head position.

Vestibular Information and Pathways

Vestibular information is used in three ways. One is to control the eye muscles so that, in spite of changes in head position, the eyes can remain fixed on the same point. ***Nystagmus*** is a large, jerky, back-and-forth movement of the eyes that can occur in response to unusual vestibular input in healthy people; it can also be a sign of pathology. Nystagmus is noticeable when a person spins in a swiveling chair for about 20 seconds, then abruptly stops the chair. For a short time after the motion ceases, the fluid in the semicircular canals continues to spin and the person's eyes will involuntarily move as though attempting to track objects spinning past the field of view. High blood alcohol concentrations disrupt functioning of the vestibular apparatus, leading to a type of nystagmus that traffic patrol officers commonly use as evidence of driving while intoxicated.

The second use of vestibular information is in reflex mechanisms for maintaining upright posture and balance. The vestibular apparatus plays a role in the support of the head during movement, orientation of the head in space, and reflexes accompanying locomotion. Very few postural reflexes, however, depend exclusively on input from the vestibular system despite the fact that the vestibular organs are sometimes called the sense organs of balance.

The third use of vestibular information is in providing conscious awareness of the position and acceleration of the body, perception of the space surrounding the body, and memory of spatial information.

Information about hair cell stimulation is relayed from the vestibular apparatus to nuclei within the brainstem via the vestibular branch of the vestibulocochlear nerve. It is transmitted via a polysynaptic pathway through the thalamus to a system of vestibular centers in the parietal lobe. Descending projections are also sent from the brainstem nuclei to the spinal cord to influence postural reflexes. Vestibular information is integrated with information from the joints, tendons, and skin, leading to the sense of posture (**proprioception**) and movement. A good example of this occurs when you try to maintain your posture while standing on a moving train or subway.

A mismatch in information from the various sensory systems can create feelings of nausea and dizziness. For example, many amusement parks feature widescreen virtual thrill rides in which your eyes take you on a dizzying helicopter ride, while your vestibular system signals that you are not moving at all. ***Motion sickness*** also involves the vestibular system, occurring when you experience unfamiliar patterns of linear and rotational acceleration and adaptation to them has not yet occurred.

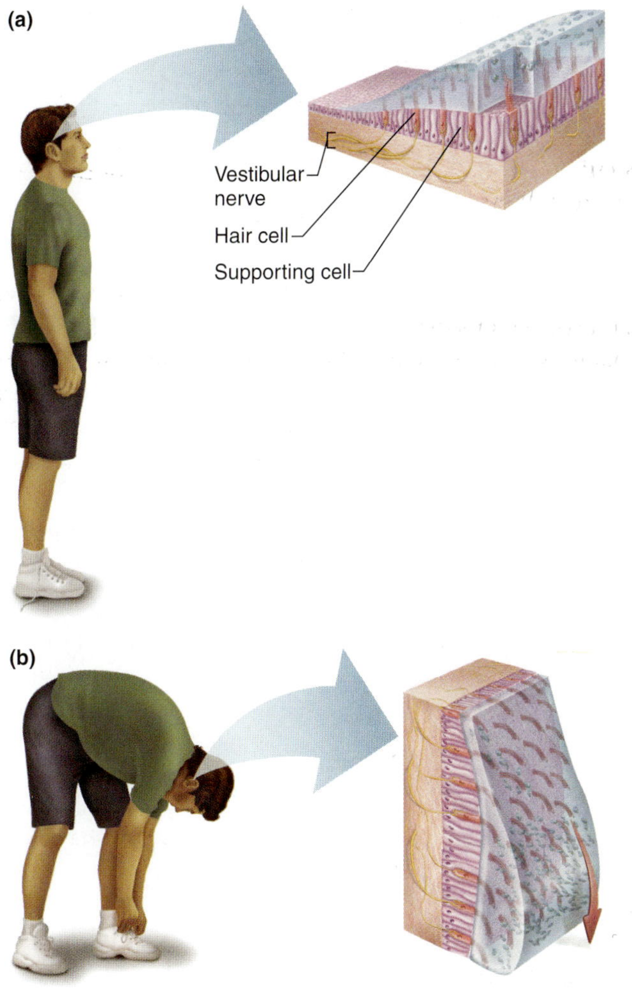

Figure 7.46 Effect of head position on otolith organ of the utricle. (a) Upright position: hair cells are not bent. (b) Gravity bends the hair cells when the head tilts forward.

7.9 Chemical Senses

Recall that receptors sensitive to specific chemicals are chemoreceptors. Some of these respond to chemical changes in the internal environment; two examples are receptors that sense oxygen and hydrogen ion concentration in the blood, which you will learn more about in Chapter 13. Others respond to external chemical changes. In this category are the receptors for taste and smell, which affect a person's appetite, saliva flow, gastric secretions, and avoidance of harmful substances.

Taste

The specialized sense organs for taste (also called **gustation**) are the 10,000 or so **taste buds** found in the mouth and throat, the vast majority on the upper surface and sides of the tongue. Taste buds are small groups of cells arranged like orange slices around a hollow pore and are found in the walls of visible structures called **lingual papillae** (**Figure 7.47**). Some of the cells serve mainly as supporting cells, but others are specialized epithelial cells that act as receptors for various chemicals in the food we eat. Small, hairlike microvilli increase the surface area of taste receptor cells and contain integral membrane proteins that transduce the presence of a given chemical into a receptor potential. At the bottom of taste buds are **basal cells**, which divide and differentiate to continually replace taste receptor cells damaged in the occasionally harsh environment of the mouth. To enter the pores of the taste buds and come into contact with taste receptor cells, food molecules must be dissolved in liquid—either ingested or provided by secretions of the salivary glands. Try placing sugar or salt on your tongue after thoroughly drying it; little or no taste sensation occurs until saliva begins to flow and dissolves the substance.

Many different chemicals can generate the sensation of taste by differentially activating a few basic types of taste receptors. Taste submodalities generally fall into five different categories according to the receptor type most strongly activated: sweet, sour, salty, bitter, and **umami** (oo-MAH-mee). This latter category gets its name from a Japanese word that can be roughly translated as "delicious." This taste is associated with the taste of glutamate and similar amino acids and is sometimes described as conveying the sense of savoriness or flavorfulness. Glutamate (or monosodium glutamate, MSG) is a common additive used to enhance the flavor of foods in traditional Asian cuisine. In addition to these known taste receptors, there are likely others yet to be discovered. For example, recent experiments suggest that a fatty

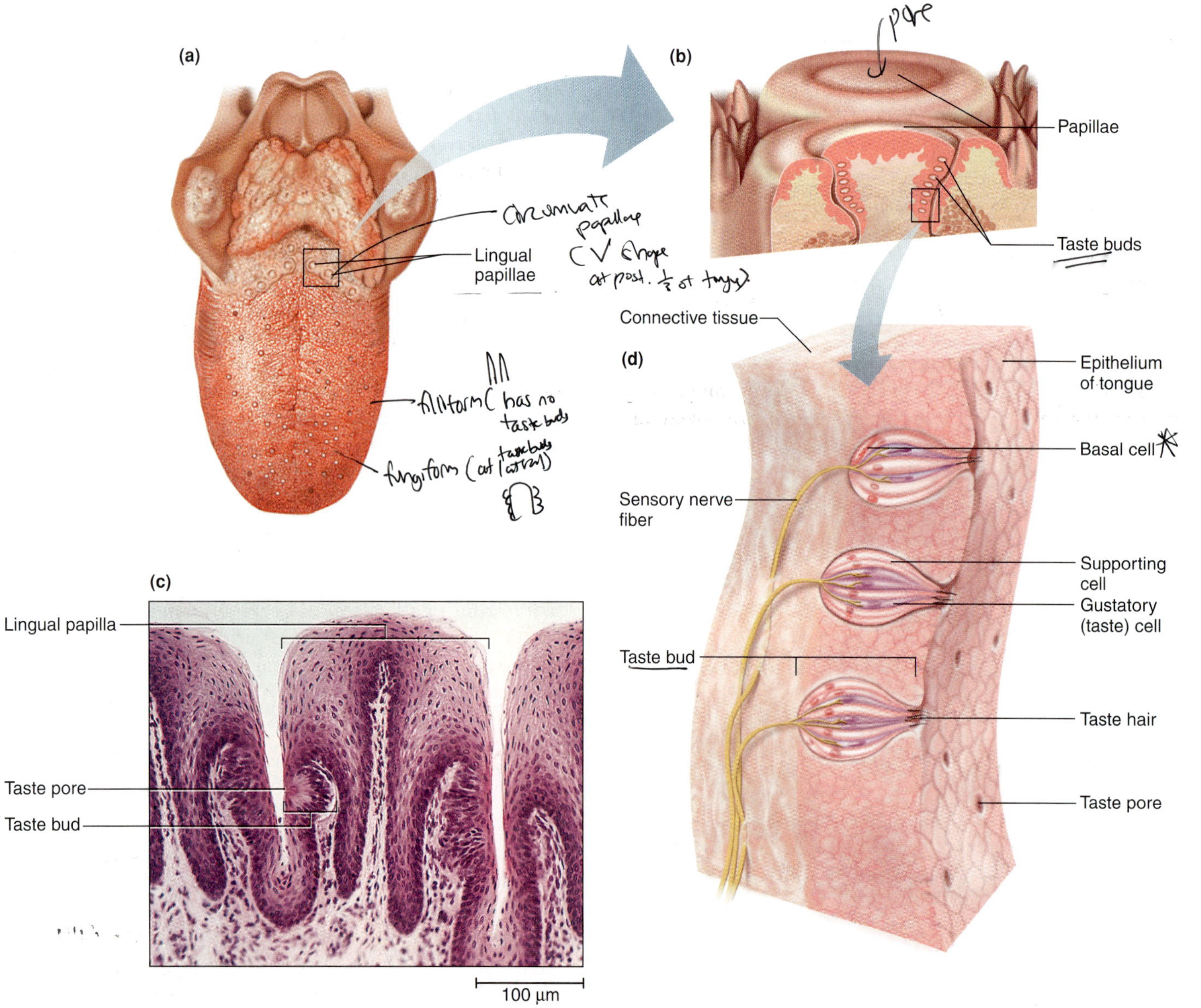

Figure 7.47 AP|R Taste receptors. (a) Top view of the tongue showing lingual papillae. (b and c) Cross section of one type of papilla with taste buds. (d) Pores in the sides of papillae open into taste buds, which are composed of supporting cells, taste receptor cells, and basal cells.

acid transport protein first identified in the lingual papillae of rodents may soon be added to the list. Research has shown that blocking these transporters inhibits the preference for the taste of foods with high lipid content and reduces the production of fat-digesting enzymes by the gastrointestinal system. If confirmed in humans, this fatty acid transporter could become the sixth member of the taste receptor family and might help explain our tendency to overindulge on high-calorie, high-fat foods.

Each group of tastes has a distinct signal transduction mechanism. Salt taste is detected by a simple mechanism in which ingested sodium ions enter channels in the receptor cell membrane, depolarizing the cell and stimulating the production of action potentials in the associated sensory neuron. Sour taste is stimulated by foods with high acid content, such as lemons, which contain citric acid. Hydrogen ions block K^+ channels in the sour receptors, and the loss of the hyperpolarizing K^+ leak current depolarizes the receptor cell. Sweet receptors have integral membrane proteins that bind natural sugars like glucose, as well as artificial sweetener molecules like saccharin and aspartame. Binding of sugars to these receptors activates a G-protein-coupled second-messenger pathway (Chapter 5) that ultimately blocks K^+ channels and thus generates a depolarizing receptor potential. Bitter flavor is associated with many poisonous substances, especially certain elements such as arsenic, and plant alkaloids like strychnine. There is an obvious evolutionary advantage in recognizing a wide variety of poisonous substances, and thus there are many varieties of bitter receptors. All of those types, however, generate receptor potentials via G-protein-mediated second-messenger pathways and ultimately evoke the negative sensation of bitter flavor. Umami receptor cells also depolarize via a G-protein-coupled receptor mechanism.

Each afferent neuron synapses with more than one receptor cell, and the taste system is organized into independent coded pathways into the central nervous system. Single receptor cells, however, respond in varying degrees to substances that fall into more than one taste category. This property is analogous to the overlapping sensitivities of photoreceptors to different wavelengths. Awareness of the specific taste of a substance depends also upon the pattern of firing in other types of sensory neurons. For example, sensations of pain (hot spices), texture, and temperature contribute to taste.

The pathways for taste in the central nervous system project to the gustatory cortex, near the "mouth" region of the somatosensory cortex (see Figure 7.13).

Smell

A major part of the flavor of food is actually contributed by the sense of smell, or **olfaction.** This is illustrated by the common experience of finding that food lacks taste when a head cold blocks your nasal passages. The odor of a substance is directly related to its chemical structure. We can recognize and identify thousands of different odors with great accuracy. Thus, neural circuits that deal with olfaction must encode information about different chemical structures, store (learn) the different code patterns that represent the different structures, and at a later time recognize a particular neural code to identify the odor.

The olfactory receptor neurons, the first cells in the pathways that give rise to the sense of smell, lie in a small patch of epithelium called the **olfactory epithelium** in the upper part of the nasal cavity (**Figure 7.48a**). Olfactory receptor neurons survive for only about 2 months, so they are constantly being replaced by new cells produced from stem cells in the olfactory epithelium. The mature cells are specialized afferent neurons that have a single, enlarged dendrite that extends to the surface of the epithelium. Several long, nonmotile cilia extend from the tip of the dendrite and lie along the surface of the olfactory

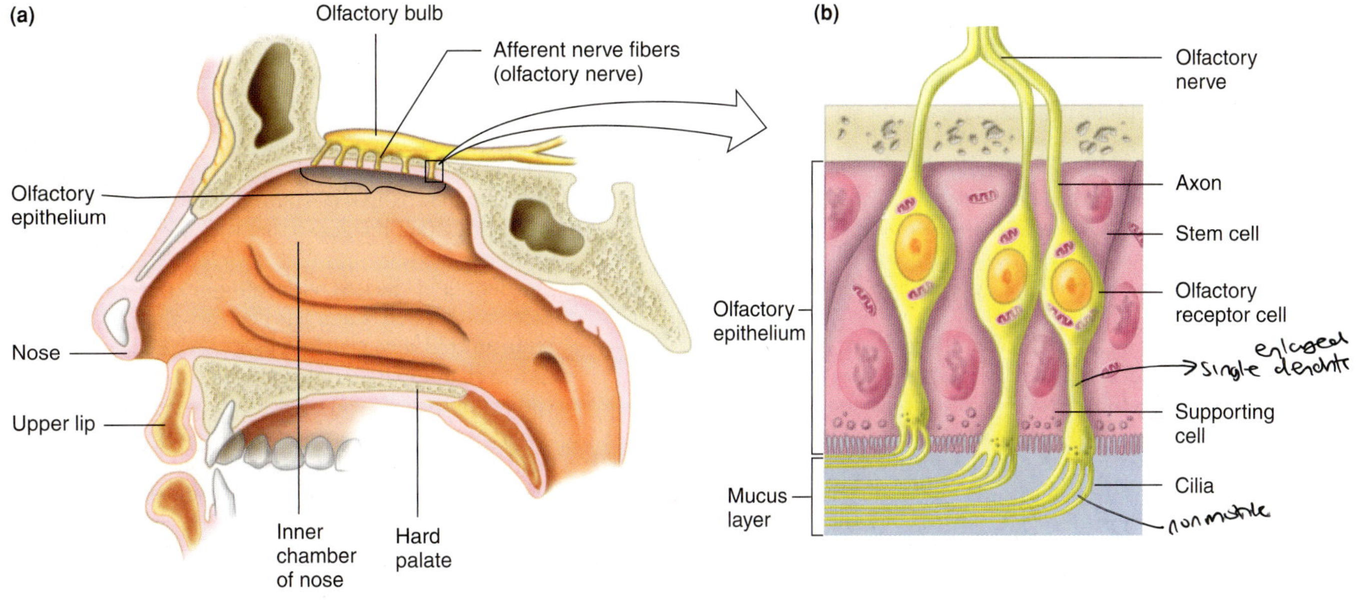

Figure 7.48 AP|R (a) Location and (b) enlargement of a portion of the olfactory epithelium showing the structure of the olfactory receptor cells. In addition to these cells, the olfactory epithelium contains stem cells, which give rise to new receptors and supporting cells.

epithelium (**Figure 7.48b**) where they are bathed in mucus. The cilia contain the receptor proteins that provide the binding sites for odor molecules. The axons of the neurons form the olfactory nerve, which is cranial nerve I.

For us to detect an odorous substance (an **odorant**), molecules of the substance must first diffuse into the air and pass into the nose to the region of the olfactory epithelium. Once there, they dissolve in the mucus that covers the epithelium and then bind to specific odorant receptors on the cilia. Proteins in the mucus may interact with the odorant molecules, transport them to the receptors, and facilitate their binding to the receptors. Stimulated odorant receptors activate a G-protein-mediated pathway that increases cAMP, which in turn opens nonselective cation channels and depolarizes the cell.

Although there are many thousands of olfactory receptor cells, each contains only one of the 1000 or so different plasma membrane odorant receptor types. In turn, each of these types responds only to a specific chemically related group of odorant molecules. Each odorant has characteristic chemical groups that distinguish it from other odorants, and each of these groups activates a different plasma membrane odorant receptor type. Thus, the identity of a particular odorant is determined by the activation of a precise combination of plasma membrane receptors, each of which is contained in a distinct group of olfactory receptor cells.

The axons of the olfactory receptor cells synapse in a pair of brain structures known as **olfactory bulbs**, which lie on the undersurface of the frontal lobes. Axons from olfactory receptor cells that share a common receptor specificity synapse together on certain olfactory bulb neurons, thereby maintaining the specificity of the original stimulus. In other words, specific odorant receptor cells activate only certain olfactory bulb neurons, allowing the brain to determine which receptors have been stimulated. The codes used to transmit olfactory information probably use both spatial (which specific neurons are firing) and temporal (the frequency of action potentials in each neuron) components.

The olfactory system is the only sensory system that does not synapse in the thalamus prior to reaching the cortex. Information passes from the olfactory bulbs directly to the olfactory cortex and parts of the limbic system. The limbic system and associated hypothalamic structures are involved with emotional, food-getting, and sexual behaviors; the direct connection from the olfactory system explains why the sense of smell has such an important influence on these activities. Some areas of the olfactory cortex then send projections to other regions of the frontal cortex. Different odors elicit different patterns of electrical activity in several cortical areas, allowing humans to discriminate between some 10,000 different odorants even though they have only 1000 or so different olfactory receptor types.

Olfactory discrimination varies with attentiveness, hunger (sensitivity is greater in hungry subjects), gender (women in general have keener olfactory sensitivities than men), smoking (decreased sensitivity has been repeatedly associated with smoking), age (the ability to identify odors decreases with age, and a large percentage of elderly persons cannot detect odors at all), and state of the olfactory mucosa (as we have mentioned, the sense of smell decreases when the mucosa is congested, as in a head cold). Some individuals are born with genetic defects resulting in a total lack of the ability to smell (***anosmia***). For example, defects in genes on the X chromosome, as well as in chromosomes 8 and 20, can cause ***Kallmann syndrome***. This is a condition in which the olfactory bulbs fail to form, as do regions of the brain associated with regulation of sex hormones.

SECTION B SUMMARY

Somatic Sensation

I. A variety of receptors sensitive to one or a few stimulus types provide sensory function of the skin and underlying tissues.

II. Information about somatic sensation enters both specific and nonspecific ascending pathways. The specific pathways cross to the opposite side of the brain.

III. The somatic sensations include touch, pressure, the senses of posture and movement, temperature, and pain.

a. Rapidly adapting mechanoreceptors of the skin give rise to sensations such as vibration, touch, and movement, whereas slowly adapting ones give rise to the sensation of pressure.

b. Skin receptors with small receptive fields are involved in fine spatial discrimination, whereas receptors with larger receptive fields signal less spatially precise touch or pressure sensations.

c. A major receptor type responsible for the senses of posture and kinesthesia is the muscle-spindle stretch receptor.

d. Cold receptors are sensitive to decreasing temperature; warmth receptors signal information about increasing temperature.

e. Tissue damage and immune cells release chemical agents that stimulate specific receptors that give rise to the sensation of pain.

f. Stimulation-produced analgesia, transcutaneous electrical nerve stimulation (TENS), and acupuncture control pain by blocking transmission in the pain pathways.

Vision

I. The color of light is defined by its wavelength or frequency.

II. The light that falls on the retina is focused by the cornea and lens.

a. Lens shape changes (accommodation) to permit viewing near or distant images so that they are focused on the retina.

b. Stiffening of the lens with aging interferes with accommodation. Cataracts decrease the amount of light transmitted through the lens.

c. An eyeball too long or too short relative to the focusing power of the lens and cornea causes nearsighted (myopic) or farsighted (hyperopic) vision, respectively.

III. The photopigments of the rods and cones are made up of a protein component (opsin) and a chromophore (retinal).

a. The rods and each of the three cone types have different opsins, which make each of the four receptor types sensitive to different ranges of light wavelengths.

b. When light strikes retinal, it changes shape, triggering a cascade of events leading to hyperpolarization of photoreceptors and decreased neurotransmitter release from them. When exposed to darkness, the rods and cones are depolarized and therefore release more neurotransmitter than in light.

IV. The rods and cones synapse on bipolar cells, which synapse on ganglion cells.
   a. Ganglion cell axons form the optic nerves, which exit the eyeballs.
   b. The optic nerve fibers from the medial half of each retina cross to the opposite side of the brain in the optic chiasm. The fibers from the optic nerves terminate in the lateral geniculate nuclei of the thalamus, which sends fibers to the visual cortex.
   c. Photoreceptors also send information to areas of the brain dealing with biological rhythms.

V. Coding in the visual system occurs along parallel pathways in which different aspects of visual information, such as color, form, movement, and depth, are kept separate from each other.

VI. The colors we perceive are related to the wavelength of light. The three cone photopigments vary in the strength of their response to light over differing ranges of wavelengths.
   a. Certain ganglion cells are excited by input from one type of cone cell and inhibited by input from a different cone type.
   b. Our sensation of color depends on the output of the various opponent color cells and the processing of this output by brain areas involved in color vision.
   c. Color blindness is due to abnormalities of the cone pigments resulting from genetic mutations.

VII. Six skeletal muscles control eye movement to scan the visual field for objects of interest, keep the fixation point focused on the fovea centralis despite movements of the object or the head, and prevent adaptation of the photoreceptors.

Hearing

I. Sound energy is transmitted by movements of pressure waves.
   a. Sound wave frequency determines pitch.
   b. Sound wave amplitude determines loudness.

II. The sequence of sound transmission follows.
   a. Sound waves enter the external auditory canal and press against the tympanic membrane, causing it to vibrate.
   b. The vibrating membrane causes movement of the three small middle ear bones; the stapes vibrates against the oval window membrane.
   c. Movements of the oval window membrane set up pressure waves in the fluid-filled scala vestibuli, which cause vibrations in the cochlear duct wall, setting up pressure waves in the fluid there.
   d. These pressure waves cause vibrations in the basilar membrane, which is located on one side of the cochlear duct.
   e. As this membrane vibrates, the hair cells of the organ of Corti move in relation to the tectorial membrane.
   f. Movement of the hair cells' stereocilia stimulates the hair cells to release glutamate, which activates receptors on the peripheral ends of the afferent nerve fibers.

III. Separate parts of the basilar membrane vibrate maximally in response to particular sound frequencies; high frequency is detected near the oval window and low frequency toward the far end of the cochlear duct.

Vestibular System

I. A vestibular apparatus lies in the temporal bone on each side of the head and consists of three semicircular canals, a utricle, and a saccule.

II. The semicircular canals detect angular acceleration during rotation of the head, which causes bending of the stereocilia on their hair cells.

III. Otoliths in the gelatinous substance of the utricle and saccule (a) move in response to changes in linear acceleration and the position of the head relative to gravity and (b) stimulate the stereocilia on the hair cells.

Chemical Senses

I. The receptors for taste lie in taste buds throughout the mouth, principally on the tongue. Different types of taste receptors have different sensory transduction mechanisms.

II. Olfactory receptors, which are part of the afferent olfactory neurons, lie in the upper nasal cavity.
   a. Odorant molecules, once dissolved in the mucus that bathes the olfactory receptors, bind to specific receptors (protein-binding sites). Each olfactory receptor cell has one or at most a few of the 1000 different receptor types.
   b. Olfactory pathways go directly to the olfactory cortex and limbic system, rather than to the thalamus.

SECTION B REVIEW QUESTIONS

1. Describe the similarities between pain and the other somatic sensations. Describe the differences.
2. Explain the mechanism of sensory transduction in temperature-sensing neurons.
3. What are the sensory implications of the different crossover points of the anterolateral and dorsal column ascending pathways in patients with injuries that damage half of the spinal cord at a given level?
4. List at least two ways the retina has adapted to minimize the potential problem caused by the photoreceptors being the last layer of the retina that light reaches.
5. Describe the events that take place during accommodation for near vision.
6. Detail the separate mechanisms activated in photoreceptor cells in the presence and in the absence of light.
7. Beginning with the photoreceptor cells of the retina, describe the interactions with bipolar and ganglion cells in the ON- and OFF-pathways of the visual system.
8. List the sequence of events that occurs between the entry of a sound wave into the external auditory canal and the firing of action potentials in the cochlear nerve.
9. Describe the functional relationship between the scala vestibuli, scala tympani, and the cochlear duct.
10. What is the relationship between head movement and cupula movement in a semicircular canal?
11. What causes the release of neurotransmitter from the utricle and saccule receptor cells?
12. In what ways are the sensory systems for taste and olfaction similar? In what ways are they different?

SECTION B KEY TERMS

accommodation 209
amacrine cell 214
ampulla 224
anterolateral pathway 206
aqueous humor 208
audition 217
basal cell 226
basilar membrane 220
binocular vision 215
bipolar cell 213
cGMP-phosphodiesterase 212
choroid 208
chromophore 211
ciliary muscle 208
cochlea 220
cochlear duct 220
cone 211
cornea 208
cupula 224
dark adaptation 212

SECTION B CLINICAL TERMS

CHAPTER 7

Clinical Case Study: Severe Dizzy Spells in a Healthy, 65-Year-Old Farmer

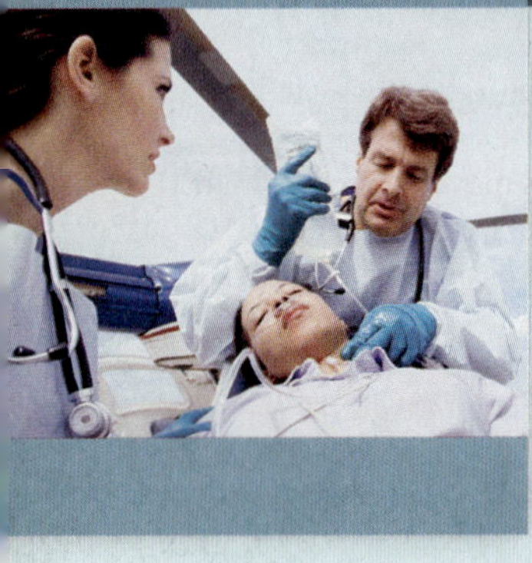

Just after 6:00 A.M. on a Sunday morning, a large man in overalls staggered into the emergency room leaning heavily for support on his wife's shoulder. He held a bloody towel pressed tightly to the right side of his head, and his skin was pale and sweaty. The towel was removed to reveal a 1-inch scalp laceration above his right ear. As the emergency room physician cleaned and stitched the wound, the man and his wife explained what had happened. A dairy farmer, he was arising to do his chores that morning when he became dizzy, fell, and struck his head on the dresser. When the doctor commented that it wasn't that unusual for a transient decrease in blood pressure to cause fainting upon standing up too quickly, the man's wife stated that this was something different. Over the past 3 months, he had experienced a number of occasions when he suddenly became dizzy. These dizzy spells also seemed to be becoming more severe, and they were not always associated with standing up; indeed, sometimes they happened even when he was lying down. Lasting anywhere from a few minutes to a few hours, the episodes were sometimes accompanied by headaches, nausea, and vomiting. Not one to complain, the man had not previously sought treatment. Because these could be signs of serious underlying illness, the physician elected to do a more thorough examination.

The patient was 65 years old and appeared relatively muscular and fit for his age. At the time of the examination, he had trouble sitting or standing without support and reported feeling dizzy and nauseated. His only known chronic medical problem was high blood pressure, which had been diagnosed 10 years earlier and had been well-controlled by medication since that time. When questioned about alcohol use, both he and his wife assured the doctor that he only drank one or two beers at a time and only on weekends.

One of the first things the physician needed to determine was whether the patient suffered from vertigo or from light-headedness. "Dizziness" is one of the most common symptoms reported by patients seeing primary care physicians, but that generic description does not discriminate between the actual underlying mechanisms of the sensation and their causes. Light-headedness is a sensation

(continued)

(continued)

of beginning to lose consciousness (becoming faint, also called ***presyncope***). Actual loss of consciousness is referred to as ***syncope.*** ***Vertigo*** is a sensation of environmental movement when lying, sitting, or standing still (e.g., a feeling that the room is spinning) and results from a disruption of the vestibular systems but usually not from disruption of cerebral blood supply. Interruption of blood flow to the brain can cause a light-headed sensation because brain cells deprived of oxygen or nutrients for even brief periods of time begin to malfunction. This is the cause of the commonly observed phenomenon in which a person can become light-headed in the moments after standing up. Lying down, the brain is level with the heart and blood delivery requires very little work, whereas in the standing position, the heart must pump more strongly to maintain blood flow to the brain against gravity. Even a slight delay in increasing cardiac contraction strength upon standing can reduce brain blood flow enough to cause light-headedness.

Reduced blood flow to the brain can also be caused by dehydration, low blood pressure, interruption of the normal rhythm of the heartbeat, and blockage of the arteries in the neck that carry blood to the brain. Even if brain blood flow is adequate, brain cells can also malfunction and cause light-headedness if the concentrations of oxygen or glucose in the blood are below normal. However, a thorough assessment of the farmer's circulatory system function, blood oxygen concentration, and blood glucose concentration showed no abnormalities. These results, combined with the fact that the patient's symptoms were not always linked to suddenly standing up, seemed to indicate that the sensation of dizziness the patient reported was most likely not light-headedness due to a problem with the blood supply to his brain.

The doctor next examined the patient's eyes, ears, nose, and throat. There was no evidence of infection of the man's nose, throat, or tympanic membranes. This suggested that he was not suffering from an infection that could cause sinus pressure or fluid buildup in the middle ear, both of which can be associated with headaches, dizziness, and nausea. Viewed with an ophthalmoscope, his retinas also appeared normal. In cases in which patients have rapidly growing brain tumors that increase the intracranial pressure and cause dizziness and disorientation, the optic discs are often observed to bulge from the surface of the retina. When asked to focus on the doctor's finger as it was held in some positions in his visual field (far left, up, down), the man's eyes remained fixated without abnormality, but they developed rapid, rhythmic, jerking movements when the finger was brought to the patient's far right. This eye-movement pattern is called nystagmus and is frequently associated with abnormalities of the vestibular apparatus of the inner ear or the neural pathways involved in reflexive integration of head and eye movements. Excess alcohol consumption can disrupt vestibular function and cause nystagmus, but the evidence did not suggest that was the cause in this case.

One condition leading to malfunction of the vestibular system is ***Ménière's disease,*** in which an abnormal buildup of pressure in the inner ear disrupts the function of the cochlea and semicircular canals. This disease often manifests as periodic bouts of vertigo and loss of balance, accompanied by nausea and vomiting; each bout may last from minutes to many hours. Because the cochlea is also involved, this condition sometimes also results in auditory symptoms including tinnitus ("ringing in the ears") and/or loss of hearing. The lack of auditory symptoms in this case led the doctor to question the patient further; when asked in more detail about what he thought triggered his dizzy spells, the patient said it tended to occur only after rapid movements of his head, especially when turning his head to the right. This statement was an essential clue leading to the correct diagnosis.

The man was suffering from ***benign paroxysmal positional vertigo*** (***BPPV***), which involves disruption of function of the vestibular apparatus or its neural pathways. This particular type of vertigo, as the name suggests, is not associated with serious or permanent damage, occurs sporadically, and is associated with changes in head position. It may occur at any age but occurs most frequently in elderly persons; this is of great concern because of the likelihood of falling when dizzy and the fragility of the bones of many elderly persons. Though the cause of BPPV is not clear in most cases, the leading hypothesis is that loose calcium carbonate crystals (otoliths) associated with the vestibular apparatus float into the semicircular canals and interrupt normal fluid movement. Otoliths may be dislodged by head injury or infection or due to the normal degeneration of aging.

One treatment that has achieved some success for reducing the symptoms of BPPV is a series of carefully choreographed manipulations of head position called the ***Epley maneuver.*** The head movements are designed to use the force of gravity to dislodge loose otoliths from the semicircular canals and move them back into the gelatinous membranes within the utricle and saccule. Patients undergoing this or similar manipulations are cured of BPPV about 80% of the time. After two times through the procedure, the farmer's vertigo went away and he was able to stand on his own. Because multiple treatments are sometimes required, he was given instructions on how to self-administer a modified Epley maneuver at home; within 3 weeks, his vertigo was gone.

Clinical terms: benign paroxysmal positional vertigo (BPPV), Epley maneuver, Ménière's disease, presyncope, syncope, vertigo

See Chapter 19 for complete, integrative case studies.

CHAPTER 7 TEST QUESTIONS

Answers found in Appendix A.

1. Choose the *true* statement:
   a. The modality of energy a given sensory receptor responds to in normal functioning is known as the "adequate stimulus" for that receptor.
   b. Receptor potentials are "all or none," that is, they have the same magnitude regardless of the strength of the stimulus.
   c. When the frequency of action potentials along sensory neurons is constant as long as a stimulus continues, it is called "adaptation."
   d. When sensory units have large receptive fields, the acuity of perception is greater.
   e. The "modality" refers to the intensity of a given stimulus.

2. Using a single intracellular recording electrode, in what part of a sensory neuron could you simultaneously record both receptor potentials and action potentials?
   a. in the cell body
   b. at the node of Ranvier nearest the peripheral end
   c. at the receptor membrane where the stimulus occurs
   d. at the central axon terminals within the CNS
   e. There is no single point where both can be measured.
3. Which best describes "lateral inhibition" in sensory processing?
   a. Presynaptic axo–axonal synapses reduce neurotransmitter release at excitatory synapses.
   b. When a stimulus is maintained for a long time, action potentials from sensory receptors decrease in frequency with time.
   c. Descending inputs from the brainstem inhibit afferent pain pathways in the spinal cord.
   d. Inhibitory interneurons decrease action potentials from receptors at the periphery of a stimulated region.
   e. Receptor potentials increase in magnitude with the strength of a stimulus.
4. What region of the brain contains the primary visual cortex?
   a. the occipital lobe
   b. the frontal lobe
   c. the temporal lobe
   d. the somatosensory cortex
   e. the parietal lobe association area
5. Which type of receptor does *not* encode a somatic sensation?
   a. muscle-spindle stretch receptor
   b. nociceptor
   c. Pacinian corpuscle
   d. thermoreceptor
   e. cochlear hair cell
6. Which best describes the vision of a person with uncorrected nearsightedness?
   a. The eyeball is too long; far objects focus on the retina when the ciliary muscle contracts.
   b. The eyeball is too long; near objects focus on the retina when the ciliary muscle is relaxed.
   c. The eyeball is too long; near objects cannot be focused on the retina.
   d. The eyeball is too short; far objects cannot be focused on the retina.
   e. The eyeball is too short; near objects focus on the retina when the ciliary muscle is relaxed.
7. If a patient suffers a stroke that destroys the optic tract on the right side of the brain, which of the following visual defects will result?
   a. Complete blindness will result.
   b. There will be no vision in the left eye, but vision will be normal in the right eye.
   c. The patient will not perceive images of objects striking the left half of the retina in the left eye.
   d. The patient will not perceive images of objects striking the right half of the retina in the right eye.
   e. Neither eye will perceive objects in the right side of the patient's field of view.
8. Which correctly describes a step in auditory signal transduction?
   a. Displacement of the basilar membrane with respect to the tectorial membrane stimulates stereocilia on the hair cells.
   b. Pressure waves on the oval window cause vibrations of the malleus, which are transferred via the stapes to the round window.
   c. Movement of the stapes causes oscillations in the tympanic membrane, which is in contact with the endolymph.
   d. Oscillations of the stapes against the oval window set up pressure waves in the semicircular canals.
   e. The malleus, incus, and stapes are found in the inner ear, within the cochlea.
9. A standing subject looking over her left shoulder suddenly rotates her head to look over her right shoulder. How does the vestibular system detect this motion?
   a. The utricle goes from a vertical to a horizontal position, and otoliths stimulate stereocilia.
   b. Stretch receptors in neck muscles send action potentials to the vestibular apparatus, which relays them to the brain.
   c. Fluid within the semicircular canals remains stationary, bending the cupula and stereocilia as the head rotates.
   d. The movement causes endolymph in the cochlea to rotate from right to left, stimulating inner hair cells.
   e. Counterrotation of the aqueous humor activates a nystagmus response.
10. Which category of taste receptor cells does MSG (monosodium glutamate) most strongly stimulate?
    a. salty
    b. bitter
    c. sweet
    d. umami
    e. sour

CHAPTER 7 GENERAL PRINCIPLES ASSESSMENT

Answers found in Appendix A.

1. A key general principle of physiology is that *homeostasis is essential for health and survival.* How might sensory receptors responsible for detecting painful stimuli (nociceptors) contribute to homeostasis?
2. How does the sensory transduction mechanism in the vestibular and auditory systems demonstrate the importance of the general principle of physiology that *controlled exchange of materials occurs between compartments and across cellular membranes?*
3. Elaboration of surface area to maximize functional capability is a common motif in the body illustrating the general principle of physiology that *structure is a determinant of—and has coevolved with—function.* Cite an example from this chapter.

CHAPTER 7 QUANTITATIVE AND THOUGHT QUESTIONS

Answers found at www.mhhe.com/widmaier13.

1. Describe several mechanisms by which pain could theoretically be controlled medically or surgically.
2. At what two sites would central nervous system injuries interfere with the perception that heat is being applied to the right side of the body? At what single site would a central nervous system injury interfere with the perception that heat is being applied to either side of the body?
3. What would vision be like after a drug has destroyed all the cones in the retina?
4. Damage to what parts of the cerebral cortex could explain the following behaviors? (a) A person walks into a chair placed in her path. (b) The person does not walk into the chair, but she does not know what the chair can be used for.
5. How could the concept of referred pain potentially complicate the clinical assessment of the source of a patient's somatic pain?

Figure 7.2 Receptor potentials would not be affected because they are not mediated by voltage-gated channels. Action potential propagation to the central nervous system would also be normal because it depends only on voltage-gated Na^+ and K^+ channels. The drug would inhibit neurotransmitter release from the central axon terminal, however, because vesicle exocytosis requires Ca^{2+} entry through voltage-gated channels.

Figure 7.6 Although the skin area of your lips is much smaller than that of your back, the much larger number of sensory neurons originating in your lips requires a larger processing area within the somatosensory cortex of your brain. See Figure 7.20 for a diagrammatic representation of cortical areas involved in sensory processing.

Figure 7.15 Pacinian corpuscles are rapidly adapting receptors, and that property is conferred by the fluid-filled connective tissue capsule that surrounds them. When pressure is initially applied, the fluid in the capsule compresses the nerve ending, opening mechanically gated nonspecific cation channels and causing depolarization and action potentials. However, fluid then redistributes within the capsule, taking the pressure off the nerve ending; consequently, the channels close and the neuron repolarizes. When the pressure is removed, redistribution of the capsule back to its original shape briefly deforms the nerve ending once again and a brief depolarization results. Without the specialized capsule, the afferent nerve ending becomes a slowly adapting receptor; as long as pressure is applied, the mechanoreceptors remain open and the receptor potential and action potentials persist.

Figure 7.18 Because the referred pain field for the lungs and diaphragm is the neck and shoulder, it is not unusual for individuals suffering from lower respiratory infections to complain of neck stiffness or pain. Lung infections are often accompanied by an accumulation of fluid in the lungs, which is detectable with a stethoscope as crackling or bubbling sounds during breathing.

Figure 7.19 Sensation of all body parts above the level of the injury would be normal. Below the level of the injury, however, there would be a mixed pattern of sensory loss. Fine touch, pressure, and body position sensation would be lost from the left side of the body below the level of the injury because that information ascends in the spinal cord on the side that it enters without crossing the midline until it reaches the brainstem. Pain and temperature sensation would be lost from the right side of the body below the injury because those pathways cross immediately upon entry and ascend in the opposite side of the spinal cord.

Figure 7.21 The frequency of this electromagnetic wave is 2×10^3 Hz (2000 cycles/sec). It would not be visible, because visible light frequencies are in the range of 10^{14} to 10^{15} Hz.

Figure 7.28 Vitamin A is the source of the chromophore retinal, which is the portion of the rhodopsin photopigment that triggers the response of rod cells to light. Because retinal is also used in cone photopigments, a severe vitamin A deficiency eventually results in impairment of vision under all lighting conditions, being generally most noticeable at night when less light is available.

Figure 7.31

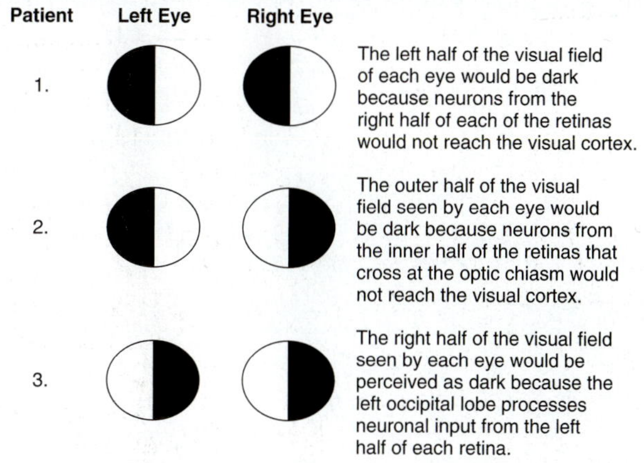

Figure 7.32 Most people who stare at the yellow background perceive an afterimage of a blue circle around the square. This is because prolonged staring at the color yellow activates most of the available retinal in the photopigments of both red and green cones (see Figure 7.32a), effectively fatiguing them into a state of reduced sensitivity. When you shift your gaze to the white background (white light contains all wavelengths of light), only the blue cones are available to respond, so you perceive a blue circle until the red and green cones recover.

Figure 7.39 Though an 80 dB warning tone is not loud enough to cause hearing damage, it can activate the contraction of the stapedius and tensor tympani muscles. With those muscles contracted, the movement of the middle ear bones is dampened during the 140 dB gun blast, thus reducing the transmission of that harmfully loud sound to the inner ear.

Figure 7.41 The transport protein responsible for reabsorbing K^+ (along with Na^+ and Cl^-) in the kidney is also present in epithelial cells surrounding the cochlear duct. It appears to play a role in generating the unusually high K^+ concentration found in the endolymph. Inhibiting this transporter with furosemide reduces the K^+ concentration in the endolymph, which reduces the ability of hair cells to depolarize when sound waves bend the tip links. Less depolarization reduces Ca^{2+} entry, glutamate release, and action potentials in the cochlear nerve, which in turn would reduce the perception of sound.

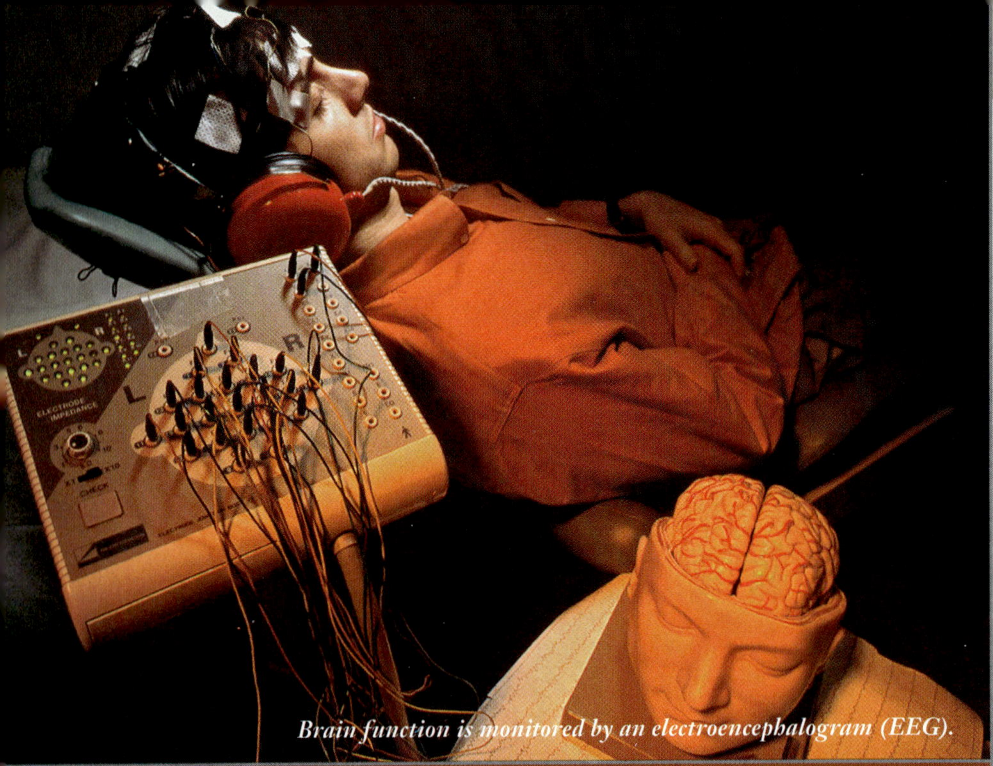

Brain function is monitored by an electroencephalogram (EEG).

8 Consciousness, the Brain, and Behavior

Chapters 6 and 7 introduced some of the fundamental mechanisms underlying the processing of information in the nervous system. The focus was on the transmission of information within neurons, between neurons, and from the peripheral nervous system (PNS) to the central nervous system (CNS). In this chapter, you will learn about higher-order functions and more complex processing of information that occurs within the CNS. We discuss the general phenomenon of consciousness and its variable states of existence, as well some of the important neural mechanisms involved in the processing of our experiences. Although advances in electrophysiological and brain-imaging techniques are yielding fascinating insights, there is still much that we do not know about these topics. If you can imagine that, for any given neuron, there may be as many as 200,000 other neurons connecting to it through synapses, you can begin to appreciate the complexity of the systems that control even the simplest behavior.

The general principle of physiology most obviously on display in this chapter is that information flow between cells, tissues, and organs is an essential feature of homoeostasis and allows for integration of physiological processes. The nervous system "information" discussed previously involved phenomena like chemical and electrical gradients, graded potentials, and action potentials. Those are the essential physiological building blocks for the higher-order processes discussed in this chapter, which include our abilities to consciously pay attention, be motivated, learn, remember, and communicate with others. These abilities are essential determinants of many complex behaviors that help us maintain homeostasis.

8.1 States of Consciousness

The term *consciousness* includes two distinct concepts: **states of consciousness** and **conscious experiences.** The first concept refers to levels of alertness such as being awake, drowsy, or asleep. The second refers to experiences a person is aware of—thoughts, feelings, perceptions, ideas, dreams, reasoning—during any of the states of consciousness.

A person's state of consciousness is defined in two ways: (1) by behavior, covering the spectrum from maximum attentiveness to comatose, and (2) by the pattern of brain activity that can be recorded electrically. This record, known as the **electroencephalogram (EEG)**, portrays the electrical potential difference between different points on the surface of the scalp. The EEG is such a useful tool in identifying the different states of consciousness that we begin with it.

Electroencephalogram

Neural activity is manifested by the electrical signals known as graded potentials and action potentials (Chapter 6). It is possible to record the electrical activity in the brain's neurons—particularly those in the cortex near the surface of the brain—from the outside of the head. Electrodes, which are wires attached to the head by a salty paste that conducts electricity, pick up electrical signals generated in the brain and transmit them to a machine that records them as the EEG.

Though we often think of electrical activity in neurons in terms of action potentials, action potentials do not usually contribute directly to the EEG. Action potentials in individual neurons are also far too small to be picked up on an EEG recording. Rather, EEG patterns are largely due to synchronous graded potentials—in this case, summed postsynaptic potentials (see Chapter 6) in the many hundreds of thousands of brain neurons that underlie the recording electrodes. The majority of the electrical signal recorded in the EEG originates in the pyramidal cells of the cortex (review Figure 6.39). The processes of these large cells lie close to and perpendicular to the surface of the brain, and the EEG records postsynaptic potentials in their dendrites.

EEG patterns are complex waveforms with large variations in both amplitude and frequency (**Figure 8.1**). (The properties of a wave are summarized in Figure 7.21.) The wave's amplitude, measured in microvolts (μV), indicates how much electrical activity of a similar type is occurring beneath the recording electrodes at any given time. A large amplitude indicates that many neurons are being activated simultaneously. In other words, it indicates the degree of synchronous firing of the neurons that are generating the synaptic activity. On the other hand, a small amplitude indicates that these neurons are less activated or are firing asynchronously. The amplitude may range from 0.5 to 100 μV, which is about 1000 times smaller than the amplitude of an action potential.

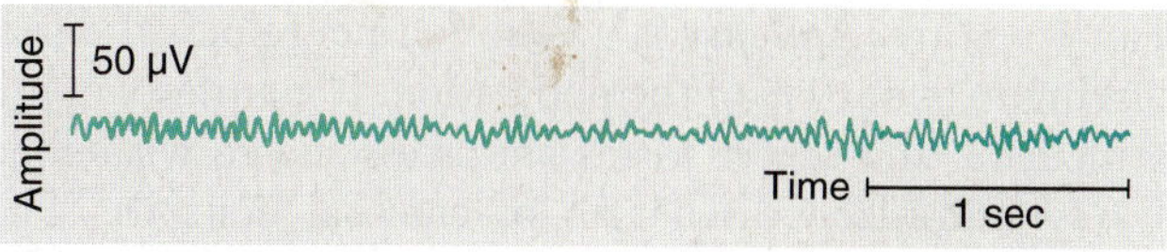

Figure 8.1 EEG patterns are wavelike. This represents a typical EEG recorded from the parietal or occipital lobe of an awake, relaxed person, with a frequency of approximately 20 Hz and an average amplitude of 20 μV.

PHYSIOLOGICAL INQUIRY

- What is the approximate duration of each wave in this recording?

Answer can be found at end of chapter.

The frequency of the wave indicates how often it cycles from the maximal to the minimal amplitude and back. The frequency is measured in hertz (Hz, or cycles per second) and may vary from 0.5 to 40 Hz or higher. Four distinct frequency ranges that define different states of consciousness are characteristic of EEG patterns. In general, lower EEG frequencies indicate less responsive states, such as sleep, whereas higher frequencies indicate increased alertness. As we will see, one stage of sleep is an exception to this general relationship.

The neuronal networks underlying the wavelike oscillations of the EEG and how they function are still not completely understood. Wave patterns vary not only as a function of state of consciousness but also according to where on the scalp they are recorded. Current thinking is that clusters of neurons in the thalamus play a critical role; they provide a fluctuating action potential frequency output through neurons leading from the thalamus to the cortex. This output, in turn, causes a rhythmic pattern of synaptic activity in the pyramidal neurons of the cortex. As noted previously, the cortical synaptic activity—not the activity of the deep thalamic structures—comprises most of a recorded EEG signal. The synchronicity of the cortical synaptic activity (in other words, the amplitude of the EEG) reflects the degree of synchronous firing of the thalamic neuronal clusters that are generating the EEG. These clusters receive input from brain areas involved in controlling the conscious state. Research is also beginning to identify and measure waves of coordinated EEG activity that spread between particular regions of the somatosensory and motor cortex in response to sensory inputs and during the performance of motor tasks.

The EEG is useful clinically in the diagnosis of and treatment of the disease epilepsy, as well as in the diagnosis of coma and brain death. It was formerly also used in the detection of brain areas damaged by tumors, blood clots, or hemorrhage. However, the much greater spatial resolution of modern imaging techniques such as ***positron emission tomography*** (***PET***) and ***magnetic resonance imaging*** (***MRI***) make them far superior for detecting and localizing damaged brain areas in such cases (see Figures 19.6 and 19.7).

A shift from a less synchronized pattern of electrical activity (small-amplitude EEG) to a highly synchronized pattern can be a prelude to the electrical storm that signifies an epileptic seizure. ***Epilepsy*** is a common neurological disease, occurring in about 1% of the population. It manifests in mild, intermediate, and severe forms and is associated with abnormally synchronized discharges of cerebral neurons. These discharges are reflected in the EEG as recurrent waves having distinctive large amplitudes (up to 1000 μV) and individual spikes or combinations of spikes and waves (**Figure 8.2**). Epilepsy is also associated with changes in behavior that vary according to the part of the brain affected and severity and can include involuntary muscle contraction and a temporary loss of consciousness. In most cases, the cause of epilepsy cannot be determined. Among the known triggers are traumatic brain injury, abnormal prenatal brain development, diseases that alter brain blood flow, heavy alcohol and illegal drug use, infectious diseases like meningitis and viral encephalitis, extreme stress, sleep deprivation, and exposure to environmental toxins such as lead or carbon monoxide.

The Waking State

Behaviorally, the waking state is far from homogeneous, reflecting the wide variety of activities you may be engaged in at any given moment. The most prominent EEG wave pattern of an awake, relaxed adult whose eyes are closed is an oscillation of 8 to 12 Hz, known as the **alpha rhythm** (**Figure 8.3a**). The alpha rhythm is recorded best over the parietal and occipital lobes and is associated with decreased levels of attention. When alpha rhythms are generated, subjects commonly report that they feel relaxed and happy. However, people who normally experience more alpha rhythm than usual have not been shown to be psychologically different from those with less.

When people are attentive to an external stimulus or are thinking hard about something, the alpha rhythm is replaced by smaller-amplitude, higher-frequency (>12 Hz) oscillations, the **beta rhythm** (**Figure 8.3b**). This transformation, known as the **EEG arousal,** is associated with the act of paying attention to a stimulus rather than with the act of perception itself. For example, if people open their eyes in a completely dark room and try to see, EEG arousal occurs even though they perceive no visual input. With decreasing attention to repeated stimuli, the EEG pattern reverts to the alpha rhythm.

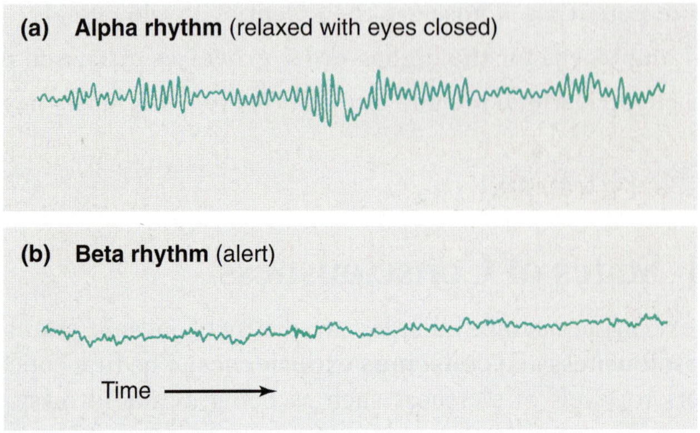

Figure 8.3 EEG recordings of (a) alpha and (b) beta rhythms. Alpha waves vary from 8 to 13 Hz and have larger amplitudes than beta waves, which have frequencies above 13 Hz. Scale is the same as Figure 8.1. Not shown are higher-frequency EEG waves known as gamma waves (30–100 Hz), which have been observed in awake individuals processing sensory inputs.

More recent research has described another EEG pattern known as **gamma rhythm.** These are high-frequency oscillations (30–100 Hz) that spread across large regions of the cortex, which seem in some cases to emanate from the thalamus. They often coincide with the occurrence of combinations of stimuli like hearing noises and seeing objects and are thought to be evidence of large numbers of neurons in the brain actively tying together disparate parts of an experienced scene or event.

Sleep

The EEG pattern changes profoundly in sleep, as demonstrated in **Figure 8.4**. As a person becomes increasingly drowsy, his or her wave pattern transitions from a beta rhythm to a predominantly alpha rhythm. When sleep actually occurs, the EEG shifts toward lower-frequency, larger-amplitude wave patterns known as the **theta rhythm** (4–8 Hz) and the **delta rhythm** (slower than 4 Hz). Relaxation of posture, decreased ease of arousal, increased threshold for sensory stimuli, and decreased motor neuron output accompany these EEG changes.

There are two phases of sleep, the names of which depend on whether or not the eyes move behind the closed eyelids: **NREM** (non–rapid eye movement) and **REM** (rapid eye movement) **sleep.** The initial phase of sleep—NREM sleep—is subdivided into three stages. Each successive stage is characterized by an EEG pattern with a lower frequency and larger amplitude than the preceding one. In stage N1 sleep, theta waves begin to be interspersed among the alpha pattern. In stage N2, high-frequency bursts called **sleep spindles** and large-amplitude **K complexes** occasionally interrupt the theta rhythm. Delta waves first appear along with the theta rhythm in stage N3 sleep; as this stage continues, the dominant

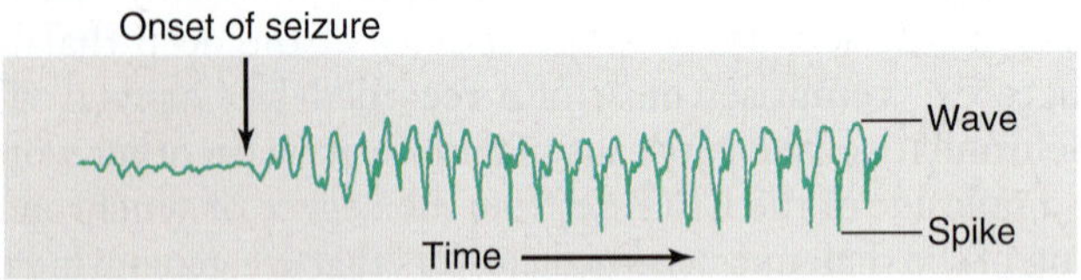

Figure 8.2 Spike-and-wave pattern in the EEG of a patient during an epileptic seizure. Scale is the same as in Figure 8.1.

PHYSIOLOGICAL INQUIRY

- Suppose the patient from which this trace was recorded had a mild form of epilepsy, with the only symptom being vivid visual hallucinations. Where on the patient's head was this measurement most likely taken?

Answer can be found at end of chapter.

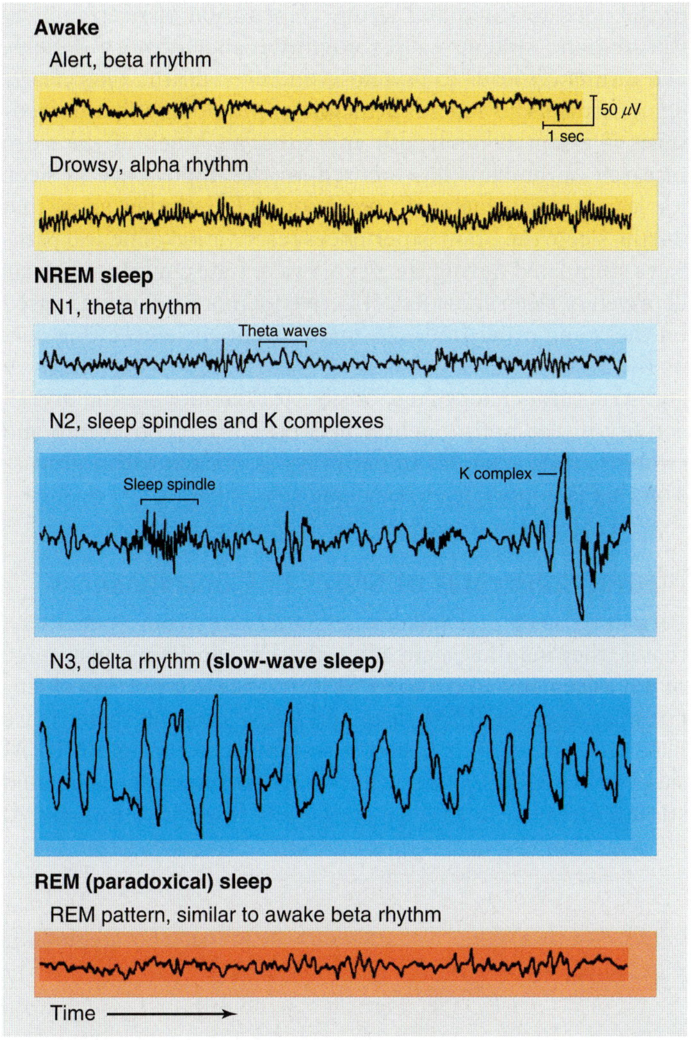

Figure 8.4 The EEG record of a person passing from an awake state through the various stages of sleep. The large-amplitude delta waves of slow-wave sleep demonstrate the synchronous activity pattern in cortical neurons. The asynchronous pattern during REM sleep is similar to that observed in awake individuals.

pattern becomes a delta rhythm N3, sometimes referred to as slow-wave sleep.

Sleep begins with the progression from stage N1 to stage N3 of NREM sleep, which normally takes 30 to 45 min. The process then reverses itself; the EEG ultimately resumes a small-amplitude, high-frequency, asynchronous pattern that looks very similar to the alert, awake state (see Figure 8.4, bottom trace). Instead of the person waking, however, the behavioral characteristics of sleep continue at this time, but this sleep also includes rapid eye movement (REM).

REM sleep is also called **paradoxical sleep,** because even though a person is asleep and difficult to arouse, his or her EEG pattern shows intense activity that is similar to that observed in the alert, awake state. In fact, brain O_2 consumption is higher during REM sleep than during the NREM or awake states. When awakened during REM sleep, subjects frequently report that they have been dreaming. This is true even in people who usually do not remember dreaming when they awaken on their own.

If uninterrupted, the stages of sleep occur in a cyclical fashion, tending to move from NREM stages N1 to N2 to N3, then back up to N2, and then to an episode of REM sleep. Continuous recordings of adults show that the average total night's sleep comprises four or five such cycles, each lasting 90 to 100 min (**Figure 8.5**). Significantly more time is spent in NREM during the first few cycles, but time spent in REM sleep increases toward the end of an undisturbed night. In young adults, REM sleep constitutes 20% to 25% of the total sleeping time; this fraction tends to decline progressively with aging. Initially, as you transition from drowsiness to stage N1 sleep, there is a considerable tension in the postural muscles, and brief muscle twitches called **hypnic jerks** sometimes occur. Eventually, the muscles become progressively more relaxed as NREM sleep progresses. Sleepers awakened during NREM sleep report dreaming less frequently than sleepers awakened during REM sleep. REM dreams also tend to seem more "real" and be more emotionally intense than those occurring in NREM sleep.

With several exceptions, skeletal muscle tension, already decreased during NREM sleep, is markedly inhibited during REM sleep. Exceptions include the eye muscles, which undergo rapid bursts of contractions and cause the sweeping eye movements that give this sleep stage its name. The significance of these eye movements is not understood. Experiments suggest that they do not seem to rigorously correlate with the content of dreams; that is, what the sleeper is "seeing" in a dream does not seem to affect the eye movements. Furthermore, eye movements also occur during REM sleep in animals and humans that have been blind since birth and thus have no experience tracking objects with eye movements. Other groups of muscles that are active during REM sleep are the respiratory muscles; in fact, the rate of breathing is frequently increased compared to the awake, relaxed state. In one form of a disease known as ***sleep apnea,*** however, stimulation of the respiratory muscles temporarily ceases, sometimes hundreds of times during a night. The resulting decreases in oxygen levels repeatedly awaken the apnea sufferer, who is deprived of both slow-wave and REM sleep. As a result, this disease is associated with excessive—and sometimes dangerous—sleepiness during the day (refer to Chapter 13 for a more complete discussion of sleep apnea).

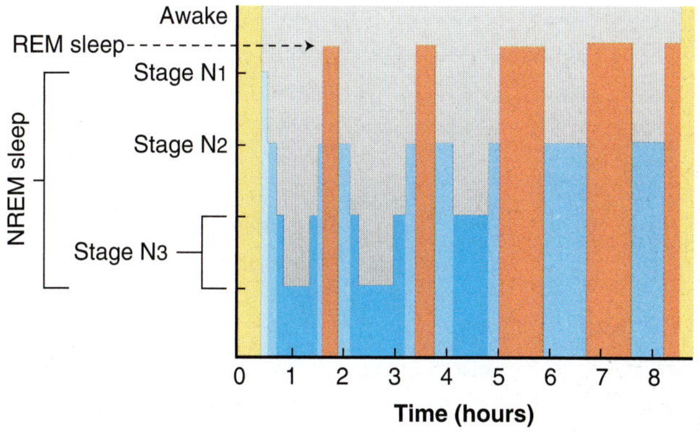

Figure 8.5 Schematic representation of the timing of sleep stages in a young adult. Bar colors correspond to the EEG traces shown in Figure 8.4.

During the sleep cycle, many changes occur throughout the body in addition to altered muscle tension, providing an excellent example of the general principle of physiology that the functions of organ systems are coordinated with each other. During NREM sleep, for example, there are pulsatile releases of hormones from the anterior pituitary gland such as growth hormone and the gonadotropic hormones (Chapter 11), so adequate sleep is essential for normal growth in children and for regulation of reproductive function in adults. Decreases in blood pressure, heart rate, and respiratory rate also occur during NREM sleep. REM sleep is associated with an increase and irregularity in blood pressure, heart rate, and respiratory rate. Moreover, twitches of the facial muscles or limb muscles may occur—despite the generalized lack of skeletal muscle tone—as may erection of the penis and engorgement of the clitoris. The occurrence of erections during REM sleep in patients being assessed for ***erectile dysfunction*** (***ED***) indicates that the cause of ED (see Chapter 17) may be psychological rather than physical.

Although we spend about one-third of our lives sleeping, the functions of sleep are not completely understood. Many lines of research, however, suggest that sleep is a fundamental necessity of a complex nervous system. Sleep, or a sleeplike state, is a characteristic found throughout the animal kingdom, including insects, reptiles, birds, mammals, and others. Studies of sleep deprivation in humans and other animals suggest that sleep is a homeostatic requirement, similar to the need for food and water. Deprivation of sleep impairs the immune system, causes cognitive and memory deficits, and ultimately leads to psychosis and even death. This clearly demonstrates the general principle of physiology that homeostasis is essential for health and survival. Much of the sleep research on humans has focused on the importance of sleep for learning and memory formation. EEG studies show that during sleep, the brain experiences reactivation of neural pathways stimulated during the prior awake state, and that subjects deprived of sleep show less effective memory retention. Based on these and other findings, many scientists believe that part of the restorative value of sleep lies in facilitating chemical and structural changes responsible for dampening the overall activity in the brain's neural networks while conserving and strengthening synapses in pathways associated with information that is important to learn and remember.

Table 8.1 summarizes the sleep states.

Neural Substrates of States of Consciousness

Periods of sleep and wakefulness alternate about once a day; that is, they manifest a circadian rhythm consisting on average of 8 h asleep and 16 h awake. Within the sleep portion of this circadian cycle, NREM sleep and REM sleep alternate, as we have seen. As we shift from the waking state through NREM sleep to REM sleep, attention shifts to internally generated stimuli (dreams) so that we are largely insensitive to external

TABLE 8.1 Sleep–Wakefulness Stages

Stage	Behavior	EEG (See Figures 8.3 and 8.4)
Alert wakefulness	Awake, alert with eyes open.	Beta rhythm (greater than 13 Hz).
Relaxed wakefulness	Awake, relaxed with eyes closed.	Mainly alpha rhythm (8–13 Hz) over the parietal and occipital lobes. Changes to beta rhythm in response to internal or external stimuli.
Relaxed drowsiness	Fatigued, tired, or bored; eyelids may narrow and close; head may start to droop; momentary lapses of attention and alertness. Sleepy but not asleep.	Decrease in alpha-wave amplitude and frequency.
NREM (slow-wave) sleep		
Stage N1	Light sleep; easily aroused by moderate stimuli or even by neck muscle jerks triggered by muscle stretch receptors as head nods; continuous lack of awareness.	Alpha waves reduced in frequency, amplitude, and percentage of time present; gaps in alpha rhythm filled with theta (4–8 Hz) and delta (slower than 4 Hz) activity.
Stage N2	Further lack of sensitivity to activation and arousal.	Alpha waves replaced by random waves of greater amplitude.
Stage N3	Deep sleep; in stage N3, activation and arousal occur only with vigorous stimulation.	Much theta and delta activity; progressive increase in amount of delta.
REM (paradoxical) sleep	Greatest muscle relaxation and difficulty of arousal; begins 50–90 min after sleep onset, episodes repeated every 60–90 min, each episode lasting about 10 min; dreaming frequently occurs, rapid eye movements behind closed eyelids; marked increase in brain O_2 consumption.	EEG resembles that of alert awake state.

stimuli. Although sleep facilitates our ability to retain memories of experiences occurring in the waking state, dreams are generally forgotten relatively quickly. The tight rules for determining reality also become relaxed during dreaming, sometimes allowing for bizarre dreams.

What physiological processes drive these cyclic changes in states of consciousness? Nuclei in both the brainstem and hypothalamus are involved.

Recall from Chapter 6 that a diverging network of neurons called the reticular formation connects the brainstem with widespread regions of the brain and spinal cord. This network is essential for life and integrates a large number of physiological functions, including motor control, cardiovascular and respiratory control, and—relevant to the present discussion—states of consciousness. The components involved in regulating consciousness are sometimes referred to as the **reticular activating system** (**RAS**). This system consists of clusters of neurons and neural pathways originating in the brainstem and hypothalamus, distinguished by both their anatomical distribution and the neurotransmitters they release (**Figure 8.6**). Neurons of the RAS project widely throughout the cortex, as well as to areas of the thalamus that influence the EEG. Varying activation and inhibition of distinct groups of these neurons mediate transitions between waking and sleeping states.

The awake state is characterized by widespread activation of the cortex and thalamus by ascending pathways of the RAS (see Figure 8.6). Neurons originating in the brainstem release the monoaminergic neurotransmitters norepinephrine, serotonin, and histamine, which in this case function principally as neuromodulators (see Chapter 6). Their nerve terminals are distributed widely throughout the brain, where they enhance excitatory synaptic activity. The drowsiness that occurs in people using antihistamines may be a result of blocking the histaminergic inputs of this system. In addition, acetylcholine from neurons in the pons and basal forebrain facilitates transmission of ascending sensory information through the thalamus and also enhances communication between the thalamus and cortex.

Recently discovered neuropeptides called **orexins** (a name meaning "to stimulate appetite") also play an important role in maintaining the awake state. They are produced by neurons in the hypothalamus that have widespread projections throughout the cortex and thalamus. (Some scientists also refer to these peptides as **hypocretins** because they are made in the *hypo*thalamus and are similar to the hormone se*cretin*.) Orexin-secreting neurons also densely innervate and stimulate action potential firing by the monoaminergic neurons of the RAS. Experimental animals and humans that lack orexins or their receptors suffer from ***narcolepsy***, a condition characterized by sudden attacks of sleepiness that unpredictably occur during the normal wakeful period. The importance of orexins in wakefulness has been recently validated by experiments showing that sleep is promoted in people ingesting a drug that blocks binding of orexins to their receptors. Loss of orexinergic neurons that occurs with age may explain why older people sometimes have difficulty sleeping.

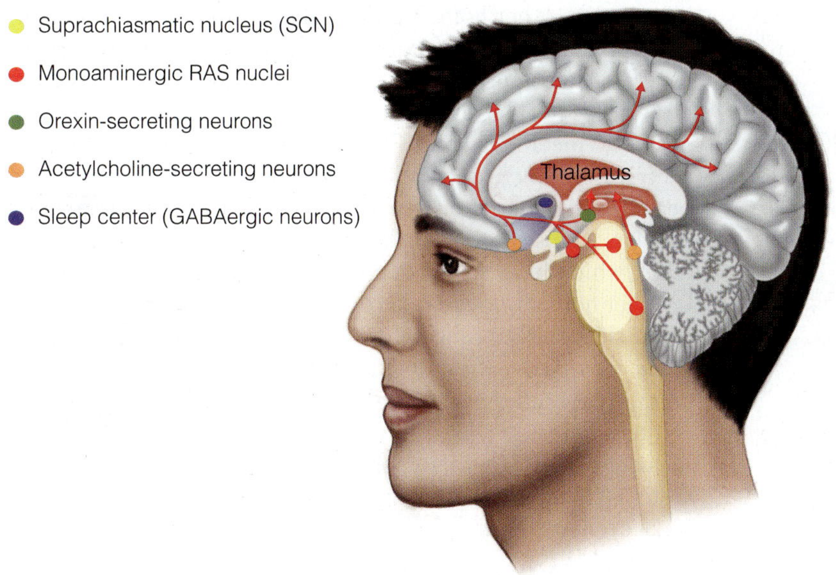

Figure 8.6 APIR Brain regions involved in regulating states of consciousness. Red arrows indicate principal pathways of ascending activation of the thalamus and cortex by the reticular activating system (RAS) during the awake state. Additional pathways not shown that are important in maintaining cortical arousal include excitatory inputs to the monoaminergic RAS nuclei from orexinergic neurons, and inhibitory inputs to the sleep center from the monoaminergic RAS nuclei. Monoamines from the RAS nuclei include histamine, norepinephrine, and serotonin. Orexin neurons and GABAergic neurons of the sleep center are hypothalamic nuclei, and the acetylcholine neurons are in the basal forebrain and pons.

PHYSIOLOGICAL INQUIRY

- Explain why some drugs prescribed to treat allergic reactions cause drowsiness as a side effect.

Answer can be found at end of chapter.

Sleep is characterized by a markedly different pattern of neuronal activity and neurotransmitter release. Of central importance is the active firing of neurons in the "sleep center," a group of neurons in the ventrolateral preoptic nucleus of the hypothalamus (see Figure 8.6). These neurons release the inhibitory neurotransmitter GABA (gamma-aminobutyric acid) onto neurons throughout the brainstem and hypothalamus, including those that secrete orexins and monoamines. Inhibition of these regions reduces the levels of orexin, norepinephrine, serotonin, and histamine throughout the brain. Each of these substances has been associated with alertness and arousal; therefore, inhibition of their secretion by GABA tends to promote sleep. This accounts for the sleep-inducing effects of ***benzodiazepines*** such as ***diazepam*** (***Valium***) and ***alprazolam*** (***Xanax***), which are GABA agonists and are used to treat anxiety and insomnia in some people.

The pattern of acetylcholine release varies in different sleep stages. It is reduced in NREM sleep, but in REM sleep it is increased to levels similar to those in the awake state. The increase in acetylcholine during REM sleep facilitates communication between the thalamus and cortex and increases the cortical activity and dreaming that occur in this state.

Figure 8.7 shows a model of factors involved in regulating the transition between waking and sleeping states. Transition to the wakeful state is favored by three main inputs to orexin-secreting cells: (1) action potential firing from the suprachiasmatic nucleus (SCN), (2) indicators of negative energy balance, and (3) arousing emotional states signaled by the limbic system (see Figure 6.40 and Section 8.3 of this chapter). The SCN is the principle circadian pacemaker of the body (see Chapters 1 and 7). Entrained to a 24-hour cycle by light and other daily stimuli, it activates orexin cells in the morning. It also triggers the secretion of melatonin at night (see Chapters 1 and 11). Although melatonin has been used as a "natural" substance for treating insomnia and jet lag, it has not yet been demonstrated unequivocally to be effective as a sleeping pill. It has, however, been shown to induce a decrease in body temperature, a key event in falling asleep.

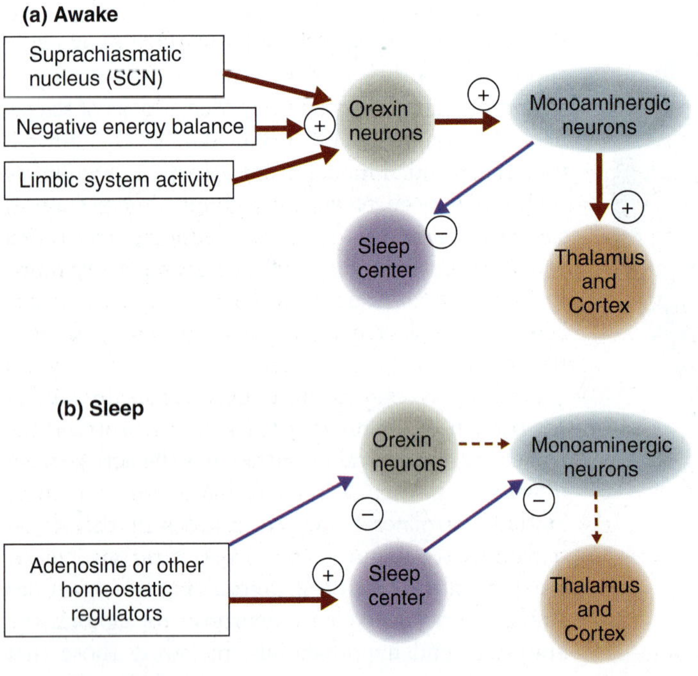

Figure 8.7 A model for the regulation of transitions to (a) the awake state and (b) sleep. Red arrows and "+" indicate stimulatory influences, blue arrows and "–" indicate inhibitory pathways. Orexin neurons and the sleep center are in the hypothalamus. Monoaminergic neurons release norepinephrine, serotonin, and histamine. Adapted from Sakurai, Takeshi. Nature Reviews, *Neuroscience* (8): pp. 171–181, March 2007.

PHYSIOLOGICAL INQUIRY

- Interleukin 1, a fever-inducing cytokine that increases in the circulation during an infection, promotes the sleep state. Speculate about some possible adaptive advantages of such a mechanism.

Answer can be found at end of chapter.

The metabolic and limbic system inputs to orexinergic neurons provide adaptive behavioral flexibility to the initiation of wakefulness, so that under special circumstances our sleep and wake patterns can vary from the typical pattern of sleeping at night and being awake during the day. Metabolic indicators of negative energy balance resulting from a prolonged fast include decreased blood glucose concentration, increased plasma concentrations of the appetite-stimulating hormone called ghrelin, and decreased concentrations of the appetite-suppressing hormone leptin (see Chapter 16 for a detailed description of these hormones). These conditions all stimulate orexin release, which may be adaptive because the resulting arousal would allow you to seek out food at times when you would otherwise be asleep. This link between metabolism and wakefulness is an excellent example of the general principle of physiology that the functions of organ systems are coordinated with each other. Limbic system inputs coding strong emotions such as fear or anger also stimulate orexin neurons. This may be adaptive by interrupting sleep at times when we need to respond to situations affecting our well-being and survival.

The factors that activate the sleep center are not completely understood, but it is thought that homeostatic regulation by one or more chemicals plays a role. The need for sleep behaves like other homeostatic demands of the body. Individuals deprived of sleep for a prolonged period will subsequently experience prolonged bouts of "catch-up" sleep, as though the body needs to rid itself of some chemical that has built up. Adenosine (a metabolite of ATP) is one likely candidate. Its concentration is increased in the brain after a prolonged waking period, and it has been shown to reduce firing by orexinergic neurons. This in part explains the stimulatory effect of caffeine, which blocks adenosine receptors. Buildup of adenosine or other homeostatic regulators can also facilitate the transition to the sleep state at times when you may normally be awake, like when you take an afternoon nap after being up late studying for an exam. Another potential sleep-inducing chemical candidate is interleukin 1, one of the cytokines in a family of intercellular messengers having an important role in the immune defense system (Chapter 18). It fluctuates in parallel with normal sleep–wake cycles and has also been shown to facilitate the sleep state.

Coma and Brain Death

The term ***coma*** describes an extreme decrease in mental function due to structural, physiological, or metabolic impairment of the brain. A person in a coma exhibits a sustained loss of the capacity for arousal even in response to vigorous stimulation. There is no outward behavioral expression of any mental function, the eyes are usually closed, and sleep–wake cycles disappear. Coma can result from extensive damage to the cerebral cortex; damage to the brainstem arousal mechanisms; interruptions of the connections between the brainstem and cortical areas; metabolic dysfunctions; brain infections; or an overdose of certain drugs, such as sedatives, sleeping pills, narcotics, or ethanol. Comas may be reversible or irreversible, depending on the type, location, and severity of brain damage. Experiments using high-density EEG arrays in some coma patients suggest that even though they exhibit no outward behaviors or responses, they may have some level of consciousness. For example, talking to a patient about tennis may evoke increased

EEG activity over motor areas of the cortex that would be active if the person were actually playing tennis.

Patients in an irreversible coma often enter a ***persistent vegetative state*** in which sleep–wake cycles are present even though the patient is unaware of his or her surroundings. Individuals in a persistent vegetative state may smile, cry, or seem to react to elements of their environment. However, there is no definitive evidence that they can comprehend these behaviors.

A coma—even when irreversible—is not equivalent to death. We are left, then, with the question, When is a person actually dead? This question often has urgent medical, legal, and social consequences. For example, with the need for viable tissues for organ transplantation, it becomes important to know just when a donor is legally dead so that the organs can be removed as soon after death as possible.

Brain death is currently accepted by the medical and legal establishment as the criterion for death, despite the viability of other organs. Brain death occurs when the brain no longer functions and appears to have no possibility of functioning again.

The problem now becomes practical. How do we know when a person (e.g., someone in a coma) is brain-dead? Although there is some variation in how different hospitals and physicians determine brain death, the criteria listed in Table 8.2 lists the generally agreed-upon standards. Notice that the cause of a coma must be known, because comas due to drug poisoning and other conditions are often reversible. Also, the criteria specify that there be no evidence of functioning neural tissues above the spinal cord because fragments of spinal reflexes may remain for several hours or longer after the brain is dead (see Chapter 10 for spinal reflex examples). The criterion for lack of spontaneous respiration (apnea) must be assessed with caution. Machines supplying artificial respiration must be turned off, and arterial blood gas levels monitored carefully (see Figure 13.21 and Table 13.6). Although arterial carbon dioxide levels must be allowed to increase above a critical point for the test to be valid, it is of course not advisable to allow arterial oxygen levels to decrease too much because of the danger of further brain damage. Therefore, apnea tests are generally limited to a duration of 8 to 10 minutes.

TABLE 8.2 Criteria for Brain Death

I. The nature and duration of the coma must be known.
   A. Known structural damage to brain or irreversible systemic metabolic disease
   B. No chance of drug intoxication, especially from paralyzing or sedative drugs
   C. No severe electrolyte, acid–base, or endocrine disorder that could be reversible
   D. Patient not suffering from hypothermia
   E. Peak arterial blood pressure above 100 mmHg

II. Cerebral and brainstem function are absent.
   A. No response to painful stimuli other than spinal cord reflexes
   B. Pupils unresponsive to light
   C. No eye movement in response to stimulation of the vestibular reflex or corneal touch
   D. Apnea (no spontaneous breathing) for 8–10 minutes when ventilator is removed and arterial carbon dioxide levels are allowed to increase above 60 mmHg
   E. No gag or cough reflex; purely spinal reflexes may be retained
   F. Confirmatory neurological exam after 6 hours

III. Supplementary (optional) criteria
   A. Flat EEG for 30 min (wave amplitudes less than 2 mV)
   B. Responses absent in vital brainstem structures
   C. Greatly reduced cerebral circulation

Table adapted from American Academy of Neurology, *Neurology* 74: 1911–1918 (2010).

8.2 Conscious Experiences

Conscious experiences are those things we are aware of—either internal, such as an idea, or external, such as an object or event. The most obvious aspect of this phenomenon is sensory awareness, but we are also aware of inner states such as fatigue, thirst, and happiness. We are aware of the passing of time, of what we are presently thinking about, and of consciously recalling a fact learned in the past. We are aware of reasoning and exerting self-control, and we are aware of directing our attention to specific events. Not least, we are aware of "self."

Basic to the concept of conscious experience is the question of attention.

Selective Attention

The term **selective attention** means avoiding the distraction of irrelevant stimuli while seeking out and focusing on stimuli that are momentarily important. Both voluntary and reflex mechanisms affect selective attention. An example of voluntary control of selective attention familiar to students is ignoring distracting events in a busy library while studying there.

Another example of selective attention occurs when a novel stimulus is presented to a relaxed subject showing an alpha EEG pattern. This causes the EEG to shift to the beta rhythm. If the stimulus has meaning for the individual, behavioral changes also occur. The person stops what he or she is doing, listens intently, and turns toward the stimulus source, a behavior called the **orienting response.** If the person is concentrating hard and is not distracted by the novel stimulus, the orienting response does not occur. It is also possible to focus attention on a particular stimulus without making any behavioral response.

For attention to be directed only toward stimuli that are meaningful, the nervous system must have the means to evaluate the importance of incoming sensory information. Thus, even before we focus attention on an object in our sensory world and become aware of it, a certain amount of processing has already occurred. This so-called **preattentive processing** directs our attention toward the part of the sensory world that is of particular interest and prepares the brain's perceptual processes for it.

If a stimulus is repeated but is found to be irrelevant, the behavioral response to the stimulus progressively decreases, a process known as **habituation.** For example, when a loud bell is sounded for the first time, it may evoke an orienting response because the person may be frightened by or curious about the novel stimulus. After several rings, however, the individual has a progressively smaller response and eventually may ignore the bell altogether. An extraneous stimulus of another type or the same stimulus at a different intensity can restore the orienting response.

Habituation involves a depression of synaptic transmission in the involved pathway, possibly related to a prolonged inactivation of Ca^{2+} channels in presynaptic axon terminals. Such inactivation results in a decreased Ca^{2+} influx during depolarization and, therefore, a decrease in the amount of neurotransmitter released by a terminal in response to action potentials.

Neural Mechanisms for Selective Attention

Directing our attention to an object involves several distinct neurological processes. First, our attention must be disengaged from its present focus. Then, attention must be moved to the new focus. Attention must then be engaged at the new focus. Finally, there must be an increased level of arousal that produces prolonged attention to the new focus.

An area that plays an important role in orienting and selective attention is in the brainstem, where the interaction of various sensory modalities in single cells can be detected experimentally. The receptive fields of the different modalities overlap. For example, a visual and auditory input from the same location in space will significantly enhance the firing rates of certain of these so-called multisensory cells, whereas the same type of stimuli originating at different places will have little effect on or may even inhibit their response. Thus, weak clues can add together to enhance each other's significance so we pay attention to the event, whereas we may ignore an isolated small clue.

The locus ceruleus is one of the monoaminergic RAS nuclei. It is located in the pons, projects to the parietal cortex and many other parts of the central nervous system, and is also implicated in selective attention. The system of fibers leading from the locus ceruleus helps determine which brain area is to gain temporary predominance in the ongoing stream of the conscious experience. These neurons release norepinephrine, which acts as a neuromodulator to enhance the signals transmitted by certain sensory inputs. The effect is to increase the difference between the sensory inputs and other, weaker signals. Thus, neurons of the locus ceruleus improve information processing during selective attention.

The thalamus is another brain region involved in selective attention. It is a synaptic relay station for the majority of ascending sensory pathways (see Figure 7.19). Inputs from regions of the cerebral cortex and brainstem can modulate synaptic activity in the thalamus, making it a filter that can selectively influence the transmission of sensory information.

There are also multisensory neurons in association areas of the cerebral cortex (see Figure 7.13). Whereas the brainstem neurons are concerned with the orienting movements associated with paying attention to a specific stimulus, the cortical multisensory neurons are more involved in the perception of the stimulus. Neuroscientists are only beginning to understand how the various areas of the attentional system interact.

Some insights into neural mechanisms of selective attention are being gained from the study of individuals diagnosed with ***attention-deficit/hyperactivity disorder*** (***AD/HD***). This condition typically begins early in childhood and is the most common neurobehavioral problem in school-aged children (estimates range from 3% to 7%). AD/HD is characterized by abnormal difficulty in maintaining selective attention and/or impulsiveness and hyperactivity. Investigation has yet to reveal clear environmental causes, but there is some evidence for a genetic basis because AD/HD tends to run in families. Functional imaging studies of the brains of children with AD/HD have indicated dysfunction of brain regions in which catecholamine signaling is prominent, including the basal nuclei and prefrontal cortex. In support of this, the most effective medication used to treat AD/HD is ***methylphenidate*** (***Ritalin***), a drug that increases synaptic concentrations of dopamine and norepinephrine.

Neural Mechanisms of Conscious Experiences

Conscious experiences are popularly attributed to the workings of the "mind," a word that conjures up the image of a nonneural "me," a phantom interposed between afferent and efferent impulses. The implication is that the mind is something more than neural activity. Most experts would agree that the mind represents a summation of neural activity at any given moment and does not require anything more. However, scientists are only beginning to understand the mechanisms that give rise to mind or to conscious experiences.

We will speculate about this problem in this section. The thinking begins with the assumption that conscious experience requires neural processes—either graded potentials or action potentials—somewhere in the brain. At any moment, certain of these processes correlate with conscious awareness, and others do not. A key question here is, What is different about the processes we are aware of?

A further assumption is that the neural activity that corresponds to a conscious experience resides not in a single anatomical cluster of "consciousness neurons" but rather in a set of neurons that are temporarily functioning together in a specific way. Because we can become aware of many different things, we further assume that this grouping of neurons can vary—shifting, for example, among parts of the brain that deal with visual or auditory stimuli, memories or new ideas, emotions, or language.

Consider the visual perception of an object. As we discussed in Chapter 7, different aspects of something we see are processed by different areas of the visual cortex—the object's color by one part, its motion by another, its location in the visual field by another, and its shape by still another—but we see *one* object. Not only do we perceive it; we may also know its name and function. Moreover, as we see an object, we can sometimes also hear or smell it, which requires participation of brain areas other than the visual cortex.

The simultaneous participation of different groups of neurons in a conscious experience can also be inferred for the olfactory system. Repugnant and alluring odors evoke different reactions, although they are both processed in the olfactory pathway. Neurons involved in emotion are also clearly involved in this type of perception.

Neurons from the various parts of the brain that simultaneously process different aspects of the information related to the object we see are said to form a "temporary set" of neurons. It is suggested that the synchronous activity of the neurons in the temporary set leads to conscious awareness of the object we are seeing.

As we become aware of still other events—perhaps a memory related to the object—the set of neurons involved in the synchronous activity shifts, and a different temporary set forms. In other words, it is suggested that specific relevant neurons in many areas of the brain function together to form the unified activity that corresponds to awareness.

What parts of the brain may be involved in such a temporary neuronal set? Clearly, the cerebral cortex is involved. Removal of specific areas of the cortex abolishes awareness of only specific types of consciousness. For example, in a syndrome called ***sensory neglect***, damage to association areas of the parietal cortex causes the injured person to neglect parts of the body or parts of the visual field as though they do not exist. Stroke patients with parietal lobe damage often do not acknowledge the presence of a paralyzed part of their body or will only be able to describe some but not all elements in a visual field. **Figure 8.8** shows an example of sensory neglect as shown in drawings made by a patient with parietal lobe damage on the right side of the brain. Patients such as these are completely unaware of the left-hand parts of the visual image. Subcortical areas such as the thalamus and basal ganglia may also be directly involved in conscious experience, but it seems that the hippocampus and cerebellum are not.

Saying that we can use one set of neurons and then shift to a new set at a later time may be the same as saying we can focus attention on—that is, bring into conscious awareness—one object or event and then shift our focus of attention to another object or event at a later time. Thus, the mechanisms of conscious awareness and attention are intimately related.

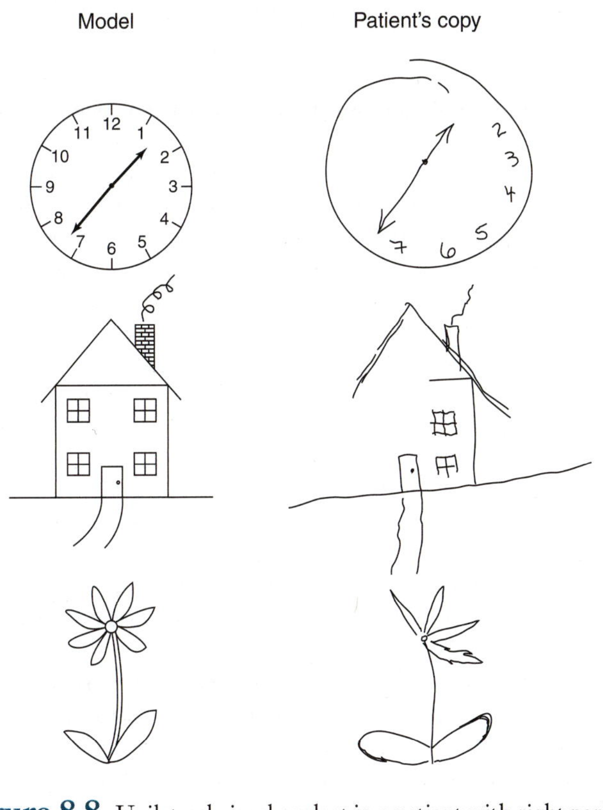

Figure 8.8 Unilateral visual neglect in a patient with right parietal lobe damage. Although patients such as these are not impaired visually, they do not perceive part of their visual world. The drawings on the right were copied by the patient from the drawings on the left.

8.3 Motivation and Emotion

Motivation is a factor in most, if not all, behaviors, and emotions accompany many of our conscious experiences. Motivated behaviors such as sexual behaviors play a part in controlling much of our day-to-day behavior, and emotions may help us to achieve the goals we set for ourselves as well as express our feelings.

Motivation

Those processes responsible for the goal-directed quality of behavior are the **motivations,** or "drives," for that behavior. Motivation can lead to hormonal, autonomic, and behavioral responses. **Primary motivated behavior** is behavior related directly to homeostasis—that is, the maintenance of a relatively stable internal environment, such as getting something to drink when you are thirsty. In such homeostatic goal-directed behavior, specific body "needs" are satisfied. Thus, in our example, the perception of need results from a decrease in total body water, and the correlate of need satisfaction is the return of body water concentration to normal. We will discuss the neurophysiological integration of much homeostatic goal-directed behavior later (thirst and drinking, Chapter 14; food intake and temperature regulation, Chapter 16).

In many kinds of behavior, however, the relation between the behavior and the primary goal is indirect. For example, the selection of a particular flavor of beverage has little if any apparent relation to homeostasis. The motivation in this case is secondary. Much of human behavior fits into this latter category and is influenced by habit, learning, intellect, and emotions—factors that can be lumped together under the term "incentives." Often, it is difficult to distinguish between primary and secondary goals. For instance, although some salt in the diet is required for survival, most of your drive to eat salt is hedonistic (for enjoyment). Sometimes the primary homeostatic goals and secondary goals conflict, as, for example, during a religious fast.

The concepts of reward and punishment are inseparable from motivation. Rewards are things that organisms work for or things that make the behavior that leads to them occur more often—in other words, positive reinforcement. Punishments are the opposite.

The neural system subserving reward and punishment is part of the reticular activating system, which you will recall arises in the brainstem and comprises several components. The component involved in motivation is known as the **mesolimbic dopamine pathway:** *meso-* because it arises in the midbrain (mesencephalon) area of the brainstem; *limbic* because it sends its fibers to areas of the limbic system, such as the prefrontal cortex, the nucleus accumbens, and the undersurface of the frontal lobe (**Figure 8.9**); and *dopamine* because its fibers release the neurotransmitter dopamine. The mesolimbic dopamine pathway is implicated in evaluating the availability of incentives and reinforcers (asking, Is it worth it? for example) and translating the evaluation into action.

Much of the available information concerning the neural substrates of motivation has been obtained by studying behavioral responses of animals to rewarding or punishing stimuli. One way in which this can be done is by using the technique of **brain self-stimulation.** In this technique, an awake experimental animal regulates the rate at which electrical stimuli are

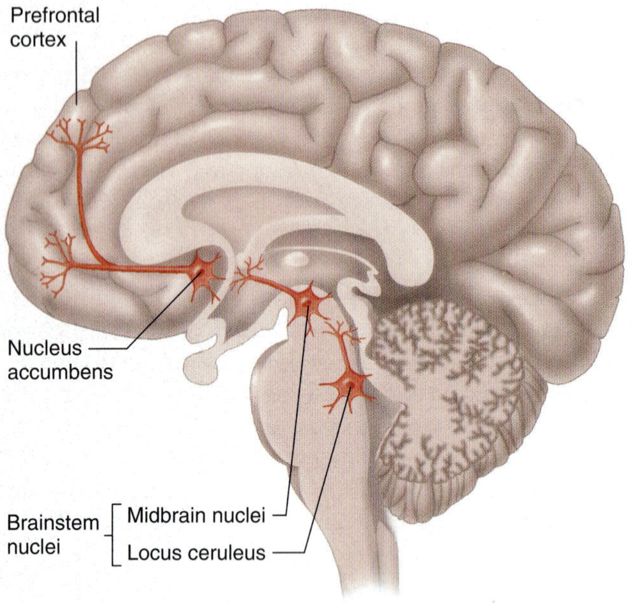

Figure 8.9 AP|R Schematic drawing of the mesolimbic dopamine pathway. Various psychoactive substances are thought to work in these areas to enhance brain reward.

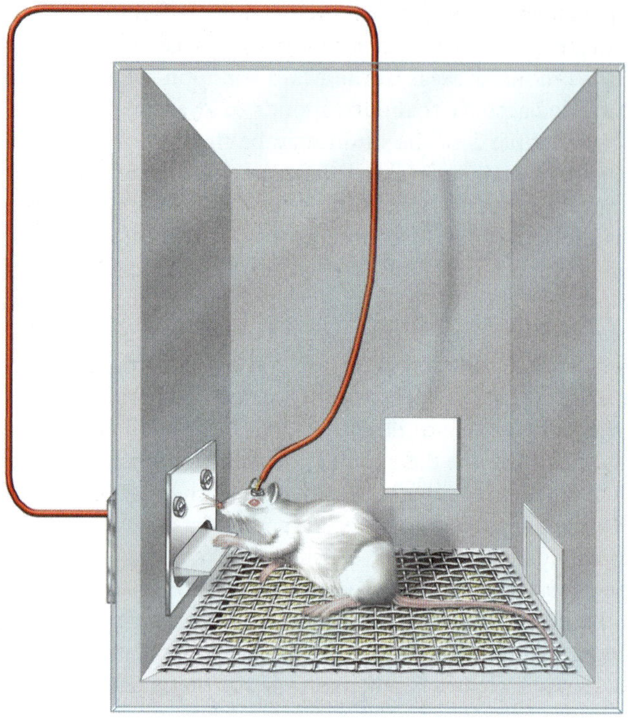

Figure 8.10 Apparatus for self-stimulation experiments. Rats like the one shown here do not appear to be bothered by the implanted electrode. In fact, they work hard to get the electrical stimulation. Adapted from Olds.

delivered through electrodes implanted in discrete brain areas. The small electrical charges given to the brain cause the local neurons to depolarize, thus mimicking what may happen if these neurons were to fire spontaneously. The experimental animal is placed in a box containing a lever it can press (**Figure 8.10**). If no stimulus is delivered to the brain when the bar is pressed, the animal usually presses it occasionally at random.

However, if a stimulus is delivered to the brain as a result of a bar press, different behaviors occur, depending on the location of the electrodes. If the animal increases the bar-pressing rate above the level of random presses, the electrical stimulus is by definition rewarding. If the animal decreases the press rate below the random level, the stimulus is punishing. Thus, the rate of bar pressing with the electrode in different brain areas is taken to be a measure of the effectiveness of the reward or punishment. Different pressing rates are found for different brain regions.

Scientists expected the hypothalamus to play a role in motivation because the neural centers for the regulation of eating, drinking, temperature control, and sexual behavior are there (Chapter 6). Indeed, it was found that brain self-stimulation of the lateral regions of the hypothalamus serves as a positive reward. Animals with electrodes in these areas have been known to press a bar to stimulate their brains 2000 times per hour continuously for 24 h until they collapse from exhaustion. In fact, electrical stimulation of the lateral hypothalamus is more rewarding than external rewards. Hungry rats, for example, often ignore available food for the sake of stimulating their brains at that location.

Although the rewarding sites—particularly those for primary motivated behavior—are more densely packed in the lateral hypothalamus than anywhere else in the brain, self-stimulation can occur in a large number of brain areas. Motivated behaviors based on learning also involve additional integrative centers, including the cortex, and limbic system, brainstem, and spinal cord—in other words, all levels of the nervous system can be involved.

Chemical Mediators

Dopamine is a major neurotransmitter in the pathway that mediates the brain reward systems and motivation. For this reason, drugs that increase synaptic activity in the dopamine pathways increase self-stimulation rates—that is, they provide positive reinforcement. Amphetamines are an example of such a drug because they increase the presynaptic release of dopamine. Conversely, drugs such as chlorpromazine, an antipsychotic drug that blocks dopamine receptors and lowers activity in the catecholamine pathways, are negatively reinforcing. The catecholamines, as we will see, are also implicated in the pathways involved in learning. This is not unexpected, because rewards and punishments are believed to constitute incentives for learning.

Emotion

Emotion can be considered in terms of a relation between an individual and the environment based on the individual's evaluation of the environment (is it pleasant or hostile?), disposition toward the environment (am I happy and attracted to the environment or fearful of it?), and the actual physical response to it. While analyzing the physiological bases of emotion, it is helpful to distinguish (1) the anatomical sites where the emotional value of a stimulus is determined; (2) the hormonal, autonomic, and outward expressions and displays of response to the stimulus (so-called **emotional behavior**); and (3) the conscious experience, or **inner emotions,** such as feelings of fear, love, anger, joy, anxiety, hope, and so on.

Emotional behavior can be studied more easily than the anatomical systems or inner emotions because it includes responses that can be measured externally (in terms of behavior). For example, stimulation of certain regions of the lateral hypothalamus causes an experimental animal to arch its back, puff out the fur on its tail, hiss, snarl, bare its claws and teeth, flatten its ears, and strike. Simultaneously, its heart rate, blood pressure, respiration, salivation, and plasma concentrations of epinephrine and fatty acids all increase. Clearly, this behavior typifies that of an enraged or threatened animal. Moreover, the animal's behavior can be changed from savage to docile and back again simply by activating different areas of the limbic system (**Figure 8.11**).

An early case study that shed light on neurological structures involved in emotional behavior was that of a patient known as S.M. This patient suffered from a rare disorder (***Urbach–Wiethe disease***) in which the anterior and medial portions of the temporal lobe atrophied, essentially destroying the amygdala bilaterally. Intelligence and memory formation remained intact. However, this individual lacked the ability to express fear in appropriate situations and could not recognize fearful expressions on other people's faces. Therefore, in humans, the amygdala is important for the emotion of fear.

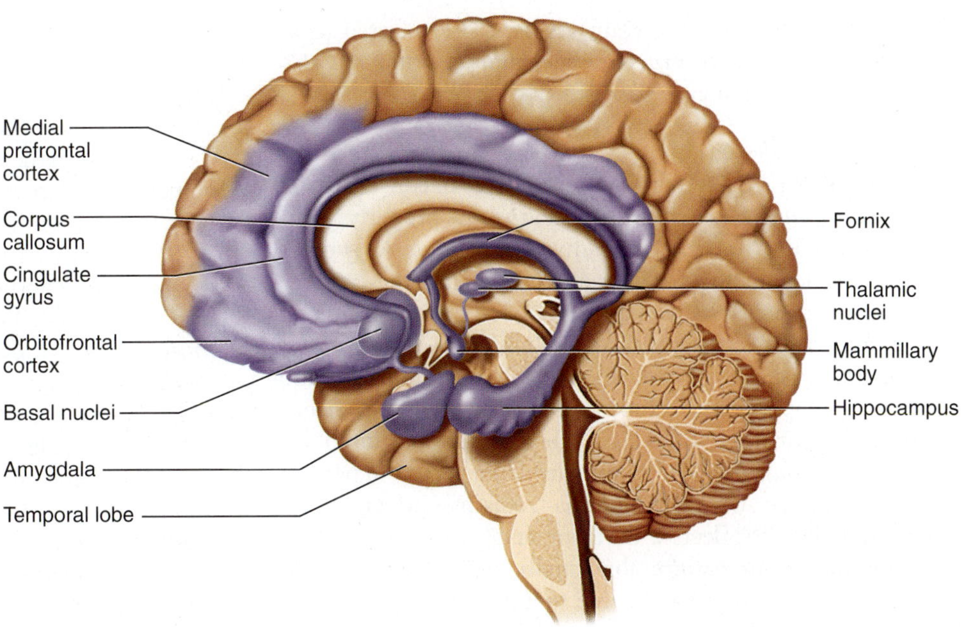

Figure 8.11 AP|R Brain structures involved in emotion, motivation, and the affective disorders. The limbic system is shaded purple; individual basal nuclei are not shown in this view.

PHYSIOLOGICAL INQUIRY

- What might have favored the evolution of emotions?

Answer can be found at end of chapter.

Emotional behavior includes such complex behaviors as the passionate defense of a political ideology and such simple actions as laughing, sweating, crying, or blushing. Emotional behavior is achieved by the autonomic and somatic nervous systems under the influence of integrating centers such as those we just mentioned, and provides an outward sign that the brain's "emotion systems" are activated.

The cerebral cortex plays a major role in directing many of the motor responses during emotional behavior (for example, whether you approach or avoid a situation). Moreover, forebrain structures, including the cerebral cortex, account for the modulation, direction, understanding, or even inhibition of emotional behaviors.

Although limbic areas of the brain seem to handle inner emotions, there is no single "emotional system." The amygdala (see Figure 8.11), and the region of association cortex on the lower surface of the frontal lobe, however, are central to most emotional states (**Figure 8.12**). The amygdala, in addition to being responsible for the emotion of fear, interacts with other parts of the brain via extensive reciprocal connections that can influence emotions about external stimuli, decision making, memory, attention, homeostatic processes, and behavioral responses. For example, it sends output to the hypothalamus, which is central to autonomic and hormonal homeostatic processes.

The limbic areas have been stimulated in awake human beings undergoing neurosurgery. These patients reported vague feelings of fear or anxiety during periods of stimulation to certain areas. Stimulation of other areas induced pleasurable sensations that the subjects found hard to define precisely. In normal functioning, the cerebral cortex allows us to connect such inner emotions with the particular experiences or thoughts that cause them.

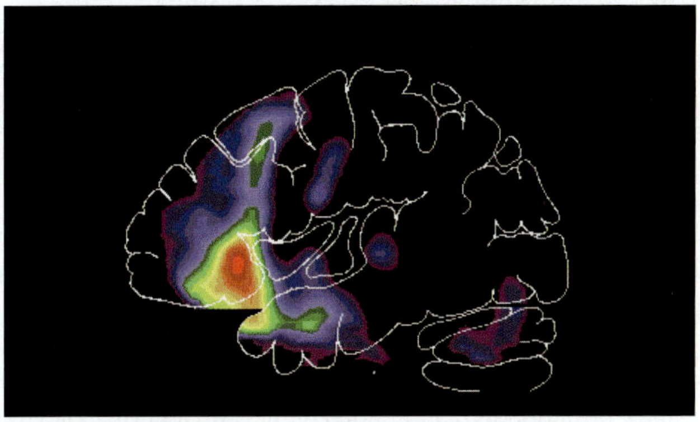

Figure 8.12 AP|R Computer image showing increased activity (red and yellow areas) in the prefrontal cortex during a sad thought. Marcus E. Raichle, M.D., Washington University School of Medicine.

8.4 Altered States of Consciousness

States of consciousness may be different from the commonly experienced ones like wakefulness and drowsiness. Other, more unusual sensations, such as those occurring with hypnosis, mind-altering drugs, and certain diseases, are referred to as ***altered states of consciousness.*** These altered states are also characteristic of psychiatric illnesses.

Schizophrenia

One of the diseases that induces altered states of consciousness is ***schizophrenia,*** in which information is not properly regulated in the brain. The amazingly diverse symptoms of schizophrenia include hallucinations, especially "hearing" voices, and delusions, such as the belief that one has been chosen for a special mission or is being persecuted by others. Schizophrenics become withdrawn, are emotionally unresponsive, and experience inappropriate moods. They may also experience abnormal motor behavior, which can include total immobilization (***catatonia***). The symptoms vary from person to person.

The causes of schizophrenia remain unclear. Studies suggest that it reflects a developmental disorder in which neurons migrate or mature abnormally during brain formation. The abnormality may be due to a genetic predisposition or multiple environmental factors such as viral infections and malnutrition during fetal life or early childhood. The brain abnormalities involve diverse neural circuits and neurotransmitter systems that regulate basic cognitive processes. A widely accepted explanation for schizophrenia suggests that certain mesocortical dopamine pathways are overactive. This hypothesis is supported by the fact that amphetamine-like drugs, which enhance dopamine signaling, make the symptoms worse, as well as by the fact that the most therapeutically beneficial drugs used in treating schizophrenia block dopamine receptors.

Schizophrenia affects approximately 1% of people over the age of 18, with the typical age of onset in the late teens or early 20s just as brain development nears completion. Currently, there is no prevention or cure for the disease, although drugs can often control the symptoms. In a small number of cases, there has been complete recovery.

The Mood Disorders: Depressions and Bipolar Disorders

The term **mood** refers to a pervasive and sustained inner emotion that affects a person's perception of the world. In addition to being part of the conscious experience of the person, others can observe it. In healthy people, moods can be normal, elevated, or depressed, and people generally feel that they have some degree of control over their moods. That sense of control is lost, however, in the ***mood disorders,*** which include depressive disorders and bipolar disorders. Along with schizophrenia, the mood disorders represent the major psychiatric illnesses.

Some of the prominent features of ***depressive disorder*** (***depression***) are a pervasive feeling of emptiness or sadness; a loss of energy, interest, or pleasure; anxiety; irritability; an increase or decrease in appetite; disturbed sleep; and thoughts of death or suicide. Depression can occur on its own, independent of any other illness, or it can arise secondary to other medical disorders. It is associated with decreased neuronal activity and metabolism in the anterior part of the limbic system and nearby prefrontal cortex. These same brain regions show abnormalities, albeit inconsistent ones, in bipolar disorders.

The term ***bipolar disorder*** describes swings between mania and depression. Episodes of ***mania*** are characterized by an abnormally and persistently elevated mood, sometimes with euphoria (that is, an exaggerated and unrealistic sense of well-being), racing thoughts, excessive energy, overconfidence, impulsiveness, significantly decreased time spent sleeping, and irritability.

Although the major biogenic amine neurotransmitters (norepinephrine, dopamine, and serotonin) and acetylcholine have all been implicated, the causes of the mood disorders are unknown.

Current treatment of the mood disorders emphasizes drugs and psychotherapy. The classical antidepressant drugs are of three types. The ***tricyclic antidepressant drugs*** such as ***amitriptyline*** (***Elavil***), ***desipramine*** (***Norpramin***), and ***doxepin*** (***Sinequan***) interfere with serotonin and/or norepinephrine reuptake by presynaptic endings. The ***monoamine oxidase inhibitors*** interfere with the enzyme responsible for the breakdown of these same two neurotransmitters. A third class of antidepressant drugs, the ***serotonin-specific reuptake inhibitors*** (***SSRIs***), includes the most widely used antidepressant drugs—including ***escitalopram*** (***Lexapro***), ***fluoxetine*** (***Prozac***), ***paroxetine*** (***Paxil***), and ***sertraline*** (***Zoloft***). As the name of this class of drugs suggests, they selectively inhibit serotonin reuptake by presynaptic terminals. In all three classes, the result is an increased concentration of serotonin and (except for the third class) norepinephrine in the extracellular fluid at synapses. SSRIs are currently the most commonly prescribed of the three types, due to a better safety record and fewer side effects and interactions with other medications. Recent research suggests that combining psychotherapy with drug therapy provides the maximum benefit to most patients with depression.

The biochemical effects of antidepressant medications occur immediately, but the beneficial antidepressant effects usually appear only after several weeks of treatment. Thus, the known biochemical effect must be only an early step in a complex sequence that leads to a therapeutic effect of these drugs. Consistent with the long latency of the antidepressant effect is the recent evidence that these drugs may ultimately stimulate the growth of new neurons in the hippocampus. Chronic stress is a known trigger of depression in some people, and it has also been shown to inhibit neurogenesis in animals. In addition, careful measurements of the hippocampus in chronically depressed patients show that it tends to be smaller than in matched, nondepressed individuals. Finally, though antidepressant drugs normally have measurable effects on behavior in animal models of depression, it was recently shown that those effects disappear completely when steps are taken to prevent neurogenesis.

Alternative treatments used when drug therapy and psychotherapy are not effective include electrical stimulation of the brain. One such treatment is ***electroconvulsive therapy*** (***ECT***). As the name suggests, pulses of electrical current applied through the skull are used to activate a large number of neurons in the brain simultaneously, thereby inducing a convulsion, or seizure. The patient is under anesthesia and prepared with a muscle relaxant to minimize the effects of the convulsion on the musculoskeletal system. A series of ECT treatments is believed to act via changes in neurotransmitter function by causing changes in the sensitivity of certain serotonin and adrenergic postsynaptic receptors. Despite good evidence that it can be an effective treatment, ECT tends to be utilized as a treatment of last resort in patients with depression or bipolar disorder who do not respond to medication.

A more recent alternative to drug therapy used to treat depression involves stimulation of the brain with electromagnets and is called ***repetitive transcranial magnetic stimulation*** (***rTMS***). In rTMS, circular or figure-eight-shaped metallic coils are placed against the skull overlying specific brain regions; then, brief, powerful electrical currents are applied at frequencies between 1 and 25 pulses per second. The resulting magnetic field induces current to flow through cortical neuronal networks directly beneath the coil. The immediate effect is similar to ECT—neural activity is transiently disordered or sometimes silenced in that brain region. However, no anesthesia is required and no pain, convulsion, or memory loss occurs. Depending on the frequency and treatment regimen applied, the lasting effects of rTMS can cause either an increase or a decrease in the overall activity of the targeted area. In recent clinical trials, 2 to 4 weeks of daily rTMS stimulation of the left prefrontal cortex resulted in marked improvement of patients with major depression who had not responded to medication. However, rTMS has not yet shown the same level of clinical effectiveness as ECT. Medical scientists are hopeful that refinements in rTMS techniques in the future could lead to breakthroughs in the treatment of obsessive-compulsive disorder, mania, schizophrenia, and other psychiatric illnesses.

Another nondrug therapy used for the type of annual depression known as ***seasonal affective depressive disorder*** (***SADD***) is ***phototherapy***, which exposes the patient to bright light for several hours per day during the winter months. Although light is thought to relieve depression by suppressing melatonin secretion from the pineal gland, as yet there is little evidence to support this claim.

A major drug used in treating patients with bipolar disorder is the chemical element ***lithium*** (***Eskalith, Lithobid***), sometimes given in combination with anticonvulsant drugs. It is highly specific, normalizing both the manic and depressed moods and slowing down thinking and motor behavior without causing sedation. In addition, it decreases the severity of the swings between mania and depression that occur in the bipolar disorders. In some cases, lithium is even effective in depression not associated with mania. Although it has been used for more than 50 years, the mechanisms of lithium action are not completely understood. It may help because it interferes with the formation of signaling molecules of the inositol phosphate family, thereby decreasing the response of postsynaptic neurons to neurotransmitters that utilize this signal transduction pathway (Chapter 5). Lithium has also been found to chronically increase the rate of glutamate uptake at excitatory synapses, which would be expected to reduce excessive nervous system activity during manic episodes.

Psychoactive Substances, Dependence, and Tolerance

In the previous sections, we mentioned several drugs used to combat altered states of consciousness. Psychoactive substances are also used as "recreational" drugs in a deliberate attempt to elevate mood and produce unusual states of consciousness ranging from meditative states to hallucinations. Virtually all the psychoactive substances exert their actions either directly or indirectly by altering neurotransmitter–receptor interactions in the biogenic amine pathways, particularly those of dopamine. For example, the primary effect of cocaine comes from its ability to block the reuptake of dopamine into the presynaptic axon terminal. Psychoactive substances are often chemically similar to neurotransmitters such as dopamine, serotonin, and norepinephrine, and they interact with the receptors activated by these transmitters (**Figure 8.13**).

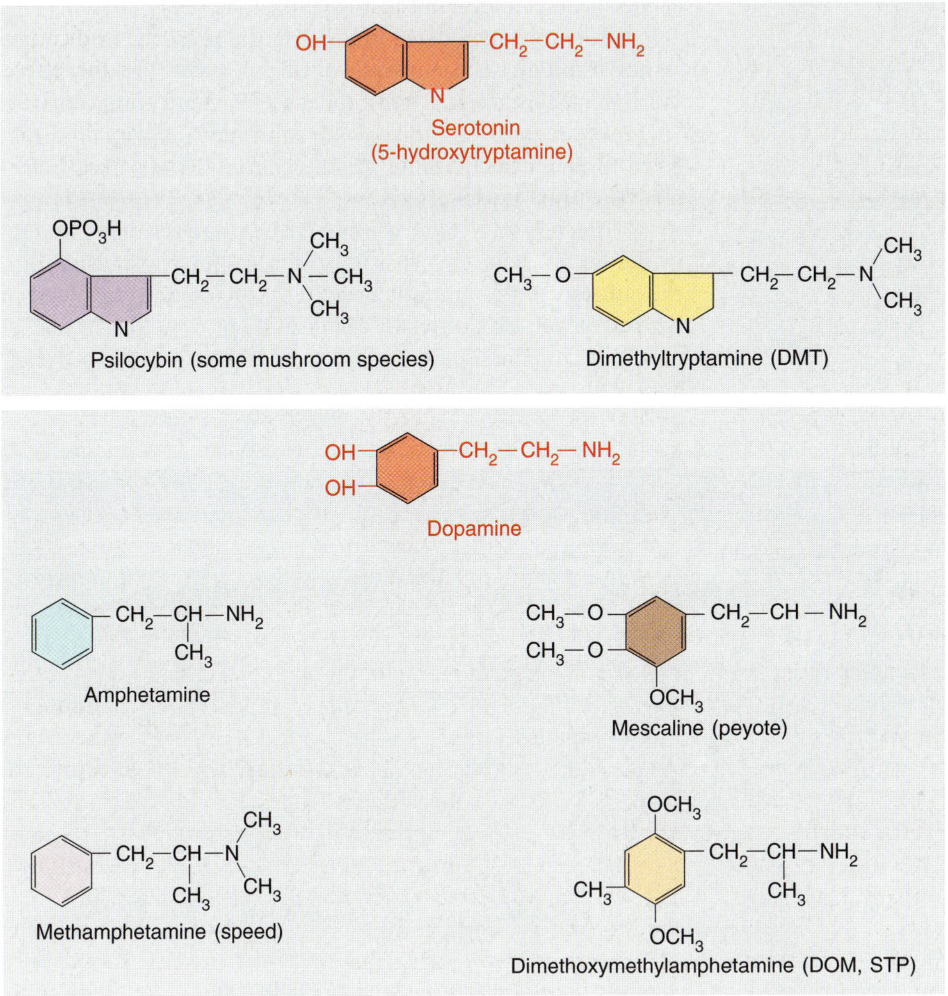

Figure 8.13 Molecular similarities between neurotransmitters (orange) and some substances that elevate mood. At high doses, these substances can cause hallucinations.

PHYSIOLOGICAL INQUIRY

- How would you expect dimethyltryptamine (DMT) to affect sleeping behavior?

Answer can be found at end of chapter.

Dependence

Substance dependence, the term now preferred to *addiction*, has two facets that may occur either together or independently: (1) a ***psychological dependence*** that is experienced as a craving for a substance and an inability to stop using the substance at will; and (2) a ***physical dependence*** that requires one to take the substance to avoid ***withdrawal,*** which is the spectrum of unpleasant physiological symptoms that occur with cessation of substance use. Substance dependence is diagnosed if three or more of the characteristics listed in **Table 8.3** occur within a 12-month period. **Table 8.4** lists rates of use and risk of dependence for some commonly used substances.

Several neuronal systems are involved in substance dependence, but most psychoactive substances act on the mesolimbic dopamine pathway (see Figure 8.9). In addition to the actions of this system mentioned earlier in the context of motivation and emotion, the mesolimbic dopamine pathway allows a person to experience pleasure in response to pleasurable events or in response to certain substances. Although the major neurotransmitter implicated in substance dependence is dopamine, other neurotransmitters, including GABA, enkephalin, serotonin, and glutamate, can also be involved.

TABLE 8.3 Diagnostic Criteria for Substance Dependence

Substance dependence is indicated when three or more of the following occur within a 12-month period.

I. Tolerance, as indicated by
   A. a need for increasing amounts of the substance to achieve the desired effect, or
   B. decreasing effects when continuing to use the same amount of the substance.

II. Withdrawal, as indicated by
   A. appearance of the characteristic withdrawal symptoms upon terminating use of the substance, or
   B. use of the substance (or one closely related to it) to relieve or avoid withdrawal symptoms.

III. Use of the substance in larger amounts or for longer periods of time than intended.

IV. Persistent desire for the substance; unsuccessful attempts to cut down or control use of the substance.

V. A great deal of time is spent in activities necessary to obtain the substance, use it, or recover from its effects.

VI. Occupational, social, or recreational activities are given up or reduced because of substance use.

VII. Use of the substance is continued despite knowledge that one has a physical or psychological problem that the substance is likely to exacerbate.

Table adapted from *The Diagnostic and Statistical Manual of Mental Disorders*, 4th ed., American Psychiatric Association, Arlington, VA, 2000.

Tolerance

Tolerance to a substance occurs when increasing doses of the substance are required to achieve effects that initially occurred in response to a smaller dose. That is, it takes more of the substance to do the same job. Moreover, tolerance can develop to another substance as a result of taking the initial substance, a phenomenon called ***cross-tolerance.*** Cross-tolerance may develop if the physiological actions of the two substances are similar. Tolerance and cross-tolerance can occur with many classes of substances, not just psychoactive substances.

Tolerance may develop because the presence of the substance stimulates the synthesis of the enzymes that degrade it. With persistent use of a substance, the concentrations of these enzymes increase, so more of the substance must be administered to produce the same plasma concentrations and, therefore, the same initial effect.

Alternatively, tolerance can develop as a result of changes in the number and/or sensitivity of receptors that respond to the substance, the amount or activity of enzymes involved in neurotransmitter synthesis, the activity of reuptake transport molecules, or the signal transduction pathways in the postsynaptic cell.

TABLE 8.4 Substance Use and Dependence

Substance	Percentage of Population Using at Least Once	Percentage of Population Who Meet Dependence Criteria	Percentage of Those Using Who Become Dependent
Tobacco	75.6	24.1	31.9
Heroin	1.5	0.4	23.1
Cocaine	16.2	2.7	16.7
Alcohol	91.5	14.1	15.4
Amphetamines	15.3	1.7	11.2
Marijuana	46.3	4.2	9.1

Table adapted from Laurence L. Brunton, John S. Lazo, and Keither L. Parker, eds., *Goodman and Gilman's The Pharmacological Basis of Therapeutics*, 11th ed., McGraw-Hill, NY, 2006.

8.5 Learning and Memory

Learning is the acquisition and storage of information as a consequence of experience. It is measured by an increase in the likelihood of a particular behavioral response to a stimulus. Generally, rewards or punishments are crucial ingredients of learning, as are contact with and manipulation of the environment. **Memory** is the relatively permanent storage form of learned information, although, as we will see, it is not a single, unitary phenomenon. Rather, the brain processes, stores, and retrieves information in different ways to suit different needs.

Memory

The term **memory encoding** defines the neural processes that change an experience into the memory of that experience—in other words, the physiological events that lead to memory formation. This section addresses three questions. First, are there different kinds of memories? Second, where do they occur in the brain? Third, what happens physiologically to make them occur?

New scientific information about memory are being generated at a tremendous pace; there is as yet no unifying theory as to how memory is encoded, stored, and retrieved. However, memory can be viewed in two broad categories called declarative and procedural memory. **Declarative memory** (sometimes also referred to as "explicit" memory) is the retention and recall of conscious experiences that can be put into words (declared). One example is the memory of having perceived an object or event and, therefore, recognizing it as familiar and maybe even knowing the specific time and place when the memory originated. A second example would be the general knowledge of the world, such as names and facts. The hippocampus, amygdala, and other parts of the limbic system are required for the formation of declarative memories.

The second broad category of memory, **procedural memory,** can be defined as the memory of how to do things (sometimes this is also called "implicit" or "reflexive" memory). This is the memory for skilled behaviors independent of conscious understanding, as, for example, riding a bicycle. Individuals can suffer severe deficits in declarative memory but have intact procedural memory. One case study describes a pianist who learned a new piece to accompany a singer at a concert but had no recollection the following morning of having performed the composition. He could remember how to play the music but could not remember having done so. The category of procedural memory also includes learned emotional responses, such as fear of spiders, and the classic example of Pavlov's dogs, which learned to salivate at the sound of a bell after the sound had previously been associated with food. The primary areas of the brain involved in procedural memory are regions of sensorimotor cortex, the basal nuclei, and the cerebellum.

Another way to classify memory is in terms of duration—does it last for a long or only a short time? **Working memory,** also known as **short-term memory,** registers and retains incoming information for a short time—a matter of seconds to minutes—after its input. In other words, it is the memory that we use when we keep information consciously "in mind." For example, you may hear a telephone number in a radio advertisement and remember it only long enough to reach for your phone and enter the number. Working memory makes possible a temporary impression of one's present environment in a readily accessible form and is an essential ingredient of many forms of higher mental activity. Short-term memories may be converted into **long-term memories,** which may be stored for days to years and recalled at a later time. The process by which short-term memories become long-term memories is called **consolidation.**

Focusing attention is essential for many memory-based skills. The longer the span of attention in working memory, the better the chess player, the greater the ability to reason, and the better a student is at understanding complicated sentences and drawing inferences from texts. In fact, there is a strong correlation between working memory and standard measures of intelligence. Conversely, the specific memory deficit that occurs in the early stages of ***Alzheimer disease*** (also called Alzheimer's disease), a condition marked by dementia and serious memory losses, may be in this attention-focusing component of working memory.

The Neural Basis of Learning and Memory

The neural mechanism and parts of the brain involved vary for different types of memory. Short-term encoding and long-term memory storage occur in different brain areas for both declarative and procedural memories (**Figure 8.14**).

What is happening during memory formation on a cellular level? Conditions such as coma, deep anesthesia, electroconvulsive shock, and insufficient blood supply to the brain, all of which interfere with the electrical activity of the brain, also interfere with working memory. Therefore, it is assumed that

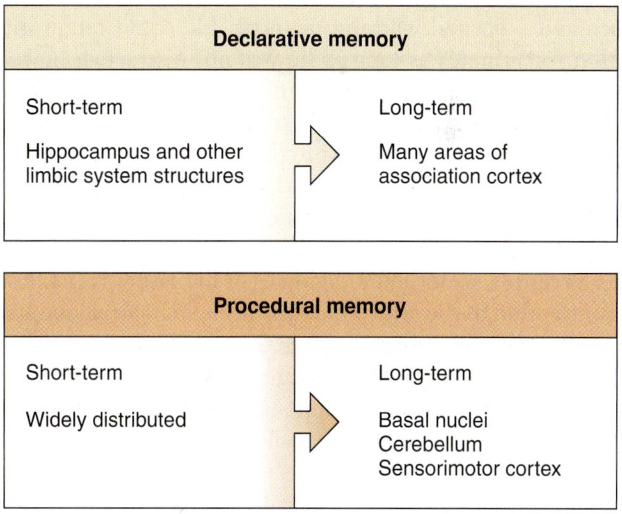

Figure 8.14 Brain areas involved in encoding and storage of declarative and procedural memories.

PHYSIOLOGICAL INQUIRY

- After a brief meeting, you are more likely to remember the name of someone you are strongly attracted to than the name of someone for whom you have no feelings. Propose a mechanism.

Answer can be found at end of chapter.

working memory requires ongoing graded or action potentials. Working memory is interrupted when a person becomes unconscious from a blow on the head, and memories are abolished for all that happened for a variable period of time before the blow, a condition called ***retrograde amnesia.*** (***Amnesia*** is the loss of memory.) Working memory is also susceptible to external interference, such as an attempt to learn conflicting information. On the other hand, long-term memory can survive deep anesthesia, trauma, or electroconvulsive shock, all of which disrupt the normal patterns of neural conduction in the brain. Thus, working memory requires electrical activity in the neurons.

Another type of amnesia is referred to as ***anterograde amnesia.*** It results from damage to the limbic system and associated structures, including the hippocampus, thalamus, and hypothalamus. Patients with this condition lose their ability to consolidate short-term declarative memories into long-term memories. Although they can remember stored information and events that occurred before their brain injury, after the injury they can only retain information as long as it exists in working memory. This type of amnesia is sometimes transiently induced pharmacologically during medical procedures for which patients are required to remain conscious, such as colonoscopy (see Chapter 15). The most common drugs used to produce this "conscious sedation" stimulate GABA receptors.

The case of a patient known as H.M. illustrates that formation of declarative and procedural memories involves distinct neural processes and that limbic system structures are essential for consolidating declarative memories. In 1953, H.M. underwent bilateral removal of the amygdala and large parts of the hippocampus as a treatment for persistent, debilitating epilepsy. Although his epileptic condition improved after this surgery, it resulted in anterograde amnesia. He still had a normal intelligence and a normal working memory. He could retain information for minutes as long as he was not distracted; however, he could not form long-term memories. If he was introduced to someone on one day, on the next day he did not recall having previously met that person. Nor could he remember any events that occurred after his surgery, although his memory for events prior to the surgery was intact. Interestingly, H.M. had normal procedural memory and could learn new puzzles and motor tasks as readily as normal individuals. This case was the first to draw attention to the critical importance of temporal lobe structures of the limbic system in consolidating short-term declarative memories into long-term memories. Additional cases since have demonstrated that the hippocampus is the primary structure involved in this process. Because H.M. retained memories from before the surgery, his case showed that the hippocampus is not involved in the *storage* of declarative memories.

The problem of exactly how memories are stored in the brain is still unsolved, but some of the pieces of the puzzle are falling into place. One model for memory is **long-term potentiation (LTP)**, in which certain synapses undergo a long-lasting increase in their effectiveness when they are heavily used. Review Figure 6.36, which details how this occurs at glutamatergic synapses. An analogous process, **long-term depression (LTD)**, *decreases* the effectiveness of synaptic contacts between neurons. The mechanism of this suppression of activity appears to be mainly via changes in the channels in the postsynaptic membrane.

It is generally accepted that long-term memory formation involves processes that alter gene expression. This is achieved by a cascade of second messengers and transcription factors that ultimately leads to the production of new cellular proteins. These new proteins may be involved in the increased number of synapses that have been demonstrated after long-term memory formation. They may also be involved in structural changes in individual synapses (e.g., by an increase in the number of receptors on the postsynaptic membrane). This ability of neural tissue to change because of activation is known as **plasticity.**

Certain types of learning depend not only on factors such as attention, motivation, and various neurotransmitters but also on certain hormones. For example, the hormones epinephrine, ACTH, and vasopressin affect the retention of learned experiences. These hormones are normally released in stressful or mildly stimulating circumstances, suggesting that the hormonal consequences of our experiences affect our memories of them.

Two of the opioid peptides, enkephalin and endorphin (see Chapter 6, Section C), interfere with learning and memory, particularly when the lesson involves a painful stimulus. They may inhibit learning simply because they decrease the emotional (fear, anxiety) component of the painful experience associated with the learning situation, thereby decreasing the motivation necessary for learning to occur.

Table 8.5 summarizes some general principles about learning and memory.

8.6 Cerebral Dominance and Language

The two cerebral hemispheres appear to be nearly symmetrical, but each has anatomical, chemical, and functional specializations. We have already mentioned that the left hemisphere deals with the somatosensory and motor functions of the right side of the body, and vice versa. In addition, specific aspects of language use tend to be controlled by predominantly one cerebral hemisphere or the other. In 90% of the population, the left hemisphere is specialized to handle specific tasks involved in

TABLE 8.5 General Principles of Learning and Memory
There are multiple memory systems in the brain.
Short-term and long-term forms of learning and memory involve changes in existing neural circuits.
These changes may involve multiple cellular mechanisms within individual neurons.
Second-messenger systems play a role in mediating cellular changes.
Changes in membrane channels are often correlated with learning and memory.
Long-term memory requires new protein synthesis, whereas short-term memory does not.

Table adapted from John H. Byrne, "Learning and Memory: Basic Mechanisms," in Larry R. Squire, Darwin Berg, Floyd E. Bloom, Sascha du Lac, Anirvan Ghosh, and Nicholas C. Spitzer, eds., *Fundamental Neuroscience*, Academic Press, San Diego, CA, 2008.

producing and comprehending language—the conceptualization of the words you want to say or write, the neural control of the act of speaking or writing, and recent verbal memory. This is even true of the sign language used by some deaf people. Conversely, the right cerebral hemisphere in most people tends to have dominance in determining the ability to understand and express affective, or emotional aspects of language.

Language is a complex code that includes the acts of listening, seeing, reading, speaking, and expressing emotion. The major centers for the technical aspects of language function are in the left hemisphere in the temporal, parietal, and frontal cortex next to the **Sylvian fissure,** which separates the temporal lobe from the frontal and parietal lobes (**Figure 8.15**). Each of the various regions deals with a separate aspect of language. For example, distinct areas are specialized for hearing, seeing, speaking, and generating words (**Figure 8.16**). There are even distinct brain networks for different categories of things, such as "animals" and "tools." Although the regions responsible for the affective components of language have not been as specifically mapped, it appears they are in the same general region of the right cerebral hemisphere. There is variation between individuals in the regional processing of language, and some research even suggests that males and females may process language slightly differently. Females are more likely to involve areas of both hemispheres for some language tasks, whereas males generally show activity mainly on the left side (**Figure 8.17**). The cerebellum is also important in speaking and writing, because those tasks involve coordinated muscle contractions.

Much of our knowledge about how language is produced has been obtained from patients who have suffered brain damage and, as a result, have one or more defects in language, including ***aphasia*** (from the Greek, "speechlessness") and ***aprosodia.*** (**Prosody** includes aspects of communication such as intonation, rhythm, pitch, emphasis, gestures, and accompanying facial expressions, so aprosodia refers to the absence of those aspects.)

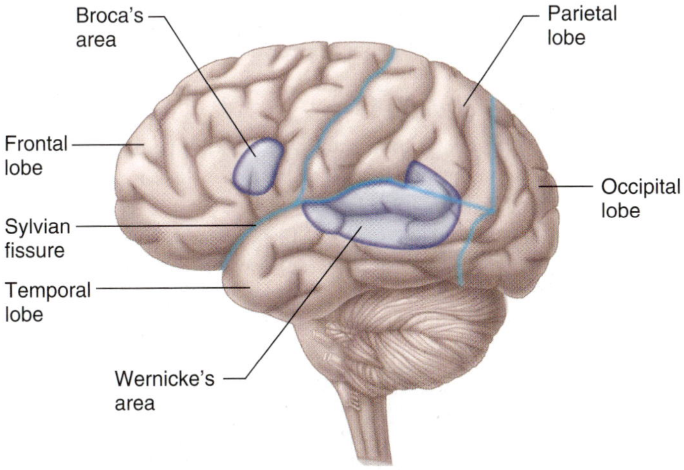

Figure 8.15 APIR Areas of the left cerebral hemisphere found clinically to be involved in the comprehension (Wernicke's area) and motor (Broca's area) aspects of language. Blue lines indicate divisions of the cortex into frontal, parietal, temporal, and occipital lobes. Similar regions on the right side of the brain are involved in understanding and expressing affective (emotional) aspects of language.

The specific defects that occur vary according to the region of the brain that is damaged. For example, damage to the left temporal region known as **Wernicke's area** (see Figure 8.15) generally results in aphasias that are more closely related to *comprehension*—the individuals have difficulty understanding spoken or written language even though their hearing and vision are unimpaired. Although they may have fluent speech, they scramble words so that their sentences make no sense, often adding unnecessary words, or even creating made-up words. For example, they may intend to ask someone on a date but say, "If when going movie by fleeble because have to watch would."

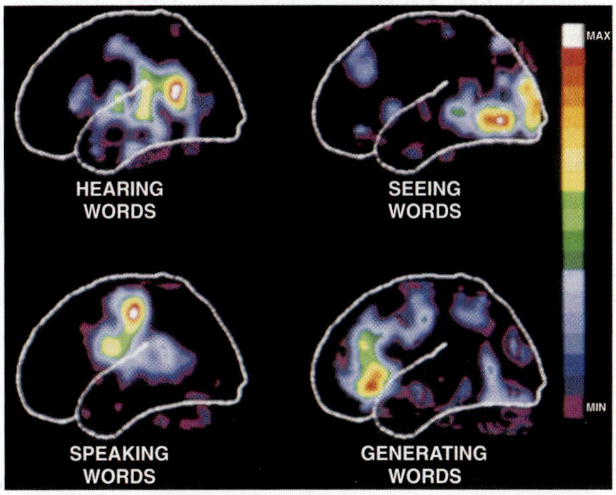

Figure 8.16 APIR PET scans reveal areas of increased blood flow in specific parts of the temporal, occipital, parietal, and frontal lobes during various language-based activities. Courtesy of Dr. Marcus E. Raichle.

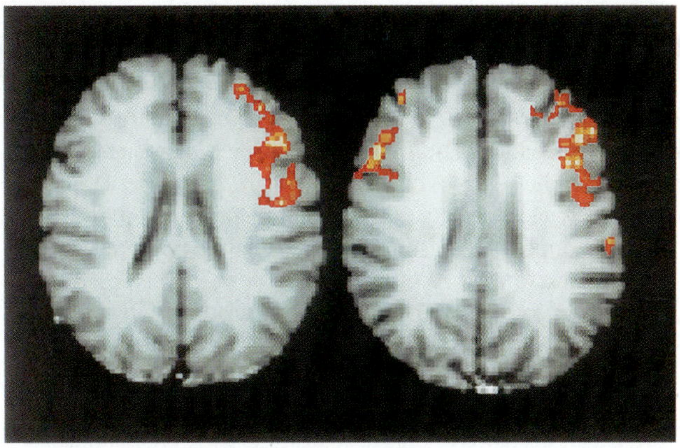

Figure 8.17 APIR Images of the active areas of the brain in a male (left) and a female (right) during a language task. (In scans of this type, the patient's left is displayed on the right of the image.) Note that both sides of the woman's brain are used in processing language, but the man's brain is more compartmentalized.
Shaywitz et al., 1995 NMR Research/Yale Medical School.

PHYSIOLOGICAL INQUIRY

- Based on typical patterns of cerebral dominance of language tasks, how may you explain the difference in how these two individuals processed this task?

Answer can be found at end of chapter.

They are often unaware that they are not speaking in clear sentences. In contrast, damage to **Broca's area,** the language area in the frontal cortex responsible for the articulation of speech, can cause *expressive* aphasias. Individuals with this condition have difficulty carrying out the coordinated respiratory and oral movements necessary for language even though they can move their lips and tongues. They understand spoken language and know what they want to say but have trouble forming words and sentences. For example, instead of fluidly saying, "I have two sisters," they may hesitantly utter, "Two . . . sister . . . sister." Patients with damage to Broca's area can become frustrated because they generally are aware that their words do not accurately convey their thoughts. Aprosodias result from damage to language areas in the right cerebral hemisphere or to neural pathways connecting the left and right hemispheres. Though they can form and understand words and sentences, people with these conditions have impaired ability to interpret or express emotional intentions, and their social interactions suffer greatly as a result. For example, they may not be able to distinguish whether a person who said "thank you very much" was expressing genuine appreciation for a thoughtful compliment or delivering a sarcastic retort after feeling insulted.

The potential for the development of language-specific mechanisms in the two hemispheres is present at birth, but the assignment of language functions to specific brain areas is fairly flexible in the early years of life. Thus, for example, damage to the language areas of the left hemisphere during infancy or early childhood causes temporary, minor language impairment until the right hemisphere can take over. However, similar damage acquired during adulthood typically causes permanent, devastating language deficits. By puberty, the brain's ability to transfer language functions between hemispheres is less successful, and often language skills are lost permanently.

Differences between the two hemispheres are usually masked by the integration that occurs via the corpus callosum and other pathways that connect the two sides of the brain. However, the separate functions of the left and right hemispheres have been uncovered by studying patients in whom the two hemispheres have been separated surgically for treatment of severe epilepsy. These so-called **split-brain** patients participated in studies in which they were asked to hold and identify an object such as a ball in their left or right hand behind a barrier that prevented them from seeing the object. Subjects who held the ball in their right hand were able to say that it was a ball, but persons who held the ball in their left hand were unable to name it. Because the processing of sensory information occurs on the side of the brain opposite to the sensation, this result demonstrated conclusively that the left hemisphere contains a language center that is not present in the right hemisphere.

Although language skills emerge spontaneously in children in all societies, there is a critical period during childhood when exposure to language is necessary for these skills to develop, just as the ability to see depends upon effective visual input early in life. The critical period is thought to end at puberty or earlier. The dramatic change at puberty in the possibility of learning language, or the ease of learning a second language, occurs as the brain attains its structural, biochemical, and functional maturity at that time.

SUMMARY

States of Consciousness

I. The electroencephalogram (EEG) provides one means of defining the states of consciousness.
   a. Electrical currents in the cerebral cortex due predominantly to summed postsynaptic potentials are recorded as the EEG.
   b. Slower EEG wave frequencies correlate with less responsive behaviors.
   c. Rhythm generators in the thalamus are probably responsible for the wavelike nature of the EEG.
   d. EEGs are used to diagnose brain disease and damage.

II. Alpha rhythms and, during EEG arousal, beta rhythms characterize the EEG of an awake person.

III. NREM sleep progresses from stage N1 (higher-frequency, smaller-amplitude waves) through stage N3 (lower-frequency, larger-amplitude waves) and then back again, followed by an episode of REM sleep. There are generally four or five of these cycles per night.

IV. Wakefulness is stimulated by regulated by groups of neurons originating in the brainstem and hypothalamus that activate cortical arousal by releasing orexins, norepinephrine, serotonin, histamine, and acetylcholine. A sleep center in the hypothalamus releases GABA and inhibits these activating centers.

V. Extensive damage to the cerebral cortex or brainstem arousal mechanisms can result in coma or brain death.

Conscious Experiences

I. Brain structures involved in selective attention determine which brain areas gain temporary predominance in the ongoing stream of conscious experience.

II. Conscious experiences may occur because a set of neurons temporarily function together, with the neurons that compose the set changing as the focus of attention changes.

Motivation and Emotion

I. Behaviors that satisfy homeostatic needs are primary motivated behaviors. Behavior not related to homeostasis is a result of secondary motivation.
   a. Repetition of a behavior indicates it is rewarding, and avoidance of a behavior indicates it is punishing.
   b. The mesolimbic dopamine pathway, which goes to prefrontal cortex and parts of the limbic system, mediates emotion and motivation.
   c. Dopamine is the primary neurotransmitter in the brain pathway that mediates motivation and reward.

II. Three aspects of emotion—anatomical and physiological bases for emotion, emotional behavior, and inner emotions—can be distinguished. The limbic system integrates inner emotions and behavior.

Altered States of Consciousness

I. Hyperactivity in a brain dopaminergic system is implicated in schizophrenia.

II. Mood disorders may be caused by disturbances in transmission at brain synapses mediated by dopamine, norepinephrine, serotonin, and acetylcholine.
III. Many psychoactive drugs, which are often chemically related to neurotransmitters, result in substance dependence, withdrawal, and tolerance. The mesolimbic dopamine pathway is implicated in substance abuse.

Learning and Memory

I. The brain processes, stores, and retrieves information in different ways to suit different needs.
II. Memory encoding involves cellular or molecular changes specific to different memories.
III. Declarative memories are involved in remembering facts and events. Procedural memories are memories of how to do things.
IV. Short-term memories are converted into long-term memories by a process known as consolidation.
V. Prefrontal cortex and limbic regions of the temporal lobe are important brain areas for some forms of memory.
VI. Formation of long-term memory probably involves changes in second-messenger systems and protein synthesis.

Cerebral Dominance and Language

I. The two cerebral hemispheres differ anatomically, chemically, and functionally. In 90% of the population, the left hemisphere dominates the technical aspects of language production and comprehension such as word meanings and sentence structure, while the right hemisphere dominates in mediating the emotional content of language.
II. The development of language functions occurs in a critical period that ends around the time of puberty.
III. After damage to the dominant hemisphere, the opposite hemisphere can acquire some language function—the younger the patient, the greater the transfer of function.

REVIEW QUESTIONS

1. State the two criteria used to define one's state of consciousness.
2. What type of neural activity is recorded as the EEG?
3. Draw EEG records that show alpha and beta rhythms, the stages of NREM sleep, and REM sleep. Indicate the characteristic wave frequencies of each.
4. Distinguish NREM sleep from REM sleep.
5. Briefly describe a neural mechanism that determines the states of consciousness.
6. Name the criteria used to distinguish brain death from coma.
7. Describe the orienting response as a form of directed attention.
8. Distinguish primary from secondary motivated behavior.
9. Explain how rewards and punishments are anatomically related to emotions.
10. Explain what brain self-stimulation can tell about emotions and rewards and punishments.
11. Name the primary neurotransmitter that mediates the brain reward systems.
12. Distinguish inner emotions from emotional behavior. Name the brain areas involved in each.
13. Describe the role of the limbic system in emotions.
14. Name the major neurotransmitters involved in schizophrenia and the mood disorders.
15. Describe a mechanism that could explain tolerance and withdrawal.
16. Distinguish the types of memory.

KEY TERMS

CLINICAL TERMS

Clinical Case Study: Head Injury in a Teenage Soccer Player

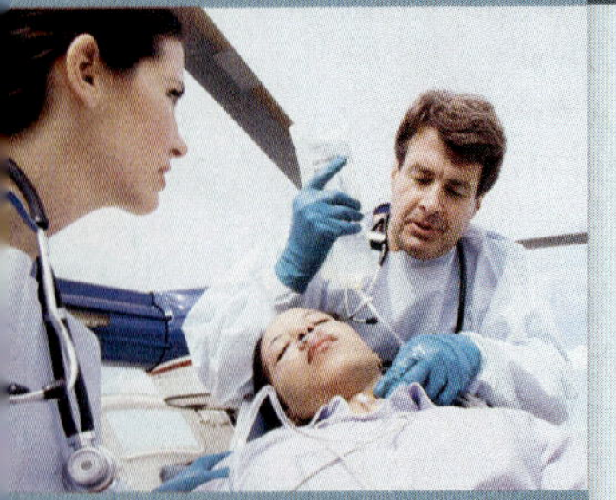

In the final minute of the high-school state championship match, with the score tied 1 to 1, the corner kick sailed toward the far post. Lunging for a header and the win, the 17-year-old midfielder was kicked solidly in the right side of her head by a defender. She crumpled to the ground and lay motionless. The team physician rushed onto the field, where the girl lay on her back with her eyes closed. She was breathing normally but failed to respond to the sound of her name or a touch on her arm. An ambulance was immediately summoned. After a few moments, her eyes fluttered open, and she looked up at the doctor and her teammates with a confused expression on her face. Asked how she was feeling, she said "fine" and attempted to sit up but winced in pain and put her hand to her head as the physician told her to remain lying down. It was an encouraging sign that all four limbs and her trunk muscles had moved normally in her attempt to sit up, suggesting she did not have a serious injury to her spinal cord.

The physician then asked her a series of questions. Did she remember how she had been injured? She responded with a blank look and a small shake of her head. Did she know what day this was and where she was? After a long pause and a look at her surroundings, she replied that it was Saturday and this was the championship soccer match. How much time was left in the game, and what was the score? Another long pause, and then "It's almost halftime, and it's zero to zero." Before he could ask the next question, her eyes rolled back in their sockets and her body stiffened for several seconds, after which she once again looked around with a confused expression.

These signs suggested that she had suffered an injury to her brain and should undergo a thorough neurological exam. The ambulance arrived, she was placed on a rigid backboard with her head supported and restrained, and she was transported to the hospital for further assessment and observation.

By the time she reached the emergency room, she was less disoriented and had no nausea but still complained that her head hurt. Her pulse rate and blood pressure were normal. A series of neurological tests was then performed. When a light was shone into either eye, both pupils constricted equally. She was also able to smoothly track a moving object with her eyes. Her sense of balance was good, and she was able to feel a vibrating tuning fork, light pinpricks, and warm and cold objects on the skin of all of her extremities. Muscle tone, strength, and reflexes were also normal. Asked again about the collision, she still was unsure what had happened. However, suddenly straightening in her chair, she said, "Wait—the game was almost over and we were tied one to one. . . . Did we win?"

The blow to this soccer player's head resulted in a ***concussion,*** an injury suffered by more than 300,000 athletes each year in the United States. Concussion is a usually brief loss of consciousness that occurs after some form of head trauma. It sometimes results in temporary retrograde amnesia, which varies in extent with the severity of the injury, and also in brief epileptic-like seizures. The mechanism of the loss of consciousness, amnesia, and seizures is thought to be a transient electrophysiological dysfunction of the reticular activating system in the upper midbrain caused by rotation of the cerebral hemispheres on the relatively fixed brainstem. The relatively large size and inertia

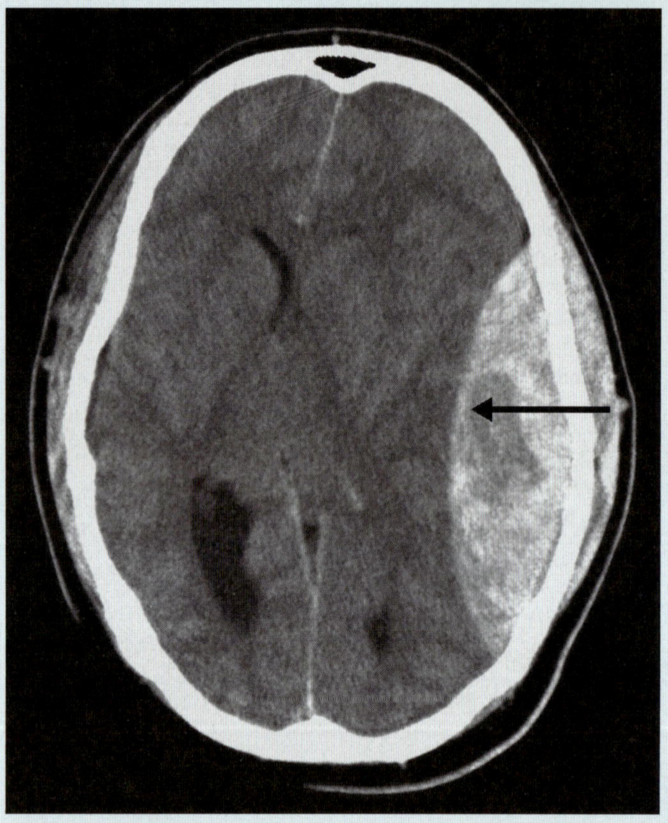

Figure 8.18 CT scan of a large, left-side epidural hematoma resulting from a motorcycle crash in which the rider was not wearing a helmet. Arrow shows where blood pooling within the cranium has compressed the brain tissue. Patient's left side is on the right side of the image. Courtesy of Lee Faucher, M.D., University of Wisconsin SMPH.

of the brains of humans and other primates make them especially susceptible to such injuries. By comparison, animals adapted for cranial impact like goats, rams, and woodpeckers are able to withstand 100-fold greater force than humans without sustaining injury. Computed tomography and magnetic resonance imaging scans of most concussion patients show no abnormal swelling or vascular injury of the brain. However, widespread reports of persistent memory and concentration problems have increasingly raised concerns that in some cases concussion injuries may involve lasting damage in the form of microscopic shearing lesions in the brain. Quantitative analysis of EEG recordings is currently under investigation for its usefulness in the acute diagnosis of concussion and for the post-concussion monitoring of brain function.

More serious than a concussion is ***intracranial hemorrhage,*** which results from damage to blood vessels in and around the brain. It can be associated with skull fracture, violent shaking, and sudden accelerative forces such as those that would occur during an automobile accident. Blood may collect between the skull and the dura mater (an ***epidural hematoma,*** **Figure 8.18**), or between the arachnoid mater and the surrounding meninges or within the brain (***subdural hematoma***). Intracranial hemorrhage often occurs without loss of consciousness; symptoms such as nausea, headache,

(continued)

(continued)

motor dysfunction, and loss of pupillary reflexes may not occur until several hours or days afterward. Another symptom of brain swelling after vascular trauma is ***Cushing's phenomenon,*** in which systemic blood pressure is markedly elevated (see Chapter 12, Section D). It is treated when necessary by drainage of the blood from the affected area. One reason that it is important to closely monitor the condition of a person with concussion for some time after the injury is to be able to recognize whether the initial trauma has resulted in an intracranial hemorrhage.

The soccer player in this case was given pain medication and kept in the hospital overnight for observation. She suffered no further seizures, and by morning her memory had completely returned and other neurological test results were normal. She was sent home with instructions to return for a follow-up examination the next week, or sooner if her headache did not steadily improve. She was also advised to avoid competing for a minimum of 2 weeks. A person who receives a second blow to the head prior to complete healing of a first concussion injury has an elevated risk of suffering life-threatening brain swelling.

Concussion injuries in sports are receiving increased attention. Some neurologists suspect that concussions have the potential to cause long-term physical, cognitive, and psychological changes, and that the risk is magnified in those who experience multiple concussions. Suspicions have been fueled by high-profile cases of professional boxers who have developed symptoms similar to those seen in the neurodegenerative conditions Parkinson disease (see Chapter 10) and Alzheimer disease (see Chapter 6). Recent histological studies of the brains of deceased professional football players have shown significant microscopic damage in those who have suffered multiple concussions. Even more disconcerting are the recent findings in teenage football players, that milder repetitive blows to the head that do not meet the clinical criteria of a concussion may also lead to lasting brain damage. To address issues such as these, research is currently under way in which athletes are being assessed for attention span, memory, processing speed, and reaction time—both before and after suffering concussions. Other initiatives include developing more sensitive diagnostic tests, creating guidelines on when to allow athletes to return to competition following a head injury, and the design of protective headgear.

Clinical terms: concussion, Cushing's phenomenon, epidural hematoma, intracranial hemorrhage, subdural hematoma

See Chapter 19 for complete, integrative case studies.

CHAPTER 8 TEST QUESTIONS

Answers found in Appendix A.

1–4: Match the state of consciousness (a–d) with the correct electroencephalogram pattern (use each answer once).

State of consciousness:

a. relaxed, awake, eyes closed
b. stage N3 non–rapid eye movement (NREM) sleep
c. rapid eye movement (REM) sleep
d. epileptic seizure

Electroencephalogram pattern:

1. Very large-amplitude, recurrent waves, associated with sharp spikes
2. Small-amplitude, high-frequency waves, similar to the attentive awake state
3. Irregular, slow-frequency, large-amplitude, "alpha" rhythm
4. Regular, very slow-frequency, very large-amplitude "delta" rhythm

5. Which pattern of neurotransmitter activity is most consistent with the awake state?
   a. high histamine, orexins and GABA; low norepinephrine
   b. high norepinephrine, histamine and serotonin; low orexins
   c. high histamine and serotonin; low GABA and orexins
   d. high histamine, GABA and orexins; low serotonin
   e. high orexins, histamine and norepinephrine; low GABA

6. Which best describes "habituation"?
   a. seeking out and focusing on momentarily important stimuli
   b. decreased behavioral response to a persistent irrelevant stimulus
   c. halting current activity and orienting toward a novel stimulus
   d. evaluation of the importance of sensory stimuli that occur prior to focusing attention
   e. strengthening of synapses that are repeatedly stimulated during learning

7. The mesolimbic dopamine pathway is most closely associated with
   a. shifting between states of consciousness.
   b. emotional behavior.
   c. motivation and reward behaviors.
   d. perception of fear.
   e. primary visual perception.

8. Antidepressant medications most commonly target what neurotransmitter?
   a. acetylcholine
   b. dopamine
   c. histamine
   d. serotonin
   e. glutamate

9. Which is a true statement about memory?
   a. Consolidation converts short-term memories into long-term memories.
   b. Working memory stores information for years, perhaps indefinitely.
   c. In retrograde amnesia, the ability to form new memories is lost.
   d. The cerebellum is an important site of storage for declarative memory.
   e. Destruction of the hippocampus erases all previously stored memories.

10. Broca's area
   a. is in the parietal association cortex and is responsible for language comprehension.
   b. is in the right frontal lobe and is responsible for memory formation.
   c. is in the left frontal lobe and is responsible for articulation of speech.
   d. is in the occipital lobe and is responsible for interpreting body language.
   e. is part of the limbic system and is responsible for the perception of fear.

CHAPTER 8 GENERAL PRINCIPLES ASSESSMENT

Answers found in Appendix A.

1. Review the general principles of physiology presented in Chapter 1. Which of those eight principles is best demonstrated by the two parts of Figure 8.7, and why?
2. How does the regulation of sleep exemplify the general principle of physiology that *homeostasis is essential for health and survival?*

CHAPTER 8 QUANTITATIVE AND THOUGHT QUESTIONS

Answers found at www.mhhe.com/widmaier13.

1. Explain why patients given drugs to treat Parkinson disease (Chapter 6) sometimes develop symptoms similar to those of schizophrenia.
2. Explain how clinical observations of individuals with various aphasias help physiologists understand the neural basis of language.

CHAPTER 8 ANSWERS TO PHYSIOLOGICAL INQUIRIES

Figure 8.1 If the frequency of the waveform is 20 Hz (20 waves per second), then the duration of each wave is 1/20 sec, or 50 msec.

Figure 8.2 The primary visual cortex and related association areas are in the occipital lobes of the brain (review Figure 7.13), so it is most likely that this abnormal rhythm was recorded by electrodes placed on the scalp at the back of the patient's head.

Figure 8.6 Among the drugs used to treat allergic reactions are antihistamines. They are prescribed because of their ability to block histamine's contributions to the inflammatory response, which include vasodilation and leakiness of small blood vessels (see Table 18.12). Because a decrease in histamine is associated with the induction of NREM sleep, drowsiness is a common side effect of antihistamines. Fortunately, antihistamines have been developed that do not cross the blood–brain barrier and thus do not have this side effect (e.g., loratadine [Claritin, Alavert]).

Figure 8.7 There are a number of possible reasons it may be adaptive for cytokines to induce sleep. For example, the decreased physical activity associated with sleep may conserve metabolic energy when running a fever and fighting an infection. Sleeping more and eating less may also help by decreasing intake and plasma concentrations of specific nutrients needed by invading organisms to replicate, like iron (see Chapter 1). From a population health perspective, more time spent in sleep may be adaptive by reducing the number of others with which an infected person comes into contact.

Figure 8.11 There are many ways emotions could potentially contribute to survival and reproduction. The perception of fear aids survival by stimulating avoidance or caution in potentially dangerous situations, like coming into contact with potentially venomous spiders or snakes or walking near the edge of a high cliff. Our tendency to be disgusted by the smell of rotting food and fecal matter might have evolved as a protection against infection by potentially harmful bacteria or pathogens. Anger and rage could contribute to both survival and reproduction by facilitating our ability to fight for mates or territory or for self-defense. Emotions like happiness and love might have been selected for because of the advantage they provided in kinship safety and pair bonding with mates.

Figure 8.13 An increase in serotonin concentrations is associated with the waking state (refer back to Figure 8.7), so sleep is inhibited by DMT and other drugs that simulate serotonin action. For this same reason, sleeplessness is also a common side effect of antidepressant medications discussed earlier in the text (e.g., serotonin-specific reuptake inhibitors) because they increase serotonin levels in the brain.

Figure 8.14 The involvement of the limbic system in the formation of declarative memories (like remembering names) provides a clue. Experiences that generate strong emotional responses cause greater activity in the limbic system and are more likely to be remembered than emotionally neutral experiences. Also, much like a rat that repeatedly presses a bar to stimulate the mesolimbic dopamine pathway (see Figure 8.10), you may internally rehearse the name of a person who attracts you.

Figure 8.17 The left side of the brain is responsible for technical aspects of language like the definitions of words, sentence construction, and motor programs for speaking; the right side of the brain is responsible for encoding and expressing affective, or emotional, aspects. The individual showing right-hemisphere activity might have invested greater emotional content in the language task than the individual showing only left-hemisphere activity.

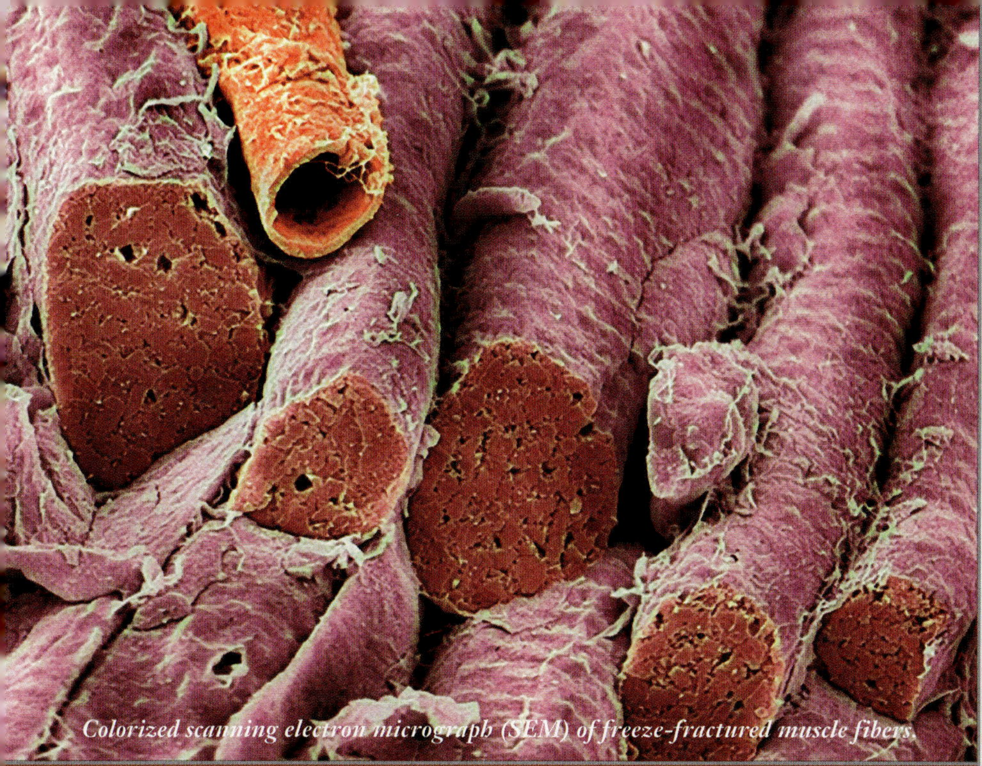

Colorized scanning electron micrograph (SEM) of freeze-fractured muscle fibers.

9 Muscle

Muscle was introduced in Chapter 1 as one of the four principal tissue types that make up the human body. The ability to use chemical energy to produce force and movement is present to a limited extent in most cells, but in muscle cells it has become dominant. Muscles generate force and movements used to regulate the internal environment, and they also produce movements of the body in relation to the external environment. In humans, the ability to communicate, whether by speech, writing, or artistic expression, also depends on muscle contractions. Indeed, it is only by controlling muscle activity that the human mind ultimately expresses itself.

Three types of muscle tissue can be identified on the basis of structure, contractile properties, and control mechanisms—skeletal muscle, smooth muscle, and cardiac muscle. Most skeletal muscle, as the name implies, is attached to bone, and its contraction is responsible for supporting and moving the skeleton. As described in Chapter 6, contraction of skeletal muscle is initiated by action potentials in neurons of the somatic motor division of the nervous system, and is usually under voluntary control.

Sheets of smooth muscle surround various hollow organs and tubes, including the stomach, intestines, urinary bladder, uterus, blood vessels, and airways in the lungs. Contraction of smooth muscle may propel the luminal contents through the hollow organs, or it may regulate internal flow by changing the tube diameter. In addition, contraction of smooth muscle cells makes the hairs of the skin stand up and the pupil of the eye change diameter. In contrast to skeletal muscle, smooth muscle contraction is not normally under voluntary control. It occurs autonomously in some cases, but frequently it occurs in response to signals from the autonomic nervous system, hormones, autocrine or paracrine signals, and other local chemical factors.

Cardiac muscle is the muscle of the heart. Its contraction generates the pressure that propels blood through the circulatory system. Like smooth muscle, it is regulated by the autonomic nervous system, hormones, and autocrine or paracrine signals; and it can undergo spontaneous contractions.

Several of the general principles of physiology described in Chapter 1 are demonstrated in this chapter. One of these principles, that structure is a determinant of—and has coevolved with—function, is apparent in the elaborate specialization of muscle cells and whole muscles that enable them to generate force and movement. The principle that controlled exchange of materials occurs between compartments and across cellular membranes is exemplified by the movements of Ca^{2+} that underlie the regulation of activation and relaxation of muscle. The laws of chemistry and physics are fundamental to the molecular mechanism by which muscle cells convert chemical energy into force, and also to the mechanics governing bone–muscle lever systems. Finally, the transfer and balance of matter and energy are demonstrated by the ability of muscle cells to generate, store, and utilize energy via multiple metabolic pathways.

This chapter will describe skeletal muscle first, followed by smooth and cardiac muscle. Cardiac muscle, which combines some of the properties of both skeletal and smooth muscle, will be described in more depth in Chapter 12 in association with its role in the circulatory system.

SECTION A

Skeletal Muscle

9.1 Structure

The most striking feature seen when viewing **skeletal muscle** through a microscope is a distinct series of alternating light and dark bands perpendicular to the long axis. Because **cardiac muscle** shares this characteristic striped pattern, these two types are both referred to as **striated muscle.** The third basic muscle type, **smooth muscle,** derives its name from the fact that it lacks this striated appearance. **Figure 9.1** compares the appearance of skeletal muscle cells to cardiac and smooth muscle cells.

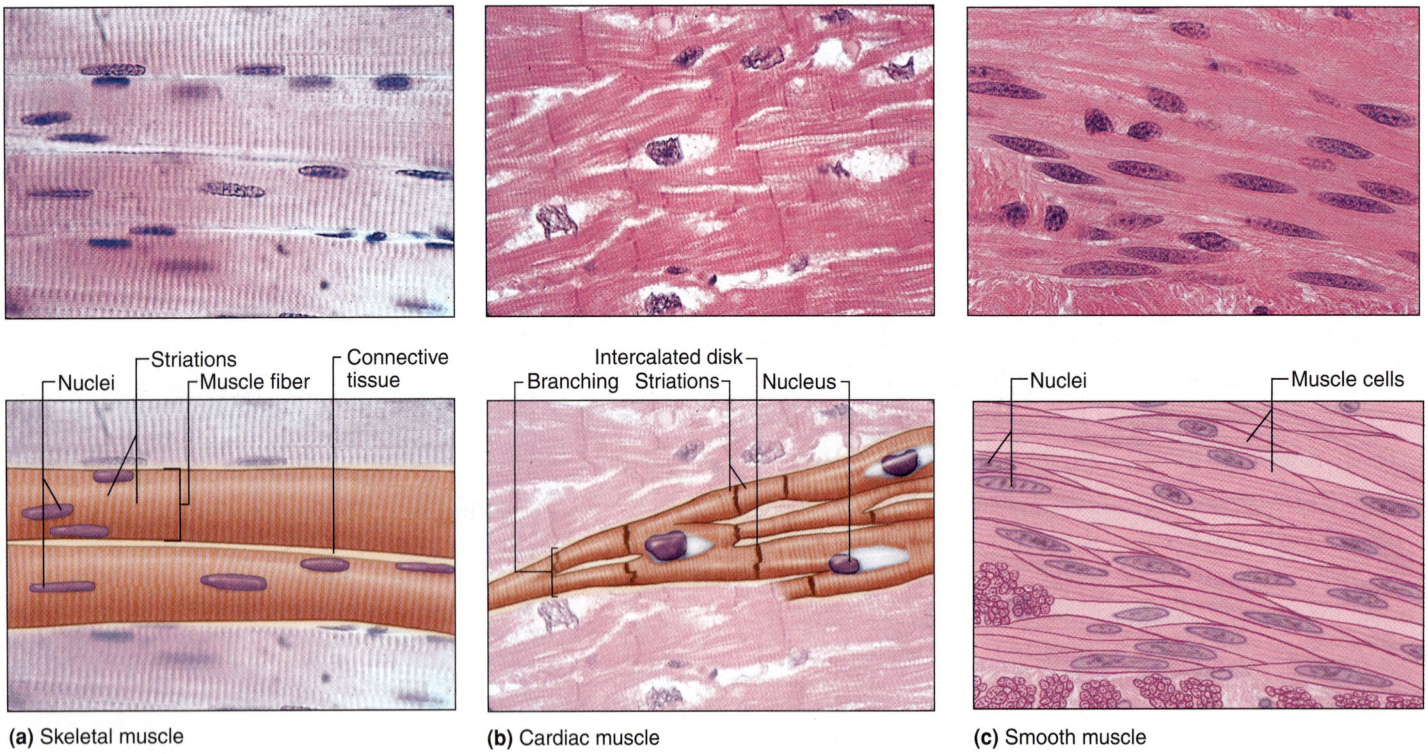

Figure 9.1 AP|R Comparison of (a) skeletal muscle to (b) cardiac and (c) smooth muscle as seen with light microscopy (top panels) and in schematic form (bottom panels). Both skeletal and cardiac muscle have a striated appearance. Cardiac and smooth muscle cells generally have a single nucleus, but skeletal muscle fibers are multinucleated.

Due to its elongated shape and the presence of multiple nuclei, a skeletal muscle cell is also referred to as a **muscle fiber.** Each muscle fiber is formed during development by the fusion of a number of undifferentiated, mononucleated cells known as **myoblasts** into a single, cylindrical, multinucleated cell. Skeletal muscle differentiation is completed around the time of birth, and these differentiated fibers continue to increase in size from infancy to adulthood. Compared to other cell types, skeletal muscle fibers are extremely large. Adult skeletal muscle fibers have diameters between 10 and 100 μm and lengths that may extend up to 20 cm. Key to the maintenance and function of such large cells is the retention of the nuclei from the original myoblasts. Spread throughout the length of the muscle fiber, each participates in regulation of gene expression and protein synthesis within its local domain.

If skeletal muscle fibers are damaged or destroyed after birth as a result of injury, they undergo a repair process involving a population of undifferentiated stem cells known as **satellite cells.** Satellite cells are normally quiescent, located between the plasma membrane and surrounding basement membrane along the length of muscle fibers. In response to strain or injury, they become active and undergo mitotic proliferation. Daughter cells then differentiate into myoblasts that can either fuse together to form new fibers or fuse with stressed or damaged muscle fibers to reinforce and repair them. The capacity for forming new skeletal muscle fibers is considerable but may not restore a severely damaged muscle to the original number of muscle fibers. Some of the compensation for a loss of muscle tissue also occurs through a satellite cell-mediated increase in the size (**hypertrophy**) of the remaining muscle fibers. Muscle hypertrophy also occurs in response to heavy exercise. Evidence suggests that this occurs through a combination of hypertrophy of existing fibers, splitting of existing fibers, and satellite cell proliferation, differentiation, and fusion. Many hormones and growth factors are involved in regulating these processes, such as growth hormone, insulin-like growth factor, and sex hormones (see Chapter 11).

The term **muscle** refers to a number of muscle fibers bound together by connective tissue (**Figure 9.2**). The relationship between a single muscle fiber and a muscle is analogous to that between a single neuron and a nerve, which is composed of

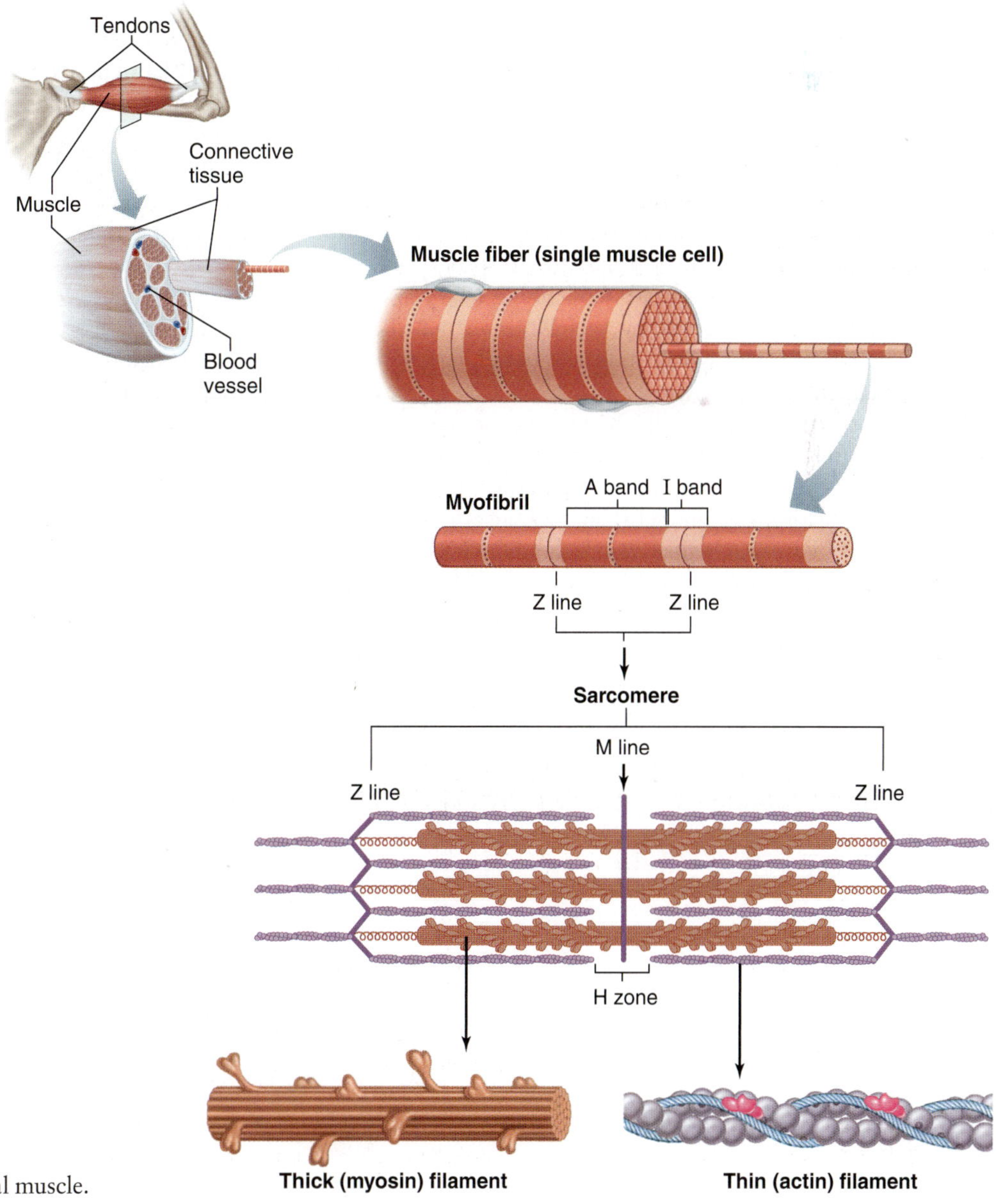

Figure 9.2 AP|R Structure of skeletal muscle.

the axons of many neurons. Skeletal muscles are usually attached to bones by bundles of collagen fibers known as **tendons.**

In some muscles, the individual fibers extend the entire length of the muscle, but in most, the fibers are shorter, often oriented at an angle to the longitudinal axis of the muscle. The transmission of force from muscle to bone is like a number of people pulling on a rope, each person corresponding to a single muscle fiber and the rope corresponding to the connective tissue and tendons.

Some tendons are very long, with the site where the tendon attaches to the bone far removed from the end of the muscle. For example, some of the muscles that move the fingers are in the forearm (wiggle your fingers and feel the movement of the muscles just below your elbow). These muscles are connected to the fingers by long tendons.

The striated pattern in skeletal (and cardiac) muscle results from the arrangement of two types of filaments within the cytoplasm, the larger referred to as **thick filaments** and the smaller as **thin filaments.** These filaments are part of cylindrical bundles called **myofibrils,** which are approximately 1 to 2 μm in diameter (see Figure 9.2). Most of the cytoplasm of a fiber is filled with myofibrils, each extending from one end of the fiber to the other and linked to the tendons at the ends of the fiber. One unit of this repeating pattern of thick and thin filaments is known as a **sarcomere** (from the Greek *sarco,* "muscle," and *mer,* "part").

The molecular structure of thick and thin filaments is shown in **Figure 9.3**. The thick filaments are composed almost entirely of the protein **myosin.** The myosin molecule is composed of two large polypeptide **heavy chains** and four smaller **light chains.** These polypeptides combine to form a molecule that consists of two globular heads (containing heavy and light chains) and a long tail formed by the two intertwined heavy chains. The tail of each myosin molecule lies along the axis of the thick filament, and the two globular heads extend out to the sides, forming **cross-bridges,** which make contact with the thin filament and exert force during muscle contraction. Each globular head contains two binding sites, one for attaching to the thin filament and one for ATP. The ATP binding site also serves as an enzyme—an ATPase that hydrolyzes the bound ATP, harnessing its energy for contraction. The thin filaments (which are about half the diameter of the thick filaments) are principally composed of the protein **actin,** as well as two other proteins—**troponin** and **tropomyosin**—that play important roles in regulating contraction. An actin molecule is a globular protein composed of a single polypeptide (a monomer) that polymerizes with other actin monomers to form a polymer made up of two intertwined, helical chains. These chains make up the core of a thin filament. Each actin molecule contains a binding site for myosin.

The alternating dark and light bands produced by the orderly, parallel arrangement of thick and thin filaments are apparent in a microscopic view of skeletal muscle (**Figure 9.4**). The thick filaments are located in the middle of each sarcomere, where they create a wide, dark band known as the **A band** (see the Figure 9.4 legend for an explanation of the naming of the bands and zones of the sarcomere).

Each sarcomere contains two sets of thin filaments, one at each end. One end of each thin filament is anchored to a network of interconnecting proteins known as the **Z line,** whereas the other end overlaps a portion of the thick filaments. Two successive Z lines define the limits of one sarcomere. Thus, thin filaments from two adjacent sarcomeres are anchored to the two sides of each Z line. (The term *line* refers to the appearance of these structures in two dimensions. Because myofibrils are cylindrical, it is more realistic to think of them as *Z disks.*) A light band known as the **I band** lies between the ends of the A bands of two adjacent sarcomeres and contains those portions of the thin filaments that do not overlap the thick filaments. The I band is bisected by the Z line. Two additional bands are present in the A-band region of each sarcomere. The **H zone** is a narrow, light band in the center of the A band. It corresponds to the space between the opposing ends of the two sets of thin filaments in each sarcomere. A narrow, dark band in the center of the H zone, known as the **M line** (also technically a disk), corresponds to proteins that link together the central region of adjacent thick filaments. In addition, filaments composed of the elastic protein **titin** extend from the Z line to the M line and are linked to both the M-line proteins and the thick filaments. Both the M-line linkage between thick filaments and the titin filaments act to maintain the alignment of thick filaments in the middle of each sarcomere. A cross section through the A bands (**Figure 9.5**) shows the regular arrangement of overlapping thick and thin filaments. Each thick filament is surrounded by a hexagonal array of six thin filaments, and each thin filament is

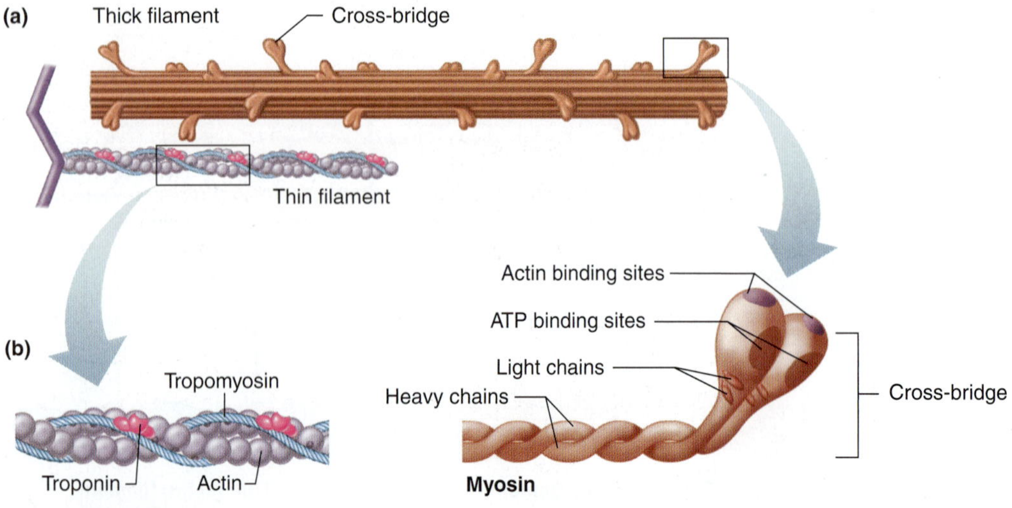

Figure 9.3 AP|R (a) The heavy chains of myosin molecules form the core of a thick filament. The myosin molecules are oriented in opposite directions in either half of a thick filament. (b) Structure of thin filament and myosin molecule. Cross-bridge binding sites on actin are covered by tropomyosin. The two globular heads of each myosin molecule extend from the sides of a thick filament, forming a cross-bridge.

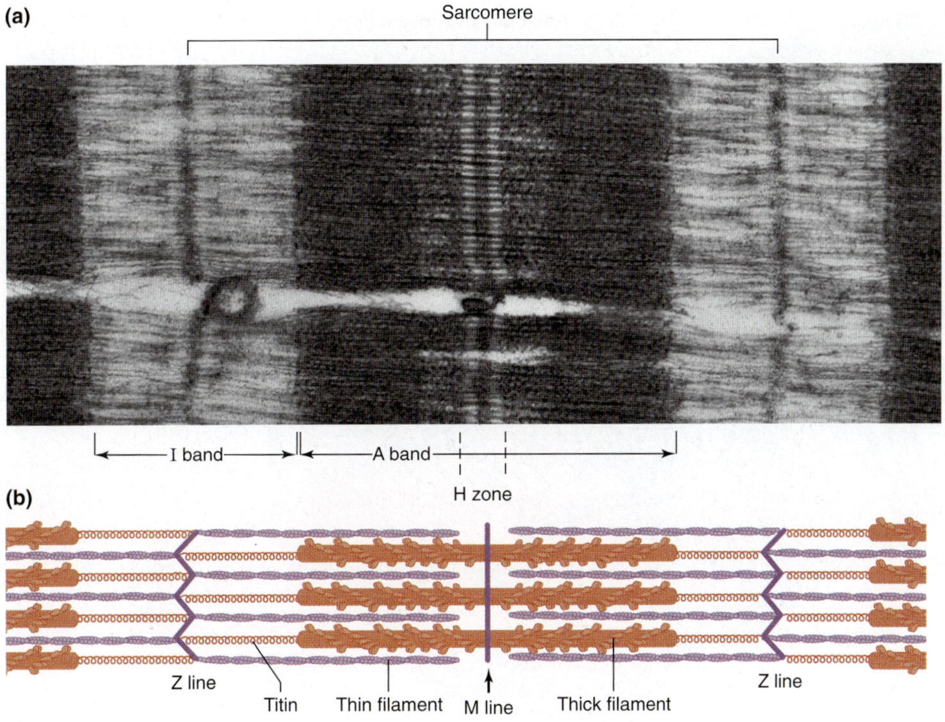

Figure 9.4 AP|R (a) High magnification of a sarcomere within myofibrils. (b) Arrangement of the thick and thin filaments in the sarcomere shown in (a). The names of the I and A bands come from "isotropy" and "anisotropy," terms from physics indicating that the I band has uniform appearance in all directions and the A band has a nonuniform appearance in different directions. The names for the Z line, M line, and H zone are from their initial descriptions in German: *zwischen* ("between"), *mittel* ("middle"), and *heller* ("light").

surrounded by a triangular arrangement of three thick filaments. Altogether, there are twice as many thin as thick filaments in the region of filament overlap.

In addition to force-generating mechanisms, skeletal muscle fibers have an elaborate system of membranes that play important roles in the activation of contraction (**Figure 9.6**). The **sarcoplasmic reticulum** in a muscle fiber is homologous to the endoplasmic reticulum found in most cells. This structure forms a series of sleevelike segments around each myofibril. At the end of each segment are two enlarged regions, known as **terminal cisternae** (sometimes also referred to as "lateral sacs"), that are connected to each other by a series of smaller tubular elements. Ca^{2+} is stored in the terminal cisternae and is released into the cytosol following membrane excitation.

A separate tubular structure, the **transverse tubule** (**T-tubule**), lies directly between—and is intimately associated with—the terminal cisternae of adjacent segments of the sarcoplasmic reticulum. The T-tubules and terminal cisternae surround the myofibrils at the region of the sarcomeres where the A bands and I bands meet. T-tubules are continuous with the plasma membrane (which in muscle cells is sometimes referred to as the **sarcolemma**), and action potentials propagating along the surface membrane also travel throughout the interior of the muscle fiber by way of the T-tubules. The lumen of the T-tubule is continuous with the extracellular fluid surrounding the muscle fiber.

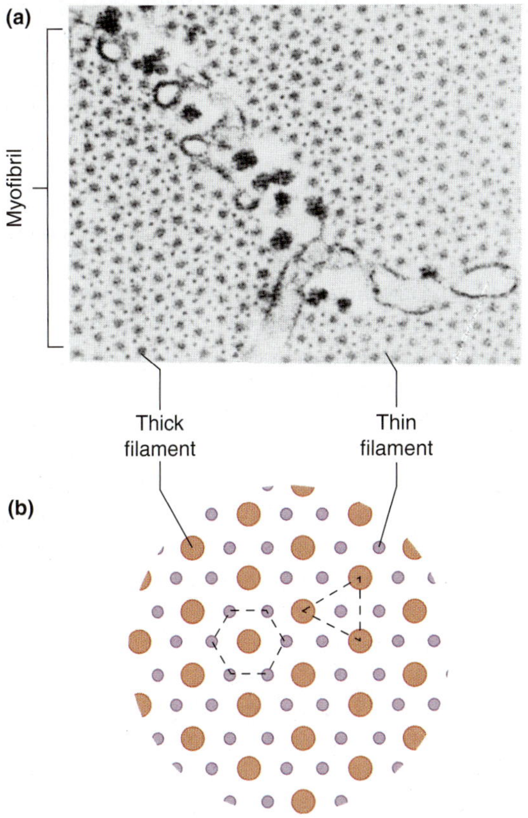

Figure 9.5 AP|R (a) Electron micrograph of a cross section through three myofibrils in a single skeletal muscle fiber. (b) Hexagonal arrangements of the thick and thin filaments in the overlap region in a single myofibril. Six thin filaments surround each thick filament, and three thick filaments surround each thin filament. Titin filaments and cross-bridges are not shown. From H. E. Huxley, *J. Mol. Biol.*, 37:507–520 (1968).

PHYSIOLOGICAL INQUIRY

- Draw a cross-section diagram like the one in part (b) for a slice taken (1) in the H zone, (2) in the I band, (3) at the M line, and (4) at the Z line (ignore titin).

Answer can be found at end of chapter.

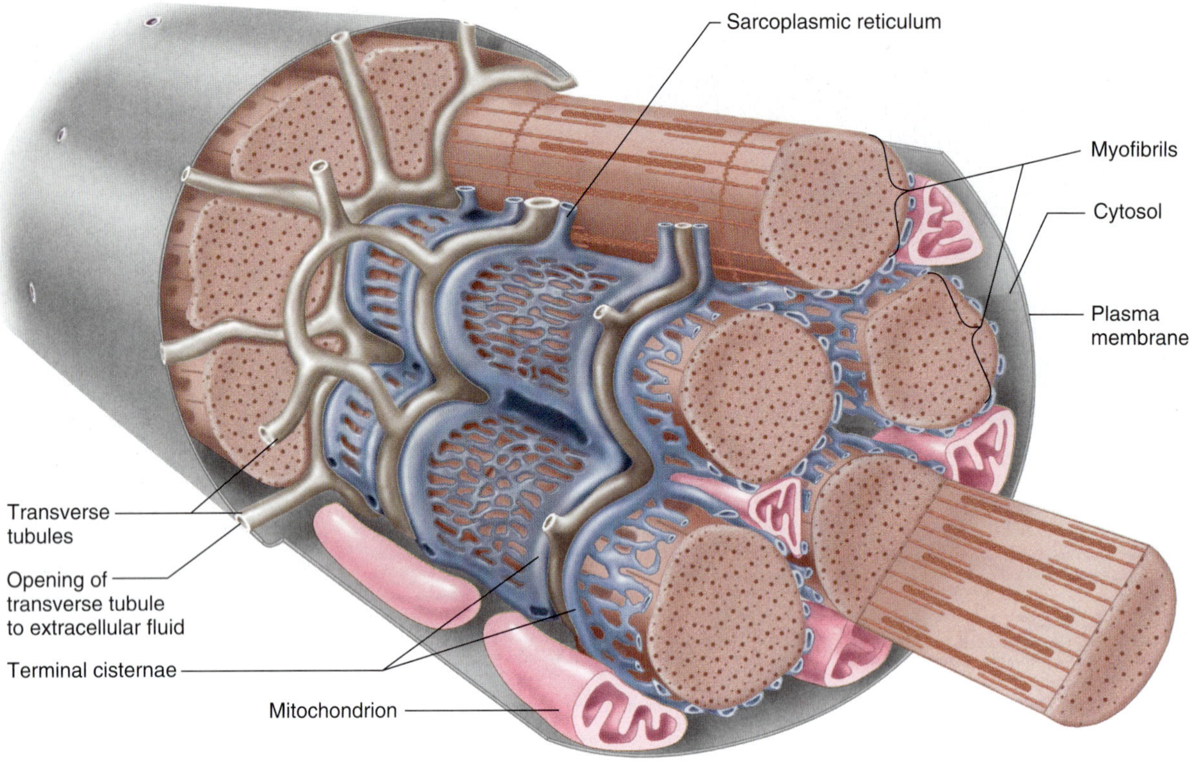

Figure 9.6 APIR Transverse tubules and sarcoplasmic reticulum in a single skeletal muscle fiber.

9.2 Molecular Mechanisms of Skeletal Muscle Contraction

The term **contraction,** as used in muscle physiology, does not necessarily mean "shortening." It simply refers to activation of the force-generating sites within muscle fibers—the cross-bridges. For example, holding a dumbbell steady with your elbow bent requires muscle contraction but not muscle shortening. Following contraction, the mechanisms that generate force are turned off and tension declines, allowing **relaxation** of muscle fibers. We now begin our explanation of how skeletal muscles contract by describing the mechanism by which they are activated by neurons.

Membrane Excitation: The Neuromuscular Junction

Stimulation of the neurons to a skeletal muscle is the only mechanism by which action potentials are initiated in this type of muscle. In subsequent sections, you will see additional mechanisms for activating cardiac and smooth muscle contraction.

The neurons whose axons innervate skeletal muscle fibers are known as **motor neurons** (or somatic efferent neurons), and their cell bodies are located in the brainstem and the spinal cord. The axons of motor neurons are myelinated (see Figure 6.2) and are the largest-diameter axons in the body. They are therefore able to propagate action potentials at high velocities, allowing signals from the central nervous system to travel to skeletal muscle fibers with minimal delay (review Figure 6.24).

Upon reaching a muscle, the axon of a motor neuron divides into many branches, each branch forming a single junction with a muscle fiber. A single motor neuron innervates many muscle fibers, but each muscle fiber is controlled by a branch from only one motor neuron. A motor neuron plus the muscle fibers it innervates is called a **motor unit** (**Figure 9.7a**). The muscle fibers in a single motor unit are located in one muscle, but they are distributed throughout the muscle and are not necessarily adjacent to each other (**Figure 9.7b**). When an action potential occurs in a motor neuron, all the muscle fibers in its motor unit are stimulated to contract.

The myelin sheath surrounding the axon of each motor neuron ends near the surface of a muscle fiber, and the axon divides into a number of short processes that lie embedded in grooves on the muscle fiber surface (**Figure 9.8a**). The axon terminals of a motor neuron contain vesicles similar to those found at synaptic junctions between two neurons. The vesicles contain the neurotransmitter **acetylcholine** (**ACh**). The region of the muscle fiber plasma membrane that lies directly under the terminal portion of the axon is known as the **motor end plate.** The junction of an axon terminal with the motor end plate is known as a **neuromuscular junction** (**Figure 9.8b**).

Figure 9.9 shows the events occurring at the neuromuscular junction. When an action potential in a motor neuron arrives at the axon terminal, it depolarizes the plasma membrane, opening voltage-sensitive Ca^{2+} channels and allowing calcium ions to diffuse into the axon terminal from the extracellular fluid. This Ca^{2+} binds to proteins that enable the membranes of acetylcholine-containing vesicles to fuse with the neuronal plasma membrane (see Figure 6.27), thereby releasing acetylcholine into the extracellular cleft separating the axon terminal and the motor end plate.

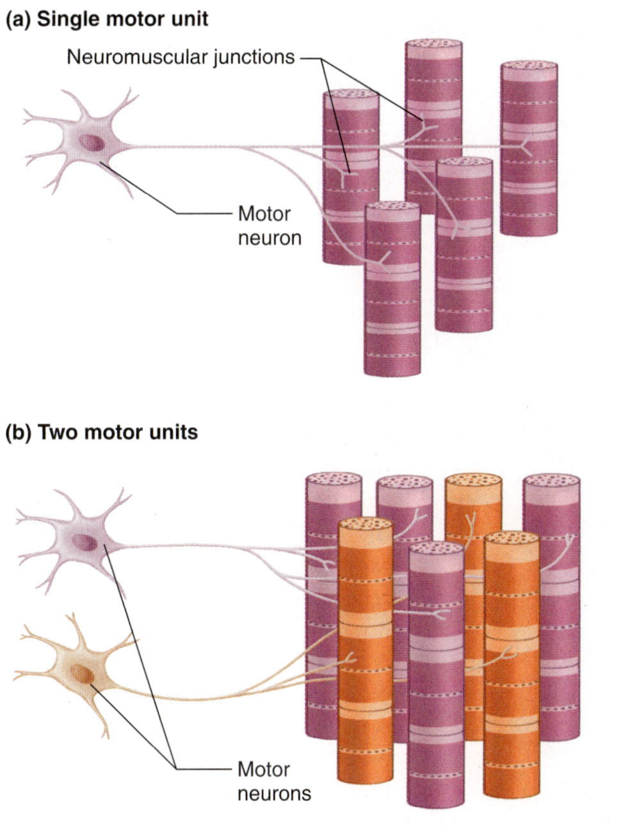

Figure 9.7 (a) Single motor unit consisting of one motor neuron and the muscle fibers it innervates. (b) Two motor units and their intermingled fibers in a muscle.

ACh diffuses from the axon terminal to the motor end plate where it binds to ionotropic receptors of the nicotinic type (see Chapter 6). The binding of ACh opens an ion channel in each receptor protein; both sodium and potassium ions can pass through these channels. Because of the differences in electrochemical gradients across the plasma membrane (see Figure 6.12), more Na^+ moves in than K^+ out, producing a local depolarization of the motor end plate known as an **end-plate potential (EPP)**. Thus, an EPP is analogous to an EPSP (excitatory postsynaptic potential) at a neuron–neuron synapse (see Figure 6.28).

The magnitude of a single EPP is, however, much larger than that of an EPSP because neurotransmitter is released over a larger surface area, binding to many more receptors, and opening many more ion channels. For this reason, one EPP is normally more than sufficient to depolarize the muscle plasma membrane adjacent to the end-plate membrane to its threshold potential, initiating an action potential. This action potential is then propagated over the surface of the muscle fiber and into the T-tubules by the same mechanism shown in Figure 6.23 for the propagation of action potentials along unmyelinated axon membranes. Most neuromuscular junctions are located near the middle of a muscle fiber, and newly generated muscle action potentials propagate from this region in both directions toward the ends of the fiber.

Every action potential in a motor neuron normally produces an action potential in each muscle fiber in its motor unit. This is quite different from synaptic junctions between

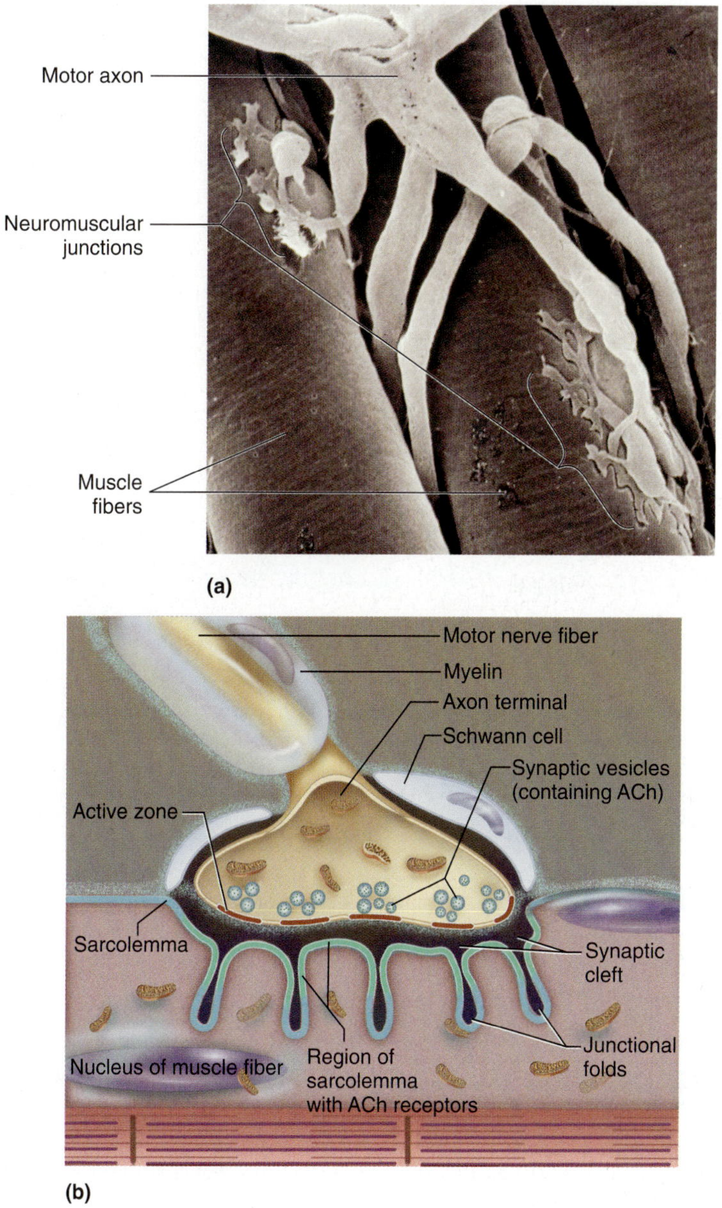

Figure 9.8 APIR The neuromuscular junction. (a) Scanning electron micrograph showing branching of motor neuron axons, with axon terminals embedded in grooves in the muscle fiber's surface. (b) Structure of a neuromuscular junction.

neurons, where multiple EPSPs must occur in order for threshold to be reached and an action potential elicited in the postsynaptic membrane.

There is another difference between interneuronal synapses and neuromuscular junctions. As we saw in Chapter 6, IPSPs (inhibitory postsynaptic potentials) are produced at some synaptic junctions. They hyperpolarize or stabilize the postsynaptic membrane and decrease the probability of its firing an action potential. In contrast, inhibitory potentials do not occur in human skeletal muscle; *all neuromuscular junctions are excitatory.*

In addition to receptors for ACh, the synaptic junction contains the enzyme **acetylcholinesterase,** which breaks down ACh, just as it does at ACh-mediated synapses in the nervous system. Choline is then transported back into the axon terminals,

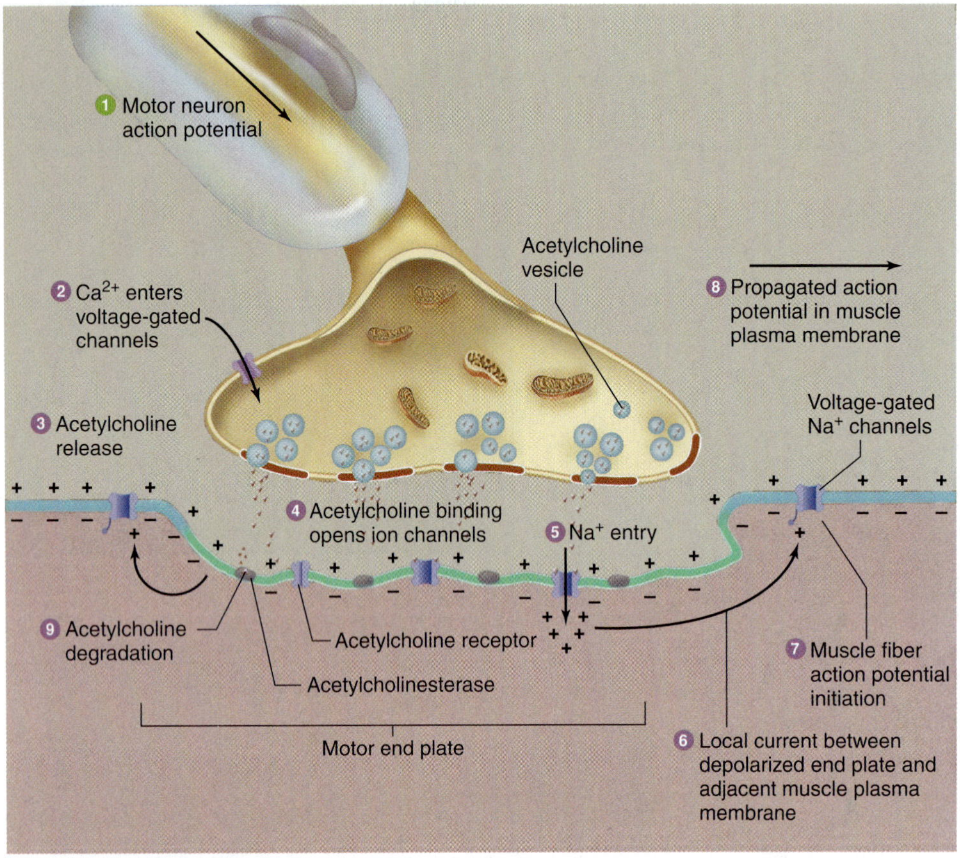

Figure 9.9 APIR Events at the neuromuscular junction that lead to an action potential in the muscle fiber plasma membrane. Although K^+ also exits the muscle cell when ACh receptors are open, Na^+ entry and depolarization dominate, as shown here.

PHYSIOLOGICAL INQUIRY

- If the ACh receptor channel is equally permeable to Na^+ and K^+, why does Na^+ influx dominate? (*Hint:* Review Figure 6.12.)

Answer can be found at end of chapter.

where it is reused in the synthesis of new ACh. ACh bound to receptors is in equilibrium with free ACh in the cleft between the neuronal and muscle membranes. As the concentration of free ACh decreases because of its breakdown by acetylcholinesterase, less ACh is available to bind to the receptors. When the receptors no longer contain bound ACh, the ion channels in the end plate close. The depolarized end plate returns to its resting potential and can respond to the subsequent arrival of ACh released by another neuron action potential.

Disruption of Neuromuscular Signaling

There are many ways by which disease or drugs can modify events at the neuromuscular junction. For example, ***curare***, a deadly arrowhead poison used by indigenous peoples of South America, binds strongly to nicotinic ACh receptors. It does not open their ion channels, however, and is resistant to destruction by acetylcholinesterase. When a receptor is occupied by curare, ACh cannot bind to the receptor. Therefore, although the motor neurons still conduct normal action potentials and release ACh, there is no resulting EPP in the motor end plate and no contraction. Because the skeletal muscles responsible for breathing, like all skeletal muscles, depend upon neuromuscular transmission to initiate their contraction, curare poisoning can cause death by asphyxiation.

Neuromuscular transmission can also be blocked by inhibiting acetylcholinesterase. Some organophosphates, which are the main ingredients in certain pesticides and "nerve gases" (the latter developed for chemical warfare), inhibit this enzyme. In the presence of these chemicals, ACh is released normally upon the arrival of an action potential at the axon terminal and binds to the end-plate receptors. The ACh is not destroyed, however, because the acetylcholinesterase is inhibited. The ion channels in the end plate therefore remain open, producing a maintained depolarization of the end plate and the muscle plasma membrane adjacent to the end plate. A skeletal muscle membrane maintained in a depolarized state cannot generate action potentials because the voltage-gated Na^+ channels in the membrane become inactivated, which requires repolarization to reverse. After prolonged exposure to ACh, the receptors of the motor end plate become insensitive to it, preventing any further depolarization. Thus, the muscle does not contract in response to subsequent nerve stimulation, and the result is skeletal muscle paralysis and death from asphyxiation. Nerve gases also cause ACh to build up at muscarinic synapses (see Chapter 6, Section C), for example, where parasympathetic neurons inhibit cardiac pacemaker cells (see Chapter 12). This can result in an extreme slowing of the heart rate, virtually halting blood flow through the body. Thus, the antidote for organophosphate and nerve gas exposure includes both ***pralidoxime***, which reactivates acetylcholinesterase, and ***atropine***, the muscarinic receptor antagonist.

Drugs that block neuromuscular transmission are sometimes used in small amounts to prevent muscular contractions during certain types of surgical procedures, when it is necessary to immobilize the surgical field. One example is ***succinylcholine***, which actually acts as an agonist to the ACh receptors and produces a depolarizing/desensitizing block similar to acetylcholinesterase inhibitors. It has a rapid onset of action (about 1 minute) and relatively short duration (7 to 8 minutes). Nondepolarizing neuromuscular junction blocking drugs that act more like curare and last longer are also used, such as ***rocuronium*** and ***vecuronium***. The use of such paralytic agents in surgery reduces the required dose of general anesthetic, allowing patients to recover faster and with fewer complications. Patients must be artificially ventilated, however, to maintain respiration until the drugs have cleared from their bodies.

Another group of substances, including the toxin produced by the bacterium *Clostridium botulinum*, blocks the release of acetylcholine from axon terminals. Botulinum toxin is an enzyme that breaks down proteins of the SNARE complex that are required for the binding and fusion of ACh vesicles with the plasma membrane of the axon terminal (review Figure 6.27). This toxin, which produces the food poisoning called ***botulism***, is one of the most potent poisons known. Application of botulinum toxin to block ACh release is increasingly being used for clinical and cosmetic procedures, including the inhibition of overactive extraocular muscles, prevention of excessive sweat gland activity, treatment of migraine headaches, and reduction of aging-related skin wrinkles.

Having described how action potentials in motor neurons initiate action potentials in skeletal muscle cells, we will now examine how that excitation results in muscle contraction.

Excitation–Contraction Coupling

Excitation–contraction coupling refers to the sequence of events by which an action potential in the plasma membrane activates the force-generating mechanisms. An action potential in a skeletal muscle fiber lasts 1 to 2 msec and is completed before any signs of mechanical activity begin (**Figure 9.10**). Once begun, the mechanical activity following an action potential may last 100 msec or more. The electrical activity in the plasma membrane does not directly act upon the contractile proteins but instead produces a state of increased cytosolic Ca^{2+} concentration, which continues to activate the contractile apparatus long after the electrical activity in the membrane has ceased.

How does the presence of Ca^{2+} in the cytoplasm initiate force generation by the thick and thin filaments? The answer requires a closer look at the thin filament proteins, troponin and tropomyosin (**Figure 9.11**). Tropomyosin is a rod-shaped molecule composed of two intertwined polypeptides with a length approximately equal to that of seven actin monomers. Chains of tropomyosin molecules are arranged end to end along the actin thin filament. These tropomyosin molecules partially cover the myosin-binding site on each actin monomer, thereby preventing the cross-bridges from making contact with actin. Each tropomyosin molecule is held in this blocking position by the smaller globular protein, troponin. Troponin, which interacts with both actin and tropomyosin, is composed of three subunits designated by the letters I (inhibitory), T (tropomyosin-binding) and C (Ca^{2+}-binding). One molecule of troponin binds to each molecule of tropomyosin and regulates the access to myosin-binding sites on the seven actin monomers in contact with that tropomyosin. This is the status of a resting muscle fiber; troponin and tropomyosin cooperatively block the interaction of cross-bridges with the thin filament.

To allow cross-bridges from the thick filament to bind to the thin filament, tropomyosin molecules must move away from their blocking positions on actin. This happens when Ca^{2+} binds to specific binding sites on the Ca^{2+}-binding subunit of troponin. The binding of Ca^{2+} produces a change in the

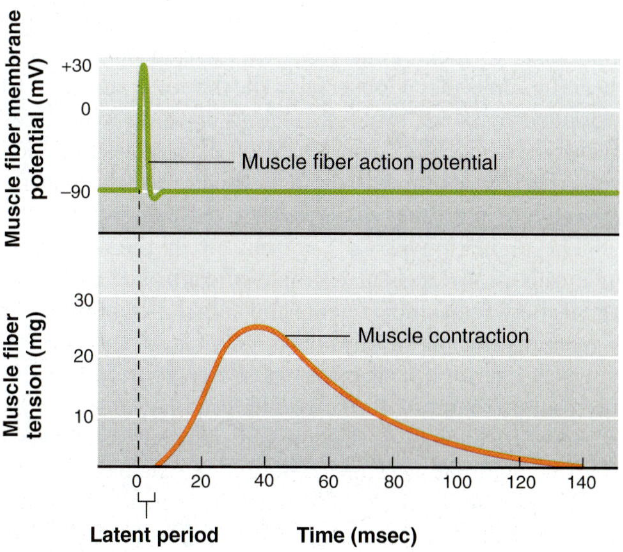

Figure 9.10 Time relationship between a skeletal muscle fiber action potential and the resulting contraction and relaxation of the muscle fiber. The latent period is the delay between the beginning of the action potential and the initial increase in tension.

PHYSIOLOGICAL INQUIRY

- Following a single action potential, cytosolic Ca^{2+} concentration increases and then decreases back to resting levels by about 50 msec. Why does the force last so much longer?

Answer can be found at end of chapter.

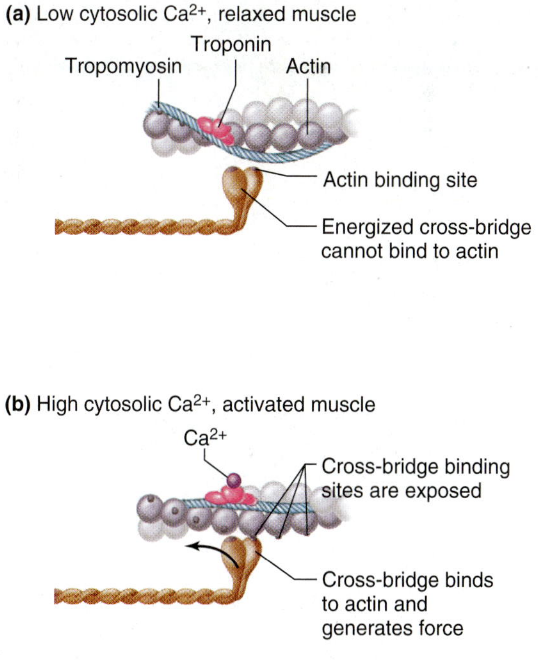

Figure 9.11 AP|R Activation of cross-bridge cycling by Ca^{2+}. (a) Without calcium ions bound, troponin holds tropomyosin over cross-bridge binding sites on actin. (b) When Ca^{2+} binds to troponin, tropomyosin is allowed to move away from cross-bridge binding sites on actin, and cross-bridges can bind to actin.

shape of troponin, which relaxes its inhibitory grip and allows tropomyosin to move away from the myosin-binding site on each actin molecule. Conversely, the removal of Ca^{2+} from troponin reverses the process, turning off contractile activity. Thus, the cytosolic Ca^{2+} concentration determines the number of troponin sites occupied by Ca^{2+}, which in turn determines the number of actin sites available for cross-bridge binding.

The regulation of Ca^{2+} movement in the activation of muscle cells is an excellent example of controlled exchange of materials between compartments and across membranes, which is a general principle of physiology (see Chapter 1). In a resting muscle fiber, the concentration of free, ionized calcium in the cytosol surrounding the thick and thin filaments is very low, only about 10^{-7} mol/L. At this low Ca^{2+} concentration, very few of the Ca^{2+}-binding sites on troponin are occupied and, thus, cross-bridge activity is blocked by tropomyosin. Following an action potential, there is a rapid increase in cytosolic Ca^{2+} concentration and Ca^{2+} binds to troponin, removing the blocking effect of tropomyosin and allowing myosin cross-bridges to bind actin. The source of the increased cytosolic Ca^{2+} is the sarcoplasmic reticulum within the muscle fiber.

A specialized mechanism couples T-tubule action potentials with Ca^{2+} release from the sarcoplasmic reticulum (**Figure 9.12**, step 2). The T-tubules are in intimate contact with the terminal cisternae of the sarcoplasmic reticulum, connected by structures known as **junctional feet,** or **foot processes.** This junction involves two integral membrane proteins, one in the T-tubule membrane and the other in the membrane of the sarcoplasmic reticulum. The T-tubule protein is a modified voltage-sensitive Ca^{2+} channel known as the **dihydropyridine (DHP) receptor** (so named because it binds the class of drugs called dihydropyridines). The main role of the DHP receptor, however, is not to conduct Ca^{2+} but rather to act as a voltage sensor. The protein embedded in the sarcoplasmic reticulum membrane is known as the **ryanodine receptor** (because it binds to the plant alkaloid ryanodine). This large molecule not only includes the foot process but also forms a Ca^{2+} channel. During a T-tubule action potential, charged amino acid residues

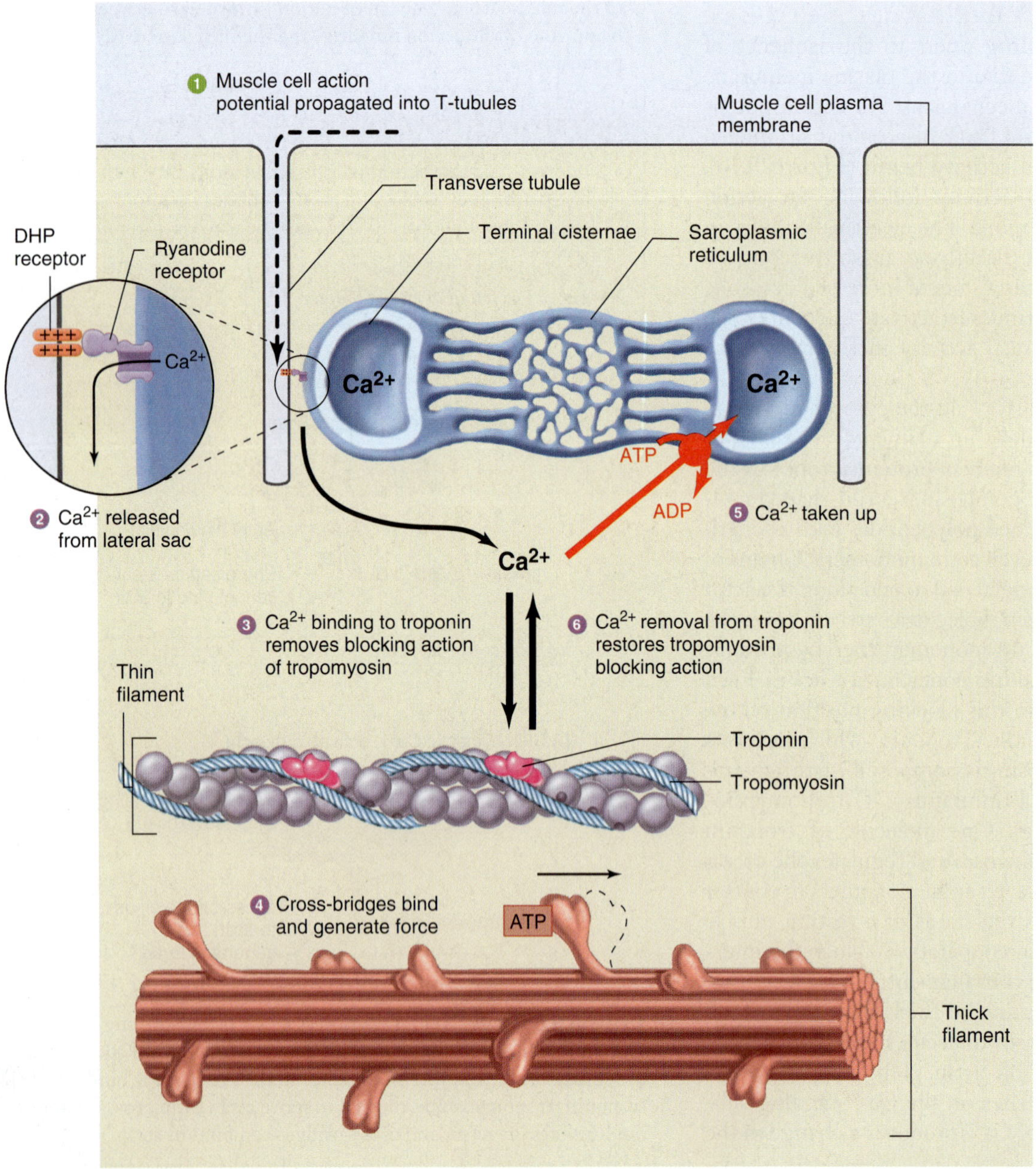

Figure 9.12 APIR
Release and uptake of Ca^{2+} by the sarcoplasmic reticulum during contraction and relaxation of a skeletal muscle fiber.

within the DHP receptor protein induce a conformational change, which acts via the foot process to open the ryanodine receptor channel. Ca^{2+} is thus released from the terminal cisternae of the sarcoplasmic reticulum into the cytosol, where it can bind to troponin. The increase in cytosolic Ca^{2+} in response to a single action potential is normally enough to briefly saturate all troponin-binding sites on the thin filaments.

A contraction is terminated by removal of Ca^{2+} from troponin, which is achieved by lowering the Ca^{2+} concentration in the cytosol back to its prerelease level. The membranes of the sarcoplasmic reticulum contain primary active-transport proteins—Ca^{2+}-ATPases—that pump calcium ions from the cytosol back into the lumen of the reticulum. As we just saw, Ca^{2+} is released from the reticulum when an action potential begins in the T-tubule, but the pumping of the released Ca^{2+} back into the reticulum requires a much longer time. Therefore, the cytosolic Ca^{2+} concentration remains elevated, and the contraction continues for some time after a single action potential.

To reiterate, just as contraction results from the release of Ca^{2+} stored in the sarcoplasmic reticulum, so contraction ends and relaxation begins as Ca^{2+} is pumped back into the reticulum (see Figure 9.12). ATP is required to provide the energy for the Ca^{2+} pump.

Sliding-Filament Mechanism

When force generation produces shortening of a skeletal muscle fiber, the overlapping thick and thin filaments in each sarcomere move past each other, propelled by movements of the cross-bridges. During this shortening of the sarcomeres, there is no change in the lengths of either the thick or thin filaments. This is known as the **sliding-filament mechanism** of muscle contraction.

During shortening, each myosin cross-bridge attached to a thin filament actin molecule moves in an arc much like an oar on a boat. This swiveling motion of many cross-bridges forces the thin filaments attached to successive Z lines to move toward the center of the sarcomere, thereby shortening the sarcomere (**Figure 9.13**). One stroke of a cross-bridge produces only a very small movement of a thin filament relative to a thick filament. As long as binding sites on actin remain exposed, however, each cross-bridge repeats its swiveling motion many times, resulting in large displacements of the filaments. It is worth noting that a common pattern of muscle shortening involves one end of the muscle remaining at a fixed position while the other end shortens toward it. In this case, as filaments slide and each sarcomere shortens internally, the center of each sarcomere also slides toward the fixed end of the muscle (this is depicted in **Figure 9.14**).

The sequence of events that occurs between the time a cross-bridge binds to a thin filament, moves, and then is set to repeat the process is known as a **cross-bridge cycle.** Each cycle consists of four steps: (1) attachment of the cross-bridge to a thin filament; (2) movement of the cross-bridge, producing tension in the thin filament; (3) detachment of the cross-bridge from the thin filament; and (4) energizing the cross-bridge so it can again attach to a thin filament and repeat the cycle. Each cross-bridge undergoes its own cycle of movement independently of other cross-bridges. At any instant during contraction, only some of the cross-bridges are attached to the thin filaments, producing tension, while others are simultaneously in a detached portion of their cycle.

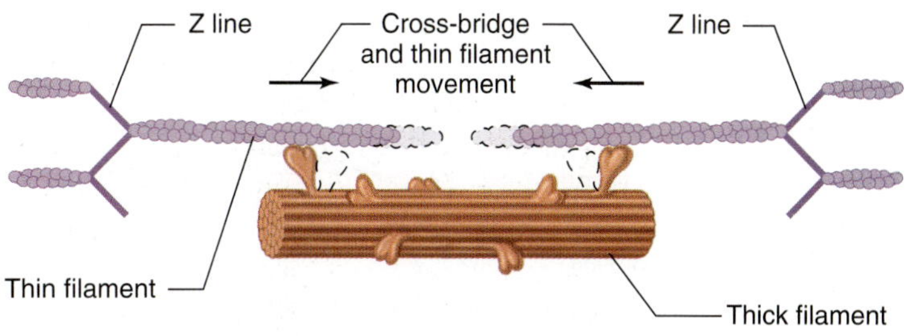

Figure 9.13 APIR Cross-bridges in the thick filaments bind to actin in the thin filaments and undergo a conformational change that propels the thin filaments toward the center of a sarcomere. (Only a few of the approximately 200 cross-bridges in each thick filament are shown.)

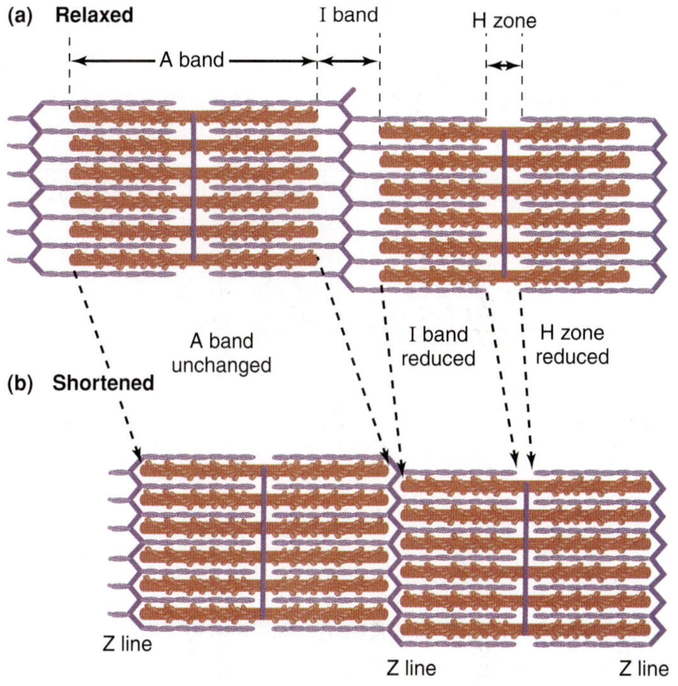

Figure 9.14 APIR The sliding of thick filaments past overlapping thin filaments shortens the sarcomere with no change in thick or thin filament length. The I band and H zone are reduced.

PHYSIOLOGICAL INQUIRY

- Sphincter muscles are circular and generally not attached to bones. How would this diagram differ if the sarcomeres shown were part of a sphincter muscle?

Answer can be found at end of chapter.

A general principle of physiology states that physiological processes are dictated by the laws of chemistry and physics (see Chapter 1), and the details of the cross-bridge mechanism are an excellent example. **Figure 9.15** illustrates the chemical and physical events during the four steps of the cross-bridge cycle. The cross-bridges in a resting muscle fiber are in an energized state resulting from the splitting of ATP, and the hydrolysis products ADP and inorganic phosphate (P_i) are still bound

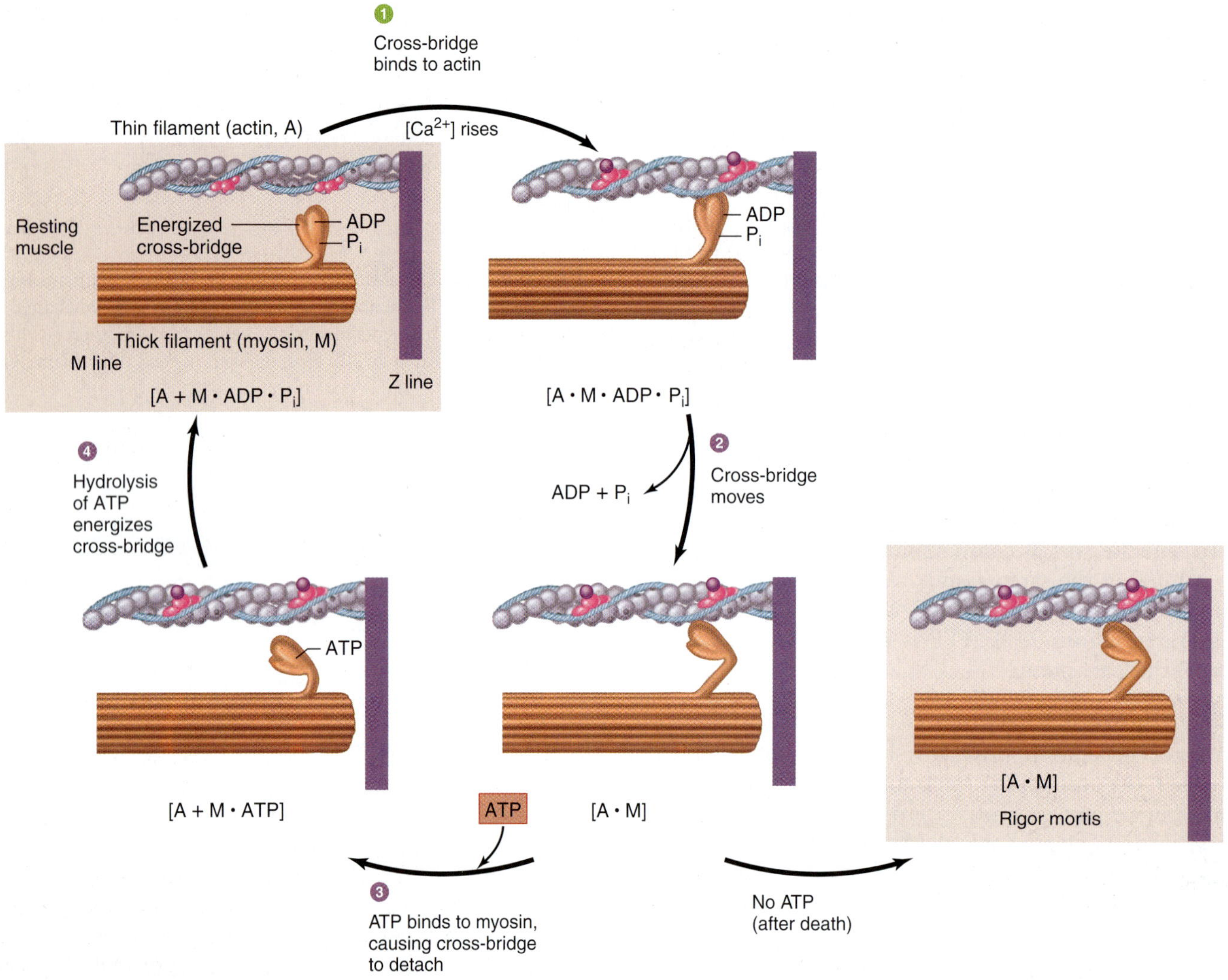

Figure 9.15 APR Chemical (shown in brackets) and mechanical representations of the four stages of a cross-bridge cycle. Cross-bridges remain in the resting state (pink box at left) when Ca^{2+} remains low. In the rigor mortis state (pink box at right), cross-bridges remain rigidly bound when ATP is absent. In the chemical representation, A = actin, M = myosin, dots are between bound components, and plus signs are between detached components.

PHYSIOLOGICAL INQUIRY

- Under certain experimental conditions, it is possible to extract the protein troponin from a skeletal muscle fiber. Predict how cross-bridge cycling in a skeletal muscle fiber would be affected in the absence of troponin.

Answer can be found at end of chapter.

to myosin (in the chemical representation, bound elements are separated by a dot, while detached elements are separated by a plus sign). This energy storage in myosin is analogous to the storage of potential energy in a stretched spring.

Cross-bridge cycling is initiated when the excitation–contraction coupling mechanism elevates cytosolic Ca^{2+} and the binding sites on actin are exposed. The cycle begins with the binding of an energized myosin cross-bridge (M) to a thin filament actin molecule (A):

$$\text{Step 1} \quad A + M \cdot ADP \cdot P_i \xrightarrow[\text{actin binding}]{} A \cdot M \cdot ADP \cdot P_i$$

The binding of energized myosin to actin triggers the release of the strained conformation of the energized cross-bridge, which produces the movement of the bound cross-bridge (sometimes called the **power stroke**) and the release of P_i and ADP:

$$\text{Step 2} \quad A \cdot M \cdot ADP \cdot P_i \xrightarrow[\text{cross-bridge movement}]{} A \cdot M + ADP + P_i$$

This sequence of energy storage and release by myosin is analogous to the operation of a mousetrap: Energy is stored in the trap by cocking the spring (ATP hydrolysis) and released after springing the trap (binding to actin).

During the cross-bridge movement, myosin is bound very firmly to actin, but this linkage must be broken to allow the cross-bridge to be reenergized and repeat the cycle. The binding of a new molecule of ATP to myosin breaks the link between actin and myosin:

$$\text{Step 3} \quad A \cdot M + ATP \xrightarrow[\text{dissociation from actin}]{} A + M \cdot ATP$$

cross-bridge dissociation from actin

The dissociation of actin and myosin by ATP is an example of allosteric regulation of protein activity (see Figure 3.32a). The binding of ATP at one site on myosin decreases myosin's affinity for actin bound at another site. Note that ATP is not split in this step; that is, it is not acting as an energy source but only as an allosteric modulator of the myosin head that weakens the binding of myosin to actin.

Following the dissociation of actin and myosin, the ATP bound to myosin is hydrolyzed, thereby re-forming the energized state of myosin and returning the cross-bridge to its pre-power-stroke position:

$$\text{Step 4} \quad A + M \cdot ATP \longrightarrow A + M \cdot ADP \cdot P_i$$

ATP hydrolysis

Note that the hydrolysis of ATP (step 4) and the movement of the cross-bridge (step 2) are not simultaneous events. If binding sites on actin are still exposed after a cross-bridge finishes its cycle, the cross-bridge can reattach to a new actin monomer in the thin filament and the cross-bridge cycle repeats. (In the event that the muscle is generating force without actually shortening, the cross-bridge will reattach to the same actin molecule as in the previous cycle.)

Thus, in addition to being used to maintain membrane excitability and regulate cytosolic Ca^{2+}, ATP performs two distinct roles in the cross-bridge cycle: (1) The energy released from ATP *hydrolysis* ultimately provides the energy for cross-bridge movement; and (2) ATP *binding* (not hydrolysis) to myosin breaks the link formed between actin and myosin during the cycle, allowing the next cycle to begin. **Table 9.1** summarizes the functions of ATP in skeletal muscle contraction.

TABLE 9.1	Functions of ATP in Skeletal Muscle Contraction
Hydrolysis of ATP by the Na^+/K^+-ATPase in the plasma membrane maintains Na^+ and K^+ gradients, which allows the membrane to produce and propagate action potentials (review Figure 6.13).	
Hydrolysis of ATP by the Ca^{2+}-ATPase in the sarcoplasmic reticulum provides the energy for the active transport of calcium ions into the reticulum, lowering cytosolic Ca^{2+} to prerelease concentrations, ending the contraction, and allowing the muscle fiber to relax.	
Hydrolysis of ATP by myosin energizes the cross-bridges, providing the energy for force generation.	
Binding of ATP to myosin dissociates cross-bridges bound to actin, allowing the bridges to repeat their cycle of activity.	

The importance of ATP in dissociating actin and myosin during step 3 of a cross-bridge cycle is illustrated by **rigor mortis,** the gradual stiffening of skeletal muscles that begins several hours after death and reaches a maximum after about 12 hours. The ATP concentration in cells, including muscle cells, declines after death because the nutrients and oxygen the metabolic pathways require to form ATP are no longer supplied by the circulation. In the absence of ATP, the breakage of the link between actin and myosin does not occur (see Figure 9.15). The thick and thin filaments remain bound to each other by immobilized cross-bridges, producing a rigid condition in which the thick and thin filaments cannot be pulled past each other. The stiffness of rigor mortis disappears about 48 to 60 hours after death as the muscle tissue decomposes.

Table 9.2 summarizes the sequence of events that lead from an action potential in a motor neuron to the contraction and relaxation of a skeletal muscle fiber.

9.3 Mechanics of Single-Fiber Contraction

The force exerted on an object by a contracting muscle is known as muscle **tension,** and the force exerted on the muscle by an object (usually its weight) is the **load.** Muscle tension and load are opposing forces. Whether a fiber shortens depends on the relative magnitudes of the tension and the load. For muscle fibers to shorten and thereby move a load, muscle tension must be greater than the opposing load.

When a muscle develops tension but does not shorten or lengthen, the contraction is said to be an **isometric** (constant length) **contraction.** Such contractions occur when the muscle supports a load in a constant position or attempts to move an otherwise supported load that is greater than the tension developed by the muscle. A contraction in which the muscle changes length while the load on the muscle remains constant is an **isotonic** (constant tension) **contraction.**

Depending on the relative magnitudes of muscle tension and the opposing load, isotonic contractions can be associated with either shortening or lengthening of a muscle. When tension exceeds the load, shortening occurs and it is referred to as **concentric contraction.** When an unsupported load is greater than the tension generated by cross-bridges, the result is an **eccentric contraction** (lengthening contraction). In this situation, the load pulls the muscle to a longer length in spite of the opposing force produced by the cross-bridges. Such lengthening contractions occur when an object being supported by muscle contraction is lowered, as when the knee extensors in your thighs are used to lower you to a seat from a standing position. It must be emphasized that in these situations the lengthening of muscle fibers is not an active process produced by the contractile proteins but a consequence of the external forces being applied to the muscle. In the absence of external lengthening forces, a fiber will only *shorten* when stimulated; it will never lengthen. All three types of contractions—isometric, concentric, and eccentric—occur in the natural course of everyday activities.

During each type of contraction, the cross-bridges repeatedly go through the four steps of the cross-bridge cycle illustrated in Figure 9.15. During step 2 of a concentric isotonic contraction,

TABLE 9.2 Sequence of Events Between a Motor Neuron Action Potential and Skeletal Muscle Fiber Contraction

1. Action potential is initiated and propagates to motor neuron axon terminals.
2. Ca^{2+} enters axon terminals through voltage-gated Ca^{2+} channels.
3. Ca^{2+} entry triggers release of ACh from axon terminals.
4. ACh diffuses from axon terminals to motor end plate in muscle fiber.
5. ACh binds to nicotinic receptors on motor end plate, increasing their permeability to Na^+ and K^+.
6. More Na^+ moves into the fiber at the motor end plate than K^+ moves out, depolarizing the membrane and producing the end-plate potential (EPP).
7. Local currents depolarize the adjacent muscle cell plasma membrane to its threshold potential, generating an action potential that propagates over the muscle fiber surface and into the fiber along the T-tubules.
8. Action potential in T-tubules induces DHP receptors to pull open ryanodine receptor channels, allowing release of Ca^{2+} from terminal cisternae of sarcoplasmic reticulum.
9. Ca^{2+} binds to troponin on the thin filaments, causing tropomyosin to move away from its blocking position, thereby uncovering cross-bridge binding sites on actin.
10. Energized myosin cross-bridges on the thick filaments bind to actin: $A + M \cdot ADP \cdot P_i \rightarrow A \cdot M \cdot ADP \cdot P_i$
11. Cross-bridge binding triggers release of ATP hydrolysis products from myosin, producing an angular movement of each cross-bridge: $A \cdot M \cdot ADP \cdot P_i \rightarrow A \cdot M + ADP + P_i$
12. ATP binds to myosin, breaking linkage between actin and myosin and thereby allowing cross-bridges to dissociate from actin: $A \cdot M + ATP \rightarrow A + M \cdot ATP$
13. ATP bound to myosin is split, energizing the myosin cross-bridge: $M \cdot ATP \rightarrow M \cdot ADP \cdot P_i$
14. Cross-bridges repeat steps 10 to 13, producing movement (sliding) of thin filaments past thick filaments. Cycles of cross-bridge movement continue as long as Ca^{2+} remains bound to troponin.
15. Cytosolic Ca^{2+} concentration decreases as Ca^{2+}-ATPase actively transports Ca^{2+} into sarcoplasmic reticulum.
16. Removal of Ca^{2+} from troponin restores blocking action of tropomyosin, the cross-bridge cycle ceases, and the muscle fiber relaxes.

the cross-bridges bound to actin rotate through their power stroke, causing shortening of the sarcomeres. In contrast, during an isometric contraction, the bound cross-bridges do exert a force on the thin filaments but they are unable to move it. Rather than the filaments sliding, the rotation during the power stroke is absorbed within the structure of the cross-bridge in this circumstance. If isometric contraction is prolonged, cycling cross-bridges repeatedly rebind to the same actin molecule. During a lengthening contraction, the load pulls the cross-bridges in step 2 backward toward the Z lines while they are still bound to actin and exerting force. The events of steps 1, 3, and 4 are the same in all three types of contractions. Thus, the chemical changes in the contractile proteins during each type of contraction are the same. The end result (shortening, no length change, or lengthening) is determined by the magnitude of the load on the muscle.

Contraction terminology applies to both single fibers and whole muscles. In this section, we describe the mechanics of single-fiber contractions. Later, we will discuss the factors controlling the mechanics of whole-muscle contraction.

Twitch Contractions

The mechanical response of a muscle fiber to a single action potential is known as a **twitch.** Figure 9.16a shows the main features of an isometric twitch. Following the action potential, there is an interval of a few milliseconds known as the **latent period** before the tension in the muscle fiber begins to increase. During this latent period, the processes associated with excitation–contraction coupling are occurring. The time interval from the beginning of tension development at the end of the latent period to the peak tension is the **contraction time.**

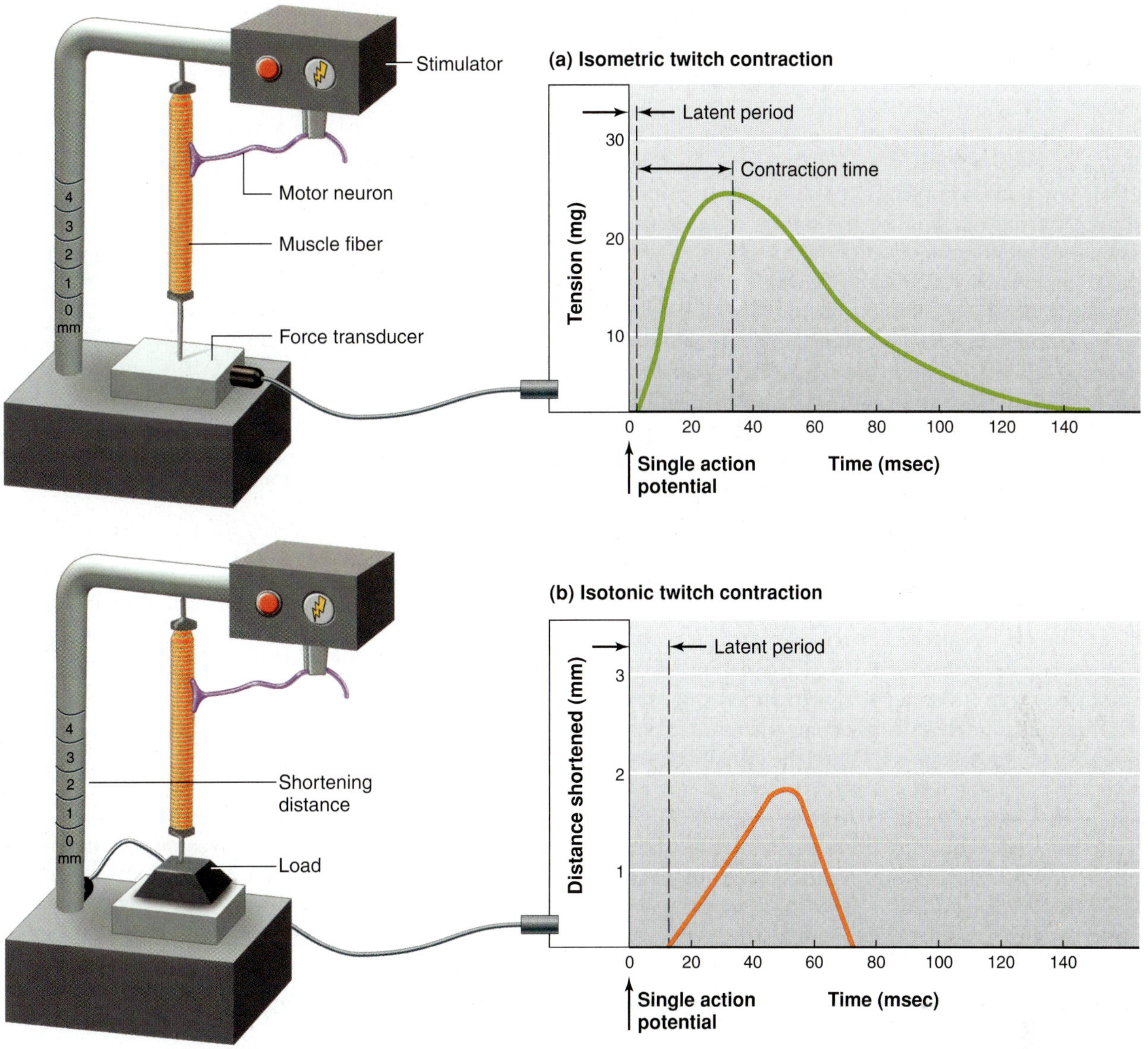

Figure 9.16 (a) Measurement of tension during a single isometric twitch contraction of a skeletal muscle fiber. (b) Measurement of shortening during a single isotonic twitch contraction of a skeletal muscle fiber.

PHYSIOLOGICAL INQUIRY

- Assuming that the same muscle fiber is used in these two experiments, estimate the magnitude of the load (in mg) being lifted in the isotonic experiment.

Answer can be found at end of chapter.

Not all skeletal muscle fibers have the same twitch contraction time. Some fibers have contraction times as short as 10 msec, whereas slower fibers may take 100 msec or longer. The total duration of a contraction depends in part on the time that cytosolic Ca^{2+} remains elevated so that cross-bridges can continue to cycle. This is closely related to the Ca^{2+}-ATPase activity in the sarcoplasmic reticulum; activity is greater in fast-twitch fibers and less in slow-twitch fibers. Twitch duration also depends on how long it takes for cross-bridges to complete their cycle and detach after the removal of Ca^{2+} from the cytosol.

Comparing isotonic and isometric twitches in the same muscle fiber, you can see from **Figure 9.16b** that the latent period in an isotonic twitch contraction is longer than that in an isometric twitch contraction. However, the duration of the mechanical event—shortening—is briefer in an isotonic twitch than the duration of force generation in an isometric twitch. The reason for these differences is most easily explained by referring to the measuring devices shown in Figure 9.16. In the isometric twitch experiment, twitch tension begins to increase as soon as the first cross-bridge attaches, so the latent period is due only to the excitation–contraction coupling delay. By contrast, in the isotonic twitch experiment, the latent period includes both the time for excitation–contraction coupling and the extra time it takes to accumulate enough attached cross-bridges to lift the load off of the platform. Similarly, at the end of the twitch, the isotonic load comes back to rest on the platform well before all of the cross-bridges have detached in the isometric experiment.

Moreover, the characteristics of an isotonic twitch depend upon the magnitude of the load being lifted (**Figure 9.17**). At heavier loads, (1) the latent period is longer, (2) the velocity of shortening (distance shortened per unit of time) is slower, (3) the duration of the twitch is shorter, and (4) the distance shortened is less.

A closer look at the sequence of events in an isotonic twitch explains this load-dependent behavior. As just explained, shortening does not begin until enough cross-bridges have attached and the muscle tension just exceeds the load on the fiber. Thus, before shortening, there is a period of *isometric* contraction during which the tension increases. The heavier the load, the longer it takes for the tension to increase to the value of the load, when shortening will begin. If the load on a fiber is increased, eventually a load is reached that the fiber is unable to lift, the velocity and distance of shortening decrease to zero, and the contraction will become completely isometric.

Load–Velocity Relation

It is a common experience that light objects can be moved faster than heavy objects. The isotonic twitch experiments illustrated in Figure 9.17 demonstrate that this phenomenon arises in part at the level of individual muscle fibers. When the initial shortening velocity (slope) of a series of isotonic twitches is plotted as a function of the load on a single fiber, the result is a hyperbolic curve (**Figure 9.18**). The shortening velocity is maximal when there is no load and is zero when the load is equal to the maximal isometric tension. At loads greater than the maximal isometric tension, the fiber will *lengthen* at a velocity that increases with load.

The unloaded shortening velocity is determined by the rate at which individual cross-bridges undergo their cyclical activity. Because one ATP is hydrolyzed during each cross-bridge cycle, the rate of ATP hydrolysis determines the shortening velocity. Increasing the load on a cross-bridge, however, slows its forward movement during the power stroke. This reduces the overall rate of ATP hydrolysis and, thus, decreases the velocity of shortening.

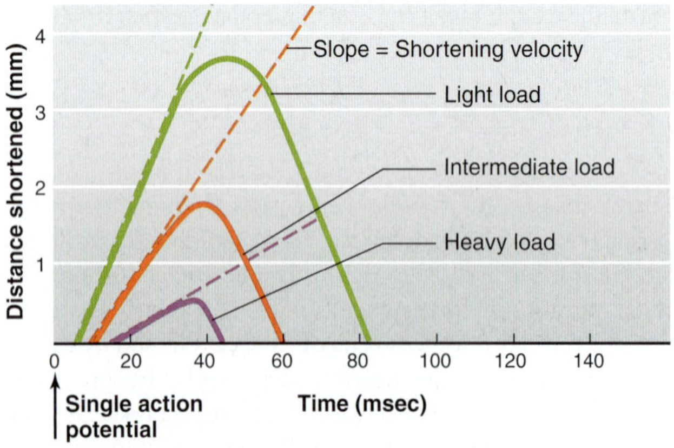

Figure 9.17 Isotonic twitch contractions with different loads. The distance shortened, velocity of shortening, and duration of shortening all decrease with increased load, whereas the time from stimulation to the beginning of shortening increases with increasing load.

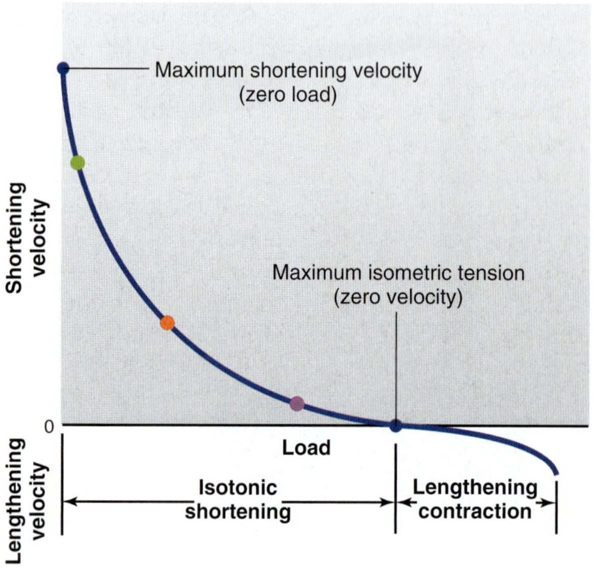

Figure 9.18 Velocity of skeletal muscle fiber shortening and lengthening as a function of load. Note that the force on the cross-bridges during a lengthening contraction is greater than the maximum isometric tension. The center three points correspond to the rate of shortening (slope) of the curves in Figure 9.17.

PHYSIOLOGICAL INQUIRY

- Multiplying the amount of a load times the velocity the load is moved gives the power a muscle fiber generates. From this plot, determine whether maximum power is generated when moving light, intermediate, or heavy loads. (*Hint:* Set maximum shortening velocity and isometric tension to an arbitrary value such as 10, and interpolate values on the load–velocity curve.)

Answer can be found at end of chapter.

Frequency–Tension Relation

Because a single action potential in a skeletal muscle fiber lasts only 1 to 2 msec but the twitch may last for 100 msec, it is possible for a second action potential to be initiated during the period of mechanical activity. **Figure 9.19** illustrates the tension generated during isometric contractions of a muscle fiber in response to multiple stimuli. The isometric twitch following the first stimulus, S_1, lasts 150 msec. The second stimulus, S_2, applied to the muscle fiber 200 msec after S_1, when the fiber has completely relaxed, causes a second identical twitch. When a stimulus is applied before a fiber has completely relaxed from a twitch, it induces a contractile response with a peak tension greater than that produced in a single twitch (S_3 and S_4). If the interval between stimuli is reduced further, the resulting peak tension is even greater (S_5 and S_6). Indeed, the mechanical response to S_6 is a smooth continuation of the mechanical response already induced by S_5.

The increase in muscle tension from successive action potentials occurring during the phase of mechanical activity is known as **summation.** Do not confuse this with the summation of neuronal postsynaptic potentials described in Chapter 6. Postsynaptic potential summation involves additive voltage effects on the membrane, whereas here we are observing the effect of additional attached cross-bridges. A maintained contraction in response to repetitive stimulation is known as a **tetanus** (tetanic contraction). At low stimulation frequencies, the tension may oscillate as the muscle fiber partially relaxes between stimuli, producing an **unfused tetanus.** A **fused tetanus,** with no oscillations, is produced at higher stimulation frequencies (**Figure 9.20**).

As the frequency of action potentials increases, the level of tension increases by summation until a maximal fused tetanic tension is reached, beyond which tension no longer increases even with further increases in stimulation frequency. This maximal tetanic tension is about three to five times greater than the isometric twitch tension. Different muscle fibers have different contraction times, so the stimulus frequency that will produce a maximal tetanic tension differs from fiber to fiber.

Why is tetanic tension so much greater than twitch tension? We can explain summation of tension in part by considering the relative timing of Ca^{2+} availability and cross-bridge binding. The isometric tension produced by a muscle fiber at any instant depends mainly on the total number of cross-bridges bound to actin and undergoing the power stroke of the cross-bridge cycle. Recall that a single action potential in a skeletal muscle fiber briefly releases enough Ca^{2+} to saturate troponin, and all the myosin-binding sites on the thin filaments are therefore *initially* available. However, the binding of energized cross-bridges to these sites (step 1 of the cross-bridge cycle) takes time, whereas the Ca^{2+} released into the cytosol begins to be pumped back into the sarcoplasmic reticulum almost immediately. Thus, after a single action potential, the Ca^{2+} concentration begins to decrease and the troponin–tropomyosin complex reblocks many binding sites before cross-bridges have had time to attach to them.

In contrast, during a tetanic contraction, the successive action potentials each release Ca^{2+} from the sarcoplasmic reticulum before all the Ca^{2+} from the previous action potential has been pumped back into the sarcoplasmic reticulum. This results in a persistent elevation of cytosolic Ca^{2+} concentration, which prevents a decline in the number of available binding sites on the thin filaments. Under these conditions, more binding sites remain available and many more cross-bridges become bound to the thin filaments.

Other causes of the lower tension seen in a single twitch are elastic structures, such as muscle tendons and the protein titin, which delay the transmission of cross-bridge force to the ends of a fiber. Because a single twitch is so brief, cross-bridge activity is already declining before force has been fully transmitted through these structures. This is less of a factor during tetanic stimulation because of the much longer duration of cross-bridge activity and force generation.

Length–Tension Relation

The springlike characteristic of the protein titin (see Figure 9.4), which is attached to the Z line at one end and the thick filaments at the other, is responsible for most of the *passive* elastic properties of relaxed muscle fibers. With increased stretch, the passive

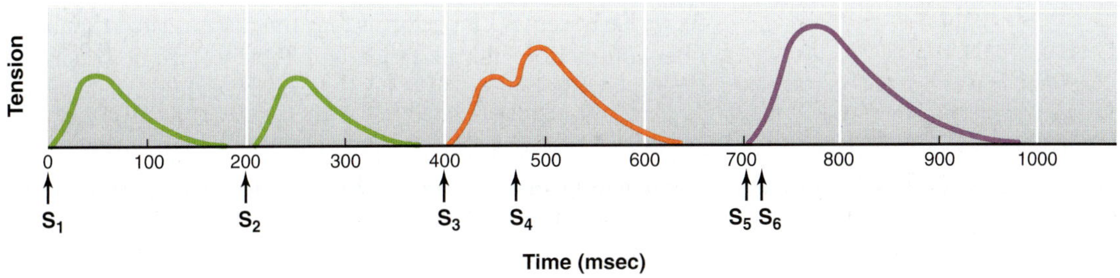

Figure 9.19 Summation of isometric contractions produced by shortening the time between stimuli.

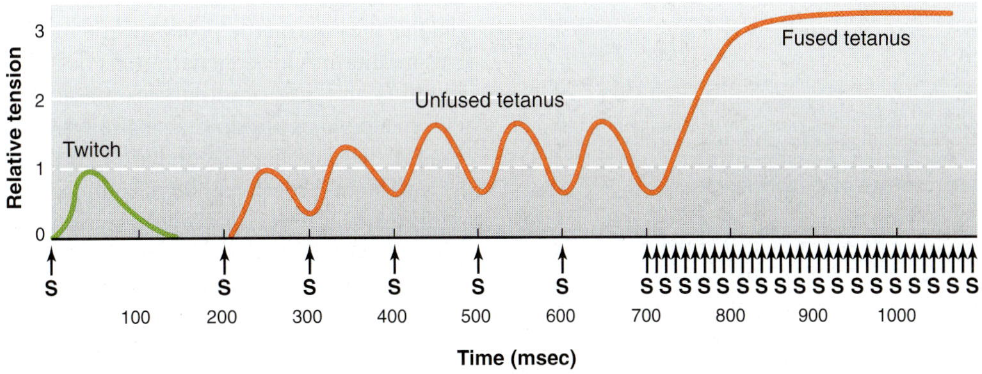

Figure 9.20 Isometric contractions produced by multiple stimuli (S) at 10 stimuli per second (unfused tetanus) and 100 stimuli per second (fused tetanus), as compared with a single twitch.

PHYSIOLOGICAL INQUIRY

- If the twitch contraction time is 35 msec and twitch duration is 150 msec, estimate the range of stimulation frequencies (stimuli per second) over which unfused tetanic contractions will occur.

Answer can be found at end of chapter.

tension in a relaxed fiber increases (**Figure 9.21**), not from active cross-bridge movements but from elongation of the titin filaments. If the stretched fiber is released, it will return to an equilibrium length, much like what occurs when releasing a stretched rubber band. By a different mechanism, the amount of *active* tension a muscle fiber develops during contraction can also be altered by changing the length of the fiber. If you stretch a muscle fiber to various lengths and tetanically stimulate it at each length, the magnitude of the active tension will vary with length, as Figure 9.21 shows. The length at which the fiber develops the greatest isometric active tension is termed the **optimal length (L_0)**.

When a muscle fiber length is 60% of L_0 or shorter, the fiber develops no tension when stimulated. As the length is increased from this point, the isometric tension at each length is increased up to a maximum at L_0. Further lengthening leads to a *decrease* in tension. At lengths of 175% of L_0 or greater, the fiber develops no active tension when stimulated (although the passive elastic tension would be quite high when stretched to this extent).

When most skeletal muscle fibers are relaxed, passive elastic properties keep their length near L_0 and thus near the optimal length for force generation. The length of a relaxed fiber can be altered by the load on the muscle or the contraction of other muscles that stretch the relaxed fibers, but the extent to which the relaxed length will change is limited by the muscle's attachments to bones. It rarely exceeds a 30% change from L_0 and is often much less. Over this range of lengths, the ability to develop tension never decreases below about half of the tension that can be developed at L_0 (see the blue-shaded region in Figure 9.21).

We can partially explain the relationship between fiber length and the fiber's capacity to develop active tension during contraction in terms of the sliding-filament mechanism. Stretching a relaxed muscle fiber pulls the thin filaments past the thick filaments, changing the amount of overlap between them. Stretching a fiber to 175% of L_0 pulls the filaments apart to the point where there is no overlap. At this point, there can be no cross-bridge binding to actin and no development of tension. As the fiber shortens toward L_0, more and more filament overlap occurs and the tension developed upon stimulation increases in proportion to the increased number of cross-bridges in the overlap region. Filament overlap is ideal at L_0, allowing the maximal number of cross-bridges to bind to the thin filaments, thereby producing maximal tension.

The tension decline at lengths less than L_0 is the result of several factors. For example, (1) the overlapping sets of thin filaments from opposite ends of the sarcomere may interfere with the cross-bridges' ability to bind and exert force; and (2) at very short lengths, the Z lines collide with the ends of the relatively rigid thick filaments, creating an internal resistance to sarcomere shortening.

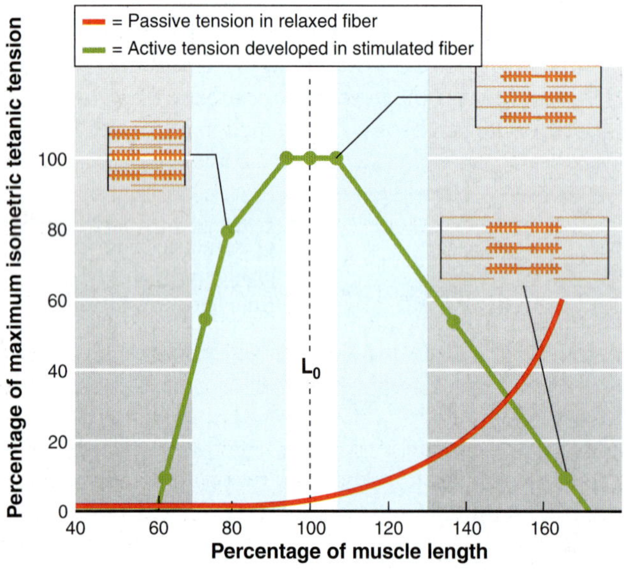

Figure 9.21 Variation in muscle tension at different lengths. Red curve shows passive (elastic) tension when cross-bridges are inactive. Green curve shows isometric tension resulting from cross-bridge activity during a fused, tetanic stimulus at the indicated length. The blue band represents the approximate range of length changes that can normally occur in the body.

PHYSIOLOGICAL INQUIRY

- If this muscle fiber is stretched to 150% of muscle length and then tetanically stimulated, what would be the *total* force measured by the transducer (as a percentage of maximum isometric tension)?

Answer can be found at end of chapter.

9.4 Skeletal Muscle Energy Metabolism

As we have seen, ATP performs four functions related to muscle fiber contraction and relaxation (see Table 9.1). In no other cell type does the rate of ATP breakdown increase so much from one moment to the next as in a skeletal muscle fiber when it goes from rest to a state of contractile activity. The ATP breakdown may change 20- to several-hundred-fold depending on the type of muscle fiber. The small supply of preformed ATP that exists at the start of contractile activity would only support a few twitches. If a fiber is to sustain contractile activity, metabolism must produce molecules of ATP as rapidly as they break down during the contractile process. The mechanisms by which muscles maintain ATP concentrations despite large variations in the intensity and time of activity are an excellent example of the general principle of physiology that physiological processes require the transfer and balance of matter and energy (see Chapter 1).

There are three ways a muscle fiber can form ATP (**Figure 9.22**): (1) phosphorylation of ADP by **creatine phosphate,** (2) oxidative phosphorylation of ADP in the mitochondria, and (3) phosphorylation of ADP by the glycolytic pathway in the cytosol.

Phosphorylation of ADP by creatine phosphate (CP) provides a very rapid means of forming ATP at the onset of contractile activity. When the chemical bond between creatine (C) and phosphate is broken, the amount of energy released is about the same as that released when the terminal phosphate bond in ATP is broken. This energy, along with the phosphate group, can be transferred to ADP to form ATP in a reversible reaction catalyzed by creatine kinase:

$$\text{CP} + \text{ADP} \xrightleftharpoons{\text{creatine kinase}} \text{C} + \text{ATP}$$

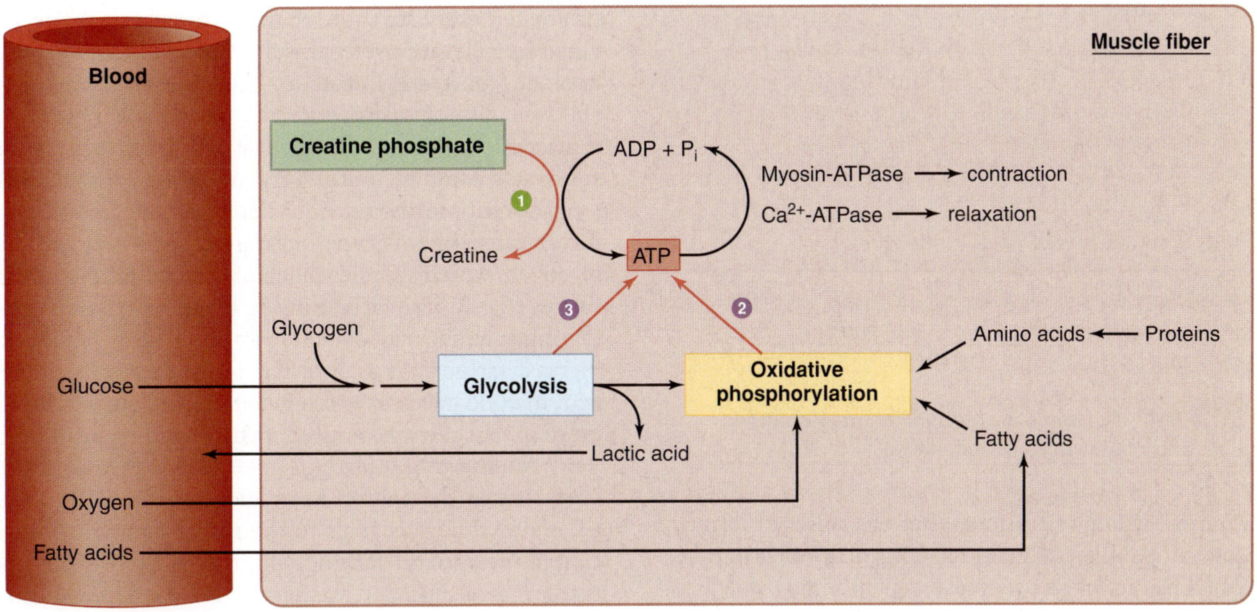

Figure 9.22 APIR The three sources of ATP production during muscle contraction: (1) creatine phosphate, (2) oxidative phosphorylation, and (3) glycolysis.

Although creatine phosphate is a high-energy molecule, its energy cannot be released by myosin to drive cross-bridge activity. During periods of rest, muscle fibers build up a concentration of creatine phosphate that is approximately five times that of ATP. At the beginning of contraction, when the ATP concentration begins to decrease and that of ADP begins to increase, owing to the increased rate of ATP breakdown by myosin, mass action favors the formation of ATP from creatine phosphate. This energy transfer is so rapid that the concentration of ATP in a muscle fiber changes very little at the start of contraction, whereas the concentration of creatine phosphate decreases rapidly.

Although the formation of ATP from creatine phosphate is very rapid, requiring only a single enzymatic reaction, the amount of ATP that this process can form is limited by the initial concentration of creatine phosphate in the cell. For this reason, many athletes in sports that require rapid power output consume creatine supplements to increase the pool of immediately available ATP in their muscles. If contractile activity is to continue for more than a few seconds, however, the muscle must be able to form ATP from the other two sources listed previously. The use of creatine phosphate at the start of contractile activity provides the few seconds necessary for the slower, multienzyme pathways of oxidative phosphorylation and glycolysis to increase their rates of ATP formation to levels that match the rates of ATP breakdown.

At moderate levels of muscular activity, most of the ATP used for muscle contraction is formed by oxidative phosphorylation, and during the first 5 to 10 min of such exercise, breakdown of muscle glycogen to glucose provides the major fuel contributing to oxidative phosphorylation. For the next 30 min or so, blood-borne fuels become dominant, blood glucose and fatty acids contributing approximately equally. Beyond this period, fatty acids become progressively more important, and the muscle's glucose utilization decreases.

If the intensity of exercise exceeds about 70% of the maximal rate of ATP breakdown, however, glycolysis contributes an increasingly significant fraction of the total ATP generated by the muscle. The glycolytic pathway, although producing only small quantities of ATP from each molecule of glucose metabolized, can produce ATP quite rapidly when enough enzymes and substrate are available, and it can do so in the absence of oxygen (anaerobic conditions). The glucose for glycolysis can be obtained from two sources: the blood or the stores of glycogen within the contracting muscle fibers. As the intensity of muscle activity increases, a greater fraction of the total ATP production is formed by anaerobic glycolysis. This is associated with a corresponding increase in the production of lactic acid (see Figure 3.41).

At the end of muscle activity, creatine phosphate and glycogen concentrations in the muscle have decreased. To return a muscle fiber to its original state, therefore, these energy-storing compounds must be replaced. Both processes require energy, so a muscle continues to consume increased amounts of oxygen for some time after it has ceased to contract. In addition, extra oxygen is required to metabolize accumulated lactate and return interstitial fluid oxygen concentrations to pre-exercise values. These processes are evidenced by the fact that you continue to breathe deeply and rapidly for a period of time immediately following intense exercise. This elevated oxygen consumption following exercise repays the **oxygen debt**—that is, the increased production of ATP by oxidative phosphorylation following exercise is used to restore the energy reserves in the form of creatine phosphate and glycogen.

Muscle Fatigue

When a skeletal muscle fiber is repeatedly stimulated, the tension the fiber develops eventually decreases even though the stimulation continues (**Figure 9.23**). This decline in muscle tension as a result of previous contractile activity is known as **muscle fatigue.** Additional characteristics of fatigued muscle are a decreased shortening velocity and a slower rate of relaxation. The onset of fatigue and its rate of development depend on the type of skeletal muscle fiber that is active, the intensity and duration of contractile activity, and the degree of an individual's fitness.

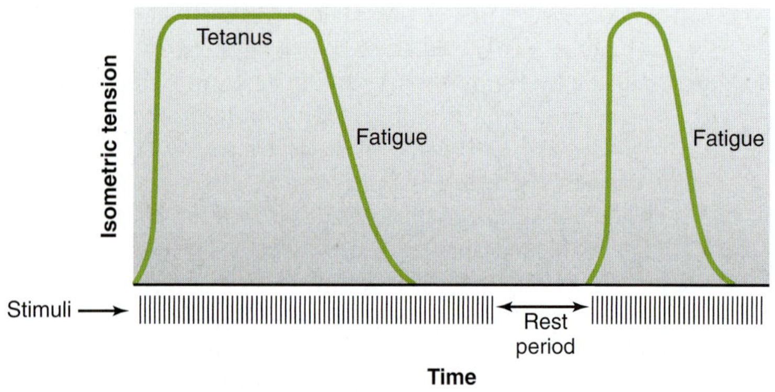

Figure 9.23 Muscle fatigue during a maintained isometric tetanus and recovery following a period of rest.

If a muscle is allowed to rest after the onset of fatigue, it can recover its ability to contract upon restimulation (see Figure 9.23). The rate of recovery also depends upon the duration and intensity of the previous activity. Some muscle fibers fatigue rapidly if continuously stimulated but also recover rapidly after only a few seconds of rest. This type of fatigue accompanies high-intensity, short-duration exercise, such as lifting up and continuously holding a very heavy weight for as long as possible. During this type of activity, blood flow through muscles can cease due to blood vessel compression. In contrast, fatigue develops more slowly with low-intensity, long-duration exercise, such as long-distance running, which includes cyclical periods of contraction and relaxation. Recovery from fatigue after such repetitive activities can take from minutes to hours. After exercise of extreme duration, like running a marathon, it may take days or weeks before muscles achieve complete recovery, likely due to a combination of fatigue and muscle damage.

The causes of acute muscle fatigue following various types of contractions in different types of muscle cells have been the subject of much research, but our understanding is still incomplete. Metabolic changes that occur in active muscle cells include a decrease in ATP concentration and increases in the concentrations of ADP, P_i, Mg^{2+}, H^+ (from lactic acid), and oxygen free radicals (see Chapter 2). Individually, and in combination, those metabolic changes have been shown to

1. decrease the rate of Ca^{2+} release, reuptake, and storage by the sarcoplasmic reticulum;
2. decrease the sensitivity of the thin filament proteins to activation by Ca^{2+}; and
3. directly inhibit the binding and power-stroke motion of the myosin cross-bridges.

Each of these mechanisms has been demonstrated to be important under particular experimental conditions, but their exact relative contributions to acute fatigue in intact human muscle has yet to be resolved.

A number of different processes have been implicated in the persistent fatigue that follows low-intensity, long-duration exercise. The acute effects just listed may play minor roles in this type of exercise as well, but at least two other mechanisms are thought to be more important. One involves changes in the regulation of the ryanodine receptor channels through which Ca^{2+} exits the sarcoplasmic reticulum. During prolonged exercise, these channels become leaky to Ca^{2+}, and persistent elevation of cytosolic Ca^{2+} activates proteases that degrade contractile proteins. The result is muscle soreness and weakness that lasts until the synthesis of new proteins can replace those that are damaged. It appears that depletion of fuel substrates could also play a role in fatigue that occurs during long-duration exercise. ATP depletion does not seem to be a direct cause of this type of fatigue, but a decrease in muscle glycogen, which supplies much of the fuel for contraction, correlates closely with fatigue onset. In addition, low blood glucose (hypoglycemia) and dehydration have been demonstrated to increase fatigue. Thus, a certain level of carbohydrate metabolism may be necessary to prevent fatigue during low-intensity exercise, but the mechanism of this requirement is unknown.

Another type of fatigue quite different from muscle fatigue occurs when the appropriate regions of the cerebral cortex fail to send excitatory signals to the motor neurons. This is called **central command fatigue,** and it may cause a person to stop exercising even though the muscles are not fatigued. An athlete's performance depends not only on the physical state of the appropriate muscles but also upon the mental ability to initiate central commands to muscles during a period of increasingly distressful sensations. Intriguingly, recent experiments have revealed a connection between fuel status and central command mechanisms. Subjects who rinse their mouths with solutions of carbohydrates are able to exercise significantly longer before exhaustion than subjects who rinse with water alone. This may represent a feedforward mechanism in which central command fatigue is inhibited when carbohydrate sensors in the mouth notify brain centers involved in motivation that more fuel is on the way.

9.5 Types of Skeletal Muscle Fibers

Skeletal muscle fibers do not all have the same mechanical and metabolic characteristics. Different types of fibers can be classified on the basis of (1) their maximal velocities of shortening—fast or slow—and (2) the major pathway they use to form ATP—oxidative or glycolytic.

Fast and slow fibers contain forms of myosin that differ in the maximal rates at which they use ATP. This, in turn, determines the maximal rate of cross-bridge cycling and thus the maximal shortening velocity. Fibers containing myosin with low ATPase activity are classified as **slow fibers** and are also sometimes referred to as type I fibers. By contrast, fibers containing myosin with higher ATPase activity are called **fast fibers** or type II fibers. Several subtypes of fast myosin can be distinguished based on small variations in their structure. Although the rate of cross-bridge cycling is about four times faster in fast fibers than in slow fibers, the force produced by both types of cross-bridges is about the same.

The second means of classifying skeletal muscle fibers is according to the type of enzymatic machinery available for synthesizing ATP. Some fibers contain numerous mitochondria and thus have a high capacity for oxidative phosphorylation. These fibers are classified as **oxidative fibers.** Most of the ATP such fibers produce is dependent upon blood flow to deliver oxygen and fuel molecules to the muscle. Not surprisingly, therefore, these fibers are surrounded by many small blood vessels.

They also contain large amounts of an oxygen-binding protein known as **myoglobin,** which increases the rate of oxygen diffusion into the fiber and provides a small store of oxygen. The large amounts of myoglobin present in oxidative fibers give the fibers a dark red color; thus, oxidative fibers are often referred to as **red muscle fibers.** Myoglobin is similar in structure and function to hemoglobin (see Figures 2.20 and 13.25 to 13.29).

In contrast, **glycolytic fibers** have few mitochondria but possess a high concentration of glycolytic enzymes and a large store of glycogen. Corresponding to their limited use of oxygen, these fibers are surrounded by relatively few blood vessels and contain little myoglobin. The lack of myoglobin is responsible for the pale color of glycolytic fibers and their designation as **white muscle fibers.**

On the basis of these two characteristics, three principal types of skeletal muscle fibers can be distinguished:

1. **Slow-oxidative fibers** (type I) combine low myosin-ATPase activity with high oxidative capacity.
2. **Fast-oxidative-glycolytic fibers** (type IIa) combine high myosin-ATPase activity with high oxidative capacity and intermediate glycolytic capacity.
3. **Fast-glycolytic fibers** (type IIb) combine high myosin-ATPase activity with high glycolytic capacity.

In addition to these biochemical differences, there are also size differences. Glycolytic fibers generally have larger diameters than oxidative fibers (**Figure 9.24**). This fact has significance for tension development. The number of thick and thin filaments per unit of cross-sectional area is about the same in all types of skeletal muscle fibers. Therefore, the larger the diameter of a muscle fiber, the greater the total number of thick and thin filaments acting in parallel to produce force, and the greater the maximum tension it can develop. Accordingly, the average glycolytic fiber, with its larger diameter, develops more tension when it contracts than does an average oxidative fiber.

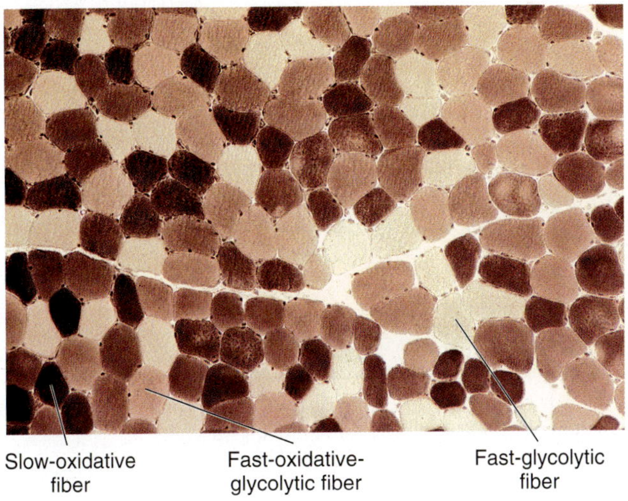

Figure 9.24 Muscle fiber types in normal human muscle, prepared using ATPase stain. Darkest fibers are slow-oxidative type; lighter-colored fibers are fast-oxidative-glycolytic and fast-glycolytic fibers. Note that the fourth theoretical possibility—slow-glycolytic fibers—is not found.

These three types of fibers also differ in their capacity to resist fatigue. Fast-glycolytic fibers fatigue rapidly, whereas slow-oxidative fibers are very resistant to fatigue, which allows them to maintain contractile activity for long periods with little loss of tension. Fast-oxidative-glycolytic fibers have an intermediate capacity to resist fatigue (**Figure 9.25**).

Table 9.3 summarizes the characteristics of the three types of skeletal muscle fibers.

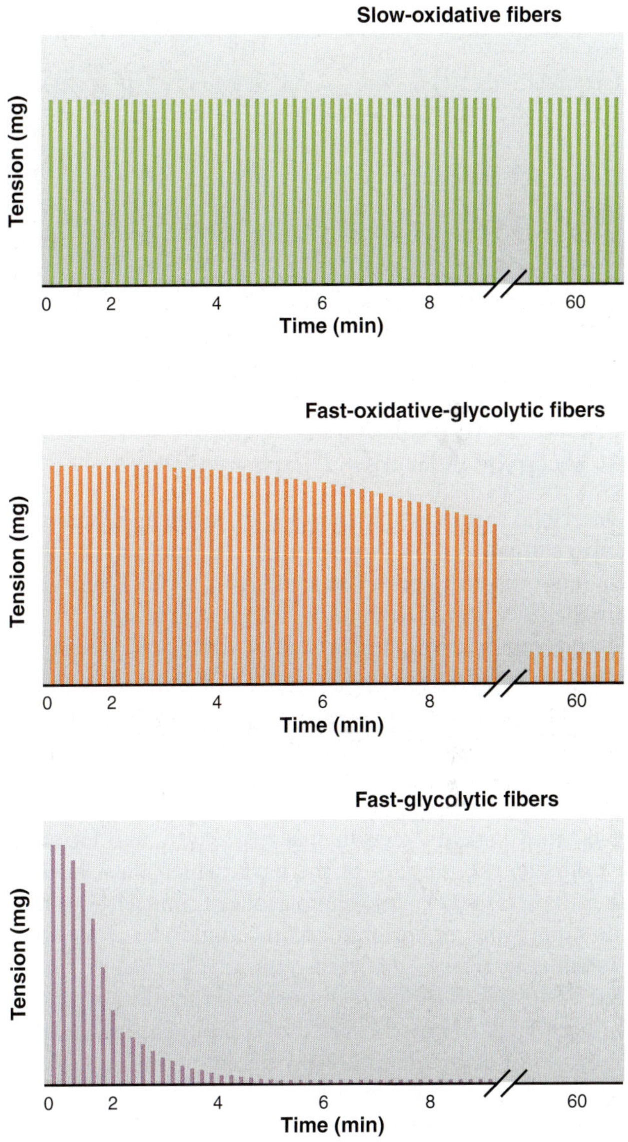

Figure 9.25 The rate of fatigue development in the three fiber types. Each vertical line is the contractile response to a brief tetanic stimulus and relaxation. The contractile responses occurring between about 9 min and 60 min are not shown on the figure.

PHYSIOLOGICAL INQUIRY

- Why is it logical that there are no muscle fibers classified as slow-glycolytic?

Answer can be found at end of chapter.

TABLE 9.3	Characteristics of the Three Types of Skeletal Muscle Fibers		
	Slow-Oxidative Fibers (Type I)	**Fast-Oxidative-Glycolytic Fibers (Type IIa)**	**Fast-Glycolytic Fibers (Type IIb)***
Primary source of ATP production	Oxidative phosphorylation	Oxidative phosphorylation	Glycolysis
Mitochondria	Many	Many	Few
Capillaries	Many	Many	Few
Myoglobin content	High (red muscle)	High (red muscle)	Low (white muscle)
Glycolytic enzyme activity	Low	Intermediate	High
Glycogen content	Low	Intermediate	High
Rate of fatigue	Slow	Intermediate	Fast
Myosin-ATPase activity	Low	High	High
Contraction velocity	Slow	Fast	Fast
Fiber diameter	Small	Large	Large
Motor unit size	Small	Intermediate	Large
Size of motor neuron innervating fiber	Small	Intermediate	Large

*Type IIb fibers are sometimes designated as type IIx in the human muscle physiology literature.

9.6 Whole-Muscle Contraction

As described earlier, whole muscles are made up of many muscle fibers organized into motor units. All the muscle fibers in a single motor unit are of the same fiber type. Thus, you can apply the fiber designation to the motor unit and refer to slow-oxidative motor units, fast-oxidative-glycolytic motor units, and fast-glycolytic motor units.

Most skeletal muscles are composed of all three motor unit types interspersed with each other (**Figure 9.26**). No muscle has only a single fiber type. Depending on the proportions of the fiber types present, muscles can differ considerably in their maximal contraction speed, strength, and fatigability. For example, the muscles of the back, which must be able to maintain their activity for long periods of time without fatigue while supporting an upright posture, contain large numbers of slow-oxidative fibers. In contrast, muscles in the arms that are called upon to produce large amounts of tension over a short time period, as when a boxer throws a punch, have a greater proportion of fast-glycolytic fibers. Leg muscles used for fast running over intermediate distances typically have a high proportion of fast-oxidative-glycolytic fibers. Significant variation occurs between individuals, however. For example, elite distance runners on average have greater than 75% slow-twitch fibers in the gastrocnemius muscle of the lower leg, whereas in elite sprinters the same muscle has 75% fast-twitch fibers.

We will next use the characteristics of single fibers to describe whole-muscle contraction and its control.

Control of Muscle Tension

The total tension a muscle can develop depends upon two factors: (1) the amount of tension developed by each fiber, and (2) the number of fibers contracting at any time. By controlling these two factors, the nervous system controls whole-muscle

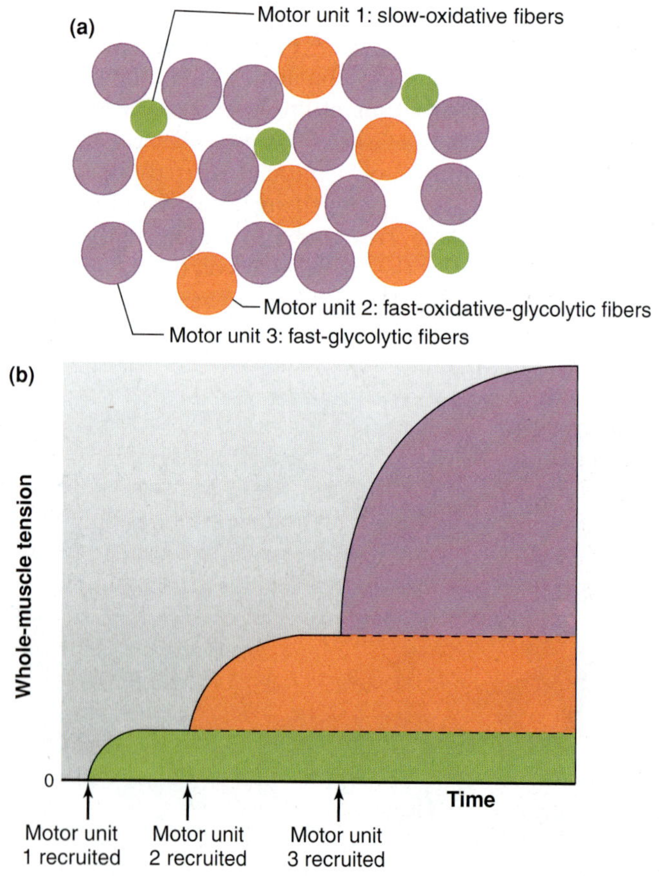

Figure 9.26 (a) Diagram of a cross section through a muscle composed of three types of motor units. (b) Tetanic muscle tension resulting from the successive recruitment of the three types of motor units. Note that motor unit 3, composed of fast-glycolytic fibers, produces the greatest increase in tension because it is composed of large-diameter fibers with the largest number of fibers per motor unit.

TABLE 9.4 Factors Determining Muscle Tension

I. Tension developed by each fiber
   A. Action potential frequency (frequency–tension relation)
   B. Fiber length (length–tension relation)
   C. Fiber diameter
   D. Fatigue

II. Number of active fibers
   A. Number of fibers per motor unit
   B. Number of active motor units

tension as well as shortening velocity. The conditions that determine the amount of tension developed in a single fiber have been discussed previously and are summarized in **Table 9.4**.

The number of fibers contracting at any time depends on (1) the number of fibers in each motor unit (motor unit size), and (2) the number of active motor units.

Motor unit size varies considerably from one muscle to another. The muscles in the hand and eye, which produce very delicate movements, contain small motor units. For example, one motor neuron innervates only about 13 fibers in an eye muscle. In contrast, in the more coarsely controlled muscles of the legs, each motor unit is large, containing hundreds and in some cases several thousand fibers. When a muscle is composed of small motor units, the total tension the muscle produces can be increased in small steps by activating additional motor units. If the motor units are large, large increases in tension will occur as each additional motor unit is activated. Thus, finer control of muscle tension is possible in muscles with small motor units.

The force a single fiber produces, as we have seen earlier, depends in part on the fiber diameter—the greater the diameter, the greater the force. We have also noted that fast-glycolytic fibers have the largest diameters. Thus, a motor unit composed of 100 fast-glycolytic fibers produces more force than a motor unit composed of 100 slow-oxidative fibers. In addition, fast-glycolytic motor units tend to have more muscle fibers. For both of these reasons, activating a fast-glycolytic motor unit will produce more force than activating a slow-oxidative motor unit.

The process of increasing the number of motor units that are active in a muscle at any given time is called **recruitment.** It is achieved by activating excitatory synaptic inputs to more motor neurons. The greater the number of active motor neurons, the more motor units recruited and the greater the muscle tension.

Motor neuron size plays an important role in the recruitment of motor units. The size of a motor neuron refers to the diameter of the neuronal cell body, which usually correlates with the diameter of its axon. Given the same number of sodium ions entering a cell at a single excitatory synapse in a large and in a small motor neuron, the small neuron will undergo a greater depolarization because these ions will be distributed over a smaller membrane surface area. Accordingly, given the same level of synaptic input, the smallest neurons will be recruited first—that is, they will begin to generate action potentials first. The larger neurons will be recruited only as the level of synaptic input increases. Because the smallest motor neurons innervate the slow-oxidative motor units (see Table 9.3), these motor units are recruited first, followed by fast-oxidative-glycolytic motor units, and finally, during very strong contractions, by fast-glycolytic motor units (see Figure 9.26).

Thus, during moderate-strength contractions, such as those that occur in most endurance types of exercise, relatively few fast-glycolytic motor units are recruited, and most of the activity occurs in the more fatigue-resistant oxidative fibers. The large, fast-glycolytic motor units, which fatigue rapidly, begin to be recruited when the intensity of contraction exceeds about 40% of the maximal tension the muscle can produce.

In summary, the neural control of whole-muscle tension involves (1) the frequency of action potentials in individual motor units (to vary the tension generated by the fibers in that unit) and (2) the recruitment of motor units (to vary the number of active fibers). Most motor neuron activity occurs in bursts of action potentials, which produce tetanic contractions of individual motor units rather than single twitches. Recall that the tension of a single fiber increases only threefold to fivefold when going from a twitch to a maximal tetanic contraction. Therefore, varying the frequency of action potentials in the neurons supplying them provides a way to make only threefold to fivefold adjustments in the tension of the recruited motor units. The force a whole muscle exerts can be varied over a much wider range than this, from very delicate movements to extremely powerful contractions, by recruiting motor units. Thus, recruitment provides the primary means of varying tension in a whole muscle. Recruitment is controlled by the central commands from the motor centers in the brain to the various motor neurons (see Chapter 10).

Control of Shortening Velocity

As we saw earlier, the velocity at which a single muscle fiber shortens is determined by (1) the load on the fiber and (2) whether the fiber is a fast or slow fiber. Translated to a whole muscle, these characteristics become (1) the load on the whole muscle and (2) the types of motor units in the muscle. For the whole muscle, however, recruitment becomes a third very important factor, one that explains how the shortening velocity can be varied from very fast to very slow even though the load on the muscle remains constant. Consider for the sake of illustration a muscle composed of only two motor units of the same size and fiber type. One motor unit by itself will lift a 4 g load more slowly than a 2 g load because the shortening velocity decreases with increasing load. When both units are active and a 4 g load is lifted, each motor unit bears only half the load and its fibers will shorten as if it were lifting only a 2 g load. In other words, the muscle will lift the 4 g load at a higher velocity when both motor units are active. Recruitment of motor units thus leads to increases in both force and velocity.

Muscle Adaptation to Exercise

The regularity with which a muscle is used—as well as the duration and intensity of its activity—affects the properties of the muscle. If the neurons to a skeletal muscle are destroyed or the neuromuscular junctions become nonfunctional, the denervated muscle fibers will become progressively smaller in diameter and the amount of contractile proteins they contain will decrease. This condition is known as ***denervation atrophy.*** A muscle can also atrophy with its nerve supply intact if the muscle is not used for a long period of time, as when a broken arm or leg is immobilized in a cast. This condition is known as ***disuse atrophy.***

In contrast to the decrease in muscle mass that results from a lack of neural stimulation, increased amounts of contractile activity—in other words, exercise—can produce an increase in the size (hypertrophy) of muscle fibers as well as changes in their capacity for ATP production.

Exercise that is of relatively low intensity but long duration (popularly called "aerobic exercise"), such as distance running, produces increases in the number of mitochondria in the fibers that are recruited in this type of activity. In addition, the number of capillaries around these fibers also increases. All these changes lead to an increase in the capacity for endurance activity with a minimum of fatigue. (Surprisingly, fiber diameter decreases slightly, and thus there is a small decrease in the maximal strength of muscles as a result of endurance training.) As we will see in later chapters, endurance exercise produces changes not only in the skeletal muscles but also in the respiratory and circulatory systems, changes that improve the delivery of oxygen and fuel molecules to the muscle.

In contrast, short-duration, high-intensity exercise (popularly called "strength training") such as weight lifting affects primarily the fast-twitch fibers, which are recruited during strong contractions. These fibers undergo an increase in diameter (hypertrophy) due to satellite cell activation and increased synthesis of actin and myosin filaments, which form more myofibrils. In addition, glycolytic activity is increased by increasing the synthesis of glycolytic enzymes. The result of such high-intensity exercise is an increase in the strength of the muscle and the bulging muscles of a conditioned weight lifter. Such muscles, although very powerful, have little capacity for endurance and they fatigue rapidly. It should be noted that not all of the gains in strength with resistance exercise are due to muscle hypertrophy. It has frequently been observed, particularly in women, that strength can almost double with training without measurable muscle hypertrophy. The most likely mechanisms are modifications of neural pathways involved in motor control. For example, regular weight training is hypothesized to cause increased synchronization in motor unit recruitment, enhanced ability to recruit fast-glycolytic motor neurons, and a reduction in inhibitory afferent inputs from tendon sensory receptors (described in Chapter 10).

Exercise produces limited change in the types of myosin enzymes the fibers form and thus little change in the proportions of fast and slow fibers in a muscle. Research suggests that even with extreme exercise training, the change in ratio between slow and fast myosin types in muscle fibers is less than 10%. As described previously, however, exercise does change the rates at which metabolic enzymes are synthesized, leading to changes in the proportion of oxidative and glycolytic fibers within a muscle. With endurance training, there is a decrease in the number of fast-glycolytic fibers and an increase in the number of fast-oxidative-glycolytic fibers as the oxidative capacity of the fibers increases.

The signals responsible for all these changes in muscle with different types of activity are just beginning to be understood by researchers. They are related to the frequency and intensity of the contractile activity in the muscle fibers and, thus, to the pattern of action potentials and tension produced in the muscle over an extended period of time. Though multiple neural and chemical factors are likely involved, evidence is accumulating that locally produced insulin-like growth factor-1 (see Chapter 11) may play a central role. Anabolic steroids (androgens) also exert an influence on muscle strength and growth, which is discussed in Chapter 17. Recently, a regulatory protein called **myostatin** was discovered in the blood, which is produced by skeletal muscle cells and binds to receptors on those same cells. It appears to exert a negative feedback effect to prevent excessive muscle hypertrophy. Humans and other mammals with genetic mutations leading to deficiencies of myostatin or its receptors show exceptional muscle growth. Researchers are currently seeking ways to block myostatin activity to treat diseases that cause muscle atrophy, like muscular dystrophy (discussed at the end of this section).

Because different types of exercise training produce quite different changes in the strength and endurance capacity of a muscle, an individual performing regular exercise to improve muscle performance must choose a type of exercise compatible with the type of activity he or she ultimately wishes to perform. For example, lifting weights will not improve the endurance of a long-distance runner, and jogging will not produce the increased strength a weight lifter desires. Most types of exercise, however, produce some effect on both strength and endurance. These changes in muscle in response to repeated periods of exercise occur slowly over a period of weeks. If regular exercise ceases, the muscles will slowly revert to their unexercised state.

The maximum force a muscle generates decreases by 30% to 40% between the ages of 30 and 80. This decrease in tension-generating capacity is due primarily to a decrease in average fiber diameter. Some of the change is simply the result of diminishing physical activity and can be prevented by regular exercise. The ability of a muscle to adapt to exercise, however, decreases with age. The same intensity and duration of exercise in an older individual will not produce the same amount of change as in a younger person.

This effect of aging, however, is only partial; there is no question that even in elderly people, increases in exercise can produce significant adaptation. Aerobic training has received major attention because of beneficial effects on the cardiovascular system (see Chapter 12). Strength training to even a modest degree, however, can partially prevent the loss of muscle tissue that occurs with aging. Moreover, it helps maintain stronger bones and joints.

Extensive exercise by an individual whose muscles have not been used in performing that particular type of exercise leads to muscle soreness the next day. This soreness is thought to be the result of structural damage to muscle cells and their membranes, which activates the inflammation response (see Chapter 18). As part of this response, substances such as histamine released by cells of the immune system activate the endings of pain neurons in the muscle. Soreness most often results from lengthening contractions, indicating that the lengthening of a muscle fiber by an external force produces greater muscle damage than does either shortening or isometric contraction. Thus, exercising by gradually lowering weights will produce greater muscle soreness than an equivalent amount of weight

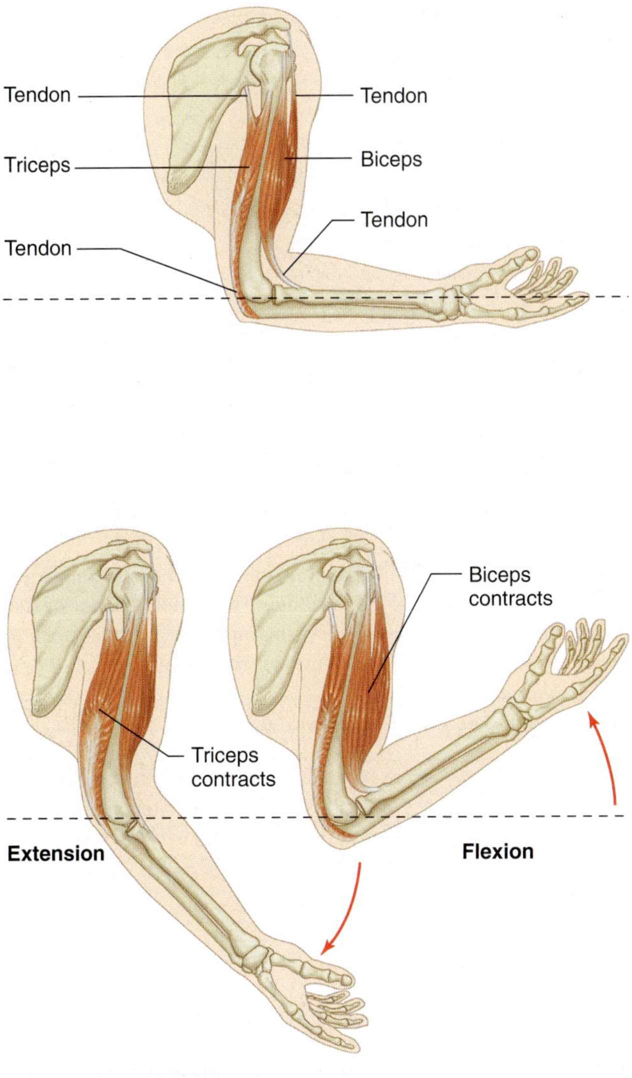

Figure 9.27 AP|R Antagonistic muscles for flexion and extension of the forearm.

lifting. This explains a phenomenon well-known to athletic trainers: The shortening contractions of leg muscles used to run *up* flights of stairs result in far less soreness than the lengthening contractions used for running *down*. Interestingly, it has been demonstrated that most of the strength gains during weight lifting is due to the eccentric portion of the movement. It therefore seems that the mechanisms underlying muscle soreness and muscle adaptation to exercise are related.

Lever Action of Muscles and Bones

A contracting muscle exerts a force on bones through its connecting tendons. When the force is great enough, the bone moves as the muscle shortens. A contracting muscle exerts only a pulling force, so that as the muscle shortens, the bones it is attached to are pulled toward each other. **Flexion** refers to the *bending* of a limb at a joint, whereas **extension** is the *straightening* of a limb (**Figure 9.27**). These opposing motions require at least two muscles, one to cause flexion and the other extension. Groups of muscles that produce oppositely directed movements at a joint are known as **antagonists.** For example, from Figure 9.27 we can see that contraction of the biceps causes flexion of the arm at the elbow, whereas contraction of the antagonistic muscle, the triceps, causes the arm to extend. Both muscles exert only a pulling force upon the forearm when they contract.

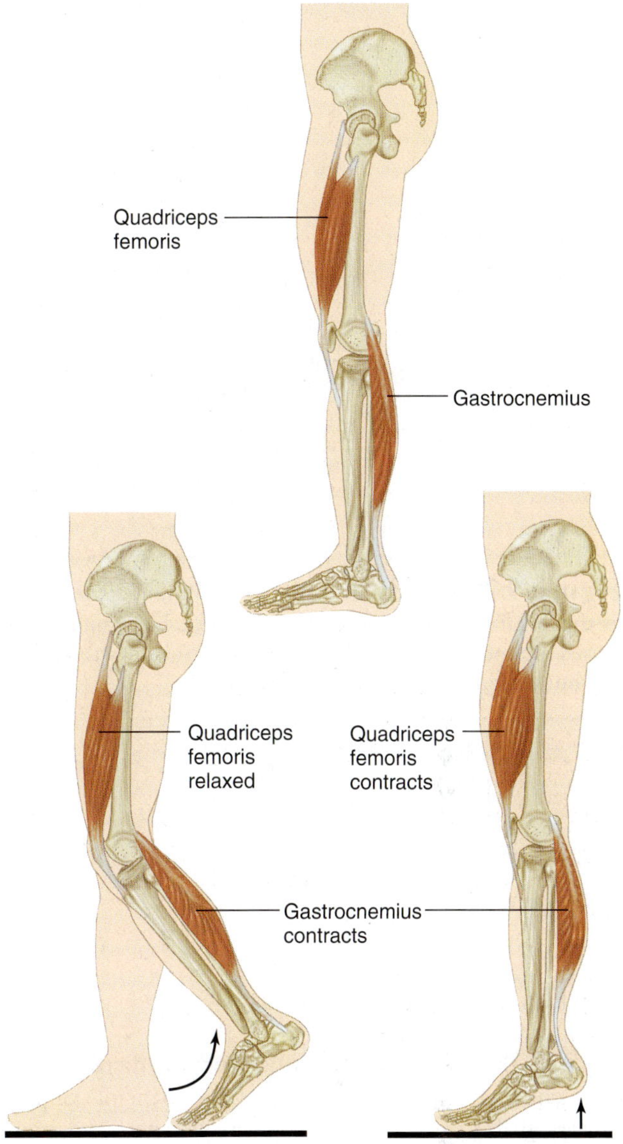

Figure 9.28 AP|R Contraction of the gastrocnemius muscle in the calf can lead either to flexion of the leg, if the quadriceps femoris muscle is relaxed, or to extension of the foot, if the quadriceps is contracting, preventing the knee joint from bending.

Sets of antagonistic muscles are required not only for flexion–extension but also for side-to-side movements or rotation of a limb. The contraction of some muscles leads to two types of limb movement, depending on the contractile state of other muscles acting on the same limb. For example, contraction of the gastrocnemius muscle in the calf causes a flexion of the leg at the knee, as in walking (**Figure 9.28**). However, contraction of the gastrocnemius muscle with the simultaneous contraction of the quadriceps femoris (which causes extension of the lower leg) prevents the knee joint from bending, leaving only the ankle joint capable of moving. The foot is extended, and the body rises on tiptoe.

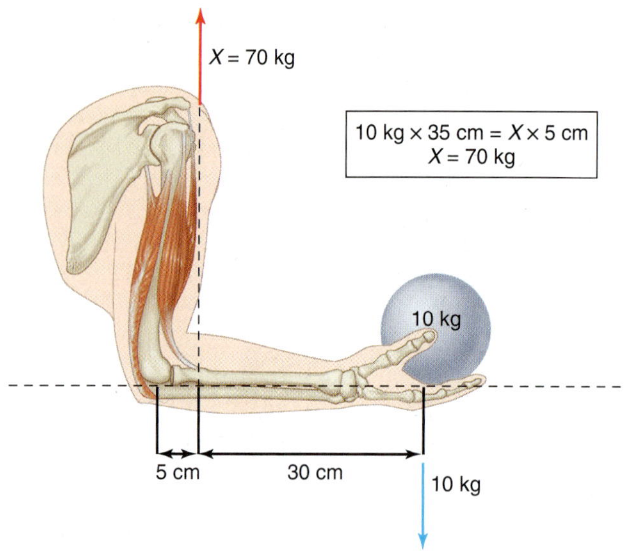

Figure 9.29 APIR Mechanical equilibrium of forces acting on the forearm while supporting a 10 kg load. For simplicity, mass is used as a measure of the force here rather than newtons, which are the standard scientific units of force.

PHYSIOLOGICAL INQUIRY

- Describe what would happen if this weight was mounted on a rod that moved it 10 cm farther away from the elbow and the tension generated by the muscle was increased to 85 kg.

Answer can be found at end of chapter.

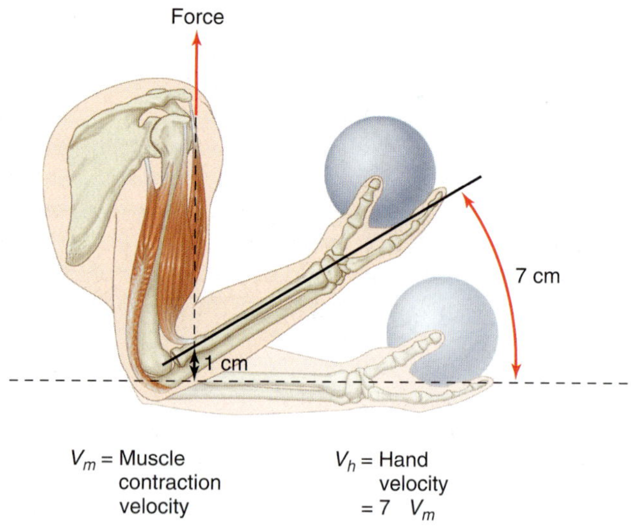

Figure 9.30 APIR The lever system of the arm amplifies the velocity of the biceps muscle, producing a greater velocity of the hand. The range of movement is also amplified (1 cm of shortening by the muscle produces 7 cm of movement by the hand).

PHYSIOLOGICAL INQUIRY

- If an individual's biceps insertion was 5 cm from the elbow joint (as shown in Figure 9.29) and the center of the hand was 45 cm from the elbow joint, how fast would an object move if the biceps shortened at 2 cm/sec?

Answer can be found at end of chapter.

The muscles, bones, and joints in the body are arranged in lever systems—a good example of the general principle of physiology that physiological processes are dictated by the laws of chemistry and physics. The basic principle of a lever is illustrated by the flexion of the arm by the biceps muscle (**Figure 9.29**), which exerts an upward pulling tension on the forearm about 5 cm away from the elbow joint. In this example, a 10 kg weight held in the hand exerts a downward load of 10 kg about 35 cm from the elbow. A law of physics tells us that the forearm is in mechanical equilibrium when the product of the downward load (10 kg) and its distance from the elbow (35 cm) is equal to the product of the isometric tension exerted by the muscle (X) and its distance from the elbow (5 cm); that is, $10 \times 35 = X \times 5$. Thus, $X = 70$ kg. The important point is that this system is working at a mechanical disadvantage because the tension exerted by the muscle (70 kg) is considerably greater than the load (10 kg) it is supporting.

However, the mechanical disadvantage that most muscle lever systems operate under is offset by increased maneuverability. As illustrated in **Figure 9.30**, when the biceps shortens 1 cm, the hand moves through a distance of 7 cm. Because the muscle shortens 1 cm in the same amount of time that the hand moves 7 cm, the velocity at which the hand moves is seven times greater than the rate of muscle shortening. The lever system amplifies the velocity of muscle shortening so that short, relatively slow movements of the muscle produce faster movements of the hand. Thus, a pitcher can throw a baseball at 90 to 100 mph even though his muscles shorten at only a small fraction of this velocity.

9.7 Skeletal Muscle Disorders

A number of conditions and diseases can affect the contraction of skeletal muscle. Many of them are caused by defects in the parts of the nervous system that control contraction of the muscle fibers rather than by defects in the muscle fibers themselves. For example, ***poliomyelitis*** is a viral disease that destroys motor neurons, leading to the paralysis of skeletal muscle, and may result in death due to respiratory failure.

Muscle Cramps

Involuntary tetanic contraction of skeletal muscles produces ***muscle cramps***. During cramping, action potentials fire at abnormally high rates, a much greater rate than occurs during maximal voluntary contraction. The specific cause of this high activity is uncertain, but it is probably related to electrolyte imbalances in the extracellular fluid surrounding both the muscle and nerve fibers. These imbalances may arise from overexercise or persistent dehydration, and they can directly induce action potentials in motor neurons and muscle fibers. Another theory is that chemical imbalances within the muscle stimulate sensory receptors in the muscle, and the motor neurons to the area are activated by reflex when those signals reach the spinal cord.

Hypocalcemic Tetany

Hypocalcemic tetany is the involuntary tetanic contraction of skeletal muscles that occurs when the extracellular Ca^{2+} concentration decreases to about 40% of its normal value. This may seem surprising, because we have seen that Ca^{2+} is required for excitation–contraction coupling. However, recall that this Ca^{2+} is sarcoplasmic reticulum Ca^{2+}, not extracellular Ca^{2+}. The effect of changes in extracellular Ca^{2+} is exerted not on the sarcoplasmic reticulum Ca^{2+} but directly on the plasma membrane. Low extracellular Ca^{2+} (**hypocalcemia**) increases the opening of Na^{+} channels in excitable membranes, leading to membrane depolarization and the spontaneous firing of action potentials. This causes the increased muscle contractions, which are similar to muscular cramping. Chapter 11 discusses the mechanisms controlling the extracellular concentration of calcium ions.

Muscular Dystrophy

Muscular dystrophy is a common genetic disease, affecting an estimated one in every 3500 males (but many fewer females). It is associated with the progressive degeneration of skeletal and cardiac muscle fibers, weakening the muscles and leading ultimately to death from respiratory or cardiac failure.

Muscular dystrophy is caused by the absence or defect of one or more proteins that make up the costameres in striated muscle. **Costameres** (*costa* = "rib") are clusters of structural and regulatory proteins that link the Z disks of the outermost myofibrils to the sarcolemma and extracellular matrix (**Figure 9.31a**). Proteins of the costameres serve multiple roles, including lateral transmission of force from the sarcomeres to the extracellular matrix and neighboring muscle fibers, stabilization of the sarcolemma against physical forces during muscle fiber contraction or stretch, and initiation of intracellular signals that link contractile activity with regulation of muscle cell remodeling. Defects in a number of specific costamere proteins have been demonstrated to cause various types of muscular dystrophy.

Duchenne muscular dystrophy is a sex-linked recessive disorder caused by a mutation in a gene on the X chromosome that codes for the protein **dystrophin.** Dystrophin was the first costamere protein discovered to be related to a muscular dystrophy, which is how it earned its name. As described in Chapter 17, females have two X chromosomes and males only one. Consequently, a female with one abnormal X chromosome and one normal one generally will not develop the disease, but males with an abnormal X chromosome always will. The defective gene can result in either a nonfunctional or missing protein. Dystrophin is an extremely large protein that normally forms a link between the contractile filament actin and proteins embedded in the overlying sarcolemma. In its absence, fibers subjected to repeated structural deformation during contraction are susceptible to membrane rupture and cell death. Therefore, the condition progresses with muscle use and age. Symptoms of weakness in the muscles of the hips and trunk become evident at about 2 to 6 years of age, and most affected individuals do not survive much beyond the age of 20 (**Figure 9.31b**). Preliminary attempts are being made to treat the disease by inserting the normal gene into dystrophic muscle cells.

Myasthenia Gravis

Myasthenia gravis is a collection of neuromuscular disorders characterized by muscle fatigue and weakness that progressively worsen as the muscle is used. Myasthenia gravis affects about one out of every 7500 Americans, occurring more often in women than men. The most common cause is the destruction of nicotinic ACh-receptor proteins of the motor end plate, mediated by antibodies of a person's own immune system (see Chapter 18 for a description of autoimmune diseases). The release of ACh from the axon terminals is normal, but

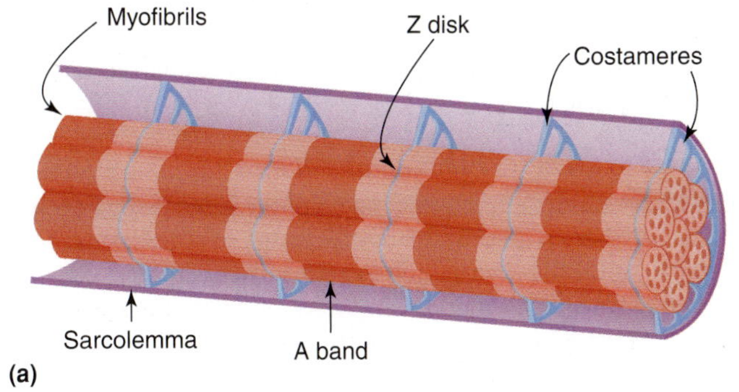

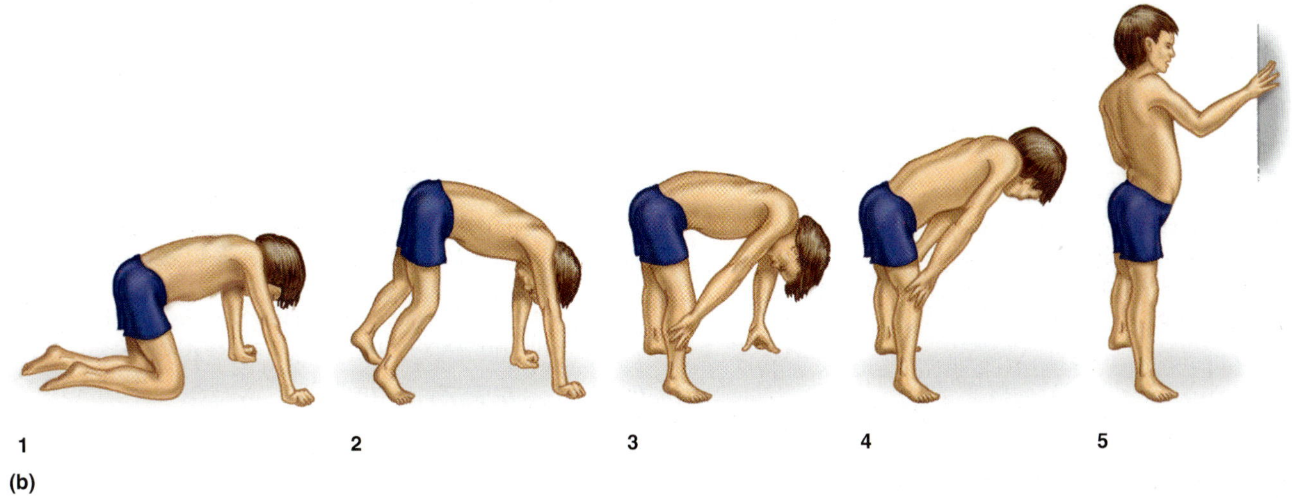

Figure 9.31 (a) Schematic diagram showing costamere proteins that link Z disks with membrane and extracellular matrix proteins. (b) Boy with Duchenne muscular dystrophy. Muscles of the hip girdle and trunk are the first to weaken, requiring patients to use their arms to "climb up" the legs in order to go from lying to standing. Part (a) is redrawn from James Ervasti, "Costameres: The Achilles' heel of Herculean muscle," *Journal of Biological Chemistry*, 278(16): 13591–13594 (2003).

the magnitude of the end-plate potential is markedly reduced because of the decreased availability of receptors. Even in normal muscle, the amount of ACh released with each action potential decreases with repetitive activity, and thus the magnitude of the resulting end-plate potential (EPP) decreases. In normal muscle, however, the EPP remains well above the threshold necessary to initiate a muscle action potential. In contrast, after a few motor nerve impulses in a myasthenia gravis patient, the magnitude of the EPP decreases below the threshold for initiating a muscle action potential.

A number of approaches are currently used to treat the disease. One is to administer acetylcholinesterase inhibitors (e.g., ***pyridostigmine***). This can partially compensate for the reduction in available ACh receptors by prolonging the time that acetylcholine is available at the synapse. Other therapies aim at blunting the immune response. Treatment with glucocorticoids is one way that immune function is suppressed (see Chapter 11). Removal of the thymus gland (***thymectomy***) reduces the production of antibodies and reverses symptoms in about 50% of patients. ***Plasmapheresis*** is a treatment that involves replacing the liquid fraction of blood (plasma) that contains the offending antibodies. A combination of these treatments has greatly reduced the mortality rate for myasthenia gravis.

SECTION A SUMMARY

There are three types of muscle—skeletal, smooth, and cardiac. Skeletal muscle is attached to bones and moves and supports the skeleton. Smooth muscle surrounds hollow cavities and tubes. Cardiac muscle is the muscle of the heart.

Structure

I. Skeletal muscles, composed of cylindrical muscle fibers (cells), are linked to bones by tendons at each end of the muscle.
II. Skeletal muscle fibers have a repeating, striated pattern of light and dark bands due to the arrangement of the thick and thin filaments within the myofibrils.
III. Actin-containing thin filaments are anchored to the Z lines at each end of a sarcomere. Their free ends partially overlap the myosin-containing thick filaments in the A band at the center of the sarcomere.
IV. Myosin molecules form the backbone of the thick filament and also have extensions called cross-bridges that span the gap between the thick and thin filaments. Each cross-bridge has two globular heads that contain a binding site for actin and an enzymatic site that splits ATP.
V. Skeletal muscle fibers have an elaborate membrane system in which the plasma membrane (sarcolemma) sends tubular extensions (T-tubules) throughout the cross section of the cell. T-tubules interact with terminal cisternae of the sarcoplasmic reticulum, in which Ca^{2+} is stored.

Molecular Mechanisms of Skeletal Muscle Contraction

I. Branches of a motor neuron axon form neuromuscular junctions with the muscle fibers in its motor unit. Each muscle fiber is innervated by a branch from only one motor neuron.
   a. Acetylcholine released by an action potential in a motor neuron binds to receptors on the motor end plate of the muscle membrane, opening ion channels that allow the passage of sodium and potassium ions, which depolarize the end-plate membrane.
   b. A single action potential in a motor neuron is sufficient to produce an action potential in a skeletal muscle fiber.
   c. Figure 9.9 summarizes events at the neuromuscular junction.
   d. Signaling at the neuromuscular junction can be disrupted by a number of different toxins, drugs, and disease processes.
II. In a resting muscle, tropomyosin molecules that are in contact with the actin subunits of the thin filaments block the attachment of cross-bridges to actin.
III. Contraction is initiated by an increase in cytosolic Ca^{2+} concentration. The calcium ions bind to troponin, producing a change in its shape that is transmitted via tropomyosin to uncover the binding sites on actin, allowing the cross-bridges to bind to the thin filaments.
   a. The increase in cytosolic Ca^{2+} concentration is triggered by an action potential in the plasma membrane. The action potential is propagated into the interior of the fiber along the transverse tubules to the region of the sarcoplasmic reticulum, where dihydropyridine receptors sense the voltage change and pull open ryanodine receptors, releasing calcium ions from the reticulum.
   b. Relaxation of a contracting muscle fiber occurs as a result of the active transport of cytosolic calcium ions back into the sarcoplasmic reticulum.
IV. When a skeletal muscle fiber actively shortens, the thin filaments are propelled toward the center of their sarcomere by movements of the myosin cross-bridges that bind to actin.
   a. The four steps occurring during each cross-bridge cycle are summarized in Figure 9.15. The cross-bridges undergo repeated cycles during a contraction, each cycle producing only a small increment of movement.
   b. The functions of ATP in muscle contraction are summarized in Table 9.1.
V. Table 9.2 summarizes the events leading to the contraction of a skeletal muscle fiber.

Mechanics of Single-Fiber Contraction

I. Contraction refers to the turning on of the cross-bridge cycle. Whether there is an accompanying change in muscle length depends upon the external forces acting on the muscle.
II. Three types of contractions can occur following activation of a muscle fiber: (1) an isometric contraction in which the muscle generates tension but does not change length; (2) an isotonic contraction in which the muscle shortens (concentric), moving a load; and (3) a lengthening (eccentric) contraction in which the external load on the muscle causes the muscle to lengthen during the period of contractile activity.
III. Increasing the frequency of action potentials in a muscle fiber increases the mechanical response (tension or shortening) up to the level of maximal tetanic tension.
IV. Maximum isometric tetanic tension is produced at the optimal sarcomere length L_0. Stretching a fiber beyond its optimal length or decreasing the fiber length below L_0 decreases the tension generated.
V. The velocity of muscle fiber shortening decreases with increases in load. Maximum velocity occurs at zero load.

Skeletal Muscle Energy Metabolism

I. Muscle fibers form ATP by the transfer of phosphate from creatine phosphate to ADP, by oxidative phosphorylation of ADP in mitochondria, and by substrate-level phosphorylation of ADP in the glycolytic pathway.
II. At the beginning of exercise, muscle glycogen is the major fuel consumed. As the exercise proceeds, glucose and fatty acids from the blood provide most of the fuel, and fatty acids

become progressively more important during prolonged exercise. When the intensity of exercise exceeds about 70% of maximum, glycolysis begins to contribute an increasing fraction of the total ATP generated.

III. A variety of factors may contribute to muscle fatigue, including a decrease in ATP concentration and increases in the concentrations of ADP, P_i, Mg^{2+}, H^+, and oxygen free radicals. Individually and in combination, those changes have effects such as decreasing Ca^{2+} uptake and storage by the sarcoplasmic reticulum, decreasing the sensitivity of the thin filaments to Ca^{2+}, and inhibiting the binding and power-stroke motion of the cross-bridges.

Types of Skeletal Muscle Fibers

I. Three types of skeletal muscle fibers can be distinguished by their maximal shortening velocities and the predominate pathway they use to form ATP: slow-oxidative, fast-oxidative-glycolytic, and fast-glycolytic fibers.
  a. Differences in maximal shortening velocities are due to different myosin enzymes with high or low ATPase activities, giving rise to fast and slow fibers.
  b. Fast-glycolytic fibers have a larger average diameter than oxidative fibers and therefore produce greater tension, but they also fatigue more rapidly.

II. All the muscle fibers in a single motor unit belong to the same fiber type, and most muscles contain all three types.

III. Table 9.3 summarizes the characteristics of the three types of skeletal muscle fibers.

Whole-Muscle Contraction

I. The tension produced by whole-muscle contraction depends on the amount of tension each fiber develops and the number of active fibers in the muscle (Table 9.4).

II. Muscles that produce delicate movements have a small number of fibers per motor unit, whereas large powerful muscles have much larger motor units.

III. Fast-glycolytic motor units not only have large-diameter fibers but also tend to have large numbers of fibers per motor unit.

IV. Increases in muscle tension are controlled primarily by increasing the number of active motor units in a muscle, a process known as recruitment. Slow-oxidative motor units are recruited first; then fast-oxidative-glycolytic motor units are recruited; and finally, fast-glycolytic motor units are recruited only during very strong contractions.

V. Increasing motor-unit recruitment increases the velocity at which a muscle will move a given load.

VI. Exercise can alter a muscle's strength and susceptibility to fatigue.
  a. Long-duration, low-intensity exercise increases a fiber's capacity for oxidative ATP production by increasing the number of mitochondria and blood vessels in the muscle, resulting in increased endurance.
  b. Short-duration, high-intensity exercise increases fiber diameter as a result of increased synthesis of actin and myosin, resulting in increased strength.

VII. Movement around a joint generally involves groups of antagonistic muscles; some flex a limb at the joint and others extend the limb.

VIII. The lever system of muscles and bones generally requires muscle tension far greater than the load in order to sustain a load in an isometric contraction, but the lever system produces a shortening velocity at the end of the lever arm that is greater than the muscle-shortening velocity.

Skeletal Muscle Disorders

I. Muscle cramps are involuntary tetanic contractions related to heavy exercise and may be due to dehydration and electrolyte imbalances in the fluid surrounding muscle and nerve fibers.

II. When extracellular Ca^{2+} concentration decreases below normal, Na^+ channels of nerve and muscle open spontaneously, which causes the excessive muscle contractions of hypocalcemic tetany.

III. Muscular dystrophies are commonly occurring genetic disorders that result from defects of muscle-membrane-stabilizing proteins such as dystrophin. Muscles of individuals with Duchenne muscular dystrophy progressively degenerate with use.

IV. Myasthenia gravis is an autoimmune disorder in which destruction of ACh receptors of the motor end plate causes progressive loss of the ability to activate skeletal muscles.

SECTION A REVIEW QUESTIONS

1. List the three types of muscle cells and their locations.
2. Diagram the arrangement of thick and thin filaments in a striated muscle sarcomere, and label the major bands that give rise to the striated pattern.
3. Describe the organization of myosin, actin, tropomyosin, and troponin molecules in the thick and thin filaments.
4. Describe the location, structure, and function of the sarcoplasmic reticulum in skeletal muscle fibers.
5. Describe the structure and function of the transverse tubules.
6. Define *motor unit* and describe its structure.
7. Describe the sequence of events by which an action potential in a motor neuron produces an action potential in the plasma membrane of a skeletal muscle fiber.
8. What is an end-plate potential, and what ions produce it?
9. Compare and contrast the transmission of electrical activity at a neuromuscular junction with that at a synapse.
10. What prevents cross-bridges from attaching to sites on the thin filaments in a resting skeletal muscle?
11. Describe the role and source of calcium ions in initiating contraction in skeletal muscle.
12. Describe the four steps of one cross-bridge cycle.
13. Describe the physical state of a muscle fiber in rigor mortis and the conditions that produce this state.
14. What three events in skeletal muscle contraction and relaxation depend on ATP?
15. Describe the events that result in the relaxation of skeletal muscle fibers.
16. Describe isometric, concentric, and eccentric contractions.
17. What factors determine the duration of an isotonic twitch in skeletal muscle? An isometric twitch?
18. What effect does increasing the frequency of action potentials in a skeletal muscle fiber have upon the force of contraction? Explain the mechanism responsible for this effect.
19. Describe the length–tension relationship in skeletal muscle fibers.
20. Describe the effect of increasing the load on a skeletal muscle fiber on the velocity of shortening.
21. What is the function of creatine phosphate in skeletal muscle contraction?
22. What fuel molecules are metabolized to produce ATP during skeletal muscle activity?
23. List the factors responsible for skeletal muscle fatigue.
24. What component of skeletal muscle fibers accounts for the differences in the fibers' maximal shortening velocities?

25. Summarize the characteristics of the three types of skeletal muscle fibers.
26. Upon what three factors does the amount of tension developed by a whole skeletal muscle depend?
27. Describe the process of motor-unit recruitment in controlling (a) whole-muscle tension and (b) velocity of whole-muscle shortening.
28. During increases in the force of skeletal muscle contraction, what is the order of recruitment of the different types of motor units?
29. What happens to skeletal muscle fibers when the motor neuron to the muscle is destroyed?
30. Describe the changes that occur in skeletal muscles following a period of (a) long-duration, low-intensity exercise training; and (b) short-duration, high-intensity exercise training.
31. How are skeletal muscles arranged around joints so that a limb can push or pull?
32. What are the advantages and disadvantages of the muscle-bone-joint lever system?

SECTION A KEY TERMS

A band 260
acetylcholine (ACh) 262
acetylcholinesterase 263
actin 260
antagonist 281
cardiac muscle 258
central command fatigue 276
concentric contraction 269
contraction 262
contraction time 270
costameres 283
creatine phosphate 274
cross-bridge 261
cross-bridge cycle 267
dihydropyridine (DHP) receptor 266
dystrophin 283
eccentric contraction 269
end-plate potential (EPP) 263
excitation–contraction coupling 265
extension 281
fast fiber 276
fast-glycolytic fiber 277
fast-oxidative-glycolytic fiber 277
flexion 281
foot process 266
fused tetanus 273
glycolytic fiber 277
H zone 260
heavy chains 260
hypertrophy 259
hypocalcemia 283
I band 260
isometric contraction 269
isotonic contraction 269
junctional feet 266
latent period 270
light chains 260
load 269
M line 260
motor end plate 262
motor neuron 262
motor unit 262
muscle 259
muscle fatigue 275
muscle fiber 259
myoblast 259
myofibril 260
myoglobin 277
myosin 260
myostatin 280
neuromuscular junction 262
optimal length (L_0) 274
oxidative fiber 276
oxygen debt 275
power stroke 268
recruitment 279
red muscle fiber 277
relaxation 262
rigor mortis 269
ryanodine receptor 266
sarcolemma 261
sarcomere 260
sarcoplasmic reticulum 261
satellite cell 259
skeletal muscle 258
sliding-filament mechanism 267
slow fiber 276
slow-oxidative fiber 277
smooth muscle 258
striated muscle 258
summation 272
tendon 260
tension 269
terminal cisternae 261
tetanus 273
thick filament 260
thin filament 260
titin 260
transverse tubule (T-tubule) 260
tropomyosin 260
troponin 261
twitch 270
unfused tetanus 273
white muscle fiber 277
Z line 260

SECTION A CLINICAL TERMS

atropine 264
botulism 265
curare 264
denervation atrophy 279
disuse atrophy 280
Duchenne muscular dystrophy 283
hypocalcemic tetany 282
muscle cramp 282
muscular dystrophy 283
myasthenia gravis 283
plasmapheresis 284
poliomyelitis 282
pralidoxime 264
pyridostigmine 284
rocuronium 264
succinylcholine 264
thymectomy 284
vecuronium 264

SECTION B

Smooth and Cardiac Muscle

We now turn our attention to the other muscle types, beginning with smooth muscle. Two characteristics are common to all smooth muscles. They lack the cross-striated banding pattern found in skeletal and cardiac fibers (which makes them "smooth"), and the nerves to them are part of the autonomic division of the nervous system rather than the somatic division. Thus, smooth muscle is not normally under direct voluntary control.

Smooth muscle, like skeletal muscle, uses cross-bridge movements between actin and myosin filaments to generate force, and calcium ions to control cross-bridge activity. However, the organization of the contractile filaments and the process of excitation–contraction coupling are quite different in smooth muscle. Furthermore, there is considerable diversity among smooth muscles with respect to the excitation–contraction coupling mechanism.

9.8 Structure of Smooth Muscle

Each smooth muscle cell is spindle-shaped, with a diameter between 2 and 10 μm, and length ranging from 50 to 400 μm. They are much smaller than skeletal muscle fibers, which are 10 to 100 μm wide and can be tens of centimeters long (see Figure 9.1). Skeletal muscle fibers are sometimes large enough to run the entire length of the muscles in which they are found, whereas many individual smooth muscle cells are generally interconnected to form sheetlike layers of cells (**Figure 9.32**). Skeletal muscle fibers are multinucleate cells with limited ability to

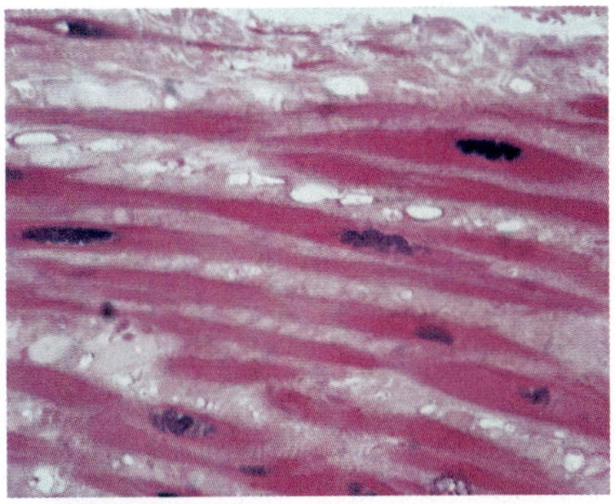

Figure 9.32 APIR Photomicrograph of a sheet of smooth muscle cells stained with a dye for visualization. Note the spindle shape, single nucleus, and lack of striations.

divide once they have differentiated; smooth muscle cells have a single nucleus and have the capacity to divide throughout the life of an individual. A variety of paracrine factors can stimulate smooth muscle cells to divide, often in response to tissue injury.

Just like skeletal muscle fibers, smooth muscle cells have thick myosin-containing filaments and thin actin-containing filaments. Although tropomyosin is present in the thin filaments, the regulatory protein troponin is absent. A protein called **caldesmon** also associates with the thin filaments; in some types of muscle, it may play a role in regulating contraction. The thin filaments are anchored either to the plasma membrane or to cytoplasmic structures known as **dense bodies,** which are functionally similar to the Z lines in skeletal muscle fibers. Note in **Figure 9.33** that the filaments are oriented diagonally to the long axis of the cell. When the fiber shortens, the regions of the plasma membrane between the points where actin is attached to the membrane balloon out. The thick and thin filaments are not organized into myofibrils, as in striated muscles, and there is no regular alignment of these filaments into sarcomeres, which accounts for the absence of a banding pattern. Nevertheless, smooth muscle contraction occurs by a sliding-filament mechanism.

The concentration of myosin in smooth muscle is only about one-third of that in striated muscle, whereas the actin content can be twice as great. In spite of these differences, the maximal tension per unit of cross-sectional area developed by smooth muscles is similar to that developed by skeletal muscle.

The isometric tension produced by smooth muscle fibers varies with fiber length in a manner qualitatively similar to that observed in skeletal muscle—tension development is highest at intermediate lengths and lower at shorter or longer lengths. However, in smooth muscle, significant force is generated over a relatively broad range of muscle lengths compared to that of skeletal muscle. This property is highly adaptive because most smooth muscles surround hollow structures and organs that undergo changes in volume with accompanying changes in the lengths of the smooth muscle fibers in their walls. Even with relatively large increases in volume, as during the accumulation of large amounts of urine in the bladder, the smooth muscle fibers in the wall retain some ability to develop tension, whereas such distortion might stretch skeletal muscle fibers beyond the point of thick and thin filament overlap.

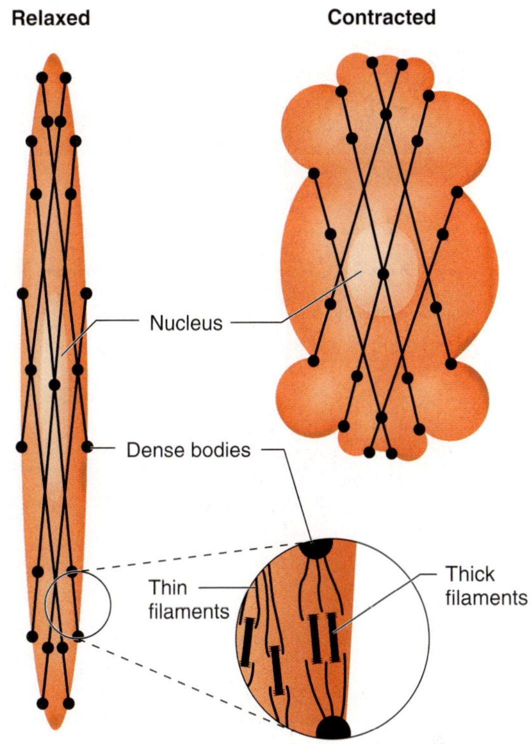

Figure 9.33 APIR Thick and thin filaments in smooth muscle are arranged in diagonal chains that are anchored to the plasma membrane or to dense bodies within the cytoplasm. When activated, the thick and thin filaments slide past each other, causing the smooth muscle fiber to shorten and thicken.

9.9 Smooth Muscle Contraction and Its Control

Changes in cytosolic Ca^{2+} concentration control the contractile activity in smooth muscle fibers, as in striated muscle. However, there are significant differences in the way Ca^{2+} activates cross-bridge cycling and in the mechanisms by which stimulation leads to alterations in Ca^{2+} concentration.

Cross-Bridge Activation

Because smooth muscle lacks the Ca^{2+}-binding protein troponin, tropomyosin is never held in a position that blocks cross-bridge access to actin. Thus, the thin filament is not the main switch that regulates cross-bridge cycling. *Instead, cross-bridge cycling in smooth muscle is controlled by a Ca^{2+}-regulated enzyme that phosphorylates myosin.* Only the phosphorylated form of smooth muscle myosin can bind to actin and undergo cross-bridge cycling.

The following sequence of events occurs after an increase in cytosolic Ca^{2+} in a smooth muscle fiber (**Figure 9.34**): (1) Ca^{2+} binds to calmodulin, a Ca^{2+}-binding protein that is present in the cytosol of most cells (see Chapter 5) and whose structure is related to that of troponin. (2) The Ca^{2+}–calmodulin complex binds to another cytosolic protein, **myosin light-chain kinase,** thereby activating the enzyme. (3) Active myosin light-chain kinase then uses ATP to phosphorylate myosin light chains in the globular head of myosin. (4) Phosphorylation of myosin drives the cross-bridge away from the thick filament backbone, allowing it to bind to actin.

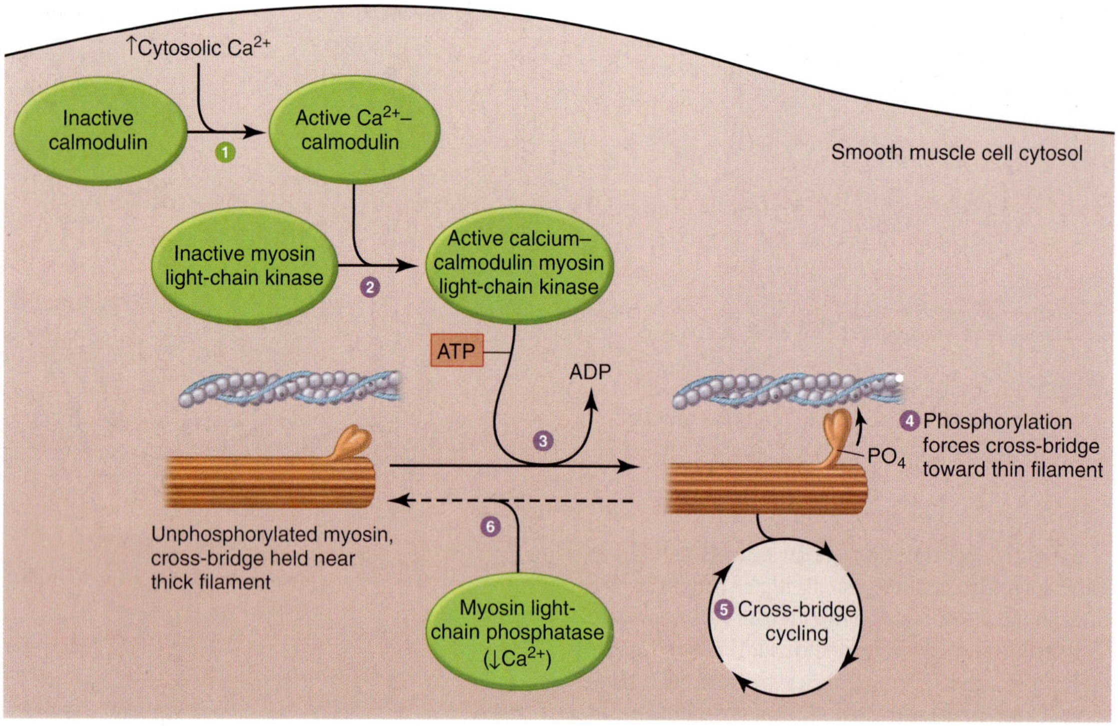

Figure 9.34 Activation of smooth muscle contraction by Ca^{2+}. See text for description of the numbered steps.

(5) Cross-bridges go through repeated cycles of force generation as long as myosin light chains are phosphorylated. A key difference here is that Ca^{2+}-mediated changes in the thick filaments turn on cross-bridge activity in smooth muscle, whereas in striated muscle, Ca^{2+} mediates changes in the thin filaments. However, recent research suggests that in some types of smooth muscle there may also be some Ca^{2+}-dependent regulation of the thin filament mediated by the protein caldesmon.

The smooth muscle form of myosin has a very low rate of ATPase activity, on the order of 10 to 100 times less than that of skeletal muscle myosin. Because the rate of ATP hydrolysis determines the rate of cross-bridge cycling and shortening velocity, smooth muscle shortening is much slower than that of skeletal muscle. Due to this slow rate of energy usage, smooth muscle does not undergo fatigue during prolonged periods of activity. Note the distinction between the two roles of ATP in smooth muscle: Hydrolyzing one ATP to transfer a phosphate onto a myosin light chain (*phosphorylation*) starts a cross-bridge cycling, after which one ATP per cycle is hydrolyzed to provide the energy for force generation.

To relax a contracted smooth muscle, myosin must be dephosphorylated because dephosphorylated myosin is unable to bind to actin. This dephosphorylation is mediated by the enzyme **myosin light-chain phosphatase,** which is continuously active in smooth muscle during periods of rest and contraction (step 6 in Figure 9.34). When cytosolic Ca^{2+} concentration increases, the rate of myosin phosphorylation by the activated kinase exceeds the rate of dephosphorylation by the phosphatase and the amount of phosphorylated myosin in the cell increases, producing an increase in tension. When the cytosolic Ca^{2+} concentration decreases, the rate of phosphorylation decreases below that of dephosphorylation and the amount of phosphorylated myosin decreases, producing relaxation.

In some smooth muscles, when stimulation is persistent and the cytosolic Ca^{2+} concentration remains elevated, the rate of ATP hydrolysis by the cross-bridges declines even though isometric tension is maintained. This condition is known as the **latch state** and a smooth muscle in this state can maintain tension in an almost rigorlike state without movement. Dissociation of cross-bridges from actin does occur in the latch state, but at a much slower rate. The net result is the ability to maintain tension for long periods of time with a very low rate of ATP consumption. A good example of the usefulness of this mechanism is seen in sphincter muscles of the gastrointestinal tract, where smooth muscle must maintain contraction for prolonged periods. **Figure 9.35** compares the activation of smooth and skeletal muscles.

Sources of Cytosolic Ca^{2+}

Two sources of Ca^{2+} contribute to the increase in cytosolic Ca^{2+} that initiates smooth muscle contraction: (1) the sarcoplasmic reticulum and (2) extracellular Ca^{2+} entering the cell through plasma membrane Ca^{2+} channels. The amount of Ca^{2+} each of these two sources contributes differs among various smooth muscles.

First, we will examine the role of the sarcoplasmic reticulum. The total quantity of this organelle in smooth muscle is smaller than in skeletal muscle, and it is not arranged in any specific pattern in relation to the thick and thin filaments. Moreover, there are no T-tubules continuous with the plasma membrane in smooth muscle. The small cell diameter and the slow rate of contraction do not require such a rapid mechanism for getting an excitatory signal into the muscle cell. Portions of the sarcoplasmic reticulum are located near the plasma membrane, however, forming associations similar to the relationship between T-tubules and the terminal cisternae

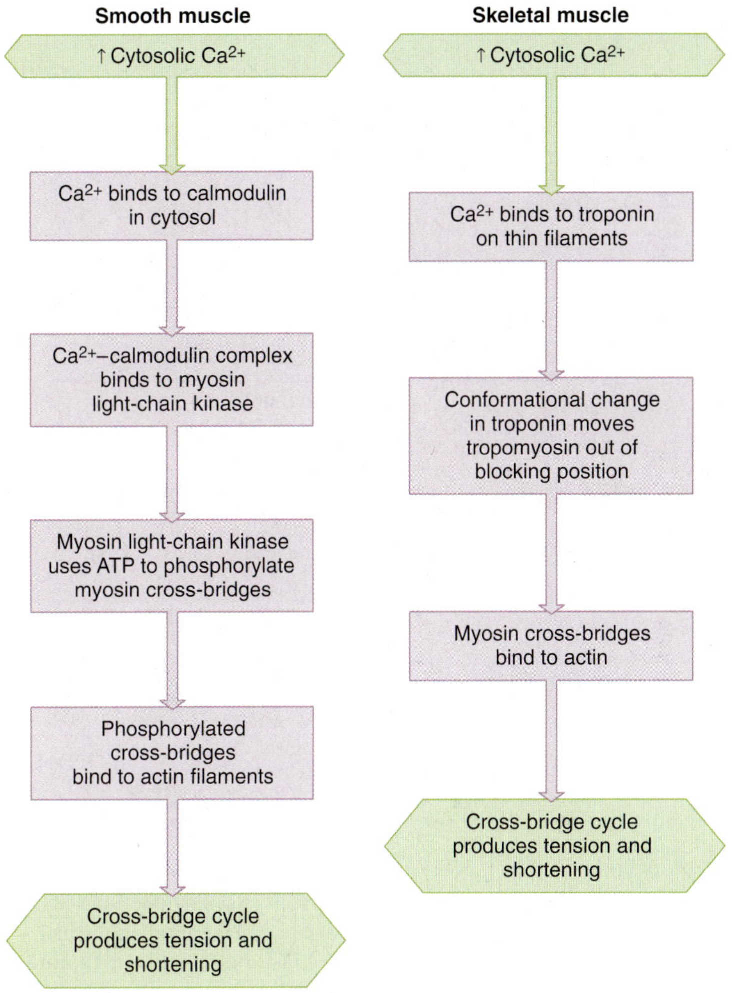

Figure 9.35 Pathways leading from increased cytosolic Ca^{2+} to cross-bridge cycling in smooth and skeletal muscle fibers.

in skeletal muscle. Action potentials in the plasma membrane can be coupled to the release of sarcoplasmic reticulum Ca^{2+} at these sites. In some types of smooth muscles, action potentials are not necessary for Ca^{2+} release. Instead, second messengers released from the plasma membrane, or generated in the cytosol in response to the binding of extracellular chemical messengers to plasma membrane receptors, can trigger the release of Ca^{2+} from the more centrally located sarcoplasmic reticulum (review Figure 5.10 for a specific example).

What about extracellular Ca^{2+} in excitation–contraction coupling? There are voltage-sensitive Ca^{2+} channels in the plasma membranes of smooth muscle cells, as well as Ca^{2+} channels controlled by extracellular chemical messengers. The Ca^{2+} concentration in the extracellular fluid is 10,000 times greater than in the cytosol; thus, the opening of Ca^{2+} channels in the plasma membrane results in an increased flow of Ca^{2+} into the cell. Because of the small cell size, the entering Ca^{2+} does not have far to diffuse to reach binding sites within the cell.

Removal of Ca^{2+} from the cytosol to bring about relaxation is achieved by the active transport of Ca^{2+} back into the sarcoplasmic reticulum as well as out of the cell across the plasma membrane. The rate of Ca^{2+} removal in smooth muscle is much slower than in skeletal muscle, with the result that a single twitch lasts several seconds in smooth muscle compared to a fraction of a second in skeletal muscle.

The degree of activation also differs between muscle types. In skeletal muscle, a single action potential releases sufficient Ca^{2+} to saturate all troponin sites on the thin filaments, whereas only a portion of the cross-bridges are activated in a smooth muscle fiber in response to most stimuli. Therefore, the tension generated by a smooth muscle cell can be *graded* by varying cytosolic Ca^{2+} concentration. The greater the increase in Ca^{2+} concentration, the greater the number of cross-bridges activated and the greater the tension.

In some smooth muscles, the cytosolic Ca^{2+} concentration is sufficient to maintain a low level of basal cross-bridge activity in the absence of external stimuli. This activity is known as **smooth muscle tone.** Factors that alter the cytosolic Ca^{2+} concentration also vary the intensity of smooth muscle tone.

Membrane Activation

Many inputs to a smooth muscle plasma membrane can alter the contractile activity of the muscle (**Table 9.5**). This contrasts with skeletal muscle, in which membrane activation depends only upon synaptic inputs from somatic neurons. Some inputs to smooth muscle increase contraction, and others inhibit it. Moreover, at any one time, the smooth muscle plasma membrane may be receiving multiple inputs, with the contractile state of the muscle dependent on the relative intensity of the various inhibitory and excitatory stimuli. All these inputs influence contractile activity by altering cytosolic Ca^{2+} concentration as described in the previous section.

Some smooth muscles contract in response to membrane depolarization, whereas others can contract in the absence of any membrane potential change. Interestingly, in smooth muscles in which action potentials occur, calcium ions, rather than sodium ions, carry a positive charge into the cell during the rising phase of the action potential—that is, depolarization of the membrane opens voltage-gated Ca^{2+} channels, producing Ca^{2+}-mediated rather than Na^{+}-mediated action potentials.

Smooth muscle is different from skeletal muscle in another important way with regard to electrical activity and cytosolic Ca^{2+} concentration. Smooth muscle cytosolic Ca^{2+} concentration can be increased (or decreased) by graded depolarizations (or hyperpolarizations) in membrane potential, which increase or decrease the number of open Ca^{2+} channels.

TABLE 9.5 Inputs Influencing Smooth Muscle Contractile Activity
Spontaneous electrical activity in the plasma membrane of the muscle cell
Neurotransmitters released by autonomic neurons
Hormones
Locally induced changes in the chemical composition (paracrine factors, acidity, oxygen, osmolarity, and ion concentrations) of the extracellular fluid surrounding the cell
Stretch

Spontaneous Electrical Activity

Some types of smooth muscle cells generate action potentials spontaneously in the absence of any neural or hormonal input. The plasma membranes of such cells do not maintain a constant resting potential. Instead, they gradually depolarize until they reach the threshold potential and produce an action potential. Following repolarization, the membrane again begins to depolarize (**Figure 9.36a**), so that a sequence of action potentials occurs, producing a rhythmic state of contractile activity. The membrane potential change occurring during the spontaneous depolarization to threshold is known as a **pacemaker potential.**

Other smooth muscle pacemaker cells have a slightly different pattern of activity. The membrane potential drifts up and down due to regular variation in ion flux across the membrane. These periodic fluctuations are called **slow waves** (**Figure 9.36b**). When an excitatory input is superimposed, slow waves are depolarized above threshold, and action potentials lead to smooth muscle contraction.

Pacemaker cells are found throughout the gastrointestinal tract; thus, gut smooth muscle tends to contract rhythmically even in the absence of neural input. Some cardiac muscle cells and some neurons in the central nervous system also have pacemaker potentials and can spontaneously generate action potentials in the absence of external stimuli.

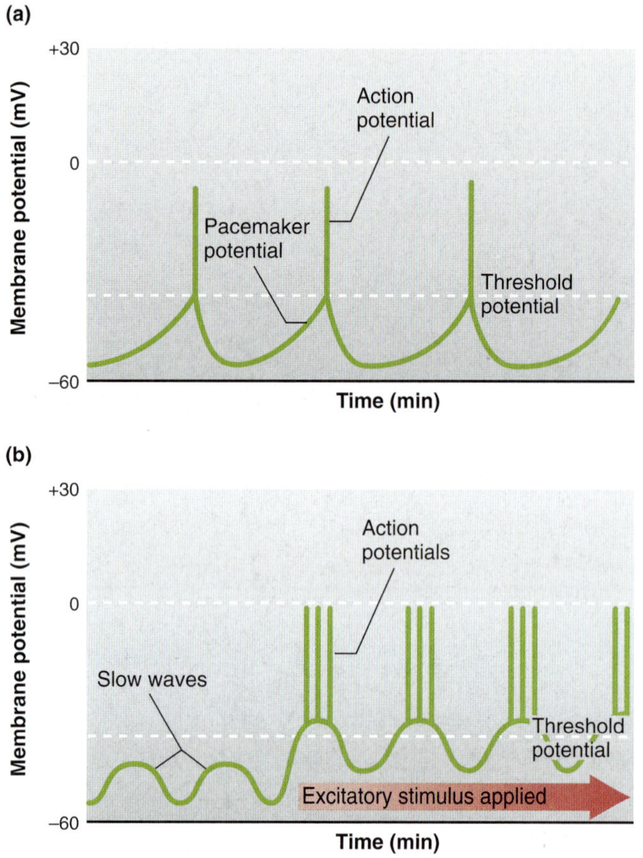

Figure 9.36 Generation of action potentials in smooth muscle fibers. (a) Some smooth muscle cells have pacemaker potentials that drift to threshold at regular intervals. (b) Pacemaker cells with a slow-wave pattern drift periodically toward threshold; excitatory stimuli can depolarize the cell to reach threshold and fire action potentials.

Nerves and Hormones

The contractile activity of smooth muscles is influenced by neurotransmitters released by autonomic neuron endings. Unlike skeletal muscle fibers, smooth muscle cells do not have a specialized motor end-plate region. As the axon of a postganglionic autonomic neuron enters the region of smooth muscle cells, it divides into many branches, each branch containing a series of swollen regions known as **varicosities** (**Figure 9.37**). Each varicosity contains many vesicles filled with neurotransmitter, some of which are released when an action potential passes the varicosity. Varicosities from a single axon may be located along several muscle cells, and a single muscle cell may be located near varicosities belonging to postganglionic fibers of both sympathetic and parasympathetic neurons. Therefore, a number of smooth muscle cells are influenced by the neurotransmitters released by a single neuron, and a single smooth muscle cell may be influenced by neurotransmitters from more than one neuron.

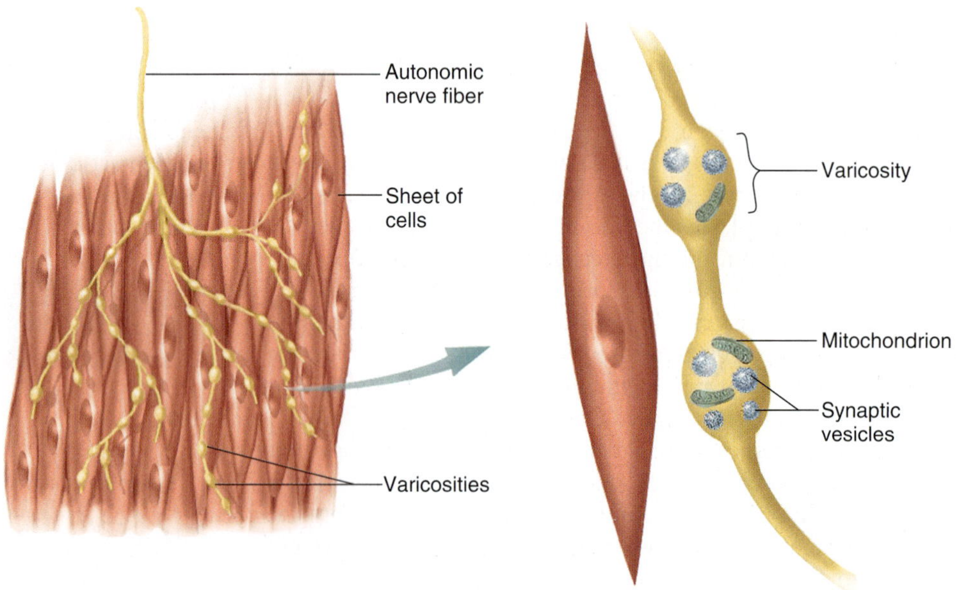

Figure 9.37 Innervation of smooth muscle by a postganglionic autonomic neuron. Neurotransmitter, released from varicosities along the branched axon, diffuses to receptors on muscle cell plasma membranes. Both sympathetic and parasympathetic neurons follow this pattern, often overlapping in their distribution. Note that the size of the varicosities is exaggerated compared to the cell at right.

Whereas some neurotransmitters enhance contractile activity, others decrease contractile activity. This is different than in skeletal muscle, which receives only excitatory input from its motor neurons; smooth muscle tension can be either increased or decreased by neural activity.

Moreover, a given neurotransmitter may produce opposite effects in different smooth muscle tissues. For example, norepinephrine, the neurotransmitter released from most postganglionic sympathetic neurons, enhances contraction of most vascular smooth muscle by acting on α-adrenergic receptors. By contrast, the same neurotransmitter produces relaxation of airway (bronchiolar) smooth muscle by acting on β_2-adrenergic receptors. Thus, the type of response (excitatory or inhibitory) depends not on the chemical messenger, per se, but on the receptors the chemical messenger binds to in the membrane and on the intracellular signaling mechanisms those receptors activate.

In addition to receptors for neurotransmitters, smooth muscle plasma membranes contain receptors for a variety of hormones. Binding of a hormone to its receptor may lead to either increased or decreased contractile activity.

Although most changes in smooth muscle contractile activity induced by chemical messengers are accompanied by a change in membrane potential, this is not always the case. Second messengers—for example, inositol trisphosphate—can cause the release of Ca^{2+} from the sarcoplasmic reticulum, producing a contraction without a change in membrane potential (review Figure 5.10).

Local Factors

Local factors, including paracrine signals, acidity, oxygen and carbon dioxide concentration, osmolarity, and the ionic composition of the extracellular fluid, can also alter smooth muscle tension. Responses to local factors provide a means for altering smooth muscle contraction in response to changes in the muscle's immediate internal environment, which can lead to regulation that is independent of long-distance signals from nerves and hormones.

Many of these local factors induce smooth muscle relaxation. Nitric oxide (NO) is one of the most commonly encountered paracrine compounds that produce smooth muscle relaxation. NO is released from some axon terminals as well as from a variety of epithelial and endothelial cells. Because of the short life span of this reactive molecule, it acts in a paracrine manner, influencing only those cells that are very near its release site.

Some smooth muscles can also respond by contracting when they are stretched. Stretching opens mechanically gated ion channels, leading to membrane depolarization. The resulting contraction opposes the forces acting to stretch the muscle.

At any given moment, smooth muscle cells in the body receive many simultaneous signals. The state of contractile activity that results depends on the net magnitude of the signals promoting contraction versus those promoting relaxation. This is a classic example of the general principle of physiology that most physiological functions are controlled by multiple regulatory systems, often working in opposition.

Types of Smooth Muscle

The great diversity of the factors that can influence the contractile activity of smooth muscles in various organs has made it difficult to classify smooth muscle fibers. Many smooth muscles can be placed, however, into one of two groups, based on the electrical characteristics of their plasma membrane: **single-unit smooth muscles** and **multiunit smooth muscles.**

Single-Unit Smooth Muscle

The muscle cells in a single-unit smooth muscle undergo synchronous activity, both electrical and mechanical; that is, the whole muscle responds to stimulation as a single unit. This occurs because each muscle cell is linked to adjacent fibers by gap junctions, which allow action potentials occurring in one cell to propagate to other cells by local currents. Therefore, electrical activity occurring anywhere within a group of single-unit smooth muscle cells can be conducted to all the other connected cells (**Figure 9.38**).

Some of the cells in a single-unit muscle are pacemaker cells that spontaneously generate action potentials. These action potentials are conducted by way of gap junctions to the rest of the cells, most of which are not capable of pacemaker activity.

Nerves, hormones, and local factors can alter the contractile activity of single-unit smooth muscles using the variety of mechanisms described previously for smooth muscles in general. The extent to which these muscles are innervated varies considerably in different organs. The axon terminals are often restricted to the regions of the muscle that contain pacemaker cells. The activity of the entire muscle can be controlled by regulating the frequency of the pacemaker cells' action potentials.

One additional characteristic of single-unit smooth muscles is that a contractile response can often be induced by stretching the muscle. In several hollow organs—the stomach, for example—stretching the smooth muscles in the walls of the organ as a result of increases in the volume of material in the lumen initiates a contractile response.

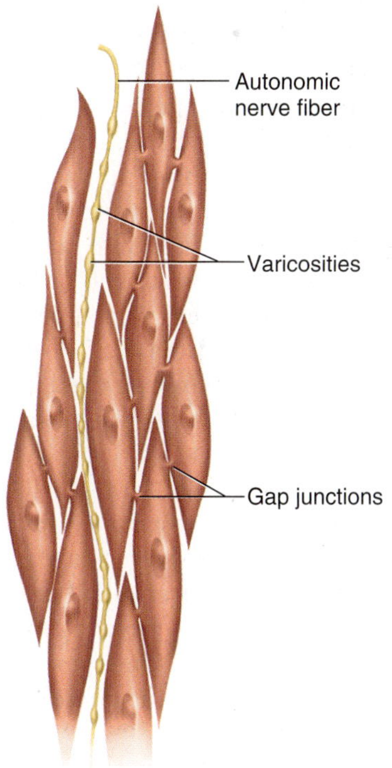

Figure 9.38 Innervation of a single-unit smooth muscle is often restricted to only a few cells in the muscle. Electrical activity is conducted from cell to cell throughout the muscle by way of the gap junctions between the cells.

The smooth muscles of the intestinal tract, uterus, and small-diameter blood vessels are examples of single-unit smooth muscles.

Multiunit Smooth Muscle

Multiunit smooth muscles have no or few gap junctions. Each cell responds independently, and the muscle behaves as multiple units. Multiunit smooth muscles are richly innervated by branches of the autonomic nervous system. The contractile response of the whole muscle depends on the number of muscle cells that are activated and on the frequency of nerve stimulation. Although stimulation of the muscle by neurons leads to some degree of depolarization and a contractile response, action potentials do not occur in most multiunit smooth muscles. Circulating hormones can increase or decrease contractile activity in multiunit smooth muscle, but stretching does not induce contraction in this type of muscle. The smooth muscles in the large airways to the lungs, in large arteries, and attached to the hairs in the skin are multiunit smooth muscles.

It must be emphasized that most smooth muscles do not show all the characteristics of either single-unit or multiunit smooth muscles. These two prototypes represent the two extremes in smooth muscle characteristics, with many smooth muscles having overlapping characteristics.

9.10 Cardiac Muscle

The third general type of muscle, cardiac muscle, is found only in the heart. Although many details about cardiac muscle will be discussed in the context of the cardiovascular system in Chapter 12, a brief explanation of its function and how it compares to skeletal and smooth muscle is presented here.

Cellular Structure of Cardiac Muscle

Cardiac muscle combines properties of both skeletal and smooth muscle. Like skeletal muscle, it has a striated appearance due to regularly repeating sarcomeres composed of myosin-containing thick filaments interdigitating with thin filaments that contain actin. Troponin and tropomyosin are also present in the thin filament, and they have the same functions as in skeletal muscle. Cellular membranes include a T-tubule system and associated Ca^{2+}-loaded sarcoplasmic reticulum. The mechanism by which these membranes interact to release Ca^{2+} is different than in skeletal muscle, however, as will be discussed shortly.

Like smooth muscle cells, individual cardiac muscle cells are relatively small (100 μm long and 20 μm in diameter) and generally contain a single nucleus. Adjacent cells are joined end to end at structures called **intercalated disks,** within which are desmosomes (see Figure 3.9) that hold the cells together and to which the myofibrils are attached (**Figure 9.39**). Also found within the intercalated disks are gap junctions similar to those found in single-unit smooth muscle. Cardiac muscle cells also are arranged in layers and surround hollow cavities—in this case, the blood-filled chambers of the heart. When muscle in the walls of cardiac chambers contracts, it acts like a squeezing fist and exerts pressure on the blood inside.

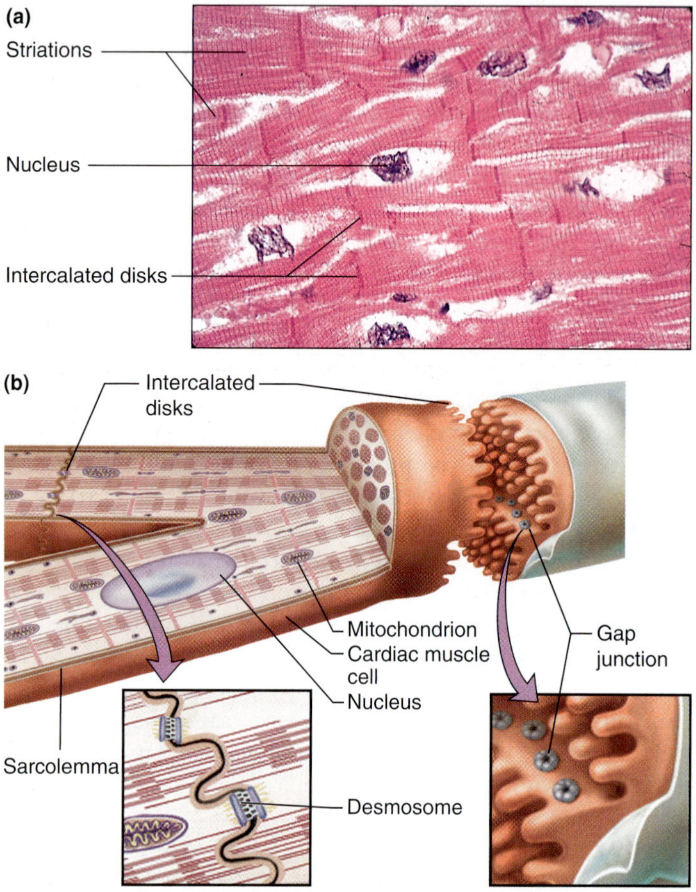

Figure 9.39 APIR Cardiac muscle. (a) Light micrograph. (b) Cardiac muscle cells and intercalated disks.

Excitation–Contraction Coupling in Cardiac Muscle

As in skeletal muscle, contraction of cardiac muscle cells occurs in response to a membrane action potential that propagates through the T-tubules, but the mechanisms linking that excitation to the generation of force exhibit features of both skeletal and smooth muscles (**Figure 9.40**). Depolarization during cardiac muscle cell action potentials is in part due to an influx of Ca^{2+} through specialized voltage-gated channels. These Ca^{2+} channels are known as **L-type Ca^{2+} channels** (named for their Long-lasting current) and are modified versions of the dihydropyridine (DHP) receptors that act as the voltage sensor in skeletal muscle cell excitation–contraction coupling. Not only does this entering Ca^{2+} participate in depolarization of the plasma membrane and cause a small increase in cytosolic Ca^{2+} concentration, but it also serves as a trigger for the release of a much larger amount of Ca^{2+} from the sarcoplasmic reticulum. This occurs because ryanodine receptors in the cardiac sarcoplasmic reticulum terminal cisternae are Ca^{2+} channels; but rather than being opened directly by voltage as in skeletal muscle, they are opened by the binding of trigger Ca^{2+} in the cytosol. Once cytosolic Ca^{2+} is elevated, thin filament activation, cross-bridge cycling, and force generation occur by the same basic mechanisms described for skeletal muscle (review Figures 9.11 and 9.15).

Thus, even though most of the Ca^{2+} that initiates cardiac muscle contraction comes from the sarcoplasmic

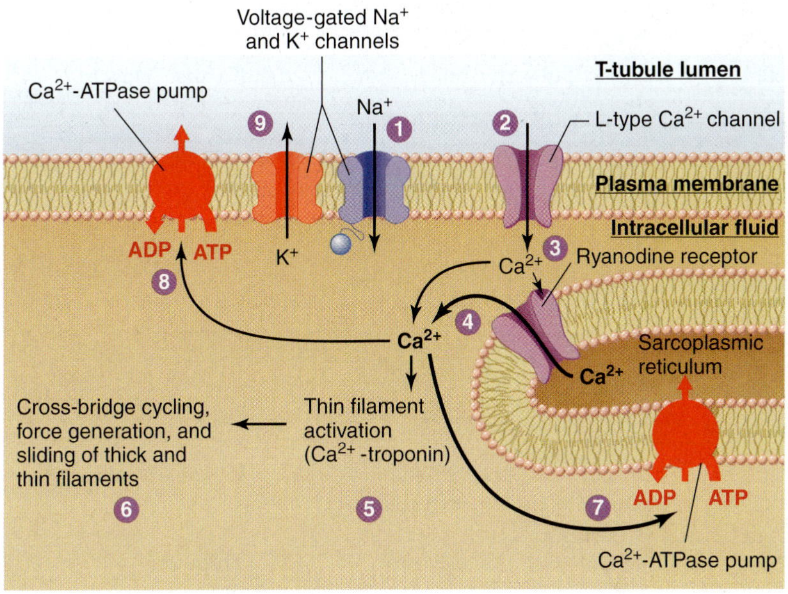

1. The membrane is depolarized by Na^+ entry as an action potential begins.
2. Depolarization opens L-type Ca^{2+} channels in the T-tubules.
3. A small amount of "trigger" Ca^{2+} enters the cytosol, contributing to cell depolarization. That trigger Ca^{2+} binds to, and opens, ryanodine receptor Ca^{2+} channels in the sarcoplasmic reticulum membrane.
4. Ca^{2+} flows into the cytosol, raising the Ca^{2+} concentration.
5. Binding of Ca^{2+} to troponin exposes cross-bridge binding sites on thin filaments.
6. Cross-bridge cycling causes force generation and sliding of thick and thin filaments.
7. Ca^{2+}-ATPase pumps return Ca^{2+} to the sarcoplasmic reticulum.
8. Ca^{2+}-ATPase pumps (and also Na^+/Ca^{2+} exchangers) remove Ca^{2+} from the cell.
9. The membrane is repolarized when K^+ exits to end the action potential.

Figure 9.40 Excitation–contraction coupling in cardiac muscle.

reticulum, the process—unlike that in skeletal muscle—is dependent on the movement of extracellular Ca^{2+} into the cytosol. Contraction ends when the cytosolic Ca^{2+} concentration is restored to its original extremely low resting value by primary active Ca^{2+}-ATPase pumps in the sarcoplasmic reticulum and sarcolemma and Na^+/Ca^{2+} countertransporters in the sarcolemma. The amount of Ca^{2+} returned to the extracellular fluid and into the sarcoplasmic reticulum exactly matches the amounts that entered the cytosol during excitation. During a single twitch contraction of cardiac muscle in a person at rest, the amount of Ca^{2+} entering the cytosol is only sufficient to expose about 30% of the cross-bridge attachment sites on the thin filament. As Chapter 12 will describe, however, hormones and neurotransmitters of the autonomic nervous system modulate the amount of Ca^{2+} released during excitation–contraction coupling, enabling the strength of cardiac muscle contractions to be varied. Cardiac muscle contractions are thus graded in a manner similar to that of smooth muscle contractions.

The prolonged duration of L-type Ca^{2+} channel current underlies an important feature of this muscle type—cardiac muscle cannot undergo tetanic contractions. Unlike skeletal muscle, in which the membrane action potential is extremely brief (1–2 msec) and force generation lasts much longer (20–100 msec), in cardiac muscle the action potential and twitch are both prolonged due to the long-lasting Ca^{2+} current (**Figure 9.41**). Because the plasma membrane remains refractory to additional stimuli as long as it is depolarized (review

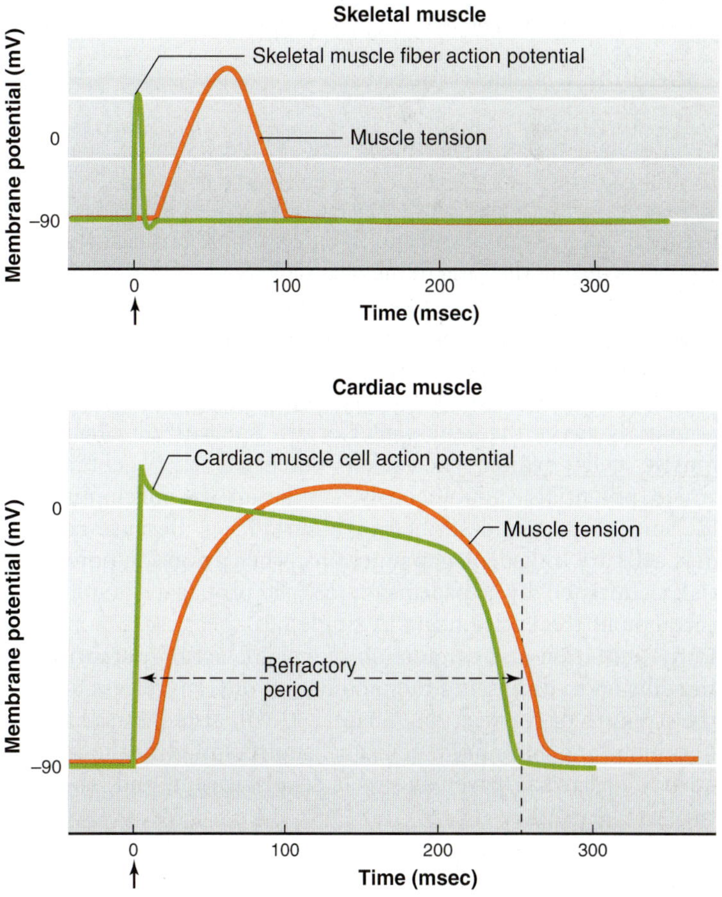

Figure 9.41 Timing of action potentials and twitch tension in skeletal and cardiac muscles. Muscle tension not drawn to scale.

PHYSIOLOGICAL INQUIRY

- The single-fiber twitch experiments shown here were generated by stimulating the muscle cell membranes to threshold with an electrode and measuring the resulting action potential and force. How would the results differ if Ca^{2+} were removed from the extracellular solution just before the electrical stimulus was applied?

Answer can be found at end of chapter.

TABLE 9.6 Characteristics of Muscle Cells

Characteristic	Skeletal Muscle	Smooth Muscle: Single Unit	Smooth Muscle: Multiunit	Cardiac Muscle
Thick and thin filaments	Yes	Yes	Yes	Yes
Sarcomeres—banding pattern	Yes	No	No	Yes
Transverse tubules	Yes	No	No	Yes
Sarcoplasmic reticulum (SR)*	++++	+	+	++
Gap junctions between cells	No	Yes	Few	Yes
Source of activating Ca^{2+}	SR	SR and extracellular	SR and extracellular	SR and extracellular
Site of Ca^{2+} regulation	Troponin	Myosin	Myosin	Troponin
Speed of contraction	Fast–slow	Very slow	Very slow	Slow
Spontaneous production of action potentials by pacemakers	No	Yes	No	Yes, in a few specialized cells, but most not spontaneously active
Tone (low levels of maintained tension in the absence of external stimuli)	No	Yes	No	No
Effect of nerve stimulation	Excitation	Excitation or inhibition	Excitation or inhibition	Excitation or inhibition
Physiological effects of hormones on excitability and contraction	No	Yes	Yes	Yes
Stretch of cell produces contraction	No	Yes	No	No

*Number of plus signs (+) indicates the relative amount of sarcoplasmic reticulum present in a given muscle type.

Figure 6.22), it is not possible to initiate multiple cardiac action potentials during the time frame of a single twitch. This is critical for the heart's function as an oscillating pump, because it must alternate between being relaxed—and filling with blood—and contracting to eject blood.

A final question to consider is, What initiates action potentials in cardiac muscle? Certain specialized cardiac muscle cells exhibit pacemaker potentials that generate action potentials spontaneously, similar to the mechanism for smooth muscle described in Figure 9.36a. Because cardiac cells are linked via gap junctions, when an action potential is initiated by a pacemaker cell, it propagates rapidly throughout the entire heart. A single heartbeat corresponds to the initiation and conduction of a single action potential. In addition to discussing the modulation of Ca^{2+} release and the strength of contraction, Chapter 12 will also discuss how hormones and autonomic neurotransmitters modify the frequency of cardiac pacemaker cell depolarization and, thus, vary the heart rate.

Table 9.6 summarizes and compares the properties of the different types of muscle.

SECTION B SUMMARY

Structure of Smooth Muscle

I. Smooth muscle cells are spindle-shaped, lack striations, have a single nucleus, and are capable of cell division. They contain actin and myosin filaments and contract by a sliding-filament mechanism.

Smooth Muscle Contraction and Its Control

I. An increase in cytosolic Ca^{2+} leads to the binding of Ca^{2+} by calmodulin. The Ca^{2+}–calmodulin complex then binds to myosin light-chain kinase, activating the enzyme, which uses ATP to phosphorylate smooth muscle myosin. Only phosphorylated myosin can bind to actin and undergo cross-bridge cycling.

II. Smooth muscle myosin has a low rate of ATP splitting, resulting in a much slower shortening velocity than in striated muscle. However, the tension produced per unit cross-sectional area is equivalent to that of skeletal muscle.

III. Two sources of the cytosolic calcium ions that initiate smooth muscle contraction are the sarcoplasmic reticulum and extracellular Ca^{2+}. The opening of Ca^{2+} channels in the smooth muscle plasma membrane and sarcoplasmic reticulum, mediated by a variety of factors, allows calcium ions to enter the cytosol.

IV. The increase in cytosolic Ca^{2+} resulting from most stimuli does not activate all the cross-bridges. Therefore, smooth muscle tension can be increased by agents that increase the concentration of cytosolic calcium ions.

V. Table 9.5 summarizes the types of stimuli that can initiate smooth muscle contraction by opening or closing Ca^{2+} channels in the plasma membrane or sarcoplasmic reticulum.

VI. Most, but not all, smooth muscle cells can generate action potentials in their plasma membrane upon membrane depolarization. The rising phase of the smooth muscle action potential is due to the influx of calcium ions into the cell through voltage-gated Ca^{2+} channels.

VII. Some smooth muscles generate action potentials spontaneously, in the absence of any external input, because of pacemaker potentials in the plasma membrane that repeatedly depolarize the membrane to threshold. Slow waves are a pattern of spontaneous, periodic depolarization of the membrane potential seen in some smooth muscle pacemaker cells.

VIII. Smooth muscle cells do not have a specialized end-plate region. A number of smooth muscle cells may be influenced by neurotransmitters released from the varicosities on a single nerve ending, and a single smooth muscle cell may be influenced by neurotransmitters from more than one neuron. Neurotransmitters may have either excitatory or inhibitory effects on smooth muscle contraction.

IX. Smooth muscles can be classified broadly as single-unit or multiunit smooth muscles.

Cardiac Muscle

I. Cardiac muscle combines features of skeletal and smooth muscles. Like skeletal muscle, it is striated, is composed of myofibrils with repeating sarcomeres, has troponin in its thin filaments, has T-tubules that conduct action potentials, and has sarcoplasmic reticulum terminal cisternae that store Ca^{2+}. Like smooth muscle, cardiac muscle cells are small and single-nucleated, arranged in layers around hollow cavities, and connected by gap junctions.

II. Cardiac muscle excitation–contraction coupling involves entry of a small amount of Ca^{2+} through L-type Ca^{2+} channels, which triggers opening of ryanodine receptors that release a larger amount of Ca^{2+} from the sarcoplasmic reticulum. Ca^{2+} activates the thin filament and cross-bridge cycling as in skeletal muscle.

III. Cardiac contractions and action potentials are prolonged, tetany does not occur, and both the strength and frequency of contraction are modulated by autonomic neurotransmitters and hormones.

IV. Table 9.6 summarizes and compares the features of skeletal, smooth, and cardiac muscles.

SECTION B REVIEW QUESTIONS

1. How does the organization of thick and thin filaments in smooth muscle fibers differ from that in striated muscle fibers?
2. Compare the mechanisms by which an increase in cytosolic Ca^{2+} concentration initiates contractile activity in skeletal, smooth, and cardiac muscle cells.
3. What are the two sources of Ca^{2+} that lead to the increase in cytosolic Ca^{2+} that triggers contraction in smooth muscle?
4. What types of stimuli can trigger an increase in cytosolic Ca^{2+} in smooth muscle cells?
5. What effect does a pacemaker potential have on a smooth muscle cell?
6. In what ways does the neural control of smooth muscle activity differ from that of skeletal muscle?
7. Describe how a stimulus may lead to the contraction of a smooth muscle cell without a change in the plasma membrane potential.
8. Describe the differences between single-unit and multiunit smooth muscles.
9. Compare and contrast the physiology of cardiac muscle with that of skeletal and smooth muscles.
10. Explain why cardiac muscle cannot undergo tetanic contractions.

SECTION B KEY TERMS

caldesmon 287
dense body 287
intercalated disk 292
latch state 288
L-type Ca^{2+} channel 292
multiunit smooth muscle 291
myosin light-chain kinase 287
myosin light-chain phosphatase 288
pacemaker potential 290
single-unit smooth muscle 291
slow waves 290
smooth muscle tone 289
varicosity 290

CHAPTER 9

Clinical Case Study: A Dangerous Increase in Body Temperature in a Boy During Surgery

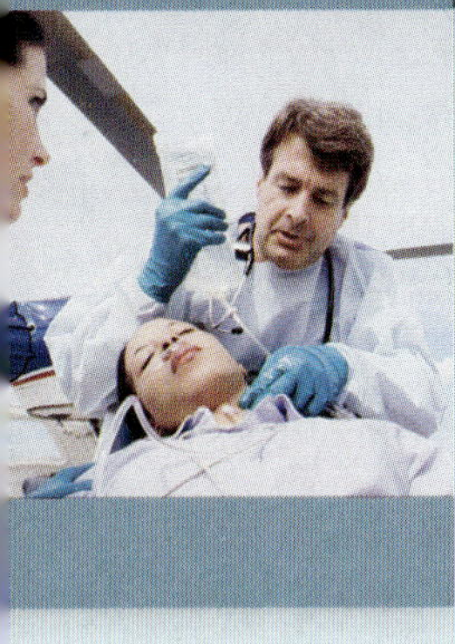

A 17-year-old boy lay on an operating table undergoing a procedure to repair a fractured jaw. In addition to receiving the local anesthetic ***lidocaine*** (which blocks voltage-gated Na^{+} channels and therefore action potential propagation), he was breathing ***sevofluorane,*** an inhaled general anesthetic that induces unconsciousness. An hour into the procedure, the anesthesiologist suddenly noticed that the patient's face was red and beads of sweat were forming on his forehead. The patient's monitors revealed that his heart rate had almost doubled since the beginning of the procedure and that there had been significant increases in his body temperature and in the carbon dioxide concentration in his exhaled breath. The oral surgeon reported that the patient's jaw muscles had gone rigid. The patient was exhibiting all of the signs of a rare but deadly condition called ***malignant hyperthermia,*** and quick action would be required to save his life.

(continued)

(continued)

Most patients who suffer from malignant hyperthermia inherit an autosomal dominant mutation of a gene found on chromosome 19. This gene encodes the ryanodine receptors—the ion channels involved in releasing calcium ions from the sarcoplasmic reticulum in skeletal muscle. Although the channels function normally under most circumstances, they malfunction when exposed to some types of inhalant anesthetics or to drugs that depolarize and block skeletal muscle neuromuscular junctions (like succinylcholine). In some cases, the malfunction does not occur until the second exposure to the triggering agent.

The mechanism of malignant hyperthermia involves an excessive opening of the ryanodine receptor channel, with massive release of Ca^{2+} from the sarcoplasmic reticulum into the cytosol of skeletal muscle cells. The rate of Ca^{2+} release is so great that sarcoplasmic reticulum Ca^{2+}-ATPase pumps are unable to work fast enough to re-sequester it. The excess Ca^{2+} results in persistent activation of cross-bridge cycling and muscle contraction and also stimulates Ca^{2+}-activated proteases that degrade muscle proteins. The metabolism of ATP by muscle cells is increased enormously during an episode, with a number of consequences, some of which will be discussed in greater detail in later chapters:

1. ATP is depleted, causing cross-bridges to enter the rigor state, and therefore muscle rigidity ensues.
2. Muscle cells must resort to anaerobic metabolism to produce ATP because oxygen cannot be delivered to muscles fast enough to maintain aerobic production of ATP, so patients develop lactic acidosis (acidified blood due to the buildup of lactic acid).
3. CO_2 production increases, generating carbonic acid that contributes to acidosis (see Chapter 13).
4. Muscles generate a tremendous amount of heat as a by-product of ATP breakdown and production, producing the hyperthermia characteristic of this condition.
5. The drive to maintain homeostasis of body temperature, pH, and oxygen and carbon dioxide levels triggers an increase in heart rate to support an increase in the rate of blood circulation (see Chapter 12).
6. Flushing of the skin and sweating occur to help dissipate excess heat (see Chapter 16).

The anesthesiologist immediately halted the surgical procedure, then substituted 100% oxygen for the sevofluorane in the boy's breathing tube. Providing a high concentration of inspired oxygen increases the blood oxygen delivery to help muscles reestablish aerobic ATP production. The patient was then hyperventilated to help rid the body of excess CO_2, and ice bags were placed on his body to keep his temperature from increasing further. He was also given multiple injections of dantrolene until his condition began to improve. ***Dantrolene,*** a drug originally developed as a muscle relaxant, blocks the flux of Ca^{2+} through the ryanodine receptor. Since its introduction as a treatment, the mortality rate from malignant hyperthermia has decreased from greater than 70% to approximately 5%.

The boy was transferred to the intensive care unit, and his condition was monitored closely. Laboratory tests showed elevated blood H^+, K^+, Ca^{2+}, creatine kinase, and myoglobin concentrations, all of which are released during the rapid breakdown of muscle tissue (***rhabdomyolysis***). Among the dangers faced by such patients are malfunction of cardiac and other excitable cells, from abnormal pH and electrolyte levels, and kidney failure resulting from the overwhelming load of waste products released from damaged muscle cells. Over the next several days, the boy's condition improved and his blood chemistries returned to normal. Because the recognition and reaction by the medical team had been swift, the boy only suffered from sore muscles for the next few weeks but had no lasting damage to vital organs.

Malignant hyperthermia has a relatively low incidence, about one in 15,000 children and one in 50,000 adults. Because of its potentially lethal nature, however, it has become common practice to assess a given patient's risk of developing the condition. Although definitive proof of malignant hyperthermia can be determined by taking a muscle biopsy and assessing its response to anesthetics, the test is invasive and only available in a few clinical laboratories, so it is not usually performed. Risk is more commonly assessed by taking a detailed history that includes whether the patient or a genetic relative has ever had an adverse reaction to anesthesia. Even if the family history is negative, surgical teams need to have dantrolene on hand and be prepared. Advances in our understanding of the genetic basis of this disease make it likely that a reliable genetic screening test for malignant hyperthermia will someday be available.

Clinical terms: dantrolene, lidocaine, malignant hyperthermia, rhabdomyolysis, sevofluorane

See Chapter 19 for complete, integrative case studies.

CHAPTER 9 TEST QUESTIONS

Answers found in Appendix A.

1. Which is a *false* statement about skeletal muscle structure?
   a. A myofibril is composed of multiple muscle fibers.
   b. Most skeletal muscles attach to bones by connective-tissue tendons.
   c. Each end of a thick filament is surrounded by six thin filaments.
   d. A cross-bridge is a portion of the myosin molecule.
   e. Thin filaments contain actin, tropomyosin, and troponin.
2. Which is correct regarding a skeletal muscle sarcomere?
   a. M lines are found in the center of the I band.
   b. The I band is the space between one Z line and the next.
   c. The H zone is the region where thick and thin filaments overlap.
   d. Z lines are found in the center of the A band.
   e. The width of the A band is equal to the length of a thick filament.

3. When a skeletal muscle fiber undergoes a concentric isotonic contraction,
   a. M lines remain the same distance apart.
   b. Z lines move closer to the ends of the A bands.
   c. A bands become shorter.
   d. I bands become wider.
   e. M lines move closer to the end of the A band.
4. During excitation–contraction coupling in a skeletal muscle fiber,
   a. the Ca^{2+}-ATPase pumps Ca^{2+} into the T-tubule.
   b. action potentials propagate along the membrane of the sarcoplasmic reticulum.
   c. Ca^{2+} floods the cytosol through the dihydropyridine (DHP) receptors.
   d. DHP receptors trigger the opening of terminal cisternae ryanodine receptor Ca^{2+} channels.
   e. acetylcholine opens the DHP receptor channel.
5. Why is the latent period longer during an isotonic twitch of a skeletal muscle fiber than it is during an isometric twitch?
   a. Excitation–contraction coupling is slower during an isotonic twitch.
   b. Action potentials propagate more slowly when the fiber is shortening, so extra time is required to activate the entire fiber.
   c. In addition to the time for excitation–contraction coupling, it takes extra time for enough cross-bridges to attach to make the tension in the muscle fiber greater than the load.
   d. Fatigue sets in much more quickly during isotonic contractions, and when muscles are fatigued the cross-bridges move much more slowly.
   e. The latent period is longer because isotonic twitches only occur in slow (type I) muscle fibers.
6. What prevents a drop in muscle fiber ATP concentration during the first few seconds of intense contraction?
   a. Because cross-bridges are pre-energized, ATP is not needed until several cross-bridge cycles have been completed.
   b. ADP is rapidly converted back to ATP by creatine phosphate.
   c. Glucose is metabolized in glycolysis, producing large quantities of ATP.
   d. The mitochondria immediately begin oxidative phosphorylation.
   e. Fatty acids are rapidly converted to ATP by oxidative glycolysis.
7. Which correctly characterizes a "fast-oxidative" type of skeletal muscle fiber?
   a. few mitochondria and high glycogen content
   b. low myosin ATPase rate and few surrounding capillaries
   c. low glycolytic enzyme activity and intermediate contraction velocity
   d. high myoglobin content and intermediate glycolytic enzyme activity
   e. small fiber diameter and fast onset of fatigue
8. Which is *false* regarding the structure of smooth muscle?
   a. The thin filament does not include the regulatory protein troponin.
   b. The thick and thin filaments are not organized in sarcomeres.
   c. Thick filaments are anchored to dense bodies instead of Z lines.
   d. The cells have a single nucleus.
   e. Single-unit smooth muscles have gap junctions connecting individual cells.
9. The role of myosin light-chain kinase in smooth muscle is to
   a. bind to calcium ions to initiate excitation–contraction coupling.
   b. phosphorylate cross-bridges, thus driving them to bind with the thin filament.
   c. split ATP to provide the energy for the power stroke of the cross-bridge cycle.
   d. dephosphorylate myosin light chains of the cross-bridge, thus relaxing the muscle.
   e. pump Ca^{2+} from the cytosol back into the sarcoplasmic reticulum.
10. Single-unit smooth muscle differs from multiunit smooth muscle because
    a. single-unit muscle contraction speed is slow, and multiunit is fast.
    b. single-unit muscle has T-tubules, and multiunit muscle does not.
    c. single-unit muscles are not innervated by autonomic nerves.
    d. single-unit muscle contracts when stretched, whereas multiunit muscle does not.
    e. single-unit muscle does not produce action potentials spontaneously, but multiunit muscle does.
11. Which of the following describes a similarity between cardiac and smooth muscle cells?
    a. An action potential always precedes contraction.
    b. The majority of the Ca^{2+} that activates contraction comes from the extracellular fluid.
    c. Action potentials are generated by slow waves.
    d. An extensive system of T-tubules is present.
    e. Ca^{2+} release and contraction strengths are graded.

CHAPTER 9 GENERAL PRINCIPLES ASSESSMENT

Answers found in Appendix A.

1. Some cardiac muscle cells are specialized to serve as pacemaker cells that generate action potentials at regular intervals. Stimulation by sympathetic neurotransmitters increases the frequency of action potentials generated, while parasympathetic stimulation reduces the frequency. Which of the general principles of physiology described in Chapter 1 does this best demonstrate?
2. A general principle of physiology states that *physiological processes are dictated by the laws of chemistry and physics.* The chemical law of mass action tells us that the rate of a chemical reaction will slow down when there is a buildup in concentration of products of the reaction. How can this principle be applied as a contributing factor in muscle fatigue?
3. Explain how the process of skeletal muscle excitation–contraction coupling demonstrates the general principle of physiology that *controlled exchange of materials occurs between compartments and across cellular membranes.*

CHAPTER 9 QUANTITATIVE AND THOUGHT QUESTIONS *Answers found at www.mhhe.com/widmaier13.*

1. Which of the following corresponds to the state of myosin (M) under resting conditions, and which corresponds to rigor mortis? (a) M · ATP (b) M · ADP · P_i (c) A · M · ADP · P_i (d) A · M
2. If the insertion of a person's biceps muscle is 3 cm from the elbow joint, and the center of her hand is 27 cm from the insertion of the biceps, how fast will her hand move when her biceps contracts at 2 m/sec?
3. When a small load is attached to a skeletal muscle that is then tetanically stimulated, the muscle lifts the load in an isotonic contraction over a certain distance but then stops shortening and enters a state of isometric contraction. With a heavier load, the distance shortened before entering an isometric contraction is shorter. Explain these shortening limits in terms of the length–tension relation of muscle.
4. What conditions will produce the maximum tension in a skeletal muscle fiber?
5. A skeletal muscle can often maintain a moderate level of active tension for long periods of time, even though many of its fibers become fatigued. Explain.
6. If the blood flow to a skeletal muscle were markedly decreased, which types of motor units would most rapidly undergo a severe reduction in their ability to produce ATP for muscle contraction? Why?
7. As a result of an automobile accident, 50% of the muscle fibers in the biceps muscle of a patient were destroyed. Ten months later, the biceps muscle was able to generate 80% of its original force. Describe the changes that took place in the damaged muscle that enabled it to recover.
8. In the laboratory, if an isolated skeletal muscle is placed in a solution that contains no calcium ions, will the muscle contract when it is stimulated (a) directly by depolarizing its membrane, or (b) by stimulating the nerve to the muscle? What would happen if it was a smooth muscle?
9. The following experiments were performed on a single-unit smooth muscle in the gastrointestinal tract.
   a. Stimulating the parasympathetic nerves to the muscle produced a contraction.
   b. Applying a drug that blocks the voltage-sensitive Na^+ channels in most plasma membranes led to a failure to contract upon stimulating the parasympathetic nerves.
   c. Applying a drug that blocks muscarinic ACh receptors (see Chapter 6) did not prevent the muscle from contracting when the parasympathetic nerve was stimulated.

   From these observations, what might you conclude about the mechanism by which parasympathetic nerve stimulation produces a contraction of the smooth muscle?
10. Some endocrine tumors secrete a hormone that leads to elevation of extracellular fluid Ca^{2+} concentrations. How might this affect cardiac muscle?
11. If a single twitch of a skeletal muscle fiber lasts 40 msec, what action potential stimulation frequency (in action potentials per second) must be exceeded to produce an unfused tetanus?

CHAPTER 9 ANSWERS TO PHYSIOLOGICAL INQUIRIES

Figure 9.5

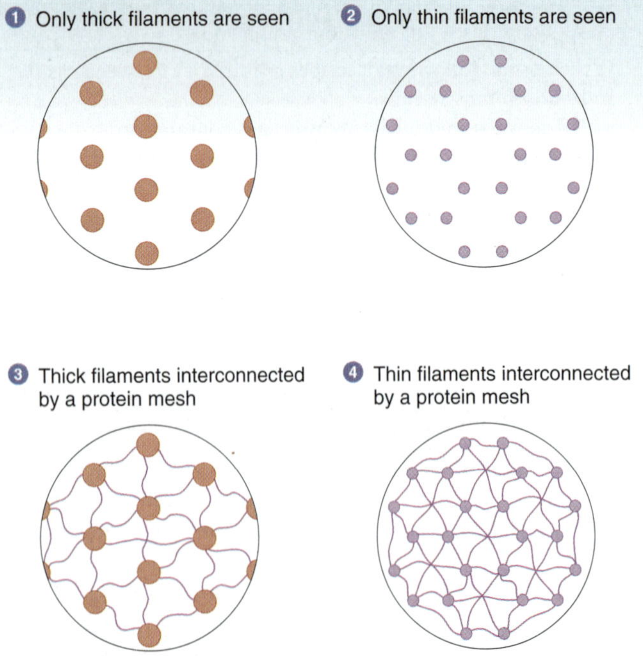

Figure 9.9 Na^+ current dominates when the ACh channels open because it has both a large inward diffusion gradient and, at the muscle cell's resting membrane potential, a large inward electrical gradient. Although the diffusion gradient for K^+ to leave the cell is large, the electrical gradient actually opposes its movement out of the cell. See Figure 6.12.

Figure 9.10 Tension takes longer to return to resting levels because all of the cross-bridges that attached to actin when Ca^{2+} was elevated require time to complete their power stroke and detach from actin.

Figure 9.14 Changes in the width of the I bands and H zone would be the same, but the sarcomeres would not slide toward the fixed Z line at the right side of the diagram. They would shorten uniformly and pull both of the outer Z lines toward the center one.

Figure 9.15 As long as ATP is available, cross-bridges would cycle continuously regardless of whether Ca^{2+} was present.

Figure 9.16 The weight in the isotonic experiment is approximately 14 mg. This can be estimated by determining the time at which the isotonic load begins to move on the lower graph (approximately 12 msec), then using the upper graph to assess the amount of tension generated by the fiber at that point in time.

Figure 9.18 Peak power generation by muscle fibers occurs at intermediate loads, usually at about one-third of their maximum isometric tension load. Using the arbitrary scale of 10 for the maximum velocity and load in this plot, for the points shown in this figure the power at the light load would be approximately $0.5 \times 7.5 = 3.75$. At the heavy load, it would be $7 \times 1 = 7$. At the intermediate load, the approximate power would be $3 \times 3 = 9$.

Figure 9.20 Unfused tetanic contractions will occur at between 6.7 and 28.6 stimuli per second. In order for an unfused tetanus to occur, the interval between stimuli must be less than 150 msec but greater than 35 msec. (If the interval was greater than 150 msec, twitches would not summate, and if less than 35 msec, a fused tetanus would occur.) To calculate the corresponding frequencies:

1 stimulus/150 msec $\times$ 1000 msec/sec = 6.7 stimuli/sec
1 stimulus/35 msec $\times$ 1000 msec/sec = 28.6 stimuli/sec

Figure 9.21 The passive tension at 150% of muscle length would be about 35% of the maximum isometric tension (see the red curve). When stimulated at that length, the active tension developed would be an additional 35% (see the green curve). The total tension measured would therefore be approximately 70% of the maximum isometric tetanic tension.

Figure 9.25 Muscle fibers containing the slow isoform of myosin contract and hydrolyze ATP relatively slowly. Their requirement for ATP can thus be satisfied by aerobic/oxidative mechanisms that, although slow, are extremely efficient (a yield of 38 ATP per glucose molecule with water and carbon dioxide as waste products—see Chapter 3). It would not be efficient for a slow fiber to produce its ATP predominantly by glycolysis, a process that is extremely rapid and relatively inefficient (only 2 ATP per glucose and lactic acid as a waste product).

Figure 9.29 The force acting upward on the forearm ($85 \times 5 = 425$) would be less than the downward-acting force ($10 \times 45 = 450$), so the muscle would undergo a lengthening (eccentric) contraction and the weight would move toward the ground.

Figure 9.30 The object would move nine times farther than the biceps in the same amount of time, or 18 cm/sec.

Figure 9.41 The skeletal muscle experiment would look the same. The calcium ions for contraction in skeletal muscle come from inside the sarcoplasmic reticulum. (*Note:* If the stimulus had been applied via a motor neuron, the lack of external Ca^{2+} would have prevented exocytosis of ACh and there would have been no action potential or contraction in the skeletal muscle cell.) Removing extracellular Ca^{2+} in the cardiac muscle experiment would eliminate both the prolonged plateau of the action potential and the contraction. Although the majority of the Ca^{2+} that activates contraction also comes from the sarcoplasmic reticulum in cardiac muscle, its release is triggered by entry of Ca^{2+} from the extracellular fluid through L-type channels during the action potential.

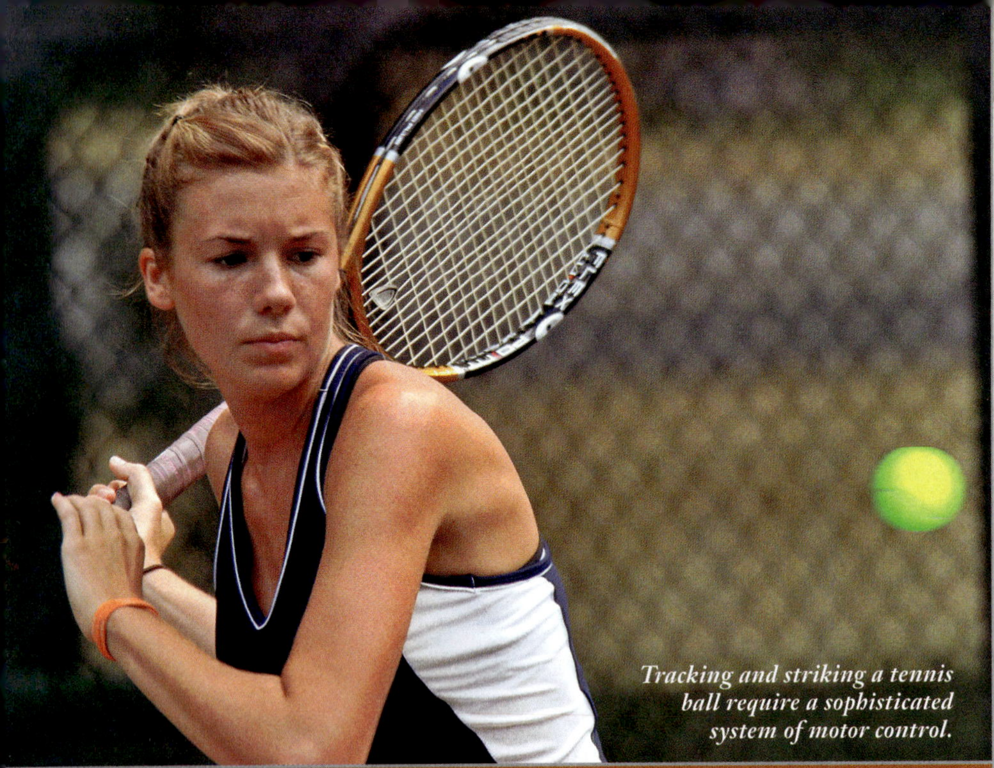

Tracking and striking a tennis ball require a sophisticated system of motor control.

10 Control of Body Movement

Previous chapters described the complex structure and functions of the nervous system (Chapters 6–8) and skeletal muscles (Chapter 9). In this chapter, you will learn how those systems interact with each other in the initiation and control of body movements. Consider the events associated with reaching out and grasping an object. The trunk is inclined toward the object, and the wrist, elbow and shoulder are extended (straightened) and stabilized to support the weight of the arm and hand, as well as the object. The fingers are extended to reach around the object and then flexed (bent) to grasp it. The degree of extension will depend upon the size of the object, and the force of flexion will depend upon its weight and consistency (for example, you would grasp an egg less tightly than a rock). Through all this, the body maintains upright posture and balance despite its continuously shifting position.

The building blocks for these movements—as for all movements—are **motor units**, each comprising one motor neuron together with all the skeletal muscle fibers innervated by that neuron (Chapter 9). The motor neurons are the final common pathway out of the central nervous system because all neural influences on skeletal muscle converge on the motor neurons and can only affect skeletal muscle through them. All the motor neurons that supply a given muscle make up the **motor neuron pool** for the muscle. The cell bodies of the pool for a given muscle are close to each other either in the ventral horn of the spinal cord or in the brainstem.

Within the brainstem or spinal cord, the axon terminals of many neurons synapse on a motor neuron to control its activity. The precision and speed of normally coordinated actions are produced by a balance of excitatory and inhibitory inputs onto motor neurons. For example, if inhibitory synaptic input to a given motor neuron is decreased, the excitatory input to that neuron will be unopposed and the motor neuron firing will increase, leading to increased contraction. It is important to realize that movements—even simple movements such as flexing a finger—are rarely achieved by just one muscle. Body movements are achieved by activation, in a precise sequence, of many motor units in various muscles.

This chapter deals with the interrelated neural inputs that converge upon motor neurons to control their activity, and features several of the general principles of physiology described in Chapter 1. Throughout the chapter, signaling along individual neurons and within complex neural networks demonstrates the general principle of physiology that information flow between cells, tissues, and organs is an essential feature of homeostasis and allows for integration of physiological processes. Inputs to motor neurons can be either excitatory or inhibitory, a good example of the general principle of physiology that most physiological functions are controlled by multiple regulatory systems, often working in opposition. Finally, the challenge of maintaining posture and balance against gravity shows the general principle of physiology that physiological processes are dictated by the laws of chemistry and physics. We first present a general model of how the motor system functions and then describe each component of the model in detail. Keep in mind throughout this chapter that many of the contractions that skeletal muscles execute—particularly the muscles involved in postural support—are isometric (Chapter 9). These isometric contractions serve to stabilize body parts rather than to move them but are included in the discussion because they are essential in the overall control of body movements.

10.1 Motor Control Hierarchy

The neurons involved in controlling skeletal muscles can be thought of as being organized in a hierarchical fashion, with each level of the hierarchy having a certain task in motor control (**Figure 10.1**). To begin a consciously planned movement, a general intention such as "pick up sweater" or "write signature" or "answer telephone" is generated at the highest level of the motor control hierarchy. These higher centers include many regions of the brain, including sensorimotor areas and others involved in memory, emotions, and motivation.

Information is relayed from these higher-center "command" neurons to parts of the brain that make up the middle level of the motor control hierarchy. The middle-level structures specify the individual postures and movements needed to carry out the intended action. In our example of picking up a sweater, structures of the middle hierarchical level coordinate the commands that tilt the body and extend the arm and hand toward the sweater and shift the body's weight to maintain balance. The middle-level hierarchical structures are located in parts of the cerebral cortex as well as in the cerebellum, subcortical nuclei, and brainstem (see Figure 10.1 and **Figure 10.2**). These structures have extensive interconnections, as the arrows in Figure 10.1 indicate.

As the neurons in the middle level of the hierarchy receive input from the command neurons, they simultaneously receive afferent information from receptors in the muscles, tendons, joints, and skin, as well as from the vestibular apparatus and eyes. These afferent signals relay information to the middle-level

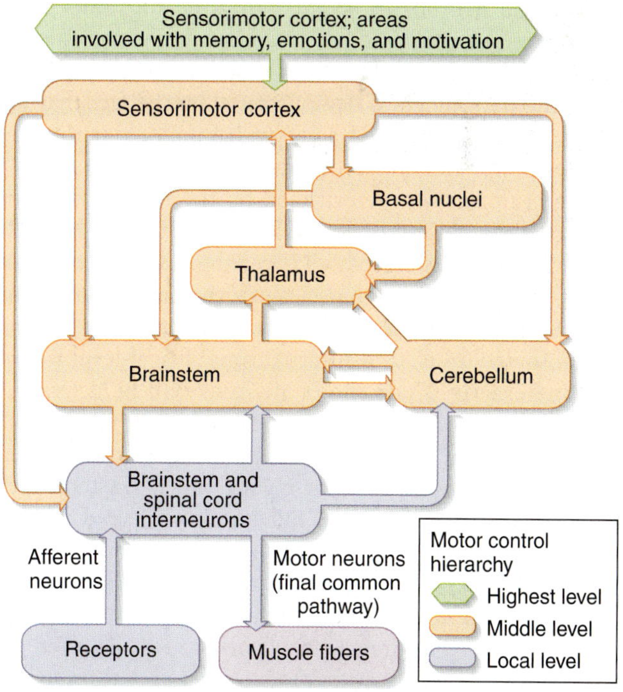

Figure 10.1 APIR The conceptual hierarchical organization of the neural systems controlling body movement. Motor neurons control all the skeletal muscles of the body. The sensorimotor cortex includes those parts of the cerebral cortex that act together to control skeletal muscle activity. The middle level of the hierarchy also receives input from the vestibular apparatus and eyes (not shown in the figure).

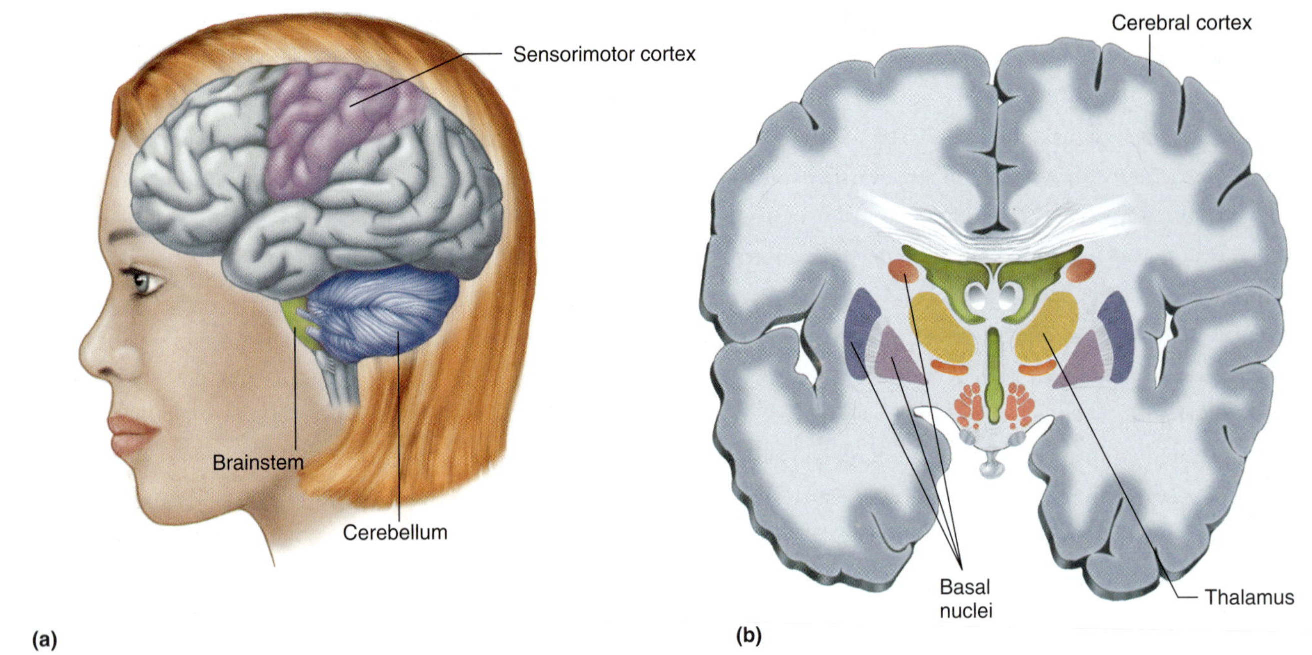

Figure 10.2 APIR (a) Side view of the brain showing three of the five components of the middle level of the motor control hierarchy. (Figure 10.10 shows details of the sensorimotor cortex.) (b) Cross section of the brain showing the thalamus and basal nuclei.

neurons about the starting positions of the body parts that are "commanded" to move. They also relay information about the nature of the space just outside the body in which a movement will take place. Neurons of the middle level of the hierarchy integrate all of this afferent information with the signals from the command neurons to create a **motor program**—defined as the pattern of neural activity required to properly perform the desired movement. The importance of sensory pathways in planning movements is demonstrated by the fact that when these pathways are impaired, a person has not only sensory deficits but also slow and uncoordinated voluntary movement.

The information determined by the motor program is transmitted via **descending pathways** to the local level of the motor control hierarchy. There, the axons of the motor neurons projecting to the muscles exit the brainstem or spinal cord. The local level of the hierarchy includes afferent neurons, motor neurons, and interneurons. Local-level neurons determine exactly which motor neurons will be activated to achieve the desired action and when this will happen. Note in Figure 10.1 that the descending pathways to the local level arise only in the sensorimotor cortex and brainstem. Other brain areas, notably the basal nuclei (also referred to as the basal ganglia), thalamus, and cerebellum, exert their effects on the local level only indirectly via the descending pathways from the cerebral cortex and brainstem.

The motor programs are continuously adjusted during the course of most movements. As the initial motor program begins and the action gets underway, brain regions at the middle level of the hierarchy continue to receive a constant stream of updated afferent information about the movements taking place. Afferent information about the position of the body and its parts in space is called **proprioception.** Say, for example, that the sweater you are picking up is wet and heavier than you expected so that the initially determined strength of muscle contraction is not sufficient to lift it. Any discrepancies between the intended and actual movements are detected, program corrections are determined, and the corrections are relayed to the local level of the hierarchy and the motor neurons. Reflex circuits acting entirely at the local level are also important in refining ongoing movements. Thus, many proprioceptive inputs are processed and influence ongoing movements without ever reaching the level of conscious perception.

If a complex movement is repeated often, learning takes place and the movement becomes skilled. Then, the initial information from the middle hierarchical level is more accurate and fewer corrections need to be made. Movements performed at high speed without concern for fine control are made solely according to the initial motor program.

Table 10.1 summarizes the structures and functions of the motor control hierarchy.

Voluntary and Involuntary Actions

Given such a highly interconnected and complicated neuroanatomical basis for the motor system, it is difficult to use the phrase **voluntary movement** with any real precision. We will use it, however, to refer to actions that have the following characteristics: (1) the movement is accompanied by a conscious awareness of what we are doing and why we are doing it, and (2) our attention is directed toward the action or its purpose.

The term *involuntary*, on the other hand, describes actions that do not have these characteristics. *Unconscious*, *automatic*, and *reflex* often serve as synonyms for *involuntary*, although in the motor system, the term *reflex* has a more precise meaning.

Despite our attempts to distinguish between voluntary and involuntary actions, almost all motor behavior involves both components, and it is not easy to make a distinction between the two. For example, even such a highly conscious act as walking involves many reflexive components, as the

TABLE 10.1 Conceptual Motor Control Hierarchy for Voluntary Movements

I. Higher centers
  A. Function: Forms complex plans according to individual's intention and communicates with the middle level via command neurons.
  B. Structures: Areas involved with memory, emotions and motivation, and sensorimotor cortex. All these structures receive and correlate input from many other brain structures.

II. The middle level
  A. Function: Converts plans received from higher centers to a number of smaller motor programs that determine the pattern of neural activation required to perform the movement. These programs are broken down into subprograms that determine the movements of individual joints. The programs and subprograms are transmitted through descending pathways to the local control level.
  B. Structures: Sensorimotor cortex, cerebellum, parts of basal nuclei, some brainstem nuclei.

III. The local level
  A. Function: Specifies tension of particular muscles and angle of specific joints at specific times necessary to carry out the programs and subprograms transmitted from the middle control levels.
  B. Structures: Brainstem or spinal cord interneurons, afferent neurons, motor neurons.

pattern of contraction of leg muscles is subconsciously varied to adapt to obstacles or uneven terrain.

Most motor behavior, therefore, is neither purely voluntary nor purely involuntary but has elements of both. Moreover, actions shift along this continuum according to the frequency with which they are performed. When a person first learns to drive a car with a manual transmission, for example, shifting gears requires a great deal of conscious attention. With practice, those same actions become automatic. On the other hand, reflex behaviors that are generally involuntary can, with special effort, sometimes be voluntarily modified or even prevented.

We now turn to an analysis of the individual components of the motor control system. We will begin with local control mechanisms because their activity serves as a base upon which the descending pathways exert their influence. Keep in mind throughout these descriptions that motor neurons always form the final common pathway to the muscles.

10.2 Local Control of Motor Neurons

The local control systems are the relay points for instructions to the motor neurons from centers higher in the motor control hierarchy. In addition, the local control systems play a major role in adjusting motor unit activity to unexpected obstacles to movement and to painful stimuli in the surrounding environment.

To carry out these adjustments, the local control systems use information carried by afferent fibers from sensory receptors in the muscles, tendons, joints, and skin of the body parts to be moved. As noted earlier, the afferent fibers also transmit information to higher levels of the hierarchy.

Interneurons

Most of the synaptic input to motor neurons from the descending pathways and afferent neurons does not go directly to motor neurons but, rather, goes to interneurons that synapse with the motor neurons. Interneurons comprise 90% of spinal cord neurons, and they are of several types. Some are near the motor neuron they synapse upon and thus are called local interneurons. Others have processes that extend up or down short distances in the spinal cord and brainstem, or even throughout much of the length of the central nervous system. The interneurons with longer processes are important for integrating complex movements such as stepping forward with your left foot as you throw a baseball with your right arm.

The interneurons are important elements of the local level of the motor control hierarchy, integrating inputs not only from higher centers and peripheral receptors but from other interneurons as well (**Figure 10.3**). They are crucial in determining which muscles are activated and when. This is especially important in coordinating repetitive, rhythmic activities like walking or running, for which spinal cord interneurons encode pattern generator circuits responsible for activating and inhibiting limb movements in an alternating sequence. Moreover, interneurons can act as "switches" that enable a movement to be turned on or off under the command of higher motor centers. For example, if you pick up a hot plate, a local reflex arc will be initiated by pain receptors in the skin of your hands, normally causing you to drop the plate. If it contains

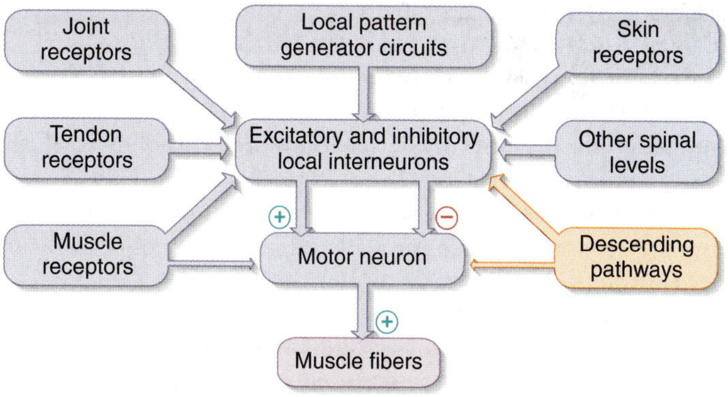

Figure 10.3 Converging inputs to local interneurons that control motor neuron activity. Plus signs indicate excitatory synapses and minus sign an inhibitory synapse. Neurons in addition to those shown may synapse directly onto motor neurons.

PHYSIOLOGICAL INQUIRY

- Many spinal cord interneurons release the neurotransmitter glycine, which opens chloride ion channels on postsynaptic cell membranes. Given that the plant-derived chemical strychnine blocks glycine receptors, predict the symptoms of strychnine poisoning.

Answer can be found at end of chapter.

your dinner, however, descending commands can inhibit the local activity, and you can hold onto the plate until you can put it down safely. The integration of various inputs by local interneurons is an excellent example of the general principle of physiology that most physiological functions are controlled by multiple regulatory systems, often working in opposition.

Local Afferent Input

As just noted, afferent fibers sometimes impinge on the local interneurons. (In one case that will be discussed shortly, they synapse directly on motor neurons.) The afferent fibers carry information from sensory receptors located in three places: (1) in the skeletal muscles controlled by the motor neurons; (2) in other nearby muscles, such as those with antagonistic actions; and (3) in the tendons, joints, and skin of body parts affected by the action of the muscle.

These receptors monitor the length and tension of the muscles, movement of the joints, and the effect of movements on the overlying skin. In other words, the movements themselves give rise to afferent input that, in turn, influences how the movement proceeds. As we will see next, their input sometimes provides negative feedback control over the muscles and also contributes to the conscious awareness of limb and body position.

Length-Monitoring Systems

Stretch receptors embedded within muscles monitor muscle length and the rate of change in muscle length. These receptors consist of peripheral endings of afferent nerve fibers wrapped around modified muscle fibers, several of which are enclosed in a connective-tissue capsule. The entire apparatus is collectively called a **muscle spindle** (**Figure 10.4**). The modified muscle fibers within the spindle are known as **intrafusal fibers.** The skeletal muscle fibers that form the bulk of the muscle and generate its force and movement are the **extrafusal fibers.**

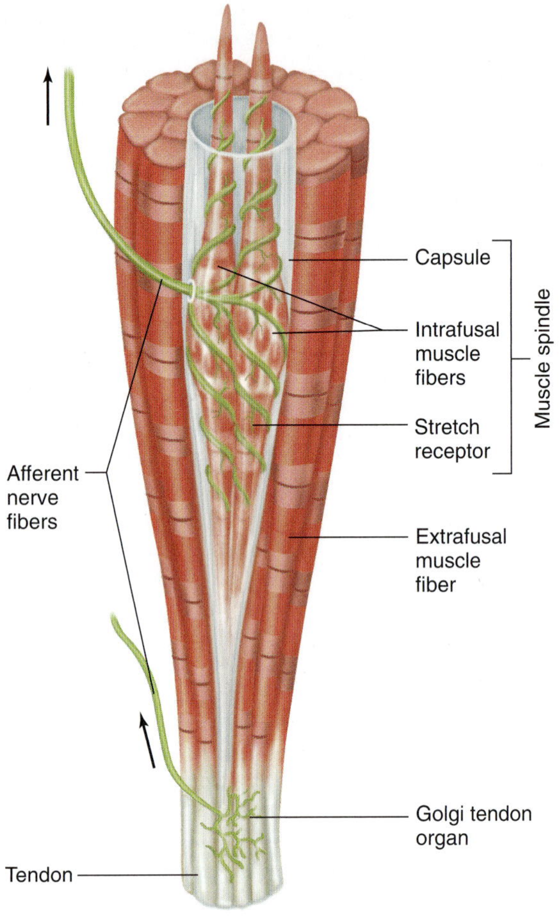

Figure 10.4 A muscle spindle and Golgi tendon organ. The muscle spindle is exaggerated in size compared to the extrafusal muscle fibers. The Golgi tendon organ will be discussed later in the chapter. Adapted from Elias, Pauly, and Burns.

Within a given spindle are two kinds of stretch receptors. One responds best to how much a muscle is stretched (**nuclear chain fibers**), whereas the other responds to both the magnitude of a stretch and the speed with which it occurs (**nuclear bag fibers**). Although the two kinds of stretch receptors are separate entities, we will refer to them collectively as the **muscle-spindle stretch receptors.**

The muscle spindles are attached by connective tissue in parallel to the extrafusal fibers. Thus, an external force stretching the muscle also pulls on the intrafusal fibers, stretching them and activating their receptor endings (**Figure 10.5a**). The more or the faster the muscle is stretched, the greater the rate of receptor firing. In contrast, if action potentials along motor neurons cause contraction of the extrafusal fibers, the resultant shortening of the muscle removes tension on the spindle and slows the rate of firing in the stretch receptor (**Figure 10.5b**).

If muscles were always activated as shown in Figure 10.5b, slackening of muscle spindles would reduce the available sensory information about muscle length during rapid shortening contractions. A mechanism called **alpha–gamma coactivation** prevents this loss of information. Extrafusal fibers of a muscle are activated by large-diameter **alpha motor neurons,** and the two ends of intrafusal muscle fibers are activated by smaller-diameter neurons called **gamma motor neurons.** The cell bodies of alpha and gamma motor neurons to a given muscle lie close together in the spinal cord or brainstem. Both types are activated by interneurons in their immediate vicinity and sometimes directly by neurons of the descending pathways. The contractile ends of intrafusal fibers are not large or strong enough to contribute to force or shortening of the whole muscle. However, they can maintain tension and stretch in the central receptor region of the intrafusal fibers. Activating gamma motor neurons alone therefore increases the sensitivity of a muscle to stretch. Coactivating gamma motor neurons along with alpha motor neurons prevents the central region of the muscle spindle from going slack during a shortening contraction (**Figure 10.5c**). This ensures that information about muscle length will be continuously available to provide for adjustment during ongoing actions and to plan and program future movements.

The Stretch Reflex

When the afferent fibers from the muscle spindle enter the central nervous system, they divide into branches that take different paths. In **Figure 10.6**, path A makes excitatory synapses directly onto motor neurons that return to the muscle that was stretched, thereby completing a reflex arc known as the **stretch reflex.**

This reflex is probably most familiar in the form of the **knee-jerk reflex,** part of a routine medical examination.

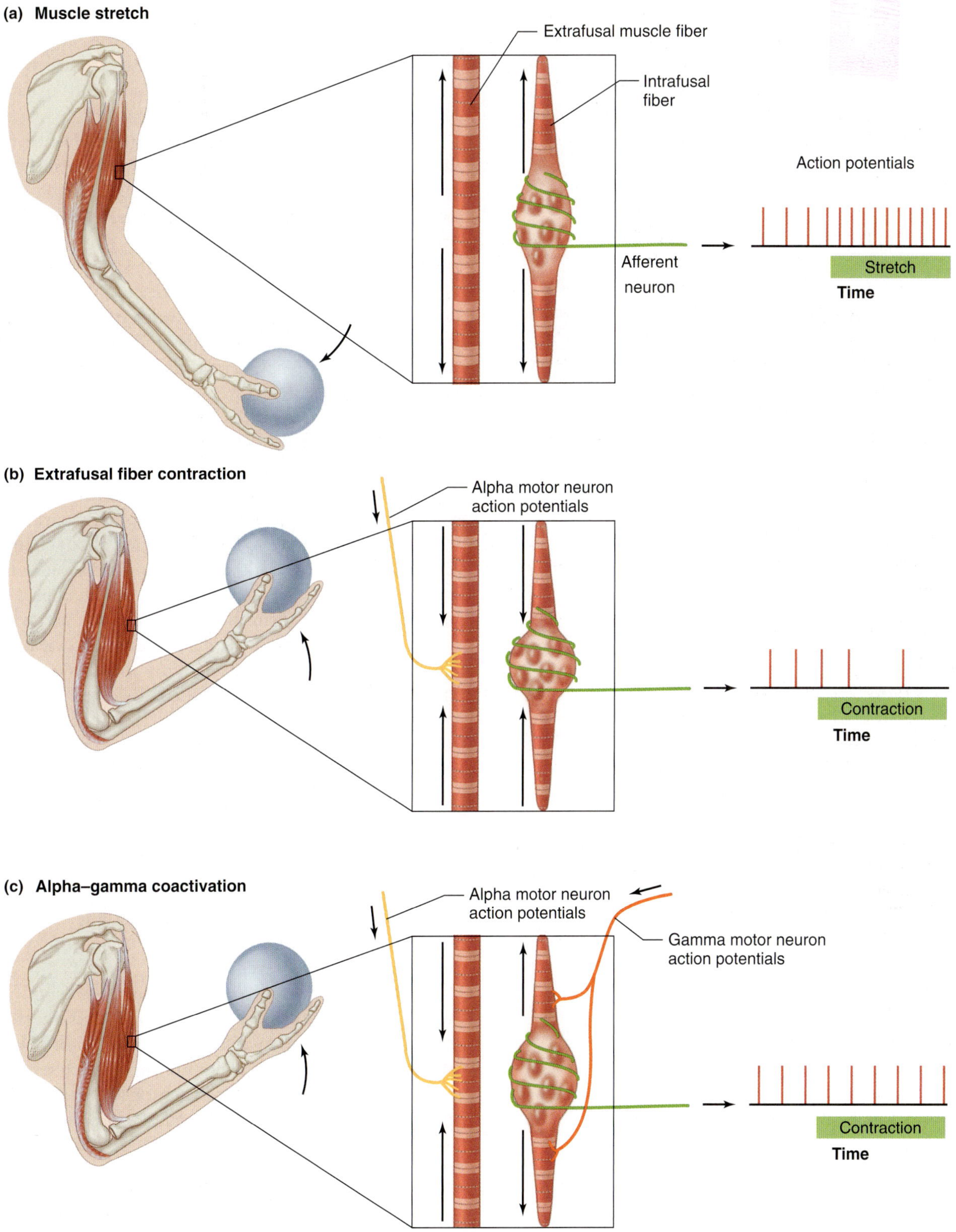

Figure 10.5 (a) Passive stretch of the muscle by an external load activates the spindle stretch receptors and causes an increased rate of action potentials in the afferent nerve. (b) Contraction of the extrafusal fibers removes tension on the stretch receptors and decreases the rate of action potential firing. (c) Simultaneous activation of alpha and gamma motor neurons results in maintained stretch of the central region of intrafusal fibers. Afferent information about muscle length continues to reach the central nervous system.

The examiner taps the patellar tendon (see Figure 10.6), which passes over the knee and connects extensor muscles in the thigh to the tibia in the lower leg. As the tendon is pushed in by tapping, the thigh muscles it is attached to are stretched, and all the stretch receptors within these muscles are activated. This stimulates a burst of action potentials in

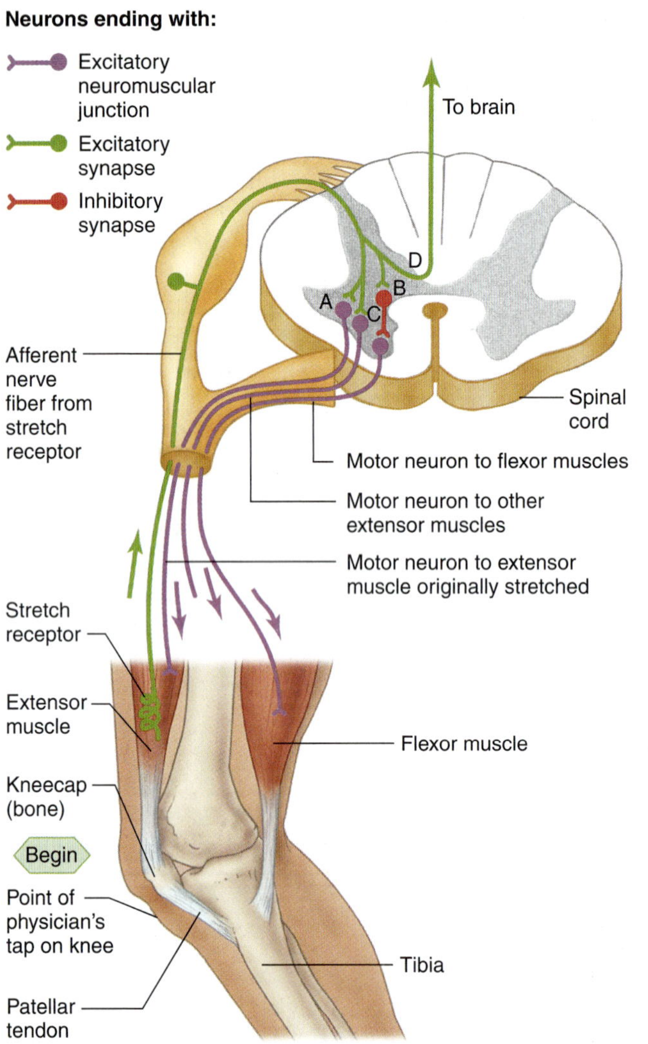

Figure 10.6 AP|R Neural pathways involved in the knee-jerk reflex. Tapping the patellar tendon stretches the extensor muscle, causing (paths A and C) compensatory contraction of this and other extensor muscles, (path B) relaxation of flexor muscles, and (path D) information about muscle length to go to the brain. Arrows indicate direction of action potential propagation.

PHYSIOLOGICAL INQUIRY

- Based on this figure and Figure 10.5, hypothesize what might happen if you could suddenly stimulate gamma motor neurons to leg flexor muscles in a resting subject.

Answer can be found at end of chapter.

the afferent nerve fibers from the stretch receptors, and these action potentials activate excitatory synapses on the motor neurons that control these same muscles. The motor units are stimulated, the thigh muscles contract, and the patient's lower leg extends to give the knee jerk. The proper performance of the knee jerk tells the physician that the afferent fibers, the balance of synaptic input to the motor neurons, the motor neurons, the neuromuscular junctions, and the muscles themselves are functioning normally.

Because the afferent nerve fibers in the stretched muscle synapse directly on the motor neurons to that muscle without any interneurons, this portion of the stretch reflex is called **monosynaptic.** Stretch reflexes have the only known monosynaptic reflex arcs. All other reflex arcs are **polysynaptic;** they have at least one interneuron—and usually many—between the afferent and efferent neurons.

In path B of Figure 10.6, the branches of the afferent nerve fibers from stretch receptors end on inhibitory interneurons. When activated, these inhibit the motor neurons controlling antagonistic muscles whose contraction would interfere with the reflex response. In the knee jerk, for example, neurons to muscles that flex the knee are inhibited. This component of the stretch reflex is polysynaptic. The activation of neurons to one muscle with the simultaneous inhibition of neurons to its antagonistic muscle is called **reciprocal innervation.** This is characteristic of many movements, not just the stretch reflex.

Path C in Figure 10.6 activates motor neurons of **synergistic muscles**—that is, muscles whose contraction assists the intended motion. In the example of the knee-jerk reflex, this would include other muscles that extend the leg.

Path D of Figure 10.6 is not explicitly part of the stretch reflex; it demonstrates that information about changes in muscle length ascends to higher centers. The axon of the afferent neuron continues to the brainstem and synapses there with interneurons that form the next link in the pathway that conveys information about the muscle length to areas of the brain dealing with motor control. This information is especially important during slow, controlled movements such as the performance of an unfamiliar action. Ascending paths also provide information that contributes to the conscious perception of the position of a limb.

Tension-Monitoring Systems

Any given set of inputs to a given set of motor neurons can lead to various degrees of tension in the muscles they innervate. The tension depends on muscle length, the load on the muscles, and the degree of muscle fatigue. Therefore, feedback is necessary to inform the motor control systems of the tension actually achieved.

Some of this feedback is provided by vision (you can see whether you are lifting or lowering an object) as well as by afferent input from skin, muscle, and joint receptors. An additional receptor type specifically monitors how much tension the contracting motor units are exerting (or is being imposed on the muscle by external forces if the muscle is being stretched).

The receptors employed in this tension-monitoring system are the **Golgi tendon organs,** which are endings of afferent nerve fibers that wrap around collagen bundles in the tendons near their junction with the muscle (see Figure 10.4). These collagen bundles are slightly bowed in the resting state. When the muscle is stretched or the attached extrafusal muscle fibers contract, tension is exerted on the tendon. This tension straightens the collagen bundles and distorts the receptor endings, activating them. The tendon is typically stretched much more by an active contraction of the muscle than when the whole muscle is passively stretched (**Figure 10.7**). Therefore, the Golgi tendon organs discharge in response to the tension generated by the contracting muscle and initiate action potentials that are transmitted to the central nervous system.

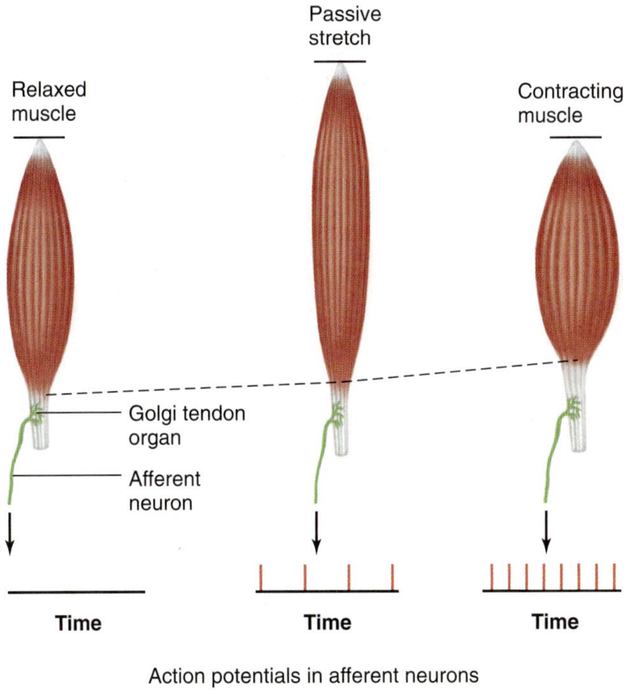

Figure 10.7 Activation of Golgi tendon organs. Compared to when a muscle is contracting, passive stretch of the relaxed muscle produces less stretch of the tendon and fewer action potentials from the Golgi tendon organ.

PHYSIOLOGICAL INQUIRY

- Which of these conditions would result in the greatest action potential frequency in afferent neurons from muscle-spindle receptors?

Answer can be found at end of chapter.

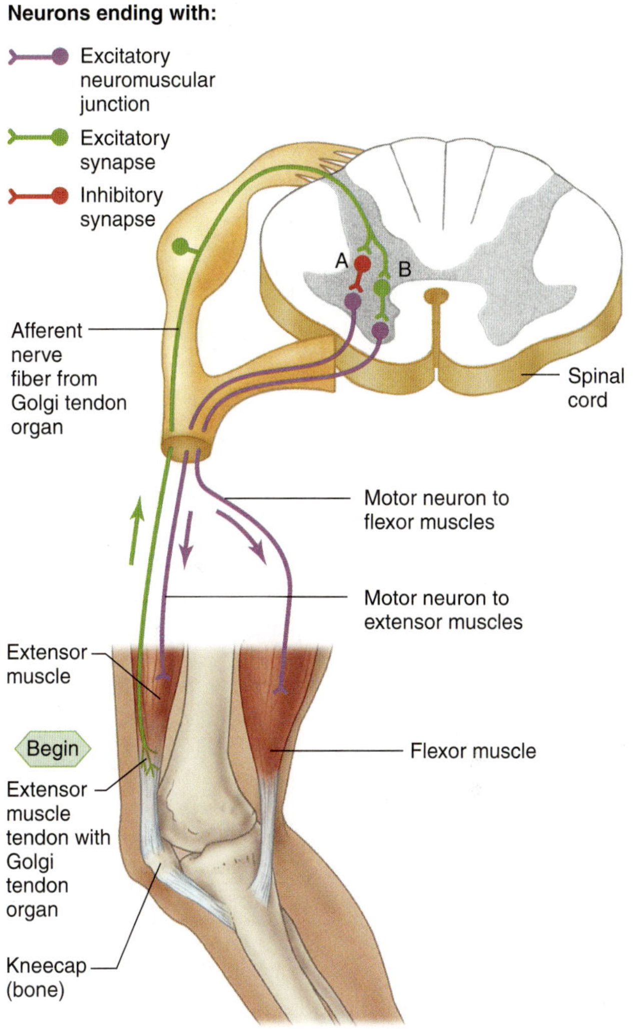

Figure 10.8 APIR Neural pathways underlying the Golgi tendon organ component of the local control system. In this diagram, contraction of the extensor muscles causes tension in the Golgi tendon organ and increases the rate of action potential firing in the afferent nerve fiber. By way of interneurons, this increased activity results in (path A) inhibition of the motor neurons of the extensor muscle and its synergists and (path B) excitation of flexor muscle motor neurons. Arrows indicate the direction of action potential propagation.

PHYSIOLOGICAL INQUIRY

- Explain how the Golgi tendon organ protects against excessive force exertion that might tear a muscle or tendon.

Answer can be found at end of chapter.

Branches of the afferent neuron from the Golgi tendon organ cause widespread inhibition of the contracting muscle and its synergists via interneurons (path A in **Figure 10.8**). They also stimulate the motor neurons of the antagonistic muscles (path B in Figure 10.8). Note that this reciprocal innervation is the opposite of that produced by the muscle-spindle afferents. This difference reflects the different functional roles of the two systems: The muscle spindle provides local homeostatic control of muscle *length*, and the Golgi tendon organ provides local homeostatic control of muscle *tension*. In addition, the activity of afferent fibers from these two receptors supplies the higher-level motor control systems with information about muscle length and tension, which can be used to modify an ongoing motor program.

The Withdrawal Reflex

In addition to the afferent information from the spindle stretch receptors and Golgi tendon organs of the activated muscle, other input is transmitted to the local motor control systems. For example, painful stimulation of the skin, as occurs from stepping on a tack, activates the flexor muscles and inhibits the extensor muscles of the ipsilateral (on the same side of the body) leg. The resulting action moves the affected limb away from the harmful stimulus and is thus known as a **withdrawal reflex** (**Figure 10.9**). The same stimulus causes just the opposite response in the contralateral leg (on the opposite side of the body from the stimulus); motor neurons to the extensors are activated while the flexor muscle motor neurons are inhibited. This **crossed-extensor reflex** enables the contralateral leg to support the body's weight as the injured foot is lifted by flexion (see Figure 10.9). This concludes our discussion of the local level of motor control.

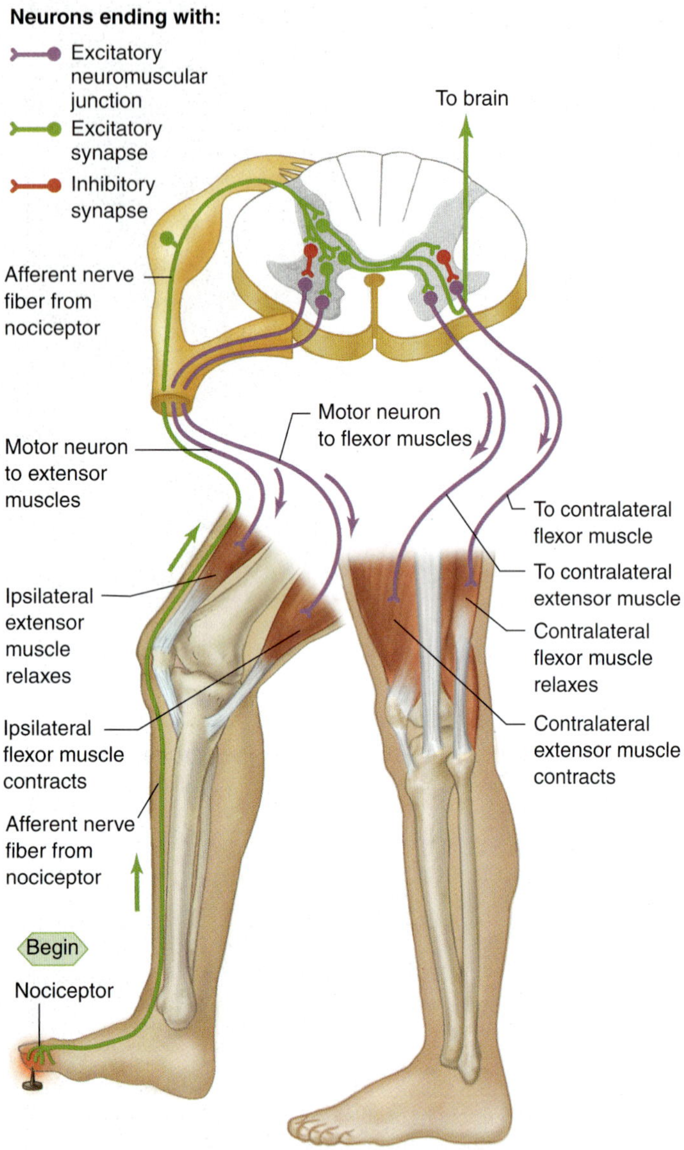

Figure 10.9 AP|R In response to pain detected by nociceptors (Chapter 7), the ipsilateral flexor muscle's motor neuron is stimulated (withdrawal reflex). In the case illustrated, the opposite limb is extended (crossed-extensor reflex) to support the body's weight. Arrows indicate direction of action potential propagation.

PHYSIOLOGICAL INQUIRY

- While crawling across a floor, a child accidentally places her right hand onto a piece of broken glass. How will the flexor muscles of her left arm respond?

Answer can be found at end of chapter.

10.3 The Brain Motor Centers and the Descending Pathways They Control

We now turn our attention to the motor centers in the brain and the descending pathways that direct the local control system (review Figure 10.1).

Cerebral Cortex

The cerebral cortex plays a critical role in both the planning and ongoing control of voluntary movements, functioning in both the highest and middle levels of the motor control hierarchy. The term **sensorimotor cortex** is used to include all those parts of the cerebral cortex that act together to control muscle movement. A large number of neurons that give rise to descending pathways for motor control come from two areas of sensorimotor cortex on the posterior part of the frontal lobe: the **primary motor cortex** (sometimes called simply the **motor cortex**) and the **premotor area** (**Figure 10.10**).

Other areas of sensorimotor cortex shown in Figure 10.10 include the **supplementary motor cortex,** which lies mostly on the surface on the frontal lobe where the cortex folds down between the two hemispheres, the **somatosensory cortex,** and parts of the **parietal-lobe association cortex.** The neurons of the motor cortex that control muscle groups in various parts of the body are arranged anatomically into a **somatotopic map,** as shown in **Figure 10.11**.

Although these areas of the cortex are anatomically and functionally distinct, they are heavily interconnected, and individual muscles or movements are represented at multiple sites. Thus, the cortical neurons that control movement form a neural network, meaning that many neurons participate in each single movement. In addition, any one neuron may function in more than one movement. The neural networks can be distributed across multiple sites in parietal and frontal cortex, including the sites named in the preceding two paragraphs. The interactions of the neurons within the networks are flexible so that the neurons are capable of responding differently under different circumstances. This adaptability enhances the possibility of integrating incoming neural signals from diverse sources and the final coordination of many parts into a smooth, purposeful movement. It probably also accounts for the remarkable variety of ways in which we can approach a goal. For example, you can comb your hair with the right hand or the left, starting at the back of your head or the front. This same adaptability also accounts for some of the learning that occurs in all aspects of motor behavior.

We have described the various areas of sensorimotor cortex as giving rise, either directly or indirectly, to pathways descending to the motor neurons. However, additional brain areas are involved in the initiation of intentional movements, such as the areas involved in memory, emotion, and motivation.

Association areas of the cerebral cortex also play other roles in motor control. For example, neurons of the parietal association cortex are important in the visual control of reaching and grasping. These neurons play an important role in matching motor signals concerning the pattern of hand action with signals from the visual system concerning the three-dimensional features of the objects to be grasped. Imagine a glass of water sitting in front of you on your desk—you could reach out and pick it up much more smoothly with your eyes tracking your arm and hand movements than you could with your eyes closed. During activation of the cortical areas involved in motor control, subcortical mechanisms also become active. We now turn to these areas of the motor control system.

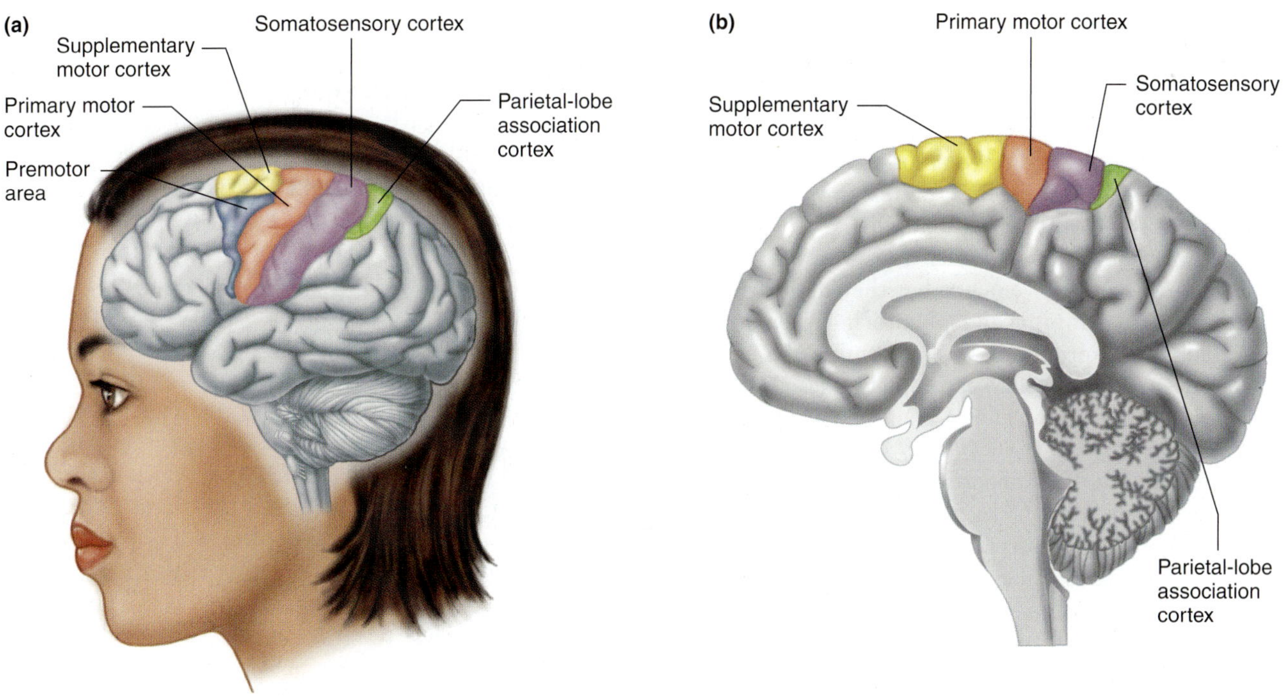

Figure 10.10 APIR (a) The major motor areas of the cerebral cortex. (b) Midline view of the right side of the brain showing the supplementary motor cortex, which lies in the part of the cerebral cortex that is folded down between the two cerebral hemispheres. Other cortical motor areas also extend onto this area. The premotor, supplementary motor, primary motor, somatosensory, and parietal-lobe association cortices together make up the sensorimotor cortex.

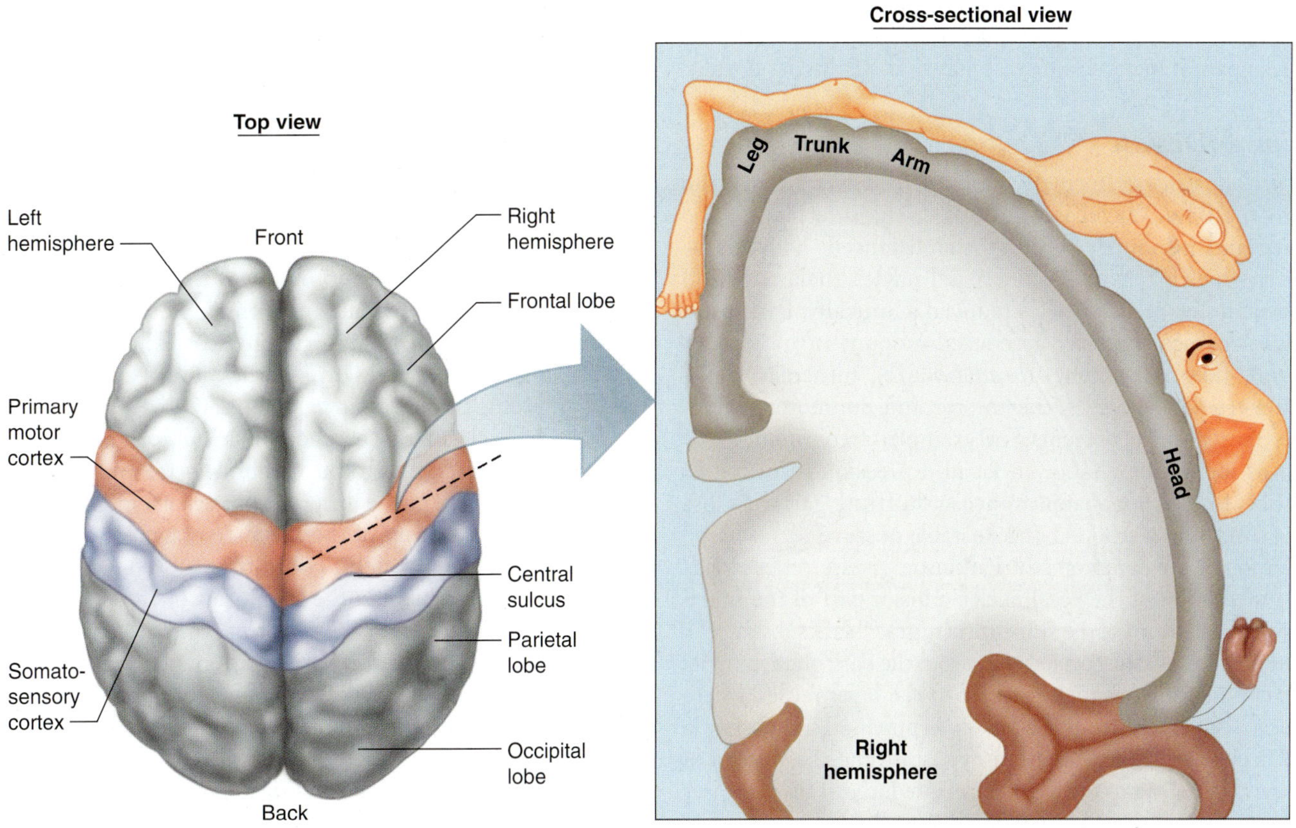

Figure 10.11 APIR Somatotopic map of major body areas in the primary motor cortex. Within the broad areas, no one area exclusively controls the movement of a single body region and there is much overlap and duplication of cortical representation. Relative sizes of body structures are proportional to the number of neurons dedicated to their motor control. Only the right motor cortex, which principally controls muscles on the left side of the body, is shown.

Subcortical and Brainstem Nuclei

Numerous highly interconnected structures lie in the brainstem and within the cerebrum beneath the cortex, where they interact with the cortex to control movements. Their influence is transmitted indirectly to the motor neurons both by pathways that ascend to the cerebral cortex and by pathways that descend from some of the brainstem nuclei.

It is not known to what extent—if any—these structures are involved in initiating movements, but they definitely play a prominent role in planning and monitoring them. Their role is to establish the programs that determine the specific sequence of movements needed to accomplish a desired action. Subcortical and brainstem nuclei are also important in learning skilled movements.

Prominent among the subcortical nuclei are the paired **basal nuclei** (see Figure 10.2b), which consist of a closely related group of separate nuclei. As described in Chapter 6, these structures are often referred to as basal ganglia, but their presence within the central nervous system makes the term *nuclei* more technically correct. They form a link in some of the looping parallel circuits through which activity in the motor system is transmitted from a specific region of sensorimotor cortex to the basal nuclei, from there to the thalamus, and then back to the cortical area where the circuit started (review Figure 10.1). Some of these circuits facilitate movements, and others suppress them. This explains why brain damage to subcortical nuclei following a stroke or trauma can result in either hypercontracted muscles or flaccid paralysis—it depends on which specific circuits are damaged. The importance of the basal nuclei is particularly apparent in certain disease states, as we discuss next.

Parkinson Disease

In ***Parkinson disease*** (formerly called *Parkinson's disease*), the input to the basal nuclei is diminished, the interplay of the facilitory and inhibitory circuits is unbalanced, and activation of the motor cortex (via the basal nuclei–thalamus limb of the circuit just mentioned) is reduced. Clinically, Parkinson disease is characterized by a reduced amount of movement (***akinesia***), slow movements (***bradykinesia***), muscular rigidity, and a tremor at rest. Other motor and nonmotor abnormalities may also be present. For example, a common set of symptoms includes a change in facial expression resulting in a masklike, unemotional appearance, a shuffling gait with loss of arm swing, and a stooped and unstable posture.

Although the symptoms of Parkinson disease reflect inadequate functioning of the basal nuclei, a major part of the initial defect arises in neurons of the **substantia nigra** ("black substance"), a brainstem nucleus that gets its name from the dark pigment in its cells. These neurons normally project to the basal nuclei, where they release dopamine from their axon terminals. The substantia nigra neurons degenerate in Parkinson disease and the amount of dopamine they deliver to the basal nuclei is reduced. This decreases the subsequent activation of the sensorimotor cortex.

It is not currently known what causes the degeneration of neurons of the substantia nigra and the development of Parkinson disease. In a small fraction of cases, there is evidence that it may have a genetic cause, based on observed changes in the function of genes associated with mitochondrial function, protection from oxidative stress, and removal of cellular proteins that have been targeted for metabolic breakdown. Scientists suspect that exposure to environmental toxins such as manganese, carbon monoxide, and some pesticides may also play a role. One chemical clearly linked to destruction of the substantia nigra is ***MPTP*** (***1-methyl-4-phenyl-1,2,3,6-tetrahydropyridine***). MPTP is an impurity sometimes created in the manufacture of a synthetic heroin-like opioid drug, which when injected leads to a Parkinson-like syndrome.

The drugs used to treat Parkinson disease are all designed to restore dopamine activity in the basal nuclei. They fall into three main categories: (1) agonists (stimulators) of dopamine receptors, (2) inhibitors of the enzymes that metabolize dopamine at synapses, and (3) precursors of dopamine itself. The most widely prescribed drug is ***Levodopa*** (***L-dopa***), which falls into the third category. L-dopa enters the bloodstream, crosses the blood–brain barrier, and is converted to dopamine. (Dopamine itself is not used as medication because it cannot cross the blood–brain barrier and it has too many systemic side effects.) The newly formed dopamine activates receptors in the basal nuclei and improves the symptoms of the disease. Side effects sometimes occurring with L-dopa include hallucinations, like those seen in individuals with schizophrenia who have excessive dopamine activity (see Chapter 8), and spontaneous, abnormal motor activity. Other therapies for Parkinson disease include the lesioning (destruction) of overactive areas of the basal nuclei and ***deep brain stimulation.*** The latter is accomplished with surgically implanted electrodes connected to an electrical pulse generator similar to a cardiac artificial pacemaker (Chapter 12); while in some cases it relieves symptoms, the mechanism is not understood. Injection of undifferentiated stem cells is also being explored as a possible treatment.

Cerebellum

The cerebellum is located dorsally to the brainstem (see Figure 10.2a). It influences posture and movement indirectly by means of input to brainstem nuclei and (by way of the thalamus) to regions of the sensorimotor cortex that give rise to pathways that descend to the motor neurons. The cerebellum receives information from the sensorimotor cortex, and also from the vestibular system, eyes, skin, muscles, joints, and tendons—that is, from some of the very receptors that movement affects.

One role of the cerebellum in motor functioning is to provide timing signals to the cerebral cortex and spinal cord for precise execution of the different phases of a motor program, in particular, the timing of the agonist/antagonist components of a movement. It also helps coordinate movements that involve several joints and stores the memories of these movements so they are easily achieved the next time they are tried.

The cerebellum also participates in planning movements—integrating information about the nature of an intended movement with information about the surrounding space. The cerebellum then provides this as a feedforward (see Chapter 1) signal to the brain areas responsible for refining the motor program. Moreover, during the course of the movement, the cerebellum compares information about what the muscles *should* be doing with information about what they actually *are* doing. If a discrepancy develops between the intended movement and the actual one, the cerebellum sends an error signal to the motor cortex and subcortical centers to correct the ongoing program.

The role of the cerebellum in programming movements can best be appreciated when observing its absence in individuals with ***cerebellar disease.*** They typically cannot perform limb or eye movements smoothly but move with a tremor—a so-called ***intention tremor*** that increases as a movement nears its final destination. This differs from patients with Parkinson disease, who have a tremor while at rest. People with cerebellar disease also cannot combine the movements of several joints into a single, smooth, coordinated motion. The role of the cerebellum in the precision and timing of movements can be appreciated when you consider the complex tasks it helps us accomplish. For example, a tennis player sees a ball fly over the net, anticipates its flight path, runs along an intersecting path, and swings the racquet through an arc that will intercept the ball with the speed and force required to return it to the other side of the court. People with cerebellar damage cannot achieve this level of coordinated, precise, learned movement.

Unstable posture and awkward gait are two other symptoms characteristic of cerebellar disease. For example, people with cerebellar damage walk with their feet wide apart, and they have such difficulty maintaining balance that their gait is similar to that seen in people who are intoxicated by ethanol. Visual input helps compensate for some of the loss of motor coordination—patients can stand on one foot with eyes open but not closed. A final symptom involves difficulty in learning new motor skills. Individuals with cerebellar disease find it hard to modify movements in response to new situations. Unlike damage to areas of sensorimotor cortex, cerebellar damage is not usually associated with paralysis or weakness.

Descending Pathways

The influence exerted by the various brain regions on posture and movement occurs via descending pathways to the motor neurons and the interneurons that affect them. The pathways are of two types: the **corticospinal pathways,** which, as their name implies, originate in the cerebral cortex; and a second group we will refer to as the **brainstem pathways,** which originate in the brainstem.

Neurons from both types of descending pathways end at synapses on alpha and gamma motor neurons or on interneurons that affect them. Sometimes these are the same interneurons that function in local reflex arcs, thereby ensuring that the descending signals are fully integrated with local information before the activity of the motor neurons is altered. In other cases, the interneurons are part of neural networks involved in posture or locomotion. The ultimate effect of the descending pathways on the alpha motor neurons may be excitatory or inhibitory.

Importantly, some of the descending fibers affect *afferent* systems. They do this via (1) presynaptic synapses on the terminals of afferent neurons as these fibers enter the central nervous system, or (2) synapses on interneurons in the ascending pathways. The overall effect of this descending input to afferent systems is to regulate their influence on either the local or brain motor control areas, thereby altering the importance of a particular bit of afferent information or sharpening its focus. For example, when performing an exceptionally delicate or complicated task, like brain surgery, descending inputs might facilitate signaling in afferent pathways carrying proprioceptive inputs monitoring hand and finger movements. This descending (motor) control over ascending (sensory) information provides another example to show that there is no real functional separation between the motor and sensory systems.

Corticospinal Pathway

The nerve fibers of the corticospinal pathways have their cell bodies in the sensorimotor cortex and terminate in the spinal cord. The corticospinal pathways are also called the **pyramidal tracts** or **pyramidal system** because of their triangular shape as they pass along the ventral surface of the medulla oblongata. In the medulla oblongata near the junction of the spinal cord and brainstem, most of the corticospinal fibers cross (known as decussation) to descend on the opposite side (**Figure 10.12**). The skeletal muscles on the left side of the body are therefore controlled largely by neurons in the right half of the brain, and vice versa.

As the corticospinal fibers descend through the brain from the cerebral cortex, they are accompanied by fibers of

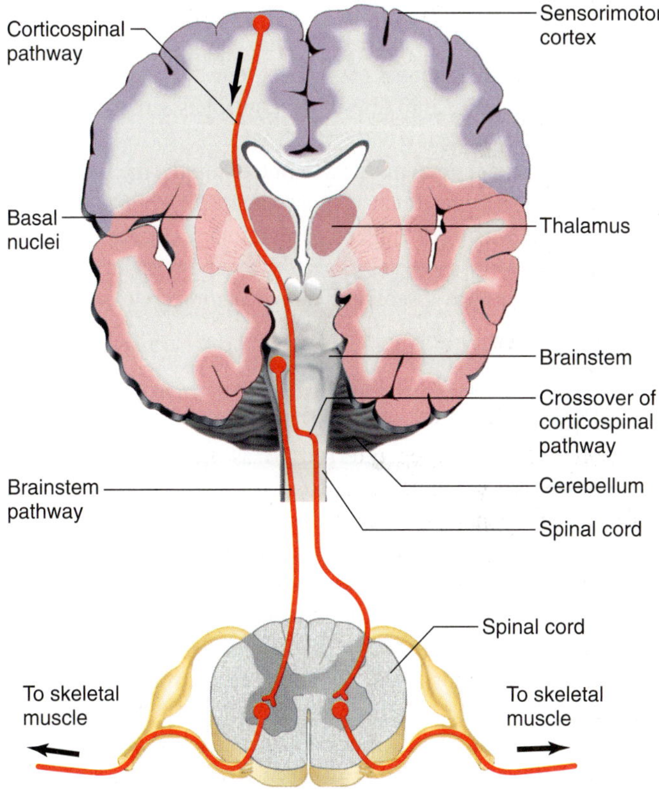

Figure 10.12 AP|R The corticospinal and brainstem pathways. Most of the corticospinal fibers cross in the brainstem to descend in the opposite side of the spinal cord, but the brainstem pathways are mostly uncrossed. The descending neurons are shown synapsing directly onto motor neurons in the spinal cord, but they commonly synapse onto local interneurons. Adapted from Gardner.

PHYSIOLOGICAL INQUIRY

- If a blood clot blocked a cerebral blood vessel supplying a small region of the right cerebral cortex just in front of the central sulcus in the deep groove between the hemispheres, what symptoms might result? (*Hint:* See Figure 10.11.)

Answer can be found at end of chapter.

the **corticobulbar pathway** (*bulbar* means "pertaining to the brainstem"), a pathway that begins in the sensorimotor cortex and ends in the brainstem. The corticobulbar fibers control, directly or indirectly via interneurons, the motor neurons that innervate muscles of the eye, face, tongue, and throat. These fibers provide the main source of control for voluntary movement of the muscles of the head and neck, whereas the corticospinal fibers serve this function for the muscles of the rest of the body. For convenience, we will include the corticobulbar pathway in the general term *corticospinal pathways.*

Convergence and divergence are hallmarks of the corticospinal pathway. For example, a great number of different neuronal sources converge on neurons of the sensorimotor cortex, which is not surprising when you consider the many factors that can affect motor behavior. As for the descending pathways, neurons from wide areas of the sensorimotor cortex converge onto single motor neurons at the local level so that multiple brain areas usually control single muscles. Also, axons of single corticospinal neurons diverge markedly to synapse with a number of different motor neuron populations at various levels of the spinal cord, thereby ensuring that the motor cortex can coordinate many different components of a movement.

This apparent "blurriness" of control is surprising when you think of the delicacy with which you can move a fingertip, because the corticospinal pathways control rapid, fine movements of the distal extremities, such as those you make when you manipulate an object with your fingers. After damage occurs to the corticospinal pathways, movements are slower and weaker, individual finger movements are absent, and it is difficult to release a grip.

Brainstem Pathways

Axons from neurons in the brainstem also form pathways that descend into the spinal cord to influence motor neurons. These pathways are sometimes referred to as the **extrapyramidal system,** or indirect pathways, to distinguish them from the corticospinal (pyramidal) pathways. However, no general term is widely accepted for these pathways; for convenience, we will refer to them collectively as the brainstem pathways.

Axons of most of the brainstem pathways remain uncrossed and affect muscles on the same side of the body (see Figure 10.12), although a few do cross over to contralateral muscles. In the spinal cord, the fibers of the brainstem pathways descend as distinct clusters, named according to their sites of origin. For example, the vestibulospinal pathway descends to the spinal cord from the vestibular nuclei in the brainstem, whereas the reticulospinal pathway descends from neurons in the brainstem reticular formation. The brainstem pathways are especially important in controlling muscles of the trunk for upright posture, balance, and walking.

As stated previously, the corticospinal neurons generally have their greatest influence over motor neurons that control muscles involved in fine, isolated movements, particularly those of the fingers and hands. The brainstem descending pathways, in contrast, are involved more with coordination of the large muscle groups used in the maintenance of upright posture, in locomotion, and in head and body movements when turning toward a specific stimulus.

There is, however, much interaction between the descending pathways. For example, some fibers of the corticospinal pathway end on interneurons that play important roles in posture, whereas fibers of the brainstem descending pathways sometimes end directly on the alpha motor neurons to control discrete muscle movements. Because of this redundancy, one system may compensate for loss of function resulting from damage to the other system, although the compensation is generally not complete.

The distinctions between the corticospinal and brainstem descending pathways are not clear-cut. All movements, whether automatic or voluntary, require the continuous coordinated interaction of both types of pathways.

10.4 Muscle Tone

Even when a skeletal muscle is relaxed, there is a slight and uniform resistance when it is stretched by an external force. This resistance is known as **muscle tone,** and it can be an important diagnostic tool for clinicians assessing a patient's neuromuscular function.

Muscle tone is due both to the passive elastic properties of the muscles and joints and to the degree of ongoing alpha motor neuron activity. When a person is very relaxed, the alpha motor neuron activity does not make a significant contribution to the resistance to stretch. As the person becomes increasingly alert, however, more activation of the alpha motor neurons occurs and muscle tone increases.

Abnormal Muscle Tone

Abnormally high muscle tone, called ***hypertonia,*** accompanies a number of diseases and is seen very clearly when a joint is moved passively at high speeds. The increased resistance is due to an increased level of alpha motor neuron activity, which keeps a muscle contracted despite the attempt to relax it. Hypertonia usually occurs with disorders of the descending pathways that normally inhibit the motor neurons.

Clinically, the descending pathways and neurons of the motor cortex are often referred to as the **upper motor neurons** (a confusing misnomer because they are not really motor neurons). Abnormalities due to their dysfunction are classified, therefore, as ***upper motor neuron disorders.*** Thus, hypertonia usually indicates an upper motor neuron disorder. In this clinical classification, the alpha motor neurons—the true motor neurons—are termed **lower motor neurons.**

Spasticity is a form of hypertonia in which the muscles do not develop increased tone until they are stretched a bit, and after a brief increase in tone, the contraction subsides for a short time. The period of "give" occurring after a time of resistance is called the ***clasp-knife phenomenon.*** (When an examiner bends the limb of a patient with this condition, it is like folding a pocketknife—at first, the spring resists the bending motion, but once bending begins, it closes easily.) Spasticity may be accompanied by increased responses of motor reflexes such as the knee jerk and by decreased coordination and strength of voluntary actions. ***Rigidity*** is a form of hypertonia in which the increased muscle contraction is continual and the resistance to passive stretch is constant (as occurs in the disease tetanus, which is described in detail in the Clinical Case Study at the end of this chapter). Two other forms of hypertonia that can occur suddenly in individual or multiple muscles sometimes originate as problems in muscle and not nervous tissue: Muscle ***spasms*** are brief contractions, and muscle ***cramps*** are prolonged and painful contractions (see Chapter 9).

Hypotonia is a condition of abnormally low muscle tone accompanied by weakness, atrophy (a decrease in muscle bulk), and decreased or absent reflex responses. Dexterity and coordination are generally preserved unless profound weakness is present. Although hypotonia may develop after cerebellar disease, it more frequently accompanies disorders of the alpha motor neurons (lower motor neurons), neuromuscular junctions, or the muscles themselves. The term ***flaccid,*** which means "weak" or "soft," is often used to describe hypotonic muscles.

10.5 Maintenance of Upright Posture and Balance

The skeleton supporting the body is a system of long bones and a many-jointed spine that cannot stand erect against the forces of gravity without the support provided through coordinated muscle activity. The muscles that maintain upright posture—that is, support the body's weight against gravity—are controlled by the brain and by reflex mechanisms "wired into" the neural networks of the brainstem and spinal cord. Many of the reflex pathways previously introduced (for example, the stretch and crossed-extensor reflexes) are active in posture control.

Added to the problem of maintaining upright posture is that of maintaining balance. A human being is a tall structure balanced on a relatively small base, with the center of gravity quite high, just above the pelvis. For stability, the center of gravity must be kept within the base of support the feet provide (**Figure 10.13**). Once the center of gravity has moved beyond this base, the body will fall unless one foot is shifted to broaden the base of support. Yet, people can operate under conditions of unstable equilibrium because complex interacting **postural reflexes** maintain their balance.

The afferent pathways of the postural reflexes come from three sources: the eyes, the vestibular apparatus, and the receptors involved in proprioception (joint, muscle, and touch receptors, for example). The efferent pathways are the alpha motor neurons to the skeletal muscles, and the integrating centers are neuron networks in the brainstem and spinal cord.

In addition to these integrating centers, there are centers in the brain that form an internal representation of the body's geometry, its support conditions, and its orientation with respect to vertical. This internal representation serves two purposes: (1) it provides a reference framework for the perception of the body's position and orientation in space and for planning actions, and (2) it contributes to stability via the motor controls involved in maintaining upright posture.

There are many familiar examples of using reflexes to maintain upright posture; one is the crossed-extensor reflex. As one leg is flexed and lifted off the ground, the other is extended more strongly to support the weight of the body, and the positions of various parts of the body are shifted to move the center of gravity over the single, weight-bearing leg. This shift in the center of gravity, as **Figure 10.14** demonstrates, is an important component in the stepping mechanism of locomotion.

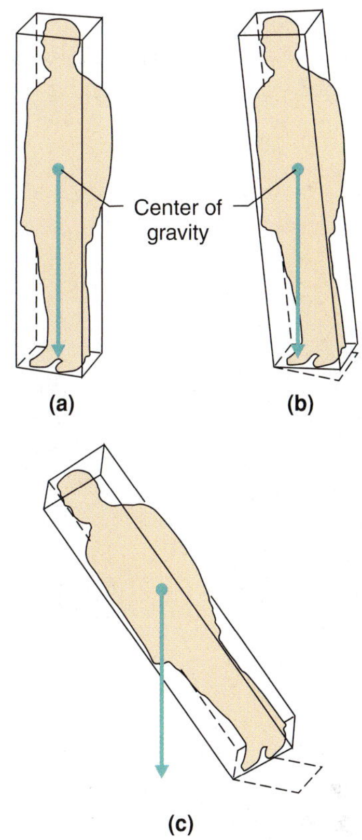

Figure 10.13 The center of gravity is the point in an object at which, if a string were attached and pulled up, all the downward force due to gravity would be exactly balanced. (a) The center of gravity must remain within the upward vertical projections of the object's base (the tall box outlined in the drawing) if stability is to be maintained. (b) Stable conditions. The box tilts a bit, but the center of gravity remains within the base area—the dashed rectangle on the floor—so the box returns to its upright position. (c) Unstable conditions. The box tilts so far that its center of gravity is not above any part of the object's base and the object will fall.

Afferent inputs from several sources are necessary for optimal postural adjustments, yet interfering with any one of these inputs alone does not cause a person to topple over. Blind people maintain their balance quite well with only a slight loss of precision, and people whose vestibular mechanisms have been destroyed can, with rehabilitation, have very little disability in everyday life as long as their visual system and somatic receptors are functioning.

The conclusion to be drawn from such examples is that the postural control mechanisms are not only effective and flexible but also highly adaptable.

10.6 Walking

Walking requires the coordination of many muscles, each activated to a precise degree at a precise time. We initiate walking by allowing the body to fall forward to an unstable position and then moving one leg forward to provide support. When the extensor muscles are activated on the supported side of the body to bear the body's weight, the contralateral extensors are inhibited by reciprocal innervation to allow the nonsupporting limb to flex and swing forward. The cyclical,

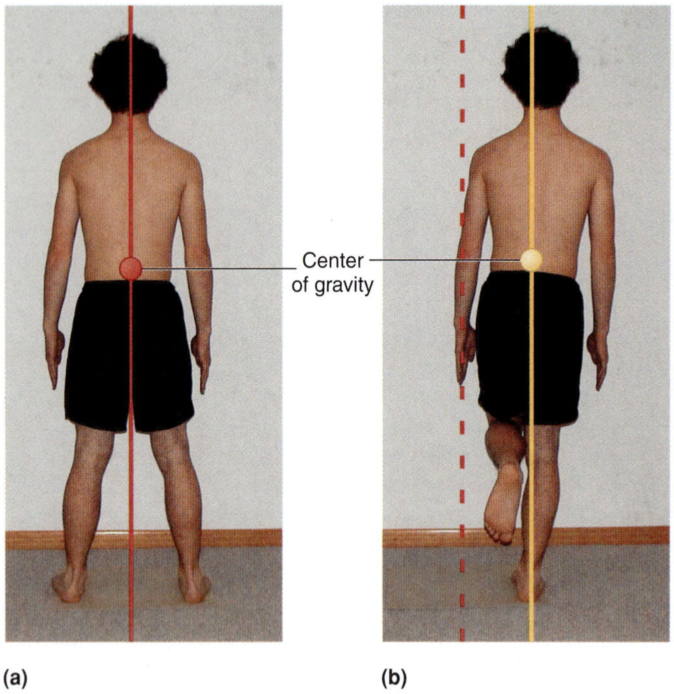

Figure 10.14 Postural changes with stepping. (a) Normal standing posture. The center of gravity falls directly between the two feet. (b) As the left foot is raised, the whole body leans to the right so that the center of gravity shifts over the right foot. Dashed line in part (b) indicates the location of the center of gravity when the subject was standing on both feet.

PHYSIOLOGICAL INQUIRY

- How might the posture shown in part (b) influence contractions of this individual's shoulder muscles?

Answer can be found at end of chapter.

alternating movements of walking are brought about largely by networks of interneurons in the spinal cord at the local level. The interneuron networks coordinate the output of the various motor neuron pools that control the appropriate muscles of the arms, shoulders, trunk, hips, legs, and feet.

The network neurons rely on both plasma membrane spontaneous pacemaker properties and patterned synaptic activity to establish their rhythms. At the same time, however, the networks are remarkably adaptable and a single network can generate many different patterns of neural activity, depending upon its inputs. These inputs come from other local interneurons, afferent fibers, and descending pathways.

These complex spinal cord neural networks can even produce the rhythmic movement of limbs in the absence of command inputs from descending pathways. This was demonstrated in classical experiments involving animals with their cerebrums surgically separated from their spinal cords just above the brainstem. Though sensory perception and voluntary movement were completely absent, when suspended in a position that brought the limbs into contact with a treadmill, normal walking and running actions were initiated by spinal reflexes arising from contact with the moving surface. This demonstrates that afferent inputs and local spinal cord neural networks contribute substantially to the coordination of locomotion.

Under normal conditions, neural activation occurs in the cerebral cortex, cerebellum, and brainstem, as well as in the spinal cord during locomotion. Moreover, middle and higher levels of the motor control hierarchy are necessary for postural control, voluntary override commands (like breaking stride to jump over a puddle), and adaptations to the environment (like walking across a stream on unevenly spaced stepping stones). Damage to even small areas of the sensorimotor cortex can cause marked disturbances in gait, which demonstrates its importance in locomotor control.

SUMMARY

Skeletal muscles are controlled by their motor neurons. All the motor neurons that control a given muscle form a motor neuron pool.

Motor Control Hierarchy

I. The neural systems that control body movements can be conceptualized as being arranged in a motor control hierarchy.
   a. The highest level determines the general intention of an action.
   b. The middle level establishes a motor program and specifies the postures and movements needed to carry out the intended action, taking into account sensory information that indicates the body's position.
   c. The local level ultimately determines which motor neurons will be activated.
   d. As the movement progresses, information about what the muscles are doing feeds back to the motor control centers, which make program corrections.
   e. Almost all actions have voluntary and involuntary components.

Local Control of Motor Neurons

I. Most direct input to motor neurons comes from local interneurons, which themselves receive input from peripheral receptors, descending pathways, and other interneurons.

II. Muscle-spindle stretch receptors monitor muscle length and the velocity of changes in length.
   a. Activation of these receptors initiates the stretch reflex, which inhibits motor neurons of ipsilateral antagonists and activates those of the stretched muscle and its synergists. This provides negative feedback control of muscle length.
   b. Tension on the stretch receptors is maintained during muscle contraction by activation of gamma motor neurons to the spindle muscle fibers.
   c. Alpha and gamma motor neurons are generally coactivated.

III. Golgi tendon organs monitor muscle tension. Through interneurons, they activate inhibitory synapses on motor neurons of the contracting muscle and excitatory synapses on motor neurons of ipsilateral antagonists. This provides negative feedback control of muscle tension.

IV. The withdrawal reflex excites the ipsilateral flexor muscles and inhibits the ipsilateral extensors. The crossed-extensor reflex excites the contralateral extensor muscles and inhibits the contralateral flexor muscles.

The Brain Motor Centers and the Descending Pathways They Control

I. Neurons in the motor cortex are anatomically arranged in a somatotopic map.

II. Different areas of sensorimotor cortex have different functions but much overlap in activity.

III. The basal nuclei form a link in a circuit that originates in and returns to sensorimotor cortex. These subcortical nuclei facilitate some motor behaviors and inhibit others.

IV. The cerebellum coordinates posture and movement and plays a role in motor learning.

V. The corticospinal pathways pass directly from the sensorimotor cortex to motor neurons in the spinal cord (or brainstem, in the case of the corticobulbar pathways) or, more commonly, to interneurons near the motor neurons.

   a. In general, neurons on one side of the brain control muscles on the other side of the body.

   b. Corticospinal pathways control predominantly fine, precise movements.

   c. Some corticospinal fibers affect the transmission of information in afferent pathways.

VI. Other descending pathways arise in the brainstem, control muscles on the same side of the body, and are involved mainly in the coordination of large groups of muscles used in posture and locomotion.

VII. There is significant interaction between the two descending pathways.

Muscle Tone

I. Hypertonia, as seen in spasticity and rigidity, usually occurs with disorders of the descending pathways.

II. Hypotonia can be seen with cerebellar disease or, more commonly, with disease of the alpha motor neurons or muscle.

Maintenance of Upright Posture and Balance

I. Maintenance of posture and balance depends upon inputs from the eyes, vestibular apparatus, and somatic proprioceptors.

II. To maintain balance, the body's center of gravity must be maintained over the body's base.

III. The crossed-extensor reflex is a postural reflex.

Walking

I. The activity of interneuron networks in the spinal cord brings about the cyclical, alternating movements of locomotion.

II. These pattern generators are controlled by corticospinal and brainstem descending pathways and affected by feedback and motor programs.

REVIEW QUESTIONS

1. Describe motor control in terms of the conceptual motor control hierarchy. Use the following terms: *highest, middle,* and *local levels; motor program; descending pathways;* and *motor neuron.*
2. List the characteristics of voluntary actions.
3. Picking up a book, for example, has both voluntary and involuntary components. List the components of this action and indicate whether each is voluntary or involuntary.
4. List the inputs that can converge on the interneurons active in local motor control.
5. Draw a muscle spindle within a muscle, labeling the spindle, intrafusal and extrafusal muscle fibers, stretch receptors, afferent fibers, and alpha and gamma efferent fibers.
6. Describe the components of the knee-jerk reflex (stimulus, receptor, afferent pathway, integrating center, efferent pathway, effector, and response).
7. Describe the major function of alpha–gamma coactivation.
8. Distinguish among the following areas of the cerebral cortex: sensorimotor, primary motor, premotor, and supplementary motor.
9. Contrast the two major types of descending motor pathways in terms of structure and function.
10. Describe the roles that the basal nuclei and cerebellum play in motor control.
11. Explain how hypertonia may result from disease of the descending pathways.
12. Explain how hypotonia may result from lower motor neuron disease.
13. Explain the role the crossed-extensor reflex plays in postural stability.
14. Explain the role of the interneuronal networks in walking, incorporating in your discussion the following terms: *interneuron, reciprocal innervation, synergist, antagonist,* and *feedback.*

KEY TERMS

alpha–gamma coactivation 304
alpha motor neuron 304
basal nuclei 310
brainstem pathway 311
corticobulbar pathway 312
corticospinal pathway 311
crossed-extensor reflex 307
descending pathway 302
extrafusal fiber 304
extrapyramidal system 312
gamma motor neuron 304
Golgi tendon organ 306
intrafusal fiber 304
knee-jerk reflex 304
lower motor neurons 312
monosynaptic 306
motor cortex 308
motor neuron pool 300
motor program 302
motor unit 300
muscle spindle 304
muscle-spindle stretch receptor 304
muscle tone 312
nuclear bag fiber 304
nuclear chain fiber 304
parietal-lobe association cortex 308
polysynaptic 306
postural reflex 313
premotor area 308
primary motor cortex 308
proprioception 302
pyramidal system 311
pyramidal tract 311
reciprocal innervation 306
sensorimotor cortex 308
somatosensory cortex 308
somatotopic map 308
stretch reflex 304
substantia nigra 310
supplementary motor cortex 308
synergistic muscle 306
upper motor neurons 312
voluntary movement 302
withdrawal reflex 307

CLINICAL TERMS

akinesia 310
bradykinesia 310
cerebellar disease 311
clasp-knife phenomenon 312
cramp 313
deep brain stimulation 310
flaccid 313
hypertonia 312
hypotonia 313
intention tremor 311
Levodopa (L-dopa) 310
MPTP (1-methyl-4-phenyl-1,2,3,6-tetrahydropyridine) 310
Parkinson disease 310
rigidity 312
spasm 313
spasticity 312
upper motor neuron disorders 312

CHAPTER 10 Clinical Case Study: A Woman Develops Stiff Jaw Muscles After a Puncture Wound

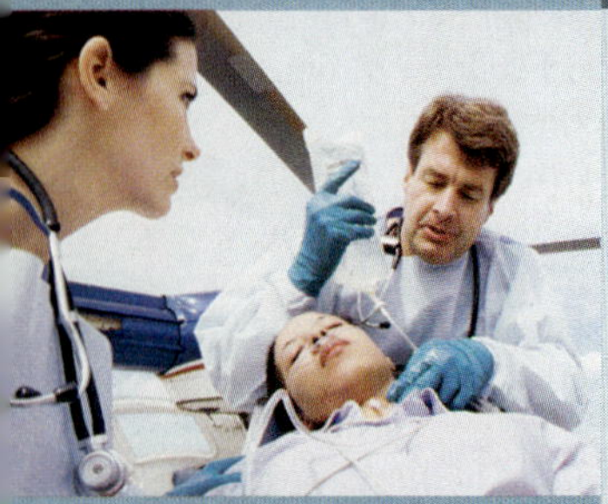

A 55-year-old woman with complaints of muscle pain was brought to an urgent-care clinic by her husband. The woman had trouble speaking, so her husband explained that over the previous 3 days, her back and jaw muscles had grown gradually stiffer and more painful. By the time of her visit, she could barely open her mouth wide enough to drink through a straw. Until that week, she had been extremely healthy, had no history of allergies or surgical procedures, and was not taking any medications. At the time of examination, her blood pressure was 122/70 mmHg and her temperature was 98.5°F. Other than a stiff jaw, findings from a head and neck exam were otherwise unremarkable, her lung sounds were clear, and her heart sounds were normal. Evaluating her extremities, the physician noticed that her right leg was bandaged just below the knee. A little over a week prior to this visit, she had been working in her garden and had stumbled and fallen onto a rake, puncturing her shin. The wound had not bled a great deal, so she had washed and bandaged it herself. Removal of the bandage revealed a raised, 5-cm-wide erythematous (reddened) region, surrounding a 1 cm puncture wound that had scabbed over. The doctor then asked a key question, When had she received her most recent tetanus booster shot? It had been so long ago that neither the woman nor her husband could remember exactly when it was—more than 20 years, they guessed. This piece of information, along with her leg wound and symptoms, led the physician to conclude that the woman had developed tetanus. Because this is a potentially fatal condition, she was admitted to the hospital.

Tetanus is a neurological disorder that results from a decrease in the inhibitory input to alpha motor neurons. It occurs when spores of *Clostridium tetani*, a bacterium commonly found in manure-treated soils, invade a poorly oxygenated wound. Proliferation of the bacterium under anaerobic conditions induces it to secrete a neurotoxin called ***tetanospasmin*** that targets inhibitory interneurons in the brainstem and spinal cord. Blockage of neurotransmitter release from these interneurons allows the normal excitatory inputs to dominate control of the alpha motor neurons, and the result is high-frequency action potential firing that causes increased muscle tone and spasms.

Because the toxin attacks interneurons by traveling backward along the axons of alpha motor neurons, muscles with short motor neurons are affected first. Muscles of the head are in this category, in particular those that move the jaw. The jaw rigidly clamps shut, because the muscles that close it are much stronger than those that open it. Appearance of this symptom early in the disease process explains the common name of this condition, ***lockjaw.*** Untreated tetanus is fatal, as progressive spastic contraction of all of the skeletal muscles eventually affects those involved in respiration, and asphyxia occurs.

Treatment for tetanus includes (1) cleaning and sterilizing wounds; (2) administering antibiotics to kill the bacteria; (3) injecting antibodies known as ***tetanus immune globulin (TIG)*** that bind the toxin, (4) providing neuromuscular blocking drugs to relax and/or paralyze spastic muscles; and (5) mechanically ventilating the lungs to maintain airflow despite spastic or paralyzed respiratory muscles. Treated promptly, 80% to 90% of tetanus victims recover completely. It can take several months, however, because inhibitory axon terminals damaged by the toxin must be regrown.

The patient in this case was fortunate to have had partial immunity from vaccinations received earlier in her life and to have received prompt treatment. Her disease was relatively mild as a result and did not require weeks of hospitalization with drug-induced paralysis and ventilation, as is necessary in more serious cases. She was immediately given intramuscular injections of TIG and a combination of strong antibiotics to be taken for the next 10 days. The leg wound was surgically opened, thoroughly cleaned, and monitored closely over the next week as the redness and swelling gradually subsided. Within 2 days, her jaw and back muscles had relaxed. She was released from the hospital with orders to continue the complete course of antibiotics and return immediately if any muscular symptoms returned. At the time of discharge, she was also vaccinated to stimulate production of her own antibodies against the tetanus toxin and was advised to receive booster shots against tetanus at least every 10 years.

Clinical terms: lockjaw, tetanospasmin, tetanus, tetanus immune globulin (TIG)

See Chapter 19 for complete, integrative case studies.

CHAPTER 10 TEST QUESTIONS

Answers found in Appendix A.

1. Which is a correct statement regarding the hierarchical organization of motor control?
   a. Skeletal muscle contraction can only be initiated by neurons in the cerebral cortex.
   b. The basal nuclei participate in the creation of a motor program that specifies the pattern of neural activity required for a voluntary movement.
   c. Neurons in the cerebellum have long axons that synapse directly on alpha motor neurons in the ventral horn of the spinal cord.
   d. The cell bodies of alpha motor neurons are found in the primary motor region of the cerebral cortex.
   e. Neurons with cell bodies in the basal nuclei can form either excitatory or inhibitory synapses onto skeletal muscle cells.
2. In the stretch reflex,
   a. Golgi tendon organs activate contraction in extrafusal muscle fibers connected to that tendon.
   b. lengthening of muscle-spindle receptors in a muscle leads to contraction in an antagonist muscle.

c. action potentials from muscle-spindle receptors in a muscle form monosynaptic excitatory synapses on motor neurons to extrafusal fibers within the same muscles.
d. slackening of intrafusal fibers within a muscle activates gamma motor neurons that form excitatory synapses with extrafusal fibers within that same muscle.
e. afferent neurons to the sensorimotor cortex stimulate the agonist muscle to contract and the antagonist muscle to be inhibited.

3. Which would result in reflex contraction of the extensor muscles of the right leg?
   a. stepping on a tack with the left foot
   b. stretching the flexor muscles in the right leg
   c. dropping a hammer on the right big toe
   d. action potentials from Golgi tendon organs in extensors of the right leg
   e. action potentials from muscle-spindle receptors in flexors of the right leg
4. If implanted electrodes were used to stimulate action potentials in gamma motor neurons to flexors of the left arm, which would be the most likely result?
   a. inhibition of the flexors of the left arm
   b. a decrease in action potentials from muscle-spindle receptors in the left arm
   c. a decrease in action potentials from Golgi tendon organs in the left arm
   d. an increase in action potentials along alpha motor neurons to flexors in the left arm
   e. contraction of flexor muscles in the right arm
5. Where is the primary motor cortex found?
   a. in the cerebellum
   b. in the occipital lobe of the cerebrum
   c. between the somatosensory cortex and the premotor area of the cerebrum
   d. in the ventral horn of the spinal cord
   e. just posterior to the parietal lobe association cortex

True or False

6. Neurons in the primary motor cortex of the right cerebral hemisphere mainly control muscles on the left side of the body.
7. Patients with upper motor neuron disorders generally have reduced muscle tone and flaccid paralysis.
8. Neurons descending in the corticospinal pathway control mainly trunk musculature and postural reflexes, whereas neurons of the brainstem pathways control fine motor movements of the distal extremities.
9. In patients with Parkinson disease, an excess of dopamine from neurons of the substantia nigra causes intention tremors when the person performs voluntary movements.
10. The disease tetanus results when a bacterial toxin blocks the release of inhibitory neurotransmitter.

CHAPTER 10 GENERAL PRINCIPLES ASSESSMENT

Answers found in Appendix A.

1. One of the general principles of physiology introduced in Chapter 1 states that *most physiological functions are controlled by multiple regulatory systems, often working in opposition.* However, skeletal muscle cells are only innervated by alpha motor neurons, which always release acetylcholine and always excite them to contract. By what mechanism are skeletal muscles induced to relax?
2. Another general principle of physiology is that *homeostasis is essential for health and survival.* How might the withdrawal reflex (see Figure 10.9) contribute to the maintenance of homeostasis?

CHAPTER 10 QUANTITATIVE AND THOUGHT QUESTIONS

Answers found at www.mhhe.com/widmaier13.

1. What changes would occur in the knee-jerk reflex after destruction of the gamma motor neurons?
2. What changes would occur in the knee-jerk reflex after destruction of the alpha motor neurons?
3. Draw a cross section of the spinal cord and a portion of the thigh (similar to Figure 10.6) and "wire up" and activate the neurons so the leg becomes a stiff pillar, that is, so the knee does not bend.
4. Hypertonia is usually considered a sign of disease of the descending motor pathways. How might it also result from abnormal function of the alpha motor neurons?
5. What neurotransmitters/receptors might be effective targets for drugs used to prevent the muscle spasms characteristic of the disease tetanus?
6. A patient is told to relax, and her patellar tendon reflex is tested (see Figure 10.6). Next, the patient is instructed to hook the fingers of her two hands together and pull outward with her arms. While she is doing this, the patellar reflex is tested again, and the knee jerk is significantly greater. What are some possible explanations for this phenomenon?

CHAPTER 10 ANSWERS TO PHYSIOLOGICAL INQUIRIES

Figure 10.3 Recall that when chloride ion channels are opened, a neuron is inhibited from depolarizing to threshold (see Figure 6.29 and accompanying text). Thus, the neurons of the spinal cord that release glycine are inhibitory interneurons. By specifically blocking glycine receptors, strychnine shifts the balance of inputs to motor neurons in favor of excitatory interneurons, resulting in excessive excitation. Poisoning victims experience excessive and uncontrollable muscle contractions body-wide, and when the respiratory muscles are affected, asphyxiation can occur. These symptoms are similar to those observed in the disease state tetanus, which is described in the Clinical Case Study at the end of this chapter.

Figure 10.6 Stimulation of gamma motor neurons to leg flexor muscles would stretch muscle-spindle receptors in those muscles. That would trigger a monosynaptic reflex that would cause contraction of the flexor muscles and, through an interneuron, the extensor muscles would be inhibited. As a result, there would be a reflexive bending of the leg—the opposite of what occurs in the typical knee-jerk reflex.

Figure 10.7 Although the contracting muscle results in the greatest stretch of the tendon, the muscle itself (and consequently the intrafusal fibers) are stretched the most under passive stretch conditions. Action potentials from muscle-spindle receptors would therefore have the greatest frequency during passive stretch.

Figure 10.8 Tendons are stretched more by actively contracting muscles than when muscles are passively stretched (see Figure 10.7). Thus, during very intense contractions that have the potential to cause injury, Golgi tendon organs are strongly activated. The resulting high-frequency action potentials arriving in the spinal cord stimulate interneurons that inhibit motor neurons to the muscle associated with that tendon, thus reducing the force and protecting the muscle.

Figure 10.9 When crawling, the crossed-extensor reflex will occur for the arms just like it does in the legs during walking. Afferent pain pathways will stimulate flexor muscles and inhibit extensor muscles in the right arm, while stimulating extensor muscles and inhibiting flexor muscles in the left arm. This withdraws the right hand from the painful stimulus while the left arm straightens to bear the child's weight.

Figure 10.12 When a region of the brain is deprived of oxygen and nutrients for even a short time, it often results in a stroke—neuronal cell death (see Chapter 6, Section D). Because the right primary motor cortex was damaged in this case, the patient would have impaired motor function on the left side of the body. Given the midline location of the lesion, the leg would be most affected (see Figure 10.11).

Figure 10.14 To stand on the right foot, the hip extensors on the right side are activated while the hip flexors on the left side are activated. This is similar to what occurs when a walking person lifts the left leg and pushes forward with the right foot. In adults, spinal cord interneurons form locomotor pattern generators that connect the arms and legs, typically activating them in reciprocal fashion. Therefore, while standing on the right foot, the right shoulder flexor muscles and the left shoulder extensor muscles will tend to be activated.

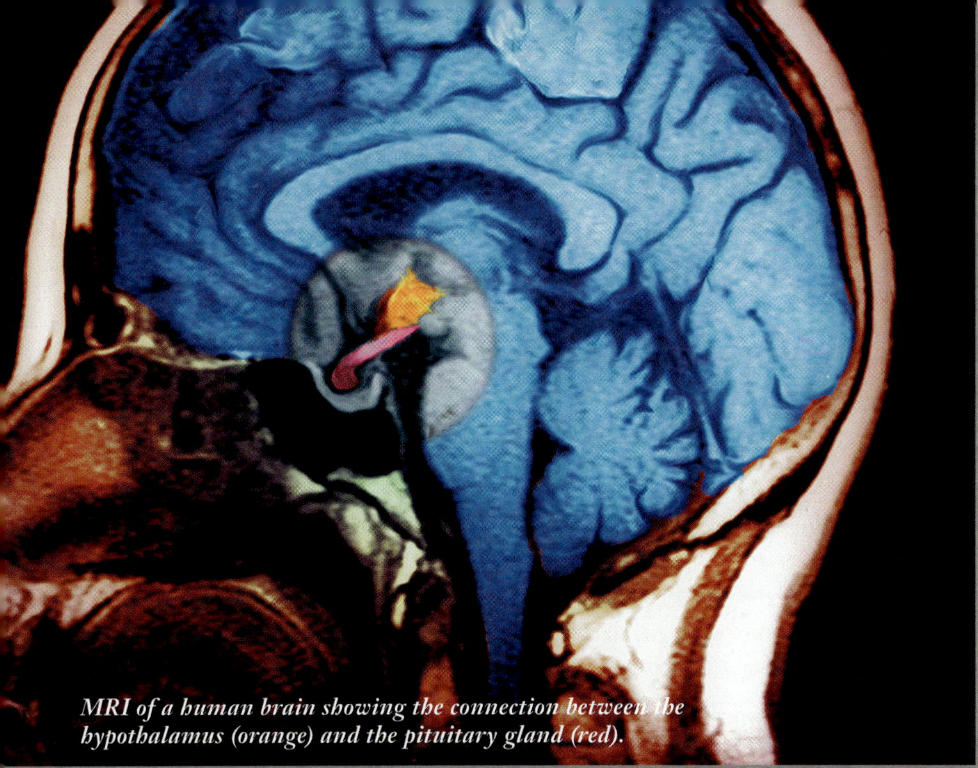

MRI of a human brain showing the connection between the hypothalamus (orange) and the pituitary gland (red).

11 The Endocrine System

In Chapters 6–8 and 10, you learned that the nervous system is one of the two major control systems of the body, and now we turn our attention to the other—the endocrine system. The endocrine system consists of all those glands, called endocrine glands, that secrete hormones, as well as hormone-secreting cells located in various organs such as the heart, kidneys, liver, and stomach. Hormones are chemical messengers that enter the blood, which carries them from their site of secretion to the cells upon which they act. The cells a particular hormone influences are known as the target cells for that hormone. The aim of this chapter is to first present a detailed overview of endocrinology—that is, a structural and functional analysis of general features of hormones—followed by a more detailed analysis of several important hormonal systems. Before continuing, you should review the principles of ligand-receptor interactions and cell signaling that were described in Chapter 3 (Section C) and Chapter 5, because they pertain to the mechanisms by which hormones exert their actions.

Hormones functionally link various organ systems together. As such, several of the general principles of physiology first introduced in Chapter 1 apply to the study of the endocrine system, including the principle that the functions of organ systems are coordinated with each other. This coordination is key to the maintenance of homeostasis, another important general principle of physiology that will be covered in Sections C, D, and F. In many cases, the actions of one hormone can be potentiated, inhibited, or counterbalanced by the actions of another. This illustrates the general principle of physiology that most physiological functions are controlled by multiple regulatory systems, often working in opposition. It will be especially relevant in the sections on the endocrine control of metabolism and the control of pituitary gland function. Finally, this chapter exemplifies the general principle of physiology that information flow between cells, tissues, and organs is an essential feature of homeostasis and allows for integration of physiological processes.

SECTION A

General Characteristics of Hormones and Hormonal Control Systems

11.1 Hormones and Endocrine Glands

Endocrine glands are distinguished from another type of gland in the body called exocrine glands. Exocrine glands secrete their products into a duct, from where the secretions either exit the body (as in sweat) or enter the lumen of another organ, such as the intestines. By contrast, endocrine glands are ductless and release hormones into the blood (**Figure 11.1**). Hormones are actually released first into interstitial fluid, from where they diffuse into the blood, but for simplicity we will often omit the interstitial fluid step in our discussion.

Table 11.1 summarizes most of the endocrine glands and other hormone-secreting organs, the hormones they secrete, and some of the major functions the hormones control. The endocrine system differs from most of the other organ systems of the body in that the various components are not anatomically connected; however, they do form a system in the functional sense. You may be puzzled to see some organs—the heart, for instance—that clearly have other functions yet are listed as part of the endocrine system. The explanation is that, in addition to the cells that carry out other functions, the organ also contains cells that secrete hormones.

Note also in Table 11.1 that the hypothalamus, a part of the brain, is considered part of the endocrine system. This is because the chemical messengers released by certain axon terminals in both the hypothalamus and its extension, the posterior pituitary, do not function as neurotransmitters affecting adjacent cells but, rather, enter the blood as hormones. The blood then carries these hormones to their sites of action.

Table 11.1 demonstrates that there are a large number of endocrine glands and hormones. This chapter is not all inclusive. Some of the hormones listed in Table 11.1 are best considered in the context of the control systems in which they participate. For example, the pancreatic hormones (insulin and glucagon) are described in Chapter 16 in the context of organic metabolism, and the reproductive hormones are extensively covered in Chapter 17.

Also evident from Table 11.1 is that a single gland may secrete multiple hormones. The usual pattern in such cases is that a single cell type secretes only one hormone, so that multiple-hormone secretion reflects the presence of different types of endocrine cells in the same gland. In a few cases, however, a single cell may secrete more than one hormone.

Finally, in some cases, a hormone secreted by an endocrine-gland cell may also be secreted by other cell types and serves in these other locations as a neurotransmitter or paracrine or autocrine substance. For example, somatostatin, a hormone produced by neurons in the hypothalamus, is also secreted by cells of the stomach and pancreas, where it has local paracrine actions.

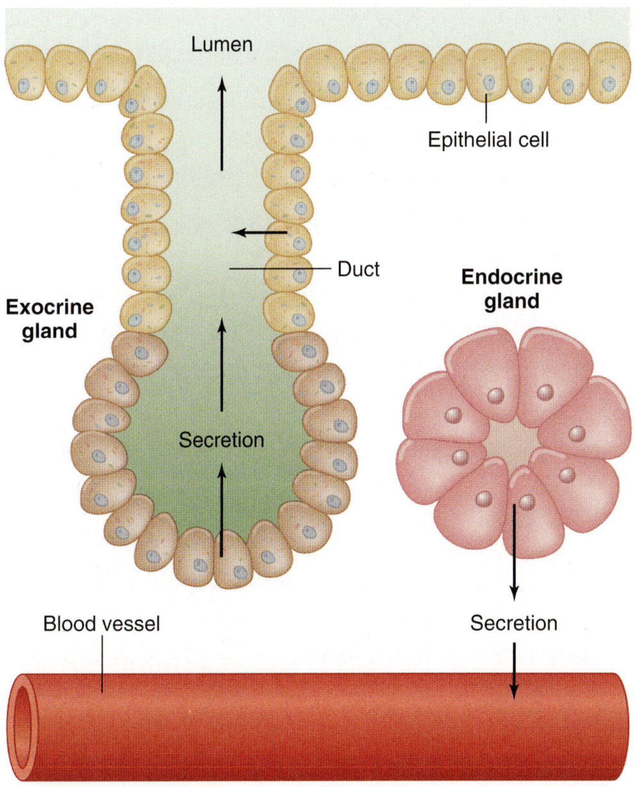

Figure 11.1 AP|R Exocrine gland secretions enter ducts from where their secretions either exit the body or, as shown here, connect to the lumen of a structure such as the intestines or to the surface of the skin. By contrast, endocrine glands secrete hormones that enter the interstitial fluid and diffuse into the blood, from where they can reach distant target cells.

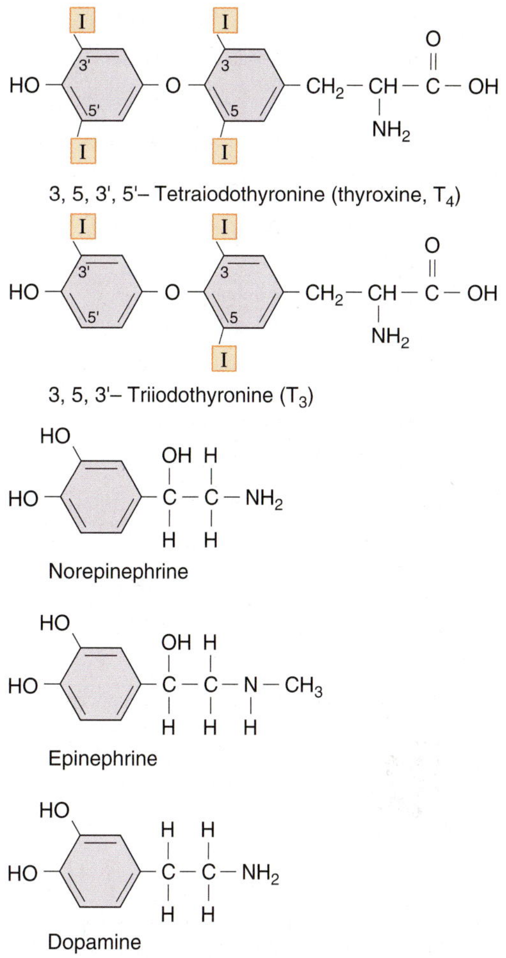

Figure 11.2 Chemical structures of the amine hormones: thyroxine, triiodothyronine, norepinephrine, epinephrine, and dopamine. The two thyroid hormones differ by only one iodine atom, a difference noted in the abbreviations T_3 and T_4. The position of the carbon atoms in the two rings of T_3 and T_4 are numbered; this provides the basis for the complete names of T_3 and T_4 as shown in the figure.

11.2 Hormone Structures and Synthesis

Hormones fall into three major structural classes: (1) amines, (2) peptides and proteins, and (3) steroids.

Amine Hormones

The **amine hormones** are derivatives of the amino acid tyrosine. They include the **thyroid hormones** (produced by the thyroid gland) and the catecholamines **epinephrine** and **norepinephrine** (produced by the adrenal medulla) and **dopamine** (produced by the hypothalamus). The structure and synthesis of the iodine-containing thyroid hormones will be described in detail in Section C of this chapter. For now, their structures are included in **Figure 11.2.** Chapter 6 described the structures of catecholamines and the steps of their synthesis; the structures are reproduced here in Figure 11.2.

There are two adrenal glands, one above each kidney. Each **adrenal gland** is composed of an inner **adrenal medulla,** which secretes amine hormones, and a surrounding **adrenal cortex,** which secretes steroid hormones. The adrenal medulla is really a modified sympathetic ganglion whose cell bodies do not have axons. Instead, they release their secretions into the blood, thereby fulfilling a criterion for an endocrine gland.

The adrenal medulla secretes mainly two amine hormones, epinephrine and norepinephrine. In humans, the adrenal medulla secretes approximately four times more epinephrine than norepinephrine. This is because the adrenal medulla expresses high amounts of an enzyme called phenylethanolamine-N-methyltransferase (PNMT), which catalyzes the reaction that converts norepinephrine to epinephrine. Epinephrine and norepinephrine exert actions similar to those of the sympathetic nerves, which, because they do not express PNMT, make only norepinephrine. These actions are described in various chapters and summarized in Section B of this chapter.

The other catecholamine hormone, dopamine, is synthesized by neurons in the hypothalamus. Dopamine is released into a special circulatory system called a portal system (see Section B), which carries the hormone to the pituitary gland; there, it acts to inhibit the activity of certain endocrine cells.

Peptide and Protein Hormones

Most hormones are polypeptides. Recall from Chapter 2 that short polypeptides with a known function are often referred to simply as peptides; longer polypeptides with

TABLE 11.1 Summary of Some Important Hormones		
Site Produced	**Hormone**	**Major Function* Is Control Of:**
Adipose tissue cells	Leptin, several others	Appetite; metabolic rate; reproduction
Adrenal glands:		
Adrenal cortex	Cortisol	Organic metabolism; response to stress; immune system; development
	Androgens	Sex drive in women; adrenarche
	Aldosterone	Na^+ and K^+ excretion by kidneys; extracellular water balance
Adrenal medulla	Epinephrine and norepinephrine	Organic metabolism; cardiovascular function; response to stress ("fight-or-flight")
Gastrointestinal tract	Gastrin	Gastrointestinal tract motility and acid secretion
	Ghrelin	Appetite
	Secretin	Exocrine and endocrine secretions from pancreas
	Cholecystokinin (CCK)†	Secretion of bile from gallbladder
	Glucose-dependent insulinotropic peptide (GIP) and glucagon-like peptide 1 (GLP-1)	Insulin secretion
	Motilin	Gastrointestinal tract motility
Gonads:		
Ovaries: female	Estrogen (estradiol in humans)	Reproductive system; secondary sex characteristics; growth and development; development of ovarian follicles
	Progesterone	Endometrium and pregnancy
	Inhibin	Follicle-stimulating hormone (FSH) secretion
	Relaxin	Relaxation of cervix and pubic ligaments
Testes: male	Androgen (testosterone and dihydrotestosterone)	Reproductive system; secondary sex characteristics; growth and development; sex drive; gamete development
	Inhibin	FSH secretion
	Müllerian-inhibiting substance (MIS)	Regression of Müllerian ducts
Heart	Atrial natriuretic peptide (ANP)	Na^+ excretion by kidneys; blood pressure
Hypothalamus	Hypophysiotropic hormones:	Secretion of hormones by the anterior pituitary gland
	Corticotropin-releasing hormone (CRH)	Secretion of adrenocorticotropic hormone (ACTH)
	Thyrotropin-releasing hormone (TRH)	Secretion of thyroid-stimulating hormone (TSH)
	Growth hormone–releasing hormone (GHRH)	Secretion of growth hormone (GH)
	Somatostatin (SST)	Secretion of growth hormone
	Gonadotropin-releasing hormone (GnRH)	Secretion of luteinizing hormone (LH) and follicle-stimulating hormone (FSH)
	Dopamine (DA)	Secretion of prolactin (PRL)
Kidneys	Erythropoietin (EPO; also made in liver)	Erythrocyte production in bone marrow
	1,25-dihydroxyvitamin D	Ca^{2+} absorption in GI tract
Liver	Insulin-like growth factor 1 (IGF-1)	Cell division and growth of bone and other tissues
Pancreas	Insulin	Plasma glucose, amino acids, and fatty acids
	Glucagon	Plasma glucose
Parathyroid glands	Parathyroid hormone (PTH, parathormone)	Plasma Ca^{2+} and phosphate ion; synthesis of 1,25-dihydroxyvitamin D

(continued)

TABLE 11.1	Summary of Some Important Hormones *(Continued)*	
Site Produced	**Hormone**	**Major Function* Is Control Of:**
Pineal	Melatonin	Possible role in circadian sleep-wake cycles
Pituitary gland:		
Anterior pituitary gland	Growth hormone (somatotropin)	Growth, mainly via local production of IGF-1; protein, carbohydrate, and lipid metabolism
	Thyroid-stimulating hormone (thyrotropin)	Thyroid gland activity and growth
	Adrenocorticotropic hormone (corticotropin)	Adrenal cortex activity and growth
	Prolactin	Milk production in breast
	Gonadotropic hormones:	
	Follicle-stimulating hormone	
	Males	Gamete production
	Females	Ovarian follicle growth
	Luteinizing hormone:	
	Males	Testicular production of testosterone
	Females	Ovarian production of estradiol; ovulation
	β-lipotropin and β-endorphin	Possibly fat mobilization and analgesia during stress
Posterior pituitary‡	Oxytocin	Milk secretion; uterine motility
	Vasopressin (antidiuretic hormone, ADH)	Blood pressure; water excretion by the kidneys
Placenta	Human chorionic gonadotropin (hCG)	Secretion of progesterone and estrogen by corpus luteum
	Estrogens	See Gonads: ovaries
	Progesterone	See Gonads: ovaries
	Human placental lactogen (hPL)	Breast development; organic metabolism
Thymus	Thymopoietin	T-lymphocyte function
Thyroid	Thyroxine (T_4) and triiodothyronine (T_3)	Metabolic rate; growth; brain development and function
	Calcitonin	Plasma Ca^{2+} in some vertebrates (role unclear in humans)
Other (produced in blood)	Angiotensin II	Blood pressure; production of aldosterone from adrenal cortex

*This table does not list all functions of all hormones.
†The names and abbreviations in parentheses are synonyms.
‡The posterior pituitary stores and secretes these hormones; they are synthesized in the hypothalamus.

tertiary structure and a known function are called proteins. Hormones in this class range in size from small peptides having only three amino acids to proteins, some of which contain carbohydrate and thus are glycoproteins. For convenience, we will simply refer to all these hormones as **peptide hormones.**

In many cases, peptide hormones are initially synthesized on the ribosomes of endocrine cells as larger molecules known as preprohormones, which are then cleaved to **prohormones** by proteolytic enzymes in the rough endoplasmic reticulum (**Figure 11.3a**). The prohormone is then packaged into secretory vesicles by the Golgi apparatus. In this process, the prohormone is cleaved to yield the active hormone and other peptide chains found in the prohormone. Consequently, when the cell is stimulated to release the contents of the secretory vesicles by exocytosis, the other peptides are secreted along with the hormone. In certain cases, these other peptides may also exert hormonal effects. In other words, instead of just one peptide hormone, the cell may secrete multiple peptide hormones—derived from the same prohormone—each of which differs in its effects on target cells. One well-studied example of this is the synthesis of insulin in the pancreas (**Figure 11.3b**). Insulin is synthesized as a single polypeptide preprohormone, then processed to the prohormone. Enzymes clip off a portion of the prohormone resulting in insulin and another product called C-peptide. Both insulin and C-peptide are secreted into the circulation in roughly equimolar amounts. Insulin is a key regulator of metabolism, while C-peptide has several actions on a variety of cell types.

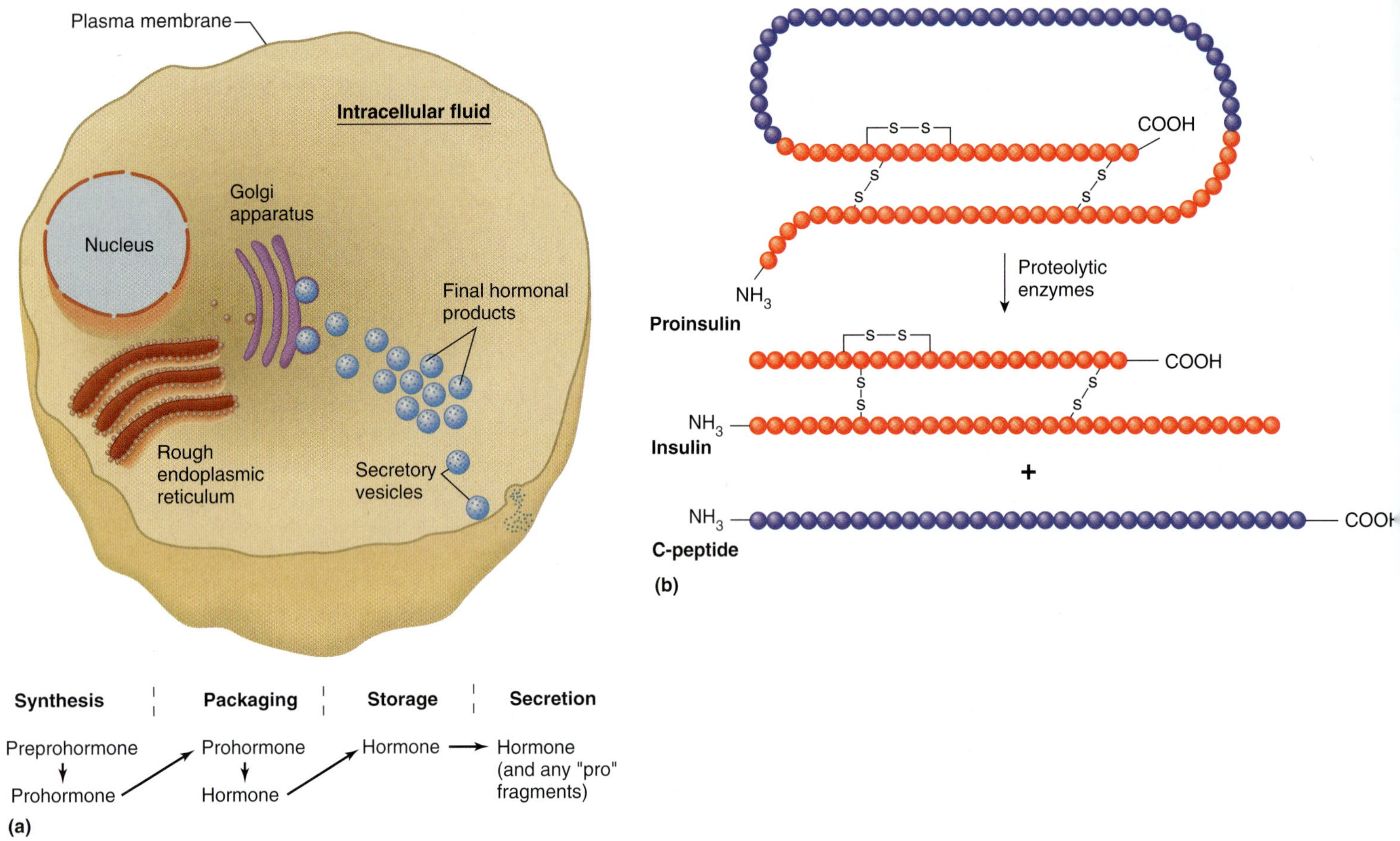

Figure 11.3 AP|R Typical synthesis and secretion of peptide hormones. (a) Peptide hormones typically are processed by enzymes from preprohormones containing a signal peptide, to prohormones; further processing results in one or more active hormones that are stored in secretory vesicles. Secretion of stored secretory vesicles occurs by the process of exocytosis. (b) An example of peptide hormone synthesis. Insulin is synthesized as a preprohormone (not shown) that is cleaved to the prohormone shown here. Each bead represents an amino acid. The action of proteolytic enzymes cleaves the prohormone into insulin and C-peptide. Note that this cleavage results in two chains of insulin, which are connected by disulfide bridges.

PHYSIOLOGICAL INQUIRY

- What is the advantage of packaging peptide hormones in secretory vesicles?

Answer can be found at end of chapter.

Steroid Hormones

Steroid hormones make up the third family of hormones. **Figure 11.4** shows some examples of steroid hormones; their ringlike structure was described in Chapter 2. Steroid hormones are primarily produced by the adrenal cortex and the **gonads** (testes and ovaries), as well as by the placenta during pregnancy. In addition, vitamin D is enzymatically converted by two hydroxylation reactions into the biologically active steroid hormone called **1,25-dihydroxyvitamin D** (also called 1,25-dihydroxycholecalciferol or calcitriol). These reactions occur in the liver and kidneys.

The general process of steroid hormone synthesis is illustrated in **Figure 11.5a.** In both the gonads and the adrenal cortex, the hormone-producing cells are stimulated by the binding of an anterior pituitary gland hormone to its plasma membrane receptor. These receptors are linked to G_s proteins (refer back to Figure 5.6), which activate adenylyl cyclase and cAMP production. The subsequent activation of protein kinase A by cAMP results in phosphorylation of numerous intracellular proteins, which facilitate the subsequent steps in the process.

All of the steroid hormones are derived from cholesterol, which is either taken up from the extracellular fluid by the cells or synthesized by intracellular enzymes. The final hormone product depends upon the cell type and the types and amounts of the enzymes it expresses. Cells in the ovary, for example, express large amounts of the enzyme needed to convert testosterone to estradiol, whereas cells in the testes do not express significant amounts of this enzyme and therefore make primarily testosterone.

Once formed, the steroid hormones cannot be stored in the cytosol in membrane-bound vesicles, because the lipophilic nature of the steroids allows them to freely diffuse across lipid bilayers. As a result, once they are synthesized, steroid hormones diffuse across the plasma membrane into the circulation. Because of their lipid nature, steroid hormones

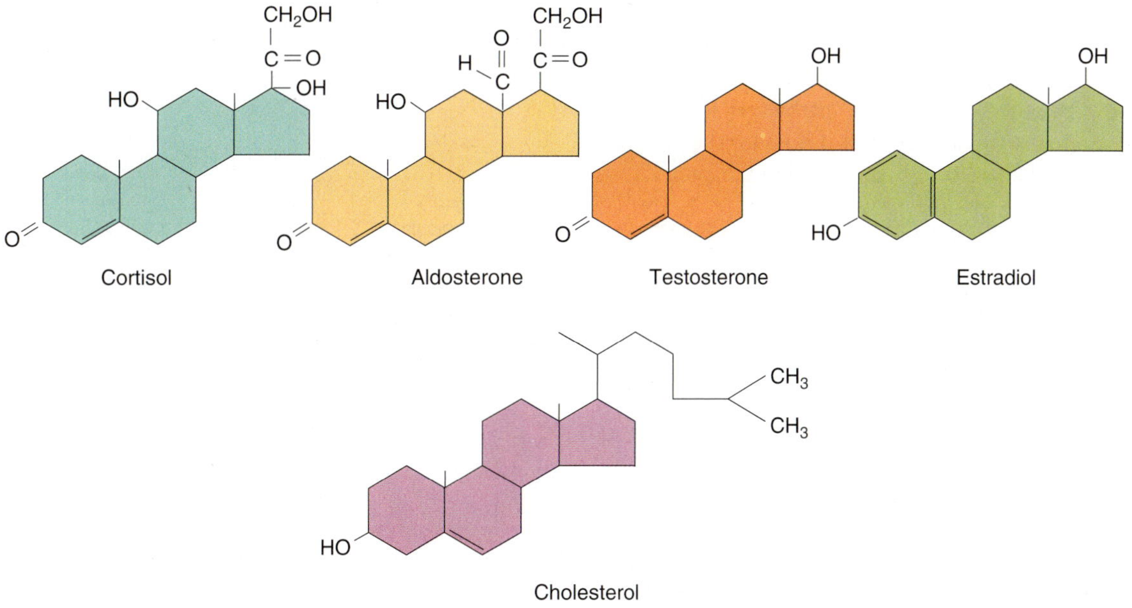

Figure 11.4 Structures of representative steroid hormones and their structural relationship to cholesterol.

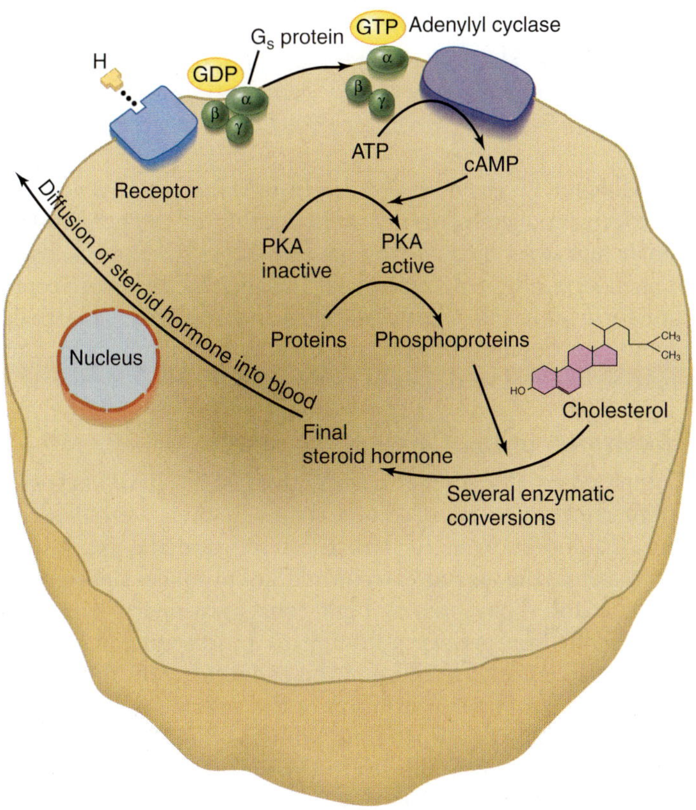

(a)

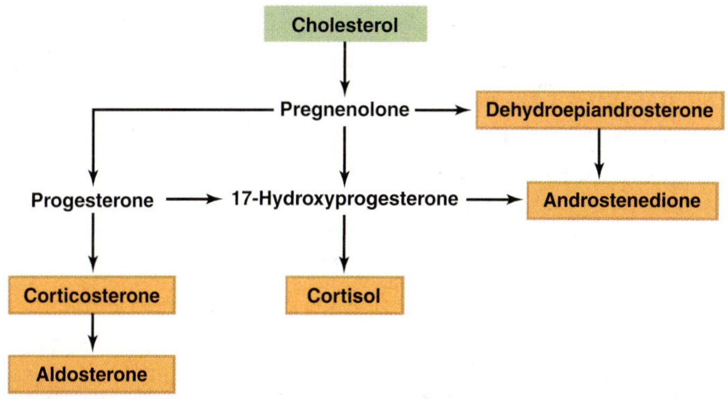

(b)

Figure 11.5 (a) Schematic overview of steps involved in steroid synthesis. (b) The five hormones shown in boxes are the major hormones secreted from the adrenal cortex. Dehydroepiandrosterone (DHEA) and androstenedione are androgens—that is, testosterone-like hormones. Cortisol and corticosterone are glucocorticoids, and aldosterone is a mineralocorticoid that is only produced by one part of the adrenal cortex. *Note:* For simplicity, not all enzymatic steps are indicated.

PHYSIOLOGICAL INQUIRY

- Why are steroid hormones not packaged into secretory vesicles, such as those depicted in Figure 11.3?

Answer can be found at end of chapter.

are not highly soluble in blood. The majority of steroid hormones are reversibly bound in plasma to carrier proteins such as albumin and various other proteins.

The next sections describe the pathways for steroid synthesis in the adrenal cortex and gonads. Those for the placenta are somewhat unusual and are briefly discussed in Chapter 17.

Hormones of the Adrenal Cortex

The five major hormones secreted by the adrenal cortex are aldosterone, cortisol, corticosterone, dehydroepiandrosterone (DHEA), and androstenedione (**Figure 11.5b**). **Aldosterone** is known as a **mineralocorticoid** because its effects are on salt (mineral) balance, mainly on the kidneys' handling of sodium, potassium, and hydrogen ions. Its actions are described in detail in Chapter 14. Briefly, production of aldosterone is under the control of another hormone called **angiotensin II,** which binds to plasma membrane receptors in the adrenal cortex to activate the inositol trisphosphate second-messenger pathway (see Chapter 5). This is different from the more common cAMP-mediated mechanism by which most steroid hormones are produced, as previously described. Once synthesized, aldosterone enters the circulation and acts on cells of the kidneys to stimulate Na^+ and H_2O retention, and K^+ and H^+ excretion in the urine.

Cortisol and corticosterone are called **glucocorticoids** because they have important effects on the metabolism of glucose and other organic nutrients. Cortisol is the predominant glucocorticoid in humans and is the only one we will discuss. In addition to its effects on organic metabolism, cortisol exerts many other effects, including facilitation of the body's responses to stress and regulation of the immune system (see Section D).

Dehydroepiandrosterone (DHEA) and androstenedione belong to the class of steroid hormones known as **androgens;** this class also includes the major male sex steroid **testosterone,** produced by the testes. All androgens have actions similar to those of testosterone. The adrenal androgens are much less potent than testosterone, and they are of little physiological significance in the adult male. They do, however, play roles in the adult female and in both sexes in the fetus and at puberty, as described in Chapter 17.

The adrenal cortex is not a homogeneous gland but is composed of three distinct layers (**Figure 11.6**). The cells of the outer layer—the zona glomerulosa—express the enzymes required to synthesize corticosterone and then convert it to aldosterone (see Figure 11.5b) but do *not* express the genes that code for the enzymes required for the formation of cortisol and androgens. Thus, this layer synthesizes and secretes aldosterone but not the other major adrenocortical hormones. In contrast, the zona fasciculata and zona reticularis have just the opposite enzyme profile. They secrete no aldosterone but do secrete cortisol and androgens. In humans, the zona fasciculata primarily produces cortisol and the zona reticularis primarily produces androgens, but both zones produce both types of steroid.

In certain diseases, the adrenal cortex may secrete decreased or increased amounts of various steroids. For example, the absence of an enzyme required for the formation of cortisol by the adrenal cortex can result in the shunting of the cortisol precursors into the androgen pathway. (Look at Figure 11.5b to imagine how this might happen.) One example of an inherited disease of this type is ***congenital adrenal hyperplasia*** (*CAH*) (see Chapter 17 for more details). In CAH, the excess adrenal androgen production results in virilization of the genitalia of female fetuses; at birth, it may not be obvious whether the baby is phenotypically male or female. Fortunately, the most common form of this disease is now routinely screened for at birth in many countries including certain states in the United States, and appropriate therapeutic measures can be initiated immediately.

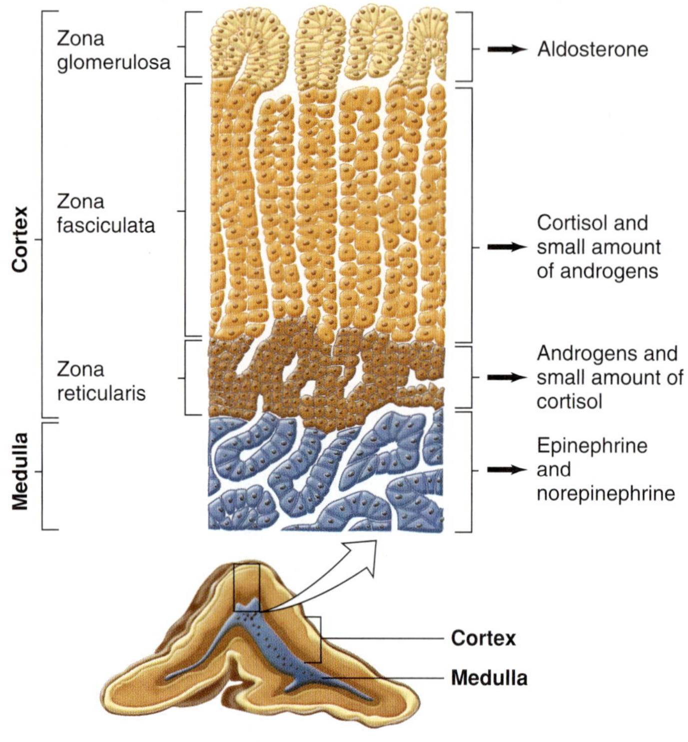

Figure 11.6 APIR Section through an adrenal gland showing both the medulla and the zones of the cortex, as well as the hormones they secrete.

Hormones of the Gonads

Compared to the adrenal cortex, the gonads have very different concentrations of key enzymes in their steroid pathways. Endocrine cells in both the testes and the ovaries do not express the enzymes required to produce aldosterone and cortisol. They possess high concentrations of enzymes in the androgen pathways leading to androstenedione, as in the adrenal cortex. In addition, the endocrine cells in the testes contain a high concentration of the enzyme that converts androstenedione to testosterone, which is therefore the major androgen secreted by the testes (**Figure 11.7**). The ovarian endocrine cells synthesize the female sex hormones, which are collectively known as **estrogens** (primarily estradiol and estrone). **Estradiol** is the predominant estrogen present during a woman's lifetime. The ovarian endocrine cells have a high concentration of the enzyme aromatase, which catalyzes the conversion of androgens to estrogens (see Figure 11.7). Consequently, estradiol—rather than testosterone—is the major steroid hormone secreted by the ovaries.

Very small amounts of testosterone do diffuse out of ovarian endocrine cells, however, and very small amounts of estradiol are produced from testosterone in the testes. Moreover, following

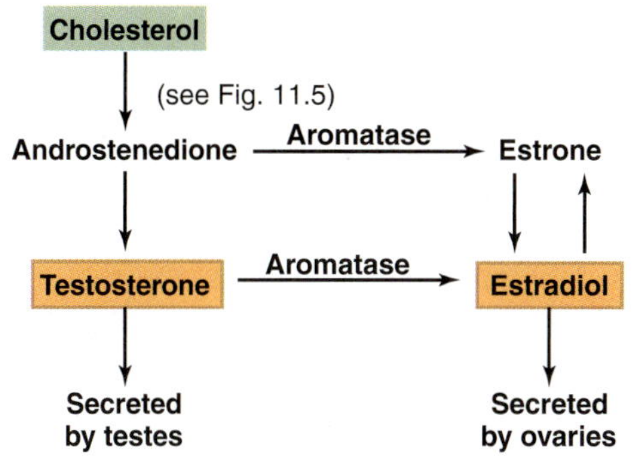

Figure 11.7 Gonadal production of steroids. Only the ovaries have high concentrations of the enzyme (aromatase) required to produce the estrogens estrone and estradiol.

their release into the blood by the gonads and the adrenal cortex, steroid hormones may undergo further conversion in other organs. For example, testosterone is converted to estradiol in some of its target cells. Consequently, the major male and female sex hormones—testosterone and estradiol, respectively—are not unique to males and females. The ratio of the concentrations of the hormones, however, is very different in the two sexes.

Finally, endocrine cells of the corpus luteum, an ovarian structure that arises following each ovulation, secrete another major steroid hormone, **progesterone.** This steroid is critically important for uterine maturation during the menstrual cycle and for maintaining a pregnancy (see Chapter 17). Progesterone is also synthesized in other parts of the body—notably, the placenta in pregnant women and in certain brain cells and the adrenal cortex in both males and females. It has been implicated in numerous functions unrelated to pregnancy, including water and ion balance; regulation of synaptic activity associated with mood, memory, and other brain activities; and immune function.

11.3 Hormone Transport in the Blood

Most peptide and all catecholamine hormones are water-soluble. Therefore, with the exception of a few peptides, these hormones are transported simply dissolved in plasma (**Table 11.2**). In contrast, the poorly soluble steroid hormones and thyroid hormones circulate in the blood largely bound to plasma proteins.

Even though the steroid and thyroid hormones exist in plasma mainly bound to large proteins, small concentrations of these hormones do exist dissolved in the plasma. The dissolved, or free, hormone is in equilibrium with the bound hormone:

$$\text{Free hormone} + \text{Binding protein} \rightleftharpoons \text{Hormone–protein complex}$$

The total hormone concentration in plasma is the sum of the free and bound hormones. However, only the *free* hormone can diffuse out of capillaries and encounter its target cells. Therefore, the concentration of the free hormone is what is biologically important rather than the concentration of the total hormone, most of which is bound. As we will see next, the degree of protein binding also influences the rate of metabolism and the excretion of the hormone.

11.4 Hormone Metabolism and Excretion

Once a hormone has been synthesized and secreted into the blood and has acted on a target tissue, the concentration of the hormone in the blood usually returns to normal. This is necessary to prevent excessive, possibly harmful effects from the prolonged exposure of target cells to hormones. A hormone's concentration in the plasma depends upon (1) its rate of secretion by the endocrine gland and (2) its rate of removal from the blood. Removal, or "clearance," of the hormone occurs either by excretion or by metabolic transformation. The liver and the kidneys are the major organs that metabolize or excrete hormones.

The liver and kidneys, however, are not the only routes for eliminating hormones. Sometimes a hormone is metabolized by the cells upon which it acts. In the case of some peptide hormones, for example, endocytosis of hormone–receptor complexes on plasma membranes enables cells to remove the hormones rapidly from their surfaces and catabolize them intracellularly. The receptors are then often recycled to the plasma membrane.

In addition, enzymes in the blood and tissues rapidly break down catecholamine and peptide hormones. These hormones therefore tend to remain in the bloodstream for only brief periods—minutes to an hour. In contrast, protein-bound

TABLE 11.2 Categories of Hormones

Chemical Class	Major Form in Plasma	Location of Receptors	Most Common Signaling Mechanisms*	Rate of Excretion/Metabolism
Peptides and catecholamines	Free (unbound)	Plasma membrane	1. Second messengers (e.g., cAMP, Ca^{2+}, IP_3) 2. Enzyme activation by receptor (e.g., JAK) 3. Intrinsic enzymatic activity of receptor (e.g., tyrosine autophosphorylation)	Fast (minutes)
Steroids and thyroid hormone	Protein-bound	Intracellular	Intracellular receptors directly alter gene transcription	Slow (hours to days)

*The diverse mechanisms of action of chemical messengers such as hormones were discussed in detail in Chapter 5.

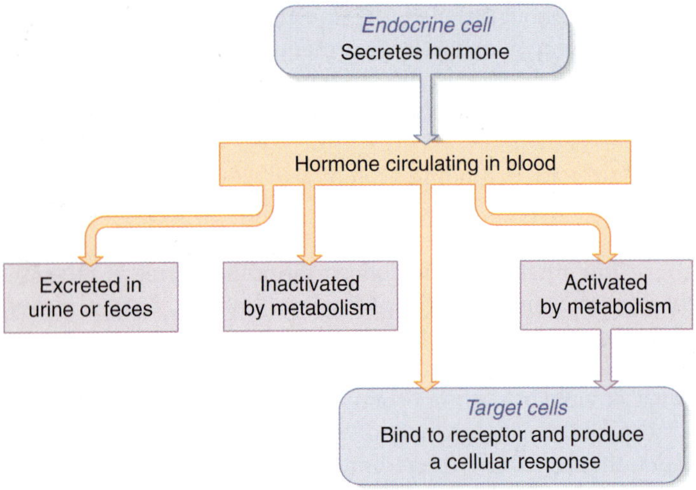

Figure 11.8 Possible fates and actions of a hormone following its secretion by an endocrine cell. Not all paths apply to all hormones.

hormones are protected from excretion or metabolism by enzymes as long as they remain bound. Therefore, removal of the circulating steroid and thyroid hormones generally takes longer, often several hours to days.

In some cases, metabolism of a hormone *activates* the hormone rather than inactivates it. In other words, the secreted hormone may be relatively inactive until metabolism transforms it. One example is one of the two major thyroid hormones, thyroxine, which is converted to a more active form upon entering a target cell.

Figure 11.8 summarizes the possible fates of hormones after their secretion.

11.5 Mechanisms of Hormone Action

Hormone Receptors

Because hormones are transported in the blood, they can reach all tissues. Yet, the response to a hormone is highly specific, involving only the target cells for that hormone. The ability to respond depends upon the presence of specific receptors for those hormones on or in the target cells.

As emphasized in Chapter 5, the response of a target cell to a chemical messenger is the final event in a sequence that begins when the messenger binds to specific cell receptors. As that chapter described, the receptors for water-soluble chemical messengers like peptide hormones and catecholamines are proteins located in the plasma membranes of the target cells. In contrast, the receptors for lipid-soluble chemical messengers like steroid and thyroid hormones are proteins located mainly *inside* the target cells.

Hormones can influence the response of target cells by regulating hormone receptors. Again, Chapter 5 described basic concepts of receptor modulation such as up-regulation and down-regulation. In the context of hormones, **up-regulation** is an increase in the number of a hormone's receptors in a cell, often resulting from a prolonged exposure to a low concentration of the hormone. This has the effect of increasing target-cell responsiveness to the hormone. **Down-regulation** is a decrease in receptor number, often from exposure to high concentrations of the hormone. This temporarily decreases target-cell responsiveness to the hormone, thereby preventing overstimulation.

In some cases, hormones can down-regulate or up-regulate not only their own receptors but the receptors for other hormones as well. If one hormone induces down-regulation of a second hormone's receptors, the result will be a reduction of the second hormone's effectiveness. On the other hand, a hormone may induce an increase in the number of receptors for a second hormone. In this case, the effectiveness of the second hormone is increased. This latter phenomenon, in some cases, underlies the important hormone–hormone interaction known as permissiveness. In general terms, **permissiveness** means that hormone A must be present in order for hormone B to exert its full effect. A low concentration of hormone A is usually all that is needed for this permissive effect, which may be due to A's ability to up-regulate B's receptors. For example, epinephrine causes a large release of fatty acids from adipose tissue, but only in the presence of permissive amounts of thyroid hormones (**Figure 11.9**). One reason is that thyroid hormones stimulate the synthesis of beta-adrenergic receptors for epinephrine in adipose tissue; as a result, the tissue becomes much more sensitive to epinephrine. However, receptor up-regulation does not explain all cases of permissiveness. Sometimes, the effect may be due to changes in the signaling pathway that mediates the actions of a given hormone.

Events Elicited by Hormone–Receptor Binding

The events initiated when a hormone binds to its receptor—that is, the mechanisms by which the hormone elicits a cellular response—are one or more of the signal transduction pathways that apply to all chemical messengers, as described in Chapter 5. In other words, there is nothing unique about the mechanisms that hormones initiate as compared to those used by neurotransmitters and paracrine or autocrine substances, and so we will only briefly review them here (see Table 11.2).

Effects of Peptide Hormones and Catecholamines

As stated previously, the receptors for peptide hormones and the catecholamine hormones are located on the outer surface of the target cell's plasma membrane. This location is important because these hormones are too hydrophilic to diffuse through the plasma membrane. When activated by hormone binding, the receptors trigger one or more of the signal transduction pathways for plasma membrane receptors described in Chapter 5. That is, the activated receptors directly influence (1) enzyme activity that is part of the receptor, (2) activity of cytoplasmic janus kinases associated with the receptor, or (3) G proteins coupled in the plasma membrane to effector proteins—ion channels and enzymes—that generate second messengers such as cAMP and Ca^{2+}. The opening or closing of ion channels changes the electrical potential across the membrane. When a Ca^{2+} channel is involved, the cytosolic concentration of this important ionic second messenger changes. The changes in enzyme activity are usually very rapid (e.g., due to phosphorylation) and produce changes in the activity of various cellular proteins. In some cases, the signal transduction pathways also lead to activation or inhibition of particular genes, causing a change in the synthesis rate of the proteins coded for by these genes. Thus, peptide hormones

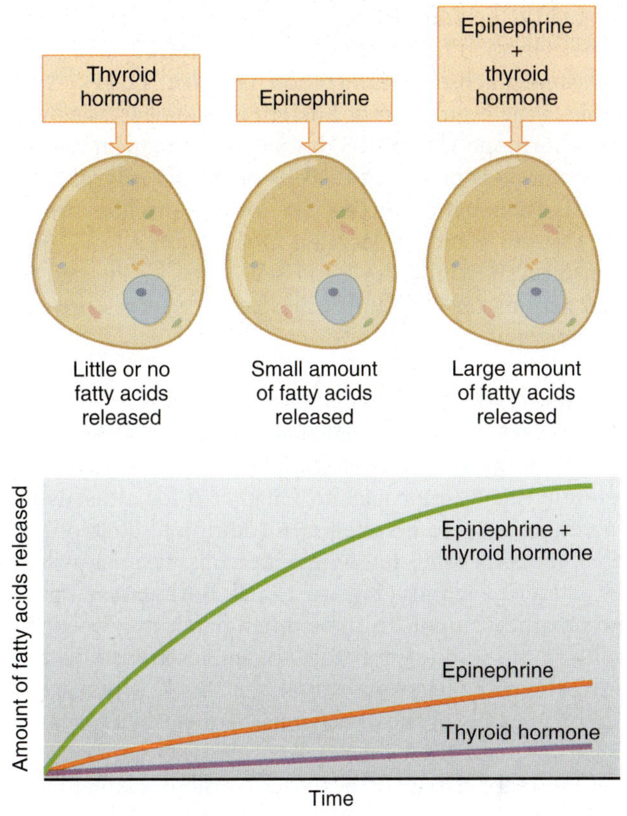

Figure 11.9 The ability of thyroid hormone to "permit" epinephrine-induced release of fatty acids from adipose tissue cells. Thyroid hormone exerts this effect by causing an increased number of beta-adrenergic receptors on the cell. Thyroid hormone by itself stimulates only a small amount of fatty acid release.

PHYSIOLOGICAL INQUIRY

- A patient is observed to have symptoms that are consistent with elevated concentrations of epinephrine in the blood, including a rapid heart rate, anxiety, and elevated fatty acid concentrations. However, the circulating epinephrine concentrations are tested and found to be in the normal range. What might explain this?

Answer can be found at end of chapter.

and catecholamines may exert both rapid (nongenomic) and slower (gene transcription) actions on the same target cell.

Effects of Steroid and Thyroid Hormone

The steroid hormones and thyroid hormone are all lipophilic, and their receptors, which are intracellular, constitute the steroid-hormone-receptor superfamily. As described for lipid-soluble messengers in Chapter 5, the binding of hormone to one of these receptors leads to the activation (or in some cases, inhibition) of the transcription of particular genes, causing a change in the synthesis rate of the proteins coded for by those genes. The ultimate result of changes in the concentrations of these proteins is an enhancement or inhibition of particular processes the cell carries out or a change in the cell's rate of protein secretion.

In addition to having intracellular receptors, some target cells also have plasma membrane receptors for certain of the steroid hormones, notably progesterone and estradiol. In such cases, the signal transduction pathways initiated by the plasma membrane receptors elicit rapid, nongenomic cell responses, whereas the intracellular receptors mediate a delayed response, requiring new protein synthesis. The physiological significance of the membrane receptors in humans is still under investigation, but it is clear from animal studies that these receptors are functional in other vertebrates.

Pharmacological Effects of Hormones

The administration of very large quantities of a hormone for medical purposes may have effects on an individual that are not usually observed in a healthy person. These ***pharmacological effects*** can also occur in diseases involving the secretion of excessive amounts of hormones. Pharmacological effects are of great importance in medicine because hormones are often used in large doses as therapeutic agents. Perhaps the most common example is that of very potent synthetic forms of cortisol, such as prednisone, which is administered to suppress allergic and inflammatory reactions. In such situations, a host of unwanted effects may be observed (as described in Section D).

11.6 Inputs That Control Hormone Secretion

Hormone secretion is mainly under the control of three types of inputs to endocrine cells (**Figure 11.10**): (1) changes in the plasma concentrations of mineral ions or organic nutrients, (2) neurotransmitters released from neurons ending on the endocrine cell, and (3) another hormone (or, in some cases, a paracrine substance) acting on the endocrine cell.

Before we look more closely at each category, we must stress that more than one input may influence hormone secretion. For example, insulin secretion is stimulated by the extracellular concentrations of glucose and other nutrients, and is either stimulated or inhibited by the different branches of the autonomic nervous system. Thus, the control of endocrine cells illustrates the general principle of physiology that most physiological functions are controlled by multiple regulatory systems, often working in opposition. The resulting output—the rate of hormone secretion—depends upon the relative amounts of stimulatory and inhibitory inputs.

The term *secretion* applied to a hormone denotes its release by exocytosis from the cell. In some cases, hormones such as steroid hormones are not secreted, per se, but instead diffuse through the cell's plasma membrane into the extracellular space. Secretion or release by diffusion is sometimes accompanied by increased synthesis of the hormone. For simplicity in this chapter and the rest of the book, we will

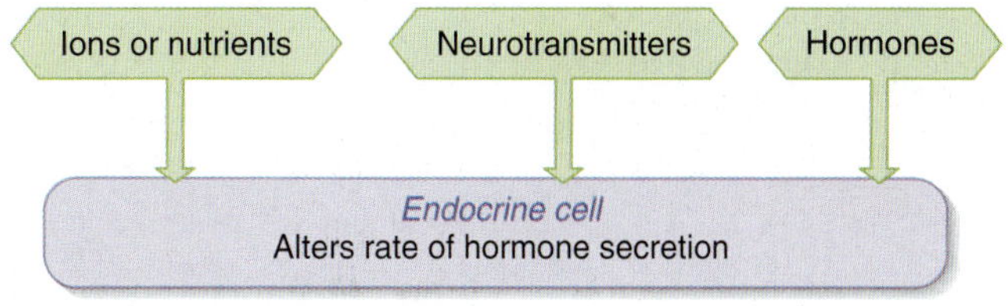

Figure 11.10 Inputs that act directly on endocrine gland cells to stimulate or inhibit hormone secretion.

generally not distinguish between these possibilities when we refer to stimulation or inhibition of hormone "secretion."

Control by Plasma Concentrations of Mineral Ions or Organic Nutrients

The secretion of several hormones is directly controlled—at least in part—by the plasma concentrations of specific mineral ions or organic nutrients. In each case, a major function of the hormone is to regulate through negative feedback (see Chapter 1) the plasma concentration of the ion or nutrient controlling its secretion. For example, insulin secretion is stimulated by an increase in plasma glucose concentration. Insulin, in turn, acts on skeletal muscle and adipose tissue to promote facilitated diffusion of glucose across the plasma membranes into the cytosol. The effect of insulin, therefore, is to decrease the plasma glucose concentration (**Figure 11.11**). Another example is the regulation of calcium ion homeostasis by parathyroid hormone (PTH), as described in detail in Section F. This hormone is produced by cells of the parathyroid glands, which, as their name implies, are located in close proximity to the thyroid gland. A decrease in the plasma Ca^{2+} concentration directly stimulates PTH secretion. PTH then exerts several actions on bone and other tissue that restore plasma Ca^{2+} to normal.

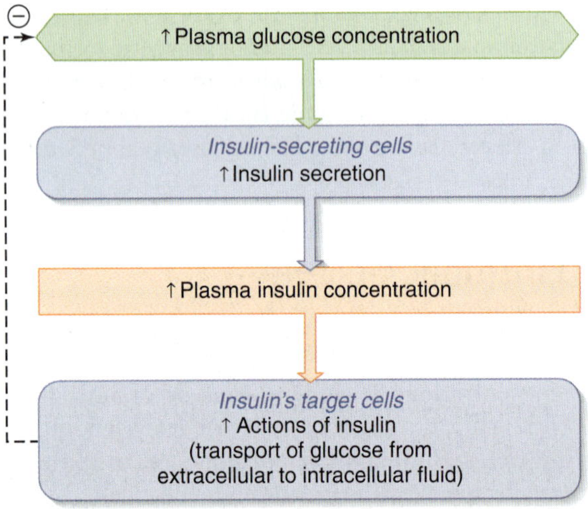

Figure 11.11 Example of how the direct control of hormone secretion by the plasma concentration of a substance—in this case, an organic nutrient—results in negative feedback control of the substance's plasma concentration. In other cases, the regulated plasma substance may be a mineral, such as Ca^{2+}.

Control by Neurons

As stated earlier, the adrenal medulla is a modified sympathetic ganglion and thus is stimulated by sympathetic preganglionic fibers (refer back to Chapter 6 for a discussion of the autonomic nervous system). In addition to controlling the adrenal medulla, the autonomic nervous system influences other endocrine glands (**Figure 11.12**). Both parasympathetic and sympathetic inputs to these other glands may occur, some inhibitory and some stimulatory. Examples are the secretions of insulin and the gastrointestinal hormones, which are stimulated by neurons of the parasympathetic nervous system and inhibited by sympathetic neurons.

One large group of hormones—those secreted by the hypothalamus and the posterior pituitary—is under the direct control not of autonomic neurons but of neurons in the brain itself (see Figure 11.12). This category will be described in detail in Section B.

Control by Other Hormones

In many cases, the secretion of a particular hormone is directly controlled by the blood concentration of another hormone. Often, the only function of the first hormone in a sequence is to stimulate the secretion of the next. A hormone that stimulates the secretion of another hormone is often referred to as a

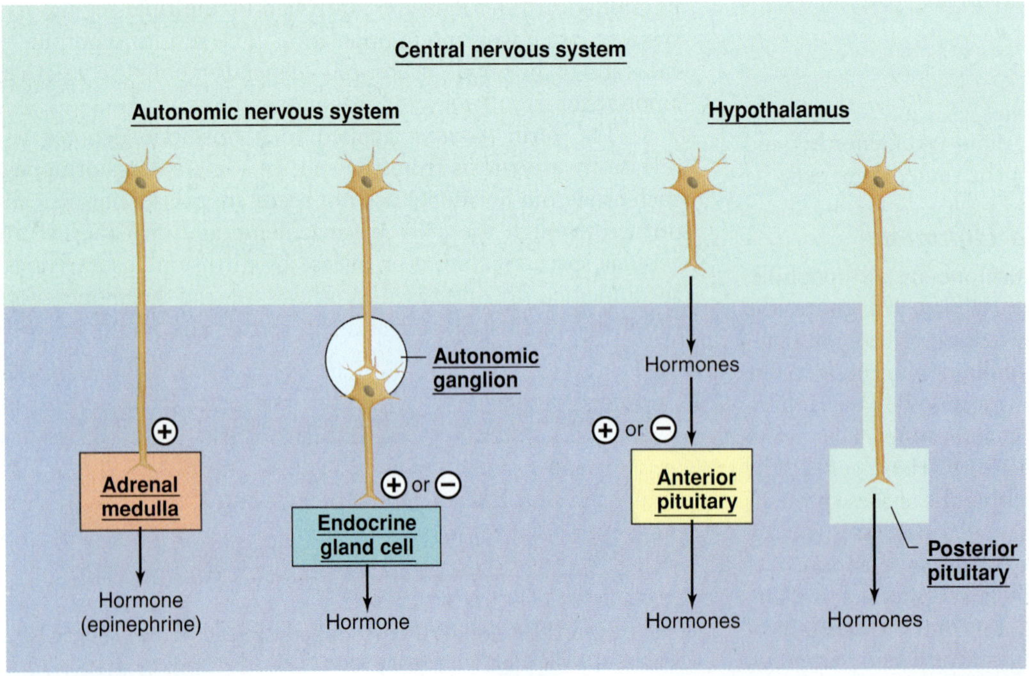

Figure 11.12 Pathways by which the nervous system influences hormone secretion. The autonomic nervous system controls hormone secretion by the adrenal medulla and many other endocrine glands. Certain neurons in the hypothalamus, some of which terminate in the posterior pituitary, secrete hormones. The secretion of hypothalamic hormones from the posterior pituitary and the effects of other hypothalamic hormones on the anterior pituitary gland are described later in this chapter. The ⊕ and ⊖ symbols indicate stimulatory and inhibitory actions, respectively.

tropic hormone. The tropic hormones usually stimulate not only secretion but also the growth of the stimulated gland. (When specifically referring to growth-promoting actions, the term *trophic* is often used, but for simplicity we will usually use only the general term *tropic*). These types of hormonal sequences are covered in detail in Section B. In addition to stimulatory actions, however, some hormones such as those in a multihormone sequence inhibit secretion of other hormones.

11.7 Types of Endocrine Disorders

Because there is such a wide variety of hormones and endocrine glands, disorders within the endocrine system may vary considerably in terms of symptoms. For example, endocrine disease may manifest as an imbalance in metabolism, leading to weight gain or loss; as a failure to grow or develop normally in early life; as an abnormally high or low blood pressure; as a loss of reproductive fertility; or as mental and emotional changes, to name a few. Despite these varied symptoms, which depend upon the particular hormone affected, essentially all endocrine diseases can be categorized in one of four ways. These include (1) too little hormone (***hyposecretion***), (2) too much hormone (***hypersecretion***), (3) decreased responsiveness of the target cells to hormone (***hyporesponsiveness***), and (4) increased responsiveness of the target cells to hormone (***hyperresponsiveness***).

Hyposecretion

An endocrine gland may be secreting too little hormone because the gland cannot function normally, a condition termed ***primary hyposecretion.*** Examples of primary hyposecretion include (1) partial destruction of a gland, leading to decreased hormone secretion; (2) an enzyme deficiency resulting in decreased synthesis of the hormone; and (3) dietary deficiency of iodine, specifically leading to decreased secretion of thyroid hormones. Many other causes, such as infections and exposure to toxic chemicals, have the common denominator of damaging the endocrine gland or reducing its ability to synthesize or secrete the hormone.

The other major cause of hyposecretion is ***secondary hyposecretion.*** In this case, the endocrine gland is not damaged but is receiving too little stimulation by its tropic hormone.

To distinguish between primary and secondary hyposecretion, one measures the concentration of the tropic hormone in the blood. If elevated, the cause is primary; if not increased, or lower than normal, the cause is secondary.

The most common means of treating hormone hyposecretion is to administer the missing hormone or a synthetic analog of the hormone. This is normally done either by oral (pill), topical (cream applied to skin), or nasal (spray) administration, or by injection. The route of administration typically depends upon the chemical nature of the hormone being replaced. For example, individuals with low thyroid hormone take a daily pill to restore normal hormone concentrations, because thyroid hormones are readily absorbed from the intestines. By contrast, people with diabetes mellitus who require insulin typically must obtain it via injection; insulin is a peptide that would be digested by the enzymes of the gastrointestinal tract if it were ingested.

Hypersecretion

A hormone can also undergo either ***primary hypersecretion*** (the gland is secreting too much of the hormone on its own) or ***secondary hypersecretion*** (excessive stimulation of the gland by its tropic hormone). One cause of primary or secondary hypersecretion is the presence of a hormone-secreting, endocrine-cell tumor. These tumors tend to produce their hormones continually at a high rate, even in the absence of stimulation.

When an endocrine tumor causes hypersecretion, the tumor can often be removed surgically or destroyed with radiation if it is confined to a small area. These procedures are also useful in certain cases where an endocrine gland is hypersecreting for reasons unrelated to the presence of a tumor. Both of these procedures can be used, for example, in treating hypersecretion from an overactive thyroid gland (see Section C). In many cases, drugs that inhibit a hormone's synthesis can block hypersecretion. Alternatively, the situation can be treated with drugs that do not alter the hormone's secretion but instead block the hormone's actions on its target cells.

Hyporesponsiveness and Hyperresponsiveness

In some cases, a component of the endocrine system may not be functioning normally, even though there is nothing wrong with hormone secretion. The problem is that the target cells do not respond normally to the hormone, a condition termed hyporesponsiveness, or hormone resistance. An important example of a disease resulting from hyporesponsiveness is the most common form of diabetes mellitus (called ***type 2 diabetes mellitus***), in which the target cells of the hormone insulin are hyporesponsive to this hormone.

One cause of hyporesponsiveness is deficiency of receptors—or abnormal, nonfunctional receptors—for the hormone. For example, some individuals who are genetically male have a defect manifested by the absence of receptors for androgens. Consequently, their target cells are unable to bind androgens, and the result is lack of development of certain male characteristics, as though the hormones were not being produced (see Chapter 17 for additional details).

In a second type of hyporesponsiveness, the receptors for a hormone may be normal but some signaling event that occurs within the cell after the hormone binds to its receptors may be defective. For example, the activated receptor may be unable to stimulate formation of cyclic AMP or another component of the signaling pathway for that hormone.

A third cause of hyporesponsiveness applies to hormones that require metabolic activation by some other tissue after secretion. There may be a deficiency of the enzymes that catalyze the activation. For example, some men secrete testosterone (the major circulating androgen) normally and have normal receptors for androgens. However, these men are missing the intracellular enzyme that converts testosterone to dihydrotestosterone, a potent metabolite of testosterone that binds to androgen receptors and mediates some of the actions of testosterone on secondary sex characteristics such as the growth of facial and body hair.

By contrast, hyperresponsiveness to a hormone can also occur and cause problems. For example, thyroid hormone causes an up-regulation of beta-adrenergic receptors for epinephrine; therefore, hypersecretion of thyroid hormone causes, in turn, a hyperresponsiveness to epinephrine. One result of this is the increased heart rate typical of people with elevated concentrations of thyroid hormones.

SECTION A SUMMARY

Hormones and Endocrine Glands

I. The endocrine system is one of the body's two major communications systems. It consists of all the glands and organs that secrete hormones, which are chemical messengers carried by the blood to target cells elsewhere in the body.

II. Endocrine glands differ from exocrine glands in that the latter secrete their products into a duct that connects with another structure, such as the intestines, or with the outside of the body.

III. A single gland may, in some cases, secrete multiple hormones.

Hormone Structures and Synthesis

I. The amine hormones are the iodine-containing thyroid hormones and the catecholamines secreted by the adrenal medulla and the hypothalamus.

II. The majority of hormones are peptides, many of which are synthesized as larger molecules, which are then cleaved into active fragments.

III. Steroid hormones are produced from cholesterol by the adrenal cortex and the gonads and by the placenta during pregnancy.
  a. The predominant steroid hormones produced by the adrenal cortex are the mineralocorticoid aldosterone; the glucocorticoid cortisol; and two androgens, DHEA and androstenedione.
  b. The ovaries produce mainly estradiol and progesterone, and the testes produce mainly testosterone.

Hormone Transport in the Blood

I. Peptide hormones and catecholamines circulate dissolved in the plasma, but steroid and thyroid hormones circulate mainly bound to plasma proteins.

Hormone Metabolism and Excretion

I. The liver and kidneys are the major organs that remove hormones from the plasma by metabolizing or excreting them.

II. The peptide hormones and catecholamines are rapidly removed from the blood, whereas the steroid and thyroid hormones are removed more slowly, in part because they circulate bound to plasma proteins.

III. After their secretion, some hormones are metabolized to more active molecules in their target cells or other organs.

Mechanisms of Hormone Action

I. The great majority of receptors for steroid and thyroid hormones are inside the target cells; those for the peptide hormones and catecholamines are on the plasma membrane.

II. Hormones can cause up-regulation and down-regulation of their own receptors and those of other hormones. The induction of one hormone's receptors by another hormone increases the first hormone's effectiveness and may be essential to permit the first hormone to exert its effects.

III. Receptors activated by peptide hormones and catecholamines utilize one or more of the signal transduction pathways available to plasma membrane receptors; the result is altered membrane potential or protein activity in the cell.

IV. Intracellular receptors activated by steroid and thyroid hormones typically function as transcription factors; the result is increased synthesis of particular proteins.

V. In pharmacological doses, hormones can have effects not seen under ordinary circumstances, some of which may be deleterious.

Inputs That Control Hormone Secretion

I. The secretion of a hormone may be controlled by the plasma concentration of an ion or nutrient that the hormone regulates, by neural input to the endocrine cells, and by one or more hormones.

II. The autonomic nervous system is the neural input controlling many hormones. Neuron endings from the sympathetic and parasympathetic nervous systems terminate directly on cells within some endocrine glands, thereby regulating hormone secretion.

Types of Endocrine Disorders

I. Endocrine disorders may be classified as hyposecretion, hypersecretion, and target-cell hyporesponsiveness or hyperresponsiveness.
  a. Primary disorders are those in which the defect is in the cells that secrete the hormone.
  b. Secondary disorders are those in which there is too much or too little tropic hormone.
  c. Hyporesponsiveness is due to an alteration in the receptors for the hormone, to disordered postreceptor events, or to failure of normal metabolic activation of the hormone in cases requiring such activation.

II. These disorders can be distinguished by measurements of the hormone and any tropic hormones under both basal conditions and during experimental stimulation of each hormone's secretion.

SECTION A REVIEW QUESTIONS

1. What distinguishes exocrine from endocrine glands?
2. What are the three general chemical classes of hormones?
3. What are the major hormones produced by the adrenal cortex? By the testes? By the ovaries?
4. Which classes of hormones are carried in the blood mainly as unbound, dissolved hormone? Mainly bound to plasma proteins?
5. Do protein-bound hormones diffuse out of capillaries?
6. Which organs are the major sites of hormone excretion and metabolic inactivation?
7. How do the rates of metabolism and excretion differ for the various classes of hormones?
8. List some metabolic transformations that prohormones and some hormones must undergo before they become biologically active.
9. Contrast the locations of receptors for the various classes of hormones.
10. How do hormones influence the concentrations of their own receptors and those of other hormones? How does this explain permissiveness in hormone action?
11. Describe the sequence of events when peptide or catecholamine hormones bind to their receptors.
12. Describe the sequence of events when steroid or thyroid hormones bind to their receptors.
13. What are the direct inputs to endocrine glands controlling hormone secretion?

14. How does control of hormone secretion by plasma mineral ions and nutrients achieve negative feedback control of these substances?
15. How would you distinguish between primary and secondary hyposecretion of a hormone? Between hyposecretion and hyporesponsiveness?

SECTION A KEY TERMS

adrenal cortex 321
adrenal gland 321
adrenal medulla 321
aldosterone 326
amine hormone 321
androgen 326
angiotensin II 326
cortisol 326
1,25-dihydroxyvitamin D 324
dopamine 321
down-regulation 328
endocrine gland 320
endocrine system 320
epinephrine 321
estradiol 326
estrogen 326
glucocorticoid 326
gonad 324
hormone 320
mineralocorticoid 326
norepinephrine 321
peptide hormone 323
permissiveness 328
progesterone 327
prohormone 323
steroid hormone 324
testosterone 326
thyroid hormone 321
tropic hormone 331
up-regulation 328

SECTION A CLINICAL TERMS

congenital adrenal hyperplasia (CAH) 326
hyperresponsiveness 331
hypersecretion 331
hyporesponsiveness 331
hyposecretion 331
pharmacological effect 329
primary hypersecretion 331
primary hyposecretion 331
secondary hypersecretion 331
secondary hyposecretion 331
type 2 diabetes mellitus 331

SECTION B The Hypothalamus and Pituitary Gland

11.8 Control Systems Involving the Hypothalamus and Pituitary Gland

The **pituitary gland,** or **hypophysis** (from a Greek term meaning "to grow underneath"), lies in a pocket (called the sella turcica) of the sphenoid bone at the base of the brain (**Figure 11.13**) just below the **hypothalamus.** The pituitary gland is connected to the hypothalamus by the **infundibulum,** or pituitary stalk, containing axons from neurons in the hypothalamus and small blood vessels. In humans, the pituitary gland is composed of two adjacent lobes called the *anterior lobe*—usually referred to as the **anterior pituitary gland** or adenohypophysis—and the *posterior lobe*—usually called the **posterior pituitary** or neurohypophysis. The anterior pituitary gland arises embryologically from an invagination of the pharynx called Rathke's pouch, whereas the posterior pituitary is not actually a gland but, rather, an extension of the neural components of the hypothalamus.

The axons of two well-defined clusters of hypothalamic neurons (the supraoptic and paraventricular nuclei) pass down the infundibulum and end within the posterior pituitary in close proximity to capillaries (small blood vessels where exchange of solutes occurs between the blood and interstitium) (**Figure 11.13b**). Therefore, these neurons do not form a synapse with other neurons. Instead, their terminals end directly on capillaries. The terminals release hormones into these capillaries, which then collect into veins and the general circulation.

In contrast to the neural connections between the hypothalamus and posterior pituitary, there are no important neural connections between the hypothalamus and anterior pituitary gland. There is, however, a special type of circulatory connection (see Figure 11.13b). The junction of the hypothalamus and infundibulum is known as the **median eminence.** Capillaries in the median eminence recombine to form the **hypothalamo–hypophyseal portal vessels** (or portal veins). The term *portal* denotes veins that connect two sets of capillaries; normally, as you will learn in Chapter 12, capillaries drain into veins that return blood to the heart. Only in portal systems does one set of capillaries drain into veins that then form a *second* set of capillaries before eventually emptying again into veins that return to the heart. The hypothalamo–hypophyseal portal vessels pass down the infundibulum and enter the anterior pituitary gland, where they drain into a second set of capillaries, the anterior pituitary gland capillaries. Thus, the hypothalamo–hypophyseal portal vessels offer a local route for blood to be delivered directly from the hypothalamus to the cells of the anterior pituitary gland. As we will see shortly, this local blood system provides a mechanism for hormones of the hypothalamus to directly alter the activity of the cells of the anterior pituitary gland, bypassing the general circulation and thus efficiently regulating hormone release from that gland.

We begin our survey of pituitary gland hormones and their major physiological actions with the two hormones of the posterior pituitary.

Posterior Pituitary Hormones

We emphasized that the posterior pituitary is really a neural extension of the hypothalamus (see Figure 11.13). The hormones are synthesized not in the posterior pituitary itself but in the hypothalamus—specifically, in the cell bodies of the supraoptic and paraventricular nuclei, whose axons pass down the infundibulum and terminate in the posterior pituitary. Enclosed in small vesicles, the hormone moves down the axons to accumulate at the axon terminals in the posterior pituitary. Various stimuli activate inputs to these neurons, causing action potentials that propagate to the axon terminals and trigger the release of the stored hormone by exocytosis. The hormone then enters capillaries to be carried away by the blood returning to the heart. In this way, the brain can receive stimuli and respond as if it were an endocrine organ.

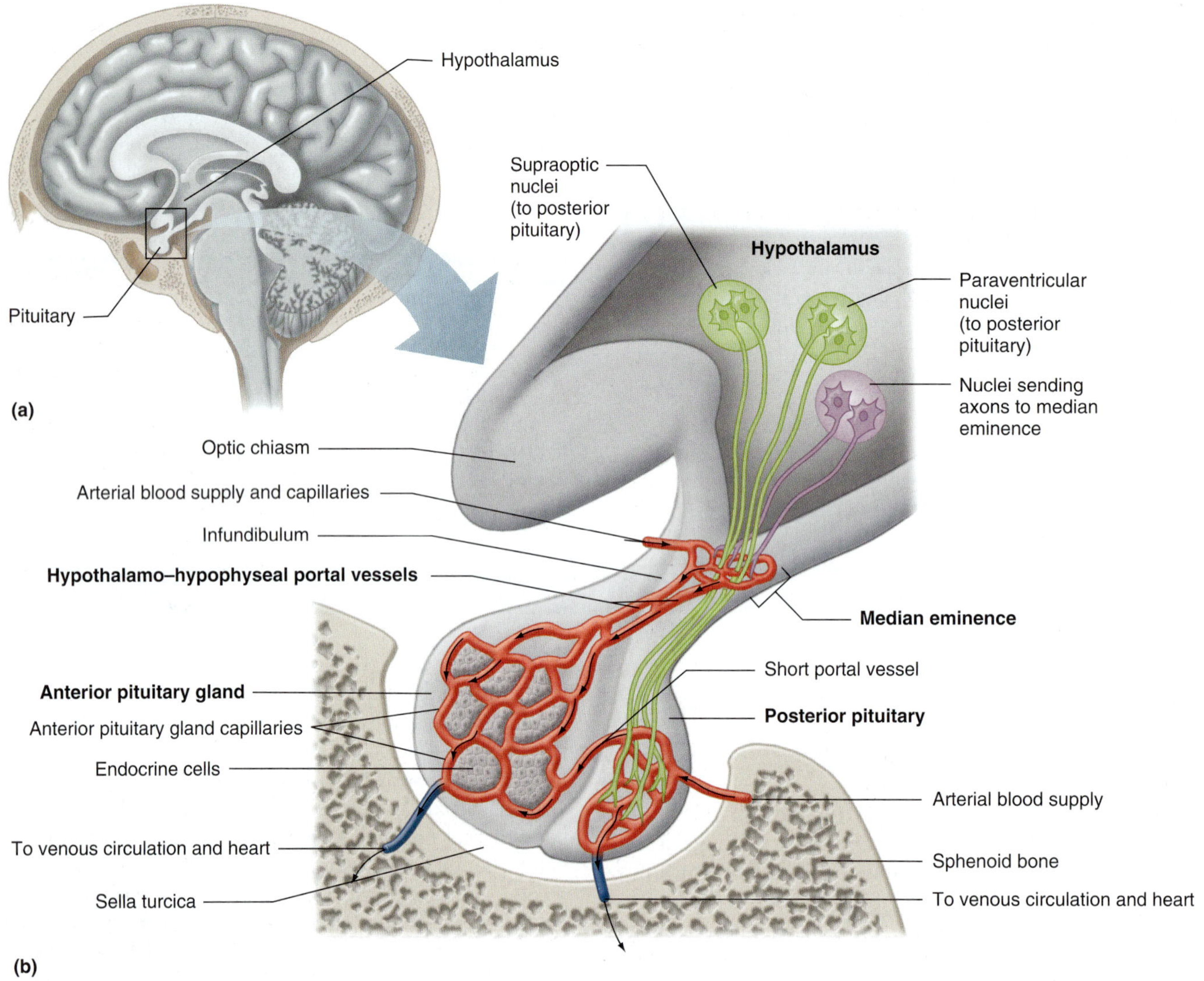

Figure 11.13 APR (a) Relation of the pituitary gland to the brain and hypothalamus. (b) Neural and vascular connections between the hypothalamus and pituitary gland. Hypothalamic neurons from the paraventricular and supraoptic nuclei travel down the infundibulum to end in the posterior pituitary, whereas others (shown for simplicity as a single nucleus, but in reality several nuclei, including some cells from the paraventricular nuclei) end in the median eminence. Almost the entire blood supply to the anterior pituitary gland comes via the hypothalamo–hypophyseal portal vessels, which originate in the median eminence. Long portal vessels connect the capillaries in the median eminence with those in the anterior pituitary gland. (The short portal vessels, which originate in the posterior pituitary, carry only a small fraction of the blood leaving the posterior pituitary and supply only a small fraction of the blood received by the anterior pituitary gland.) Arrows indicate direction of blood flow.

PHYSIOLOGICAL INQUIRY

- Why does it take only very small quantities of hypophysiotropic hormones to regulate anterior pituitary gland hormone secretion?

Answer can be found at end of chapter.

By releasing its hormones into the general circulation, the posterior pituitary can modify the functions of distant organs.

The two posterior pituitary hormones are the peptides **oxytocin** and **vasopressin.** Oxytocin is involved in two reflexes related to reproduction. In one case, oxytocin stimulates contraction of smooth muscle cells in the breasts, which results in milk ejection during lactation. This occurs in response to stimulation of the nipples of the breast during nursing of the infant. Sensory cells within the nipples send stimulatory neural signals to the brain that terminate on the hypothalamic cells that make oxytocin, causing their activation and thus release of the hormone. In a second reflex, one that occurs during labor in a pregnant woman, stretch receptors in the cervix send neural signals back to the hypothalamus, which releases oxytocin in response. Oxytocin then stimulates contraction of uterine smooth muscle cells, until eventually the baby is born (see Chapter 17 for details). Although oxytocin is also present in males, its systemic endocrine functions in males are uncertain. Recent research suggests that oxytocin may be involved in various aspects of behavior in male and female mammals, possibly including humans. These include such things as pair bonding, maternal behavior, and emotions such as love. If true in humans, this is likely due to oxytocin-containing neurons in other parts of the brain, as it is unclear whether any systemic oxytocin can cross the blood–brain barrier and enter the brain.

The other posterior pituitary hormone, vasopressin, acts on smooth muscle cells around blood vessels to cause their contraction, which constricts the blood vessels and thereby increases blood pressure. This may occur, for example, in response to a decrease in blood pressure that resulted from a loss of blood due to an injury. Vasopressin also acts within the kidneys to decrease water excretion in the urine, thereby retaining fluid in the body and helping to maintain blood volume. One way in which this would occur would be if a person were to become dehydrated. Because of its kidney function, vasopressin is also known as **antidiuretic hormone** (**ADH**). (A loss of excess water in the urine is known as a *diuresis*, and because vasopressin decreases water loss in the urine, it has *anti*diuretic properties.)

Anterior Pituitary Gland Hormones and the Hypothalamus

Other nuclei of hypothalamic neurons secrete hormones that control the secretion of all the anterior pituitary gland hormones. For simplicity's sake, Figure 11.13 depicts these neurons as arising from a single nucleus, but in fact several hypothalamic nuclei send axons whose terminals end in the median eminence. The hypothalamic hormones that regulate anterior pituitary gland function are collectively termed **hypophysiotropic hormones** (recall that another name for the pituitary gland is *hypophysis*); they are also commonly called hypothalamic releasing or inhibiting hormones.

With one exception (dopamine), each of the hypophysiotropic hormones is the first in a three-hormone sequence: (1) A hypophysiotropic hormone controls the secretion of (2) an anterior pituitary gland hormone, which controls the secretion of (3) a hormone from some other endocrine gland (**Figure 11.14**). This last hormone then acts on its target cells. The adaptive value of such sequences is that they permit a variety of types of important hormonal feedback. They also allow amplification of a response of a small number of hypothalamic neurons into a large peripheral hormonal signal. We begin our description of these sequences in the middle—that is, with the anterior pituitary gland hormones—because the names of the hypophysiotropic hormones are mostly based on the names of the anterior pituitary gland hormones.

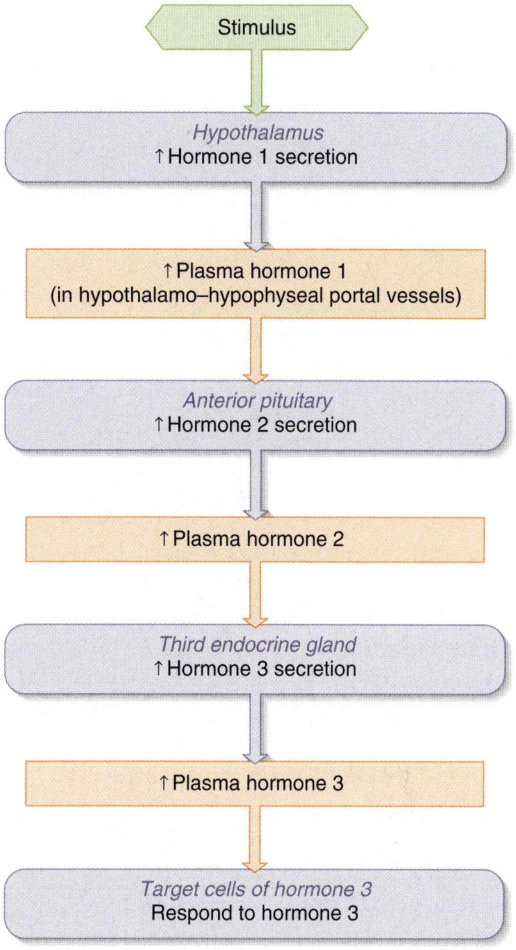

Figure 11.14 Typical sequential pattern by which a hypophysiotropic hormone (hormone 1 from the hypothalamus) controls the secretion of an anterior pituitary gland hormone (hormone 2), which in turn controls the secretion of a hormone by a third endocrine gland (hormone 3). The hypothalamo–hypophyseal portal vessels are illustrated in Figure 11.13.

Overview of Anterior Pituitary Gland Hormones

As shown in Table 11.1, the anterior pituitary gland secretes at least eight hormones, but only six have well-established functions in humans. These six hormones—all peptides—are **follicle-stimulating hormone** (**FSH**), **luteinizing hormone** (**LH**), **growth hormone** (**GH,** also known as *somatotropin*), **thyroid-stimulating hormone** (**TSH,** also known as *thyrotropin*), **prolactin,** and **adrenocorticotropic hormone** (**ACTH,** also known as *corticotropin*). Each of the last four is secreted by a distinct cell type in the anterior pituitary gland, whereas FSH and LH, collectively termed **gonadotropic hormones** (or gonadotropins) because they stimulate the gonads, are often secreted by the same cells.

The other two peptides—**beta-lipotropin** and **beta-endorphin**—are both derived from the same prohormone as ACTH, but in humans their physiological roles, if any, are unclear. In animal studies, however, beta-endorphin has been shown to have potent pain-killing effects, and beta-lipotropin can mobilize fats in the circulation to provide a source of energy. Both of these functions may contribute to the ability to cope with stressful challenges.

Figure 11.15 summarizes the target organs and major functions of the six classical anterior pituitary gland hormones. Note that the only major function of two of the six is to stimulate their target cells to synthesize and secrete other hormones (and to maintain the growth and function of these cells). Thyroid-stimulating hormone induces the thyroid to secrete the two major thyroid hormones, thyroxine and triiodothyronine. Adrenocorticotropic hormone stimulates the adrenal cortex to secrete cortisol.

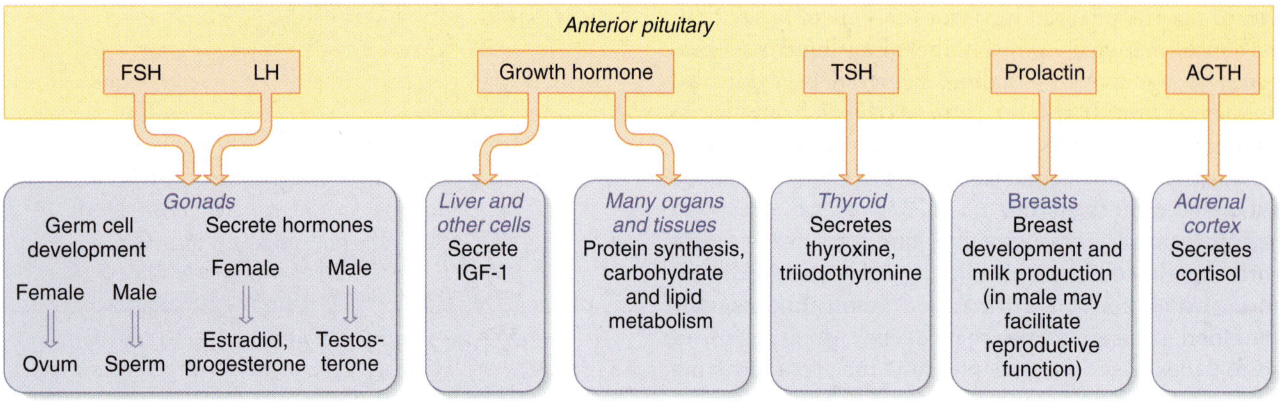

Figure 11.15 Targets and major functions of the six classical anterior pituitary gland hormones.

Three other anterior pituitary gland hormones also stimulate the secretion of another hormone but have additional functions as well. Growth hormone stimulates the liver to secrete a growth-promoting peptide hormone known as **insulin-like growth factor 1** (**IGF-1**) and, in addition, exerts direct effects on bone and on metabolism (Section E in this chapter). Follicle-stimulating hormone and luteinizing hormone stimulate the gonads to secrete the sex hormones—estradiol and progesterone from the ovaries, or testosterone from the testes; in addition, however, they regulate the growth and development of ova and sperm. The actions of FSH and LH are described in detail in Chapter 17 and therefore are not covered further here.

Prolactin is unique among the six classical anterior pituitary gland hormones in that its major function is not to exert control over the secretion of a hormone by another endocrine gland. Its most important action is to stimulate development of the mammary glands during pregnancy and milk production when a woman is nursing (lactating); this occurs by direct effects upon gland cells in the breasts. During lactation, prolactin exerts a secondary action to inhibit gonadotropin secretion, thus decreasing fertility when a woman is nursing. In the male, the physiological functions of prolactin are still under investigation.

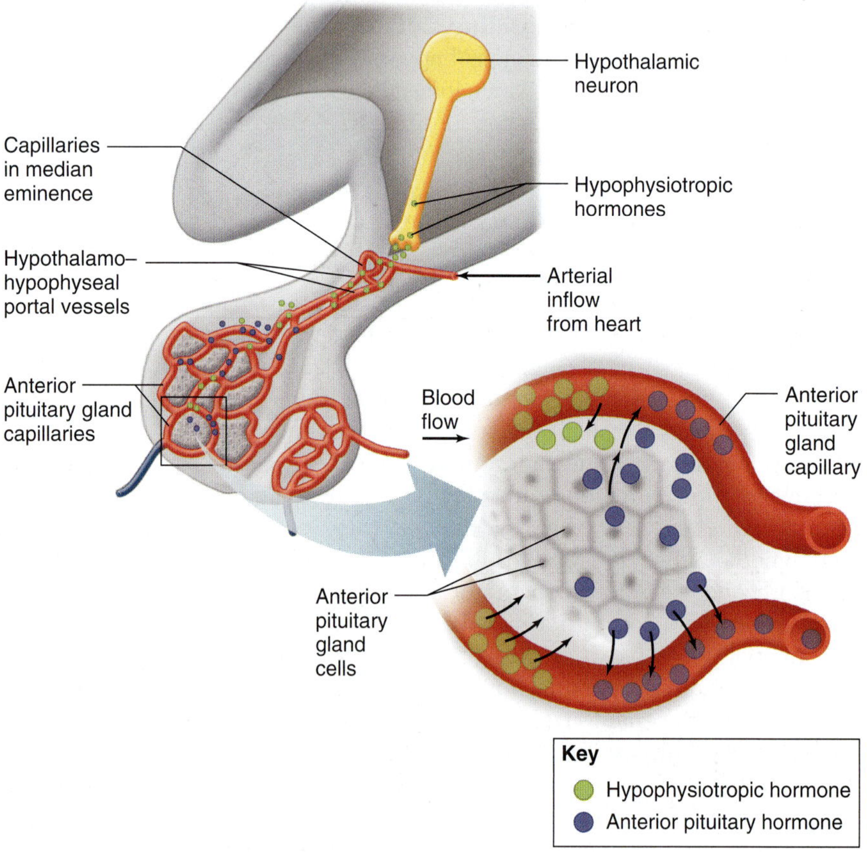

Figure 11.16 AP|R Hormone secretion by the anterior pituitary gland is controlled by hypophysiotropic hormones released by hypothalamic neurons and reaching the anterior pituitary gland by way of the hypothalamo–hypophyseal portal vessels.

Hypophysiotropic Hormones

As stated previously, secretion of the anterior pituitary gland hormones is largely regulated by hormones produced by the hypothalamus and collectively called hypophysiotropic hormones. These hormones are secreted by neurons that originate in discrete nuclei of the hypothalamus and terminate in the median eminence around the capillaries that are the origins of the hypothalamo–hypophyseal portal vessels. The generation of action potentials in these neurons causes them to secrete their hormones by exocytosis, much as action potentials cause other neurons to release neurotransmitters by exocytosis. Hypothalamic hormones, however, enter the median eminence capillaries and are carried by the hypothalamo–hypophyseal portal vessels to the anterior pituitary gland (**Figure 11.16**). There, they diffuse out of the anterior pituitary gland capillaries into the interstitial fluid surrounding the various anterior pituitary gland cells. Upon binding to specific membrane-bound receptors, the hypothalamic hormones act to stimulate or inhibit the secretion of the different anterior pituitary gland hormones.

Thus, these hypothalamic neurons secrete hormones in a manner identical to that described previously for the hypothalamic neurons whose axons end in the posterior pituitary. In both cases, the hormones are synthesized in hypothalamic neurons, pass down axons to the neuron terminals, and are released in response to action potentials in the neurons. Two crucial differences, however, distinguish the two systems. First, the axons of the hypothalamic neurons that secrete the posterior pituitary hormones leave the hypothalamus and end in the posterior pituitary, whereas those that secrete the hypophysiotropic hormones remain in the hypothalamus, ending in the median eminence. Second, most of the capillaries into which the posterior pituitary hormones are secreted immediately drain into the general circulation, which carries the hormones to the heart for distribution to the entire body. In contrast, the hypophysiotropic hormones enter capillaries in the median eminence of the hypothalamus that do not directly join the main bloodstream but empty into the hypothalamo–hypophyseal portal vessels, which carry them to the cells of the anterior pituitary gland.

When an anterior pituitary gland hormone is secreted, it will diffuse into the same capillaries that delivered the hypophysiotropic hormone. These capillaries then drain into veins, which enter the general blood circulation, where the anterior pituitary gland hormones can come into contact with their target cells. The portal circulatory system ensures that hypophysiotropic hormones can reach the cells of the anterior pituitary gland with very little delay. It also allows extremely small amounts of hypophysiotropic hormones from relatively few hypothalamic neurons to control the secretion of anterior pituitary hormones without dilution in the systemic circulation.

There are multiple hypophysiotropic hormones, each influencing the release of one or, in at least one case, two of the anterior pituitary gland hormones. For simplicity, **Figure 11.17** and the text of this chapter summarize only those hypophysiotropic hormones that have clearly documented physiological roles in humans.

Several of the hypophysiotropic hormones are named for the anterior pituitary gland hormone whose secretion they control. Thus, secretion of ACTH (corticotropin) is stimulated by **corticotropin-releasing hormone** (**CRH**), secretion of growth hormone is stimulated by **growth hormone–releasing hormone** (**GHRH**), secretion of thyroid-stimulating hormone (thyrotropin) is stimulated by **thyrotropin-releasing hormone** (**TRH**), and secretion of both luteinizing hormone and follicle-stimulating hormone (the gonadotropins) is stimulated by **gonadotropin-releasing hormone** (**GnRH**).

However, note in Figure 11.17 that two of the hypophysiotropic hormones do not *stimulate* the release of an anterior pituitary gland hormone but, rather, *inhibit* its release. One of them, **somatostatin** (**SST**), inhibits the secretion of growth hormone. The other, **dopamine** (**DA**), inhibits the secretion of prolactin.

As Figure 11.17 shows, growth hormone is controlled by *two* hypophysiotropic hormones—somatostatin, which inhibits its release, and growth hormone–releasing hormone, which stimulates it. The rate of growth hormone secretion depends, therefore, upon the relative amounts of the opposing hormones released by the hypothalamic neurons, as well as upon the relative sensitivities of the GH-producing cells of the anterior pituitary gland to them. This is a key example of the general principle of physiology that most physiological

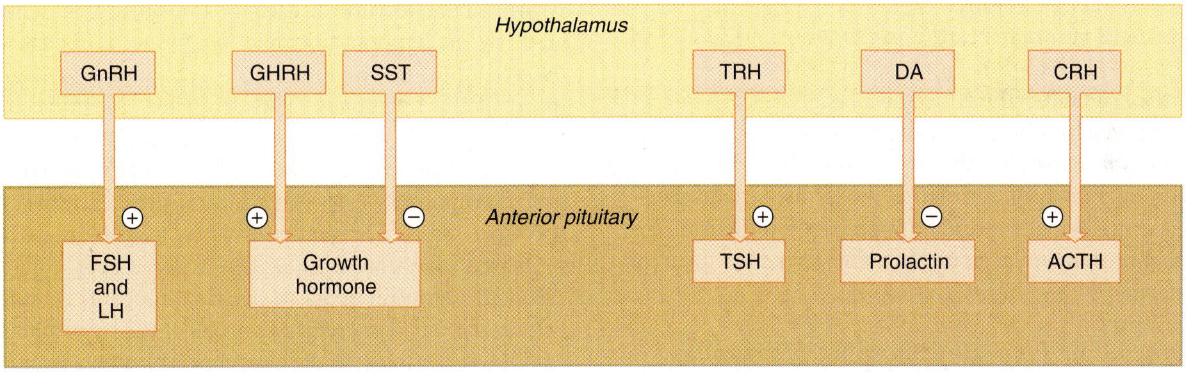

Major known hypophysiotropic hormones	Major effect on anterior pituitary
Corticotropin-releasing hormone (CRH) →	Stimulates secretion of ACTH
Thyrotropin-releasing hormone (TRH) →	Stimulates secretion of TSH
Growth hormone–releasing hormone (GHRH) →	Stimulates secretion of GH
Somatostatin (SST) →	Inhibits secretion of GH
Gonadotropin-releasing hormone (GnRH) →	Stimulates secretion of LH and FSH
Dopamine (DA)* →	Inhibits secretion of prolactin

*Dopamine is a catecholamine; all the other hypophysiotropic hormones are peptides. Evidence exists for PRL-releasing hormones, but they have not been unequivocally identified in humans. One possibility is that TRH serves this role in addition to its actions on TSH.

Figure 11.17 The effects of definitively established hypophysiotropic hormones on the anterior pituitary gland. The hypophysiotropic hormones reach the anterior pituitary gland via the hypothalamo–hypophyseal portal vessels. The ⊕ and ⊖ symbols indicate stimulatory and inhibitory actions, respectively.

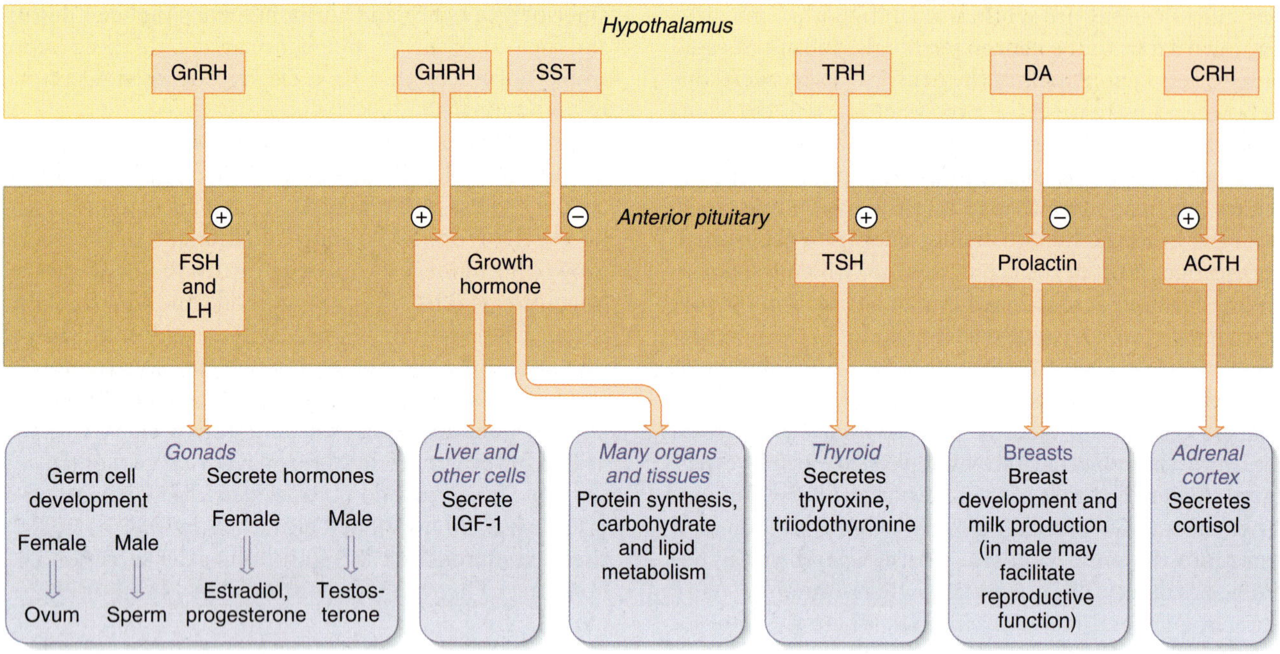

Figure 11.18 A combination of Figures 11.15 and 11.17 summarizes the hypothalamic–anterior pituitary gland system. The ⊕ and ⊖ symbols indicate stimulatory and inhibitory actions, respectively.

functions are controlled by multiple regulatory systems, often working in opposition. Such dual controls may also exist for the other anterior pituitary gland hormones. This is particularly true in the case of prolactin where the evidence for a prolactin-releasing hormone in laboratory animals is reasonably strong (the importance of such control for prolactin in humans, if it exists, is uncertain).

Figure 11.18 summarizes the information presented in Figures 11.15 and 11.17 to illustrate the full sequence of hypothalamic control of endocrine function.

Given that the hypophysiotropic hormones control anterior pituitary gland function, we must now ask, What controls secretion of the hypophysiotropic hormones themselves? Some of the neurons that secrete hypophysiotropic hormones may possess spontaneous activity, but the firing of most of them requires neural and hormonal input.

Neural Control of Hypophysiotropic Hormones

Neurons of the hypothalamus receive stimulatory and inhibitory synaptic input from virtually all areas of the central nervous system, and specific neural pathways influence the secretion of the individual hypophysiotropic hormones. A large number of neurotransmitters, such as the catecholamines and serotonin, are released at synapses on the hypothalamic neurons that produce hypophysiotropic hormones. Not surprisingly, therefore, drugs that influence these neurotransmitters can alter the secretion of the hypophysiotropic hormones.

In addition, there is a strong circadian influence (see Chapter 1) over the secretion of certain hypophysiotropic hormones. The neural inputs to these cells arise from other regions of the hypothalamus, which in turn are linked to inputs from visual pathways that recognize the presence or absence of light. A good example of this type of neural control is that of CRH, the secretion of which is tied to the day/night cycle in mammals. This pattern results in ACTH and cortisol concentrations in the blood that begin to increase just prior to the waking period.

Hormonal Feedback Control of the Hypothalamus and Anterior Pituitary Gland

A prominent feature of each of the hormonal sequences initiated by a hypophysiotropic hormone is negative feedback exerted upon the hypothalamo–hypophyseal system by one or more of the hormones in its sequence. Negative feedback is a key component of most homeostatic control systems, as introduced in Chapter 1. In this case, it is effective in dampening hormonal responses—that is, in limiting the extremes of hormone secretory rates. For example, when a stressful stimulus elicits increased secretion, in turn, of CRH, ACTH, and cortisol, the resulting elevation in plasma cortisol concentration feeds back to inhibit the CRH-secreting neurons of the hypothalamus and the ACTH-secreting cells of the anterior pituitary gland. Therefore, cortisol secretion does not increase as much as it would without negative feedback. As you will see in Section D, this is important because of the potentially damaging effects of excess cortisol on immune function and metabolic reactions, among others.

The situation described for cortisol, in which the hormone secreted by the third endocrine gland in a sequence exerts a negative feedback effect over the anterior pituitary gland and/or hypothalamus, is known as a **long-loop negative feedback** (**Figure 11.19**). This type of feedback exists for each of the three-hormone sequences initiated by a hypophysiotropic hormone.

Long-loop feedback does not exist for prolactin because this is one anterior pituitary gland hormone that does not have major control over another endocrine gland—that is, it does not participate in a three-hormone sequence. Nonetheless, there is negative feedback in the prolactin system, for this

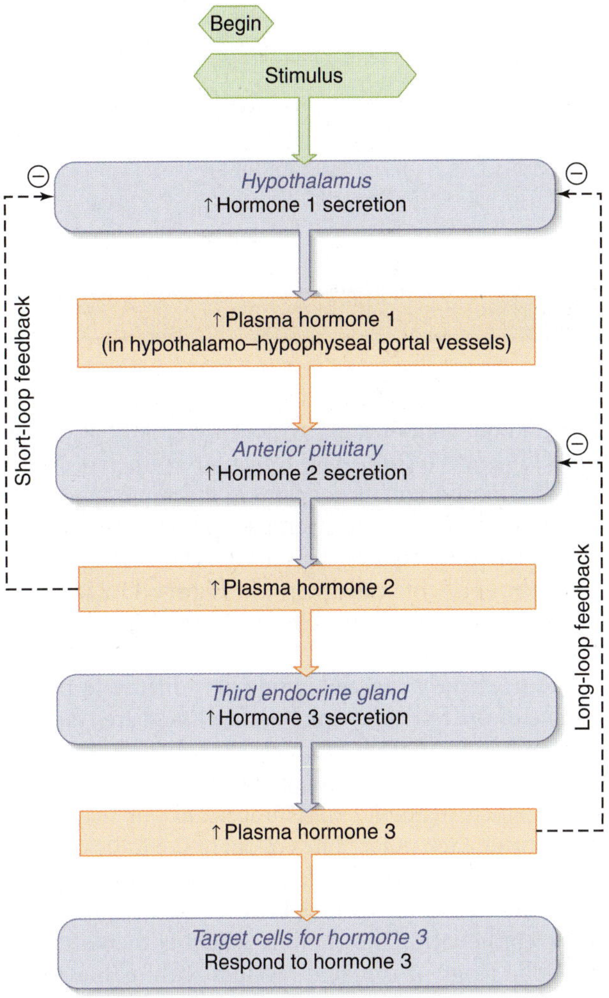

Figure 11.19 Short-loop and long-loop feedbacks. Long-loop feedback is exerted on the hypothalamus and/or anterior pituitary gland by the third hormone in the sequence. Short-loop feedback is exerted by the anterior pituitary gland hormone on the hypothalamus.

hormone itself acts upon the hypothalamus to *stimulate* the secretion of dopamine, which then *inhibits* the secretion of prolactin. The influence of an anterior pituitary gland hormone on the hypothalamus is known as a **short-loop negative feedback** (see Figure 11.19). Like prolactin, several other anterior pituitary gland hormones, including growth hormone, also exert such feedback on the hypothalamus.

The Role of "Nonsequence" Hormones on the Hypothalamus and Anterior Pituitary Gland

There are many stimulatory and inhibitory hormonal influences on the hypothalamus and/or anterior pituitary gland other than those that fit the feedback patterns just described. In other words, a hormone that is not itself in a particular hormonal sequence may nevertheless exert important influences on the secretion of the hypophysiotropic or anterior pituitary gland hormones in that sequence. For example, estradiol markedly enhances the secretion of prolactin by the anterior pituitary gland, even though estradiol secretion is not normally controlled by prolactin. Thus, the sequences we have been describing should not be viewed as isolated units.

SECTION B SUMMARY

Control Systems Involving the Hypothalamus and Pituitary Gland

I. The pituitary gland, comprising the anterior pituitary gland and the posterior pituitary, is connected to the hypothalamus by an infundibulum, or stalk, containing neuron axons and blood vessels.

II. Specific axons, whose cell bodies are in the hypothalamus, terminate in the posterior pituitary and release oxytocin and vasopressin.

III. The anterior pituitary gland secretes growth hormone (GH), thyroid-stimulating hormone (TSH), adrenocorticotropic hormone (ACTH), prolactin, and two gonadotropic hormones—follicle-stimulating hormone (FSH) and luteinizing hormone (LH). The functions of these hormones are summarized in Figure 11.15.

IV. Secretion of the anterior pituitary gland hormones is controlled mainly by hypophysiotropic hormones secreted into capillaries in the median eminence of the hypothalamus and reaching the anterior pituitary gland via the portal vessels connecting the hypothalamus and anterior pituitary gland. The actions of the hypophysiotropic hormones on the anterior pituitary gland are summarized in Figure 11.17.

V. The secretion of each hypophysiotropic hormone is controlled by neuronal and hormonal input to the hypothalamic neurons producing it.
   a. In each of the three-hormone sequences beginning with a hypophysiotropic hormone, the third hormone exerts negative feedback effects on the secretion of the hypothalamic and/or anterior pituitary gland hormone.
   b. The anterior pituitary gland hormone may exert a short-loop negative feedback inhibition of the hypothalamic releasing hormone(s) controlling it.
   c. Hormones not in a particular sequence can also influence secretion of the hypothalamic and/or anterior pituitary gland hormones in that sequence.

SECTION B REVIEW QUESTIONS

1. Describe the anatomical relationships between the hypothalamus and the pituitary gland.
2. Name the two posterior pituitary hormones and describe the site of synthesis and mechanism of release of each.
3. List all six well-established anterior pituitary gland hormones and their major functions.
4. List the major hypophysiotropic hormones and the anterior pituitary gland hormone(s) whose release each controls.
5. What kinds of inputs control secretion of the hypophysiotropic hormones?
6. What is the difference between long-loop and short-loop negative feedback in the hypothalamo–anterior pituitary gland system?

SECTION B KEY TERMS

adrenocorticotropic hormone (ACTH) 335
anterior pituitary gland 333
antidiuretic hormone (ADH) 335
beta-endorphin 335
beta-lipotropin 335
corticotropin-releasing hormone (CRH) 337
dopamine (DA) 337
follicle-stimulating hormone (FSH) 335
gonadotropic hormone 335
gonadotropin-releasing hormone (GnRH) 337
growth hormone (GH) 335
growth hormone–releasing hormone (GHRH) 337

SECTION C

The Thyroid Gland

11.9 Synthesis of Thyroid Hormone

Thyroid hormone exerts diverse effects throughout much of the body. The actions of this hormone are so widespread—and the consequences of imbalances in its concentration so significant—that it is worth examining thyroid gland function in additional detail.

The thyroid gland produces two iodine-containing molecules of physiological importance, **thyroxine** (called T_4 because it contains four iodines) and **triiodothyronine** (**T_3**, three iodines; review Figure 11.2). T_4 generally is converted into T_3 by enzymes known as deiodinases in target cells. We will therefore consider T_3 to be the major thyroid hormone, even though the concentration of T_4 in the blood is usually greater than that of T_3. (You may think of T_4 as a sort of reservoir for additional T_3.)

The thyroid gland sits within the neck straddling the trachea (**Figure 11.20a**). It first becomes functional early in fetal life. Within the thyroid gland are numerous **follicles,** each composed of an enclosed sphere of epithelial cells surrounding a core containing a protein-rich material called the **colloid** (**Figure 11.20b**). The follicular epithelial cells participate in almost all phases of thyroid hormone synthesis and secretion. Synthesis begins when circulating iodide is actively cotransported with sodium ions across the basolateral membranes of the epithelial cells (step 1 in **Figure 11.21**), a process known as **iodide trapping.** The Na^+ is pumped back out of the cell by Na^+/K^+-ATPases.

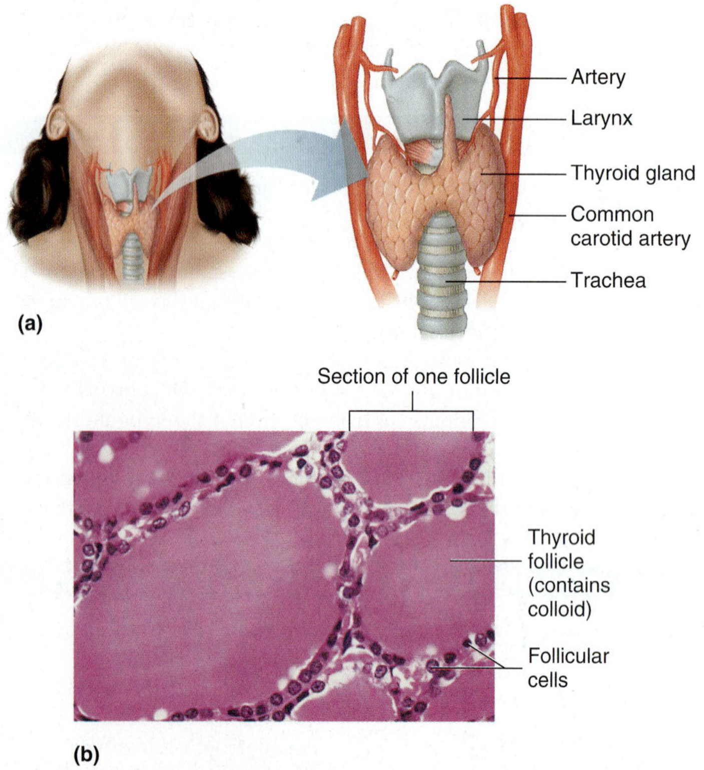

Figure 11.20 AP|R (a) Location of the bilobed thyroid gland. (b) A cross section through several adjoining follicles filled with colloid. (b): © Biophoto Associates/Photo Researchers

The negatively charged iodide ions diffuse to the apical membrane of the follicular epithelial cells and are transported into the colloid by a mechanism that is believed to require an integral membrane protein called **pendrin** (step 2). The mechanism by which pendrin acts is uncertain but may be as an iodide/chloride exchanger. The colloid of the follicles contains large amounts of a protein called **thyroglobulin.** Once in the colloid, iodide is rapidly oxidized at the luminal surface of the follicular epithelial cells to iodine, which is then attached to the phenolic rings of tyrosine residues within thyroglobulin (step 3). Thyroglobulin itself is synthesized by the follicular epithelial cells and secreted by exocytosis into the colloid. The enzyme responsible for oxidizing iodides and attaching them to tyrosines on thyroglobulin in the colloid is called **thyroid peroxidase,** and it, too, is synthesized by follicular epithelial cells. Iodine may be added to either of two positions on a given tyrosine within thyroglobulin. A tyrosine with one iodine attached is called **monoiodotyrosine** (**MIT**); if two iodines are attached, the product is **diiodotyrosine** (**DIT**). The precise mechanism of what happens next is still somewhat unclear. The phenolic ring of a molecule of MIT or DIT is removed from the remainder of its tyrosine and coupled to another DIT on the thyroglobulin molecule (step 4). This reaction may also be mediated by thyroid peroxidase. If two DIT molecules are coupled, the result is thyroxine (T_4). If one MIT and one DIT are coupled, the result is T_3.

Finally, for thyroid hormone to be secreted into the blood, extensions of the colloid-facing membranes of follicular epithelial cells engulf portions of the colloid (with its iodinated thyroglobulin) by endocytosis (step 5). The thyroglobulin, with its coupled MITs and DITs, is brought into contact with lysosomes in the cell interior (step 6). Proteolysis of thyroglobulin releases T_3 and T_4, which then diffuse out of the follicular epithelial cell into the interstitial fluid and from there to the blood (step 7). There is sufficient iodinated thyroglobulin stored within the follicles of the thyroid to provide thyroid hormone for several weeks even in the absence of dietary iodine. This storage capacity makes the thyroid gland

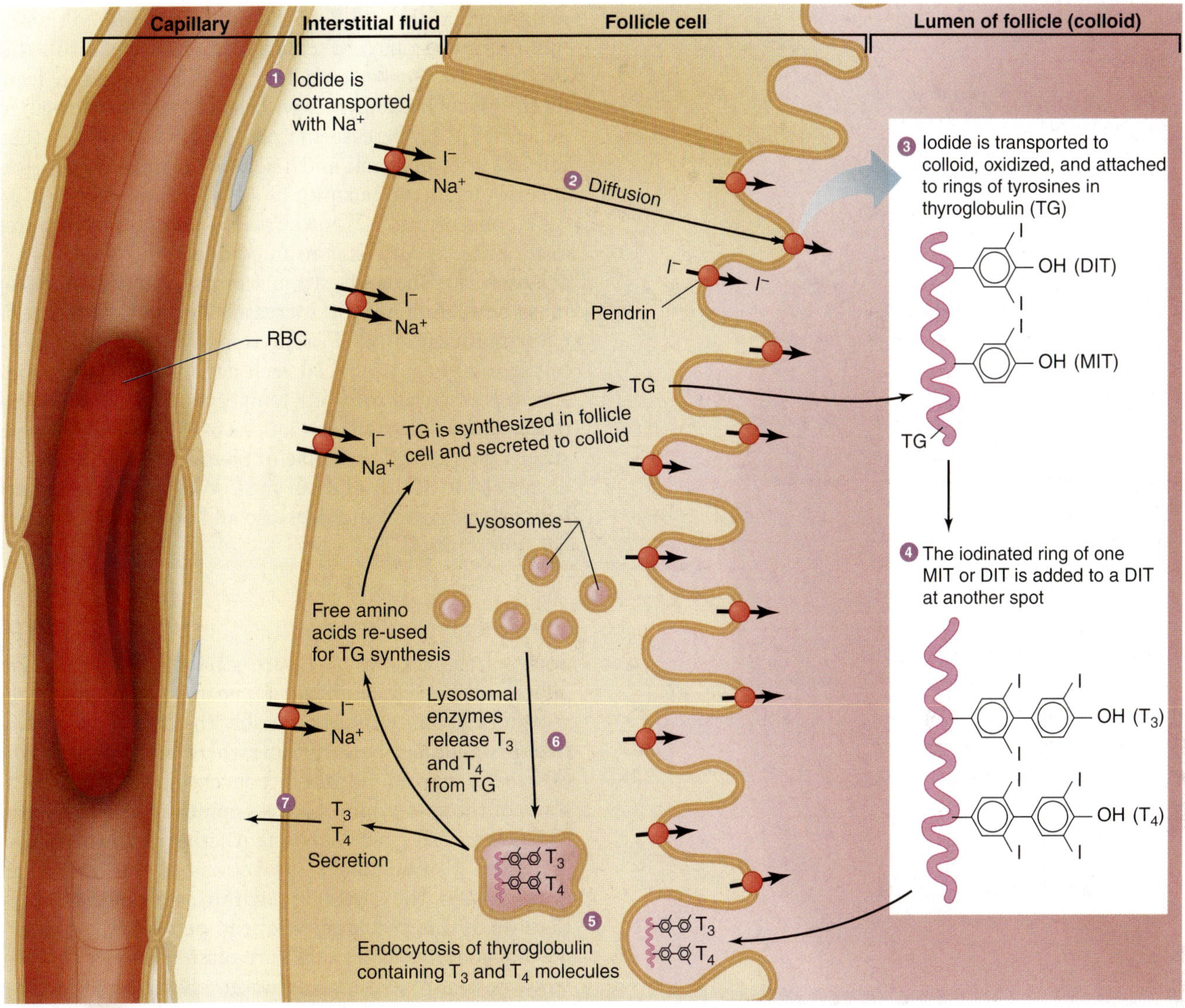

Figure 11.21 AP|R Steps involved in T_3 and T_4 formation. Steps are keyed to the text.

PHYSIOLOGICAL INQUIRY

- What is the benefit of storing iodinated thyroglobulin in the colloid?

Answer can be found at end of chapter.

unique among endocrine glands but is an essential adaptation considering the unpredictable intake of iodine in the diets of most animals.

11.10 Control of Thyroid Function

Essentially all of the actions of the follicular epithelial cells just described are stimulated by TSH, which, as we have seen, is stimulated by TRH. The basic control mechanism of TSH production is the negative feedback action of T_3 and T_4 on the anterior pituitary gland and, to a lesser extent, the hypothalamus (**Figure 11.22**). However, TSH does more than just stimulate T_3 and T_4 production. TSH also increases protein synthesis in follicular epithelial cells, increases DNA replication and cell division, and increases the amount of rough endoplasmic reticulum and other cellular machinery required by follicular epithelial cells for protein synthesis. Therefore, if thyroid cells are exposed to greater TSH concentrations than normal, they will undergo **hypertrophy;** that is, they will increase in size. An enlarged thyroid gland from any cause is called a ***goiter.*** There are several ways in which goiters can occur, in addition to increased exposure of the thyroid gland to TSH, as will be described later in this section and in one of the case studies in Chapter 19.

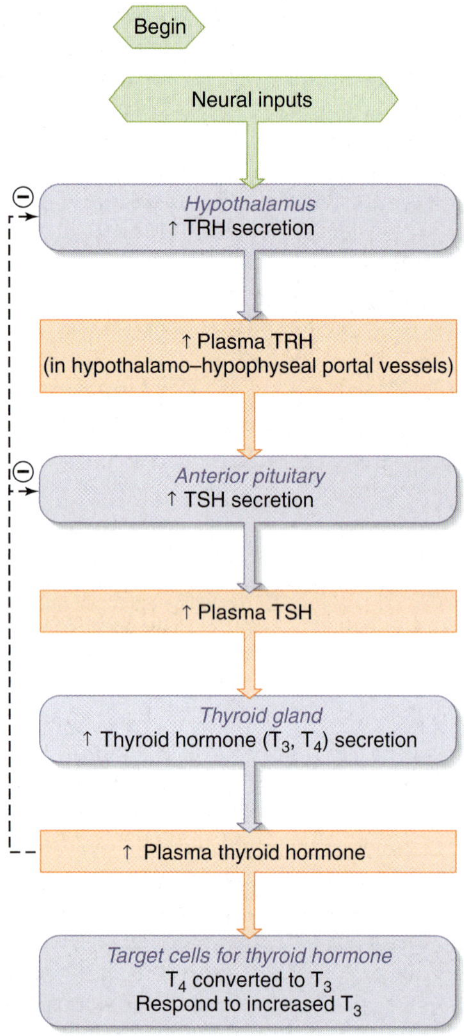

Figure 11.22 TRH-TSH-thyroid hormone sequence. T_3 and T_4 inhibit secretion of TSH and TRH by negative feedback, indicated by the ⊖ symbol.

11.11 Actions of Thyroid Hormone

Receptors for thyroid hormone are present in the nuclei of most of the cells of the body, unlike receptors for many other hormones, whose distribution is more limited. Thus, the actions of T_3 are widespread and affect many organs and tissues. Like steroid hormones, T_3 acts by inducing gene transcription and protein synthesis.

Metabolic Actions

T_3 has several effects on carbohydrate and lipid metabolism, although not to the extent as other hormones such as insulin. Nonetheless, T_3 stimulates carbohydrate absorption from the small intestine and increases fatty acid release from adipocytes. These actions provide energy that helps maintain metabolism at a high rate. Much of that energy is used to support the activity of Na^+/K^+-ATPases throughout the body; these enzymes are stimulated by T_3. The cellular concentration of ATP, therefore, is critical for the ability of cells to maintain Na^+/K^+-ATPase activity in response to thyroid hormone stimulation. ATP concentrations are controlled in part by a negative feedback mechanism; ATP negatively feeds back on the glycolytic enzymes within cells that participate in ATP generation. A decrease in cellular stores of ATP, therefore, releases the feedback and triggers an increase in glycolysis; this results in the burning of additional glucose that restores ATP concentrations. One of the by-products of this process is heat. Thus, as ATP is consumed in cells by Na^+/K^+-ATPases at a high rate due to T_3 stimulation, the cellular stores of ATP must be maintained by increased metabolism of fuels. This **calorigenic** action of T_3 represents a very significant fraction of the total heat produced each day in a typical person. This action is essential for body temperature homeostasis, just one of many ways in which the actions of thyroid hormone demonstrates the general principle of physiology that homeostasis is essential for health and survival. Without thyroid hormone, heat production would decrease and body temperature would be compromised.

Permissive Actions

Some of the actions of T_3 are attributable to its permissive effects on catecholamines. T_3 up-regulates beta-adrenergic receptors in many tissues, notably the heart and nervous system. It should not be surprising, therefore, that the symptoms of excess thyroid hormone concentration closely resemble some of the symptoms of excess epinephrine and norepinephrine (sympathetic nervous system activity). That is because the increased T_3 potentiates the actions of the catecholamines, even though the latter are within normal concentrations. Because of this potentiating effect, people with greater-than-normal concentrations of T_3 are often treated with drugs that block beta-adrenergic receptors to alleviate the anxiety, nervousness, and "racing heart" associated with excessive sympathetic activity.

Growth and Development

T_3 is required for normal production of growth hormone from the anterior pituitary gland. Therefore, in the absence of T_3, growth in children is decreased. In addition, though, T_3 is among the most important developmental hormones for the nervous system. During fetal life, T_3 exerts many effects on central nervous system development, including the formation of axon terminals and the production of synapses, the growth of dendrites and dendritic extensions (called "spines"), and the formation of myelin. Absence of T_3 during fetal life results in the syndrome called ***congenital hypothyroidism.*** This syndrome is characterized by a poorly developed nervous system and severely compromised intellectual function (mental retardation). The most common cause of congenital hypothyroidism around the world (but rare in the United States) is dietary iodine deficiency in the mother. Without iodine in her diet, iodine is not available to the fetus. Thus, even though the fetal thyroid gland may be normal, it cannot manufacture sufficient T_3. If the condition is discovered and corrected with iodine and thyroid hormone administration shortly after birth, mental and physical abnormalities can be prevented. Some evidence suggests, however, that completely normal mental function may not be restored. Furthermore, if the treatment is not initiated in the early neonatal period, the intellectual impairment resulting from congenital hypothyroidism cannot be reversed. The availability of iodized salt products has essentially eliminated congenital hypothyroidism in many countries, but it is still a common disorder in some parts of the world where iodized salt is not available.

The effects of T_3 on nervous system function are not limited to fetal and neonatal life. For example, T_3 is required for proper nerve and muscle reflexes and for normal cognition in adults.

11.12 Hypothyroidism and Hyperthyroidism

Any condition characterized by plasma concentrations of T_3 that are chronically below normal is known as ***hypothyroidism.*** Most cases of hypothyroidism—about 95%—are primary defects resulting from damage to or loss of functional thyroid tissue or from inadequate iodine consumption.

In iodine deficiency, the synthesis of T_3 is compromised, leading to a decrease in the plasma concentration of this hormone. This, in turn, releases negative feedback on the hypothalamus and anterior pituitary gland, and TRH concentrations become chronically increased in the portal circulation that leads to the anterior pituitary gland. Plasma TSH concentration is increased due to the increased TRH and loss of thyroid hormone negative feedback on the anterior pituitary gland. The resulting overstimulation of the thyroid gland can produce goiters that can achieve astounding sizes if untreated (**Figure 11.23**). This form of hypothyroidism is reversible if iodine is added to the diet. As noted earlier, it is extremely rare in the United States because of the widespread use of iodized salt, in which a small fraction of NaCl molecules is replaced with NaI.

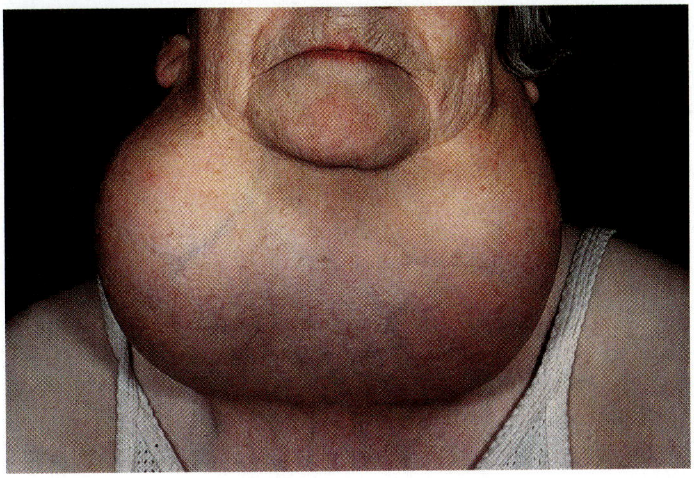

Figure 11.23 Goiter at an advanced stage.

The most common cause of hypothyroidism in the United States is autoimmune disruption of the normal function of the thyroid gland, a condition known as ***autoimmune thyroiditis.*** One form of autoimmune thyroiditis results from ***Hashimoto's disease,*** in which cells of the immune system attack and destroy thyroid tissue. Like many other autoimmune diseases, Hashimoto's disease is more common in women and can slowly progress with age. As thyroid hormone begins to decrease because of destruction of thyroid tissue, TSH concentrations increase due to the decreased negative feedback. The overstimulation of the thyroid gland results in cellular hypertrophy, and a goiter can develop. The usual treatment for autoimmune thyroiditis from any cause is daily replacement with a pill containing T_4 (most of which gets converted in the body to T_3). This causes the TSH concentration to decrease to normal due to negative feedback.

The signs and symptoms of hypothyroidism in adults may be mild or severe, depending on the degree of hormone deficiency. These include an increased sensitivity to cold (***cold intolerance***) and a tendency toward weight gain. Both of these symptoms are related to the decreased calorigenic actions normally produced by thyroid hormone. Many of the other symptoms appear to be diffuse and nonspecific, such as fatigue and changes in skin tone, hair, appetite, gastrointestinal function, and neurological function (for example, depression). The basis of the last effect in humans is uncertain, but it is now clear from work on laboratory animals that thyroid hormone has widespread effects on the adult mammalian brain. For example, thyroid hormone appears to be essential for maintaining cellular responsiveness to the neurotransmitter serotonin, and for stimulating neurogenesis in the adult hippocampus. Both serotonin and the hippocampus have been implicated in depressive disorders in humans (see Chapter 8).

In severe, untreated hypothyroidism, certain hydrophilic polymers called glycosaminoglycans accumulate in the interstitial space in scattered regions of the body. Normally, thyroid hormone acts to prevent overexpression of these extracellular compounds that are secreted by connective tissue cells. In the absence of T_3, therefore, these hydrophilic molecules accumulate and water tends to be trapped with them. This combination causes a characteristic puffiness of the face and other regions that is known as ***myxedema.***

As in the case of hypothyroidism, there are a variety of ways in which ***hyperthyroidism,*** or ***thyrotoxicosis,*** can develop. Among these are hormone-secreting tumors of the thyroid gland (rare), but the most common form of hyperthyroidism is an autoimmune disease called ***Graves' disease.*** This disease is characterized by the production of antibodies that bind to and activate the TSH receptors on thyroid gland cells, leading to chronic overstimulation of the growth and activity of the thyroid gland (see Chapter 19 for a case study related to this disease).

The signs and symptoms of thyrotoxicosis can be predicted in part from the previous discussion about hypothyroidism. Hyperthyroid patients tend to have ***heat intolerance,*** weight loss, and increased appetite, and often show signs of increased sympathetic nervous system activity (anxiety, tremors, jumpiness, increased heart rate).

Hyperthyroidism can be very serious, particularly because of its effects on the cardiovascular system (largely secondary to its permissive actions on catecholamines). It may be treated with drugs that inhibit thyroid hormone synthesis, by surgical removal of the thyroid gland, or by destroying a portion of the thyroid gland using radioactive iodine. In the last case, the radioactive iodine is ingested. Because the thyroid gland is the chief region of iodine uptake in the body, most of the radioactive iodine appears within the gland, where its high-energy radiation partly destroys the tissue.

SECTION C SUMMARY

Synthesis of Thyroid Hormone

I. T_3 and T_4 are synthesized by sequential iodinations of thyroglobulin in the thyroid follicle lumen, or colloid. Iodinated tyrosines on thyroglobulin are coupled to produce either T_3 or T_4. T_3 is the active hormone.

II. The enzyme responsible for T_3 and T_4 synthesis is thyroid peroxidase.

Control of Thyroid Function

I. All of the synthetic steps involved in T_3 synthesis are stimulated by TSH. TSH also stimulates uptake of iodide, where it is trapped in the follicle.

II. TSH causes growth (hypertrophy) of thyroid tissue. Excessive exposure of the thyroid gland to TSH can cause goiter.

Actions of Thyroid Hormone

I. T_3 increases the metabolic rate and therefore promotes consumption of calories (calorigenic effect). This results in heat production.

II. The actions of the sympathetic nervous system are potentiated by T_3. This is called the permissive action of T_3.

III. Thyroid hormone is essential for normal growth and development—particularly of the nervous system—during fetal life and childhood.

Hypothyroidism and Hyperthyroidism

I. Hypothyroidism most commonly results from autoimmune destruction of all or part of the thyroid gland. It is characterized by weight gain, fatigue, cold intolerance, and changes in skin tone and cognition. It may also result in goiter.

II. Hyperthyroidism is also typically the result of an autoimmune disorder. It is characterized by weight loss, heat intolerance, irritability and anxiety, and often goiter.

SECTION C REVIEW QUESTIONS

1. Describe the steps leading to T_3 and T_4 production, beginning with the transport of iodide into the thyroid follicular epithelial cell.
2. What are the major actions of TSH on thyroid function and growth?
3. What is the major way in which the TRH-TSH-TH pathway is regulated?
4. Explain why the symptoms of hyperthyroidism may be confused with a disorder of the autonomic nervous system.

SECTION C KEY TERMS

calorigenic 342
colloid 340
diiodotyrosine (DIT) 340
follicle 340
hypertrophy 341
iodide trapping 340
monoiodotyrosine (MIT) 340
pendrin 340
thyroglobulin 340
thyroid peroxidase 340
thyroxine (T_4) 340
triiodothyronine (T_3) 340

SECTION C CLINICAL TERMS

autoimmune thyroiditis 343
cold intolerance 343
congenital hypothyroidism 342
goiter 341
Graves' disease 343
Hashimoto's disease 343
heat intolerance 343
hyperthyroidism 343
hypothyroidism 343
myxedema 343
thyrotoxicosis 343

SECTION D
The Endocrine Response to Stress

Much of this book is concerned with the body's response to **stress** in its broadest meaning as a real or perceived threat to homeostasis. Thus, any change in external temperature, water intake, or other homeostatic factors sets into motion mechanisms designed to prevent a significant change in some physiological variable. In this section, the basic endocrine response to stress is described. These threats to homeostasis comprise an immense number of situations, including physical trauma, prolonged exposure to cold, prolonged heavy exercise, infection, shock, decreased oxygen supply, sleep deprivation, pain, and emotional stresses.

It may seem is obvious that the physiological response to cold exposure must be very different from that to infection or emotional stresses such as fright, but in one respect the response to all these situations is the same: Invariably, the secretion from the adrenal cortex of the glucocorticoid hormone cortisol is increased. Activity of the sympathetic nervous system, including release of the hormone epinephrine from the adrenal medulla, also increases in response to most types of stress.

The increased cortisol secretion during stress is mediated by the hypothalamus–anterior pituitary gland system described earlier. As illustrated in **Figure 11.24**, neural input to the hypothalamus from portions of the nervous system responding to a particular stress induces secretion of CRH. This hormone is carried by the hypothalamo–hypophyseal portal vessels to the anterior pituitary gland, where it stimulates ACTH secretion. ACTH in turn circulates through the blood, reaches the adrenal cortex, and stimulates cortisol release.

The secretion of ACTH, and therefore of cortisol, is also stimulated to a lesser extent by vasopressin, which usually

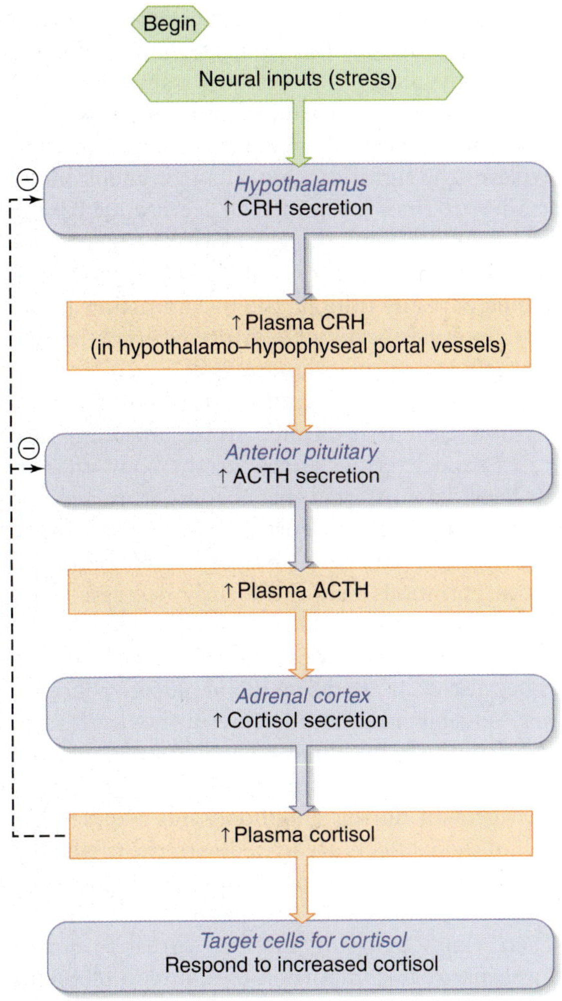

Figure 11.24 CRH-ACTH-cortisol pathway. Neural inputs include those related to stressful stimuli and nonstress inputs like circadian rhythms. Cortisol exerts a negative feedback control (⊖ symbols) over the system by acting on (1) the hypothalamus to inhibit CRH synthesis and secretion and (2) the anterior pituitary gland to inhibit ACTH production.

PHYSIOLOGICAL INQUIRY

- What hormonal changes in this pathway would be expected if a patient developed a benign tumor of the left adrenal cortex that secreted extremely large amounts of cortisol in the absence of external stimulation? What might happen to the right adrenal gland?

Answer can be found at end of chapter.

increases in response to stress and which may reach the anterior pituitary gland either from the general circulation or by the short portal vessels shown in Figure 11.13. Some of the cytokines (secretions from cells that comprise the immune system, Chapter 18) also stimulate ACTH secretion both directly and by stimulating the secretion of CRH. These cytokines provide a means for eliciting an endocrine stress response when the immune system is stimulated in, for example, systemic infection. The possible significance of this relationship for immune function is described next and in additional detail in Chapter 18.

11.13 Physiological Functions of Cortisol

Although the effects of cortisol are most dramatically illustrated during the response to stress, cortisol is always produced by the adrenal cortex and exerts many important actions even in nonstress situations. For example, cortisol has permissive actions on the reactivity to epinephrine and norepinephrine of smooth muscle cells that surround the lumen of blood vessels such as arterioles. Partly for this reason, therefore, cortisol helps maintain normal blood pressure. Likewise, cortisol is required to maintain the cellular concentrations of certain enzymes involved in metabolic homeostasis. These enzymes are expressed primarily in the liver, and they act to increase hepatic glucose production between meals, thereby preventing plasma glucose concentrations from significantly decreasing below normal.

Two important systemic actions of cortisol are its anti-inflammatory and anti-immune functions. The mechanisms by which cortisol inhibits immune system function are numerous and complex. Cortisol inhibits the production of leukotrienes and prostaglandins, both of which are involved in inflammation. Cortisol also stabilizes lysosomal membranes in damaged cells, preventing the release of their proteolytic contents. In addition, cortisol reduces capillary permeability in injured areas (thereby reducing fluid leakage to the interstitium), and it suppresses the growth and function of certain key immune cells such as lymphocytes. Thus, cortisol may serve as a "brake" on the immune system, which may overreact to minor infections in the absence of cortisol. Indeed, in diseases in which cortisol concentrations in the blood are greatly decreased, an increased incidence of autoimmune disease has been reported. Such diseases are characterized by a person's immune system launching an attack against one or more tissues of one's own body.

During fetal and neonatal life, cortisol is also an extremely important developmental hormone. It has been implicated in the proper differentiation of numerous tissues and glands, including various parts of the brain, the adrenal medulla, the intestine, and the lungs. In the last case, cortisol is very important for the production of surfactant, a substance that reduces surface tension in the lungs, thereby making it easier for the lungs to inflate (see Chapter 13).

Thus, although it is common to define the actions of cortisol in the context of the stress response, it is worth remembering that the maintenance of homeostasis in the absence of external stresses is also a critical function of cortisol.

11.14 Functions of Cortisol in Stress

Table 11.3 summarizes the major effects of increased plasma concentrations of cortisol during stress. The effects on organic metabolism are to mobilize energy sources to increase the plasma concentrations of amino acids, glucose, glycerol, and free fatty acids. These effects are ideally suited to meet a stressful situation. First, an animal faced with a potential threat is often forced to forgo eating, making these metabolic changes adaptive for coping with stress while fasting. Second, the amino acids liberated by catabolism of body protein not

TABLE 11.3	Effects of Increased Plasma Cortisol Concentration During Stress
I. Effects on organic metabolism A. Stimulation of protein catabolism in bone, lymph, muscle, and elsewhere B. Stimulation of liver uptake of amino acids and their conversion to glucose (gluconeogenesis) C. Maintenance of plasma glucose concentrations D. Stimulation of triglyceride catabolism in adipose tissue, with release of glycerol and fatty acids into the blood	
II. Enhanced vascular reactivity (increased ability to maintain vasoconstriction in response to norepinephrine and other stimuli)	
III. Unidentified protective effects against the damaging influences of stress	
IV. Inhibition of inflammation and specific immune responses	
V. Inhibition of nonessential functions (e.g., reproduction and growth)	

only provide a potential source of glucose, via hepatic gluconeogenesis, but also constitute a potential source of amino acids for tissue repair should injury occur.

A few of the medically important implications of these cortisol-induced effects on organic metabolism are as follows. (1) Any patient who is ill or is subjected to surgery catabolizes considerable quantities of body protein; (2) a person with diabetes mellitus who suffers an infection requires more insulin than usual; and (3) a child subjected to severe stress of any kind may show a decreased rate of growth.

Cortisol has important effects during stress other than those on organic metabolism. For example, it increases the ability of vascular smooth muscle to contract in response to norepinephrine, thereby improving cardiovascular performance.

As item III in Table 11.3 notes, we still do not know the other reasons that increased cortisol is so important for the body's optimal response to stress, that is, for its ability to resist the damaging influences of stress. What is clear is that a person exposed to severe stress can die, usually of circulatory failure, if his or her plasma cortisol concentration is abnormally low; the complete absence of cortisol is always fatal.

Effect IV in Table 11.3 reflects the fact that administration of large amounts of cortisol or its synthetic analogs profoundly reduces the inflammatory response to injury or infection. Because of this effect, cortisol and its synthetic analogs are a valuable tool in the treatment of ***allergy***, ***arthritis*** (inflammation of the joints), other inflammatory diseases, and graft rejection (all of which are discussed in detail in Chapter 18). These anti-inflammatory and anti-immune effects have generally been classified among the various pharmacological effects of cortisol because it was assumed they could be achieved only by very large doses of administered glucocorticoids. It is now clear, however, that such effects also occur, albeit to a lesser degree, at the plasma concentrations achieved during stress. Thus, the increased plasma cortisol typical of infection or trauma exerts a dampening effect on the body's immune responses, protecting against possible damage from excessive inflammation. This effect explains the significance of the fact, mentioned earlier, that certain cytokines (immune cell secretions) stimulate the secretion of ACTH and thereby cortisol. Such stimulation is part of a negative feedback system in which the increased cortisol then partially inhibits the inflammatory processes in which the cytokines participate. Moreover, cortisol normally dampens the fever an infection causes.

Whereas the acute cortisol responses to stress are adaptive, it is now clear that chronic stress, including emotional stress, can have deleterious effects on the body. In some studies, it has been demonstrated that chronic stress results in sustained increases in plasma cortisol concentrations (but this is not always observed). In such a case, the abnormally high cortisol concentrations may sufficiently decrease the activity of the immune system to reduce the body's resistance to infection and, perhaps, cancer. It can also worsen the symptoms of diabetes because of its effects on blood glucose concentrations, and it may possibly cause an increase in the death rate of certain neurons in the brain. Finally, chronic stress may be associated with decreased reproductive fertility, delayed puberty, and suppressed growth during childhood and adolescence. Some but not all of these effects are linked with the catabolic actions of glucocorticoids.

In summary, stress is a broadly defined situation in which there exists a real or potential threat to homeostasis. In such a scenario, it is important to maintain blood pressure, to provide extra energy sources in the blood, and to temporarily shut down nonessential functions. Cortisol is the most important hormone that carries out these activities. Cortisol enhances vascular reactivity, catabolizes protein and fat to provide energy, and inhibits growth and reproduction. The price the body pays during stress is that cortisol is strongly catabolic. Thus, cells of the immune system, bone, muscles, skin, and numerous other tissues undergo catabolism to provide substrates for gluconeogenesis. In the short term, this is not of any major consequence. Chronic exposure to stress, however, can lead to severe decreases in bone density, immune function, and reproductive fertility.

11.15 Adrenal Insufficiency and Cushing's Syndrome

Cortisol is one of several hormones essential for life. The absence of cortisol leads to the body's inability to maintain homeostasis, particularly when confronted with a stress such as infection, which is usually fatal within days without cortisol. The general term for any situation in which plasma concentrations of cortisol are chronically lower than normal is ***adrenal insufficiency***. Patients with adrenal insufficiency have a diffuse array of symptoms, depending on the severity and cause of the disease. These patients typically report weakness, fatigue, and loss of appetite and weight.

Examination may reveal low blood pressure (in part because cortisol is needed to permit the full extent of the cardiovascular actions of epinephrine) and low blood sugar, especially after fasting (because of the loss of the normal metabolic actions of cortisol).

There are several causes of adrenal insufficiency. ***Primary adrenal insufficiency*** is due to a loss of adrenal cortical function, as may rarely occur, for example, when infectious diseases such as ***tuberculosis*** infiltrate the adrenal glands and destroy them. The adrenals can also (rarely) be destroyed by invasive tumors. Most commonly by far, however, the syndrome is due to autoimmune attack in which the immune system mistakenly recognizes some component of a person's own adrenal cells as "foreign." The resultant immune reaction causes inflammation and eventually the destruction of many of the cells of the adrenal glands. Because of this, all of the zones of the adrenal cortex are affected. Thus, not only cortisol but also aldosterone concentrations are decreased below normal in primary adrenal insufficiency. This decrease in aldosterone concentration creates the additional problem of an imbalance in Na^+, K^+, and water in the blood because aldosterone is a key regulator of those variables. The loss of salt and water balance may lead to ***hypotension*** (low blood pressure). Primary adrenal insufficiency from any of these causes is also known as ***Addison's disease,*** after the nineteenth-century physician who first discovered the syndrome.

The diagnosis of primary adrenal insufficiency is made by measuring plasma concentrations of cortisol. In primary adrenal insufficiency, cortisol concentrations are well below normal, whereas ACTH concentrations are greatly increased due to the loss of the negative feedback actions of cortisol. Treatment of this disease requires daily oral administration of glucocorticoids and mineralocorticoids. In addition, the patient must carefully monitor his or her diet to ensure an adequate consumption of carbohydrates and controlled K^+ and Na^+ intake.

Adrenal insufficiency can also be due to a deficiency of ACTH—***secondary adrenal insufficiency,*** which may arise from pituitary disease. Its symptoms are often less dramatic than primary adrenal insufficiency because aldosterone secretion, which does not rely on ACTH, is maintained by other mechanisms.

Adrenal insufficiency can be life threatening if not treated aggressively. The flip side of this disorder—*excess* glucocorticoids—is usually not as immediately dangerous but can also be very severe. In ***Cushing's syndrome,*** even the nonstressed individual has excess cortisol in the blood. The cause may be a primary defect (e.g., a cortisol-secreting tumor of the adrenal) or may be secondary (usually due to an ACTH-secreting tumor of the anterior pituitary gland). In the latter case, the condition is known as ***Cushing's disease,*** which accounts for most cases of Cushing's syndrome. The increased blood concentrations of cortisol, particularly at night when cortisol is usually low, tend to promote uncontrolled catabolism of bone, muscle, skin, and other organs. As a result, bone strength diminishes and can even lead to ***osteoporosis*** (loss of bone mass), muscles weaken, and the skin becomes thinned and easily bruised. The increased catabolism may produce such a large quantity of precursors for hepatic gluconeogenesis that the blood sugar concentration increases to that observed in diabetes mellitus. A person with Cushing's syndrome, therefore, may show some of the same symptoms as a person with diabetes. Equally troubling is the possibility of ***immunosuppression,*** which may be brought about by the anti-immune actions of cortisol. Cushing's syndrome is often associated with loss of fat mass from the extremities and with redistribution of the fat in the trunk, face, and the back of the neck. Combined with an increased appetite, often triggered by high concentrations of cortisol, this results in obesity and a characteristic facial appearance in many patients (**Figure 11.25**). A further problem associated with Cushing's syndrome is the possibility of developing ***hypertension*** (high blood pressure). This is due not to increased aldosterone production but instead to the pharmacological effects of cortisol, because at high concentrations, cortisol exerts aldosterone-like actions on the kidney, resulting in salt and water retention, which contributes to hypertension.

Treatment of Cushing's syndrome depends on the cause. In Cushing's disease, for example, surgical removal of the pituitary tumor, if possible, is the best alternative.

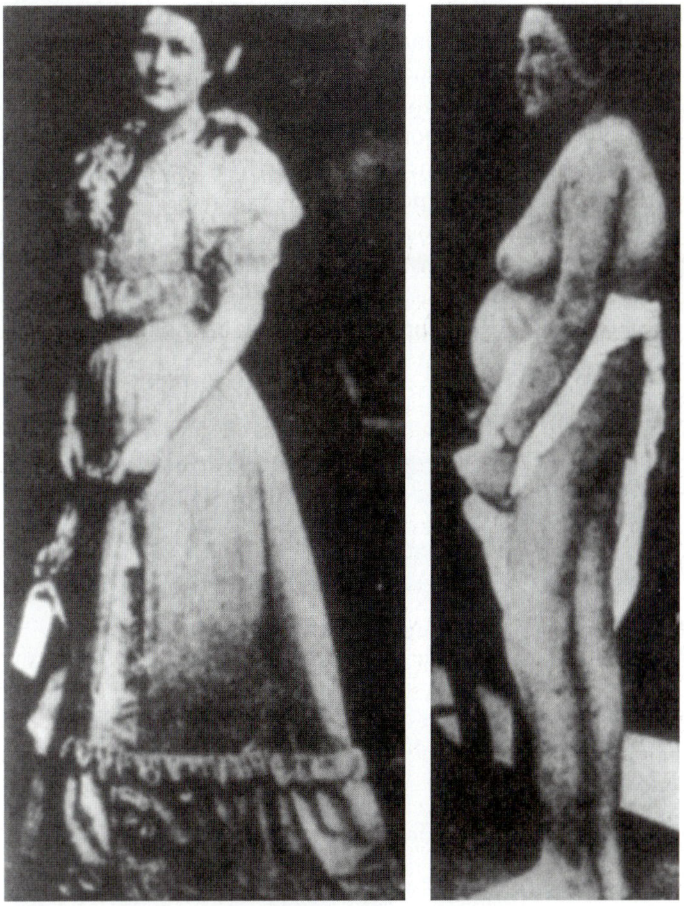

Figure 11.25 A young patient from the original series of Harvey Cushing. *Left:* Before onset of disease. *Right:* After development of Cushing's syndrome.

Of importance is the fact that glucocorticoids are often used therapeutically to treat inflammation, lung disease, and other disorders. If glucocorticoids are administered at a high enough dosage for long periods, the side effect of such treatment can be Cushing's syndrome.

11.16 Other Hormones Released During Stress

Other hormones that are usually released during many kinds of stress are aldosterone, vasopressin, growth hormone, glucagon, and beta-endorphin (which is coreleased from the anterior pituitary gland with ACTH). Insulin secretion usually decreases. Vasopressin and aldosterone act to retain water and Na^+ within the body, an important response in the face of potential losses by dehydration, hemorrhage, or sweating. The overall effects of the changes in growth hormone, glucagon, and insulin are, like those of cortisol and epinephrine, to mobilize energy stores and increase the plasma concentration of glucose. The role, if any, of beta-endorphin in stress may be related to its painkilling effects.

In addition, the sympathetic nervous system plays a key role in the stress response. Activation of the sympathetic nervous system during stress is often termed the fight-or-flight response, as described in Chapter 6. A list of the major effects of increased sympathetic activity, including secretion of epinephrine from the adrenal medulla, almost constitutes a guide to how to meet emergencies in which physical activity may be required and bodily damage may occur (**Table 11.4**).

This list of hormones whose secretion rates are altered by stress is by no means complete. It is likely that the secretion of almost every known hormone may be influenced by stress. For example, prolactin is increased, although the adaptive significance of this change is unclear. By contrast, the pituitary gonadotropins and the sex steroids are decreased. As noted previously, reproduction is not an essential function during a crisis.

TABLE 11.4	Actions of the Sympathetic Nervous System, Including Epinephrine Secreted by the Adrenal Medulla, During Stress
Increased hepatic and muscle glycogenolysis (provides a quick source of glucose)	
Increased breakdown of adipose tissue triglyceride (provides a supply of glycerol for gluconeogenesis and of fatty acids for oxidation)	
Increased cardiac function (e.g., increased heart rate)	
Diversion of blood from viscera to skeletal muscles by means of vasoconstriction in the former beds and vasodilation in the latter	
Increased lung ventilation by stimulating brain breathing centers and dilating airways	

SECTION D SUMMARY

Physiological Functions of Cortisol

I. Cortisol is released from the adrenal cortex upon stimulation with ACTH. ACTH, in turn, is stimulated by the release of corticotropin-releasing hormone (CRH) from the hypothalamus.

II. The physiological functions of cortisol are to maintain the responsiveness of target cells to epinephrine and norepinephrine, to provide a "check" on the immune system, to participate in energy homeostasis, and to promote normal differentiation of tissues during fetal life.

Functions of Cortisol in Stress

I. The stimulus that activates the CRH-ACTH-cortisol pathway is stress, which encompasses a wide array of sensory and physical inputs that disrupt, or potentially disrupt, homeostasis.

II. In response to stress, the usual physiological functions of cortisol are enhanced as cortisol concentrations in the plasma increase. Thus, gluconeogenesis, lipolysis, and inhibition of insulin actions increase. This results in increased blood concentrations of energy sources (glucose, fatty acids) required to cope with stressful situations.

III. High cortisol concentrations also inhibit "nonessential" processes, such as reproduction, during stressful situations and inhibit immune function.

Adrenal Insufficiency and Cushing's Syndrome

I. Adrenal insufficiency may result from adrenal destruction (primary adrenal insufficiency, or Addison's disease) or from hyposecretion of ACTH (secondary adrenal insufficiency).

II. Adrenal insufficiency is associated with decreased ability to maintain blood pressure (due to loss of aldosterone) and blood sugar. It may be fatal if untreated.

III. Cushing's syndrome is the result of chronically elevated plasma cortisol concentration. When the cause of the increased cortisol is secondary to an ACTH-secreting pituitary tumor, the condition is known as Cushing's disease.

IV. Cushing's syndrome is associated with hypertension, high blood sugar, redistribution of body fat, obesity, and muscle and bone weakness. If untreated, it can also lead to immunosuppression.

Other Hormones Released During Stress

I. In addition to CRH, ACTH, and cortisol, several other hormones are released during stress. Beta-endorphin is coreleased with ACTH and may act to reduce pain. Vasopressin stimulates ACTH secretion and also acts on the kidney to increase water retention. Other hormones that are increased in the blood by stress are aldosterone, growth hormone, and glucagon. Insulin secretion, by contrast, decreases during stress.

II. Epinephrine is secreted from the adrenal medulla during stress in response to stimulation from the sympathetic nervous system. The norepinephrine from sympathetic neuron terminals, combined with the circulating epinephrine, prepare the body for stress in several ways. These include increased heart rate and heart pumping strength, increased ventilation, increased shunting of blood to skeletal muscle, and increased generation of energy sources that are released into the blood.

SECTION D REVIEW QUESTIONS

1. Diagram the CRH-ACTH-cortisol pathway.
2. List the physiological functions of cortisol.

3. Define *stress*, and list the functions of cortisol during stress.
4. List the major effects of activation of the sympathetic nervous system during stress.
5. Contrast the symptoms of adrenal insufficiency and Cushing's syndrome.

SECTION D KEY TERMS

SECTION D CLINICAL TERMS

SECTION E
Endocrine Control of Growth

One of the major functions of the endocrine system is to control growth. At least a dozen hormones directly or indirectly (e.g., hypophysiotropic hormones) play important roles in stimulating or inhibiting growth. This complex process is also influenced by genetics and a variety of environmental factors, including nutrition, and provides an illustration of the general principle of physiology that most physiological functions are controlled by multiple regulatory systems, often working in opposition. The growth process involves cell division and net protein synthesis throughout the body, but a person's height is determined specifically by bone growth, particularly of the vertebral column and legs. We first provide an overview of bone and the growth process before describing the roles of hormones in determining growth rates.

11.17 Bone Growth

Bone is a living tissue consisting of a protein (collagen) matrix upon which calcium salts, particularly calcium phosphates, are deposited. A growing long bone is divided, for descriptive purposes, into the ends, or **epiphyses,** and the remainder, the **shaft.** The portion of each epiphysis in contact with the shaft is a plate of actively proliferating cartilage (connective tissue composed of collagen and other fibrous proteins) called the **epiphyseal growth plate** (Figure 11.26). **Osteoblasts,** the bone-forming cells at the shaft edge of the epiphyseal growth plate, convert the cartilaginous tissue at this edge to bone, while cells called **chondrocytes** simultaneously lay down new cartilage in the interior of the plate. In this manner, the epiphyseal growth plate widens and is gradually pushed away from the center of the bony shaft as the shaft lengthens.

Linear growth of the shaft can continue as long as the epiphyseal growth plates exist but ceases when the growth plates themselves are converted to bone as a result of other hormonal influences at puberty. This is known as **epiphyseal closure** and occurs at different times in different bones. Thus, a person's **bone age** can be determined by x-raying the bones and determining which ones have undergone epiphyseal closure.

As shown in Figure 11.27, children manifest two periods of rapid increase in height, the first during the first 2 years of life and the second during puberty. Note that increase in height is not necessarily correlated with the rates of growth of specific organs.

The pubertal growth spurt lasts several years in both sexes, but growth during this period is greater in boys. In addition,

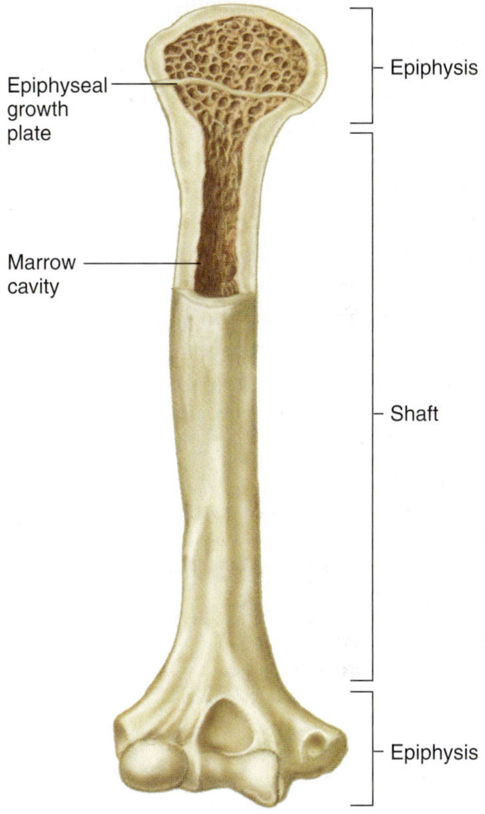

Figure 11.26 AP|R Anatomy of a long bone during growth.

boys grow more before puberty because they begin puberty approximately 2 years later than girls. These factors account for the differences in average height between men and women.

11.18 Environmental Factors Influencing Growth

Adequate nutrition and good health are the primary environmental factors influencing growth. Lack of sufficient amounts of protein, fatty acids, vitamins, or minerals interferes with growth.

The growth-inhibiting effects of malnutrition can be seen at any time of development but are most profound when they occur early in life. For this reason, maternal malnutrition may cause growth retardation in the fetus. Because low birth

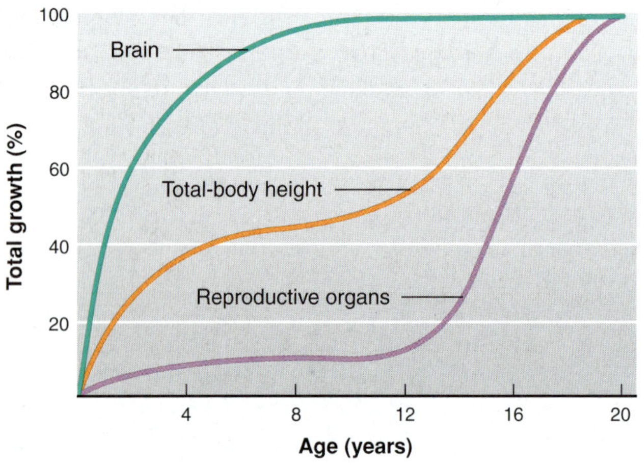

Figure 11.27 Relative growth in brain, total-body height (a measure of long-bone and vertebral growth), and reproductive organs. Note that brain growth is nearly complete by age 5, whereas maximal height (maximal bone lengthening) and reproductive-organ size are not reached until the late teens.

weight is strongly associated with increased infant mortality, prenatal malnutrition causes increased numbers of prenatal and early postnatal deaths. Moreover, irreversible stunting of brain development may be caused by prenatal malnutrition. During infancy and childhood, too, malnutrition can interfere with both intellectual development and total-body growth.

Following a temporary period of stunted growth due to malnutrition or illness, and given proper nutrition and recovery from illness, a child can manifest a remarkable growth spurt called **catch-up growth** that brings the child to within the range of normal heights expected for his or her age. The mechanisms that account for this accelerated growth are unknown, but recent evidence suggests that it may be related to the rate of stem cell differentiation within the growth plates.

11.19 Hormonal Influences on Growth

The hormones most important to human growth are growth hormone, insulin-like growth factors 1 and 2, T_3, insulin, testosterone, and estradiol, all of which exert widespread effects. In addition to all these hormones, a large group of peptide **growth factors** exert effects, most of them acting in a paracrine or autocrine manner to stimulate differentiation and/or cell division of certain cell types. The general term for a molecule that stimulates cell division is mitogen.

The various hormones and growth factors do not all stimulate growth at the same periods of life. For example, fetal growth is less dependent on fetal growth hormone, the thyroid hormones, and the sex steroids than are the growth periods that occur during childhood and adolescence.

Growth Hormone and Insulin-Like Growth Factors

Growth hormone, secreted by the anterior pituitary gland, has little effect on fetal growth but is the most important hormone for postnatal growth. Its major growth-promoting effect is stimulation of cell division in its many target tissues. Thus, growth hormone promotes bone lengthening by stimulating maturation and cell division of the chondrocytes in the epiphyseal plates, thereby continuously widening the plates and providing more cartilaginous material for bone formation.

Importantly, growth hormone exerts most of its mitogenic effect not *directly* on cells but *indirectly* through the mediation of the mitogenic hormone IGF-1, whose synthesis and release by the liver are induced by growth hormone. Despite some structural similarities to insulin (from which its name is derived), this messenger has its own unique effects distinct from those of insulin. Under the influence of growth hormone, IGF-1 is secreted by the liver, enters the blood, and functions as a hormone. In addition, growth hormone stimulates many other types of cells, including bone, to secrete IGF-1, where it functions as an autocrine or paracrine substance.

Current concepts of how growth hormone and IGF-1 interact on the epiphyseal plates of bone are as follows. (1) Growth hormone stimulates the chondrocyte precursor cells (prechondrocytes) and/or young differentiating chondrocytes in the epiphyseal plates to differentiate into chondrocytes. (2) During this differentiation, the cells begin both to secrete IGF-1 and to become responsive to IGF-1. (3) The IGF-1 then acts as an autocrine or paracrine substance (probably along with blood-borne IGF-1) to stimulate the differentiating chondrocytes to undergo cell division.

The importance of IGF-1 in mediating the major growth-promoting effect of growth hormone is illustrated by the fact that ***short stature*** can be caused not only by decreased growth hormone secretion but also by decreased production of IGF-1 or failure of the tissues to respond to IGF-1. For example, one rare form of short stature (called ***growth hormone–insensitivity syndrome***) is due to a genetic mutation that causes a change in the growth hormone receptor such that it fails to respond to growth hormone (an example of hyporesponsiveness). The result is failure to produce IGF-1 in response to growth hormone, and a consequent decreased growth rate in a child.

The secretion and activity of IGF-1 can be influenced by the nutritional status of the individual and by many hormones other than growth hormone. For example, malnutrition during childhood inhibits the production of IGF-1 even if plasma growth hormone concentration is increased.

In addition to its specific growth-promoting effect on cell division via IGF-1, growth hormone directly stimulates protein synthesis in various tissues and organs, particularly muscle. It does this by increasing amino acid uptake and both the synthesis and activity of ribosomes. All of these events are essential for protein synthesis. This anabolic effect on protein metabolism facilitates the ability of tissues and organs to enlarge. Growth hormone also plays a role in energy homeostasis. It does this in part by facilitating the breakdown of triglycerides that are stored in adipose cells, which then release fatty acids into the blood. It also stimulates gluconeogenesis in the liver and inhibits the ability of insulin to promote glucose transport into cells. Growth hormone, therefore, tends to increase circulating energy sources. Not surprisingly, therefore, situations such as exercise, stress, or fasting, for which increased energy availability is beneficial, result in stimulation of growth hormone secretion into the blood. The metabolic effects of growth hormone are important throughout life and continue in adulthood long after bone growth has ceased. **Table 11.5** summarizes some of the major effects of growth hormone.

Figure 11.28 shows the control of growth hormone secretion. Briefly, the control system begins with two of the hormones secreted by the hypothalamus. Growth hormone secretion is stimulated by growth hormone–releasing hormone (GHRH) and inhibited by somatostatin (SST). As a result of changes in these two signals, which are usually 180 degrees out of phase with each other (i.e., one is high when the other is low), growth hormone secretion occurs in episodic bursts and manifests a striking daily rhythm. During most of the day, little or no growth hormone is secreted, although bursts may be elicited by certain stimuli, including stress, hypoglycemia, and exercise. In contrast, 1 to 2 hours after a person falls asleep, one or more larger, prolonged bursts of secretion may occur. The negative feedback controls that growth hormone and IGF-1 exert on the hypothalamus and anterior pituitary gland are summarized in Figure 11.28.

In addition to the hypothalamic controls, a variety of hormones—notably, the sex steroids, insulin, and thyroid hormones—influence the secretion of growth hormone. The net result of all these inputs is that the secretion rate of growth hormone is highest during adolescence (the period of most rapid growth), next highest in children, and lowest in adults. The decreased growth hormone secretion associated with aging is responsible, in part, for the decrease in lean-body and bone mass, the expansion of adipose tissue, and the thinning of the skin that occur as people age.

The ready availability of human growth hormone produced by recombinant DNA technology has greatly facilitated the treatment of children with short stature due to growth hormone deficiency. Controversial at present is the administration of growth hormone to short children who do not have growth hormone deficiency, to athletes in an attempt to increase muscle mass, and to elderly persons to reverse growth hormone–related aging changes. It should be clear from Table 11.5 that administration of GH to an otherwise healthy individual (such as an athlete) can lead to serious side effects. Abuse of GH in such situations can lead to symptoms similar to those of diabetes mellitus, as well as numerous other problems. The consequences of chronically elevated growth

TABLE 11.5	Major Effects of Growth Hormone
I.	Promotes growth: Induces precursor cells in bone and other tissues to differentiate and secrete insulin-like growth factor 1 (IGF-1), which stimulates cell division. Also stimulates liver to secrete IGF-1.
II.	Stimulates protein synthesis, predominantly in muscle.
III.	Anti-insulin effects (particularly at high concentrations): A. Renders adipocytes more responsive to stimuli that induce breakdown of triglycerides, releasing fatty acids into the blood. B. Stimulates gluconeogenesis. C. Reduces the ability of insulin to stimulate glucose uptake by adipose and muscle cells, resulting in higher blood glucose concentrations.

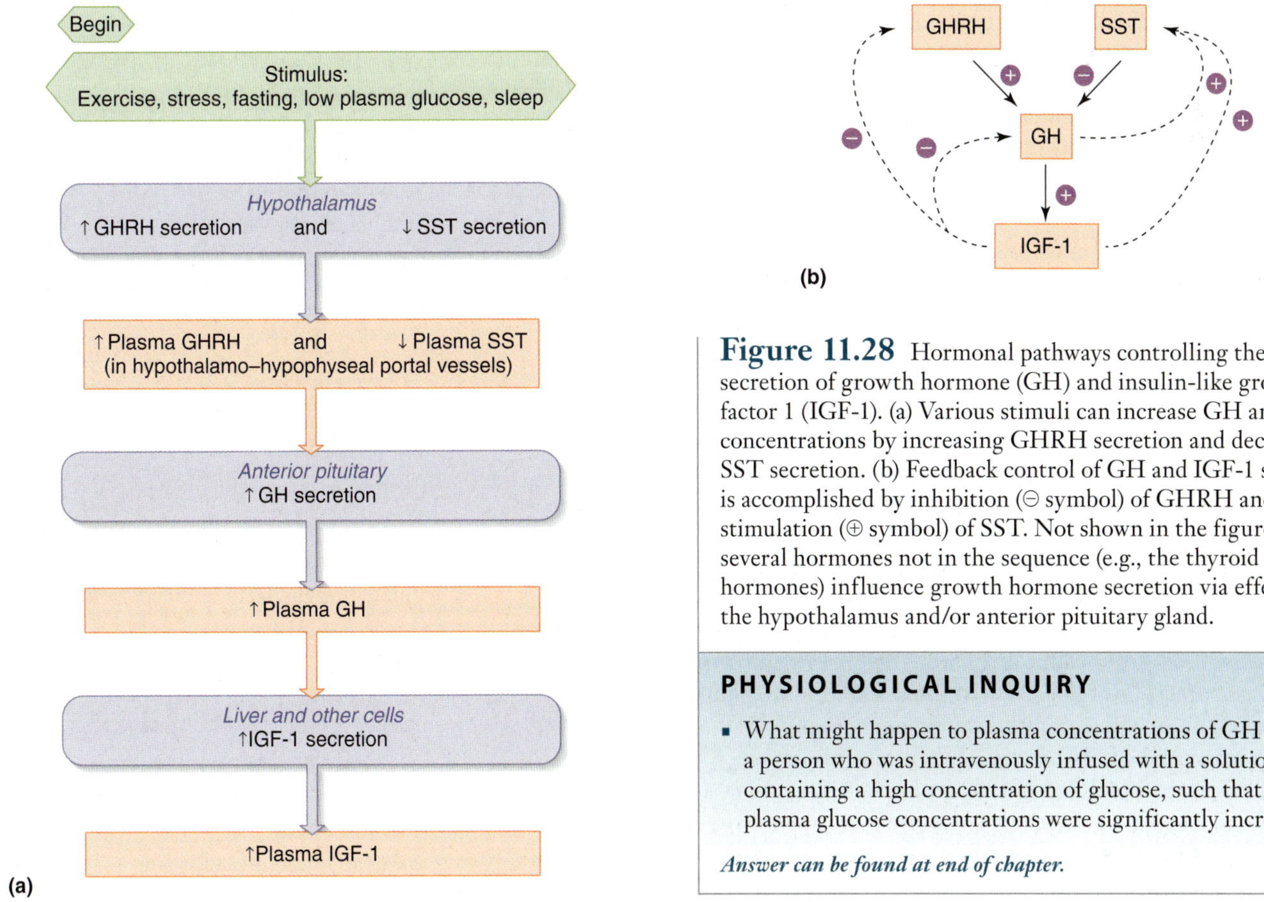

Figure 11.28 Hormonal pathways controlling the secretion of growth hormone (GH) and insulin-like growth factor 1 (IGF-1). (a) Various stimuli can increase GH and IGF-1 concentrations by increasing GHRH secretion and decreasing SST secretion. (b) Feedback control of GH and IGF-1 secretion is accomplished by inhibition (⊖ symbol) of GHRH and GH, and stimulation (⊕ symbol) of SST. Not shown in the figure is that several hormones not in the sequence (e.g., the thyroid hormones) influence growth hormone secretion via effects on the hypothalamus and/or anterior pituitary gland.

PHYSIOLOGICAL INQUIRY

- What might happen to plasma concentrations of GH in a person who was intravenously infused with a solution containing a high concentration of glucose, such that his plasma glucose concentrations were significantly increased?

Answer can be found at end of chapter.

hormone concentrations are dramatically illustrated in the disease called acromegaly (described later in this chapter).

As noted earlier, the role of GH in fetal growth, while still under investigation, appears not to be nearly as significant as at later stages of postnatal life. IGF-1, however, is required for normal fetal total-body growth and, specifically, for normal maturation of the fetal nervous system. The chief stimulus for IGF-1 secretion during prenatal life appears to be placental lactogen, a hormone released by cells of the placenta, which shares sequence similarity with growth hormone.

Finally, it should be noted that there is another messenger—**insulin-like growth factor 2 (IGF-2)**, which is closely related to IGF-1. IGF-2, the secretion of which is *independent* of growth hormone, is also a crucial mitogen during the prenatal period. It continues to be secreted throughout life, but its postnatal function is not definitively known. Recent evidence suggests a link between IGF-2 concentrations and the maintenance of skeletal muscle mass and strength in elderly persons.

Thyroid Hormone

Thyroid hormone is essential for normal growth because it is required for the synthesis of growth hormone. T_3 also has direct actions on bone, where it stimulates chondrocyte differentiation, growth of new blood vessels in developing bone, and responsiveness of bone cells to other growth factors such as fibroblast growth factor. Consequently, infants and children with hypothyroidism have slower growth rates than would be predicted.

Insulin

The major actions of insulin are described in Chapter 16. Insulin is an anabolic hormone that promotes the transport of glucose and amino acids from the extracellular fluid into adipose tissue and skeletal and cardiac muscle cells. Insulin stimulates storage of fat and inhibits protein degradation. Thus, it is not surprising that adequate amounts of insulin are necessary for normal growth. Its inhibitory effect on protein degradation is particularly important with regard to growth. In addition to this general anabolic effect, however, insulin exerts direct growth-promoting effects on cell differentiation and cell division during fetal life and, possibly, during childhood.

Sex Steroids

As Chapter 17 will explain, sex steroid secretion (testosterone in the male and estrogens in the female) begins to increase between the ages of 8 and 10 and reaches a plateau over the next 5 to 10 years. A normal pubertal growth spurt, which reflects growth of the long bones and vertebrae, requires this increased production of the sex steroids. The major growth-promoting effect of the sex steroids is to stimulate the secretion of growth hormone and IGF-1.

Unlike growth hormone, however, the sex steroids not only *stimulate* bone growth but ultimately *stop* it by inducing epiphyseal closure. The dual effects of the sex steroids explain the pattern seen in adolescence—rapid lengthening of the bones culminating in complete cessation of growth for life.

In addition to these dual effects on bone, testosterone—but not estrogen—exerts a direct anabolic effect on protein synthesis in many nonreproductive organs and tissues of the body. This accounts, at least in part, for the increased muscle mass of men in comparison to women. This effect of testosterone is also why athletes sometimes use androgens called ***anabolic steroids*** in an attempt to increase muscle mass and strength. These steroids include testosterone, synthetic androgens, and the hormones dehydroepiandrosterone (DHEA) and androstenedione. However, these steroids have multiple potential toxic side effects, such as liver damage, increased risk of prostate cancer, and infertility. Moreover, in females, they can produce virilization.

Cortisol

Cortisol, the major hormone the adrenal cortex secretes in response to stress, can have potent *antigrowth* effects under certain conditions. When present in high concentrations, it inhibits DNA synthesis and stimulates protein catabolism in many organs, and it inhibits bone growth. Moreover, it breaks down bone and inhibits the secretion of growth hormone. For all these reasons, in children, the increase in plasma cortisol that accompanies infections and other stressors is, at least in part, responsible for the decreased growth that occurs with chronic illness. One of the hallmarks of Cushing's syndrome in children is a dramatic decrease in the rate of linear growth. Furthermore, the administration of pharmacological glucocorticoid therapy for asthma or other disorders may decrease linear growth in children in a dose-related way.

This completes our survey of the major hormones that affect growth. Table 11.6 summarizes their actions.

TABLE 11.6 Major Hormones Influencing Growth

Hormone	Principal Actions
Growth hormone	Major stimulus of postnatal growth: Induces precursor cells to differentiate and secrete insulin-like growth factor 1 (IGF-1), which stimulates cell division Stimulates liver to secrete IGF-1 Stimulates protein synthesis
Insulin	Stimulates fetal growth Stimulates postnatal growth by stimulating secretion of IGF-1 Stimulates protein synthesis
Thyroid hormone	Permissive for growth hormone's secretion and actions Permissive for development of the central nervous system
Testosterone	Stimulates growth at puberty, in large part by stimulating the secretion of growth hormone Causes eventual epiphyseal closure Stimulates protein synthesis in male
Estrogen	Stimulates the secretion of growth hormone at puberty Causes eventual epiphyseal closure
Cortisol	Inhibits growth Stimulates protein catabolism

SECTION E SUMMARY

Bone Growth

I. A bone lengthens as osteoblasts at the shaft edge of the epiphyseal growth plates convert cartilage to bone while new cartilage is simultaneously being laid down in the plates.

II. Growth ceases when the plates are completely converted to bone.

Environmental Factors Influencing Growth

I. The major environmental factors influencing growth are nutrition and disease.

II. Maternal malnutrition during pregnancy may produce irreversible growth stunting and mental deficiency in offspring.

Hormonal Influences on Growth

I. Growth hormone is the major stimulus of postnatal growth.
   a. It stimulates the release of IGF-1 from the liver and many other cells, and IGF-1 then acts locally (and perhaps also as a hormone) to stimulate cell division.
   b. Growth hormone also acts directly on cells to stimulate protein synthesis.
   c. Growth hormone secretion is highest during adolescence.

II. Because thyroid hormone is required for growth hormone synthesis and the growth-promoting effects of this hormone, it is essential for normal growth during childhood and adolescence. It is also permissive for brain development during infancy.

III. Insulin stimulates growth mainly during fetal life.

IV. Mainly by stimulating growth hormone secretion, testosterone and estrogen promote bone growth during adolescence, but these hormones also cause epiphyseal closure. Testosterone also stimulates protein synthesis.

V. High concentrations of cortisol inhibit growth and stimulate protein catabolism.

SECTION E REVIEW QUESTIONS

1. Describe the process by which bone lengthens.
2. What are the effects of malnutrition on growth?
3. List the major hormones that control growth.
4. Describe the relationship between growth hormone and IGF-1 and the roles of each in growth.
5. What are the effects of growth hormone on protein synthesis?
6. What is the status of growth hormone secretion at different stages of life?
7. State the effects of the thyroid hormones on growth.
8. Describe the effects of testosterone on growth, cessation of growth, and protein synthesis. Which of these effects does estrogen also exert?
9. What is the effect of cortisol on growth?
10. Give two ways in which short stature can occur.

SECTION E KEY TERMS

SECTION E CLINICAL TERMS

SECTION F

Endocrine Control of Ca^{2+} Homeostasis

Many of the hormones of the body control functions that, though important, are not necessarily vital for survival, such as growth. By contrast, some hormones control functions so vital that the absence of the hormone would be catastrophic, even life threatening. One such function is calcium homeostasis. Calcium exists in the body fluids in its soluble, ionized form (Ca^{2+}) and bound to proteins. For simplicity in this chapter, we will refer hereafter to the physiologically active, ionic form of Ca^{2+}.

Extracellular Ca^{2+} concentration normally remains within a narrow homeostatic range. Large deviations in either direction can disrupt neurological and muscular activity, among others. For example, a low plasma Ca^{2+} concentration increases the excitability of neuronal and muscle plasma membranes. A high plasma Ca^{2+} concentration causes cardiac arrhythmias and depresses neuromuscular excitability via effects on membrane potential. In this section, we discuss the mechanisms by which Ca^{2+} homeostasis is achieved and maintained by actions of hormones.

11.20 Effector Sites for Ca^{2+} Homeostasis

Ca^{2+} homeostasis depends on the interplay among bone, the kidneys, and the gastrointestinal tract. The activities of the gastrointestinal tract and kidneys determine the net intake and output of Ca^{2+} for the entire body and, thereby, the overall Ca^{2+} balance. In contrast, interchanges of Ca^{2+} between extracellular fluid and bone do not alter total-body balance but instead change the *distribution* of Ca^{2+} within the body. We begin, therefore, with a discussion of the cellular and mineral composition of bone.

Bone

Approximately 99% of total-body calcium is contained in bone. Therefore, the movement of Ca^{2+} into and out of bone is critical in controlling the plasma Ca^{2+} concentration.

Bone is a connective tissue made up of several cell types surrounded by a collagen matrix called **osteoid,** upon which

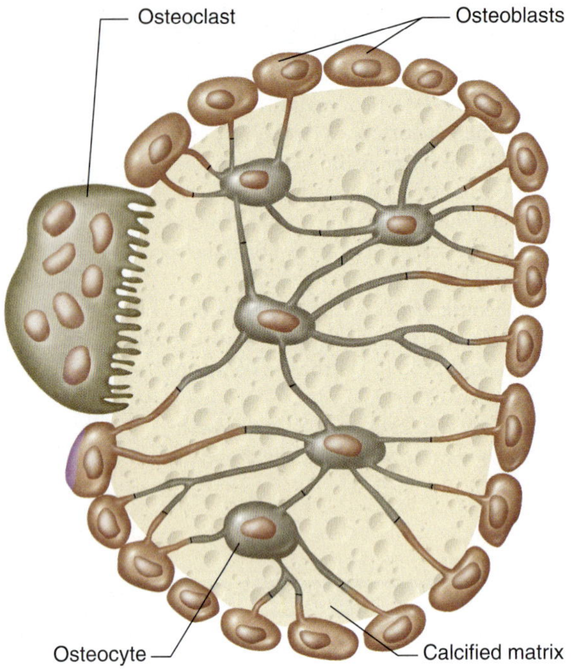

Figure 11.29 APR Cross section through a small portion of bone. The light tan area is mineralized osteoid. The osteocytes have long processes that extend through small canals and connect with each other and to osteoblasts via tight junctions. Adapted from Goodman.

are deposited minerals, particularly the crystals of calcium, phosphate, and hydroxyl ions known as **hydroxyapatite.** In some instances, bones have central marrow cavities where blood cells form. Approximately one-third of a bone, by weight, is osteoid, and two-thirds is mineral (the bone cells contribute negligible weight).

The three types of bone cells involved in bone formation and breakdown are osteoblasts, osteocytes, and osteoclasts (**Figure 11.29**). As described in Section E, osteoblasts are the bone-forming cells. They secrete collagen to form a surrounding matrix, which then becomes calcified, a process called **mineralization.** Once surrounded by calcified matrix, the osteoblasts are called **osteocytes.** The osteocytes have long cytoplasmic processes that extend throughout the bone and form tight junctions with other osteocytes. **Osteoclasts** are large, multinucleated cells that break down (resorb) previously formed bone by secreting hydrogen ions, which dissolve the crystals, and hydrolytic enzymes, which digest the osteoid.

Throughout life, bone is constantly remodeled by the osteoblasts (and osteocytes) and osteoclasts working together. Osteoclasts resorb old bone, and then osteoblasts move into the area and lay down new matrix, which becomes mineralized. This process depends in part on the stresses that gravity and muscle tension impose on the bones, stimulating osteoblastic activity. Many hormones, as summarized in **Table 11.7,** and a variety of autocrine or paracrine growth factors produced locally in the bone also play a role. Of the hormones listed, only parathyroid hormone (described later) is controlled primarily by the plasma Ca^{2+} concentration. Nonetheless, changes in the other listed hormones have important influences on bone mass and plasma Ca^{2+} concentration.

TABLE 11.7 Summary of Major Hormonal Influences on Bone Mass

Hormones That Favor Bone Formation and Increased Bone Mass
Insulin
Growth hormone
Insulin-like growth factor 1 (IGF-1)
Estrogen
Testosterone
Calcitonin
Hormones That Favor Increased Bone Resorption and Decreased Bone Mass
Parathyroid hormone (chronic elevations)
Cortisol
Thyroid hormone T_3

Kidneys

As you will learn in Chapter 14, the kidneys filter the blood and eliminate soluble wastes. In the process, cells in the tubules that make up the functional units of the kidneys recapture (reabsorb) most of the necessary solutes that were filtered, which minimizes their loss in the urine. Therefore, the urinary excretion of Ca^{2+} is the difference between the amount filtered into the tubules and the amount reabsorbed and returned to the blood. The control of Ca^{2+} excretion is exerted mainly on reabsorption. Reabsorption decreases when plasma Ca^{2+} concentration increases, and it increases when plasma Ca^{2+} decreases.

The hormonal controllers of Ca^{2+} also regulate phosphate ion balance. Phosphate ions, too, are subject to a combination of filtration and reabsorption, with the latter hormonally controlled.

Gastrointestinal Tract

The absorption of such solutes as Na^+ and K^+ from the gastrointestinal tract into the blood is normally about 100%. In contrast, a considerable amount of ingested Ca^{2+} is not absorbed from the small intestine and leaves the body along with the feces. Moreover, the active transport system that achieves Ca^{2+} absorption from the small intestine is under hormonal control. Thus, large regulated increases or decreases can occur in the amount of Ca^{2+} absorbed from the diet. Hormonal control of this absorptive process is the major means for regulating total-body-calcium balance, as we see next.

11.21 Hormonal Controls

The two major hormones that regulate plasma Ca^{2+} concentration are parathyroid hormone and 1,25-dihydroxyvitamin D. A third hormone, calcitonin, plays a limited role in humans, if any.

Parathyroid Hormone

Bone, kidneys, and the gastrointestinal tract are subject, directly or indirectly, to control by a protein hormone called **parathyroid hormone (PTH),** which is produced

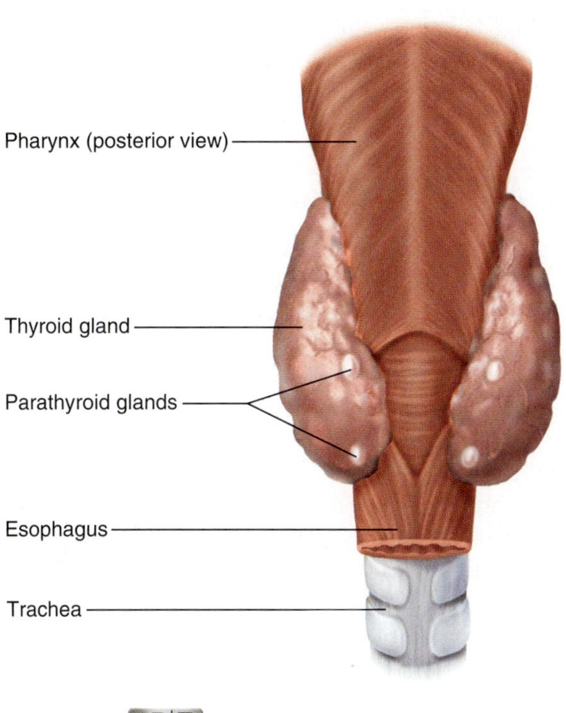

Figure 11.30 AP|R The parathyroid glands. There are usually four parathyroid glands embedded in the posterior surface of the thyroid gland.

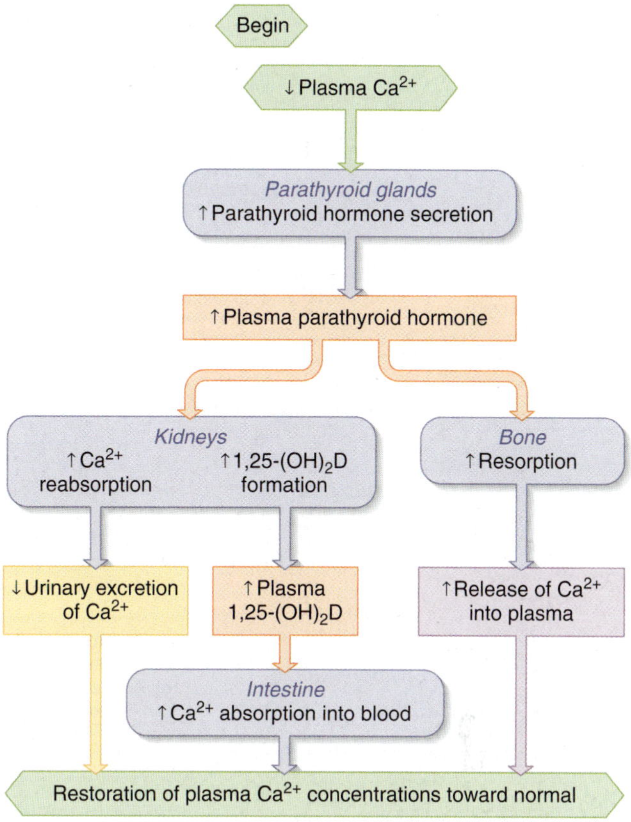

Figure 11.31 Mechanisms that allow parathyroid hormone to reverse a reduction in plasma Ca^{2+} concentration toward normal. See Figure 11.32 for a more complete description of 1,25-$(OH)_2$D (1,25-dihydroxyvitamin D). Parathyroid hormone and 1,25- $(OH)_2$D are also involved in the control of phosphate ion concentrations.

by the **parathyroid glands.** These endocrine glands are in the neck, embedded in the posterior surface of the thyroid gland, but are distinct from it (**Figure 11.30**). Parathyroid hormone production is controlled by the extracellular Ca^{2+} concentration acting directly on the secretory cells via a plasma membrane Ca^{2+} receptor. *Decreased* plasma Ca^{2+} concentration *stimulates* parathyroid hormone secretion, and an *increased* plasma Ca^{2+} concentration does just the opposite.

Parathyroid hormone exerts multiple actions that increase extracellular Ca^{2+} concentration, thereby compensating for the decreased concentration that originally stimulated secretion of this hormone (**Figure 11.31**):

1. It directly increases the resorption of bone by osteoclasts, which causes calcium (and phosphate) ions to move from bone into extracellular fluid.
2. It directly stimulates the formation of 1,25-dihydroxyvitamin D, which then increases intestinal absorption of calcium (and phosphate) ions. Thus, the effect of parathyroid hormone on the intestines is indirect.
3. It directly increases Ca^{2+} reabsorption in the kidneys, thereby decreasing urinary Ca^{2+} excretion.
4. It directly *decreases* the reabsorption of phosphate ions in the kidneys, thereby increasing its excretion in the urine. This keeps plasma phosphate ions from increasing when parathyroid hormone causes an increased release of both calcium and phosphate ions from bone, and an increased production of 1,25-dihydroxyvitamin D leading to calcium and phosphate ion absorption in the intestine.

1,25-Dihydroxyvitamin D

The term **vitamin D** denotes a group of closely related compounds. **Vitamin D_3 (cholecalciferol)** is formed by the action of ultraviolet radiation from sunlight on a cholesterol derivative (7-dehydrocholesterol) in skin. **Vitamin D_2 (ergocalciferol)** is derived from plants. Both can be found in vitamin pills and enriched foods and are collectively called vitamin D.

Because of clothing, climate, and other factors, people are often dependent upon dietary vitamin D. For this reason, it was originally classified as a vitamin. Regardless of source, vitamin D is metabolized by the addition of hydroxyl groups, first in the liver by the enzyme 25-hydroxylase and then in certain kidney cells by 1-hydroxylase (**Figure 11.32**). The end result of these changes is 1,25-dihydroxyvitamin D (abbreviated **1,25-$(OH)_2$D**), the active hormonal form of vitamin D.

The major action of 1,25-$(OH)_2$D is to stimulate the intestinal absorption of Ca^{2+}. Thus, the major consequence of vitamin D deficiency is decreased intestinal Ca^{2+} absorption, resulting in decreased plasma Ca^{2+}.

The blood concentration of 1,25-$(OH)_2$D is subject to physiological control. The major control point is the second hydroxylation step that occurs primarily in the kidneys by the action of 1-hydroxylase, and which is stimulated by parathyroid hormone. Because a low plasma Ca^{2+} concentration stimulates the secretion of parathyroid hormone, the production of

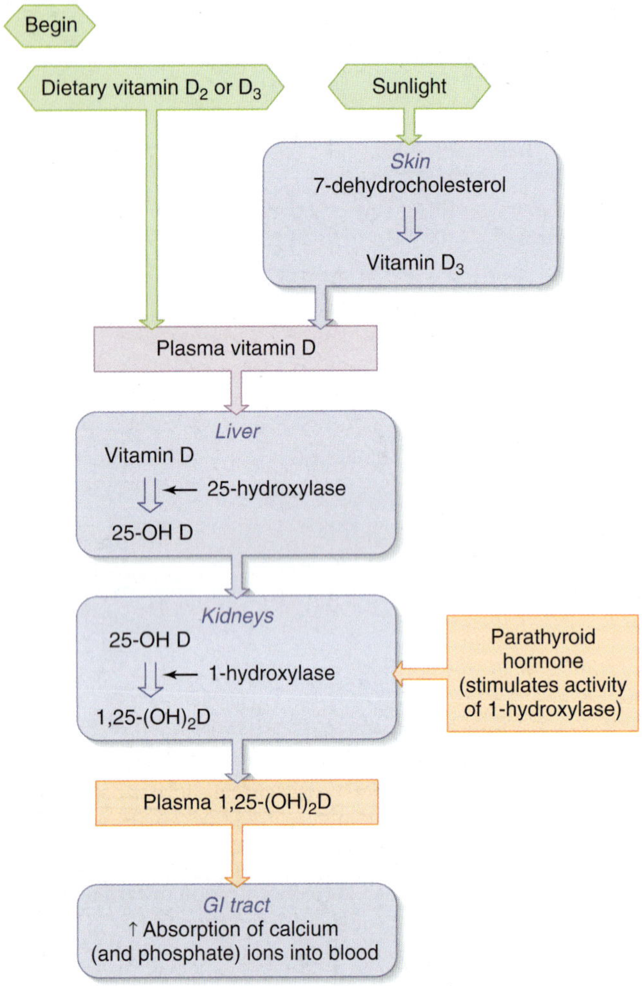

Figure 11.32 Metabolism of vitamin D to the active form, 1,25-$(OH)_2$D.

PHYSIOLOGICAL INQUIRY

- Sarcoidosis is a disease that affects a variety of organs (usually the lungs). It is characterized by the development of nodules of inflamed tissue known as granulomas. These granulomas can express significant 1-hydroxylase activity that is not controlled by parathyroid hormone. What will happen to plasma Ca^{2+} and parathyroid hormone concentrations under these circumstances?

Answer can be found at end of chapter.

1,25-$(OH)_2$D is increased as well under such conditions. Both hormones work together to restore plasma Ca^{2+} to normal.

Calcitonin

Calcitonin is a peptide hormone secreted by cells called parafollicular cells that are within the thyroid gland but are distinct from the thyroid follicles. Calcitonin decreases plasma Ca^{2+} concentration, mainly by inhibiting osteoclasts, thereby reducing bone resorption. Its secretion is stimulated by an increased plasma Ca^{2+} concentration, just the opposite of the stimulus for parathyroid hormone secretion. Unlike parathyroid hormone and 1,25-$(OH)_2$D, however, calcitonin appears to play no role in the normal day-to-day regulation of plasma Ca^{2+} in humans. It may be a factor in decreasing bone resorption when the plasma Ca^{2+} concentration is very high.

11.22 Metabolic Bone Diseases

Various diseases reflect abnormalities in the metabolism of bone. ***Rickets*** (in children) and ***osteomalacia*** (in adults) are conditions in which mineralization of bone matrix is deficient, causing the bones to be soft and easily fractured. In addition, a child suffering from rickets is typically severely bowlegged due to weight bearing on the weakened developing leg bones. A major cause of rickets and osteomalacia is deficiency of vitamin D.

In contrast to these diseases, in ***osteoporosis,*** both matrix and minerals are lost as a result of an imbalance between bone resorption and bone formation. The resulting decrease in bone mass and strength leads to an increased incidence of fractures. Osteoporosis can occur in people who are immobilized ("disuse osteoporosis"), in people who have an *excessive* plasma concentration of a hormone that favors bone resorption, and in people who have a *deficient* plasma concentration of a hormone that favors bone formation (see Table 11.7). It is most commonly seen, however, with aging. Everyone loses bone as he or she ages, but osteoporosis is more common in elderly women than in men for several reasons. Women have a smaller bone mass to begin with, and the loss that occurs with aging occurs more rapidly, particularly after menopause removes the bone-promoting influence of estrogen.

Prevention is the focus of attention for osteoporosis. Treatment of postmenopausal women with estrogen or its synthetic analogs is very effective in reducing the rate of bone loss, but long-term estrogen replacement can have serious consequences in some women (e.g., increasing the likelihood of breast cancer). A regular weight-bearing exercise program, such as brisk walking and stair climbing, is also helpful. Adequate dietary Ca^{2+} and vitamin D intake throughout life are important to build up and maintain bone mass. Several substances also provide effective therapy once osteoporosis is established. Most prominent is a group of drugs called ***bisphosphonates*** that interfere with the resorption of bone by osteoclasts. Other antiresorptive substances include calcitonin and ***selective estrogen receptor modulators*** (***SERMs***), which, as their name implies, act by interacting with (and activating) estrogen receptors, thereby compensating for the low estrogen after menopause.

A variety of pathophysiological disorders lead to abnormally high or low plasma Ca^{2+} concentrations—*hypercalcemia* or *hypocalcemia*, respectively— as described next.

Hypercalcemia

A relatively common cause of **hypercalcemia** is ***primary hyperparathyroidism.*** This is usually caused by a benign tumor (known as an adenoma) of one of the four parathyroid glands. These tumors are composed of abnormal cells that are not adequately suppressed by extracellular Ca^{2+}. As a result, the adenoma secretes parathyroid hormone in excess, leading to an increase in Ca^{2+} resorption from bone, increased kidney reabsorption of Ca^{2+}, and the increased production of 1,25-$(OH)_2$D from the kidney. This results in an increase in Ca^{2+} absorption from the small intestine. Primary hyperparathyroidism is most effectively treated by surgical removal of the parathyroid tumor.

Certain types of cancer can lead to ***humoral hypercalcemia of malignancy.*** The cause of the hypercalcemia is often the release of a molecule that is structurally similar to PTH, called ***PTH-related peptide*** (***PTHrp***), that has effects similar to those of PTH. This peptide is produced by certain types of cancerous cells (e.g., some breast-cancer cells). However, authentic PTH release from the normal parathyroid glands is decreased due to the hypercalcemia caused by PTHrp released from the cancer cells. The most effective treatment of humoral hypercalcemia of malignancy is to treat the cancer that is releasing PTHrp. In addition, drugs such as bisphosphonates that decrease bone resorption can also provide effective treatment.

Finally, excessive ingestion of vitamin D can lead to hypercalcemia, as may happen in some individuals who consume vitamin D supplements far in excess of what is required.

Regardless of the cause, hypercalcemia causes significant symptoms primarily from its effects on excitable tissues. Among these symptoms are tiredness and lethargy with muscle weakness, as well as nausea and vomiting (due to effects on the GI tract).

Hypocalcemia

Hypocalcemia can result from a loss of parathyroid gland function (***primary hypoparathyroidism***). One cause of this is the removal of parathyroid glands, which may occur (though rarely) when a person with thyroid disease has his or her thyroid gland surgically removed. Because the concentration of PTH is low, 1,25-$(OH)_2$D production from the kidney is also decreased. Decreases in both hormones lead to decreases in bone resorption, kidney Ca^{2+} reabsorption, and intestinal Ca^{2+} absorption.

Resistance to the effects of PTH in target tissue (hyporesponsiveness) can also lead to the symptoms of hypoparathyroidism, even though in such cases PTH concentrations in the blood tend to be elevated. This condition is called ***pseudohypoparathyroidism*** (see Chapter 5 Clinical Case Study).

Another interesting hypocalcemic state is ***secondary hyperparathyroidism.*** Failure to absorb vitamin D from the gastrointestinal tract, or decreased kidney 1,25-$(OH)_2$D production, which can occur in kidney disease, can lead to secondary hyperparathyroidism. The decreased plasma Ca^{2+} that results from decreased intestinal absorption of Ca^{2+} results in stimulation of the parathyroid glands. Although the increased concentration of parathyroid hormone does act to restore plasma Ca^{2+} toward normal, it does so at the expense of significant loss of Ca^{2+} from bone and the acceleration of metabolic bone disease.

The symptoms of hypocalcemia are also due to its effects on excitable tissue. It increases the excitability of nerves and muscles, which can lead to CNS effects (seizures), muscle spasms (***hypocalcemic tetany***), and neuronal excitability. Long-term treatment of hypoparathyroidism involves giving calcium salts and 1,25-$(OH)_2$D or vitamin D.

SECTION F SUMMARY

Effector Sites for Ca^{2+} Homeostasis

I. The effector sites for the regulation of plasma Ca^{2+} concentration are bone, the gastrointestinal tract, and the kidneys.
II. Approximately 99% of total-body Ca^{2+} is contained in bone as minerals on a collagen matrix. Bone is constantly remodeled as a result of the interaction of osteoblasts and osteoclasts, a process that determines bone mass and provides a means for raising or lowering plasma Ca^{2+} concentration.
III. Ca^{2+} is actively absorbed by the gastrointestinal tract, and this process is under hormonal control.
IV. The amount of Ca^{2+} excreted in the urine is the difference between the amount filtered and the amount reabsorbed, the latter process being under hormonal control.

Hormonal Controls

I. Parathyroid hormone (PTH) increases plasma Ca^{2+} concentration by influencing all of the effector sites.
   a. It stimulates kidney reabsorption of Ca^{2+}, bone resorption with release of Ca^{2+} into the blood, and formation of the hormone 1,25-dihydroxyvitamin D, which stimulates Ca^{2+} absorption by the intestine.
   b. It also inhibits the reabsorption of phosphate ions in the kidneys, leading to increased excretion of phosphate ions in the urine.
II. Vitamin D is formed in the skin or ingested and then undergoes hydroxylations in the liver and kidneys. The kidneys express the enzyme that catalyzes the production of the active form, 1,25-dihydroxyvitamin D. This process is greatly stimulated by parathyroid hormone.

Metabolic Bone Diseases

I. Osteomalacia (adults) and rickets (children) are diseases in which the mineralization of bone is deficient—usually due to inadequate vitamin D intake, absorption, or activation.
II. Osteoporosis is a loss of bone density (loss of matrix and minerals).
   a. Bone resorption exceeds formation.
   b. It is most common in postmenopausal (estrogen-deficient) women.
   c. It can be prevented by exercise, adequate Ca^{2+} and vitamin D intake, and medications (such as bisphosphonates).
III. Hypercalcemia (chronically elevated plasma Ca^{2+} concentrations) can occur from several causes.
   a. Primary hyperparathyroidism is usually caused by a benign adenoma, which produces too much PTH. Increased PTH causes hypercalcemia by increasing bone resorption of Ca^{2+}, increasing kidney reabsorption of Ca^{2+}, and increasing kidney production of 1,25-$(OH)_2$D, which increases Ca^{2+} absorption in the intestines.
   b. Humoral hypercalcemia of malignancy is often due to the production of PTH-related peptide (PTHrp) from cancer cells. PTHrp acts like PTH.
   c. Excessive vitamin D intake may also result in hypercalcemia.

IV. Hypocalcemia (chronically decreased plasma Ca^{2+} concentrations) can also be traced to several causes.
   a. Low PTH concentrations from primary hypoparathyroidism (loss of parathyroid function) lead to hypocalcemia by decreasing bone resorption of Ca^{2+}, decreasing urinary reabsorption of Ca^{2+}, and decreasing renal production of 1,25-$(OH)_2$D.
   b. Pseudohypoparathyroidism is caused by target-organ resistance to the action of PTH.
   c. Secondary hyperparathyroidism is caused by vitamin D deficiency due to inadequate intake, absorption, or activation in the kidney (e.g., in kidney disease).

SECTION F REVIEW QUESTIONS

1. Describe bone remodeling.
2. Describe the handling of Ca^{2+} by the kidneys and gastrointestinal tract.
3. What controls the secretion of parathyroid hormone, and what are the major effects of this hormone?
4. Describe the formation and action of 1,25-$(OH)_2$D. How does parathyroid hormone influence the production of this hormone?

SECTION F KEY TERMS

calcitonin 356
1,25-$(OH)_2$D 355
hydroxyapatite 354
hypercalcemia 356
hypocalcemia 357
mineralization 354
osteoclast 354
osteocyte 354
osteoid 353
parathyroid gland 355
parathyroid hormone (PTH) 354
vitamin D 355
vitamin D_2 (ergocalciferol) 355
vitamin D_3 (cholecalciferol) 355

SECTION F CLINICAL TERMS

bisphosphonate 356
humoral hypercalcemia of malignancy 357
hypocalcemic tetany 357
osteomalacia 356
osteoporosis 356
primary hyperparathyroidism 356
primary hypoparathyroidism 357
pseudohypoparathyroidism 357
PTH-related peptide (PTHrp) 357
rickets 356
secondary hyperparathyroidism 357
selective estrogen receptor modulator (SERM) 356

CHAPTER 11

Clinical Case Study: Mouth Pain, Sleep Apnea, and Enlargement of the Hands in a 35-Year-Old Man

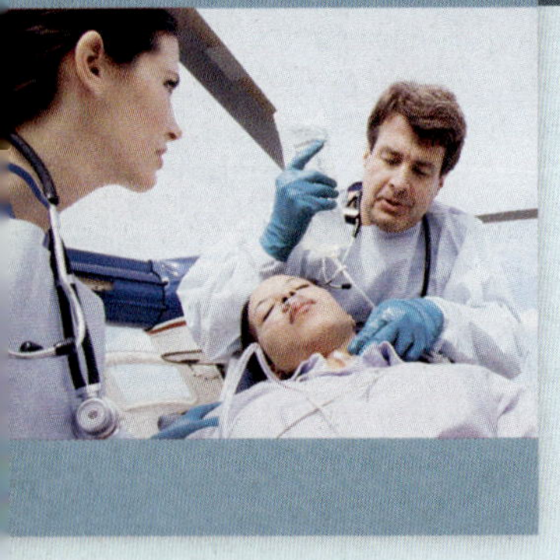

A 35-year-old man visited his dentist with a complaint of chronic mouth pain and headaches. After examining the patient, the dentist concluded that there was no dental disease but that the patient's jaw appeared enlarged and his tongue was thickened and large. The dentist referred the patient to a physician. The physician noted enlargement of the jaw and tongue, enlargement of the fingers and toes, and a very deep voice. The patient acknowledged that his voice seemed to have deepened over the past few years and that he no longer wore his wedding ring because it was too tight. The patient's height and weight were within normal ranges. His blood pressure was significantly elevated, as was his fasting plasma glucose concentration. The patient also mentioned that his wife could no longer sleep in the same room as he because of his loud snoring and sleep apnea. Based on these signs and symptoms, the physician referred the patient to an endocrinologist, who ordered a series of tests to better elucidate the cause of the diverse symptoms.

The enlarged bones and facial features suggested the possibility of ***acromegaly*** (from the Greek *akros,* "extreme" or "extremities," and *megalos,* "large"), a disease characterized by excess growth hormone and IGF-1 concentrations in the blood. This was confirmed with a blood test that revealed greatly elevated concentrations of both hormones. Based on these results, an MRI scan was ordered to look for a possible tumor of the anterior pituitary gland. A 1.5 cm mass was discovered in the sella turcica, consistent with the possibility of a growth hormone–secreting tumor. Because the patient was of normal height, it was concluded that the tumor arose at some point after puberty, when linear growth ceased because of closure of the epiphyseal plates. Had the tumor developed prior to puberty, the man would have been well above normal height because of the growth-promoting actions of growth hormone and IGF-1. Such individuals are known as pituitary giants and have a condition called ***gigantism.*** In many cases, the affected person develops both gigantism and later acromegaly, as occurred in the individual shown in **Figure 11.33**.

Acromegaly and gigantism arise when chronic, excess amounts of growth hormone are secreted into the blood. In almost all cases, acromegaly and gigantism are caused by benign (noncancerous) tumors of the anterior pituitary gland that secrete growth hormone at very high rates, which in turn results in elevated IGF-1 concentrations in the blood. Because these tumors are abnormal tissue, they are not suppressed adequately by normal negative feedback inhibitors like IGF-1, so the growth hormone concentrations remain elevated. These tumors are typically very slow growing, and, if they arise after puberty, it may be many years before a person realizes that there is something wrong. In our patient, the changes in his appearance were gradual enough that he attributed them simply to "aging," despite his relative youth.

Even when linear growth is no longer possible (after the growth plates have fused), very high plasma concentrations of

(continued)

(continued)

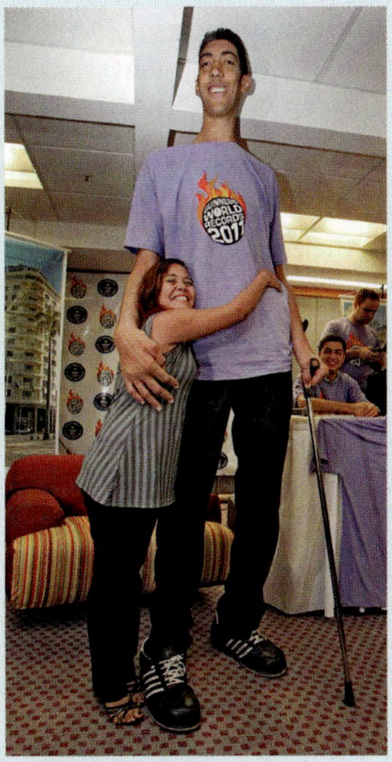

Figure 11.33 Appearance of an individual with gigantism and acromegaly.

growth hormone and IGF-1 result in the thickening of many bones in the body, most noticeably in the hands, feet, and head. The jaw, particularly, enlarges to give the characteristic facial appearance called ***prognathism*** (from the Greek *pro,* "forward," and *gnathos,* "jaw") that is associated with acromegaly. This was likely the cause of our patient's chronic mouth pain. The enlarged sinuses that resulted from the thickening of his skull bones may have been responsible in part for his headaches. In addition, many internal organs—such as the heart—also become enlarged due to growth hormone and IGF-1-induced hypertrophy, and this can interfere with their ability to function normally. In some acromegalics, the tissues comprising the larynx enlarge, resulting in a deepening of the voice as in our subject. The enlarged and deformed tongue was likely a contributor to the sleep apnea and snoring reported by the patient; this is called obstructive sleep apnea because the tongue base weakens and, consequently, the tongue obstructs the upper airway (see Chapter 13 for a discussion of sleep apnea). Finally, roughly half of all people with acromegaly have elevated blood pressure (hypertension). The cause of the hypertension is uncertain, but it is a serious medical condition that requires treatment with antihypertensive drugs.

As described earlier, adults continue to make and secrete growth hormone even after growth ceases. That is because growth hormone has metabolic actions in addition to its effects on growth. The major actions of growth hormone in metabolism are to increase the concentrations of glucose and fatty acids in the blood and decrease the sensitivity of skeletal muscle and adipose tissue to insulin. Not surprisingly, therefore, one of the stimuli that increases growth hormone concentrations in the healthy adult is a decrease in blood glucose or fatty acids. The secretion of growth hormone during these metabolic crises, however, is transient; once glucose or fatty acid concentrations are restored to normal, growth hormone concentrations decrease to baseline. In acromegaly, however, growth hormone concentrations are almost always increased. Consequently, acromegaly is often associated with increased plasma concentrations of glucose and fatty acids, in some cases even reaching the concentrations observed in diabetes mellitus. As in Cushing's syndrome (Section D), therefore, the presence of chronically increased concentrations of growth hormone may result in diabetes-like symptoms. This explains why our patient had a high fasting plasma glucose concentration.

Our subject was fortunate to have had a quick diagnosis. This case study illustrates one of the confounding features of endocrine disorders. The rarity of some endocrine diseases (e.g., acromegaly occurs in roughly 4 per million individuals), together with the fact that the symptoms of a given endocrine disease can be varied and insidious in their onset, often results in a delayed diagnosis. This means that in many cases, a patient is subjected to numerous tests for more common disorders before a diagnosis of endocrine disease is made.

Treatment of gigantism and acromegaly usually requires surgical removal of the pituitary tumor. The residual normal pituitary tissue is then sufficient to maintain baseline growth hormone concentrations. If this treatment is impossible or not successful, treatment with long-acting analogs of somatostatin is sometimes necessary. (Recall that somatostatin is the hypothalamic hormone that inhibits GH secretion.) Our patient elected to have surgery. This resulted in a reduction in his plasma growth hormone and IGF-1 concentrations. With time, several of his symptoms were reduced, including the increased plasma glucose concentrations. However, within 2 years, his growth hormone and IGF-1 concentrations were three times higher than the normal range for his age and a follow-up MRI revealed that the tumor had regrown. Not wanting a second surgery, the patient was treated with radiation therapy focused on the pituitary tumor, followed by regular administration of somatostatin analogs. This treatment decreased but did not completely normalize his hormone concentrations. His blood pressure remained elevated and was treated with two different antihypertensive drugs (see Chapter 12).

Clinical terms: acromegaly, gigantism, prognathism

See Chapter 19 for complete, integrative case studies.

CHAPTER 11 TEST QUESTIONS

Answers found in Appendix A.

1–5: Match the hormone with the function or feature (choices a–e).

Hormone:

1. vasopressin
2. ACTH
3. oxytocin
4. prolactin
5. luteinizing hormone

Function:

a. tropic for the adrenal cortex
b. is controlled by an amine-derived hormone of the hypothalamus
c. antidiuresis
d. stimulation of testosterone production
e. stimulation of uterine contractions during labor

6. In the following figure, which hormone (A or B) binds to receptor X with higher affinity?

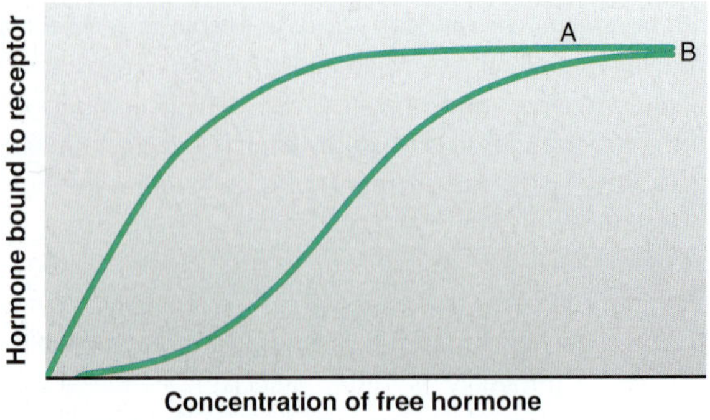

7. Which is *not* a symptom of Cushing's disease?
   a. high blood pressure
   b. bone loss
   c. suppressed immune function
   d. goiter
   e. hyperglycemia (increased blood glucose)
8. Tremors, nervousness, and increased heart rate can all be symptoms of
   a. increased activation of the sympathetic nervous system.
   b. excessive secretion of epinephrine from the adrenal medulla.
   c. hyperthyroidism.
   d. hypothyroidism.
   e. answers a, b, and c (all are correct).
9. Which of the following could theoretically result in short stature?
   a. pituitary tumor making excess thyroid-stimulating hormone
   b. mutations that result in inactive IGF-1 receptors
   c. delayed onset of puberty
   d. decreased hypothalamic concentrations of somatostatin
   e. normal plasma GH but decreased feedback of GH on GHRH
10. Choose the correct statement.
    a. During times of stress, cortisol acts as an anabolic hormone in muscle and adipose tissue.
    b. A deficiency of thyroid hormone would result in increased cellular concentrations of Na^+/K^+-ATPase pumps in target tissues.
    c. The posterior pituitary is connected to the hypothalamus by long portal vessels.
    d. Adrenal insufficiency often results in increased blood pressure and increased plasma glucose concentrations.
    e. A lack of iodide in the diet will have no significant effect on the concentration of circulating thyroid hormone for at least several weeks.
11. A lower-than-normal concentration of plasma Ca^{2+} causes
    a. a PTH-mediated increase in 25-OH D.
    b. a decrease in renal 1-hydroxylase activity.
    c. a decrease in the urinary excretion of Ca^{2+}.
    d. a decrease in bone resorption.
    e. an increase in vitamin D release from the skin.
12. Which of the following is *not* consistent with primary hyperparathyroidism?
    a. hypercalcemia
    b. elevated plasma 1,25-$(OH)_2D$
    c. increased urinary excretion of phosphate ions
    d. a decrease in Ca^{2+} resorption from bone
    e. an increase in Ca^{2+} reabsorption in the kidney

True or False

13. T_4 is the chief circulating form of thyroid hormone but is less active than T_3.
14. Acromegaly is usually associated with hypoglycemia and hypotension.
15. Thyroid hormone and cortisol are both permissive for the actions of epinephrine.

CHAPTER 11 GENERAL PRINCIPLES ASSESSMENT

Answers found in Appendix A.

1. Referring back to Tables 11.3, 11.4, and 11.5, explain how certain of the actions of epinephrine, cortisol, and growth hormone illustrate in part the general principle of physiology that *most physiological functions are controlled by multiple regulatory systems, often working in opposition.*
2. Another general principle of physiology is that *structure is a determinant of—and has coevolved with—function.* The structure of the thyroid gland is very unlike other endocrine glands. How is the structure of this gland related to its function?
3. *Homeostasis is essential for health and survival.* How do parathyroid hormone, ADH, and thyroid hormone contribute to homeostasis? What might be the consequence of having too little of each of those hormones?

CHAPTER 11 QUANTITATIVE AND THOUGHT QUESTIONS

Answers found at www.mhhe.com/widmaier13.

1. In an experimental animal, the sympathetic preganglionic fibers to the adrenal medulla are cut. What happens to the plasma concentration of epinephrine at rest and during stress?
2. During pregnancy, there is an increase in the liver's production and, consequently, the plasma concentration of the major plasma binding protein for thyroid hormone. This causes a sequence of events involving feedback that results in an increase in the plasma concentrations of T_3 but no evidence of hyperthyroidism. Describe the sequence of events.
3. A child shows the following symptoms: deficient growth, failure to show sexual development, decreased ability to respond to stress. What is the most likely cause of all these symptoms?
4. If all the neural connections between the hypothalamus and pituitary gland below the median eminence were severed, the secretion of which pituitary gland hormones would be affected? Which pituitary gland hormones would not be affected?
5. Typically, an antibody to a peptide combines with the peptide and renders it nonfunctional. If an animal were given an antibody to somatostatin, the secretion of which anterior pituitary gland hormone would change and in what direction?
6. A drug that blocks the action of norepinephrine is injected directly into the hypothalamus of an experimental animal, and the secretion rates of several anterior pituitary gland hormones are observed to change. How is this possible, given the fact that norepinephrine is not a hypophysiotropic hormone?

7. A person is receiving very large doses of a synthetic glucocorticoid to treat her arthritis. What happens to her secretion of cortisol?
8. A person with symptoms of hypothyroidism (i.e., sluggishness and intolerance to cold) is found to have abnormally low plasma concentrations of T_4, T_3, and TSH. After an injection of TRH, the plasma concentrations of all three hormones increase. Where is the site of the defect leading to the hypothyroidism?
9. A full-term newborn infant is abnormally small. Is this most likely due to deficient growth hormone, deficient thyroid hormones, or deficient nutrition during fetal life?
10. Why might the administration of androgens to stimulate growth in a short, 12-year-old male turn out to be counterproductive?

CHAPTER 11 ANSWERS TO PHYSIOLOGICAL INQUIRIES

Figure 11.3 By storing large amounts of hormone in an endocrine cell, the plasma concentration of the hormone can be increased within seconds when the cell is stimulated. Such rapid responses may be critical for an appropriate response to a challenge to homeostasis. Packaging peptides in this way also prevents intracellular degradation.

Figure 11.5 Because steroid hormones are derived from cholesterol, they are lipophilic. Consequently, they can freely diffuse through lipid bilayers, including those that constitute secretory vesicles. Therefore, once a steroid hormone is synthesized, it diffuses out of the cell.

Figure 11.9 One explanation for this patient's symptoms may be that his or her circulating concentration of thyroid hormone was elevated. This might occur if the person's thyroid was overstimulated due, for example, to thyroid disease. The increased concentration of thyroid hormone would cause an even greater potentiation of the actions of epinephrine, making it appear as if the patient had excess concentrations of epinephrine.

Figure 11.13 Because the amount of blood into which the hypophysiotropic hormones are secreted is far less than would be the case if they were secreted into the general circulation of the body, the absolute amount of hormone required to achieve a given concentration is much less. This means that the cells of the hypothalamus need only synthesize a tiny amount of hypophysiotropic hormone to reach concentrations in the portal blood vessels that are physiologically active (i.e., can activate receptors on pituitary cells). This allows for the tight control of the anterior pituitary gland by a very small number of discrete neurons within the hypothalamus.

Figure 11.21 Iodine is not widely found in foods; in the absence of iodized salt, an acute or chronic deficiency in dietary iodine is possible. The colloid permits a long-term store of iodinated thyroglobulin that can be used during times when dietary iodine intake is reduced or absent.

Figure 11.24 Plasma cortisol concentrations would increase. This would result in decreased ACTH concentrations in the systemic blood, and CRH concentrations in the portal vein blood, due to increased negative feedback at the pituitary gland and hypothalamus, respectively. The right adrenal gland would shrink in size (atrophy) as a consequence of the decreased ACTH concentrations (decreased "trophic" stimulation of the adrenal cortex).

Figure 11.28 Note from the figure that a decrease in plasma glucose concentrations results in an increase in growth hormone concentrations. This makes sense, because one of the metabolic actions of growth hormone is to increase the concentrations of glucose in the blood. By the same reasoning, an *increase* in the concentration of glucose in the blood due to any cause, including an intravenous infusion as described here, would be expected to *decrease* circulating concentrations of growth hormone.

Figure 11.32 The 1-hydroxylase activity will stimulate the conversion of 25-OH D to 1,25-$(OH)_2$D in the granulomas themselves; the 1,25-$(OH)_2$D will then diffuse out of the granuloma cells and enter the plasma, leading to increased Ca^{2+} absorption in the gastrointestinal tract. This will increase plasma Ca^{2+}, which in turn will suppress parathyroid hormone production; consequently, plasma parathyroid hormone concentrations will decrease. This is a form of secondary hypoparathyroidism.

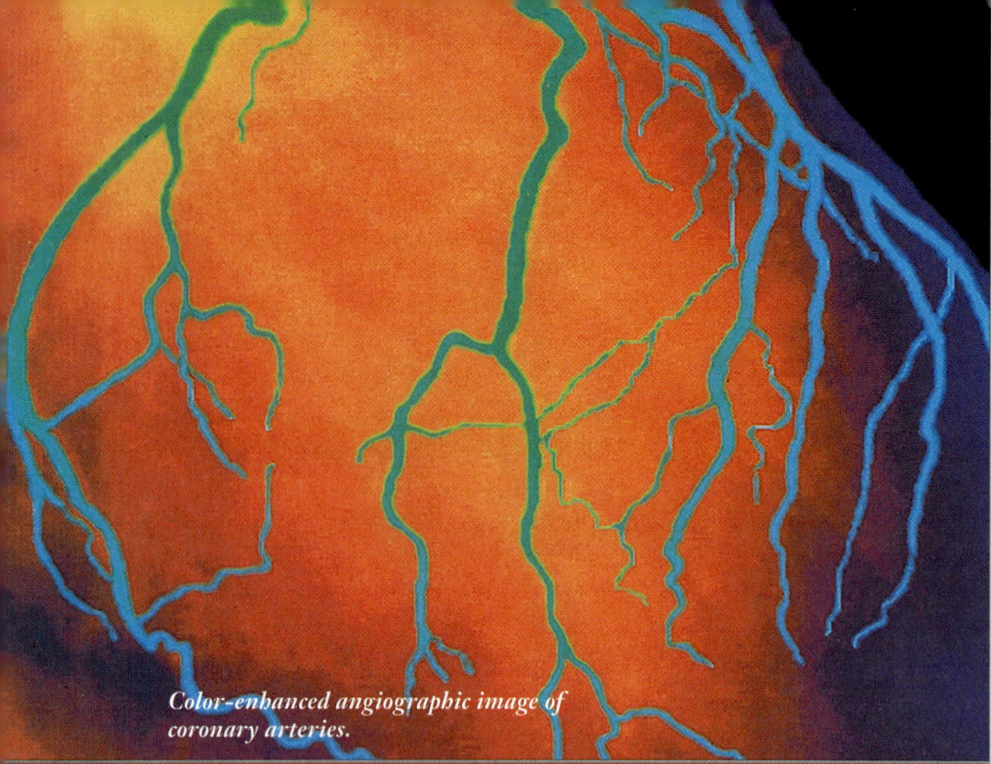

Color-enhanced angiographic image of coronary arteries.

12 Cardiovascular Physiology

Beyond a distance of a few cell diameters, the random movement of substances from a region of higher concentration to one of lower concentration (diffusion) is too slow to meet the metabolic requirements of cells. Because of this, our large, multicellular bodies require an organ system to transport molecules and other substances rapidly over the long distances between cells, tissues, and organs. This purpose is achieved by the **circulatory system** (also known as the **cardiovascular system**), which includes a pump (the **heart**); a set of interconnected tubes (**blood vessels** or **vascular system**); and a fluid connective tissue containing water, solutes, and cells that fills the tubes (the **blood**). Chapter 9 described the detailed mechanisms by which the cardiac and smooth muscle cells found in the heart and blood vessel walls, respectively, contract and generate force; in this chapter, you will learn how these contractions create pressures and move blood within the circulatory system.

The general principles of physiology described in Chapter 1 are abundantly represented in this chapter. In Section A, for example, you will learn about the relationships between blood pressure, blood flow, and resistance to blood flow, a classic illustration of the general principle of physiology that physiological processes are dictated by the laws of chemistry and physics. The general principle of physiology that structure is a determinant of—and has coevolved with—function is apparent throughout the chapter; as one example, you will learn how the structures of different types of blood vessels determine whether they participate in fluid exchange, regulate blood pressure, or provide a reservoir of blood (Section C). The general principle of physiology that most physiological functions are controlled by multiple regulatory systems, often working in opposition, is exemplified by the hormonal and neural regulation of blood vessel diameter and blood volume (Sections C and D), as well as by the opposing mechanisms that create and dissolve blood clots (Section F). Sections D and E explain how regulation of arterial blood pressure exemplifies that homeostasis is essential for health and survival, yet another general principle of physiology. Finally, multiple examples demonstrate the general principle of physiology that the functions of organ systems are coordinated with each other; for example, the circulatory and urinary systems work together to control blood pressure, blood volume, and sodium balance.

SECTION A

Overview of the Circulatory System

12.1 Components of the Circulatory System

We will begin with an overview of the components of the circulatory system and a discussion of some of the physical factors that determine its function.

Blood is composed of **formed elements** (cells and cell fragments) suspended in a liquid called **plasma.** Dissolved in the plasma are a large number of proteins, nutrients, metabolic wastes, and other molecules being transported between organ systems. The cells are the **erythrocytes** (red blood cells) and the **leukocytes** (white blood cells), and the cell fragments are the **platelets.** More than 99% of blood cells are erythrocytes, which carry oxygen. The leukocytes protect against infection and cancer, and the platelets function in blood clotting. The constant motion of the blood keeps all the cells dispersed throughout the plasma.

The **hematocrit** is defined as the percentage of blood volume that is erythrocytes. It is measured by centrifuging (spinning at high speed) a sample of blood. The erythrocytes are forced to the bottom of the centrifuge tube, the plasma remains on top, and the leukocytes and platelets form a very thin layer between them called the buffy coat (**Figure 12.1**). The normal hematocrit is approximately 45% in men and 42% in women.

The volume of blood in a 70 kg (154 lb) person is approximately 5.5 L. If we take the hematocrit to be 45%, then

$$\text{Erythrocyte volume} = 0.45 \times 5.5\ \text{L} = 2.5\ \text{L}$$

Because the volume occupied by leukocytes and platelets is usually negligible, the plasma volume equals the difference between blood volume and erythrocyte volume; therefore, in our 70 kg person,

$$\text{Plasma volume} = 5.5\ \text{L} - 2.5\ \text{L} = 3.0\ \text{L}$$

The rapid flow of blood throughout the body is produced by pressures created by the pumping action of the heart. This type of flow is known as **bulk flow** because all constituents of the blood move together. The extraordinary degree of branching of blood vessels ensures that almost all cells in the body are within a few cell diameters of at least one of the smallest branches, the capillaries. Nutrients and metabolic end products move between capillary blood and the interstitial fluid by diffusion. Movements between the interstitial fluid and the cell interior are accomplished by both diffusion and mediated transport across the plasma membrane.

At any given moment, only about 5% of the total circulating blood is actually in the capillaries. Yet, it is this 5% that is performing the ultimate functions of the entire circulatory system: the supplying of nutrients and hormonal signals and the removal of metabolic end products and other cell secretions. All other components of the system serve the overall function of getting adequate blood flow through the capillaries.

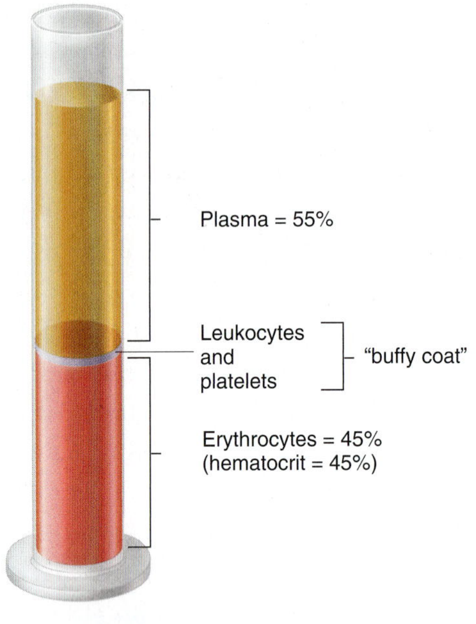

Figure 12.1 APIR Measurement of the hematocrit by centrifugation. The values shown are typical for a healthy male. Due to the presence of a thin layer of leukocytes and platelets between the plasma and red cells, the value for plasma is actually slightly less than 55%.

PHYSIOLOGICAL INQUIRY

- Estimate the hematocrit of a person with a plasma volume of 3 L and total blood volume of 4.5 L.

Answer can be found at end of chapter.

As British physiologist William Harvey reported in 1628, the circulatory system forms a closed loop, so that blood pumped out of the heart through one set of vessels returns to the heart by a different set. There are actually two circuits (**Figure 12.2**), both originating and terminating in the heart, which is divided longitudinally into two functional halves. Each half of the heart contains two chambers: an upper chamber—the **atrium**—and a lower chamber—the **ventricle.** The atrium on each side empties into the ventricle on that side, but there is usually no direct blood flow between the two atria or the two ventricles in the heart of a healthy adult.

The **pulmonary circulation** includes blood pumped from the right ventricle through the lungs and then to the left atrium. It is then pumped through the **systemic circulation** from the left ventricle through all the organs and tissues of the body—except the lungs—and then to the right atrium. In both circuits, the vessels carrying blood away from the heart are called **arteries;** those carrying blood from body organs and tissues back toward the heart are called **veins.**

In the systemic circuit, blood leaves the left ventricle via a single large artery, the **aorta** (see Figure 12.2). The arteries of the systemic circulation branch off the aorta, dividing into progressively smaller vessels. The smallest arteries branch into **arterioles,** which branch into a huge number (estimated at 10 billion) of very small vessels, the **capillaries,** which unite to form larger-diameter vessels, the **venules.** The arterioles, capillaries, and venules are collectively termed the **microcirculation.**

The venules in the systemic circulation then unite to form larger vessels, the veins. The veins from the various peripheral organs and tissues unite to produce two large veins, the **inferior vena cava,** which collects blood from below the heart, and the **superior vena cava,** which collects blood from above the heart (for simplicity, these are depicted as a single vessel in Figure 12.2). These two veins return the blood to the right atrium.

The pulmonary circulation is composed of a similar circuit. Blood leaves the right ventricle via a single large artery, the **pulmonary trunk,** which divides into the two **pulmonary arteries,** one supplying the right lung and the other the left. In the lungs, the arteries continue to branch and connect to arterioles, leading to capillaries that unite into venules and then veins. The blood leaves the lungs via four **pulmonary veins,** which empty into the left atrium.

As blood flows through the lung capillaries, it picks up oxygen supplied to the lungs by breathing. Therefore, the blood in the pulmonary veins, left side of the heart, and systemic arteries has a high oxygen content. As this blood flows through the capillaries of peripheral tissues and organs, some of this oxygen leaves the blood to enter and be used by cells, resulting in the lower oxygen content of systemic venous blood.

As shown in Figure 12.2, blood can pass from the systemic veins to the systemic arteries only by first being pumped through the lungs. Thus, the blood returning from the body's peripheral organs and tissues via the systemic veins is oxygenated before it is pumped back to them.

Note that the lungs receive all the blood pumped by the right side of the heart, whereas the branching of the systemic arteries results in a parallel pattern so that each of the peripheral organs and tissues receives only a fraction of the blood pumped by the left ventricle (see the three capillary beds shown in Figure 12.2). This arrangement (1) guarantees that all systemic tissues receive freshly oxygenated blood and (2) allows for independent variation in blood flow through different tissues as their metabolic activities change. For reference, the typical distribution of the blood pumped by the left ventricle in an adult at rest is given in **Figure 12.3**.

Finally, there are some exceptions to the usual anatomical pattern described in this section for the systemic circulation—for example, the liver and the anterior pituitary gland. In those organs, blood passes through two capillary beds, arranged in series and connected by veins, before returning to the heart. As described in Chapters 11 and 15, this pattern is known as a **portal system.**

12.2 Pressure, Flow, and Resistance

An important feature of the circulatory system is the relationship among blood pressure, blood flow, and the resistance to blood flow. As applied to blood, these factors are collectively referred to as **hemodynamics,** and they demonstrate the general principle of physiology that physiological processes are dictated by the laws of chemistry and physics. In all parts of the system, blood flow (F) is always from a region of higher pressure to one of lower pressure. The pressure exerted by any fluid is called a **hydrostatic pressure**, but this is usually shortened simply to "pressure" in descriptions of the cardiovascular system,

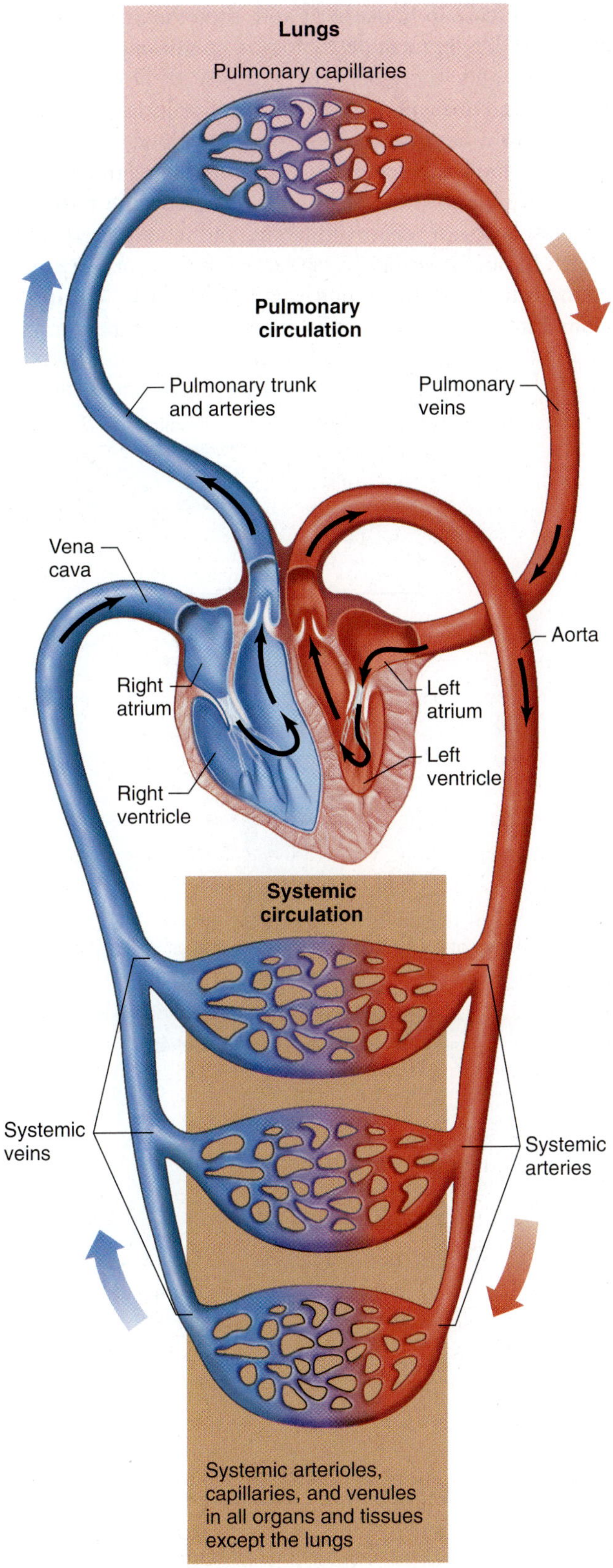

Organ	Flow at rest (mL/min)
Brain	650 (13%)
Heart	215 (4%)
Skeletal muscle	1030 (20%)
Skin	430 (9%)
Kidneys	950 (20%)
Abdominal organs	1200 (24%)
Other	525 (10%)
Total	5000 (100%)

Figure 12.3 Distribution of systemic blood flow to the various organs and tissues of the body at rest. (To see how blood flow changes during exercise, look ahead to Figure 12.61.) Adapted from Chapman and Mitchell.

PHYSIOLOGICAL INQUIRY

- Predict how the blood flow to these various areas might change in a resting person just after eating a large meal.

Answer can be found at end of chapter.

and it denotes the force exerted by the blood. This force is generated in the blood by the contraction of the heart, and its magnitude varies throughout the system for reasons that will be described later. The units for the rate of flow are volume per unit time, usually liters per minute (L/min). The units for the pressure difference (ΔP) driving the flow are millimeters of mercury (mmHg) because historically blood pressure was measured by determining how high the blood pressure could force a column of mercury. It is not the absolute pressure at any point in the cardiovascular system that determines flow rate but the difference in pressure between the relevant points (**Figure 12.4**).

Knowing only the pressure difference between two points will not tell you the flow rate, however. For this, you also need to know the **resistance** (***R***) to flow—that is, how difficult it is for blood to flow between two points at any given

Figure 12.2 APR The systemic and pulmonary circulations. As depicted by the color change from blue to red, blood becomes fully oxygenated (red) as it flows through the lungs and then loses some oxygen (red to blue) as it flows through the other organs and tissues. Deoxygenated blood is shown as blue by convention throughout this book. In reality, it is more dark red or purple in color. Veins appear blue beneath the skin only because long-wavelength red light is absorbed by skin cells and subcutaneous fat, whereas short-wavelength blue light is transmitted. For simplicity, the arteries and veins leaving and entering the heart are depicted as single vessels; in reality, this is true for the arteries but there are multiple pulmonary veins and two venae cavae (see Figure 12.6).

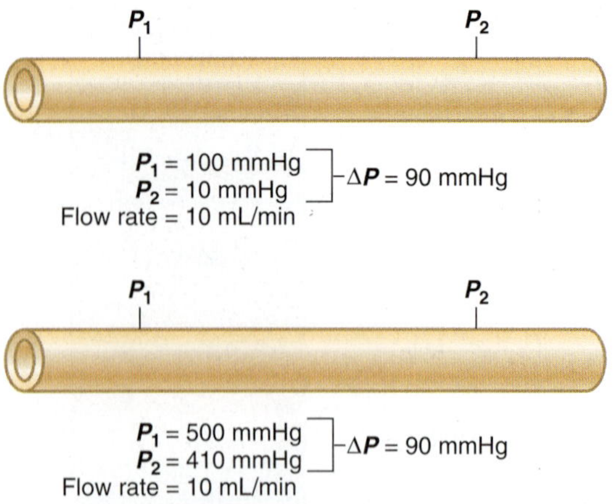

Figure 12.4 Flow between two points within a tube is proportional to the pressure difference between the points. The flows in these two identical tubes are the same (10 mL/min) because the pressure *differences* are the same.

pressure difference. Resistance is the measure of the friction that impedes flow. The basic equation relating these variables is

$$F = \Delta P / R \qquad (12\text{–}1)$$

In words, flow rate is directly proportional to the pressure difference between two points and inversely proportional to the resistance. This equation applies not only to the cardiovascular system but to any system in which liquid or air moves by bulk flow (for example, in the urinary and respiratory systems).

Resistance cannot be measured directly, but it can be calculated from the directly measured F and ΔP. For example, in Figure 12.4, the resistances in both tubes can be calculated:

$$90 \text{ mmHg} \div 10 \text{ mL/min} = 9 \text{ mmHg/mL/min}$$

This example illustrates how resistance can be calculated, but what is it that actually determines the resistance? One determinant of resistance is the fluid property known as **viscosity,** which is a function of the friction between molecules of a flowing fluid; the greater the friction, the greater the viscosity. The other determinants of resistance are the length and radius of the tube through which the fluid is flowing, because these characteristics affect the surface area inside the tube and thus determine the amount of contact between the moving fluid and the stationary wall of the tube. The following equation defines the contributions of these three determinants:

$$R = \frac{8L\eta}{\pi r^4} \qquad (12\text{–}2)$$

where η = fluid viscosity
L = length of the tube
r = inside radius of the tube
$8/\pi$ = a mathematical constant

In other words, resistance is directly proportional to both the fluid viscosity and the vessel's length, and inversely proportional to the fourth power of the vessel's radius.

Blood viscosity is not fixed but increases as hematocrit increases. Changes in hematocrit, therefore, can have significant effects on resistance to flow in certain situations. In extreme dehydration, for example, the reduction in body water leads to a relative increase in hematocrit and, therefore, in the viscosity of the blood. Under most physiological conditions, however, the hematocrit—and, therefore, the viscosity of blood—does not vary much and does not play a role in controlling resistance.

Similarly, because the lengths of the blood vessels remain constant in the body, length is also not a factor in the control of resistance along these vessels. In contrast, the radii of the blood vessels do not remain constant, and so vessel radius—the $1/r^4$ term in our equation—is the most important determinant of changes in resistance along the blood vessels. **Figure 12.5** demonstrates how radius influences the resistance and, as a

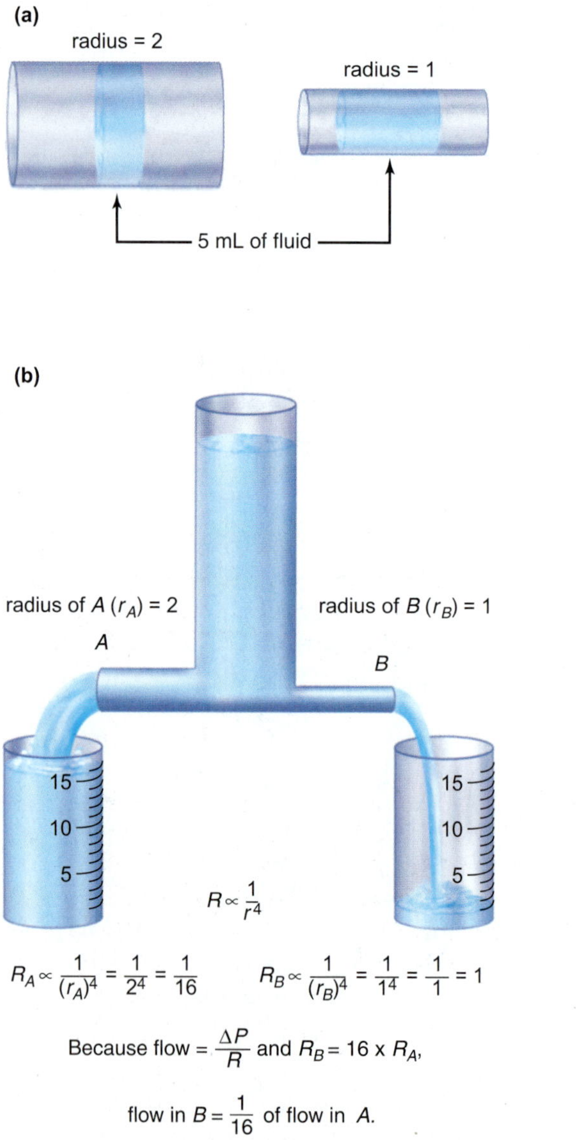

Figure 12.5 Effect of tube radius (r) on resistance (R) and flow. (a) A given volume of fluid is exposed to far more wall surface area and frictional resistance to blood flow in a smaller tube. (b) Given the same pressure gradient, flow through a tube is 16-fold less when the radius is half as large.

PHYSIOLOGICAL INQUIRY

- If outlet B in Figure 12.5b had two individual outlet tubes, each with a radius of 1, would the flow be equal to side A?

Answer can be found at end of chapter.

TABLE 12.1 The Circulatory System

Component	Function
Heart	
Atria	Chambers through which blood flows from veins to ventricles. Atrial contraction adds to ventricular filling but is not essential for it.
Ventricles	Chambers whose contractions produce the pressures that drive blood through the pulmonary and systemic vascular systems and back to the heart.
Vascular system	
Arteries	Low-resistance tubes conducting blood to the various organs with little loss in pressure. They also act as pressure reservoirs for maintaining blood flow during ventricular relaxation.
Arterioles	Major sites of resistance to flow; responsible for the pattern of blood-flow distribution to the various organs; participate in the regulation of arterial blood pressure.
Capillaries	Major sites of nutrient, metabolic end product, and fluid exchange between blood and tissues.
Venules	Sites of nutrient, metabolic end product, and fluid exchange between blood and tissues.
Veins	Low-resistance conduits for blood flow back to the heart. Their capacity for blood is adjusted to facilitate this flow.
Blood	
Plasma	Liquid portion of blood that contains dissolved nutrients, ions, wastes, gases, and other substances. Its composition equilibrates with that of the interstitial fluid at the capillaries.
Cells	Includes erythrocytes that function mainly in gas transport, leukocytes that function in immune defenses, and platelets (cell fragments) for blood clotting.

consequence, the flow of fluid through a tube. Decreasing the radius of a tube twofold increases its resistance 16-fold. If ΔP is held constant in this example, flow through the tube decreases 16-fold because $F = \Delta P/R$.

The equation relating pressure, flow, and resistance applies not only to flow through blood vessels but also to the flows into and out of the various chambers of the heart. These flows occur through valves, and the resistance of a valvular opening determines the flow through the valve at any given pressure difference across it.

As you read on, remember that *the ultimate function of the circulatory system is to ensure adequate blood flow through the capillaries of various organs*. Refer to the summary in **Table 12.1** as you read the description of each component to focus on how each contributes to this goal.

SECTION A SUMMARY

Components of the Circulatory System

I. The key components of the circulatory system are the heart, blood vessels, and blood.

II. The circulatory system consists of two circuits: the pulmonary circulation—from the right ventricle to the lungs and then to the left atrium—and the systemic circulation—from the left ventricle to all peripheral organs and tissues and then to the right atrium.

III. Arteries carry blood away from the heart, and veins carry blood toward the heart.

   a. In the systemic circuit, the large artery leaving the left side of the heart is the aorta, and the large veins emptying into the right side of the heart are the superior vena cava and inferior vena cava. The analogous vessels in the pulmonary circulation are the pulmonary trunk and the four pulmonary veins.

   b. The microcirculation consists of the vessels between arteries and veins: the arterioles, capillaries, and venules.

Pressure, Flow, and Resistance

I. Flow between two points in the cardiovascular system is directly proportional to the pressure difference between those points and inversely proportional to the resistance.

II. Resistance is directly proportional to the viscosity of a fluid and to the length of the tube. It is inversely proportional to the fourth power of the tube's radius, which is the major variable controlling changes in resistance.

SECTION A REVIEW QUESTIONS

1. What is the oxygen status of arterial and venous blood in the systemic versus the pulmonary circulation?
2. State the formula relating flow, pressure difference, and resistance.
3. What are the three determinants of resistance?
4. Which determinant of resistance is varied physiologically to alter blood flow?
5. How does variation in hematocrit influence the hemodynamics of blood flow?
6. Trace the path of a red blood cell through the entire circulatory system, naming all structures and vessel types it flows through, beginning and ending in a capillary of the left big toe.

SECTION A KEY TERMS

aorta 364
arteriole 364
artery 364
atrium 364
blood 363
blood vessels 363
bulk flow 363
capillary 364
cardiovascular system 363
circulatory system 363
erythrocytes 363
formed elements 363
heart 363
hematocrit 363
hemodynamics 364
hydrostatic pressure 364
inferior vena cava 364
leukocytes 363
microcirculation 364
plasma 363
platelet 363
portal system 364
pulmonary artery 364
pulmonary circulation 364
pulmonary trunk 364
pulmonary vein 364
resistance (*R*) 365
superior vena cava 364
systemic circulation 364
vascular system 363
vein 364
ventricle 364
venule 364
viscosity 366

SECTION B The Heart

12.3 Anatomy

The heart is a muscular organ enclosed in a protective fibrous sac, the **pericardium,** and located in the chest (**Figure 12.6**). A fibrous layer is also closely affixed to the heart and is called the **epicardium.** The extremely narrow space between the pericardium and the epicardium is filled with a watery fluid that serves as a lubricant as the heart moves within the sac.

The wall of the heart, the **myocardium,** is composed primarily of cardiac muscle cells. The inner surface of the cardiac chambers, as well as the inner wall of all blood vessels, is lined by a thin layer of cells known as **endothelial cells,** or **endothelium.**

As noted earlier, the human heart is divided into right and left halves, each consisting of an atrium and a ventricle. The two ventricles are separated by a muscular wall, the **interventricular septum.** Located between the atrium and ventricle in each half of the heart are the one-way **atrioventricular (AV) valves,** which permit blood to flow from atrium to ventricle but not backward from ventricle to atrium. The right AV valve is called the **tricuspid valve** because it has three fibrous flaps, or cusps (**Figure 12.7**). The left AV valve has two flaps and is therefore called the **bicuspid valve.** Its resemblance to a bishop's headgear (a "mitre") has earned the left AV valve another commonly used name, **mitral valve.**

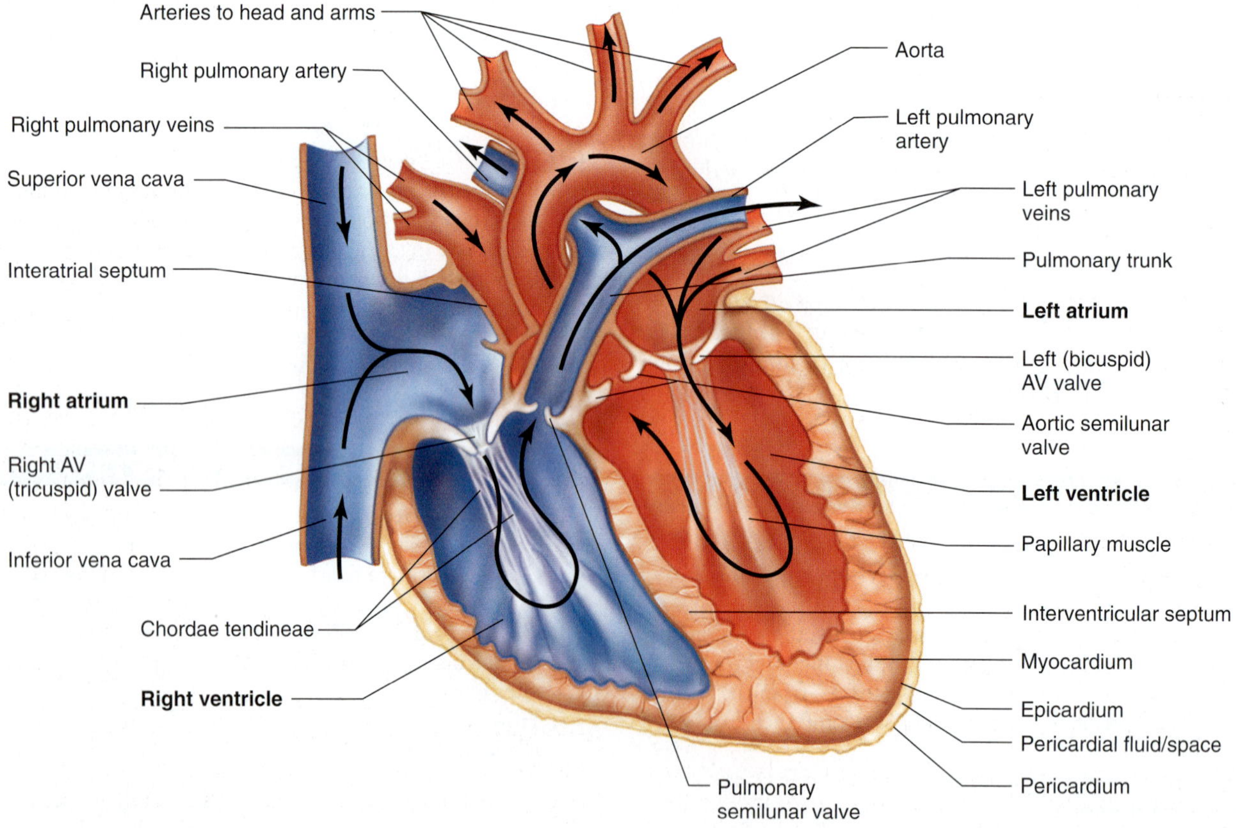

Figure 12.6 AP|R Diagrammatic section of the heart. The arrows indicate the direction of blood flow.

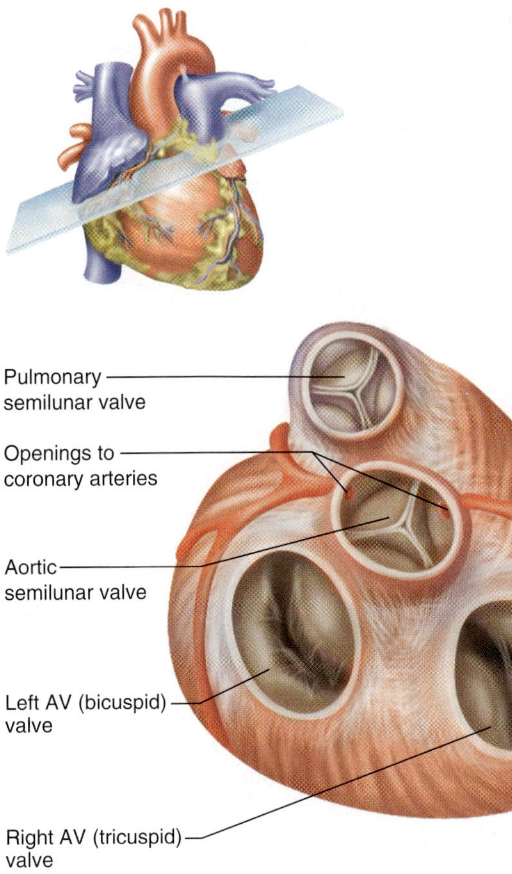

Figure 12.7 APIR Superior view of the heart with the atria removed, showing the heart valves. From R. Carola, J. P. Harley, and C. R. Noback, *Human Anatomy and Physiology*, McGraw-Hill, New York.

The opening and closing of the AV valves are passive processes resulting from pressure differences across the valves. When the blood pressure in an atrium is greater than in the corresponding ventricle, the valve is pushed open and blood flows from atrium to ventricle. In contrast, when a contracting ventricle achieves an internal pressure greater than that in its connected atrium, the AV valve between them is forced closed. Therefore, blood does not normally move back into the atria but is forced into the pulmonary trunk from the right ventricle and into the aorta from the left ventricle.

To prevent the AV valves from being pushed up and opening backward into the atria when the ventricles are contracting (a condition called ***prolapse***), the valves are fastened to muscular projections (**papillary muscles**) of the ventricular walls by fibrous strands (**chordae tendineae**). The papillary muscles do not open or close the valves. They act only to limit the valves' movements and prevent the backward flow of blood. Injury and disease of these tendons or muscles are two ways in which prolapse may occur in some individuals.

The openings of the right ventricle into the pulmonary trunk and of the left ventricle into the aorta also contain valves, the **pulmonary** and **aortic valves,** respectively (see Figures 12.6 and 12.7). These valves are also referred to as the semilunar valves, due to the half-moon shape of the cusps. These valves permit blood to flow into the arteries during ventricular contraction but prevent blood from moving in the opposite direction during ventricular relaxation. Like the AV valves, they act in a purely passive manner. Whether they are open or closed depends upon the pressure differences across them.

Another important point concerning the heart valves is that, when open, they offer very little resistance to flow. Consequently, very small pressure differences across them suffice to produce large flows. In disease states, however, a valve may become narrowed or not open fully so that it offers a high resistance to flow even when open. In such a state, the contracting cardiac chamber must produce an unusually high pressure to cause flow across the valve.

There are no valves at the entrances of the superior and inferior venae cavae (plural of *vena cava*) into the right atrium, and of the pulmonary veins into the left atrium. However, atrial contraction pumps very little blood back into the veins because atrial contraction constricts their sites of entry into the atria, greatly increasing the resistance to backflow. (Actually, a little blood is ejected back into the veins, and this accounts for the venous pulse that can often be seen in the neck veins when the atria are contracting.)

Figure 12.8 summarizes the path of blood flow through the entire cardiovascular system.

Cardiac Muscle

The bulk of the heart is comprised of specialized muscle cells with amazing resiliency and stamina. The cardiac muscle cells of the myocardium are arranged in layers that are tightly bound together and completely encircle the blood-filled chambers. When the walls of a chamber contract, they come together like a squeezing fist and exert pressure on the blood they enclose. Unlike skeletal muscle cells, which can be rested for prolonged periods and only a fraction of which are activated in a given muscle during most contractions, every heart cell contracts with every beat of the heart. Beating about once every second, cardiac muscle cells may contract almost 3 billion times in an average life span without resting! Remarkably, despite this enormous workload, the human heart has a limited ability to replace its muscle cells. Recent experiments suggest that only about 1% of heart muscle cells are replaced per year.

In other ways, cardiac muscle is similar to smooth and skeletal muscle. It is an electrically excitable tissue that converts chemical energy stored in the bonds of ATP into force generation. Action potentials propagate along cell membranes, Ca^{2+} enters the cytosol, and the cycling of force-generating cross-bridges is activated. Some details of the cellular structure and function of cardiac muscle were discussed in Chapter 9.

Approximately 1% of cardiac cells do not function in contraction but have specialized features that are essential for normal heart excitation. These cells constitute a network known as the **conducting system** of the heart and are in electrical contact with the cardiac muscle cells via gap junctions. The conducting system initiates the heartbeat and helps spread an action potential rapidly throughout the heart.

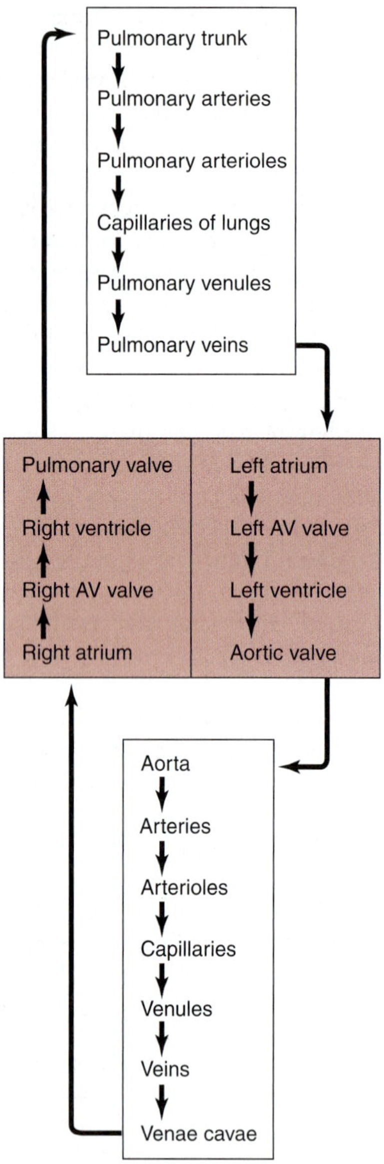

Figure 12.8 APR Path of blood flow through the entire cardiovascular system. All the structures within the colored box are located in the heart.

PHYSIOLOGICAL INQUIRY

- How would this diagram be different if it included a systemic portal vessel?

Answer can be found at end of chapter.

Innervation

The heart receives a rich supply of sympathetic and parasympathetic nerve fibers, the latter contained in the vagus nerves (**Figure 12.9**). The sympathetic postganglionic fibers innervate the entire heart and release norepinephrine, whereas the parasympathetic fibers terminate mainly on cells found in the atria and release primarily acetylcholine. The receptors for norepinephrine on cardiac muscle are mainly β-adrenergic. The hormone epinephrine, from the adrenal medulla, binds to the same receptors as norepinephrine and exerts the same actions on the heart. The receptors for acetylcholine are of the muscarinic type. Details about the autonomic nervous system and its receptors were discussed in Chapter 6.

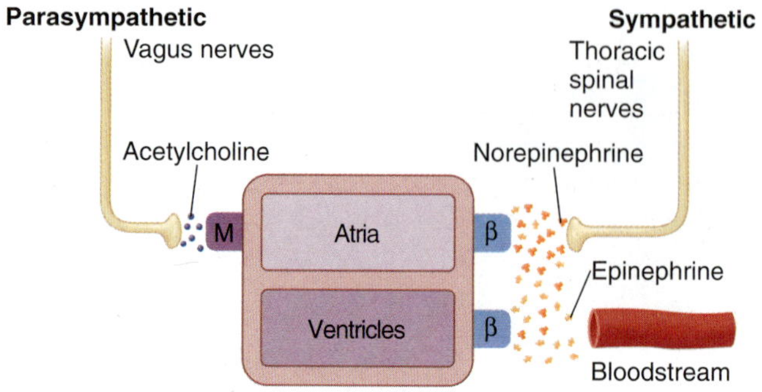

Figure 12.9 Autonomic innervation of heart. Neurons shown represent postganglionic neurons in the pathways. M = muscarinic-type ACh receptor; β = β-adrenergic receptor.

Blood Supply

The blood being pumped through the heart chambers does not exchange nutrients and metabolic end products with the myocardial cells. They, like the cells of all other organs, receive their blood supply via arteries that branch from the aorta. The arteries supplying the myocardium are the **coronary arteries,** and the blood flowing through them is the **coronary blood flow.** The coronary arteries exit from behind the aortic valve cusps in the very first part of the aorta (see Figure 12.7) and lead to a branching network of small arteries, arterioles, capillaries, venules, and veins similar to those in other organs. Most of the cardiac veins drain into a single large vein, the coronary sinus, which empties into the right atrium.

12.4 Heartbeat Coordination

The heart is a dual pump in that the left and right sides of the heart pump blood separately—but simultaneously—into the systemic and pulmonary vessels. Efficient pumping of blood requires that the atria contract first, followed almost immediately by the ventricles. Contraction of cardiac muscle, like that of skeletal muscle and many smooth muscles, is triggered by depolarization of the plasma membrane. Gap junctions interconnect myocardial cells and allow action potentials to spread from one cell to another. The initial excitation of one cardiac cell therefore eventually results in the excitation of all cardiac cells. This initial depolarization normally arises in a small group of conducting-system cells called the **sinoatrial (SA) node,** located in the right atrium near the entrance of the superior vena cava (**Figure 12.10**). The action potential then spreads from the SA node throughout the atria and then into and throughout the ventricles. This raises two questions: (1) What is the path of spread of excitation? (2) How does the SA node initiate an action potential? We will deal initially with the first question and then return to the second question in the next section.

Sequence of Excitation

The SA node is normally the pacemaker for the entire heart. Its depolarization generates the action potential that leads to depolarization of all other cardiac muscle cells. As we will see later, electrical excitation of the heart is coupled with contraction of cardiac muscle. Therefore, the discharge rate of the SA node determines the **heart rate,** the number of times the heart contracts per minute.

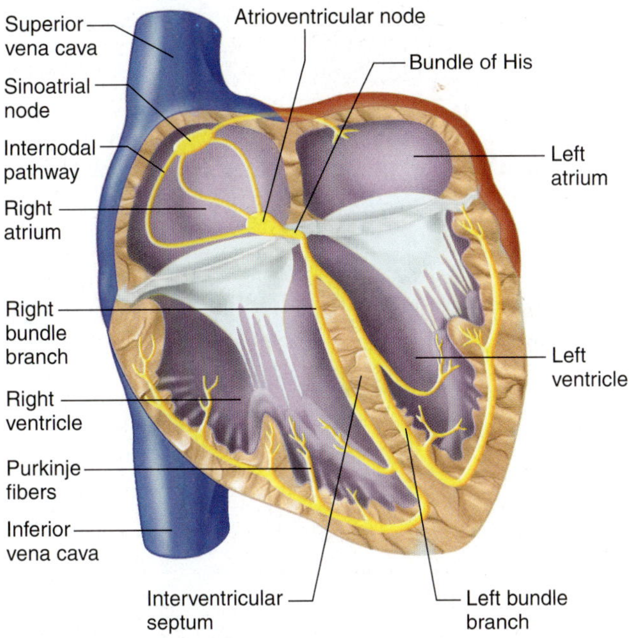

Figure 12.10 AP|R Conducting system of the heart (shown in yellow).

The action potential initiated in the SA node spreads throughout the myocardium, passing from cell to cell by way of gap junctions. Depolarization first spreads through the muscle cells of the atria, with conduction rapid enough that the right and left atria contract at essentially the same time.

The spread of the action potential to the ventricles involves a more complicated conducting system (see Figure 12.10 and **Figure 12.11**), which consists of modified cardiac cells that have lost contractile capability but that conduct action potentials with low resistance. The link between atrial depolarization and ventricular depolarization is a portion of the conducting system called the **atrioventricular (AV) node,** located at the base of the right atrium. The action potential is conducted relatively rapidly from the SA node to the AV node through **internodal pathways.** The AV node is an elongated structure with a particularly important characteristic: *The propagation of action potentials through the AV node is relatively slow* (requiring approximately 0.1 sec). This delay allows atrial contraction to be completed before ventricular excitation occurs.

After the AV node has become excited, the action potential propagates down the interventricular septum. This pathway has conducting-system fibers called the **bundle of His** (pronounced "hiss"), or atrioventricular bundle. The AV node and the bundle of His constitute the only electrical connection between the atria and the ventricles. Except for this pathway, the atria are completely separated from the ventricles by a layer of nonconducting connective tissue.

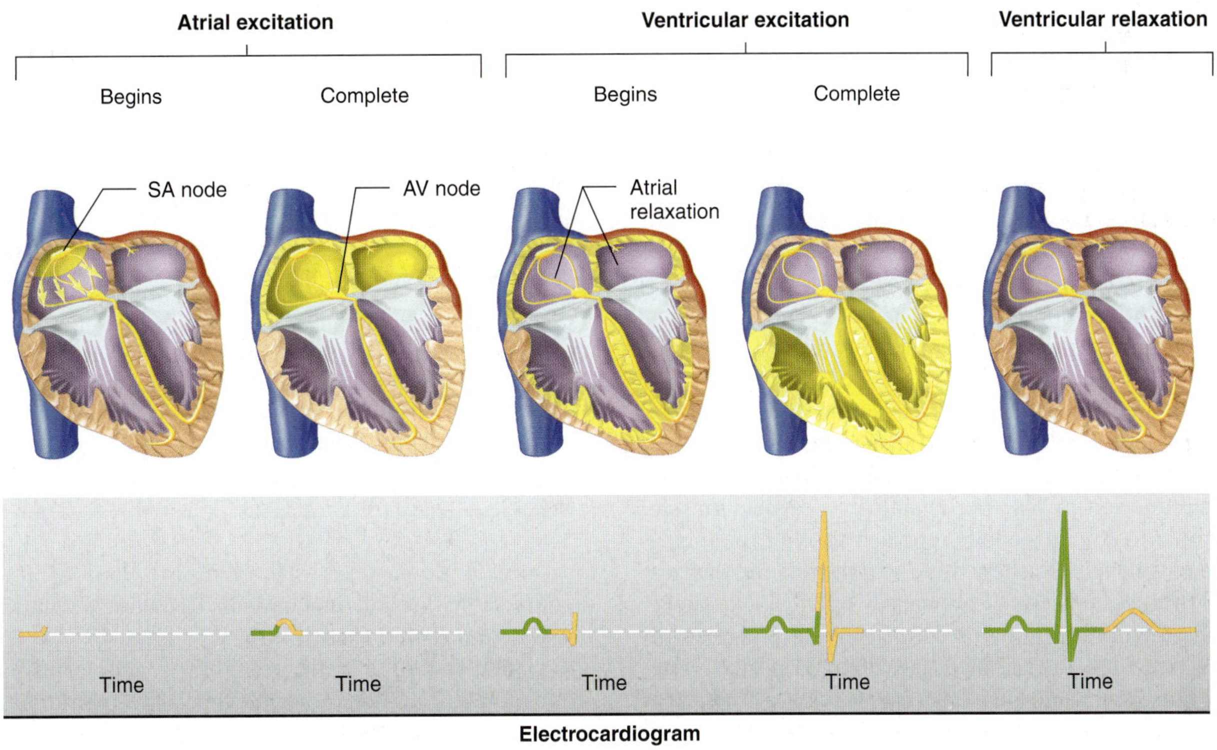

Figure 12.11 AP|R Sequence of cardiac excitation. The yellow color denotes areas that are depolarized. The electrocardiogram monitors the spread of the signal. Adapted from Rushmer.

Within the interventricular septum, the bundle of His divides into right and left **bundle branches,** conducting fibers that separate at the bottom (apex) of the heart and enter the walls of both ventricles. These fibers in turn make contact with **Purkinje fibers,** large-diameter conducting cells that rapidly distribute the impulse throughout much of the ventricles. Finally, the Purkinje fibers make contact with ventricular myocardial cells, which spread the action potential through the rest of the ventricles.

The rapid conduction along the Purkinje fibers and the diffuse distribution of these fibers cause depolarization of all right and left ventricular cells to occur nearly simultaneously and ensure a single coordinated contraction. Actually, though, depolarization and contraction do begin slightly earlier in the apex of the ventricles and then spread upward. The result is an efficient contraction that moves blood toward the exit valves, like squeezing a tube of toothpaste from the bottom up.

Cardiac Action Potentials and Excitation of the SA Node

The mechanism by which action potentials are conducted along the membranes of heart cells is basically similar to other excitable tissues like neurons and skeletal muscle cells. As was described in Chapters 6 and 9, it involves the controlled exchange of materials (ions) across cellular membranes, which is one of the general principles of physiology introduced in Chapter 1. However, different types of heart cells express unique combinations of ion channels that produce different action potential shapes. In this way, they are specialized for particular roles in the spread of excitation through the heart.

Figure 12.12a illustrates an idealized ventricular myocardial cell action potential. The changes in plasma membrane permeability that underlie it are shown in **Figure 12.12b**. As in skeletal muscle cells and neurons, the resting membrane is much more permeable to K^+ than to Na^+. Therefore, the resting membrane potential is much closer to the K^+ equilibrium potential (−90 mV) than to the Na^+ equilibrium potential (+60 mV). Similarly, the depolarizing phase of the action potential is due mainly to the opening of voltage-gated Na^+ channels. Sodium ion entry depolarizes the cell and sustains the opening of more Na^+ channels in positive feedback fashion.

Also, as in skeletal muscle cells and neurons, the increased Na^+ permeability is very transient because the Na^+ channels inactivate quickly. However, unlike other excitable tissues, the reduction in Na^+ permeability in cardiac muscle is not accompanied by immediate repolarization of the membrane to resting levels. Rather, there is a partial repolarization caused by a special class of transiently open K^+ channels, and then the membrane remains depolarized at a plateau of about 0 mV (see Figure 12.12a) for a prolonged period. The reasons for this continued depolarization are (1) K^+ permeability declines below the resting value due to the closure of the K^+ channels that were open in the resting state, and (2) a large increase in the cell membrane permeability to Ca^{2+} occurs. This second mechanism does not occur in skeletal muscle, and the explanation for it follows.

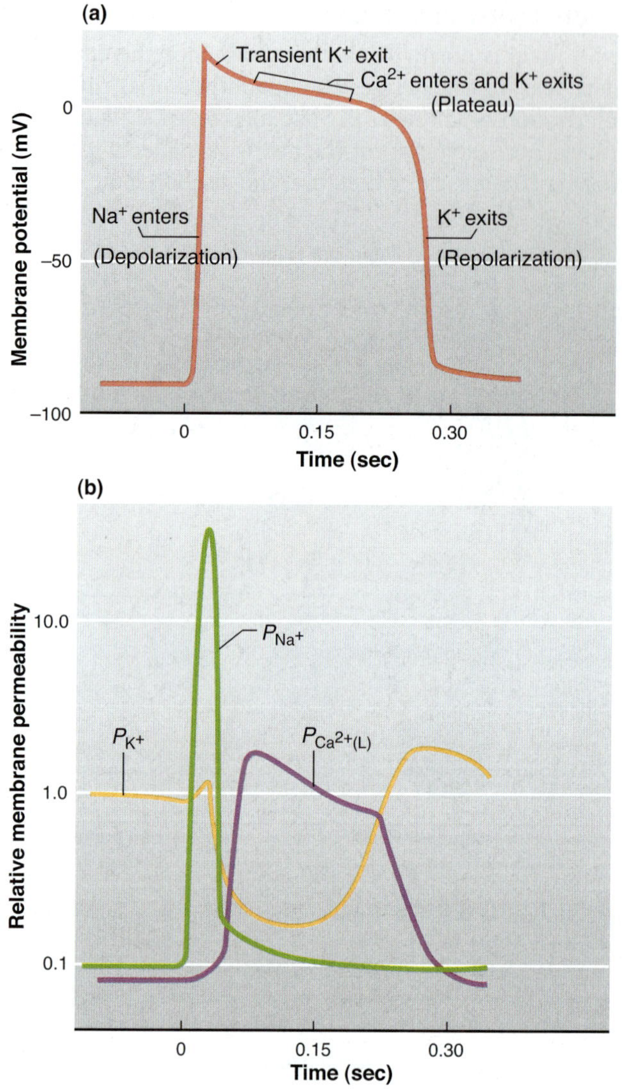

Figure 12.12 (a) Membrane potential recording from a ventricular muscle cell. Labels indicate key ionic movements in each phase. (b) Simultaneously measured permeabilities (P) to K^+, Na^+, and Ca^{2+} during the action potential of (a). Several subtypes of K^+ channels contribute to P_{K^+}.

PHYSIOLOGICAL INQUIRY

- The current due to outward K^+ movement is nearly equal to the current due to inward Ca^{2+} movement during the plateau of the action potential, and yet the membrane permeability to Ca^{2+} is much greater. How can the currents be similar despite the permeability difference?

Answer can be found at end of chapter.

In myocardial cells, membrane depolarization causes voltage-gated Ca^{2+} channels in the plasma membrane to open, which results in a flow of Ca^{2+} ions down their electrochemical gradient into the cell. These channels open much more slowly than do Na^+ channels, and, because they remain open for a prolonged period, they are often referred to as **L-type Ca^{2+} channels** (L = long lasting). These channels are modified versions of the dihydropyridine (DHP) receptors that function as voltage sensors in excitation–contraction coupling of skeletal muscle (see Figure 9.12). The flow of positive calcium ions into the cell just balances the flow of positive potassium ions out of the cell and keeps the membrane depolarized at the plateau value.

Ultimately, repolarization does occur due to the eventual inactivation of the L-type Ca^{2+} channels and the opening of another subtype of K^+ channels. These K^+ channels are similar to the ones described in neurons and skeletal muscle; they open in response to depolarization (but after a delay) and close once the K^+ current has repolarized the membrane to negative values.

The action potentials of atrial muscle cells are similar in shape to those just described for ventricular cells, but the duration of their plateau phase is shorter.

In contrast, there are extremely important differences between action potentials of cardiac muscle cells and those in nodal cells of the conducting system. **Figure 12.13a** illustrates the action potential of a cell from the SA node. Note that the SA node cell does not have a steady resting potential but, instead, undergoes a slow depolarization. This gradual depolarization is known as a **pacemaker potential;** it brings the membrane potential to threshold, at which point an action potential occurs.

Three ion channel mechanisms, which are shown in **Figure 12.13b**, contribute to the pacemaker potential. The first is a progressive reduction in K^+ permeability. The K^+ channels that opened during the repolarization phase of the previous action potential gradually close due to the membrane's return to negative potentials. Second, pacemaker cells have a unique set of channels that, unlike most voltage-gated channels, open when the membrane potential is at *negative* values. These nonspecific cation channels conduct mainly an inward, depolarizing, Na^+ current and, because of their unusual gating behavior, have been termed "funny," or **F-type channels.** The third pacemaker channel is a type of Ca^{2+} channel that opens only briefly but contributes inward Ca^{2+} current and an important final depolarizing boost to the pacemaker potential. These channels are called **T-type Ca^{2+} channels** (T = transient). Although SA node and AV node action potentials are basically similar in shape, the pacemaker currents of SA node cells bring them to threshold more rapidly than AV node cells, which is why SA node cells normally initiate action potentials and determine the pace of the heart.

Once the pacemaker mechanisms have brought a nodal cell to threshold, an action potential occurs. The depolarizing phase is caused not by Na^+ but rather by Ca^{2+} influx through L-type Ca^{2+} channels. These Ca^{2+} currents depolarize the membrane more slowly than voltage-gated Na^+ channels, and one result is that action potentials propagate more slowly along nodal-cell membranes than in other cardiac cells. This explains the slow transmission of cardiac excitation through the AV node. As in cardiac muscle cells, the long-lasting L-type Ca^{2+} channels prolong the nodal action potential, but eventually they close and K^+ channels open and the membrane is repolarized. The return to negative potentials activates the pacemaker mechanisms once again, and the cycle repeats.

Thus, the pacemaker potential provides the SA node with **automaticity,** the capacity for spontaneous, rhythmic self-excitation. The slope of the pacemaker potential—that is, how quickly the membrane potential changes per unit

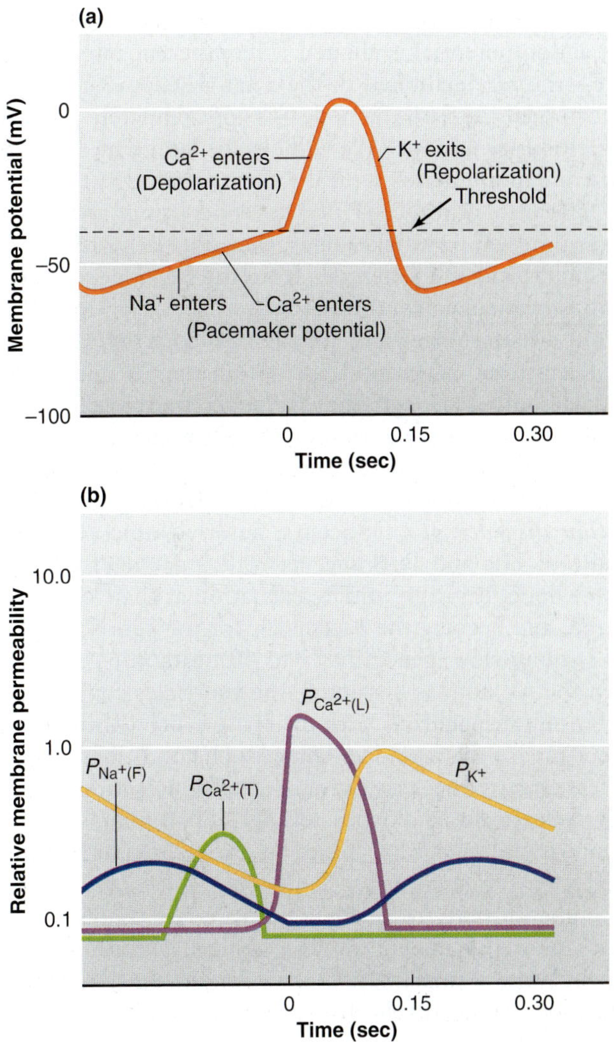

Figure 12.13 (a) Membrane potential recording from a cardiac nodal cell. Labels indicate key ionic movements in each phase. A gradual reduction in K^+ permeability also contributes to the pacemaker potential (not shown), and the Na^+ entry in this phase is through nonspecific cation channels. (b) Simultaneously measured permeabilities through four different ion channels during the action potential shown in (a).

PHYSIOLOGICAL INQUIRY

- Conducting cells of the ventricles contain all of the ion channel types found in both cardiac muscle cells and node cells. Draw a graph showing a Purkinje cell action potential.

Answer can be found at end of chapter.

time—determines how quickly threshold is reached and the next action potential is elicited. The inherent rate of the SA node—the rate exhibited in the total absence of any neural or hormonal input to the node—is approximately 100 depolarizations per minute. (We will discuss later why the resting heart rate in humans is typically slower than that.)

Because other cells of the conducting system have slower inherent pacemaker rates, they normally are driven to threshold by action potentials from the SA node and do not manifest their own rhythm. However, they can do so under certain circumstances and are then called ***ectopic pacemakers.*** Recall that excitation travels from the SA node to both ventricles only through the AV node; therefore, drug- or disease-induced malfunction of the AV node may reduce or completely eliminate the transmission of action potentials from the atria to the ventricles. This is known as an ***AV conduction disorder.*** If this occurs, autorhythmic cells in the bundle of His and Purkinje network, no longer driven by the SA node, begin to initiate excitation at their own inherent rate and become the pacemaker for the ventricles. Their rate is quite slow, generally 25 to 40 beats/min. Therefore, when the AV node is disrupted, the ventricles contract completely out of synchrony with the atria, which continue at the higher rate of the SA node. Under such conditions, the atria are less effective because they are often contracting when the AV valves are closed. Fortunately, atrial pumping is relatively unimportant for cardiac function except during strenuous exercise.

The current treatment for severe AV conduction disorders, as well as for many other abnormal rhythms, is permanent surgical implantation of an ***artificial pacemaker*** that electrically stimulates the ventricular cells at a normal rate.

The Electrocardiogram

The **electrocardiogram** (**ECG,** also abbreviated *EKG*—the *k* is from the German *elektrokardiogramm*) is a tool for evaluating the electrical events within the heart. When action potentials occur simultaneously in many individual myocardial cells, currents are conducted through the body fluids around the heart and can be detected by recording electrodes at the surface of the skin. **Figure 12.14a** illustrates an idealized normal ECG recorded as the potential difference between the right and left wrists. (Review Figure 12.11 for an illustration of how this waveform corresponds in time with the spread of an action potential through the heart.) The first deflection, the **P wave,** corresponds to current flow during atrial depolarization. The second deflection, the **QRS complex,** occurring approximately 0.15 sec later, is the result of ventricular depolarization. It is a complex deflection because the paths taken by the wave of depolarization through the thick ventricular walls differ from instant to instant, and the currents generated in the body fluids change direction accordingly. Regardless of its form (for example, the Q and/or S portions may be absent), the deflection is still called a QRS complex. The final deflection, the **T wave,** is the result of ventricular repolarization. Atrial repolarization is usually not evident on the ECG because it occurs at the same time as the QRS complex.

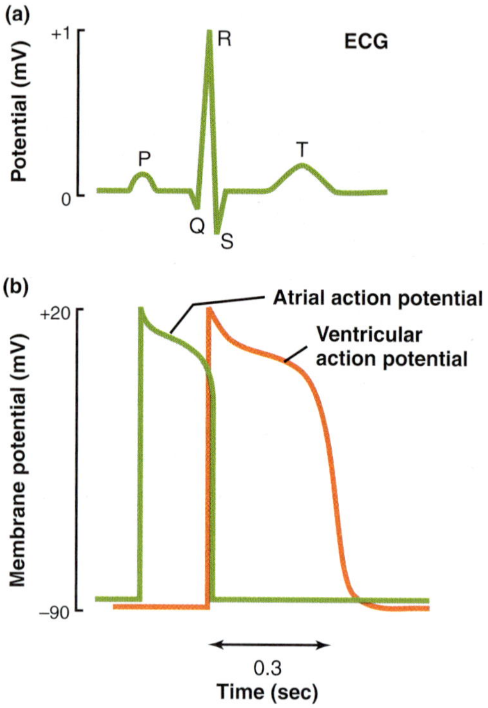

Figure 12.14 APR (a) Idealized electrocardiogram recorded from electrodes placed on the wrists. (b) Action potentials recorded from a single atrial muscle cell and a single ventricular muscle cell, synchronized with the ECG trace in panel (a). Note the correspondence of the P wave with atrial depolarization, the QRS complex with ventricular depolarization, and the T wave with ventricular repolarization.

PHYSIOLOGICAL INQUIRY

- How would the timing of the waves in (a) be changed by a drug that reduces the L-type Ca^{2+} current in AV node cells?

Answer can be found at end of chapter.

A typical ECG makes use of multiple combinations of recording locations on the limbs and chest (called **ECG leads**) so as to obtain as much information as possible concerning different areas of the heart. The shapes and sizes of the P wave, QRS complex, and T wave vary with the electrode locations. For reference, see **Figure 12.15** and **Table 12.2**, which describe the placement of electrodes for the different ECG leads.

To reiterate, the ECG is not a direct record of the changes in membrane potential across individual cardiac muscle cells. Instead, it is a measure of the currents generated in the extracellular fluid by the changes occurring simultaneously in many cardiac cells. To emphasize this point, **Figure 12.14b** shows the simultaneously occurring changes in membrane potential in single atrial and ventricular muscle cells.

Because many myocardial defects alter normal action potential propagation, and thereby the shapes and timing of the waves, the ECG is a powerful tool for diagnosing certain

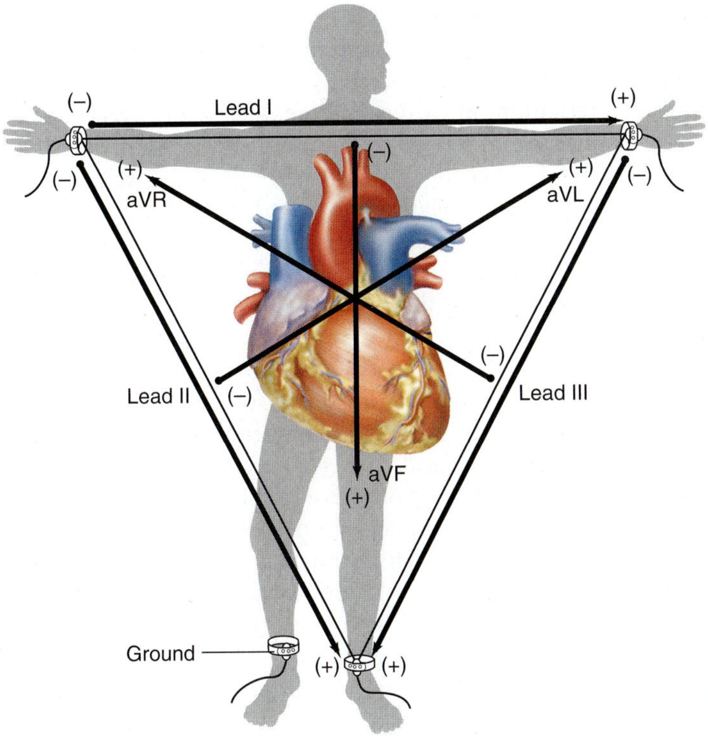

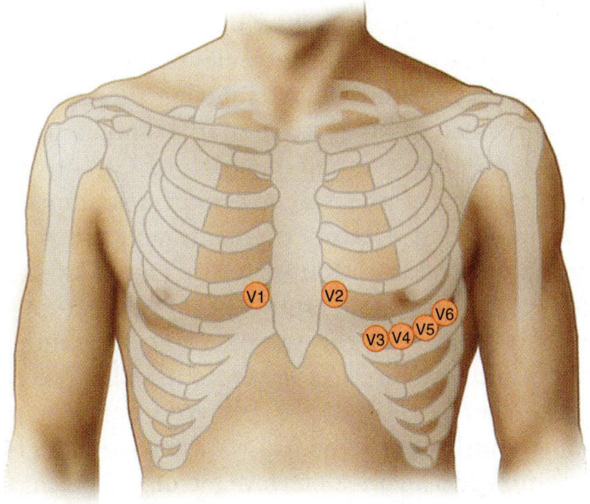

(a) (b)

Figure 12.15 Placement of electrodes in electrocardiography. Each of the 12 leads uses a different combination of reference (negative pole) and recording (positive pole) electrodes, thus providing different angles for "viewing" the electrical activity of the heart. (a) The standard limb leads (I, II, and III) form a triangle between electrodes on the wrists and left leg (the right leg is a ground electrode). Augmented leads bisect the angles of the triangle by combining two electrodes as reference. (For example, for lead aVL, the right wrist and foot are combined as the negative pole, thus creating a reference point along the line between them, pointing toward the recording electrode on the left wrist.) (b) The precordial leads (V1 – V6) are recording electrodes placed on the chest as shown, with the limb leads combined into a reference point at the center of the heart.

TABLE 12.2 Electrocardiography Leads

Name of Lead	Electrode Placement	
Standard Limb Leads	*Reference (–) Electrode*	*Recording (+) Electrode*
Lead I	Right arm	Left arm
Lead II	Right arm	Left leg
Lead III	Left arm	Left leg
Augmented Limb Leads		
aVR	Left arm and left leg	Right arm
aVL	Right arm and left leg	Left arm
aVF	Right arm and left arm	Left leg
Precordial (Chest) Leads		
V1	Combined limb leads	4th intercostal space, right of sternum
V2	" " "	4th intercostal space, left of sternum
V3	" " "	5th intercostal space, left of sternum
V4	" " "	5th intercostal space, centered on clavicle
V5	" " "	5th intercostal space, left of V4
V6	" " "	5th intercostal space, under left arm

types of heart disease. **Figure 12.16** gives one example. However, note that the ECG provides information concerning only the electrical activity of the heart. If something is wrong with the heart's mechanical activity and the defect does not give rise to altered electrical activity, the ECG will be of limited diagnostic value.

Excitation–Contraction Coupling

The mechanisms linking cardiac muscle cell action potentials to contraction were described in detail in the chapter on muscle physiology (Chapter 9; review Figure 9.40). The small amount of extracellular Ca^{2+} entering through L-type Ca^{2+} channels during the plateau of the action potential triggers the release of a larger quantity of Ca^{2+} from the ryanodine receptors in the sarcoplasmic reticulum membrane. Ca^{2+} activation of thin filaments and cross-bridge cycling then lead to generation of force, just as in skeletal muscle (review Figures 9.15 and 9.11). Contraction ends when Ca^{2+} is returned to the sarcoplasmic reticulum and extracellular fluid by Ca^{2+}-ATPase pumps and Na^+/Ca^{2+} countertransporters.

The amount that cytosolic Ca^{2+} concentration increases during excitation is a major determinant of the strength of cardiac muscle contraction. You may recall that in skeletal muscle, a single action potential releases sufficient Ca^{2+} to fully saturate the troponin sites that activate contraction. By contrast, the amount of Ca^{2+} released from the sarcoplasmic reticulum in cardiac muscle during a resting heartbeat is not usually sufficient to saturate all troponin sites. Therefore, the number of active cross-bridges—and thus the strength of contraction—can be increased if more Ca^{2+} is released from the sarcoplasmic reticulum (as would occur, for example, in exercise). The mechanisms that vary cytosolic Ca^{2+} concentration will be discussed later.

Refractory Period of the Heart

Cardiac muscle is incapable of undergoing summation of contractions like that occurring in skeletal muscle (review Figure 9.19), and this is a very good thing. If a prolonged, tetanic contraction were to occur in the heart, it would cease to function as a pump because the ventricles can only fill with blood while they are relaxed. The inability of the heart to generate tetanic contractions is the result of the long **absolute refractory period** of cardiac muscle, defined as the period during and following an action potential when an excitable membrane cannot be re-excited. As in the case of neurons and skeletal muscle fibers, the main mechanism is the inactivation of Na^+ channels. The absolute refractory period of skeletal muscle is much shorter (1 to 2 msec) than the duration of contraction (20 to 100 msec), and a second action potential can therefore be elicited while the contraction resulting from the first action potential is still under way (see Figure 9.10). In contrast, because of the prolonged, depolarized plateau in the cardiac muscle action potential, the absolute refractory period of cardiac muscle lasts almost as long as the contraction (approximately 250 msec), and the muscle cannot be re-excited multiple times during an ongoing contraction (**Figure 12.17**; also review Figure 9.41).

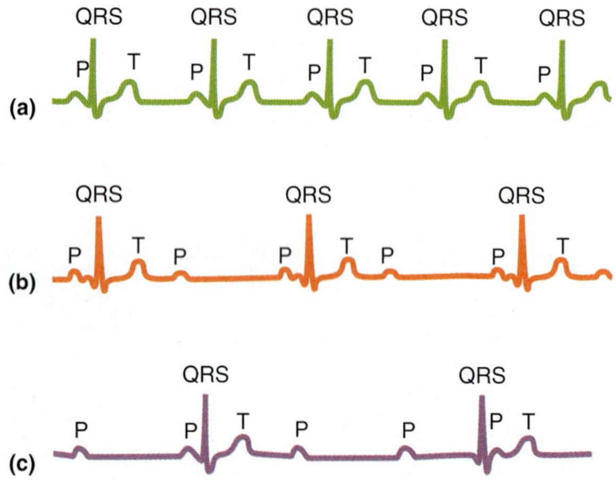

Figure 12.16 Electrocardiograms from a healthy person and from two people suffering from atrioventricular block. (a) A normal ECG. (b) Partial block. Damage to the AV node permits only every other atrial impulse to be transmitted to the ventricles. Note that every second P wave is not followed by a QRS and T. (c) Complete block. There is no synchrony between atrial and ventricular electrical activities, and the ventricles are being driven by a very slow pacemaker cell in the bundle of His.

PHYSIOLOGICAL INQUIRY

- Some people have a potentially lethal defect of ventricular muscle, in which the current through voltage-gated K^+ channels responsible for repolarization is delayed and reduced. How could this defect be detected on their ECG recordings?

Answer can be found at end of chapter.

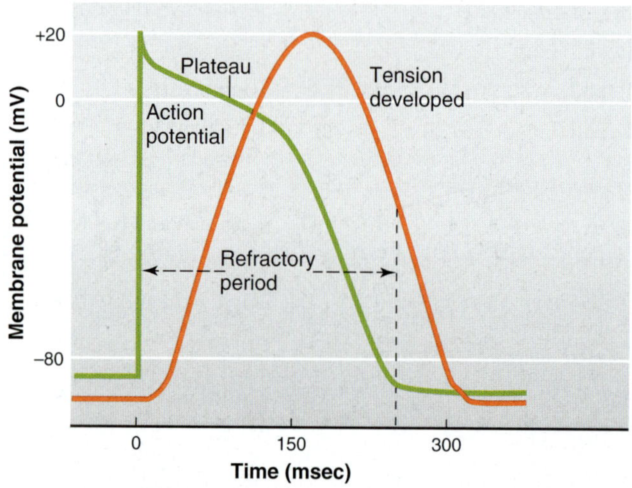

Figure 12.17 Relationship between membrane potential changes and contraction in a ventricular muscle cell. The refractory period lasts almost as long as the contraction. Tension scale not shown.

12.5 Mechanical Events of the Cardiac Cycle

The orderly process of depolarization described in the previous sections triggers a recurring **cardiac cycle** of atrial and ventricular contractions and relaxations (**Figure 12.18**). First, we will present an overview of the cycle, naming the phases and key events. A closer look at the cycle will follow, with a discussion of the pressure and volume changes that cause the events.

The cycle is divided into two major phases, both named for events in the ventricles: the period of ventricular contraction and blood ejection called **systole,** and the alternating period of ventricular relaxation and blood filling, **diastole.** For a typical heart rate of 72 beats/min, each cardiac cycle lasts approximately 0.8 sec, with 0.3 sec in systole and 0.5 sec in diastole.

As Figure 12.18 illustrates, both systole and diastole can be subdivided into two discrete periods. During the first part of systole, the ventricles are contracting but all valves in the heart are closed and so no blood can be ejected. This period is termed **isovolumetric ventricular contraction** because the ventricular volume is constant ("iso" means "equal" or in this context "unchanging"). The ventricular

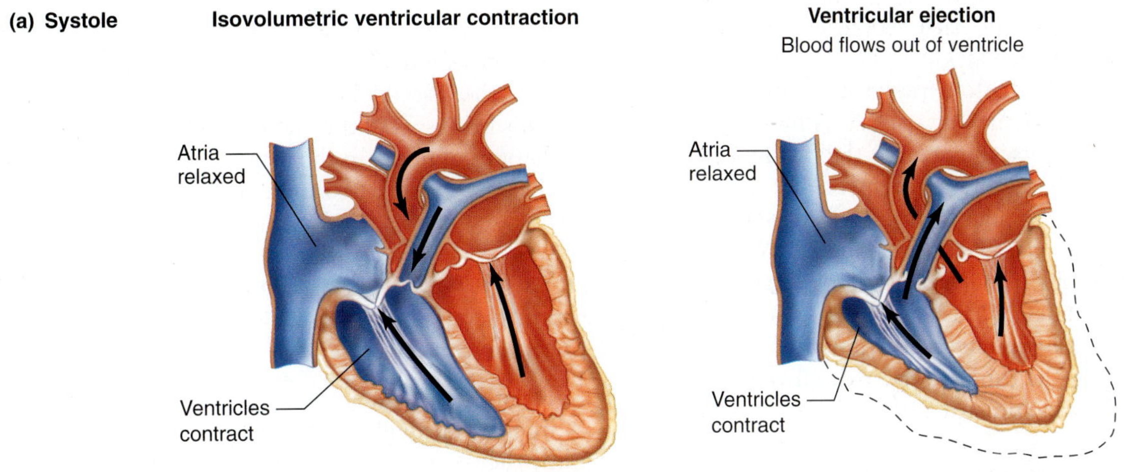

	Isovolumetric ventricular contraction	Ventricular ejection
AV valves:	Closed	Closed
Aortic and pulmonary valves:	Closed	Open

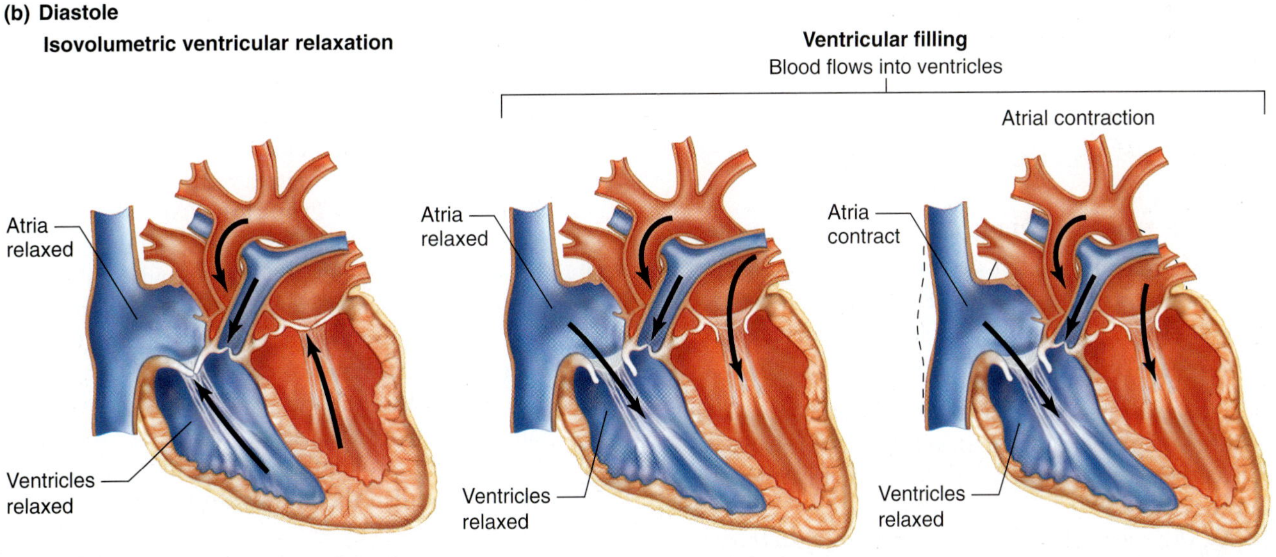

	Isovolumetric ventricular relaxation	Ventricular filling	Atrial contraction
AV valves:	Closed	Open	Open
Aortic and pulmonary valves:	Closed	Closed	Closed

Figure 12.18 APR Divisions of the cardiac cycle: (a) systole; (b) diastole. The phases of the cycle are identical in both halves of the heart. The direction in which the pressure difference *favors* flow is denoted by an arrow; note, however, that flow will not actually occur if a valve prevents it.

walls are developing tension and squeezing on the blood they enclose, increasing the ventricular blood pressure. However, because the volume of blood in the ventricles is constant and because blood, like water, is essentially incompressible, the ventricular muscle fibers cannot shorten. Thus, isovolumetric ventricular contraction is analogous to an isometric skeletal muscle contraction; the muscle develops tension, but it does not shorten.

Once the increasing pressure in the ventricles exceeds that in the aorta and pulmonary trunk, the aortic and pulmonary valves open and the **ventricular ejection** period of systole occurs. Blood is forced into the aorta and pulmonary trunk as the contracting ventricular muscle fibers shorten. The volume of blood ejected from each ventricle during systole is called the **stroke volume (*SV*)**.

During the first part of diastole, the ventricles begin to relax and the aortic and pulmonary valves close. (Physiologists and clinical cardiologists do not all agree on the dividing line between systole and diastole; as presented here, the dividing line is the point at which ventricular contraction stops and the pulmonary and aortic valves close.) At this time, the AV valves are also closed; therefore, no blood is entering or leaving the ventricles. Ventricular volume is not changing, and this period is called **isovolumetric ventricular relaxation.** Note, then, that the only times during the cardiac cycle that all valves are closed are the periods of isovolumetric ventricular contraction and relaxation.

Next, the AV valves open and **ventricular filling** occurs as blood flows in from the atria. Atrial contraction occurs at the end of diastole, after most of the ventricular filling has taken place. The ventricle receives blood throughout most of diastole, not just when the atrium contracts. Indeed, in a person at rest, approximately 80% of ventricular filling occurs before atrial contraction.

This completes the basic orientation. Using **Figure 12.19**, we can now analyze the pressure and volume changes that occur in the left atrium, left ventricle, and aorta during the cardiac cycle. Events on the right side of the heart are very similar except for the absolute pressures.

Mid-Diastole to Late Diastole

Our analysis of events in the left atrium and ventricle and the aorta begins at the far left of Figure 12.19 with the events of mid- to late diastole. The numbers that follow correspond to the numbered events shown in that figure.

1. The left atrium and ventricle are both relaxed, but atrial pressure is slightly higher than ventricular pressure because the atrium is filled with blood that is entering from the veins.
2. The AV valve is held open by this pressure difference, and blood entering the atrium from the pulmonary veins continues on into the ventricle.

To reemphasize a point made earlier, all the valves of the heart offer very little resistance when they are open, so very small pressure differences across them are required to produce relatively large flows.

3. Note that at this time, and throughout all of diastole, the aortic valve is closed because the aortic pressure is higher than the ventricular pressure.
4. Throughout diastole, the aortic pressure is slowly decreasing because blood is moving out of the arteries and through the vascular system.
5. In contrast, ventricular pressure is increasing slightly because blood is entering the relaxed ventricle from the atrium, thereby expanding the ventricular volume.
6. Near the end of diastole, the SA node discharges and the atria depolarize, as signified by the P wave of the ECG.
7. Contraction of the atrium causes an increase in atrial pressure.
8. The elevated atrial pressure forces a small additional volume of blood into the ventricle, sometimes referred to as the "atrial kick."
9. This brings us to the end of ventricular diastole, so the amount of blood in the ventricle at this time is called the **end-diastolic volume (*EDV*)**.

Systole

Thus far, the ventricle has been relaxed as it fills with blood. But immediately following the atrial contraction, the ventricles begin to contract.

10. From the AV node, the wave of depolarization passes into and throughout the ventricular tissue—as signified by the QRS complex of the ECG—and this triggers ventricular contraction.
11. As the ventricle contracts, ventricular pressure increases rapidly; almost immediately, this pressure exceeds the atrial pressure.
12. This change in pressure gradient forces the AV valve to close, thus preventing the backflow of blood into the atrium.
13. Because the aortic pressure still exceeds the ventricular pressure at this time, the aortic valve remains closed and the ventricle cannot empty despite its contraction. For a brief time, then, all valves are closed during this phase of isovolumetric ventricular contraction. Backward bulging of the closed AV valves causes a small upward deflection in the atrial pressure wave.
14. This brief phase ends when the rapidly increasing ventricular pressure exceeds aortic pressure.
15. The pressure gradient now forces the aortic valve to open, and ventricular ejection begins.
16. The ventricular volume curve shows that ejection is rapid at first and then slows down.
17. The amount of blood remaining in the ventricle after ejection is called the **end-systolic volume (*ESV*)**.

Note that the ventricle does not empty completely. The amount of blood that does exit during each cycle is the difference between what it contained at the end of diastole and what remains at the end of systole. Thus,

$$\underset{SV}{\text{Stroke volume}} = \underset{EDV}{\text{End-diastolic volume}} - \underset{ESV}{\text{End-systolic volume}}$$

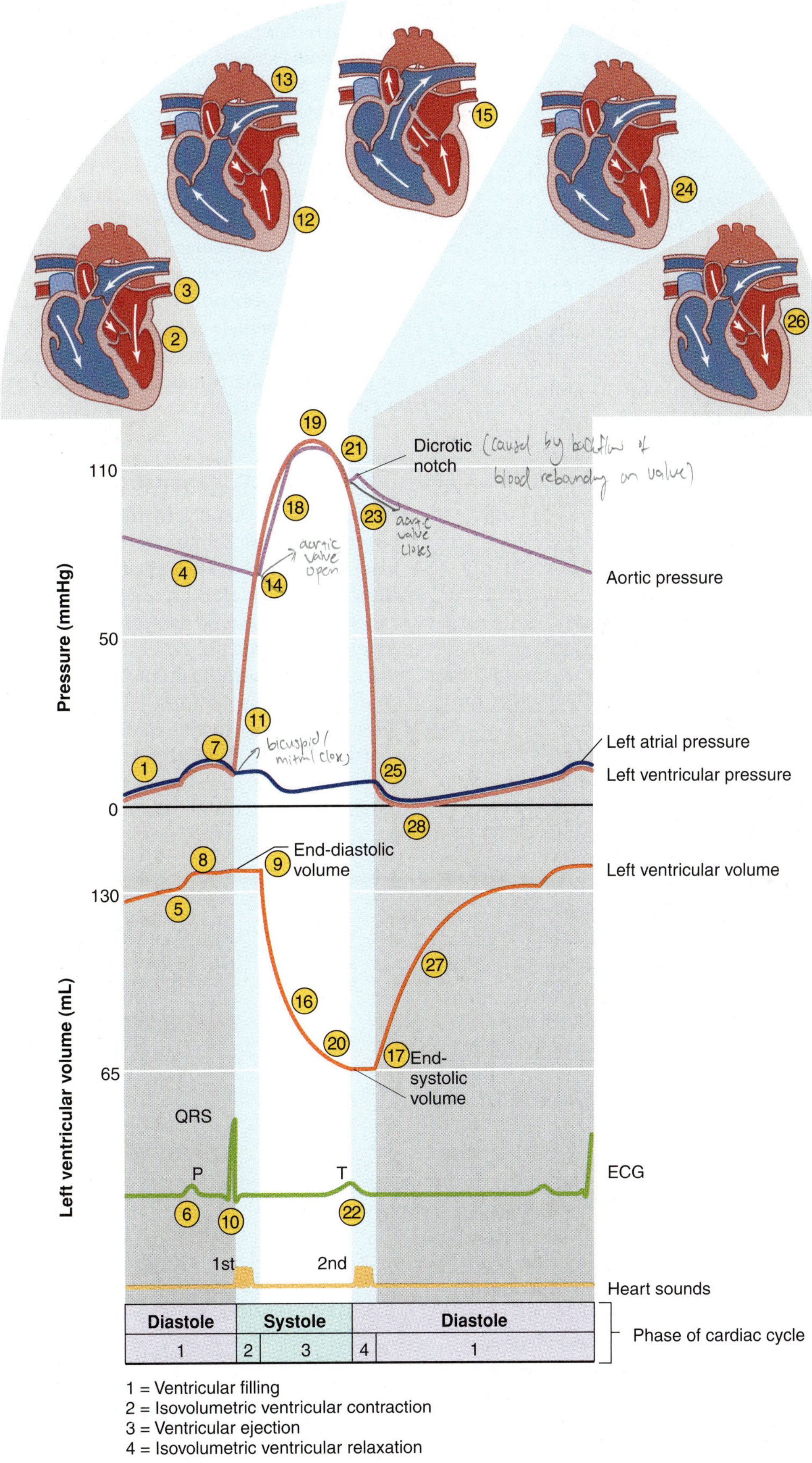

Figure 12.19 APIR Summary of events in the left atrium, left ventricle, and aorta during the cardiac cycle (sometimes called the "Wiggers" diagram). See text for a description of the numbered steps.

As Figure 12.19 shows, typical values for an adult at rest are end-diastolic volume = 135 mL, end-systolic volume = 65 mL, and stroke volume = 70 mL.

(18) As blood flows into the aorta, the aortic pressure increases along with the ventricular pressure. Throughout ejection, very small pressure differences exist between the ventricle and aorta because the open aortic valve offers little resistance to flow.

(19) Note that peak ventricular and aortic pressures are reached before the end of ventricular ejection; that is, these pressures start to decrease during the last part of systole despite continued ventricular contraction. This is because the strength of ventricular contraction diminishes during the last part of systole.

(20) This force reduction is evidenced by the reduced rate of blood ejection during the last part of systole.

(21) The volume and pressure in the aorta decrease as the rate of blood ejection from the ventricles becomes slower than the rate at which blood drains out of the arteries into the tissues.

Early Diastole

This phase of diastole begins as the ventricular muscle relaxes and ejection comes to an end.

(22) Recall that the T wave of the ECG corresponds to ventricular repolarization.

(23) As the ventricles relax, the ventricular pressure decreases below aortic pressure, which remains significantly elevated due to the volume of blood that just entered. The change in the pressure gradient forces the aortic valve to close. The combination of elastic recoil of the aorta and blood rebounding against the valve causes a rebound of aortic pressure called the **dicrotic notch.**

(24) The AV valve also remains closed because the ventricular pressure is still higher than atrial pressure. For a brief time, then, all valves are again closed during this phase of isovolumetric ventricular relaxation.

(25) This phase ends as the rapidly decreasing ventricular pressure decreases below atrial pressure.

(26) This change in pressure gradient results in the opening of the AV valve.

(27) Venous blood that had accumulated in the atrium since the AV valve closed flows rapidly into the ventricles.

(28) The rate of blood flow is enhanced during this initial filling phase by a rapid decrease in ventricular pressure. This occurs because the ventricle's previous contraction compressed the elastic elements of the chamber in such a way that the ventricle actually tends to recoil outward once systole is over. This expansion, in turn, lowers ventricular pressure more rapidly than would otherwise occur and may even create a negative (subatmospheric) pressure. Thus, some energy is stored within the myocardium during contraction, and its release during the subsequent relaxation aids filling.

The fact that most ventricular filling is completed during early diastole is of great importance. It ensures that filling is not seriously impaired during periods when the heart is beating very rapidly, and the duration of diastole and, therefore, total filling time are reduced. However, when heart rates of approximately 200 beats/min or more are reached, filling time becomes inadequate and the volume of blood pumped during each beat decreases. The clinical significance of this will be described in Section E.

Early ventricular filling also explains why the conduction defects that eliminate the atria as effective pumps do not seriously impair ventricular filling, at least in otherwise healthy individuals at rest. This is true, for example, of ***atrial fibrillation,*** a state in which the cells of the atria contract in a completely uncoordinated manner and so the atria fail to work as effective pumps.

Pulmonary Circulation Pressures

The pressure changes in the right ventricle and pulmonary arteries (**Figure 12.20**) are qualitatively similar to those just described for the left ventricle and aorta. There are striking quantitative differences, however. Typical pulmonary arterial systolic and diastolic pressures are 25 and 10 mmHg, respectively, compared to systemic arterial pressures of 120 and 80 mmHg. Thus, the pulmonary circulation is a low-pressure system, for reasons to be described later. This difference is clearly reflected in the ventricular anatomy—the right ventricular wall is much thinner than the left. Despite the difference in pressure during contraction, however, the stroke volumes of the two ventricles are the same.

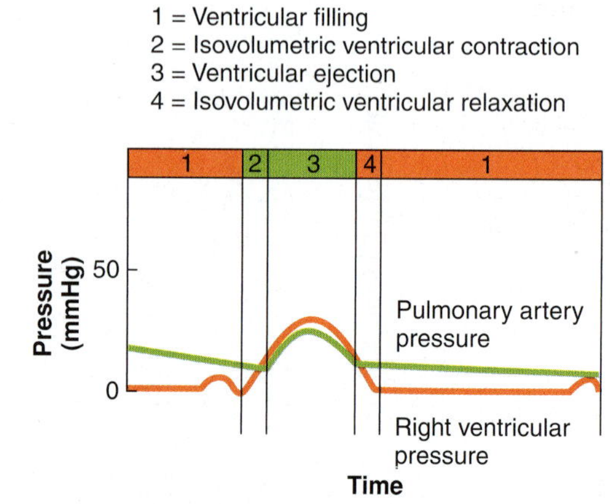

Figure 12.20 APR Pressures in the right ventricle and pulmonary artery during the cardiac cycle. Note that the pressures are lower than in the left ventricle and aorta.

PHYSIOLOGICAL INQUIRY

- If a person had a hole in the interventricular septum, would the blood ejected into the aorta have lower than normal oxygen levels?

Answer can be found at end of chapter.

Heart Sounds

Two **heart sounds** resulting from cardiac contraction are normally heard through a stethoscope placed on the chest wall. The first sound, a soft, low-pitched *lub*, is associated with closure of the AV valves; the second sound, a louder *dup*, is associated with closure of the pulmonary and aortic valves. Note in Figure 12.19 that the *lub* marks the onset of systole and the *dup* occurs at the onset of diastole. These sounds, which result from vibrations caused by the closing valves, are perfectly normal, but other sounds, known as ***heart murmurs,*** can be a sign of heart disease.

Murmurs can be produced by heart defects that cause blood flow to be turbulent. Normally, blood flow through valves and vessels is **laminar flow**—that is, it flows in smooth concentric layers (**Figure 12.21**). Turbulent flow can be caused by blood flowing rapidly in the usual direction through an abnormally narrowed valve (***stenosis***); by blood flowing backward through a damaged, leaky valve (***insufficiency***); or by blood flowing between the two atria or two ventricles through a small hole in the wall separating them (called a ***septal defect***).

The exact timing and location of the murmur provide the physician with a powerful diagnostic clue. For example, a murmur heard throughout systole suggests a stenotic pulmonary or aortic valve, an insufficient AV valve, or a hole in the interventricular septum. In contrast, a murmur heard during diastole suggests a stenotic AV valve or an insufficient pulmonary or aortic valve.

12.6 The Cardiac Output

The volume of blood each ventricle pumps as a function of time, usually expressed in liters per minute, is called the **cardiac output** (*CO*). In the steady state, the cardiac output flowing through the systemic and the pulmonary circuits is the same.

The cardiac output is calculated by multiplying the heart rate (*HR*)—the number of beats per minute—and the stroke volume (*SV*)—the blood volume ejected by each ventricle with each beat:

$$CO = HR \times SV$$

For example, if each ventricle has a rate of 72 beats/min and ejects 70 mL of blood with each beat, the cardiac output is

$$CO = 72 \text{ beats/min} \times 0.07 \text{ L/beat} = 5.0 \text{ L/min}$$

These values are typical for a resting, average-sized adult. Given that the average total blood volume is about 5.5 L, nearly all the blood is pumped around the circuit once each minute. During periods of strenuous exercise in well-trained athletes, the cardiac output may reach 35 L/min; the entire blood volume is pumped around the circuit almost seven times per minute! Even sedentary, untrained individuals can reach cardiac outputs of 20–25 L/min during exercise.

The following description of the factors that alter the two determinants of cardiac output—heart rate and stroke volume—applies in all respects to both the right and left sides of the heart because stroke volume and heart rate are the same for both under steady-state conditions. Heart rate and stroke volume do not always change in the same direction. For example, stroke volume decreases following blood loss, whereas heart rate increases. These changes produce opposing effects on cardiac output.

Control of Heart Rate

Rhythmic beating of the heart at a rate of approximately 100 beats/min will occur in the complete absence of any nervous or hormonal influences on the SA node. This is the inherent autonomous discharge rate of the SA node. The heart rate may be slower or faster than this, however, because the SA node is normally under the constant influence of nerves and hormones.

A large number of parasympathetic and sympathetic postganglionic neurons end on the SA node. Activity in the parasympathetic neurons (which travel within the vagus nerve) causes the heart rate to decrease, whereas activity in the sympathetic neurons causes an increase. In the resting state, there is considerably more parasympathetic activity to the heart than sympathetic, so the normal resting heart rate of about 70 beats/min is well below the inherent rate of 100 beats/min.

Figure 12.22 illustrates how sympathetic and parasympathetic activity influence SA node function. Sympathetic stimulation increases the slope of the pacemaker potential by increasing the F-type channel permeability. Because the

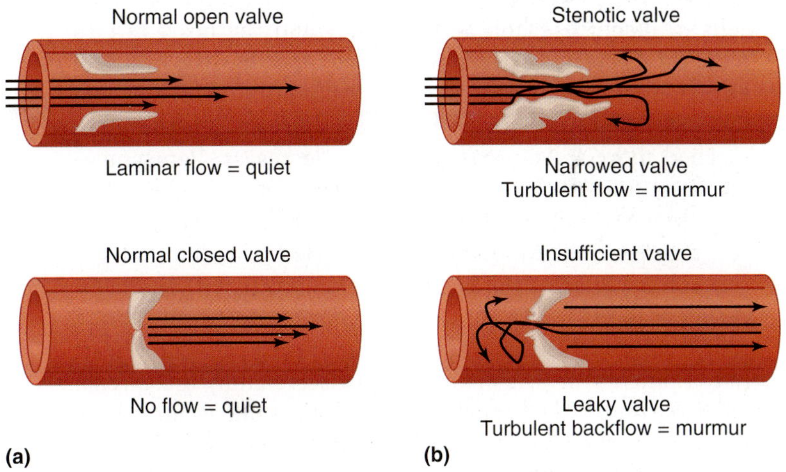

Figure 12.21 Heart valve defects causing turbulent blood flow and murmurs. (a) Normal valves allow smooth, laminar flow of blood in the forward direction when open and prevent backward flow of blood when closed. No sound is heard in either state. (b) Stenotic valves cause rapid, turbulent forward flow of blood, making a high-pitched, whistling murmur. Valve insufficiency results in turbulent backward flow when the valve should be closed, causing a low-pitched gurgling murmur.

PHYSIOLOGICAL INQUIRY

- What valve defect(s) would be indicated by the following sequence of heart sounds: *lub-whistle-dup-gurgle?*

Answer can be found at end of chapter.

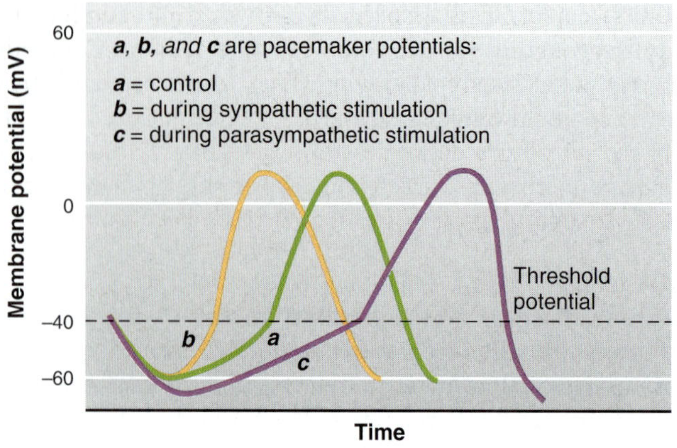

Figure 12.22 Effects of sympathetic and parasympathetic nerve stimulation on the slope of the pacemaker potential of an SA nodal cell. Note that parasympathetic stimulation not only reduces the slope of the pacemaker potential but also causes the membrane potential to be more negative before the pacemaker potential begins. Adapted from Hoffman and Cranefield.

PHYSIOLOGICAL INQUIRY

- Parasympathetic stimulation also increases the delay between atrial and ventricular contractions. What is the ionic mechanism?

Answer can be found at end of chapter.

main current through these channels is Na^+ entering the cell, faster depolarization results. This causes the SA node cells to reach threshold more rapidly and the heart rate to increase. Increasing parasympathetic input has the opposite effect—the slope of the pacemaker potential decreases due to a reduction in the inward current. Threshold is therefore reached more slowly, and heart rate decreases. Parasympathetic stimulation also hyperpolarizes the plasma membranes of SA node cells by increasing their permeability to K^+. The pacemaker potential thus starts from a more negative value (closer to the K^+ equilibrium potential) and has a reduced slope.

Factors other than the cardiac nerves can also alter heart rate. Epinephrine, the main hormone secreted by the adrenal medulla, speeds the heart by acting on the same β-adrenergic receptors in the SA node as norepinephrine released from neurons. The heart rate is also sensitive to changes in body temperature, plasma electrolyte concentrations, hormones other than epinephrine, and adenosine—a metabolite produced by myocardial cells. These factors are normally of lesser importance, however, than the cardiac nerves. **Figure 12.23** summarizes the major determinants of heart rate.

As stated in the previous section on innervation, sympathetic and parasympathetic neurons innervate not only the SA node but other parts of the conducting system as well. Sympathetic stimulation increases conduction velocity through the entire cardiac conducting system, whereas parasympathetic stimulation decreases the rate of spread of excitation through the atria and the AV node. Autonomic regulation of heart rate is one of the best examples of the general principle of physiology that most physiological

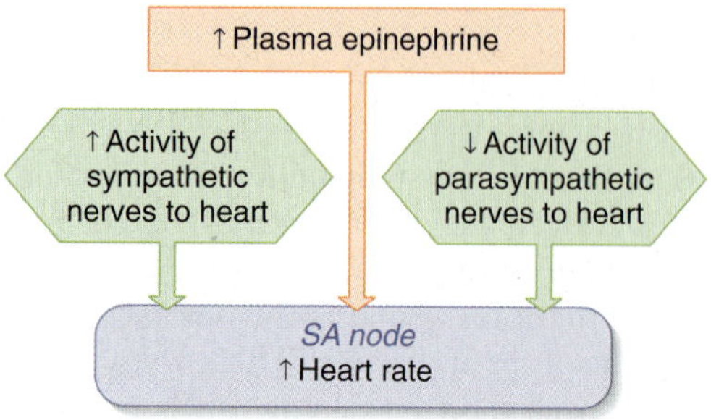

Figure 12.23 Major factors influencing heart rate. All effects are exerted upon the SA node. The figure shows how heart rate is increased; reversal of all the arrows in the boxes would illustrate how heart rate is decreased.

functions are controlled by multiple regulatory systems, often working in opposition.

Control of Stroke Volume

The second variable that determines cardiac output is stroke volume—the volume of blood each ventricle ejects during each contraction. Recall that the ventricles do not completely empty themselves during contraction. Therefore, a more forceful contraction can produce an increase in stroke volume by causing greater emptying. Changes in the force during ejection of the stroke volume can be produced by a variety of factors, but three are dominant under most physiological and pathophysiological conditions: (1) changes in the end-diastolic volume (the volume of blood in the ventricles just before contraction, sometimes referred to as the **preload**); (2) changes in the magnitude of sympathetic nervous system input to the ventricles; and (3) changes in **afterload** (i.e., the arterial pressures against which the ventricles pump).

Relationship Between Ventricular End-Diastolic Volume and Stroke Volume: The Frank–Starling Mechanism

The mechanical properties of cardiac muscle form the basis for an inherent mechanism for altering the strength of contraction and stroke volume; the ventricle contracts more forcefully during systole when it has been filled to a greater degree during diastole. In other words, all other factors being equal, the stroke volume increases as the end-diastolic volume increases. This is illustrated graphically as a **ventricular-function curve** (**Figure 12.24**). This relationship between stroke volume and end-diastolic volume is known as the **Frank–Starling mechanism** (also called *Starling's law of the heart*) in recognition of the two physiologists who identified it.

What accounts for the Frank–Starling mechanism? Basically, it is a length–tension relationship, as described for skeletal muscle in Figure 9.21, because end-diastolic volume is a major determinant of how stretched the ventricular sarcomeres are just before contraction: The greater the end-diastolic volume, the greater the stretch and the more forceful the contraction. However, a comparison of Figure 12.24 with Figure 9.21 reveals an important difference in the length–tension relationship between skeletal and cardiac muscle. The normal point for cardiac muscle in a resting individual is not at its optimal length for contraction, as it is for most resting

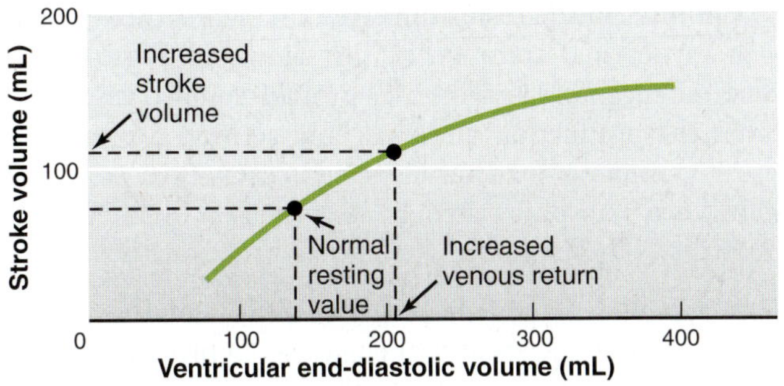

Figure 12.24 A ventricular-function curve, which expresses the relationship between end-diastolic ventricular volume and stroke volume (the Frank–Starling mechanism). The horizontal axis could have been labeled "sarcomere length" and the vertical "contractile force." In other words, this is a length–tension curve, analogous to that for skeletal muscle (see Figure 9.21). At very high volumes, force (and, therefore, stroke volume) declines as in skeletal muscle (not shown).

skeletal muscles, but is on the rising phase of the curve. For this reason, greater filling causes additional stretching of the cardiac muscle fibers and increases the force of contraction.

The mechanisms linking changes in muscle length to changes in muscle force are more complex in cardiac muscle than in skeletal muscle. In addition to changing the overlap of thick and thin filaments, stretching cardiac muscle cells toward their optimum length decreases the spacing between thick and thin filaments (allowing more cross-bridges to bind during a twitch), increases the sensitivity of troponin for binding Ca^{2+}, and increases Ca^{2+} release from the sarcoplasmic reticulum.

The significance of the Frank–Starling mechanism is as follows: At any given heart rate, an increase in the **venous return**—the flow of blood from the veins into the heart—automatically forces an increase in cardiac output by increasing end-diastolic volume and, therefore, stroke volume. One important function of this relationship is maintaining the equality of right and left cardiac outputs. For example, if the right side of the heart suddenly begins to pump more blood than the left, the increased blood flow returning to the left ventricle will automatically produce an increase in left ventricular output. This ensures that blood will not accumulate in the pulmonary circulation.

Sympathetic Regulation

Sympathetic nerves are distributed to the entire myocardium. The sympathetic neurotransmitter norepinephrine acts on β-adrenergic receptors to increase ventricular **contractility,** defined as the strength of contraction *at any given end-diastolic volume.* Plasma epinephrine acting on these receptors also increases myocardial contractility. Thus, the increased force of contraction and stroke volume resulting from sympathetic nerve stimulation or epinephrine are independent of a change in end-diastolic ventricular volume.

A change in contraction force due to increased end-diastolic volume (the Frank–Starling mechanism) does not reflect increased contractility. Increased contractility is specifically defined as an increased contraction force at *any* given end-diastolic volume.

The distinction between the Frank–Starling mechanism and sympathetic stimulation is illustrated in **Figure 12.25a.** The green ventricular-function curve is the same as that shown in Figure 12.24. The orange ventricular-function curve was

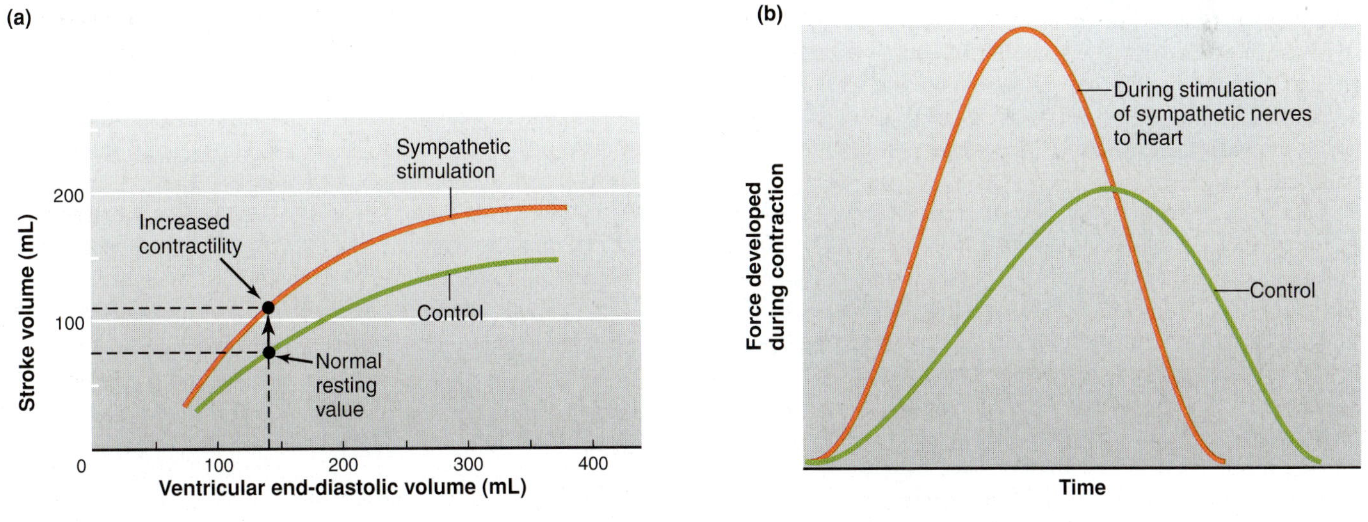

Figure 12.25 Sympathetic stimulation causes increased contractility of ventricular muscle. (a) Stroke volume is increased at any given end-diastolic volume. (b) Both the rate of force development and the rate of relaxation increase, as does the maximum force developed.

PHYSIOLOGICAL INQUIRY

- Estimate the ejection fraction and end-systolic volumes under control and sympathetic stimulation conditions at an end-diastolic volume of 140 mL.

Answer can be found at end of chapter.

obtained for the same heart during sympathetic nerve stimulation. The Frank–Starling mechanism still applies, but during sympathetic stimulation, the stroke volume is greater at any given end-diastolic volume. In other words, the increased contractility leads to a more complete ejection of the end-diastolic ventricular volume.

One way to quantify contractility is through the **ejection fraction** (***EF***), defined as the ratio of stroke volume (*SV*) to end-diastolic volume (*EDV*):

$$EF = SV/EDV$$

Expressed as a percentage, the ejection fraction normally averages between 50% and 75% under resting conditions. Increased contractility causes an increased ejection fraction.

Not only does increased sympathetic stimulation of the myocardium cause a more powerful contraction, it also causes both the contraction and relaxation of the ventricles to occur more quickly (**Figure 12.25b**). These latter effects are quite important because, as described earlier, increased sympathetic activity to the heart also increases heart rate. As heart rate increases, the time available for diastolic filling decreases, but the quicker contraction and relaxation induced simultaneously by the sympathetic neurons partially compensate for this problem by permitting a larger fraction of the cardiac cycle to be available for filling.

Cellular mechanisms involved in sympathetic regulation of myocardial contractility are shown in **Figure 12.26**. Adrenergic receptors activate a G-protein-coupled cascade that includes the production of cAMP and activation of a protein kinase. A number of proteins involved in excitation–contraction coupling are phosphorylated by the kinase, which enhances contractility. These proteins include

1. L-type Ca^{2+} channels in the plasma membrane;
2. the ryanodine receptor and associated proteins in the sarcoplasmic reticulum membrane;
3. thin filament proteins—in particular, troponin;
4. thick filament proteins associated with the cross-bridges; and
5. proteins involved in pumping Ca^{2+} back into the sarcoplasmic reticulum.

Due to these alterations, cytosolic Ca^{2+} concentration increases more quickly and reaches a greater value during excitation, Ca^{2+} returns to its pre-excitation value more quickly following excitation, and the rates of cross-bridge activation and cycling are accelerated. The net result is the stronger, faster contraction observed during sympathetic activation of the heart.

There is little parasympathetic innervation of the ventricles, so the parasympathetic system normally has a negligible direct effect on ventricular contractility.

Table 12.3 summarizes the effects of the autonomic nerves on cardiac function.

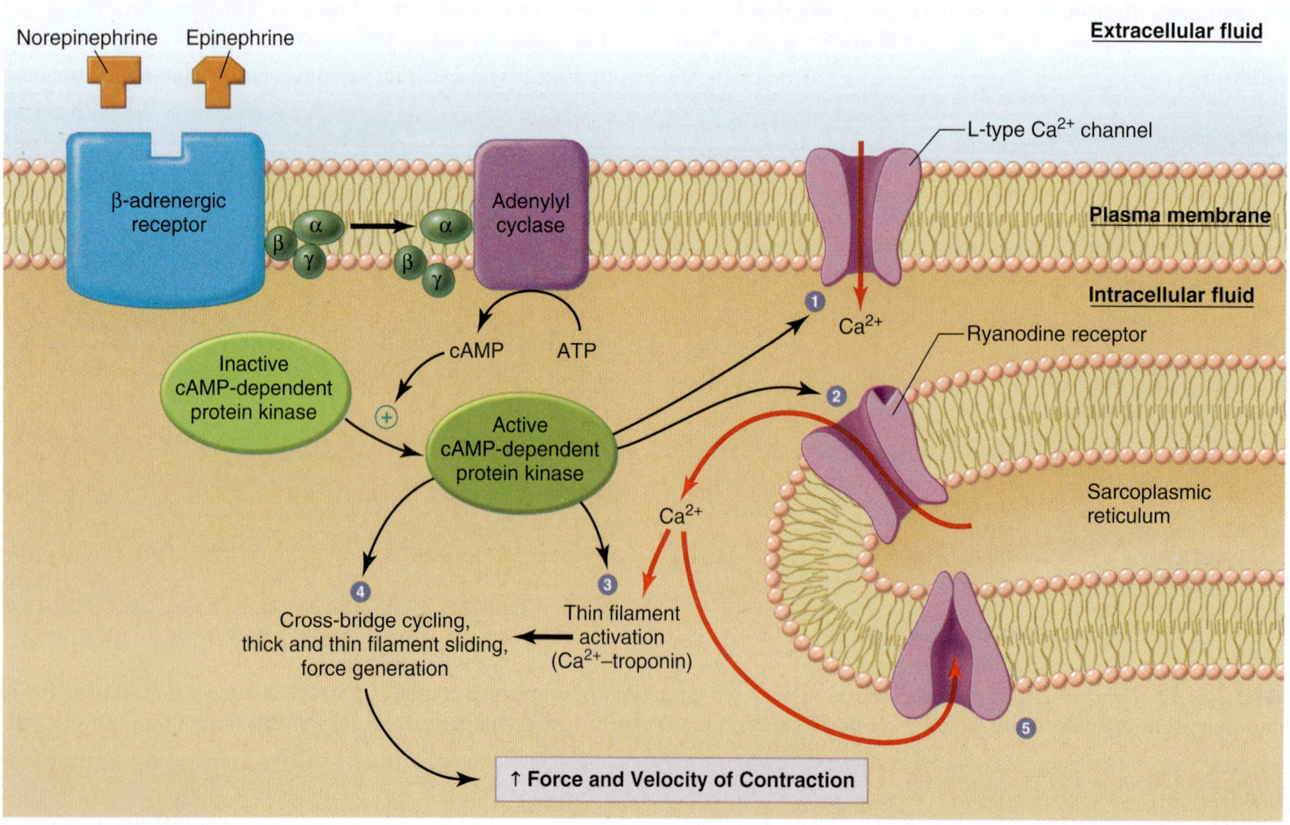

Figure 12.26 APIR Mechanisms of sympathetic effects on cardiac muscle cell contractility. In some of the pathways, the kinase phosphorylates accessory proteins that are not shown.

TABLE 12.3 Effects of Autonomic Nerves on the Heart		
Area Affected	**Sympathetic Nerves (Norepinephrine on β-Adrenergic Receptors)**	**Parasympathetic Nerves (ACh on Muscarinic Receptors)**
SA node	Increased heart rate	Decreased heart rate
AV node	Increased conduction rate	Decreased conduction rate
Atrial muscle	Increased contractility	Decreased contractility
Ventricular muscle	Increased contractility	No significant effect

Afterload

An increased arterial pressure tends to reduce stroke volume. This is because, like a skeletal muscle lifting a weight, the arterial pressure constitutes a "load" that contracting ventricular muscle must work against when it is ejecting blood. A term used to describe how hard the heart must work to eject blood is *afterload.* The greater the load, the less contracting muscle fibers can shorten at a given contractility (review Figure 9.17). This factor will not be dealt with further, because in the normal heart, several inherent adjustments minimize the overall influence of arterial pressure on stroke volume. However, in the sections on high blood pressure and heart failure, we will see that alterations in vascular resistance and long-term elevations of arterial pressure can weaken the heart and thereby influence stroke volume.

Figure 12.27 integrates the factors that determine stroke volume and heart rate into a summary of the control of cardiac output.

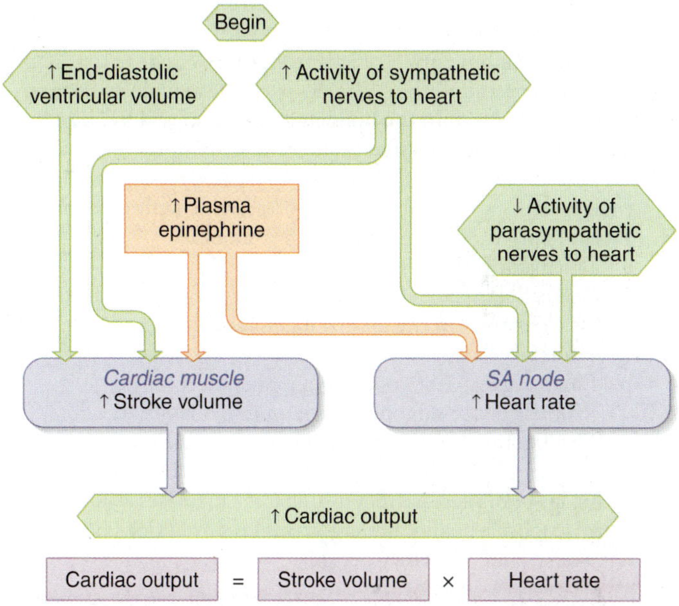

Figure 12.27 Major factors determining cardiac output. Reversal of all arrows in the boxes would illustrate how cardiac output is decreased.

PHYSIOLOGICAL INQUIRY

- Recall from Figure 12.9 that parasympathetic nerves do not innervate the ventricles. Is it therefore impossible for parasympathetic activity to influence stroke volume?

Answer can be found at end of chapter.

12.7 Measurement of Cardiac Function

Human cardiac output and heart function can be measured by a variety of methods. For example, ***echocardiography*** can be used to obtain two- and three-dimensional images of the heart throughout the entire cardiac cycle. In this procedure, ultrasonic waves are beamed at the heart and returning echoes are electronically plotted by computer to produce continuous images of the heart. It can detect the abnormal functioning of cardiac valves or contractions of the cardiac walls, and it can also be used to measure ejection fraction.

Echocardiography is a noninvasive technique because everything used remains external to the body. Other visualization techniques are invasive. One, ***cardiac angiography,*** requires the temporary threading of a thin, flexible tube called a catheter through an artery or vein into the heart. A liquid containing radiopaque contrast material is then injected through the catheter during high-speed x-ray videography. This technique is useful not only for evaluating cardiac function but also for identifying narrowed coronary arteries.

SECTION B SUMMARY

Anatomy

I. The atrioventricular (AV) valves prevent flow from the ventricles back into the atria.

II. The pulmonary and aortic valves prevent backflow from the pulmonary trunk into the right ventricle and from the aorta into the left ventricle, respectively.

III. Cardiac muscle cells are joined by gap junctions that permit the conduction of action potentials from cell to cell.

IV. The myocardium also contains specialized cells that constitute the conducting system of the heart, initiating cardiac action potentials and speeding their spread through the heart.

Heartbeat Coordination

I. Action potentials must be initiated in cardiac cells for contraction to occur.
   a. The rapid depolarization of the action potential in atrial and ventricular muscle cells is due mainly to a positive feedback increase in Na^+ permeability.
   b. Following the initial rapid depolarization, the cardiac muscle cell membrane remains depolarized (the plateau phase) for almost the entire duration of the contraction because of prolonged entry of Ca^{2+} into the cell through plasma membrane L-type Ca^{2+} channels.

II. The SA node generates the action potential that leads to depolarization of all other cardiac cells.
   a. The SA node manifests a pacemaker potential involving F-type cation channels and T-type Ca^{2+} channels, which brings its membrane potential to threshold and initiates an action potential.
   b. The action potential spreads from the SA node throughout both atria and to the AV node, where a small delay occurs. It then passes into the bundle of His, right and left bundle branches, Purkinje fibers, and ventricular muscle cells.

III. Ca^{2+}, mainly released from the sarcoplasmic reticulum (SR), functions in cardiac excitation–contraction coupling, as in skeletal muscle, by combining with troponin.
   a. The major signal for Ca^{2+} release from the SR is extracellular Ca^{2+} entering through voltage-gated L-type Ca^{2+} channels in the plasma membrane during the action potential.
   b. This "trigger" Ca^{2+} opens ryanodine receptor Ca^{2+} channels in the sarcoplasmic reticulum membrane.
   c. The amount of Ca^{2+} released does not usually saturate all troponin binding sites, so the number of active cross-bridges can increase if cytosolic Ca^{2+} increases still further.

IV. Cardiac muscle cannot undergo tetanic contractions because it has a very long refractory period.

Mechanical Events of the Cardiac Cycle

I. The cardiac cycle is divided into systole (ventricular contraction) and diastole (ventricular relaxation).
   a. At the onset of systole, ventricular pressure rapidly exceeds atrial pressure and the AV valves close. The aortic and pulmonary valves are not yet open, however, so no ejection occurs during this isovolumetric ventricular contraction.
   b. When ventricular pressures exceed aortic and pulmonary trunk pressures, the aortic and pulmonary valves open and the ventricles eject the blood.
   c. When the ventricles relax at the beginning of diastole, the ventricular pressures decrease significantly below those in the aorta and pulmonary trunk and the aortic and pulmonary valves close. Because the AV valves are also still closed, no change in ventricular volume occurs during this isovolumetric ventricular relaxation.
   d. When ventricular pressures decrease below the pressures in the right and the left atria, the AV valves open and the ventricular filling phase of diastole begins.
   e. Filling occurs very rapidly at first so that atrial contraction, which occurs at the very end of diastole, usually adds only a small amount of additional blood to the ventricles.

II. The amount of blood in the ventricles just before systole is the end-diastolic volume. The volume remaining after ejection is the end-systolic volume, and the volume ejected is the stroke volume.

III. Pressure changes in the systemic and pulmonary circulations have similar patterns, but the pulmonary pressures are much lower.

IV. The first heart sound is due to the closing of the AV valves, and the second is due to the closing of the aortic and pulmonary valves.

V. Murmurs can result from narrowed or leaky valves, as well as from holes in the interventricular septum.

The Cardiac Output

I. The cardiac output is the volume of blood each ventricle pumps per unit time, and equals the product of heart rate and stroke volume.
   a. Heart rate is increased by stimulation of the sympathetic neurons to the heart and by epinephrine; it is decreased by stimulation of the parasympathetic neurons to the heart.
   b. Stroke volume is increased mainly by an increase in end-diastolic volume (the Frank–Starling mechanism) and by an increase in contractility due to sympathetic stimulation or to epinephrine. Increased afterload can reduce stroke volume in certain situations.

Measurement of Cardiac Function

I. Methods of measuring cardiac function include echocardiography, for assessing wall and valve function, and cardiac angiography, for determining coronary blood flow.

SECTION B REVIEW QUESTIONS

1. List the structures through which blood passes from the systemic veins to the systemic arteries.
2. Contrast and compare the structure of cardiac muscle with that of skeletal and smooth muscle.
3. Describe the autonomic innervation of the heart, including the types of receptors involved.
4. Draw a ventricular muscle cell action potential. Describe the changes in membrane permeability that underlie the membrane potential changes.
5. Contrast action potentials in ventricular muscle cells with SA node action potentials. What is the pacemaker potential due to, and what is its inherent rate? By what mechanism does the SA node function as the pacemaker for the entire heart?
6. Describe the spread of excitation from the SA node through the rest of the heart.
7. Draw and label a normal ECG. Relate the P, QRS, and T waves to the atrial and ventricular action potentials.
8. Explain how the electrical activity of the heart can be viewed from different angles with electrocardiography.
9. What prevents the heart from undergoing summation of contractions?
10. Draw a diagram of the pressure changes in the left atrium, left ventricle, and aorta throughout the cardiac cycle. Show when the valves open and close, when the heart sounds occur, and the pattern of ventricular ejection.
11. Contrast the pressures in the right ventricle and pulmonary trunk with those in the left ventricle and aorta.
12. What causes heart murmurs in diastole? In systole?
13. Write the formula relating cardiac output, heart rate, and stroke volume; give normal values for a resting adult.
14. Describe the effects of sympathetic and parasympathetic neuronal stimulation on heart rate. Which is dominant at rest?
15. What are the major factors influencing force of contraction?
16. Draw a ventricular-function curve illustrating the Frank–Starling mechanism.

17. Describe the effects of sympathetic neuron stimulation on cardiac muscle during contraction and relaxation.
18. Draw a pair of curves relating end-diastolic volume and stroke volume, with and without sympathetic stimulation.
19. Summarize the effects of the autonomic nervous system on the heart.
20. Draw a flow diagram summarizing the factors determining cardiac output.

SECTION B KEY TERMS

SECTION B CLINICAL TERMS

SECTION C The Vascular System

Although the action of the muscular heart provides the overall driving force for blood movement, the vascular system plays an active role in regulating blood pressure and distributing blood flow to the various tissues. Elaborate branching and regional specializations of blood vessels enable efficient matching of blood flow to metabolic demand in individual tissues. This section will highlight repeatedly the general principle of physiology that structure is a determinant of function, as we examine the specialization of the different types of vessels that comprise the vascular system.

The structural characteristics of the blood vessels vary by region, as shown in **Figure 12.28**. However, the entire circulatory system, from the heart to the smallest capillary, has one structural component in common: a smooth, single-celled layer of endothelial cells (endothelium) that is in contact with the flowing blood. Capillaries consist only of endothelium and associated extracellular basement membrane, whereas all other vessels have one or more layers of connective tissue and smooth muscle. Endothelial cells have a large number of functions, which are summarized for reference in **Table 12.4** and are described in relevant sections of this chapter and others.

We have previously described the pressures in the aorta and pulmonary arteries during the cardiac cycle. **Figure 12.29** illustrates the pressure changes that occur along the rest of the systemic and pulmonary circulations. Text sections dealing with the individual vascular segments will describe the reasons for these changes in pressure. For the moment, note only that by the time the blood has completed its journey back to the atrium in each circuit, most of the pressure originally generated by the ventricular contraction has dissipated. The reason the average pressure at any point in the two circuits is lower than that upstream toward the heart is that the blood vessels offer resistance to the flow from one point to the next (review Figure 12.5).

12.8 Arteries

The aorta and other systemic arteries have thick walls containing large quantities of elastic tissue (see Figure 12.28). Although they also have smooth muscle, arteries can be viewed most conveniently as elastic tubes. The large radii of arteries suit their primary function of serving as low-resistance tubes conducting blood to the various organs. Their second major function, related to their elasticity, is to act as a "pressure reservoir" for maintaining blood flow through the tissues during diastole, as described next.

Arterial Blood Pressure

What are the factors determining the pressure within an elastic container, such as a balloon filled with water? The pressure inside the balloon depends on (1) the volume of water and (2) how easily the balloon can stretch. If the balloon is thin and stretchable, large quantities of water can be added with only a small increase in pressure. Conversely, the addition of even a small quantity of water causes a large pressure increase

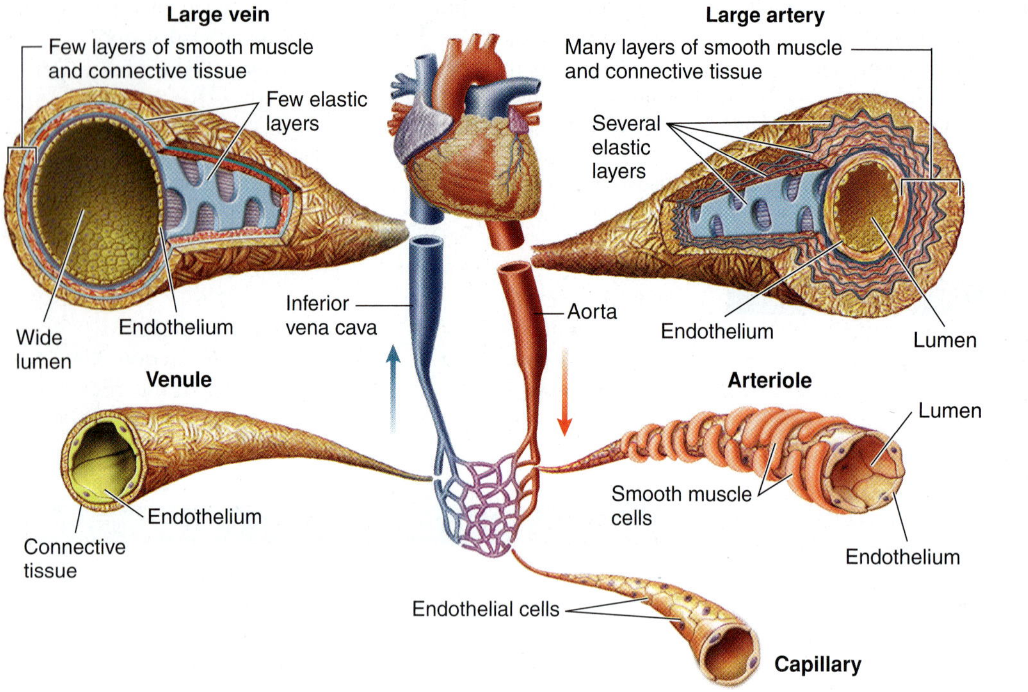

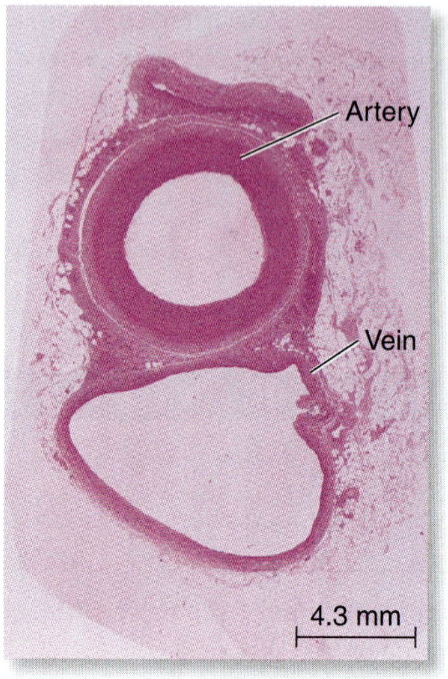

Figure 12.28 APR Comparative features of blood vessels. Sizes are not drawn to scale. *Inset:* Light micrograph (enlarged four times) of a medium-sized artery near a vein. Note the difference between the two vessels in wall thickness and lumen diameter.

TABLE 12.4 Functions of Endothelial Cells
Serve as a physical lining that blood cells do not normally adhere to in heart and blood vessels
Serve as a permeability barrier for the exchange of nutrients, metabolic end products, and fluid between plasma and interstitial fluid; regulate transport of macromolecules and other substances
Secrete paracrine agents that act on adjacent vascular smooth muscle cells, including vasodilators such as prostacyclin and nitric oxide (endothelium-derived relaxing factor [EDRF]), and vasoconstrictors such as endothelin-1
Mediate angiogenesis (new capillary growth)
Play a central role in vascular remodeling by detecting signals and releasing paracrine agents that act on adjacent cells in the blood vessel wall
Contribute to the formation and maintenance of extracellular matrix
Produce growth factors in response to damage
Secrete substances that regulate platelet clumping, clotting, and anticlotting
Synthesize active hormones from inactive precursors (Chapter 14)
Extract or degrade hormones and other mediators (Chapters 11, 13)
Secrete cytokines during immune responses (Chapter 18)
Influence vascular smooth muscle proliferation in the disease atherosclerosis (Chapter 12, Section E)

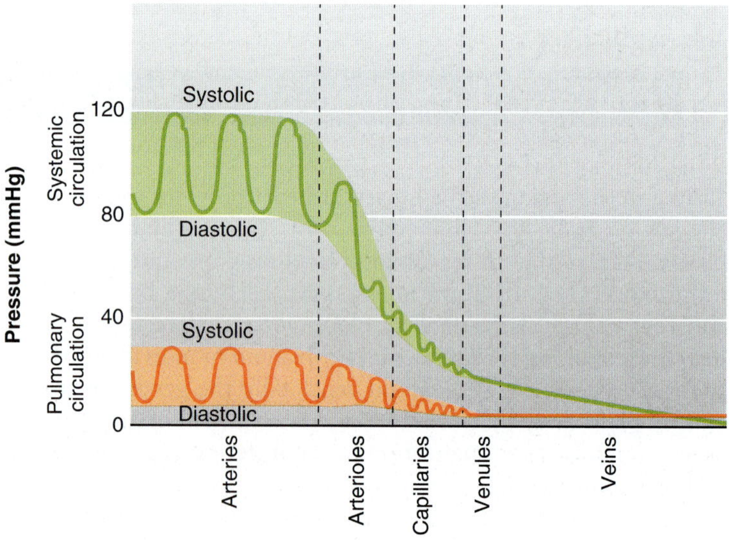

Figure 12.29 Pressures in the systemic and pulmonary vessels.

in a balloon that is thick and difficult to stretch. The term used to denote how easily a structure stretches is **compliance:**

$$\text{Compliance} = \Delta\text{Volume}/\Delta\text{Pressure}$$

The greater the compliance of a structure, the more easily it can be stretched.

These principles apply to an analysis of arterial blood pressure. The contraction of the ventricles ejects blood into the arteries during systole. If a precisely equal quantity of blood were to simultaneously drain out of the arteries into the arterioles during systole, the total volume of blood in the arteries would remain constant and arterial pressure would not change.

Such is not the case, however. As shown in **Figure 12.30**, a volume of blood equal to only about one-third of the stroke volume leaves the arteries during systole. The rest of the stroke volume remains in the arteries during systole, distending them and increasing the arterial pressure. When ventricular contraction ends, the stretched arterial walls recoil passively like a deflating balloon, and blood continues to be driven into the arterioles during diastole. As blood leaves the arteries, the arterial volume and pressure slowly decrease. The next ventricular contraction occurs while the artery walls are still stretched by the remaining blood. Therefore, the arterial pressure does not decrease to zero.

The aortic pressure pattern shown in **Figure 12.31a** is typical of the pressure changes that occur in all the large systemic arteries. The maximum arterial pressure reached during peak ventricular ejection is called **systolic pressure** (*SP*). The minimum arterial pressure occurs just before ventricular ejection begins and is called **diastolic pressure** (*DP*). Arterial pressure is generally recorded as systolic/diastolic, which would be 120/80 mmHg in the example shown. See **Figure 12.31b** for average values at different ages in the population of the United States. Both systolic pressure and diastolic pressure average about 10 mmHg lower in females than in males.

The difference between systolic pressure and diastolic pressure (120 − 80 = 40 mmHg in the example) is called the **pulse pressure.** It can be felt as a pulsation or throb in the arteries of the wrist or neck with each heartbeat. During diastole, nothing is felt over the artery, but the rapid increase in pressure at the next systole pushes out the artery wall; it is this expansion of the vessel that produces the detectable pulse.

The most important factors determining the magnitude of the pulse pressure are (1) stroke volume, (2) speed of ejection of the stroke volume, and (3) arterial compliance. Specifically, the pulse pressure produced by a ventricular ejection is greater if the volume of blood ejected increases, if the speed at which it is ejected increases, or if the arteries are less compliant. This last phenomenon occurs in ***arteriosclerosis***, a stiffening of the arteries that progresses with age and accounts for the increasing pulse pressure that often occurs in older people (see Figure 12.31b).

It is evident from Figure 12.31a that arterial pressure is continuously changing throughout the cardiac cycle. The average pressure during the cycle, referred to as the **mean arterial pressure** (*MAP*), is not merely the value halfway between systolic pressure and diastolic pressure, because diastole lasts about twice as long as systole. The exact mean arterial pressure can be obtained by complex mathematical methods, but

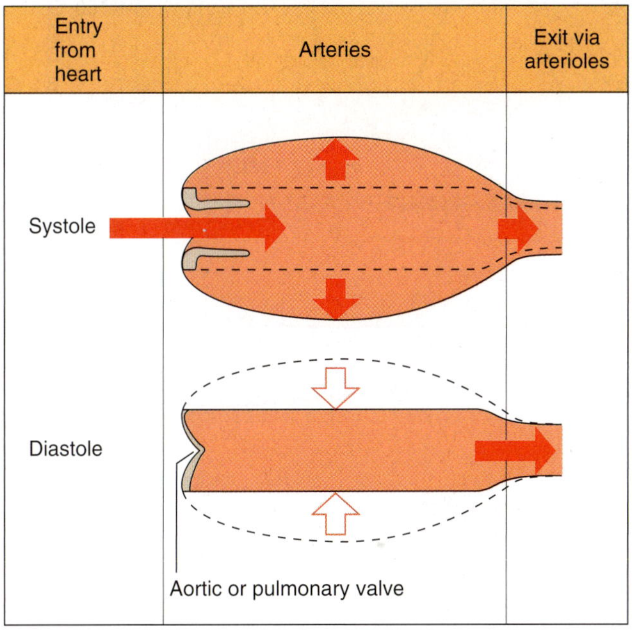

Figure 12.30 Movement of blood into and out of the arteries during the cardiac cycle. The lengths of the arrows denote relative quantities flowing into and out of the arteries and remaining in the arteries.

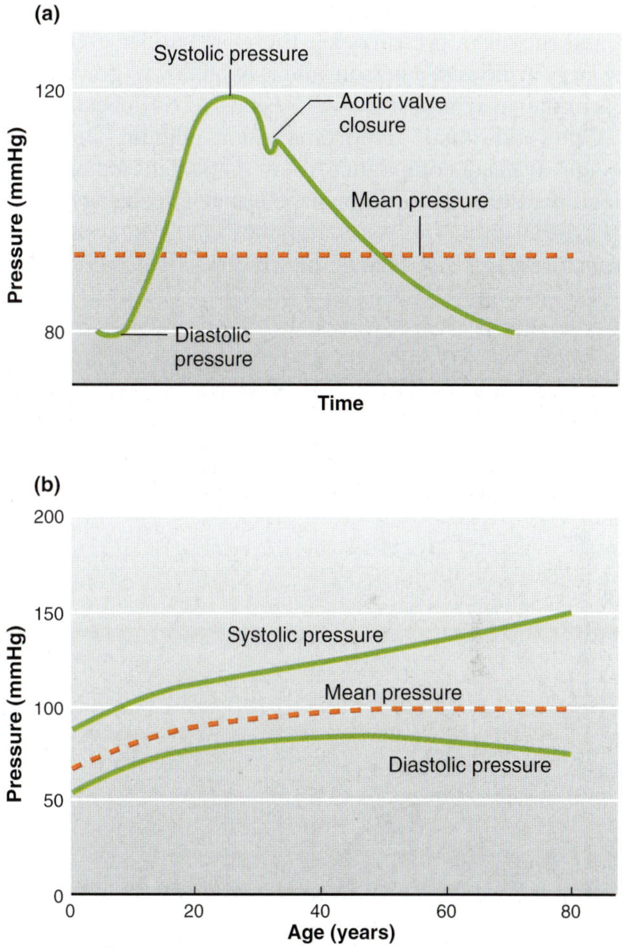

Figure 12.31 (a) Typical arterial pressure fluctuations during the cardiac cycle for a young adult male. Pressures average about 10 mmHg lower in females. (b) Changes in arterial pressure with age in the U.S. population. Adapted from National Institutes of Health Publication #04-5230, August 2004.

PHYSIOLOGICAL INQUIRY

- At an elevated heart rate, the amount of time spent in diastole is reduced more than the amount of time spent in systole. How would you estimate the mean arterial blood pressure at a heart rate elevated to the point at which the times spent in systole and diastole are roughly equal?

Answer can be found at end of chapter.

at a typical resting heart rate it is approximately equal to the diastolic pressure plus one-third of the pulse pressure:

$$MAP = DP + \frac{1}{3}(SP - DP)$$

Thus, in Figure 12.31a,

$$MAP = 80 + \frac{1}{3}(40) = 93 \text{ mmHg}$$

The *MAP* is important because it is the pressure driving blood into the tissues averaged over the entire cardiac cycle. We can say mean "arterial" pressure without specifying which artery we are referring to because the aorta and other large arteries have such large diameters that they offer negligible resistance to flow, and the mean pressures are therefore similar everywhere in the large arteries of a person who is lying down (gravitational effects in the upright posture will be considered in Section E).

One additional important point should be made: Although arterial compliance is an important determinant of pulse pressure, it does not have a major influence on the mean arterial pressure. As compliance changes, systolic and diastolic pressures also change but in opposite directions. For example, a person with a low arterial compliance (due to arteriosclerosis) but an otherwise normal cardiovascular system will have a large pulse pressure due to elevated systolic pressure and lowered diastolic pressure. The net result, however, is a mean arterial pressure that is close to normal. Pulse pressure is therefore a better diagnostic indicator of arteriosclerosis than mean arterial pressure. The determinants of mean arterial pressure are described in Section D. The method for measuring blood pressure is described next.

Measurement of Systemic Arterial Pressure

Both systolic and diastolic blood pressures are readily measured in human beings with the use of a device called a sphygmomanometer. An inflatable cuff containing a pressure gauge is wrapped around the upper arm, and a stethoscope is placed over the brachial artery just below the cuff.

The cuff is then inflated with air to a pressure greater than systolic blood pressure (**Figure 12.32**). The high pressure in the cuff is transmitted through the tissue of the arm and completely compresses the artery under the cuff, thereby preventing blood flow through the artery. The air in the cuff is then slowly released, causing the pressure in the cuff and on the artery to decrease. When cuff pressure has decreased

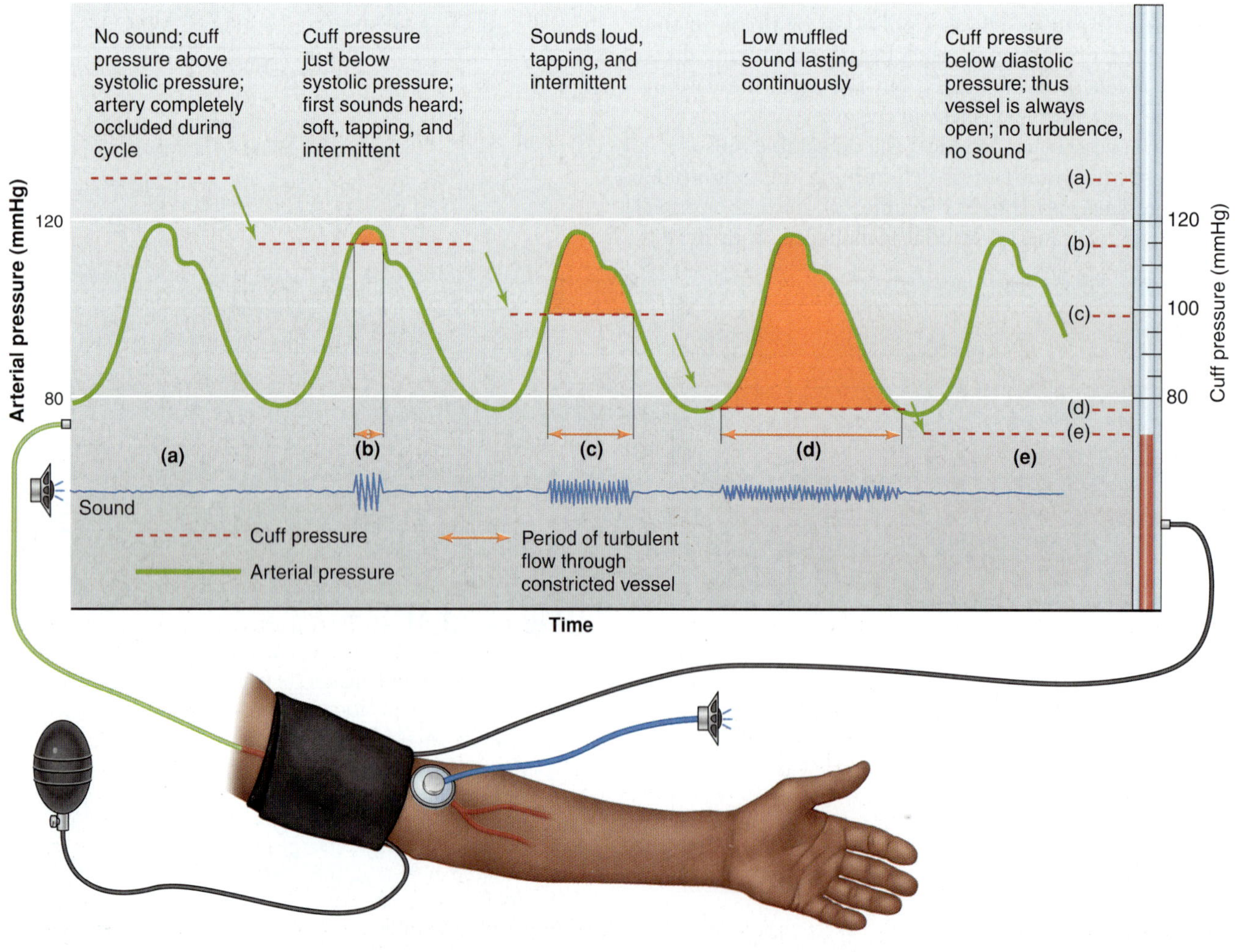

Figure 12.32 Sounds heard through a stethoscope as the cuff pressure of a sphygmomanometer is gradually lowered. Sounds are first heard when cuff falls just below systolic pressure, and they cease when cuff pressure falls below diastolic pressure.

to a value just below the systolic pressure, the artery opens slightly and allows blood flow for a brief time at the peak of systole. During this interval, the blood flow through the partially compressed artery occurs at a very high velocity because of the small opening and the large pressure difference across the opening. The high-velocity blood flow is turbulent and, therefore, produces vibrations called **Korotkoff's sounds** that can be heard through the stethoscope. Thus, the pressure at which sounds are first heard as the cuff pressure decreases is identified as the systolic blood pressure.

As the pressure in the cuff decreases further, the duration of blood flow through the artery in each cycle becomes longer. When the cuff pressure reaches the diastolic blood pressure, all sound stops because flow is continuous and nonturbulent through the open artery. Therefore, diastolic pressure is identified as the cuff pressure at which sounds disappear.

It should be clear from this description that the sounds heard during measurement of blood pressure are not the same as the heart sounds described earlier, which are due to closing of cardiac valves.

12.9 Arterioles

The arterioles play two major roles. (1) The arterioles in individual organs are responsible for determining the relative blood flows to those organs at any given mean arterial pressure. (2) The arterioles, all together, are the major factor in determining mean arterial pressure itself. The first function will be described now and the second in Section D.

Figure 12.33 illustrates the major principles of blood-flow distribution in terms of a simple model, a fluid-filled tank with a series of compressible outflow tubes. What determines the rate of flow through each exit tube? As stated in Section A of this chapter, flow (*F*) is a function of the pressure gradient (ΔP) and the resistance to flow (*R*):

$$F = \Delta P/R$$

Because the driving pressure (the height of the fluid column in the tank) is identical for each tube, differences in flow are completely determined by differences in the resistance to flow offered by each tube. The lengths of the tubes are the same and the viscosity of the fluid is constant, so differences in resistance are due solely to differences in the radii of the tubes. The widest tubes have the lowest resistance and, therefore, the greatest flows. If the radius of each tube can be independently altered, the blood flow through each is independently controlled.

This analysis can now be applied to the circulatory system. The tank is analogous to the major arteries, which serve as a pressure reservoir but are so large that they contribute little resistance to flow. Therefore, all the large arteries of the body can be considered a single pressure reservoir.

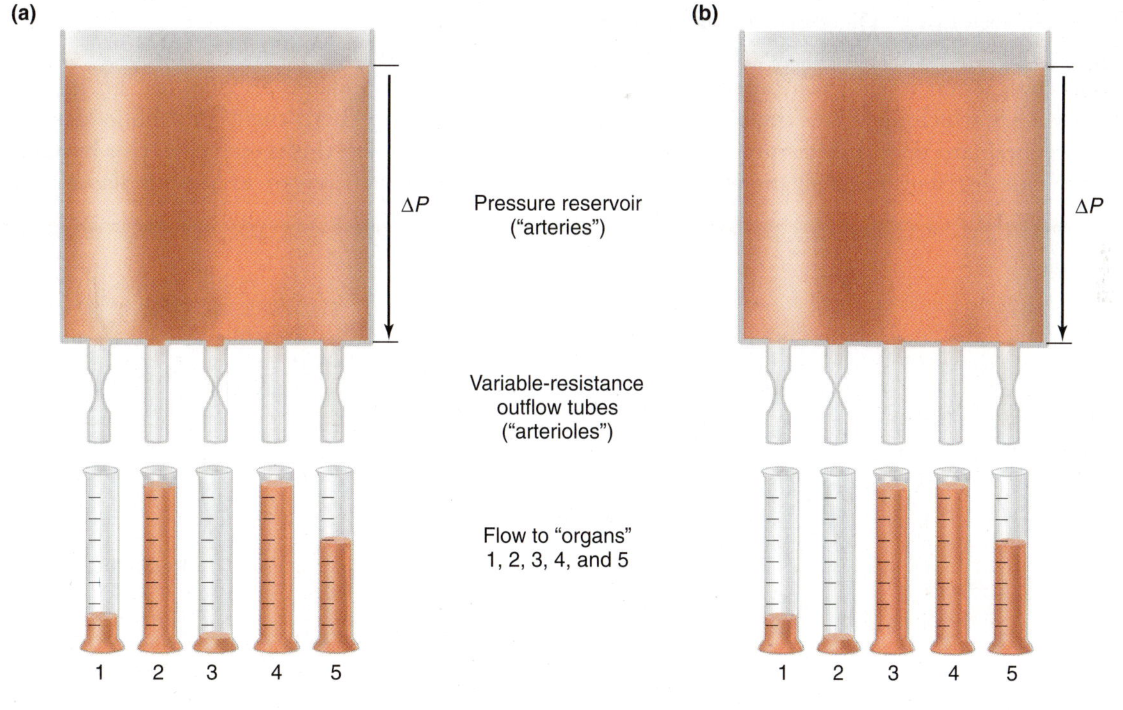

Figure 12.33 Physical model of the relationship between arterial pressure, arteriolar radius in different organs, and blood-flow distribution. In (a), blood flow is high through tube 2 and low through tube 3, whereas just the opposite is true for (b). This shift in blood flow was achieved by constricting tube 2 and dilating tube 3.

PHYSIOLOGICAL INQUIRY

- Assuming the reservoir is refilled at a constant rate, how would the flows shown in (b) be different if tube 2 remained the same as it was in condition (a)?

Answer can be found at end of chapter.

The arteries branch within each organ into progressively smaller arteries, which then branch into arterioles. The smallest arteries are narrow enough to offer significant resistance to flow, but the still narrower arterioles are the major sites of resistance in the vascular tree and are therefore analogous to the outflow tubes in the model. This explains the large decrease in mean pressure—from about 90 mmHg to 35 mmHg—as blood flows through the arterioles (see Figure 12.29). Pulse pressure also decreases in the arterioles, so flow is much less pulsatile in downstream capillaries, venules, and veins.

Like the model's outflow tubes (see Figure 12.33), the arteriolar radii in individual organs are subject to independent adjustment. The blood flow (F) through any organ is represented by the following equation:

$$F_{\text{organ}} = (MAP - \text{Venous pressure})/\text{Resistance}_{\text{organ}}$$

Venous pressure is normally close to zero, so we may write

$$F_{\text{organ}} = MAP/\text{Resistance}_{\text{organ}}$$

Because the *MAP* is the same throughout the body, differences in flows between organs depend entirely on the relative resistances of their respective arterioles. Arterioles contain smooth muscle, which can either relax and cause the vessel radius to increase (**vasodilation**), or contract and decrease the vessel radius (**vasoconstriction**). Therefore, the pattern of blood-flow distribution depends upon the degree of arteriolar smooth muscle contraction within each organ and tissue. Look back at Figure 12.3, which illustrates the distribution of blood flows at rest; these are due to differing resistances in the various organs. This distribution can change greatly when the various resistances are changed, as occurs during exercise (discussed in Section E).

How can resistance be changed? Arteriolar smooth muscle possesses a large degree of spontaneous activity (that is, contraction independent of any neural, hormonal, or paracrine input). This spontaneous contractile activity is called **intrinsic tone** (also called basal tone). It sets a baseline level of contraction that can be increased or decreased by external signals, such as neurotransmitters. These signals act by inducing changes in the cytosolic Ca^{2+} concentration of the smooth muscle cells (see Chapter 9 for a description of excitation–contraction coupling in smooth muscle). An increase in contractile force above the intrinsic tone causes vasoconstriction, whereas a decrease in contractile force causes vasodilation. The mechanisms controlling vasoconstriction and vasodilation in arterioles fall into two general categories: (1) local controls and (2) extrinsic (or reflex) controls.

Local Controls

The term **local controls** denotes mechanisms independent of nerves or hormones by which organs and tissues alter their own arteriolar resistances, thereby self-regulating their blood flows. This includes changes caused by autocrine and paracrine agents. This self-regulation is apparent in phenomena such as active hyperemia, flow autoregulation, reactive hyperemia, and local response to injury, which are described next.

Active Hyperemia

Most organs and tissues manifest an increased blood flow (**hyperemia**) when their metabolic activity is increased (**Figure 12.34a**); this is termed **active hyperemia.** For example, the blood flow to exercising skeletal muscle increases

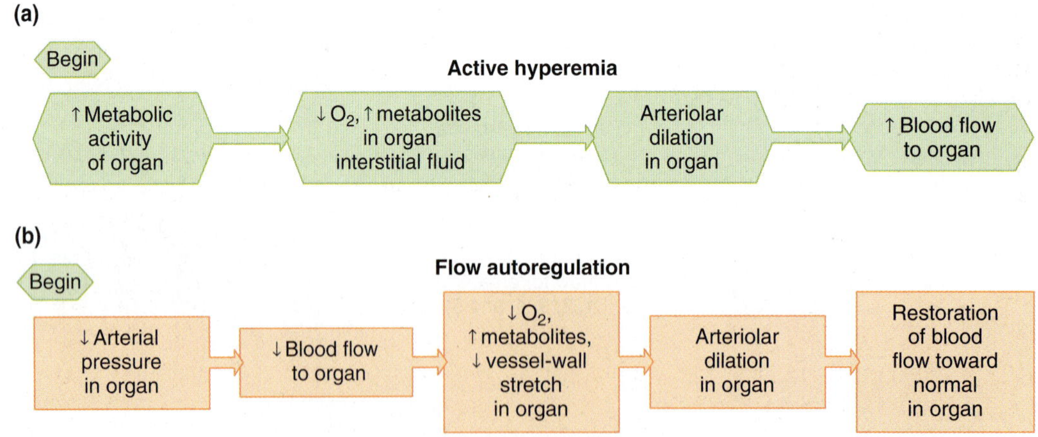

Figure 12.34 Local control of organ blood flow in response to (a) increases in metabolic activity and (b) decreases in blood pressure. Decreases in metabolic activity or increases in blood pressure would produce changes opposite those shown here.

PHYSIOLOGICAL INQUIRY

- An experiment is performed in which the blood flow through a single arteriole is measured. Initially, arterial pressure and flow through the arteriole are constant, but then the arterial pressure is experimentally increased and maintained at a higher level. How will blood flow through the arteriole change in the minutes that follow the increase in arterial pressure?

Answer can be found at end of chapter.

in direct proportion to the increased activity of the muscle. Active hyperemia is the direct result of arteriolar dilation in the more active organ or tissue.

The factors that cause arteriolar smooth muscle to relax in active hyperemia are local chemical changes in the extracellular fluid surrounding the arterioles. These result from the increased metabolic activity in the cells near the arterioles. The relative contributions of the different factors implicated vary, depending upon the organs involved and on the duration of the increased activity. Therefore, we will list—but not attempt to quantify—the local chemical changes that occur in the extracellular fluid.

Perhaps the most obvious change that occurs when tissues become more active is a decrease in the local concentration of oxygen, which is used in the production of ATP by oxidative phosphorylation. A number of other chemical factors *increase* when metabolism increases, including

1. carbon dioxide, an end product of oxidative metabolism;
2. hydrogen ions (decrease in pH), for example, from lactic acid;
3. adenosine, a breakdown product of ATP;
4. K^+ ions, accumulated from repeated action potential repolarization;
5. eicosanoids, breakdown products of membrane phospholipids;
6. osmotically active products from the breakdown of high-molecular-weight substances;
7. **bradykinin,** a peptide generated locally from a circulating protein called **kininogen** by the action of an enzyme, **kallikrein,** secreted by active gland cells; and
8. **nitric oxide,** a gas released by endothelial cells, which acts on the immediately adjacent vascular smooth muscle. Its action will be discussed in an upcoming section.

Local changes in all these chemical factors have been shown to cause arteriolar dilation under controlled experimental conditions, and they all probably contribute to the active-hyperemia response in one or more organs. It is likely, moreover, that additional important local factors remain to be discovered. All these chemical changes in the extracellular fluid act locally upon the arteriolar smooth muscle, causing it to relax. No nerves or hormones are involved.

It should not be too surprising that active hyperemia is most highly developed in skeletal muscle, cardiac muscle, and glands—tissues that show the widest range of normal metabolic activities in the body. It is highly efficient that their supply of blood is primarily determined locally.

Flow Autoregulation

During active hyperemia, increased metabolic activity of the tissue or organ is the initial event leading to local vasodilation. However, locally mediated changes in arteriolar resistance can also occur when a tissue or organ experiences a change in its blood supply resulting from a change in blood pressure (**Figure 12.34b**). The change in resistance is in the direction of maintaining blood flow nearly constant despite the pressure change, and is therefore termed **flow autoregulation.** For example, if arterial pressure to an organ is reduced because of a partial blockage in the artery supplying the organ, blood flow is reduced. In response, local controls cause arteriolar vasodilation, which tends to increase blood flow back toward normal levels.

What is the mechanism of flow autoregulation? One mechanism comprises the same metabolic factors described for active hyperemia. When a decrease in arterial pressure reduces blood flow to an organ, the supply of oxygen to the organ diminishes and the local extracellular oxygen concentration decreases. Simultaneously, the extracellular concentrations of carbon dioxide, hydrogen ions, and metabolites all increase because the blood cannot remove them as fast as they are produced. Therefore, the local metabolic changes occurring during decreased blood supply at constant metabolic activity are similar to those that occur during increased metabolic activity. This is because in both situations there is an imbalance between blood supply and level of cellular metabolic activity. Thus, the vasodilations of active hyperemia and of flow autoregulation in response to low arterial pressure involve the same metabolic mechanisms, even though they have different initiating events.

Flow autoregulation is not limited to circumstances in which arterial pressure decreases. The opposite events occur when, for various reasons, arterial pressure increases: The initial increase in flow due to the increase in pressure removes the local vasodilator chemical factors faster than they are produced and also increases the local concentration of oxygen. This causes the arterioles to constrict, thereby maintaining a relatively constant local flow despite the increased pressure.

Although our description has emphasized the role of local chemical factors in mediating flow autoregulation, another mechanism also participates in this phenomenon in certain tissues and organs. Arteriolar smooth muscle also responds directly, by contracting when increased arterial pressure causes increased wall stretch. Conversely, decreased stretch because of decreased arterial pressure causes this vascular smooth muscle to decrease its tone. These direct responses of arteriolar smooth muscle to stretch are termed **myogenic responses.** They are caused by changes in Ca^{2+} movement into the smooth muscle cells through Ca^{2+} channels in the plasma membrane.

Reactive Hyperemia

When an organ or tissue has had its blood supply completely occluded, a profound transient increase in its blood flow occurs if flow is reestablished. This phenomenon, known as **reactive hyperemia,** is essentially an extreme form of flow autoregulation. During the period of no blood flow, the arterioles in the affected organ or tissue dilate, owing to the local factors described previously. As soon as the occlusion to arterial flow is removed, blood flow increases greatly through these wide-open arterioles. This effect can be demonstrated by wrapping a string tightly around the base of your finger for 1–2 minutes. When it is removed, your finger will turn bright red due to the increase in blood flow.

Response to Injury

Tissue injury causes eicosanoids and a variety of other substances to be released locally from cells or generated from plasma precursors. These substances make arteriolar smooth muscle relax and cause vasodilation in an injured area. This phenomenon, a part of the general process known as inflammation, will be described in detail in Chapter 18.

Extrinsic Controls

Sympathetic Neurons

Most arterioles are richly innervated by sympathetic postganglionic neurons. These neurons release mainly norepinephrine, which binds to α-adrenergic receptors on the vascular smooth muscle to cause vasoconstriction.

In contrast, recall that the receptors for norepinephrine on heart muscle, including the conducting system, are mainly β-adrenergic. This permits the pharmacological use of β-adrenergic antagonists to block the actions of norepinephrine on the heart but not the arterioles, and vice versa for α-adrenergic antagonists.

Control of the sympathetic neurons to arterioles can also be used to produce vasodilation. Because the sympathetic neurons are seldom completely quiescent but discharge at some intermediate rate that varies from organ to organ, they always are causing some degree of tonic constriction in addition to the vessels' intrinsic tone. Dilation can be achieved by decreasing the rate of sympathetic activity to below this basal level.

The skin offers an excellent example of the role played by sympathetic regulation. At room temperature, skin arterioles are already under the influence of a moderate rate of sympathetic discharge. An appropriate stimulus—cold, fear, or loss of blood, for example—causes reflex enhancement of this sympathetic discharge, and the arterioles constrict further. In contrast, an increased body temperature reflexively inhibits sympathetic input to the skin, the arterioles dilate, and you radiate body heat.

In contrast to active hyperemia and flow autoregulation, the primary functions of sympathetic neurons to blood vessels are concerned not with the coordination of local metabolic needs and blood flow but with reflexes that serve whole-body needs. The most common reflex employing these pathways is that which regulates arterial blood pressure by influencing arteriolar resistance throughout the body (discussed in detail in the next section). Other reflexes redistribute blood flow to achieve a specific function (as in the previous example, to increase heat loss through the skin).

Parasympathetic Neurons

With few exceptions, there is little or no important parasympathetic innervation of arterioles. In other words, the great majority of blood vessels receive sympathetic but not parasympathetic input. This contrasts with the pattern of dual autonomic innervation of most tissues.

Noncholinergic, Nonadrenergic, Autonomic Neurons

As described in Chapter 6, there is a population of autonomic postganglionic neurons that are referred to as noncholinergic, nonadrenergic neurons because they release neither acetylcholine nor norepinephrine. Instead, they release other vasodilator substances—nitric oxide, in particular. These neurons are particularly prominent in the enteric nervous system, which plays a significant role in the control of the gastrointestinal system's blood vessels (see Chapter 15).

These neurons also innervate arterioles in other locations, for example, in the penis and clitoris, where they mediate erection. Some drugs used to treat erectile dysfunction in men, including ***sildenafil*** (***Viagra***) and ***tadalafil*** (***Cialis***), work by enhancing the nitric oxide signaling pathway and thus facilitating vasodilation.

Hormones

Epinephrine, like norepinephrine released from sympathetic neurons, can bind to α-adrenergic receptors on arteriolar smooth muscle and cause vasoconstriction. The story is more complex, however, because many arteriolar smooth muscle cells possess the β_2 subtype of adrenergic receptors as well as α-adrenergic receptors, and the binding of epinephrine to β_2 receptors causes the muscle cells to relax rather than contract (**Figure 12.35**).

In most vascular beds, the existence of β_2-adrenergic receptors on vascular smooth muscle is of little if any importance because the α-adrenergic receptors greatly outnumber them. The arterioles in skeletal muscle are an important exception, however. Because they have a significant number of β_2-adrenergic receptors, circulating epinephrine can contribute to vasodilation in muscle vascular beds.

Another hormone important for arteriolar control is **angiotensin II,** which constricts most arterioles. This peptide is part of the renin–angiotensin system, and drugs that prevent its action or formation are a major therapy for treating high blood pressure. Another hormone that causes arteriolar constriction is **vasopressin,** which is released into the blood by the posterior pituitary in response to a decrease in

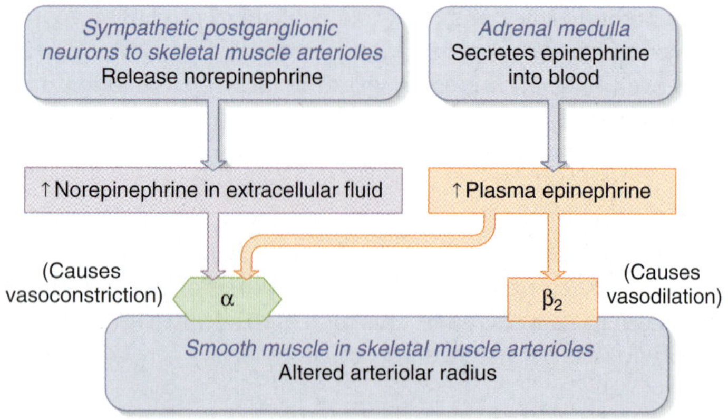

Figure 12.35 Effects of sympathetic nerves and plasma epinephrine on the arterioles in skeletal muscle. After its release from neuron terminals, norepinephrine diffuses to the arterioles, whereas epinephrine, a hormone, is blood-borne. Note that activation of α-adrenergic receptors and β_2-adrenergic receptors produces opposing effects. For simplicity, norepinephrine is shown binding only to α-adrenergic receptors; it can also bind to β_2-adrenergic receptors on the arterioles, but this occurs to a lesser extent.

blood pressure (Chapter 11). The functions of vasopressin and angiotensin II will be described more fully in Chapter 14.

Finally, the hormone secreted by the cardiac atria—**atrial natriuretic peptide**—is a potent vasodilator. It has not been established how important this effect is in the overall physiological control of arterioles. However, atrial natriuretic peptide does influence blood pressure by regulating Na^+ balance and blood volume, which also is described in Chapter 14.

Endothelial Cells and Vascular Smooth Muscle

It should be clear from the previous sections that many substances can induce the contraction or relaxation of vascular smooth muscle. Many of these substances do so by acting directly on the arteriolar smooth muscle, but others act indirectly via the endothelial cells adjacent to the smooth muscle. Endothelial cells, in response to these latter substances as well as certain mechanical stimuli, secrete several paracrine agents that diffuse to the adjacent vascular smooth muscle and induce either relaxation or contraction, resulting in vasodilation or vasoconstriction, respectively.

One very important paracrine vasodilator released by endothelial cells is nitric oxide. (*Note:* This refers to nitric oxide released from endothelial cells, not from neuronal endings as described earlier. Before the identity of the vasodilator paracrine factor released by the endothelium was determined to be nitric oxide, it was called endothelium-derived relaxing factor [EDRF], and this name is still often used because substances other than nitric oxide may also fit this general definition.) Nitric oxide is released continuously in significant amounts by endothelial cells in the arterioles and contributes to arteriolar vasodilation in the basal state. In addition, its secretion rapidly and markedly increases in response to a large number of the chemical mediators involved in both reflex and local control of arterioles. For example, nitric oxide release is stimulated by bradykinin and histamine, substances produced locally during inflammation.

Another vasodilator the endothelial cells release is the eicosanoid **prostacyclin** (also called **prostaglandin I_2 [PGI_2]**). Unlike the case for nitric oxide, there is little basal secretion of PGI_2, but secretion can increase markedly in response to various inputs. The roles of PGI_2 in the vascular responses to blood clotting are described in Section F of this chapter.

One of the important *vasoconstrictor* paracrine agents that the endothelial cells release in response to certain mechanical and chemical stimuli is **endothelin-1 (ET-1)**. Not only does ET-1 have paracrine actions, but under certain circumstances it can also achieve high enough concentrations in the blood to function as a hormone, causing widespread arteriolar vasoconstriction.

Arteriolar Control in Specific Organs

Figure 12.36 summarizes the factors that determine arteriolar radius. The importance of local and reflex controls varies from organ to organ, and **Table 12.5** lists for reference the key features of arteriolar control in specific organs. The variety of influences on arteriolar radius and their importance under various circumstances demonstrate the general principle of physiology that most physiological functions are controlled by multiple regulatory systems, often working in opposition.

12.10 Capillaries

As mentioned at the beginning of Section A, at any given moment, approximately 5% of the total circulating blood is flowing through the capillaries. It is this 5% that is performing the ultimate purpose of the entire cardiovascular system—the exchange of nutrients, metabolic end products, and cell secretions. Some exchange also occurs in the venules, which can be viewed as extensions of capillaries.

The capillaries permeate every tissue of the body except the cornea, the clear structure that allows light to enter the eye (see Chapter 7). Because most cells are no more than 0.1 mm (only a few cell widths) from a capillary, diffusion distances are very small and exchange is highly efficient. An adult has an estimated 25,000 miles (40,000 km) of capillaries, each individual capillary being only about 1 mm long with an inner diameter of about 8 μm, just wide enough for an erythrocyte

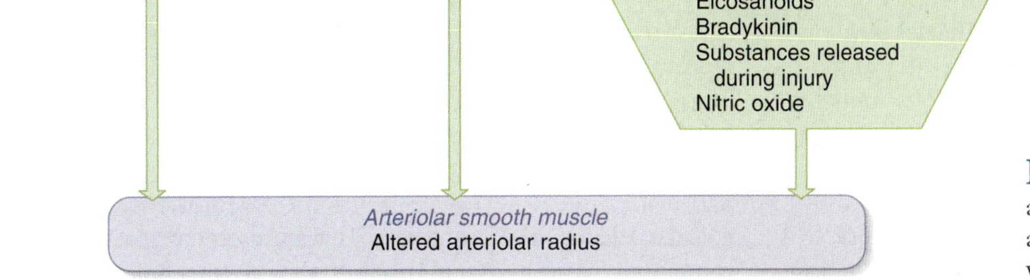

Figure 12.36 Major factors affecting arteriolar radius. Note that epinephrine can be a vasodilator or vasoconstrictor, depending on which adrenergic receptor subtype is present.

TABLE 12.5 Reference Summary of Arteriolar Control in Specific Organs

Heart	High intrinsic tone; oxygen extraction is very high at rest, so flow must increase when oxygen consumption increases if adequate oxygen supply is to be maintained. Controlled mainly by local metabolic factors, particularly adenosine, and flow autoregulation; direct sympathetic influences are minor and normally overridden by local factors. During systole, aortic semilunar cusps block the entrances to the coronary arteries, and vessels within the muscle wall are compressed; therefore, coronary flow occurs mainly during diastole.
Skeletal Muscle	Controlled by local metabolic factors during exercise. Sympathetic activation causes vasoconstriction (mediated by α-adrenergic receptors) in reflex response to decreased arterial pressure. Epinephrine causes vasodilation via β_2-adrenergic receptors when present in low concentration, and vasoconstriction via α-adrenergic receptors when present in high concentration.
GI Tract, Spleen, Pancreas, and Liver ("Splanchnic Organs")	Actually two capillary beds partially in series with each other; blood from the capillaries of the GI tract, spleen, and pancreas flows via the portal vein to the liver. In addition, the liver receives a separate arterial blood supply. Sympathetic activation causes vasoconstriction, mediated by α-adrenergic receptors, in reflex response to decreased arterial pressure and during stress. In addition, venous constriction causes displacement of a large volume of blood from the liver to the veins of the thorax. Increased blood flow occurs following ingestion of a meal and is mediated by local metabolic factors, neurons, and hormones secreted by the GI tract.
Kidneys	Flow autoregulation is a major factor. Sympathetic stimulation causes vasoconstriction, mediated by α-adrenergic receptors, in reflex response to decreased arterial pressure and during stress. Angiotensin II is also a major vasoconstrictor. These reflexes help conserve sodium and water.
Brain	Excellent flow autoregulation. Distribution of blood within the brain is controlled by local metabolic factors. Vasodilation occurs in response to increased concentration of carbon dioxide in arterial blood. Influenced relatively little by the autonomic nervous system.
Skin	Controlled mainly by sympathetic nerves, mediated by α-adrenergic receptors; reflex vasoconstriction occurs in response to decreased arterial pressure and cold, whereas vasodilation occurs in response to heat. Substances released from sweat glands and noncholinergic, nonadrenergic neurons also cause vasodilation. Venous plexus contains large volumes of blood, which contributes to skin color.
Lungs	Very low resistance compared to systemic circulation. Controlled mainly by gravitational forces and passive physical forces within the lung. Constriction mediated by local factors in response to low oxygen concentration—just the opposite of what occurs in the systemic circulation.

to squeeze through. (For comparison, a human hair is about 100 μm in diameter.)

The essential role of capillaries in tissue function has stimulated many questions concerning how capillaries develop and grow (**angiogenesis**). For example, what activates angiogenesis during wound healing and how do cancers stimulate growth of the new blood vessels required for continued tumor growth? It is known that the vascular endothelial cells play a central role in the building of a new capillary network by cell locomotion and cell division. They are stimulated to do so by a variety of **angiogenic factors** (e.g., vascular endothelial growth factor [VEGF]) secreted locally by various tissue cells like fibroblasts and by the endothelial cells themselves. Cancer cells also secrete angiogenic factors. The development of therapies to interfere with the secretion or action of these factors is a promising research area in anticancer therapy. For example, ***angiostatin*** is a peptide that occurs naturally in the body and inhibits blood vessel growth. Administering exogenous angiostatin has been found to reduce the size of tumors in mice. As another example, a drug recently approved for the treatment of colorectal cancer is an antibody that binds and traps VEGF in the bloodstream, reducing its ability to support angiogenesis.

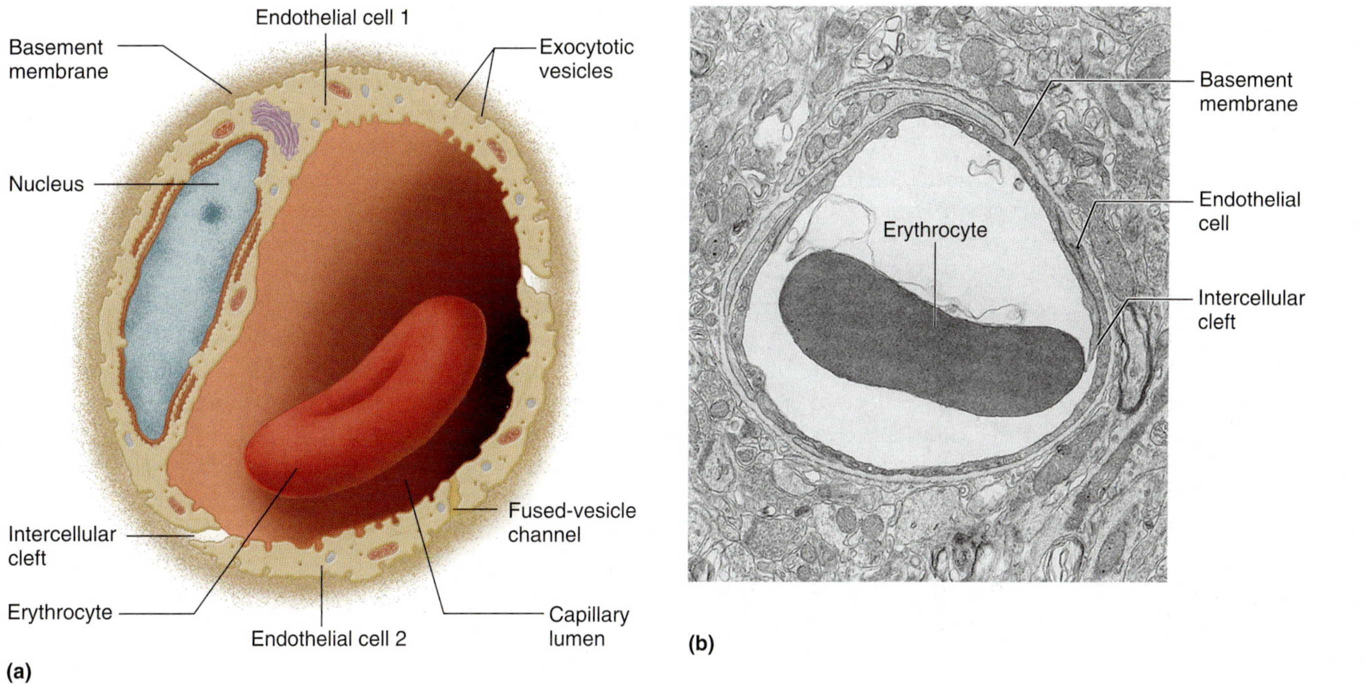

Figure 12.37 (a) Diagram of a capillary cross section. There are two endothelial cells in the figure, but the nucleus of only one is seen because the other is out of the plane of section. The fused-vesicle channel is part of endothelial cell 2. (b) Electron micrograph of a capillary containing a single erythrocyte; no nuclei are shown in this section. The long dimension of the blood cell is approximately 7 μm. Figure adapted from Lentz. EM courtesy of Dr. Michael Hart.

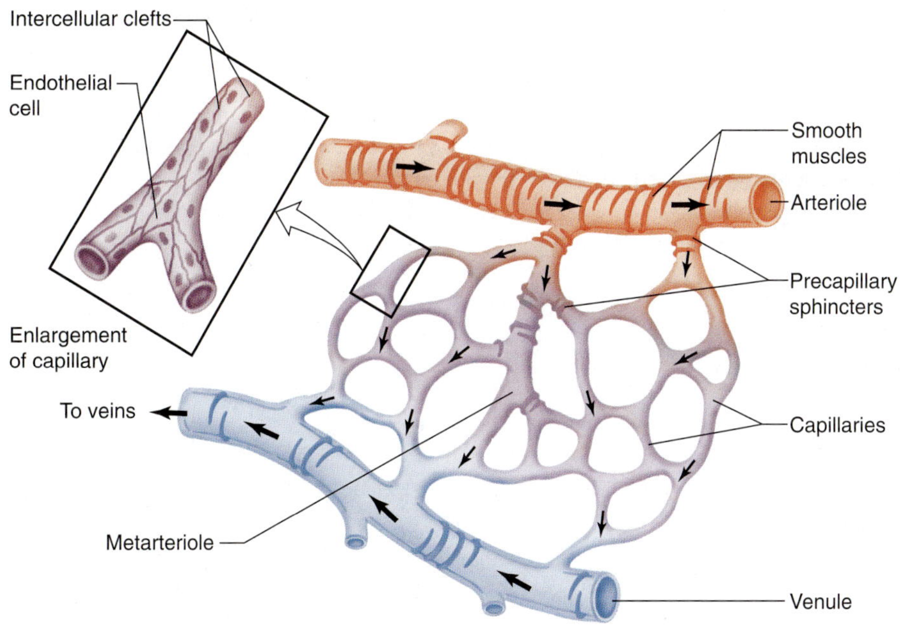

Figure 12.38 APR Diagram of microcirculation. Note the absence of smooth muscle in the capillaries. Adapted from Chaffee and Lytle.

Anatomy of the Capillary Network

Capillary structure varies considerably from organ to organ, but the typical capillary (**Figure 12.37**) is a thin-walled tube of endothelial cells one layer thick resting on a basement membrane, without any surrounding smooth muscle or elastic tissue (review Figure 12.28). Capillaries in several organs (e.g., the brain) can have a second set of cells that surround the basement membrane that affect the ability of substances to diffuse across the capillary wall.

The flat cells that constitute the endothelial wall of a capillary are not attached tightly to each other but are separated by narrow, water-filled spaces termed **intercellular clefts.** The endothelial cells generally contain large numbers of endocytotic and exocytotic vesicles, and sometimes these fuse to form continuous **fused-vesicle channels** across the cell (**Figure 12.37a**).

Blood flow through capillaries depends very much on the state of the other vessels that constitute the microcirculation (**Figure 12.38**). For example, vasodilation of the arterioles supplying the capillaries causes increased capillary flow, whereas arteriolar vasoconstriction reduces capillary flow.

In addition, in some tissues and organs, blood enters capillaries not directly from arterioles but from vessels called **metarterioles,** which connect arterioles to venules. Metarterioles, like arterioles, contain scattered smooth muscle cells. The site at which a capillary exits from a metarteriole is surrounded by a ring of smooth muscle, the **precapillary sphincter,** which relaxes or contracts in response to local metabolic factors. When contracted, the precapillary sphincter closes the entry to the capillary completely. The more active the tissue, the more precapillary sphincters are open at any moment and the more capillaries in the network are receiving blood. Precapillary sphincters may also exist where the capillaries exit from arterioles.

Velocity of Capillary Blood Flow

Figure 12.39a is a simple mechanical model that illustrates how the branching of a tubular structure influences the velocity of fluid flow. A series of 1 cm diameter balls is being pushed down a single tube that branches into six narrower tubes. Although each individual tributary tube has a smaller cross section than the wide tube, the sum of the tributary cross sections is greater than that of the wide tube. In the wide tube, each ball moves 3 cm/min, but because the collective cross-sectional area of the small tubes is three times larger, the forward movement is only one-third as fast, or 1 cm/min.

This example illustrates the following important principle: When a continuous stream moves through consecutive sets of tubes arranged in parallel, the velocity of flow decreases as the sum of the cross-sectional areas of the tubes increases. This is precisely the case in the cardiovascular system (**Figure 12.39b**). The blood velocity is fast in the aorta, slows progressively in the arteries and arterioles, and then slows markedly as the blood passes through the huge cross-sectional area of the capillaries. Slow forward flow through the capillaries maximizes the time available for substances to exchange between the blood and interstitial fluid. The velocity of blood then progressively increases in the venules and veins because the cross-sectional area decreases. To reemphasize, blood velocity is dependent not on proximity to the heart but rather on total cross-sectional area of the vessel type.

Diffusion Across the Capillary Wall: Exchanges of Nutrients and Metabolic End Products

The extremely slow forward movement of blood through the capillaries maximizes the time for substance exchange across the capillary wall. Three basic mechanisms allow substances to move between the interstitial fluid and the plasma: diffusion, vesicle transport, and bulk flow. Mediated transport (see Chapter 4) constitutes a fourth mechanism in the capillaries of some tissues, including the brain. Diffusion and vesicle transport are described in this section, and bulk flow will be described in the next.

In all capillaries, excluding those in the brain, diffusion is the only important means by which net movement of nutrients, oxygen, and metabolic end products occurs across the capillary walls. The importance of diffusion in the exchange of substances between the blood and cells illustrates the general principle of physiology that physiological processes are dictated by the laws of chemistry and physics. As described in the next section, there is some movement of these substances by bulk flow, but the amount is negligible.

Chapter 4 described the factors determining diffusion rates. Lipid-soluble substances, including oxygen and carbon dioxide, easily diffuse through the plasma membranes of the capillary endothelial cells. In contrast, ions and other polar molecules are poorly soluble in lipid and must pass through small, water-filled channels in the endothelial lining.

The presence of water-filled channels in the capillary walls allows the rate of movement of ions and small polar molecules across the wall to be quite high, although not as high as that of lipid-soluble molecules. One location where these channels exist is in the intercellular clefts—that is, the narrow, water-filled spaces between adjacent cells. The fused-vesicle channels that penetrate the endothelial cells provide another set of water-filled channels.

The water-filled channels allow only small amounts of protein to diffuse through them. Small amounts of specific proteins—some hormones, for example—may also cross the endothelial cells by vesicle transport (endocytosis of plasma at the luminal border and exocytosis of the endocytotic vesicle at the interstitial side).

Variations in the size of the water-filled channels account for great differences in the "leakiness" of capillaries in

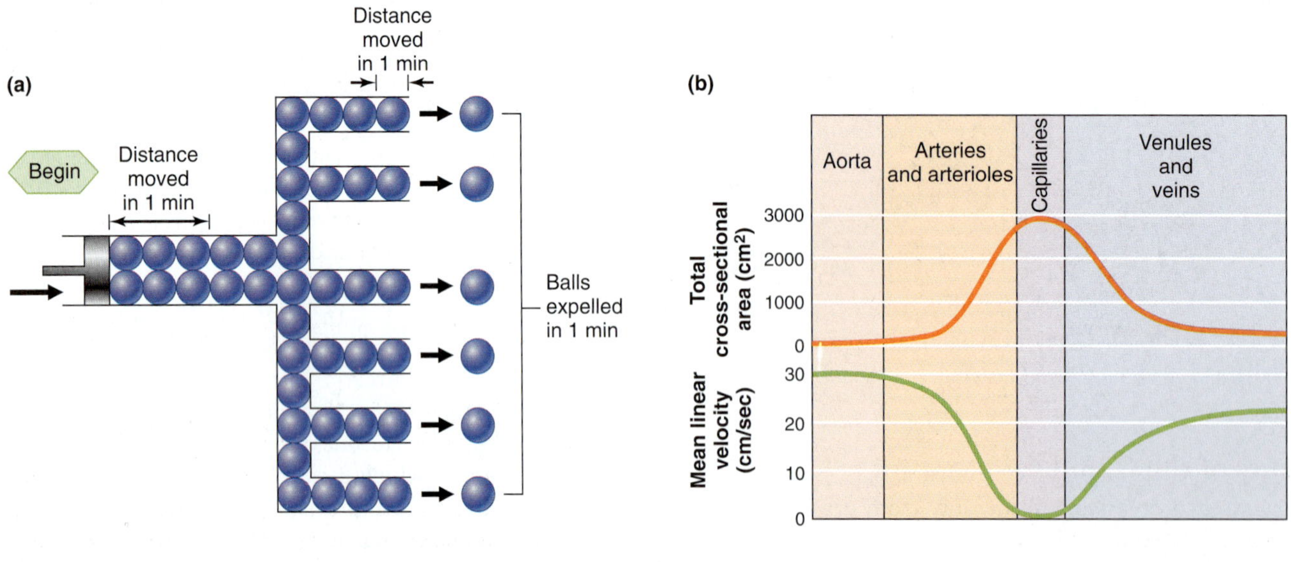

Figure 12.39 Relationship between total cross-sectional area and flow velocity. (a) The total cross-sectional area of the small tubes is three times greater than that of the large tube. Accordingly, flow velocity is one-third as great in the small tubes. (b) Cross-sectional area and velocity in the systemic circulation.

different organs. At one extreme are the "tight" capillaries of the brain, which have no intercellular clefts, only tight junctions. Therefore, water-soluble substances, even those of low molecular weight, can enter or exit the brain interstitial space only by carrier-mediated transport through the blood–brain barrier (see Chapter 6).

At the other end of the spectrum are liver capillaries, which have large intercellular clefts as well as large fused-vesicle channels through the endothelial cells, so that even protein molecules can readily pass across them. This is important because two of the major functions of the liver are the synthesis of plasma proteins and the metabolism of substances bound to plasma proteins. The leakiness of capillaries in most organs and tissues lies between these extremes of brain and liver capillaries.

Transcapillary diffusion gradients for oxygen and nutrients occur as a result of cellular utilization of the substance. Those for metabolic end products arise as a result of cellular production of the substance. Consider three examples: glucose, oxygen, and carbon dioxide in muscle (**Figure 12.40**). Glucose is continuously transported from interstitial fluid into the muscle cell by carrier-mediated transport mechanisms, and oxygen moves in the same direction by diffusion. The removal of glucose and oxygen from interstitial fluid lowers the interstitial fluid concentrations below those in capillary plasma and creates the gradient for their diffusion from the capillary into the interstitial fluid.

Simultaneously, carbon dioxide is continuously produced by muscle cells and diffuses into the interstitial fluid. This causes the carbon dioxide concentration in interstitial fluid to be greater than that in capillary plasma, producing a gradient for carbon dioxide diffusion from the interstitial fluid into the capillary.

Note that for substances moving in both directions, the local metabolic rate ultimately establishes the transcapillary diffusion gradients.

If a tissue increases its metabolic rate, it must obtain more nutrients from the blood and must eliminate more metabolic end products. One mechanism for achieving that is active hyperemia. The second important mechanism is increased diffusion gradients between plasma and tissue; increased cellular utilization of oxygen and nutrients lowers their tissue concentrations, whereas increased production of carbon dioxide and other end products raises their tissue concentrations. In both cases, the substance's transcapillary concentration difference increases, which also increases the rate of diffusion.

Bulk Flow Across the Capillary Wall: Distribution of the Extracellular Fluid

At the same time that the diffusional exchange of nutrients, oxygen, and metabolic end products is occurring across the capillaries, another, completely distinct process is also taking place across the capillary—the bulk flow of protein-free plasma. The function of this process is not the exchange of nutrients and metabolic end products but rather the distribution of the extracellular fluid volume (**Figure 12.41**). Recall that extracellular fluid includes the plasma and interstitial fluid. Normally, there is almost four times more interstitial fluid than plasma—11 L versus 3 L—in a 70 kg person. This distribution is not fixed, however, and the interstitial fluid functions as a reservoir that can supply fluid to or receive fluid from the plasma.

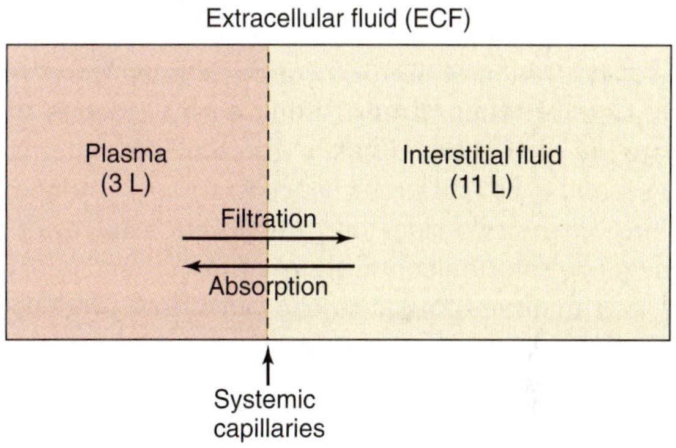

Figure 12.41 Distribution of the extracellular fluid by bulk flow.

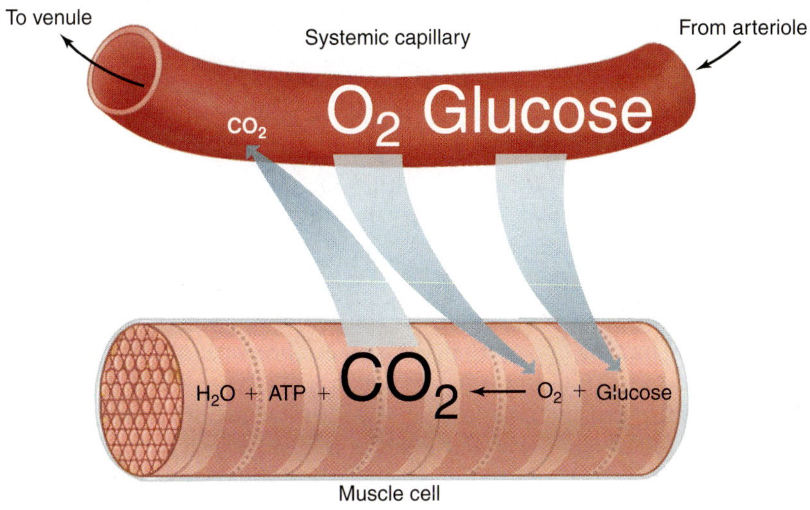

Figure 12.40 APIR Diffusion gradients at a systemic capillary.

PHYSIOLOGICAL INQUIRY

- If cellular metabolism was not changed but the blood flow through a tissue's capillaries was reduced, how would the venous blood leaving that tissue differ compared to that before flow reduction?

Answer can be found at end of chapter.

As described in the previous section, most capillary walls are highly permeable to water and to almost all plasma solutes, except plasma proteins. Therefore, in the presence of a hydrostatic pressure difference across it, the capillary wall behaves like a porous filter, permitting protein-free plasma to move by bulk flow from capillary plasma to interstitial fluid through the water-filled channels. (This is technically termed *ultrafiltration*, but we will refer to it simply as *filtration*.) *The concentrations of all the plasma solutes except protein are virtually the same in the filtered fluid as in plasma.*

The magnitude of the bulk flow is determined, in part, by the difference between the capillary blood pressure and the interstitial fluid hydrostatic pressure. Normally, the former is much higher than the latter. Therefore, a considerable hydrostatic pressure difference exists to filter protein-free plasma out of the capillaries into the interstitial fluid, with the protein remaining behind in the plasma.

Why doesn't all the plasma filter out into the interstitial space? The explanation is that the hydrostatic pressure difference favoring filtration is offset by an osmotic force opposing filtration. To understand this, we must review the principle of osmosis.

In Chapter 4, we described how a net movement of water occurs across a semipermeable membrane from a solution of high water concentration to a solution of low water concentration. Stated another way, water moves from a region with a low concentration of nonpenetrating solute to a region with a high concentration of nonpenetrating solute. Moreover, this osmotic flow of water "drags" along with it solutes that can penetrate the membrane. Thus, a difference in water concentration secondary to different concentrations of nonpenetrating solute on the two sides of a membrane can result in the movement of a solution containing both water and penetrating solutes in a manner similar to the bulk flow produced by a hydrostatic pressure difference. Units of pressure (mmHg) are used in expressing this osmotic force across a membrane, just as for hydrostatic pressures.

This analysis can now be applied to osmotically induced flow across capillaries. The plasma within the capillary and the interstitial fluid outside it contain large quantities of low-molecular-weight solutes (also termed **crystalloids**) that easily penetrate capillary pores. Examples include Na^+, Cl^-, and K^+. Because these crystalloids pass easily through the capillary wall, their concentrations in the plasma and interstitial fluid are essentially identical. Consequently, the presence of the crystalloids causes no significant difference in water concentration. In contrast, the plasma proteins (also termed **colloids**) are unable to move through capillary pores (nonpenetrating) and have a very low concentration in the interstitial fluid. The difference in protein concentration between the plasma and the interstitial fluid means that the water concentration of the plasma is slightly lower (by about 0.5%) than that of interstitial fluid, creating an osmotic force that tends to cause the flow of water from the interstitial compartment into the capillary. Because the crystalloids in the interstitial fluid move along with water, flow that is driven by either osmotic or hydrostatic pressures across the capillary wall does not alter crystalloid concentrations in either plasma or interstitial fluid.

A key word in this last sentence is *concentrations*. The amount of water (the volume) and the amount of crystalloids in the two locations do change. Thus, an increased filtration of fluid from plasma to interstitial fluid increases the volume of the interstitial fluid and decreases the volume of the plasma, even though no changes in crystalloid concentrations occur.

In summary, opposing forces act to move fluid across the capillary wall (**Figure 12.42a**): (1) The difference between capillary blood hydrostatic pressure and interstitial fluid hydrostatic pressure favors filtration out of the capillary; and (2) the water-concentration difference between plasma and interstitial fluid, which results from differences in protein concentration, favors the **absorption** of interstitial fluid into the capillary. Therefore, the **net filtration pressure** (***NFP***) depends directly upon the algebraic sum of four variables: capillary hydrostatic pressure, P_c (favoring fluid movement out of the capillary); interstitial hydrostatic pressure, P_{IF} (favoring fluid movement into the capillary); the osmotic force due to plasma protein concentration, π_c (favoring fluid movement into the capillary); and the osmotic force due to interstitial fluid protein concentration, π_{IF} (favoring fluid movement out of the capillary). Thus,

$$NFP = P_c + \pi_{IF} - P_{IF} - \pi_c$$

Note that we have arbitrarily assigned a positive value to the forces directed out of the capillary and negative values to the inward-directed forces. The four factors that determine net filtration pressure are termed the **Starling forces** because Starling, the same physiologist who helped elucidate the Frank–Starling mechanism of the heart, was the first to describe these forces.

We may now consider this movement quantitatively in the systemic circulation (**Figure 12.42b**). Much of the arterial blood pressure has already dissipated as the blood flows through the arterioles, so that hydrostatic pressure tending to push fluid out of the arterial end of a typical capillary is only about 35 mmHg. The interstitial fluid protein concentration at this end of the capillary would produce a flow of fluid out of the capillary equivalent to a hydrostatic pressure of 3 mmHg. Because the interstitial fluid hydrostatic pressure is virtually zero, the only inward-directed pressure at this end of the capillary is the osmotic pressure due to plasma proteins, with a value of 28 mmHg. At the arterial end of the capillary, therefore, the net outward pressure exceeds the inward pressure by 10 mmHg, so bulk filtration of fluid will occur.

The only substantial difference in the Starling forces at the venous end of the capillary is that the hydrostatic blood pressure (P_c) has decreased from 35 to approximately 15 mmHg due to the resistance encountered as blood flowed along the capillary wall. The other three forces are virtually the same as at the arterial end, so the net inward pressure is about 10 mmHg greater than the outward pressure, and bulk absorption of fluid into the capillaries will occur. Thus, net movement of fluid from the plasma into the interstitial space at the arterial end of capillaries tends to be balanced by fluid flow in the opposite direction at the venous end of the capillaries. In

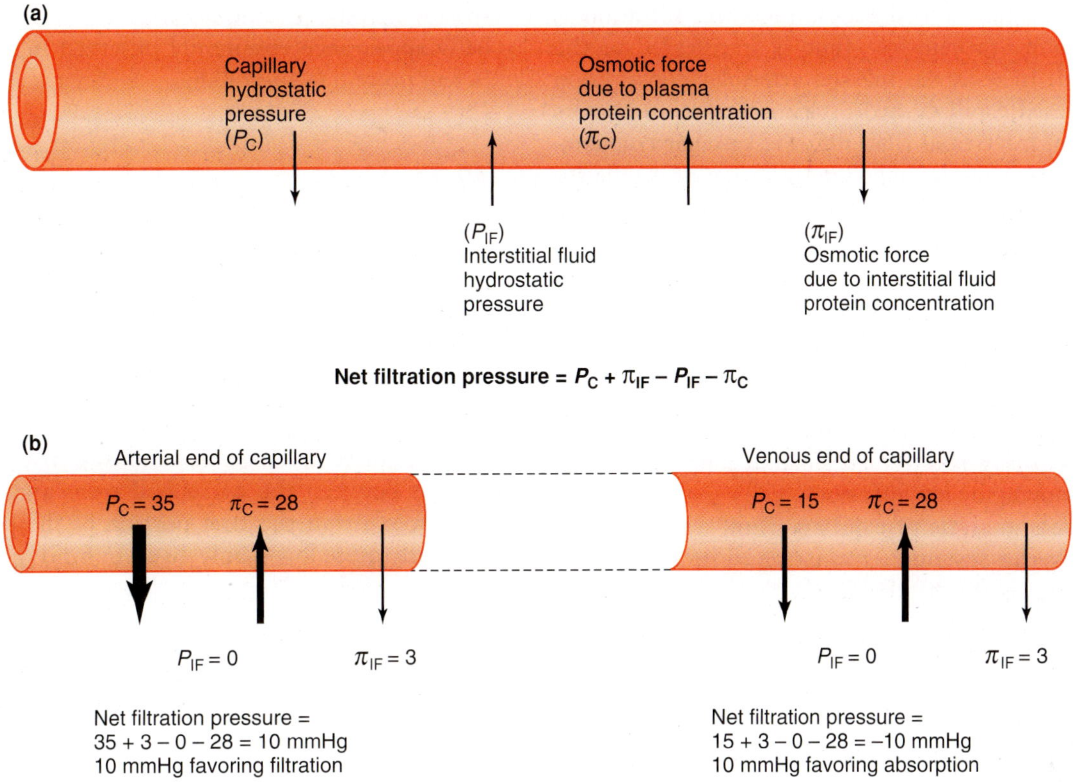

Figure 12.42 APIR (a) The four factors determining fluid movement across capillaries. (b) Quantification of forces causing filtration at the arterial end of the capillary and absorption at the venous end. Outward forces are arbitrarily assigned positive values, so a positive net filtration pressure favors filtration, whereas a negative pressure indicates that net absorption of fluid will occur. Arrows in (b) denote magnitude of forces. No arrow is shown for interstitial fluid hydrostatic pressure (P_{IF}) in (b) because it is approximately zero.

PHYSIOLOGICAL INQUIRY

- If an accident victim loses 1 L of blood, why would an intravenous injection of a liter of plasma be more effective for replacing the lost volume than injecting a liter of an equally concentrated crystalloid solution?

Answer can be found at end of chapter.

actuality, for the aggregate of capillaries in the body, the net outward force is normally slightly larger than the inward, so there is a net filtration amounting to approximately 4 L/day (this number does not include the capillaries in the kidneys). The fate of this fluid will be described in the section on the lymphatic system.

In our example, we have assumed a typical capillary hydrostatic pressure varying from 35 mmHg down to 15 mmHg. In reality, capillary hydrostatic pressures vary in different regions of the body and, as will be described in a later section, are strongly influenced by whether the person is lying down, sitting, or standing. Moreover, capillary hydrostatic pressure in any given region is subject to physiological regulation, mediated mainly by changes in the resistance of the arterioles in that region. As **Figure 12.43** shows, dilating the arterioles in a particular tissue raises capillary hydrostatic pressure in that region because less pressure is lost overcoming resistance between the arteries and the capillaries. Because

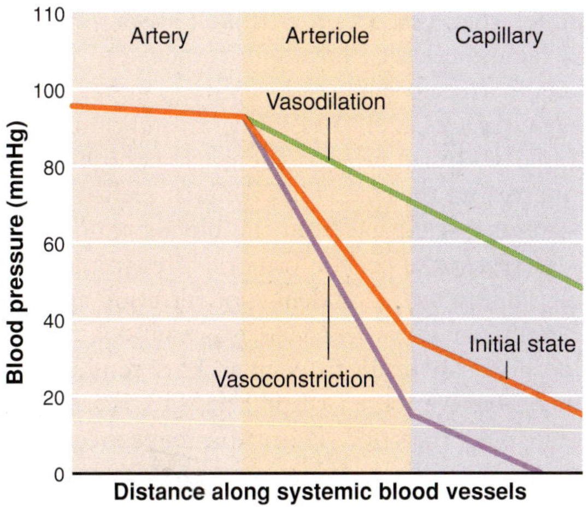

Figure 12.43 Effects of arteriolar vasodilation or vasoconstriction on capillary blood pressure in a single organ (under conditions of constant arterial pressure).

of the increased capillary hydrostatic pressure, filtration is increased and more protein-free fluid is transferred to the interstitial fluid. In contrast, marked arteriolar constriction produces decreased capillary hydrostatic pressure and favors net movement of interstitial fluid into the vascular compartment. Indeed, the arterioles supplying a group of capillaries may be so dilated or so constricted that the capillaries manifest only filtration or only absorption, respectively, along their entire length.

To reiterate an important point, capillary filtration and absorption play a minimal role in the exchange of nutrients and metabolic end products between capillaries and tissues. The reason is that the total quantity of a substance, such as glucose or carbon dioxide, moving into or out of a capillary as a result of net bulk flow is extremely small in comparison with the quantities moving by net diffusion.

Finally, this analysis of capillary fluid dynamics has considered only the systemic circulation. The same Starling forces apply to the capillaries in the pulmonary circulation, but the relative values of the four variables differ. In particular, because the pulmonary circulation is a low-resistance, low-pressure circuit, the normal pulmonary capillary hydrostatic pressure—the major force favoring movement of fluid out of the pulmonary capillaries into the interstitium—averages only about 7 mmHg. This is offset by a greater accumulation of proteins in lung interstitial fluid than is found in other tissues. Overall, the Starling forces in the lung slightly favor filtration as in other tissues, but extensive and active lymphatic drainage prevents the accumulation of extracellular fluid in the interstitial spaces and airways.

In some pathophysiological circumstances, imbalances in the Starling forces can lead to ***edema***—an abnormal accumulation of fluid in the interstitial spaces. Heart failure (discussed in detail in Section E) is a condition in which increased venous pressure reduces blood flow out of the capillaries, and the increased hydrostatic pressure (P_c) causes excess filtration and accumulation of interstitial fluid. The resulting edema can occur in either systemic or pulmonary tissues. A more common experience is the swelling that occurs with injury—for example, when you sprain an ankle. Histamine and other chemical factors released locally in response to injury dilate arterioles and therefore increase capillary pressure and filtration (review Figures 12.42 and 12.43). In addition, the chemicals released within injured tissue cause endothelial cells to distort, increasing the size of intercellular clefts and allowing plasma proteins to escape from the bloodstream more readily. This increases the protein osmotic force in the interstitial fluid (π_{IF}), adding to the tendency for filtration and edema to occur. Finally, an abnormal decrease in plasma protein concentration also can result in edema. This condition reduces the main absorptive force at capillaries (π_c), thereby allowing an increase in net filtration. Plasma protein concentration can be reduced by liver disease (decreased plasma protein production) or by kidney disease (loss of protein in the urine). In addition, as with liver disease, protein malnutrition (***kwashiorkor***) compromises the manufacture of plasma proteins. The resulting edema is particularly marked in the interstitial spaces within the abdominal cavity, producing the swollen-belly appearance commonly observed in people with insufficient protein in their diets.

12.11 Veins

Blood flows from capillaries into venules and then into veins. Some exchange of materials occurs between the interstitial fluid and the venules, just as in capillaries. Indeed, permeability to macromolecules is often greater for venules than for capillaries, particularly in damaged areas.

The veins are the last set of tubes through which blood flows on its way back to the heart. In the systemic circulation, the force driving this venous return is the pressure difference between the peripheral veins and the right atrium. The pressure in the first portion of the peripheral veins is generally quite low—only 10 to 15 mmHg—because most of the pressure imparted to the blood by the heart is dissipated by resistance as blood flows through the arterioles, capillaries, and venules. The right atrial pressure is normally close to 0 mmHg. Therefore, the total driving pressure for flow from the **peripheral veins** to the right atrium is only 10 to 15 mmHg on average. (The peripheral veins include all veins not contained within the chest cavity.) This pressure difference is adequate because of the low resistance to flow offered by the veins, which have large diameters. Thus, a major function of the veins is to act as low-resistance conduits for blood flow from the tissues to the heart. The peripheral veins of the arms and legs contain valves that permit flow only toward the heart.

In addition to their function as low-resistance conduits, the veins perform a second important function: Their diameters are reflexively altered in response to changes in blood volume, thereby maintaining peripheral venous pressure and venous return to the heart. In a previous section, we emphasized that the rate of venous return to the heart is a major determinant of end-diastolic ventricular volume and thereby stroke volume. We now see that peripheral venous pressure is an important determinant of stroke volume. We next describe how venous pressure is determined.

Determinants of Venous Pressure

The factors determining pressure in any elastic tube are the volume of fluid within it and the compliance of its walls. Consequently, total blood volume is one important determinant of venous pressure because, as we will see, most blood is in the veins. Also, the walls of veins are thinner and much more compliant than those of arteries (see Figure 12.28). Thus, veins can accommodate large volumes of blood with a relatively small increase in internal pressure. Approximately 60% of the total blood volume is present in the systemic veins (**Figure 12.44**), but the venous pressure is only about 10 mmHg on average. (In contrast, the systemic arteries contain less than 15% of the blood, at a pressure of nearly 100 mmHg.)

The walls of the veins contain smooth muscle innervated by sympathetic neurons. Stimulation of these neurons releases

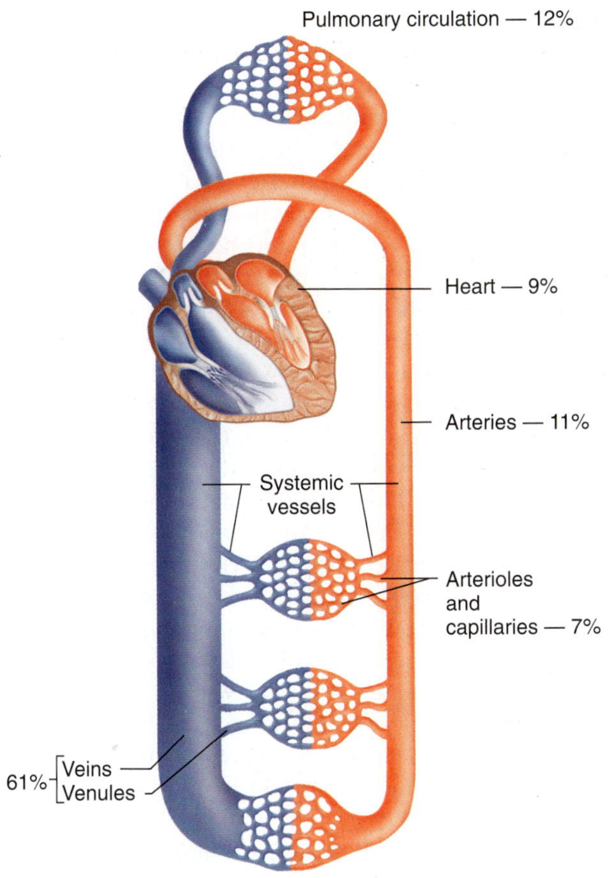

Figure 12.44 Distribution of the total blood volume in different parts of the cardiovascular system. Adapted from Guyton.

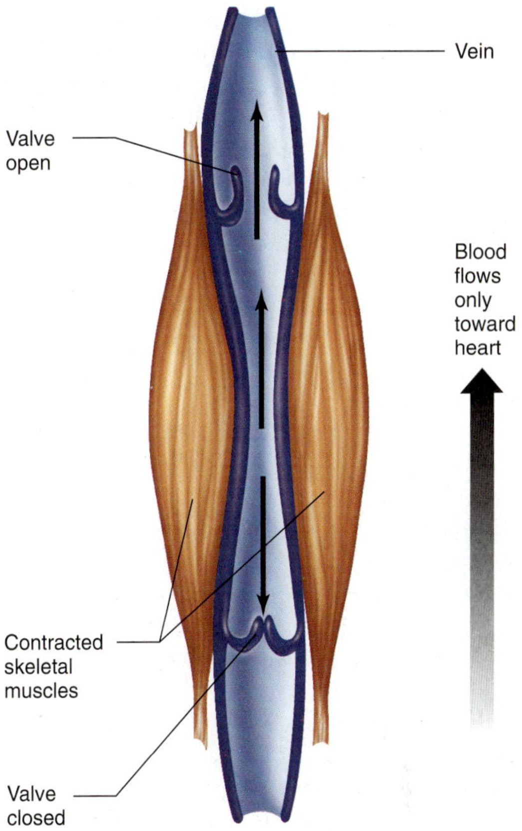

Figure 12.45 APR The skeletal muscle pump. During muscle contraction, venous diameter decreases and venous pressure increases. The increase in pressure forces the flow only toward the heart because backward pressure forces the valves in the veins to close.

norepinephrine, which causes contraction of the venous smooth muscle, decreasing the diameter and compliance of the vessels and increasing the pressure within them. Increased venous pressure then drives more blood out of the veins into the right side of the heart. Note the different effect of venous constriction compared to that of arterioles; when arterioles constrict, the constriction *reduces* forward flow through the systemic circuit, whereas constriction of veins *increases* forward flow. Although sympathetic neurons are the most important input, venous smooth muscle, like arteriolar smooth muscle, also responds to hormonal and paracrine vasodilators and vasoconstrictors.

Two other mechanisms, in addition to contraction of venous smooth muscle, can increase venous pressure and facilitate venous return. These mechanisms are the **skeletal muscle pump** and the **respiratory pump.** During skeletal muscle contraction, the veins running through the muscle are partially compressed, which reduces their diameter and forces more blood back to the heart. Now we can describe a major function of the peripheral vein valves; when the skeletal muscle pump increases local venous pressure, the valves permit blood flow only toward the heart and prevent flow back toward the capillaries (**Figure 12.45**).

The respiratory pump is somewhat more difficult to visualize. As Chapter 13 describes, at the base of the chest cavity (thorax) is a large muscle called the diaphragm, which separates the thorax from the abdomen. During inspiration of air, the diaphragm descends, pushing on the abdominal contents and increasing abdominal pressure. This pressure increase is transmitted passively to the intra-abdominal veins. Simultaneously, the pressure in the thorax decreases, thereby decreasing the pressure in the intrathoracic veins and right atrium. The net effect of the pressure changes in the abdomen and thorax is to increase the pressure difference between the peripheral veins and the heart. Thus, venous return is enhanced during inspiration (expiration would reverse this effect if not for the venous valves), and breathing deeply and frequently, as in exercise, helps blood flow toward the heart.

You might get the incorrect impression from these descriptions that venous return and cardiac output are independent entities. Rather, any change in venous return almost immediately causes equivalent changes in cardiac output, largely through the Frank–Starling mechanism. *Venous return and cardiac output therefore must be the same except for transient changes over brief periods of time.*

In summary (**Figure 12.46**), venous smooth muscle contraction, the skeletal muscle pump, and the respiratory pump all work to facilitate venous return and thereby enhance cardiac output by the same amount.

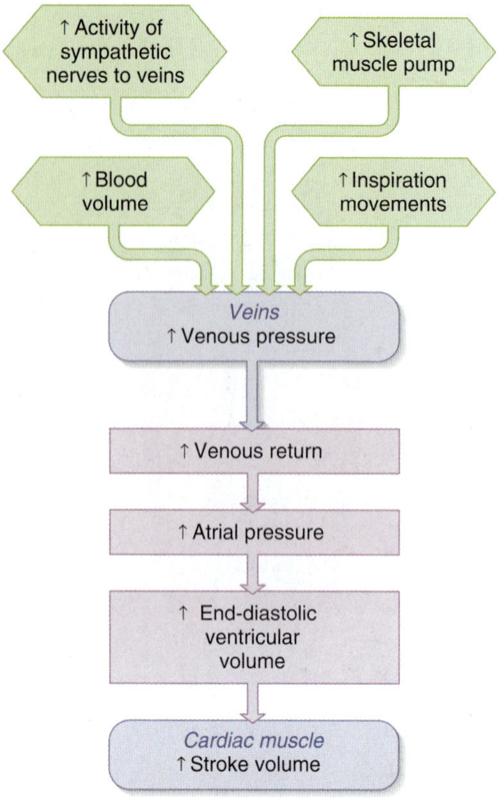

Figure 12.46 Major factors determining peripheral venous pressure, venous return, and stroke volume. Reversing the arrows in the boxes would indicate how these factors can decrease. The effects of increased inspiration on end-diastolic ventricular volume are actually quite complex, but for the sake of simplicity, they are shown here only as increasing venous pressure.

PHYSIOLOGICAL INQUIRY

- Figure 12.44 shows the typical distribution of blood in a normal, resting individual. How would the percentages change during vigorous exercise?

Answer can be found at end of chapter.

12.12 The Lymphatic System

The **lymphatic system** is a network of small organs (lymph nodes) and tubes (**lymphatic vessels** or simply "lymphatics") through which **lymph**—a fluid derived from interstitial fluid—flows. The lymphatic system is not technically part of the circulatory system, but it is described in this chapter because its vessels provide a route for the movement of interstitial fluid to the circulatory system (**Figure 12.47a**).

Present in the interstitium of virtually all organs and tissues are numerous **lymphatic capillaries** that are completely distinct from blood vessel capillaries. Like the latter, they are tubes made of only a single layer of endothelial cells resting on a basement membrane, but they have large water-filled channels that are permeable to all interstitial fluid constituents, including protein. The lymphatic capillaries are the first of the lymphatic vessels, for unlike the blood vessel capillaries, no tubes flow into them.

Small amounts of interstitial fluid continuously enter the lymphatic capillaries by bulk flow. This lymph fluid flows from the lymphatic capillaries into the next set of lymphatic vessels, which converge to form larger and larger lymphatic vessels. At various points in the body—in particular, the neck, armpits, groin, and around the intestines—the lymph flows through lymph nodes (**Figure 12.47b**), which are part of the immune system and are described in Chapter 18. Ultimately, the entire network ends in two large lymphatic ducts that drain into the veins near the junction of the jugular and subclavian veins in the upper chest. Valves at these junctions permit only one-way flow from lymphatic ducts into the veins. Thus, the lymphatic vessels carry interstitial fluid to the cardiovascular system.

The movement of interstitial fluid from the lymphatics to the cardiovascular system is very important because, as noted earlier, the amount of fluid filtered out of all the blood vessel capillaries (except those in the kidneys) exceeds that absorbed by approximately 4 L each day. This 4 L is returned to the blood via the lymphatic system. In the process, small amounts of protein that may leak out of blood vessel capillaries into the interstitial fluid are also returned to the cardiovascular system.

Under some circumstances, the lymphatic system can become occluded, which allows the accumulation of excessive interstitial fluid. For example, occlusion of lymph flow by infectious organisms can result in a condition called ***elephantiasis***, in which there is massive edema of the involved area (**Figure 12.48**). Surgical removal of lymph nodes and vessels during the treatment of breast cancer can similarly allow interstitial fluid to pool in affected tissues.

In addition to draining excess interstitial fluid, the lymphatic system provides the pathway by which fat absorbed from the gastrointestinal tract reaches the blood (see Chapter 15). The lymphatics can also be the route by which cancer cells spread from their area of origin to other parts of the body (which is why cancer treatment sometimes includes the removal of lymph nodes).

Mechanism of Lymph Flow

In large part, the lymphatic vessels beyond the lymphatic capillaries propel the lymph within them by their own contractions. The smooth muscle in the wall of the lymphatics exerts a pumplike action by inherent rhythmic contractions. Because the lymphatic vessels have valves similar to those in veins, these contractions produce a one-way flow toward the point at which the lymphatics enter the circulatory system. The lymphatic vessel smooth muscle is responsive to stretch, so when no interstitial fluid accumulates and, therefore, no lymph enters the lymphatics, the smooth muscle is inactive. However, when increased fluid filtration out of capillaries occurs, the increased fluid entering the lymphatics stretches the walls and triggers rhythmic contractions of the smooth muscle. This constitutes a negative feedback mechanism for adjusting the rate of lymph flow to the rate of lymph formation and thereby preventing edema.

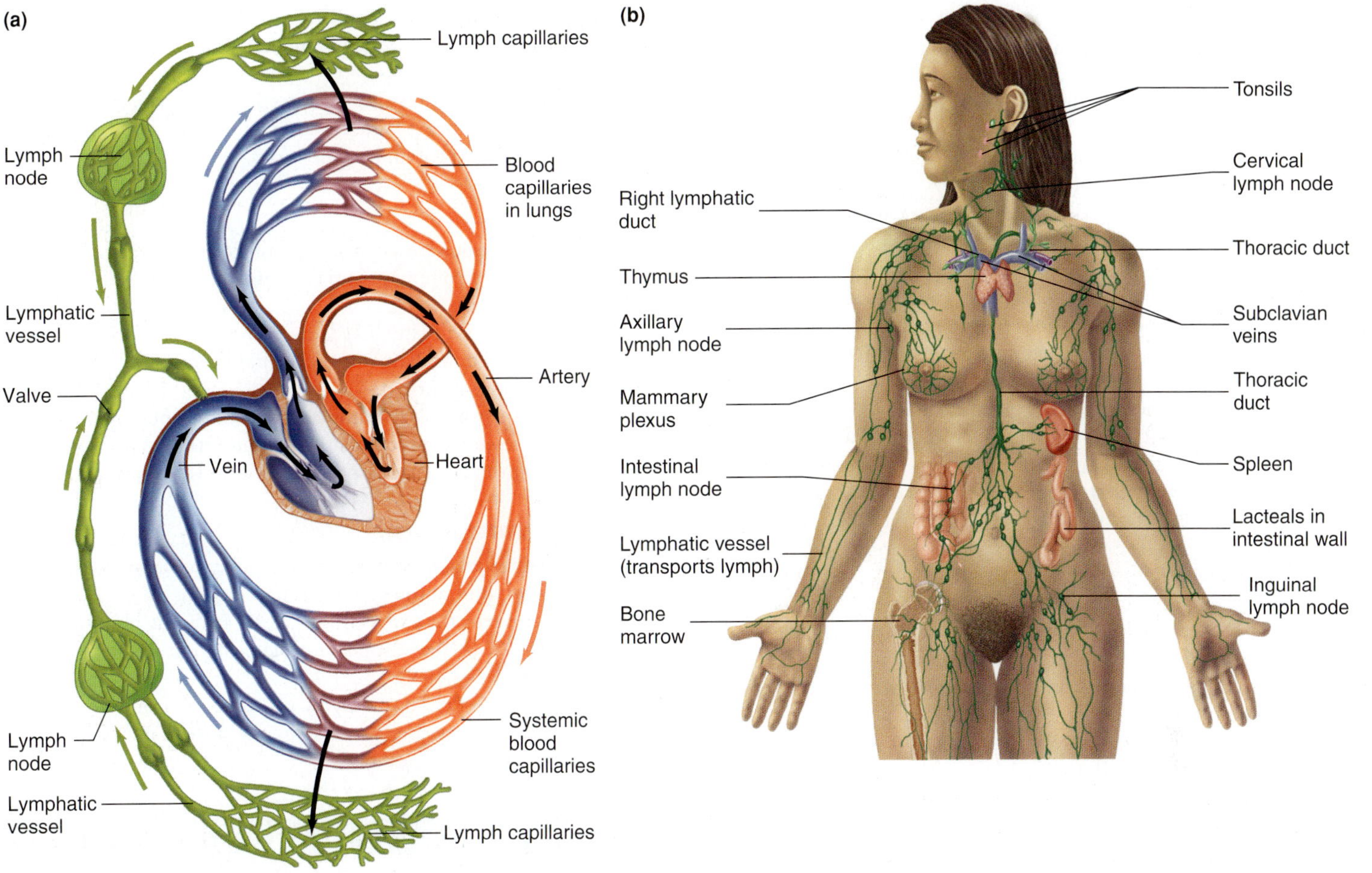

Figure 12.47 APR The lymphatic system (green) in relation to the cardiovascular system (blue and red). (a) The lymphatic system is a one-way system from interstitial fluid to the cardiovascular system. (b) Prior to reentering the blood at the subclavian veins, lymph flows through lymph nodes in the neck, armpits, groin, and around the intestines.

PHYSIOLOGICAL INQUIRY

- How might periodic ingestion of extra fluids be expected to increase the flow of lymph?

Answer can be found at end of chapter.

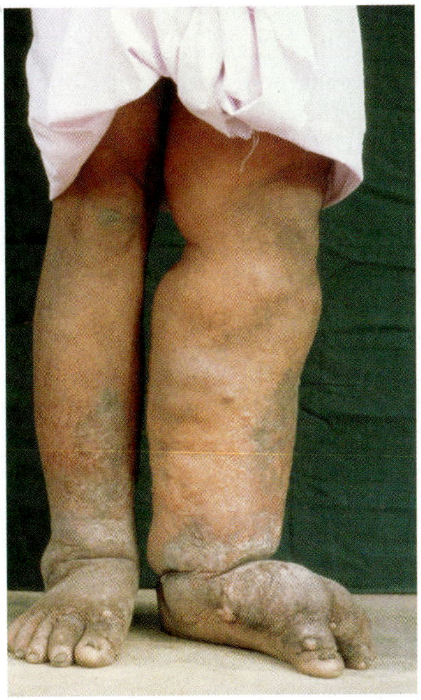

Figure 12.48 Elephantiasis is a disease resulting when mosquito-borne filarial worms block the return of lymph to the vascular system.

In addition, the smooth muscle of the lymphatic vessels is innervated by sympathetic neurons, and excitation of these neurons in various physiological states such as exercise may contribute to increased lymph flow. Forces external to the lymphatic vessels also enhance lymph flow. These include the same external forces we described for veins—the skeletal muscle pump and respiratory pump.

SECTION C SUMMARY

Arteries

I. The arteries function as low-resistance conduits and as pressure reservoirs for maintaining blood flow to the tissues during ventricular relaxation.

II. The difference between maximal arterial pressure (systolic pressure) and minimal arterial pressure (diastolic pressure) during a cardiac cycle is the pulse pressure.

III. Mean arterial pressure can be estimated as diastolic pressure plus one-third of the pulse pressure.

Arterioles

I. Arterioles are the dominant site of resistance to flow in the vascular system and play major roles in determining mean arterial pressure and in distributing flows to the various organs and tissues.

II. Arteriolar resistance is determined by local factors and by reflex neural and hormonal input.
  a. Local factors that change with the degree of metabolic activity cause the arteriolar vasodilation and increased flow of active hyperemia.
  b. Flow autoregulation involves local metabolic factors and arteriolar myogenic responses to stretch, and it changes arteriolar resistance to maintain a constant blood flow when arterial blood pressure changes.
  c. Sympathetic neurons innervate most arterioles and cause vasoconstriction via α-adrenergic receptors. In certain cases, noncholinergic, nonadrenergic neurons that release nitric oxide or other vasodilators also innervate blood vessels.
  d. Epinephrine causes vasoconstriction or vasodilation, depending on the proportion of α-adrenergic and β_2-adrenergic receptors in the organ.
  e. Angiotensin II and vasopressin cause vasoconstriction.
  f. Some chemical inputs act by stimulating endothelial cells to release vasodilator or vasoconstrictor paracrine agents, which then act on adjacent smooth muscle. These paracrine agents include the vasodilators nitric oxide (endothelium-derived relaxing factor), prostacyclin, and the vasoconstrictor endothelin-1.

III. Table 12.5 summarizes arteriolar control in specific organs.

Capillaries

I. Capillaries are the site at which nutrients and waste products are exchanged between blood and tissues.

II. Blood flows through the capillaries more slowly than through any other part of the vascular system because of the huge cross-sectional area of the capillaries.

III. Capillary blood flow is determined by the resistance of the arterioles supplying the capillaries and by the number of open precapillary sphincters.

IV. Diffusion is the mechanism that exchanges nutrients and metabolic end products between capillary plasma and interstitial fluid.
  a. Lipid-soluble substances can move through the endothelial cells, whereas ions and polar molecules only move through water-filled intercellular clefts or fused-vesicle channels.
  b. Plasma proteins do not easily move across capillary walls; specific proteins like certain hormones can be moved by vesicle transport.
  c. The diffusion gradient for a substance across capillaries arises as a result of cell utilization or production of the substance. Increased metabolism increases the diffusion gradient and increases the rate of diffusion.

V. Bulk flow of protein-free plasma or interstitial fluid across capillaries determines the distribution of extracellular fluid between these two fluid compartments.
  a. Filtration from plasma to interstitial fluid is favored by the hydrostatic pressure difference between the capillary and the interstitial fluid. Absorption from interstitial fluid to plasma is favored by the protein concentration difference between the plasma and the interstitial fluid.
  b. Filtration and absorption do not change the concentrations of crystalloids in the plasma and interstitial fluid because these substances move together with water.
  c. There is normally a small excess of filtration over absorption, which returns fluids to the bloodstream via lymphatic vessels.
  d. Disease states that alter the Starling forces can result in edema (e.g., heart failure, tissue injury, liver disease, kidney disease, and protein malnutrition).

Veins

I. Veins serve as low-resistance conduits for venous return.

II. Veins are very compliant and contain most of the blood in the vascular system.
  a. Sympathetically mediated vasoconstriction reflexively reduces venous diameter to maintain venous pressure and venous return.
  b. The skeletal muscle pump and respiratory pump increase venous pressure and enhance venous return. Venous valves permit the pressure to produce flow only toward the heart.

The Lymphatic System

I. The lymphatic system provides a one-way route to return interstitial fluid to the cardiovascular system.

II. Lymph returns the excess fluid filtered from the blood vessel capillaries, as well as the protein that leaks out of the blood vessel capillaries.

III. Lymph flow is driven mainly by contraction of smooth muscle in the lymphatic vessels but also by the skeletal muscle pump and the respiratory pump.

SECTION C REVIEW QUESTIONS

1. Draw the pressure changes along the systemic and pulmonary vascular systems during the cardiac cycle.
2. What are the two main functions of the arteries?
3. What are normal values for systolic, diastolic, and mean arterial pressures in young adult males? Females? How is mean arterial pressure estimated?
4. What are two major factors that determine pulse pressure?
5. What denotes systolic and diastolic pressure in the measurement of arterial pressure with a sphygmomanometer?
6. What are the major sites of resistance in the systemic vascular system?
7. Name two functions of arterioles.
8. Write the formula relating flow through an organ to mean arterial pressure and to the resistance to flow that organ offers.
9. List the chemical factors that mediate active hyperemia.
10. Name a mechanism other than chemical factors that contributes to flow autoregulation.
11. What is the only autonomic innervation of most arterioles? What are the major adrenergic receptors influenced by these nerves? How can control of sympathetic nerves to arterioles achieve vasodilation?
12. Name four hormones that cause vasodilation or vasoconstriction of arterioles, and specify their effects.
13. Describe the role of endothelial paracrine agents in mediating arteriolar vasoconstriction and vasodilation, and give three examples.
14. Draw a flow diagram summarizing the factors affecting arteriolar radius.
15. What are the relative velocities of flow through the various vessel types of the systemic circulation?
16. Contrast diffusion and bulk flow. Which mechanism is most important in the exchange of nutrients, oxygen, and metabolic end products across the capillary wall?

17. What is the only solute that has a significant concentration difference across the capillary wall? How does this difference influence water concentration?
18. What four variables determine the net filtration pressure across the capillary wall? Give representative values for each of them at the arteriolar and venous ends of a systemic capillary.
19. How do changes in local arteriolar resistance influence downstream capillary pressure?
20. What is the relationship between cardiac output and venous return in the steady state? What is the force driving venous return?
21. Contrast the compliances and blood volumes of the veins and arteries.
22. What four factors influence venous pressure?
23. Approximately how much fluid do the lymphatics return to the blood each day?
24. Describe the mechanisms that cause lymph flow.

SECTION C KEY TERMS

SECTION C CLINICAL TERMS

SECTION D
Integration of Cardiovascular Function: Regulation of Systemic Arterial Pressure

In Chapter 1, we described the fundamental components of homeostatic control systems: (1) an internal environmental variable maintained in a relatively narrow range, (2) receptors sensitive to changes in this variable, (3) afferent pathways from the receptors, (4) an integrating center that receives and integrates the afferent inputs, (5) efferent pathways from the integrating center, and (6) effectors that act to change the variable when signals arrive along efferent pathways. The control and integration of cardiovascular function will be described in these terms.

The major cardiovascular variable being regulated is the mean arterial pressure in the systemic circulation. This should not be surprising because this pressure is the driving force for blood flow through all the organs except the lungs. Maintaining it is therefore a prerequisite for ensuring adequate blood flow to these organs. The importance of maintaining blood pressure within a normal range demonstrates the general principle of physiology that homeostasis is essential for health and survival. Without a homeostatic control system operating to maintain blood pressure, the tissues of the body would quickly die if pressure were to decrease significantly.

The mean systemic arterial pressure is the arithmetic product of two factors: (1) the cardiac output and (2) the **total peripheral resistance (*TPR*)**, which is the combined resistance to flow of all the systemic blood vessels.

$$\begin{matrix}\text{Mean systemic} & & \text{Cardiac} & & \text{Total peripheral} \\ \text{arterial pressure} & = & \text{output} & \times & \text{resistance} \\ (MAP) & & (CO) & & (TPR)\end{matrix}$$

Cardiac output and total peripheral resistance set the mean systemic arterial pressure because they determine the average volume of blood in the systemic arteries over time; it is this blood volume that causes the pressure. This relationship cannot be emphasized too strongly: *All changes in mean arterial pressure must be the result of changes in cardiac output and/or total peripheral resistance.* Keep in mind that mean arterial pressure will change only if the arithmetic product of cardiac output and total peripheral resistance changes. For example, if cardiac output doubles and total peripheral resistance decreases by half, mean arterial pressure will not change because the product of cardiac output and total peripheral resistance has not changed. Because cardiac output is the volume of blood pumped into the arteries per unit time, it is fairly intuitive that it should be one of the two determinants of mean arterial volume and pressure. The contribution of total peripheral resistance to mean arterial pressure is less obvious, but it can be illustrated with the model introduced previously in Figure 12.33.

As shown in **Figure 12.49**, a pump pushes fluid into a container at the rate of 1 L/min. At steady state, fluid also leaves through the outflow tubes at a total rate of 1 L/min. Therefore, the height of the fluid column (ΔP), which is the driving pressure for outflow, remains stable. We then disturb the steady state by dilating outflow tube 1, thereby increasing its radius, reducing its resistance, and increasing its flow. The total outflow for the system immediately becomes greater than 1 L/min, and more fluid leaves the reservoir than enters

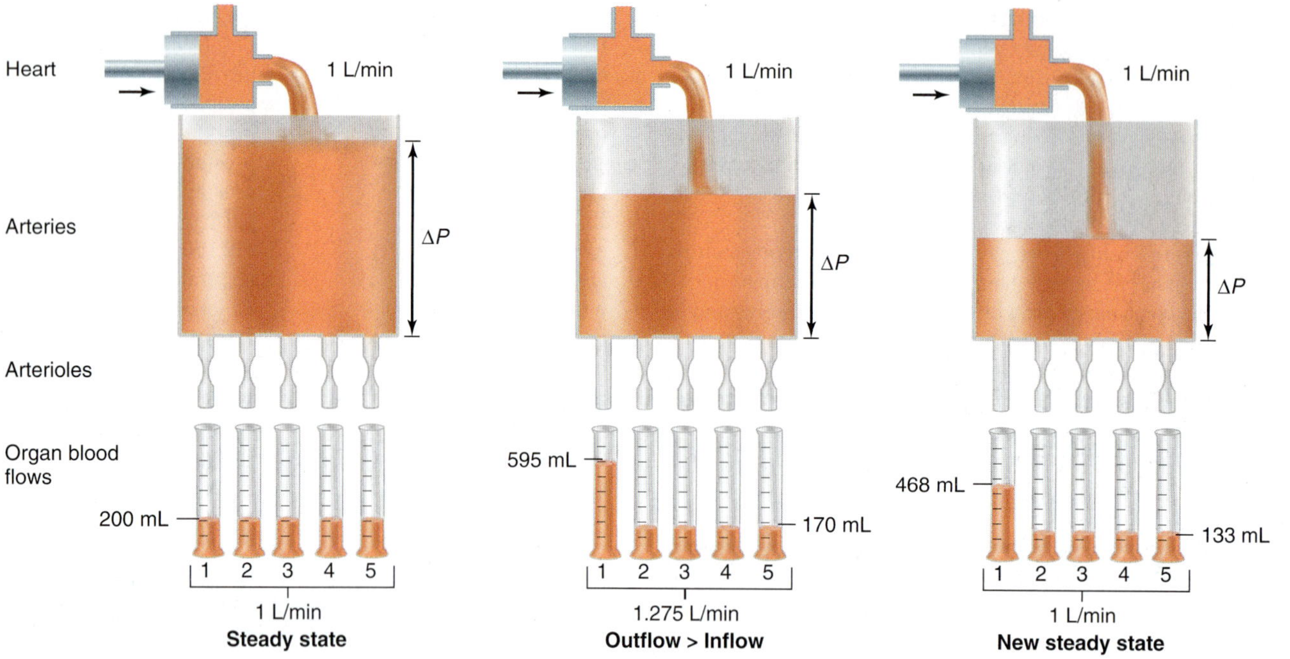

Figure 12.49 Dependence of arterial blood pressure upon total arteriolar resistance. Dilating one arteriolar bed affects arterial pressure and organ blood flow if no compensatory adjustments occur. The middle panel indicates a transient state before the new steady state occurs.

from the pump. Therefore, the volume and height of the fluid column begin to decrease until a new steady state between inflow and outflow is reached. In other words, at any given pump input, a change in total outflow resistance must produce changes in the volume and height (pressure) in the reservoir.

This analysis can be applied to the circulatory system by again equating the pump with the heart, the reservoir with the arteries, and the outflow tubes with various arteriolar beds. As described earlier, the major sites of resistance in the systemic circuit are the arterioles. Moreover, changes in total resistance are normally due to changes in the resistance of arterioles. Therefore, total peripheral resistance is determined by total arteriolar resistance.

A physiological analogy to opening outflow tube 1 is exercise. During exercise, the skeletal muscle arterioles dilate, thereby decreasing resistance. If the cardiac output and the arteriolar diameters of all other vascular beds were to remain unchanged, the increased runoff through the skeletal muscle arterioles would cause a decrease in systemic arterial pressure.

We must reemphasize that it is the *total* arteriolar resistance that influences systemic arterial blood pressure. The distribution of resistances among organs is irrelevant in this regard. **Figure 12.50** illustrates this point. On the right, outflow tube 1 has been opened, as in the previous example, while tubes 2 to 4 have been simultaneously constricted. The increased resistance in tubes 2 to 4 compensates for the decreased resistance in tube 1. Therefore, total resistance remains unchanged, and the reservoir pressure is unchanged. Total outflow remains 1 L/min, although the distribution of flows is such that flow through tube 1 increases, flow through tubes 2 to 4 decreases, and flow through tube 5 is unchanged. This is analogous to the alteration of systemic vascular resistances that occurs during exercise. When the skeletal muscle arterioles (tube 1) dilate, the total resistance of the systemic

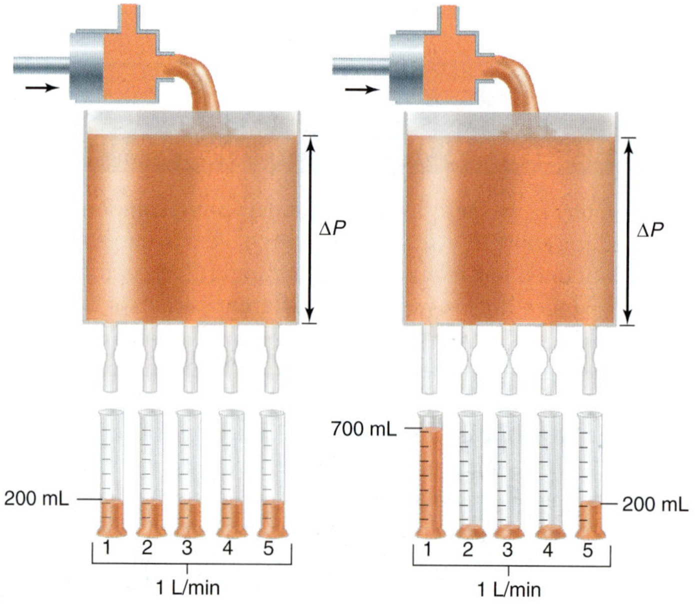

Figure 12.50 Compensation for dilation in one bed by constriction in others. When outflow tube 1 is opened, outflow tubes 2 to 4 are simultaneously tightened so that total outflow resistance, total runoff rate, and reservoir pressure all remain constant.

circulation can still be maintained if arterioles constrict in other organs, such as the kidneys, stomach, and intestine (tubes 2 to 4). In contrast, the brain arterioles (tube 5) remain unchanged, ensuring constant brain blood supply.

This type of resistance juggling can maintain total resistance only within limits, however. Obviously, if tube 1 opens too wide, even complete closure of the other tubes potentially might not prevent total outflow resistance from decreasing. In that situation, cardiac output must be

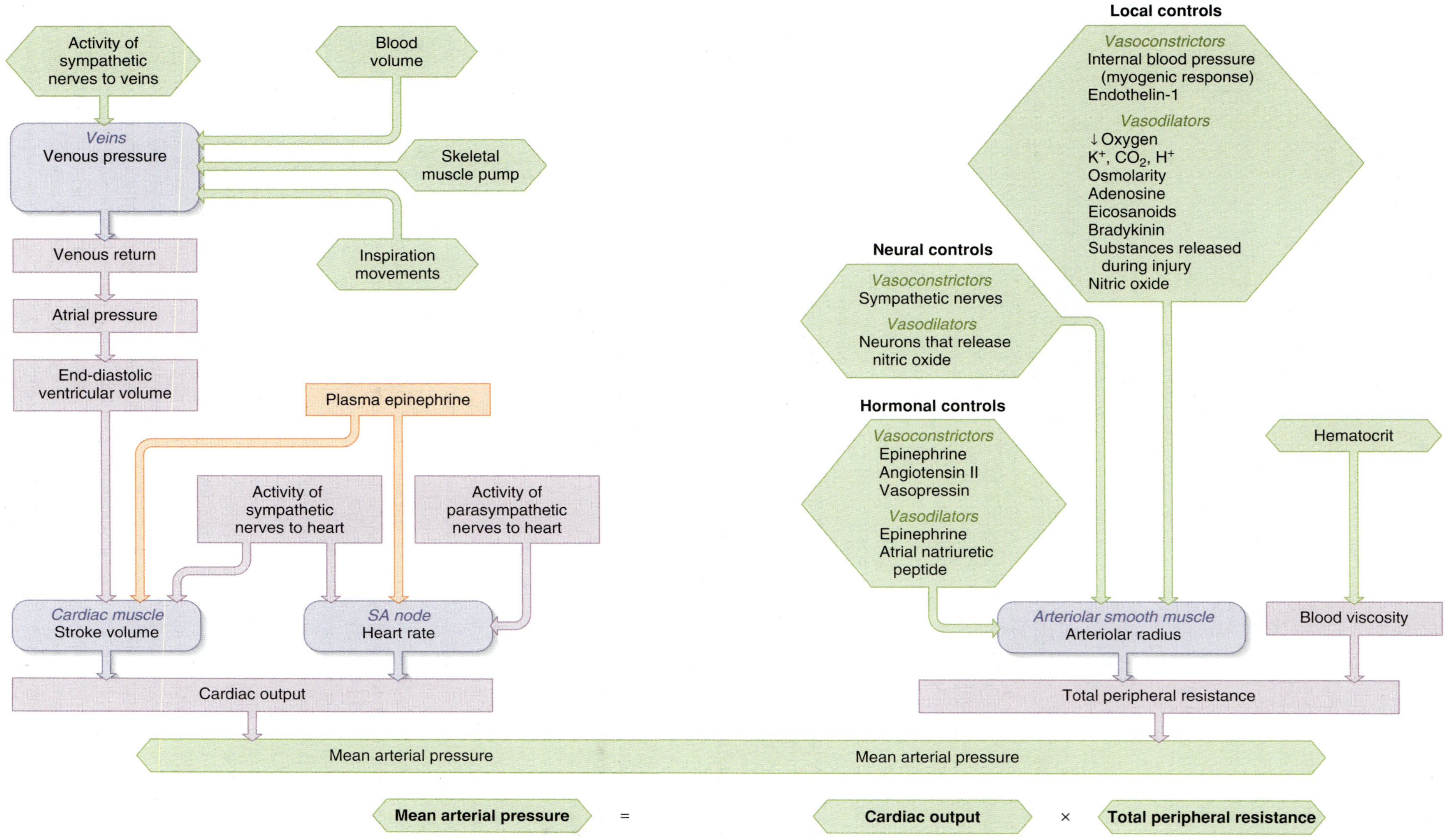

Figure 12.51 Summary of factors that determine systemic arterial pressure, a composite of Figures 12.27, 12.36, and 12.46, with the addition of the effect of hematocrit on resistance.

increased to maintain pressure in the arteries. We will see that this is actually the case during exercise.

We have so far explained in an intuitive way why cardiac output (CO) and total peripheral resistance (TPR) are the two variables that determine mean systemic arterial pressure. This intuitive approach, however, does not explain specifically why MAP is the arithmetic product of CO and TPR. This relationship can be derived formally from the basic equation relating flow, pressure, and resistance:

$$F = \Delta P/R$$

Rearranging terms algebraically,

$$\Delta P = F \times R$$

Because the systemic vascular system is a continuous series of tubes, this equation holds for the entire system—that is, from the arteries to the right atrium. Therefore, the ΔP term is mean systemic arterial pressure (MAP) minus the pressure in the right atrium, F is the cardiac output (CO), and R is the total peripheral resistance (TPR):

$$MAP - \text{Right atrial pressure} = CO \times TPR$$

Because the pressure in the right atrium is close to zero, we can drop this term and we are left with the equation presented earlier:

$$MAP = CO \times TPR$$

This equation is the fundamental equation of cardiovascular physiology. An analogous equation can also be applied to the pulmonary circulation:

$$\begin{matrix}\text{Mean pulmonary} \\ \text{arterial pressure}\end{matrix} = CO \times \begin{matrix}\text{Total pulmonary} \\ \text{vascular resistance}\end{matrix}$$

These equations provide a way to integrate information presented in this chapter. For example, we can now explain why mean pulmonary arterial pressure is much lower than mean systemic arterial pressure (**Table 12.6**). The blood flow (that is, the cardiac output) through the pulmonary and systemic arteries is the same. Therefore, the pressures can differ only if the resistances differ. Thus, we can deduce that the pulmonary vessels offer much less resistance to flow than do the systemic vessels. In other words, the total pulmonary vascular resistance is lower than the total peripheral resistance.

Figure 12.51 presents the grand scheme of factors that determine mean systemic arterial pressure. None of this information is new—all of it was presented in previous figures. A change in only a single variable will produce a change in mean systemic arterial pressure by altering either cardiac output or total peripheral resistance. For example, **Figure 12.52** illustrates how bleeding that results in significant blood loss (***hemorrhage***) leads to a decrease in mean arterial pressure. Conversely, any deviation in mean arterial pressure, such as that occurring during hemorrhage, will elicit homeostatic reflexes so that cardiac output and/or total peripheral resistance will change in the direction required to minimize the initial change in arterial pressure.

TABLE 12.6 Comparison of Hemodynamics in the Systemic and Pulmonary Circuits

	Systemic Circulation	Pulmonary Circulation
Cardiac output (L/min)	5	5
Systolic pressure (mmHg)	120	25
Diastolic pressure (mmHg)	80	10
Mean arterial pressure (mmHg)	93	15

PHYSIOLOGICAL INQUIRY

- Calculate the magnitude of the difference in total resistance between the systemic and pulmonary circuits.

Answer can be found at end of chapter.

In the short term—seconds to hours—these homeostatic adjustments to mean arterial pressure are brought about by reflexes called the *baroreceptor reflexes.* They utilize mainly changes in the activity of the autonomic neurons supplying the heart and blood vessels, as well as changes in the secretion of the hormones that influence these structures (epinephrine, angiotensin II, and vasopressin). Over longer time spans, the baroreceptor reflexes become less important and factors controlling blood volume play a dominant role in determining blood pressure. The next two sections describe these phenomena.

12.13 Baroreceptor Reflexes

Arterial Baroreceptors

The reflexes that homeostatically regulate arterial pressure originate primarily with arterial receptors that respond to changes in pressure. Two of these receptors are found where the left and right common carotid arteries divide into two smaller arteries that supply the head with blood (**Figure 12.53**). At this division, the wall of the artery is thinner than usual and contains a large number of branching, sensory neuronal processes. This portion of the artery is called the carotid sinus (the term *sinus* denotes a recess, space, or dilated channel), and the sensory neurons are highly sensitive to stretch or distortion. The degree of wall stretching is directly related to the pressure within the artery. Therefore, the carotid sinuses serve as pressure receptors, or **baroreceptors.** An area functionally similar to the carotid sinuses is found in the arch of the aorta and is termed the **aortic arch baroreceptor.** The two carotid sinuses and the aortic arch baroreceptor constitute the **arterial baroreceptors.** Afferent neurons travel from them to the brainstem and provide input to the neurons of cardiovascular control centers there.

Action potentials recorded in single afferent neurons from the carotid sinus demonstrate the pattern of baroreceptor response (**Figure 12.54a**). In this experiment, the pressure

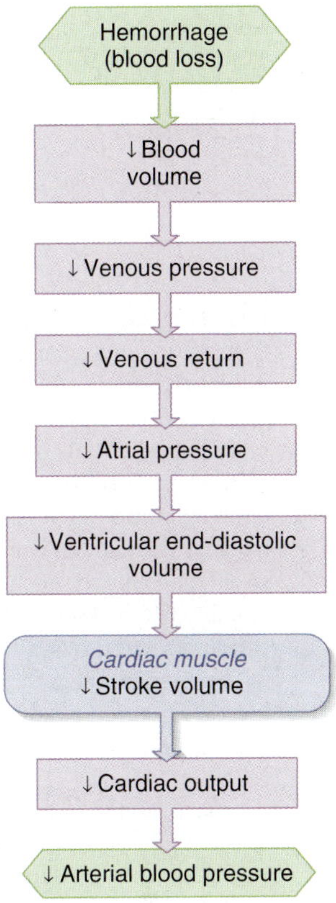

Figure 12.52 Sequence of events by which a decrease in blood volume leads to a decrease in mean arterial pressure.

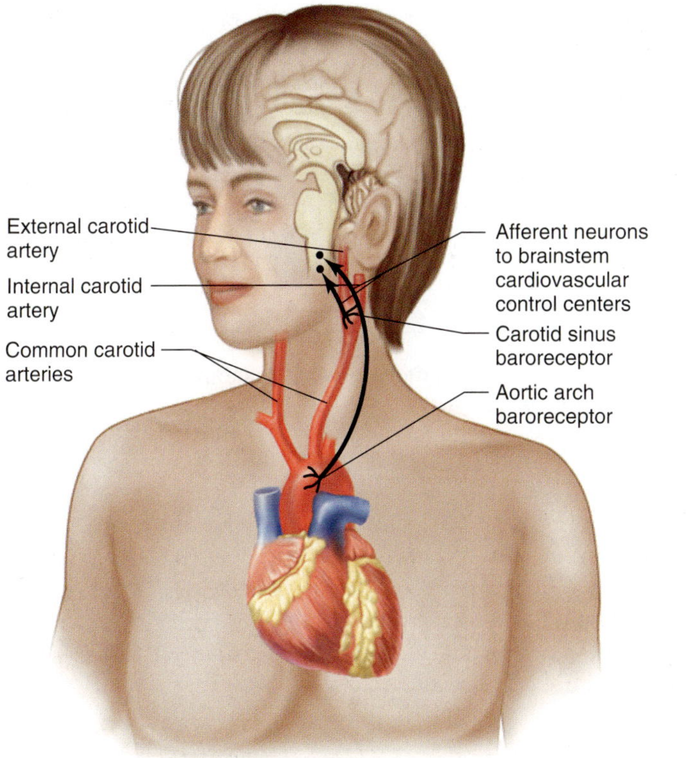

Figure 12.53 APR Locations of arterial baroreceptors.

PHYSIOLOGICAL INQUIRY

- When you first stand up after getting out of bed, how does the pressure detected by the carotid baroreceptors change?

Answer can be found at end of chapter.

in the carotid sinus is artificially controlled so that the pressure is steady, not pulsatile (i.e., not varying as usual between systolic and diastolic pressure). At a particular steady pressure, for example, 100 mmHg, there is a certain rate of discharge by the neuron. This rate can be increased by raising the arterial pressure, or it can be decreased by lowering the pressure. The rate of discharge of the carotid sinus is therefore directly proportional to the mean arterial pressure.

If the experiment is repeated using the same mean pressures as before but allowing pressure pulsations (**Figure 12.54b**), it is found that at any given mean pressure, the larger the pulse pressure, the faster the rate of firing by the carotid sinus. This responsiveness to pulse pressure adds a further element of information to blood pressure regulation, because small changes in factors such as blood volume may cause changes in arterial pulse pressure with little or no change in mean arterial pressure.

The Medullary Cardiovascular Center

The primary integrating center for the baroreceptor reflexes is a diffuse network of highly interconnected neurons called the **medullary cardiovascular center,** located in the medulla oblongata. The neurons in this center receive input from the various baroreceptors. This input determines the action potential frequency from the cardiovascular center along neural pathways that terminate upon the cell bodies and dendrites of the vagus (parasympathetic) neurons to the heart and the sympathetic neurons to the heart, arterioles, and veins. When the arterial baroreceptors increase their rate of discharge, the result is a decrease in sympathetic neuron activity and an increase in parasympathetic neuron activity (**Figure 12.55**). A decrease in baroreceptor firing rate results in the opposite pattern.

Angiotensin II generation and vasopressin secretion are also altered by baroreceptor activity and help restore blood pressure. Decreased arterial pressure elicits increased plasma concentrations of both these hormones, which increase arterial pressure by constricting arterioles.

Operation of the Arterial Baroreceptor Reflex

Our description of the arterial baroreceptor reflex is now complete. If arterial pressure decreases, as during a hemorrhage (**Figure 12.56**), the discharge rate of the arterial baroreceptors also decreases. Fewer action potentials travel up the afferent nerves to the medullary cardiovascular center, and this induces (1) increased heart rate because of increased sympathetic activity and decreased parasympathetic activity to the heart, (2) increased ventricular contractility because of increased sympathetic activity to the ventricular myocardium, (3) arteriolar constriction because of increased sympathetic activity to the arterioles (and increased plasma concentrations of angiotensin II and vasopressin), and (4) increased venous constriction because of increased sympathetic activity to the veins. The net result is an increased

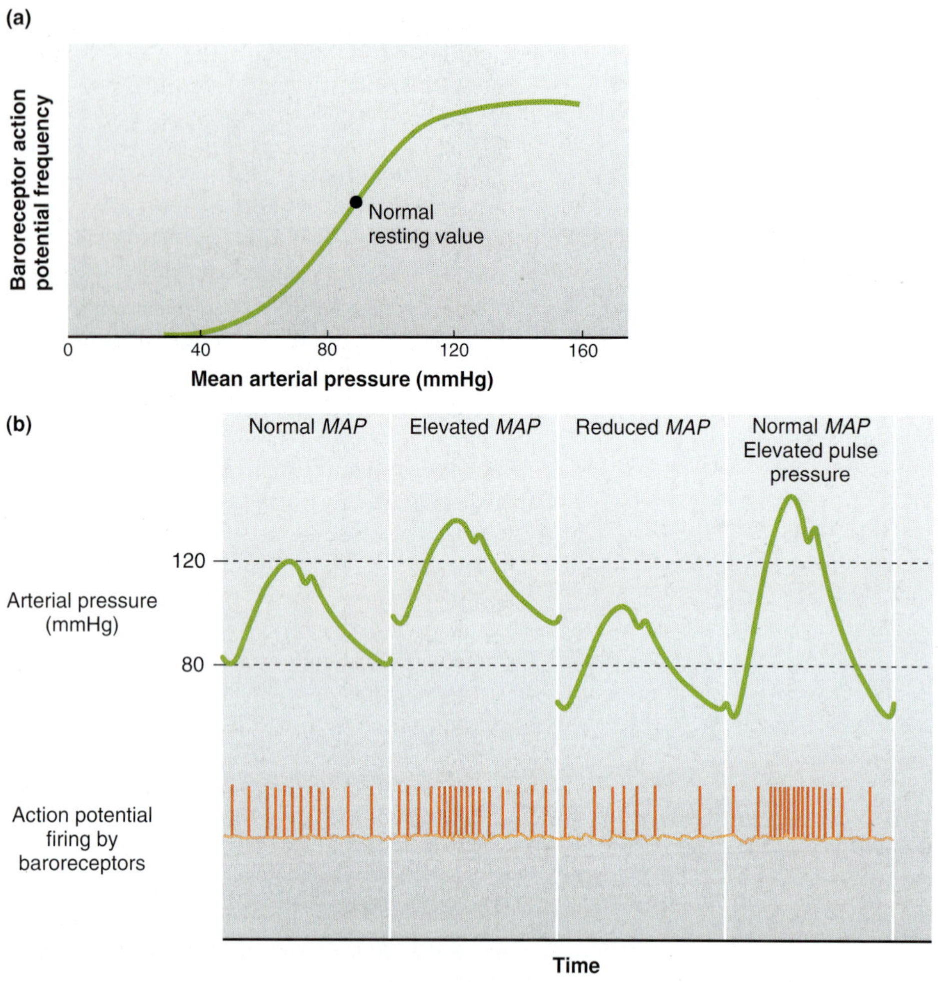

Figure 12.54 AP|R Baroreceptor firing frequency changes with changes in blood pressure. (a) Effect of changing mean arterial pressure (*MAP*) on the firing of action potentials by afferent neurons from the carotid sinus. This experiment is done by pumping blood in a nonpulsatile manner through an isolated carotid sinus so as to be able to set the pressure inside it at any value desired. (b) Baroreceptor action potential firing frequency fluctuates with pressure. Increase in pulse pressure increases overall action potential frequency even at a normal *MAP*.

PHYSIOLOGICAL INQUIRY

- Note in part (a) that the normal resting value on this pressure–frequency curve is on the steepest, center part of the curve. What might be the physiological significance of this?

Answer can be found at end of chapter.

cardiac output (increased heart rate and stroke volume), increased total peripheral resistance (arteriolar constriction), and return of blood pressure toward normal. Conversely, an increase in arterial blood pressure for any reason causes increased firing of the arterial baroreceptors, which reflexively induces compensatory decreases in cardiac output and total peripheral resistance.

Having emphasized the importance of the arterial baroreceptor reflex, we must now add an equally important qualification. The baroreceptor reflex functions primarily as a short-term regulator of arterial blood pressure. It is activated instantly by any blood pressure change and functions to restore blood pressure rapidly toward normal. However, if arterial pressure remains increased from its normal set point for more than a few days, the arterial baroreceptors adapt to this new pressure and decrease their frequency of action potential firing at any given pressure. Thus, in patients who have chronically elevated blood pressure, the arterial baroreceptors continue to oppose minute-to-minute changes in blood pressure, but at a higher set point.

Other Baroreceptors

The large systemic veins, the pulmonary vessels, and the walls of the heart also contain baroreceptors, most of which function in a manner analogous to the arterial baroreceptors. By keeping brain cardiovascular control centers constantly informed about changes in the systemic venous, pulmonary, atrial, and ventricular pressures, these other baroreceptors provide a further degree of regulatory sensitivity. In essence, they contribute a feedforward component of arterial pressure control. For example, a slight decrease in ventricular pressure reflexively increases the activity of the sympathetic nervous system even before the change decreases cardiac output and arterial pressure enough to be detected by the arterial baroreceptors.

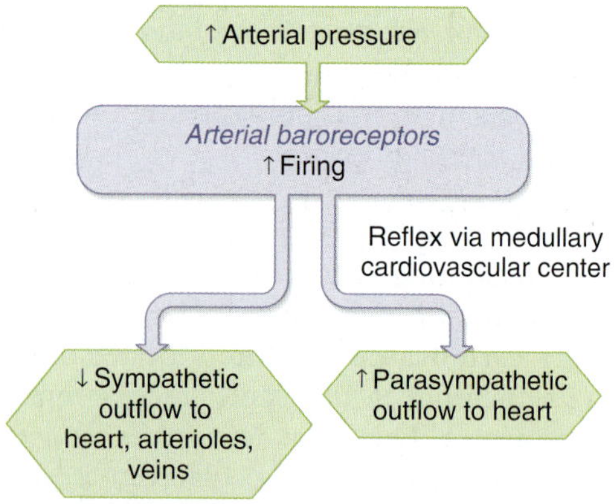

Figure 12.55 AP|R Neural components of the arterial baroreceptor reflex. If the initial change were a decrease in arterial pressure, all the arrows in the boxes would be reversed.

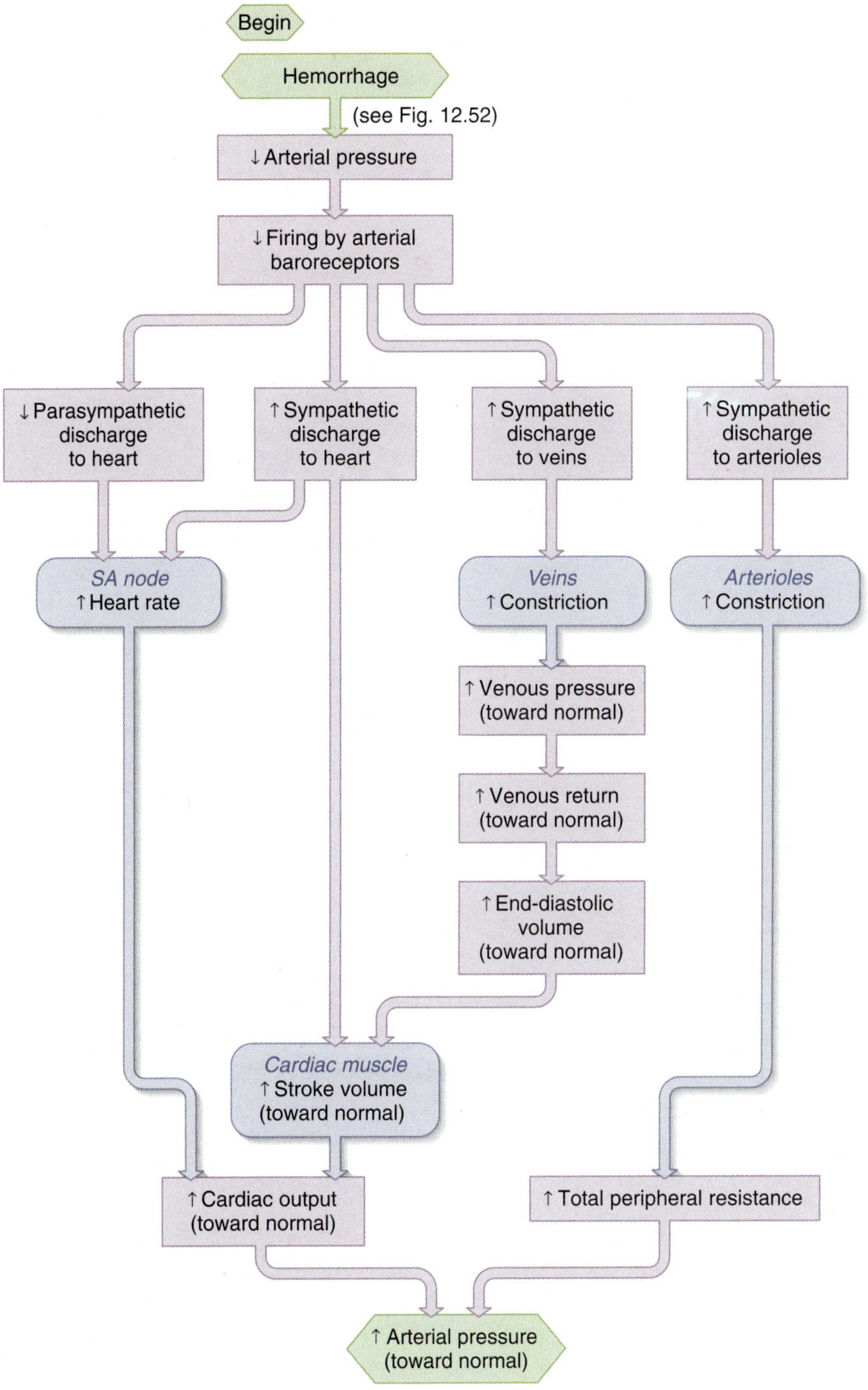

Figure 12.56 APIR Arterial baroreceptor reflex compensation for hemorrhage. The compensatory mechanisms do not restore arterial pressure completely to normal. The increases designated "toward normal" are relative to prehemorrhage values; for example, the stroke volume is increased reflexively "toward normal" relative to the low point caused by the hemorrhage (i.e., before the reflex occurs), but it does not reach the level it had prior to the hemorrhage. For simplicity, the fact that plasma angiotensin II and vasopressin are also reflexively increased and help constrict arterioles is not shown.

12.14 Blood Volume and Long-Term Regulation of Arterial Pressure

The fact that the arterial baroreceptors (and other baroreceptors as well) adapt to prolonged changes in pressure means that the baroreceptor reflexes cannot set long-term arterial pressure. The major mechanism for long-term regulation occurs through the blood volume. As described earlier, blood volume is a major determinant of arterial pressure because it influences venous pressure, venous return, end-diastolic volume, stroke volume, and cardiac output. Thus, increased blood volume increases arterial pressure. However, the opposite causal chain also exists—an increased arterial pressure reduces blood volume (more specifically, the plasma component of the blood volume) by increasing the excretion of salt and water by the kidneys, as will be described in Chapter 14.

Figure 12.57 illustrates how these two causal chains constitute negative feedback loops that determine both blood volume and arterial pressure. An increase in blood pressure for any reason causes a decrease in blood volume, which tends to bring the blood pressure back down. An increase in the blood volume for any reason increases the blood pressure, which tends to bring the blood volume back down. The important point is this: Because arterial pressure influences blood volume but blood volume also influences arterial pressure, blood pressure can stabilize, in the long run, only at a value at which blood volume is also stable. Consequently, changes in steady-state blood volume are the single most important long-term determinant of blood pressure. The cooperation of the urinary and circulatory systems in the maintenance of blood volume and pressure is an excellent example of how the functions of organ systems are coordinated with each other—one of the general principles of physiology introduced in Chapter 1.

12.15 Other Cardiovascular Reflexes and Responses

Stimuli acting upon receptors other than baroreceptors can initiate reflexes that cause changes in arterial pressure. For example, the following stimuli all cause an increase in blood pressure: decreased arterial oxygen concentration, increased arterial carbon dioxide concentration, decreased blood flow to the brain, and pain originating in the skin. In contrast, pain originating in the viscera or joints may cause *decreases* in arterial pressure.

Many physiological states such as eating and sexual activity are also associated with changes in blood pressure. For example, attending a stressful business meeting may increase mean blood pressure by as much as 20 mmHg, walking increases it 10 mmHg, and sleeping decreases it 10 mmHg. Mood also has a significant effect on blood pressure, which tends to be lower when people report that they are happy than when they are angry or anxious.

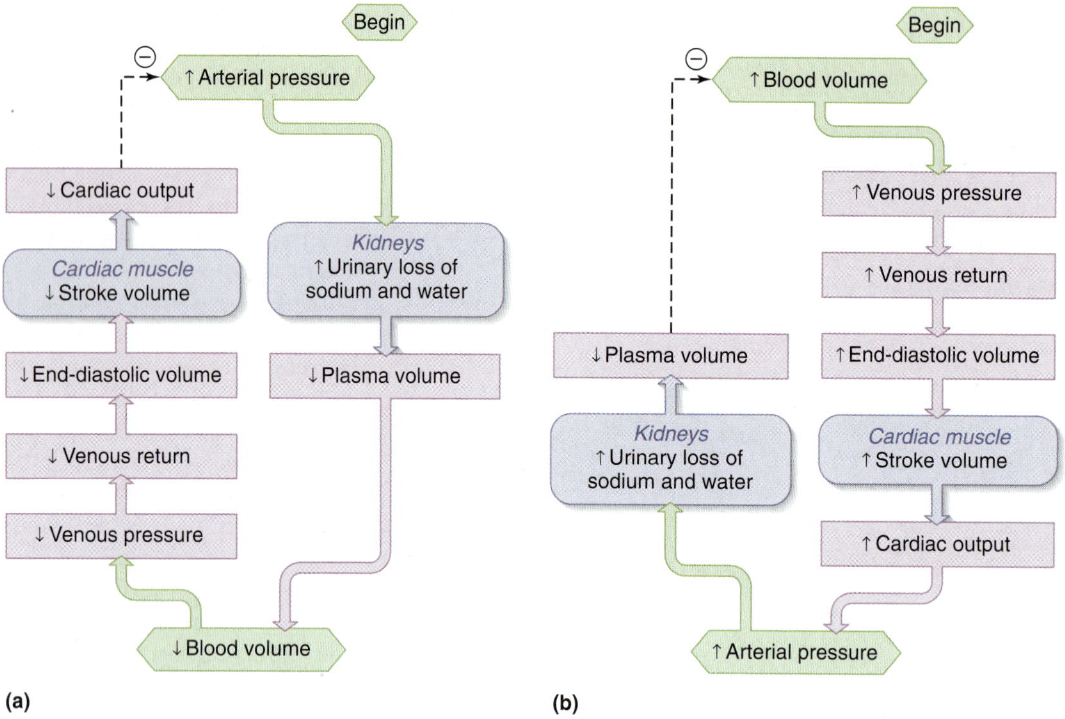

Figure 12.57 Causal relationships between arterial pressure and blood volume. (a) An increase in arterial pressure due, for example, to an increased cardiac output induces a decrease in blood volume by promoting fluid excretion by the kidneys. This tends to restore arterial pressure to its original value. (b) An increase in blood volume due, for example, to increased fluid ingestion induces an increase in arterial pressure, which tends to restore blood volume to its original value by promoting fluid excretion by the kidneys. Because of these relationships, blood volume is a major determinant of arterial pressure.

These changes are triggered by input from receptors or higher brain centers to the medullary cardiovascular center or, in some cases, to pathways distinct from these centers. For example, the fibers of certain neurons whose cell bodies are in the cerebral cortex and hypothalamus synapse directly on the sympathetic neurons in the spinal cord, bypassing the medullary center altogether.

An important clinical situation involving reflexes that regulate blood pressure is Cushing's phenomenon (not to be confused with Cushing's syndrome and disease, which are endocrine diseases discussed in Chapter 11). ***Cushing's phenomenon*** is a situation in which increased intracranial pressure causes a dramatic increase in mean arterial pressure. A number of different circumstances can cause increased pressure in the brain, including the presence of a rapidly growing cancerous tumor or a traumatic head injury that triggers internal hemorrhage or edema. What distinguishes these situations from similar problems elsewhere in the body is the fact that the enclosed bony cranium does not allow physical swelling toward the outside, so pressure is directed inward. This inward pressure exerts a collapsing force on intracranial vasculature, and the reduction in radius greatly increases the resistance to blood flow (recall that resistance increases as the fourth power of a decrease in radius). Blood flow is reduced below the level needed to satisfy metabolic requirements, brain oxygen concentration decreases, and carbon dioxide and other metabolic wastes increase. Accumulated metabolites in the brain interstitial fluid powerfully stimulate sympathetic neurons controlling systemic arterioles, resulting in a large increase in *TPR* and, consequently, a large increase in mean arterial pressure ($MAP = CO \times TPR$). In principle, this increased systemic pressure is adaptive, in that it can overcome the collapsing pressures and force blood to flow through the brain once again. However, if the original problem was an intracranial hemorrhage, restoring blood flow to the brain might only cause more bleeding and exacerbate the problem. To restore brain blood flow at a normal mean arterial pressure, the brain tumor or accumulated intracranial fluid must be removed.

SECTION D SUMMARY

I. Mean arterial pressure, the primary regulated variable in the cardiovascular system, equals the product of cardiac output and total peripheral resistance. MAP= CO × TPR

II. The factors that determine cardiac output and total peripheral resistance are summarized in Figure 12.51.

Baroreceptor Reflexes

I. The primary baroreceptors are the arterial baroreceptors, including the two carotid sinuses and the aortic arch. Other baroreceptors are located in the systemic veins, pulmonary vessels, and walls of the heart.

II. The firing rates of the arterial baroreceptors are proportional to mean arterial pressure and to pulse pressure.

III. An increase in firing of the arterial baroreceptors due to an increase in pressure causes, by way of the medullary cardiovascular center, an increase in parasympathetic outflow to the heart and a decrease in sympathetic outflow to the heart, arterioles, and veins. The result is a decrease in cardiac output, total peripheral resistance, and mean arterial pressure. The opposite occurs when the initial change is a decrease in arterial pressure.

Blood Volume and Long-Term Regulation of Arterial Pressure

I. The baroreceptor reflexes are short-term regulators of arterial pressure but adapt to a maintained change in pressure.
II. The most important long-term regulator of arterial pressure is the blood volume.

Other Cardiovascular Reflexes and Responses

I. Blood pressure can be influenced by many factors other than baroreceptors, including arterial blood gas concentrations, pain, emotions, and sexual activity.
II. Cushing's phenomenon is a clinical condition in which elevated intracranial pressure leads to decreased brain blood flow and a large increase in arterial blood pressure.

SECTION D REVIEW QUESTIONS

1. Write the equation relating mean arterial pressure to cardiac output and total peripheral resistance.
2. What variable accounts for the fact that mean pulmonary arterial pressure is lower than mean systemic arterial pressure?
3. Draw a flow diagram illustrating the factors that determine mean arterial pressure.
4. Identify the receptors, afferent pathways, integrating center, efferent pathways, and effectors in the arterial baroreceptor reflex.
5. When the arterial baroreceptors decrease or increase their rate of firing, what changes in autonomic outflow and cardiovascular function occur?
6. Describe the role of blood volume in the long-term regulation of arterial pressure.
7. Describe the cardiovascular response to a head injury that causes cerebral edema.

SECTION D KEY TERMS

aortic arch baroreceptor 409
arterial baroreceptors 409
baroreceptors 409
medullary cardiovascular center 412
total peripheral resistance (*TPR*) 407

SECTION D CLINICAL TERMS

Cushing's phenomenon 414
hemorrhage 409

SECTION E Cardiovascular Patterns in Health and Disease

12.16 Hemorrhage and Other Causes of Hypotension

The term ***hypotension*** means a low blood pressure, regardless of cause. One general cause of hypotension is a significant loss of blood volume as, for example, in a hemorrhage, which produces hypotension by the sequence of events shown previously in Figure 12.52. The most serious consequence of hypotension is reduced blood flow to the brain and cardiac muscle. The immediate counteracting response to hemorrhage is the arterial baroreceptor reflex, as summarized in Figure 12.56.

Figure 12.58, which shows how five variables change over time when blood volume decreases, adds a further degree of clarification to Figure 12.56. The values of factors changed as a direct result of the hemorrhage—stroke volume, cardiac output, and mean arterial pressure—are restored by the baroreceptor reflex toward, but not all the way to, normal. In contrast, values not altered directly by the hemorrhage but only by the reflex response to hemorrhage—heart rate and total peripheral resistance—increase above their prehemorrhage values. The increased peripheral resistance results from increases in sympathetic outflow to the arterioles in many vascular beds (but not those of the heart and brain). Thus, skin blood flow may decrease considerably because of arteriolar vasoconstriction; this is why the skin can become pale and cold following a significant hemorrhage. Kidney and intestinal blood flow also decrease because the usual functions of these organs are not immediately essential for life.

A second important type of compensatory mechanism (one not shown in Figure 12.56) involves the movement of interstitial fluid into capillaries. This occurs because both the decrease in blood pressure and the increase in arteriolar constriction decrease capillary hydrostatic pressure, thereby favoring the absorption of interstitial fluid (**Figure 12.59**). Thus, the initial events—blood loss and decreased blood volume—are in part compensated for by the movement of interstitial fluid into the vascular system. This mechanism, referred to as **autotransfusion,** can restore the blood volume to virtually normal levels within 12 to 24 hours after a moderate hemorrhage (**Table 12.7**). At this time, the entire restoration of blood volume is due to expansion of the plasma volume; therefore, the hematocrit actually decreases.

The early compensatory mechanisms for hemorrhage (the baroreceptor reflexes and interstitial fluid absorption) are

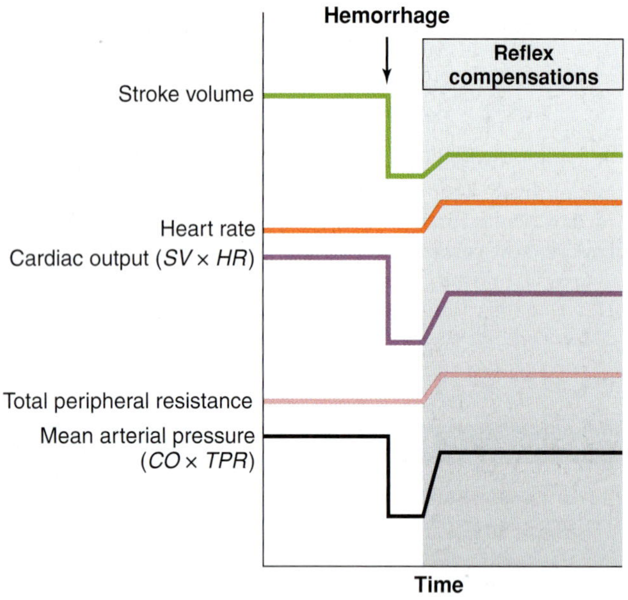

Figure 12.58 Five simultaneous graphs showing the time course of cardiovascular effects of hemorrhage. Note that the entire decrease in arterial pressure immediately following hemorrhage is secondary to the decrease in stroke volume and, therefore, cardiac output. This figure emphasizes the relative proportions of the "increase" and "decrease" arrows of Figure 12.56. All variables shown are increased relative to the state immediately following the hemorrhage, but they are not all increased compared to the state prior to the hemorrhage.

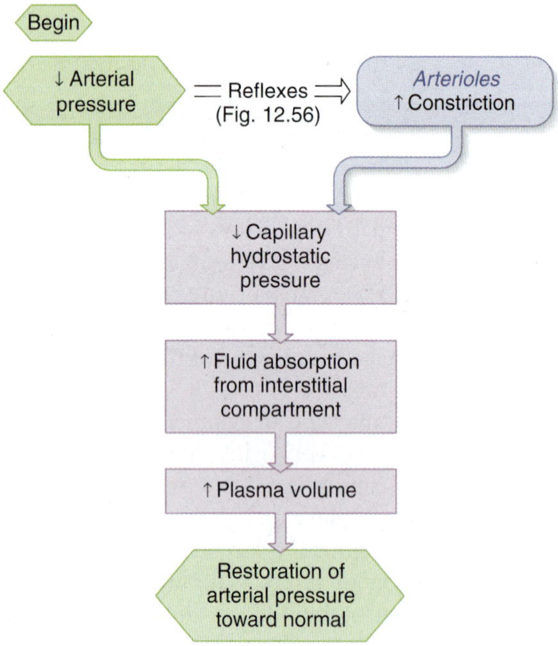

Figure 12.59 The autotransfusion mechanism compensates for blood loss by causing interstitial fluid to move into the capillaries.

highly efficient, so that losses of as much as 30% of total blood volume can be sustained with only slight reductions of mean arterial pressure or cardiac output.

We must emphasize that absorption of interstitial fluid only *redistributes* the extracellular fluid. Ultimate restoration of blood volume involves the control of fluid ingestion and

TABLE 12.7 Fluid Shifts After Hemorrhage

	Normal	Immediately After Hemorrhage	18 Hours After Hemorrhage
Total blood volume (mL)	5000	4000	4900
Erythrocyte volume (mL)	2300	1840	1840
Plasma volume (mL)	2700	2160	3060

PHYSIOLOGICAL INQUIRY

- Calculate the hematocrit before and 18 hours after the hemorrhage, and explain the changes that are observed.

Answer can be found at end of chapter.

minimizing water loss via the kidneys. These slower-acting compensations include an increase in thirst and a reduction in the excretion of salt and water in the urine. They are mediated by hormones, including renin, angiotensin, and aldosterone, and are described in Chapter 14. Replacement of the lost erythrocytes requires the hormone erythropoietin to stimulate erythropoiesis (maturation of immature red blood cells); this is described in detail in Section F of this chapter. These replacement processes require days to weeks in contrast to the rapidly occurring reflex compensations illustrated in Figure 12.59.

Hemorrhage is a striking example of hypotension due to a decrease in blood volume. There is a second way, however, that hypotension can occur due to volume depletion that does not result from loss of whole blood. It may occur through the skin, as in severe sweating or burns, or through the gastrointestinal tract, as in diarrhea or vomiting, or through the kidneys, as with unusually large urinary losses. By these various routes, the body can be depleted of water and ions such as Na^+, Cl^-, K^+, H^+, and HCO_3^-. Regardless of the route, the loss of fluid decreases circulating blood volume and produces symptoms and compensatory cardiovascular changes similar to those seen in hemorrhage.

Hypotension may also be caused by events other than blood or fluid loss. One major cause is a decrease in cardiac contractility (for example, during a heart attack). Another cause is strong emotion, which in rare cases can cause hypotension and fainting. The higher brain centers involved with emotions inhibit sympathetic activity to the cardiovascular system and enhance parasympathetic activity to the heart, resulting in a markedly decreased arterial pressure and brain blood flow. This whole process, known as ***vasovagal syncope***, is usually transient. It should be noted that the fainting that sometimes occurs in a person donating blood is usually due to hypotension brought on by emotion, not due to the blood loss, because losing 0.5 L of blood will not generally cause serious hypotension. Massive release of endogenous substances that relax arteriolar smooth muscle may also cause hypotension by reducing total peripheral resistance. An important example is the hypotension that occurs during severe allergic responses (Chapter 18).

Shock

The term ***shock*** denotes any situation in which a decrease in blood flow to the organs and tissues damages them. Arterial pressure is usually, but not always, low in shock, and the classification of shock is quite similar to that used for hypotension. ***Hypovolemic shock*** is caused by a decrease in blood volume secondary to hemorrhage or loss of fluid other than blood. ***Low-resistance shock*** is due to a decrease in total peripheral resistance secondary to excessive release of vasodilators, as in allergy and infection. ***Cardiogenic shock*** is due to an extreme decrease in cardiac output from any of a variety of factors (for example, during a heart attack).

The circulatory system, especially the heart, suffers damage if shock is prolonged. As the heart deteriorates, cardiac output further declines and shock becomes progressively worse. Ultimately, shock may become irreversible even though blood transfusions and other appropriate therapy may temporarily restore blood pressure. See Chapter 19 for a case study of a person who experiences shock.

12.17 The Upright Posture

A decrease in the effective circulating blood volume occurs in the circulatory system when moving from a lying, horizontal position to a standing, vertical one. Why this is so requires an understanding of the action of gravity upon the long, continuous columns of blood in the vessels between the heart and the feet.

The pressures described in previous sections of this chapter are for an individual in the horizontal position, in which all blood vessels are at nearly the same level as the heart. In this position, the weight of the blood produces negligible pressure. In contrast, when a person is standing, the intravascular pressure everywhere becomes equal to the pressure generated by cardiac contraction plus an additional pressure equal to the weight of a column of blood from the heart to the point of measurement. In an average adult, for example, the weight of a column of blood extending from the heart to the feet would amount to 80 mmHg. In a foot capillary, therefore, the pressure could potentially increase from 25 (the average capillary pressure resulting from cardiac contraction) to 105 mmHg, the extra 80 mmHg being due to the weight of the column of blood.

This increase in pressure due to gravity influences the effective circulating blood volume in several ways. First, the increased hydrostatic pressure that occurs in the legs (as well as the buttocks and pelvic area) when a person is standing pushes outward on the highly distensible vein walls, causing marked distension. The result is pooling of blood in the veins; that is, some of the blood emerging from the capillaries simply goes into expanding the veins rather than returning to the heart. Simultaneously, the increase in capillary pressure caused by the gravitational force produces increased filtration of fluid out of the capillaries into the interstitial space. This is why our feet can swell during prolonged standing. The combined effects of venous pooling and increased capillary filtration reduce the effective circulating blood volume very similarly to the effects caused by a mild hemorrhage. Venous pooling explains why a person may sometimes feel faint when standing up suddenly. The reduced venous return causes a transient decrease in end-diastolic volume and therefore decreased stretch of the ventricles. This reduces stroke volume, which in turn reduces cardiac output and blood pressure. This feeling is normally very transient, however, because the decrease in arterial pressure immediately causes baroreceptor-reflex-mediated compensatory adjustments similar to those shown in Figure 12.56 for hemorrhage.

The effects of gravity can be offset by contraction of the skeletal muscles in the legs. Even gentle contractions of the leg muscles without movement produce intermittent, complete emptying of deep leg veins so that uninterrupted columns of venous blood from the heart to the feet no longer exist (**Figure 12.60**). The result is a decrease in both venous distension and pooling plus a significant reduction in capillary hydrostatic pressure and fluid filtration out of the capillaries. This phenomenon is illustrated by the fact that soldiers may faint while standing at attention for long periods of time

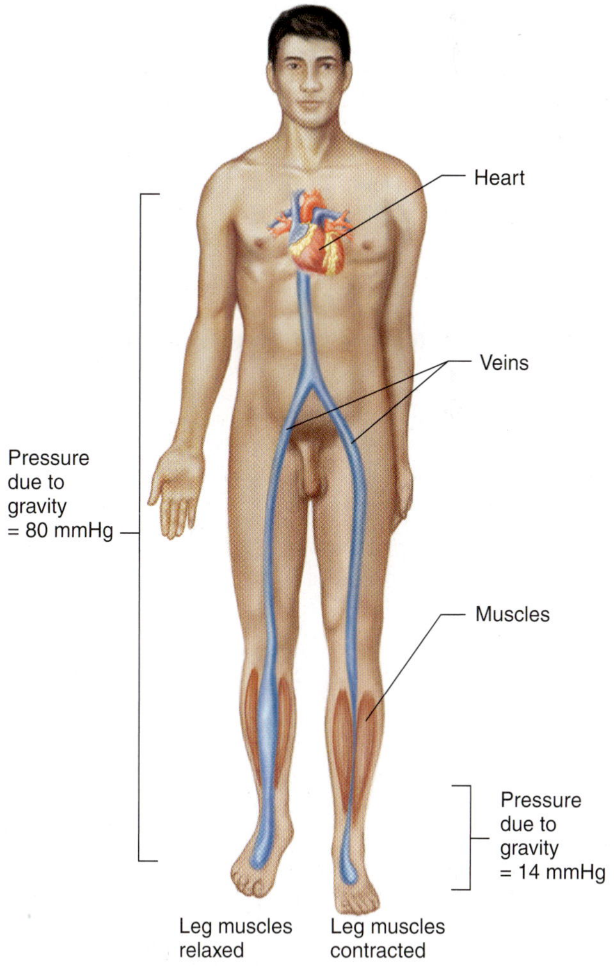

Figure 12.60 AP|R Role of contraction of the leg skeletal muscles in reducing capillary pressure and filtration in the upright position. The skeletal muscle contraction compresses the veins, causing intermittent emptying so that the columns of blood are interrupted.

because of minimal leg muscle contractions. Fainting may be considered adaptive in this circumstance, because the venous and capillary pressure changes induced by gravity are eliminated. When a person who has fainted becomes horizontal, pooled venous blood is mobilized and fluid is absorbed back into the capillaries from the interstitial fluid of the legs and feet. Consequently, the wrong thing to do for a person who has fainted is to hold him or her upright.

12.18 Exercise

During exercise, cardiac output may increase from a resting value of about 5 L/min to a maximal value of about 35 L/min in trained athletes. **Figure 12.61** illustrates the distribution of this cardiac output during strenuous exercise. As expected, most of the increase in cardiac output goes to the exercising muscles. However, there are also increases in flow to the heart, to provide for the increased metabolism and workload as cardiac output increases, and to the skin, if it becomes necessary to dissipate heat generate by metabolism. The increases in flow through these three vascular beds are the result of arteriolar vasodilation in them. In both skeletal and cardiac muscle, local metabolic factors mediate the vasodilation, whereas the vasodilation in skin is achieved mainly by a decrease in the firing of the sympathetic neurons to the skin. At the same time that arteriolar vasodilation is occurring in these three beds, arteriolar vasoconstriction is occurring in the kidneys and gastrointestinal organs. This vasoconstriction is caused by increased activity of sympathetic neurons and manifests as decreased blood flow in Figure 12.61.

Vasodilation of arterioles in skeletal muscle, cardiac muscle, and skin causes a decrease in total peripheral resistance to blood flow. This decrease is partially offset by vasoconstriction of arterioles in other organs. This compensatory change in resistance, however, is not capable of compensating for the huge dilation of the muscle arterioles, and the net result is a decrease in total peripheral resistance.

What happens to arterial blood pressure during exercise? As always, the mean arterial pressure is simply the arithmetic product of cardiac output and total peripheral resistance. During most forms of exercise (**Figure 12.62** illustrates the case for mild exercise), the cardiac output tends to increase somewhat more than the total peripheral resistance decreases so that mean arterial pressure usually increases a small amount. Pulse pressure, in contrast, significantly increases because an increase in both stroke volume and the speed at which the stroke volume is ejected significantly increases systolic pressure. It should be noted that by "exercise," we are referring to cyclic contraction and relaxation of muscles occurring over a

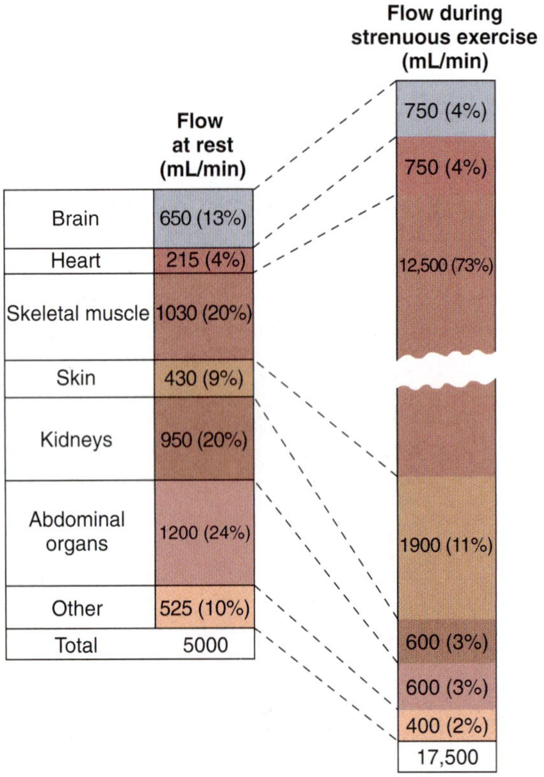

Figure 12.61 Distribution of the systemic cardiac output at rest and during strenuous exercise. The values at rest were previously presented in Figure 12.3. Adapted from Chapman and Mitchell.

PHYSIOLOGICAL INQUIRY

- Why might exercising on a very hot day result in fainting?

Answer can be found at end of chapter.

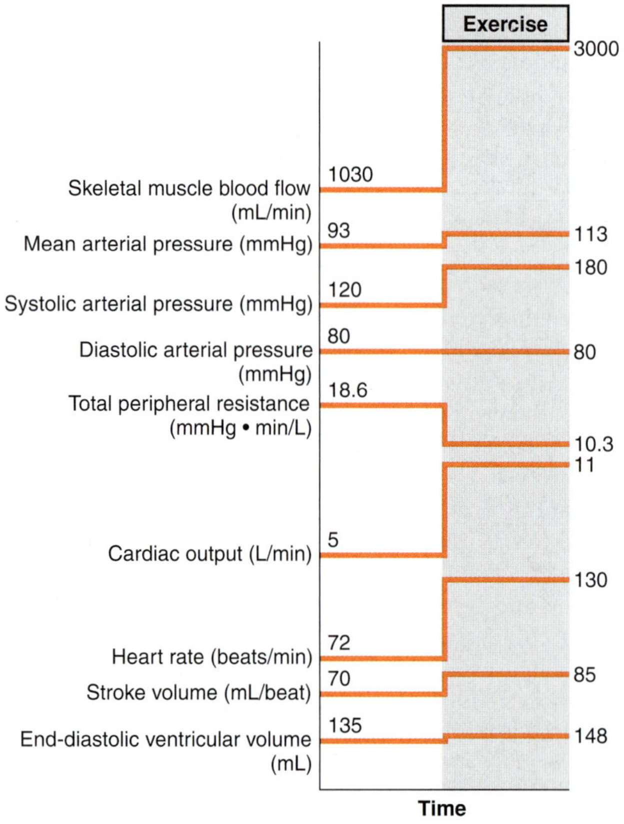

Figure 12.62 Summary of cardiovascular changes during mild upright exercise like jogging. The person was sitting quietly prior to the exercise. Total peripheral resistance was calculated from mean arterial pressure and cardiac output.

period of time, like jogging. A single, intense isometric contraction of muscles has a very different effect on blood pressure and will be described shortly.

The increase in cardiac output during exercise is supported by a large increase in heart rate and a small increase in stroke volume. The increase in heart rate is caused by a combination of decreased parasympathetic activity to the SA node and increased sympathetic activity. The increased stroke volume is due mainly to an increased ventricular contractility, manifested by an increased ejection fraction and mediated by the sympathetic neurons to the ventricular myocardium. Note in Figure 12.62, however, that there is a small increase (about 10%) in end-diastolic ventricular volume. Because of this increased filling, the Frank–Starling mechanism also contributes to the increased stroke volume, although not to the same degree as the increased contractility. We have focused our attention on factors that act directly upon the heart to alter cardiac output during exercise. By themselves, however, these factors are insufficient to account for the increased cardiac output. The fact is that cardiac output can be increased to high levels only if the peripheral processes favoring venous return to the heart are simultaneously activated to the same degree. Otherwise, the shortened filling time resulting from the high heart rate would decrease end-diastolic volume and, therefore, stroke volume (by the Frank–Starling mechanism).

Factors promoting venous return during exercise are (1) increased activity of the skeletal muscle pump, (2) increased depth and frequency of inspiration (the respiratory pump), (3) sympathetically mediated increase in venous tone, and (4) greater ease of blood flow from arteries to veins through the dilated skeletal muscle arterioles. **Figure 12.63** provides a summary of the control mechanisms that elicit the cardiovascular changes in exercise. As described previously, vasodilation of arterioles in skeletal and cardiac muscle once exercise is under way represents active hyperemia as a result of local metabolic factors within the muscle. But what drives the enhanced sympathetic outflow to most other arterioles, the heart, and the veins and the decreased parasympathetic outflow to the heart? The control of this autonomic outflow during exercise offers an excellent example of a preprogrammed pattern, modified by continuous afferent input. One or more discrete control centers in the brain are activated during exercise by output from the cerebral cortex, and descending pathways from these centers to the appropriate autonomic preganglionic neurons elicit the firing pattern typical of exercise. These centers become active, and changes to cardiac and vascular function occur even before exercise begins. Thus, this constitutes a feedforward system.

Once exercise is under way, if there is imperfect matching between blood flow and metabolic demands, local chemical changes in the muscle can develop, particularly during intense exercise. These changes activate chemoreceptors in the muscle. Afferent input from these receptors goes to the medullary cardiovascular center and facilitates the output reaching the autonomic neurons from higher brain centers. The result is a further increase in heart rate, myocardial contractility, and vascular resistance in the nonactive organs. Such a system permits a fine degree of matching between cardiac pumping and total oxygen and nutrients required by the exercising muscles. Mechanoreceptors in the exercising muscles are also stimulated and provide input to the medullary cardiovascular center.

Finally, the arterial baroreceptors also play a role in the altered autonomic outflow. Knowing that the mean and pulsatile pressures increase during exercise, you may logically assume that the arterial baroreceptors will respond to these elevated pressures and signal for increased parasympathetic and decreased sympathetic outflow, a pattern designed to counter the increase in arterial pressure. In reality, however, exactly the opposite occurs; the arterial baroreceptors play an important role in *increasing* the arterial pressure over that existing at rest. The reason is that one neural component of the

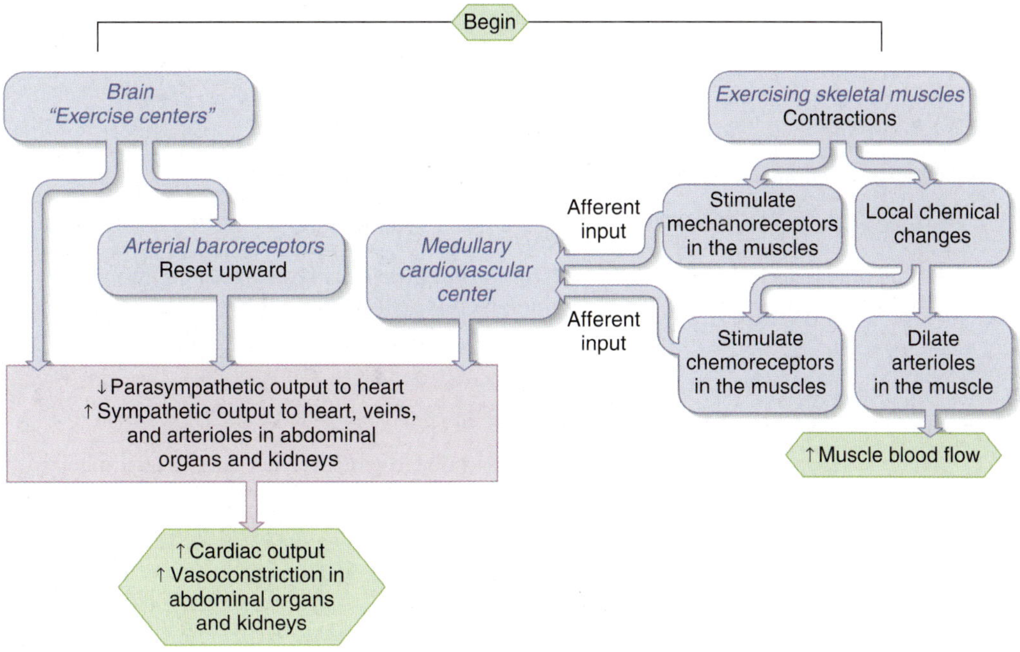

Figure 12.63 Control of the cardiovascular system during exercise. The primary outflow to the sympathetic and parasympathetic neurons is via pathways from "exercise centers" in the brain. Afferent input from mechanoreceptors and chemoreceptors in the exercising muscles and from reset arterial baroreceptors also influences the autonomic neurons by way of the medullary cardiovascular center.

central command output travels to the arterial baroreceptors and "resets" them upward as exercise begins. This resetting causes the baroreceptors to respond as though arterial pressure had decreased, and their output (decreased action potential frequency) signals for decreased parasympathetic and increased sympathetic outflow. **Table 12.8** summarizes the changes that occur during moderate exercise—that is, exercise (like jogging, swimming, or fast walking) that involves large muscle groups for an extended period of time.

In closing, we return to the other major category of exercise, which involves maintained high-force, slow-shortening-velocity contractions, as in weight lifting. Here, too, cardiac output and arterial blood pressure increase, and the arterioles in the exercising muscles undergo vasodilation due to local metabolic factors. However, there is a crucial difference. During maintained contractions, once the contracting muscles exceed 10% to 15% of their maximal force, the blood flow to the muscle is greatly reduced because the muscles are physically compressing the blood vessels that run through them. In other words, the arteriolar vasodilation is completely overcome by the physical compression of the blood vessels. Thus, the cardiovascular changes are ineffective in causing increased blood flow to the muscles, and these contractions can be maintained only briefly before fatigue sets in. Moreover, because of the compression of blood vessels, total peripheral resistance may increase considerably (instead of decreasing as it does in endurance exercise), contributing to a large increase in mean arterial pressure during the contraction. Frequent exposure of the heart to only this type of exercise can cause maladaptive changes in the left ventricle, including wall hypertrophy and diminished chamber volume.

Maximal Oxygen Consumption and Training

As the intensity of any endurance exercise increases, oxygen consumption also increases in exact proportion until reaching a point when it fails to increase despite a further increment in workload. This is known as **maximal oxygen consumption** ($\dot{V}_{O_2}$ **max**). After this point has been reached, work can be increased and sustained only briefly by anaerobic metabolism in the exercising muscles.

Theoretically, $\dot{V}_{O_2}$ max could be limited by (1) the cardiac output, (2) the respiratory system's ability to deliver oxygen to the blood, or (3) the exercising muscles' ability to use oxygen. In fact, in typical, healthy people (except for very highly trained athletes), cardiac output is the factor that determines $\dot{V}_{O_2}$ max. With increasing workload (**Figure 12.64**), heart rate increases progressively until it reaches a maximum. Stroke volume increases much less and tends to level off at 75% of $\dot{V}_{O_2}$ max (it actually starts to go back down in elderly people). The major factors responsible for limiting the increase in stroke volume and, therefore, cardiac output are (1) the very rapid heart rate, which decreases diastolic filling time; and (2) inability of the peripheral factors favoring venous return (skeletal muscle pump, respiratory pump, venous vasoconstriction, arteriolar vasodilation) to increase ventricular filling further during the very short time available.

TABLE 12.8 Cardiovascular Changes During Moderate Exercise

Variable	Change	Explanation
Cardiac output	Increases	Heart rate and stroke volume both increase, the former to a much greater extent.
Heart rate	Increases	Sympathetic stimulation of the SA node increases, and parasympathetic stimulation decreases.
Stroke volume	Increases	Contractility increases due to increased sympathetic stimulation of the ventricular myocardium; increased ventricular end-diastolic volume also contributes to increased stroke volume by the Frank–Starling mechanism.
Total peripheral resistance	Decreases	Resistance in heart and skeletal muscles decreases more than resistance in other vascular beds increases.
Mean arterial pressure	Increases	Cardiac output increases more than total peripheral resistance decreases.
Pulse pressure	Increases	Stroke volume and velocity of ejection of the stroke volume increase.
End-diastolic volume	Increases	Filling time is decreased by the high heart rate, but the factors favoring venous return—venoconstriction, skeletal muscle pump, and increased inspiratory movements—more than compensate for it.
Blood flow to heart and skeletal muscle	Increases	Active hyperemia occurs in both vascular beds, mediated by local metabolic factors.
Blood flow to skin	Increases	Sympathetic activation of skin blood vessels is inhibited reflexively by the increase in body temperature.
Blood flow to viscera	Decreases	Sympathetic activation of blood vessels in the abdominal organs and kidneys is increased.
Blood flow to brain	Increases slightly	Autoregulation of brain arterioles maintains constant flow despite the increased mean arterial pressure.

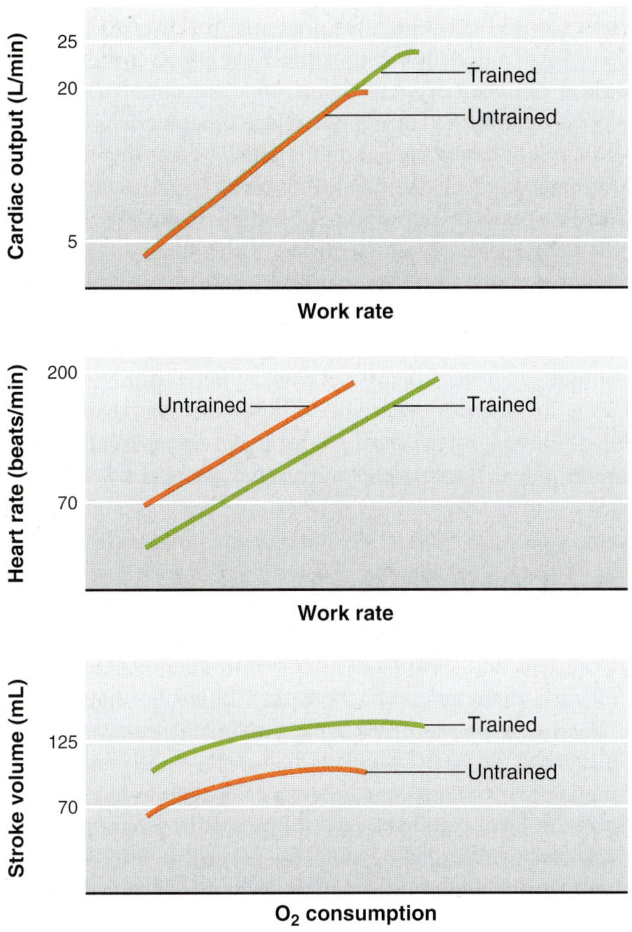

Figure 12.64 Changes in cardiac output, heart rate, and stroke volume with increasing workload in untrained and trained individuals.

An individual's $\dot{V}_{O_2}$ max is not fixed at any given value but can be altered by his or her habitual level of physical activity. For example, prolonged bed rest may decrease $\dot{V}_{O_2}$ max by 15% to 25%, whereas intense, long-term physical training may increase it by a similar amount. To be effective, the training must be endurance-type exercise and must reach certain minimal levels of duration, frequency, and intensity. For example, running 20 to 30 min three times weekly at 5 to 8 mi/h produces a significant training effect in most people.

At rest, compared to values prior to training, the trained individual has an increased stroke volume and decreased heart rate with no change in cardiac output (see Figure 12.64). At $\dot{V}_{O_2}$ max, cardiac output is increased compared to pretraining values; this is due entirely to an increased maximal stroke volume because training does not alter maximal heart rate (see Figure 12.64). The increase in stroke volume is due to a combination of (1) effects on the heart (remodeling of the ventricular walls produces moderate hypertrophy and an increase in chamber size); and (2) peripheral effects, including increased blood volume and increases in the number of blood vessels in skeletal muscle, which permit increased muscle blood flow and venous return.

Training also increases the concentrations of oxidative enzymes and mitochondria in the exercised muscles. These changes increase the speed and efficiency of metabolic reactions in the muscles and permit 200% to 300% increases in exercise endurance, but they do not increase $\dot{V}_{O_2}$ max because they were not limiting it in the untrained individuals.

Aging is associated with significant changes in the heart's performance during exercise. Most striking is a decrease in the maximum heart rate (and, therefore, cardiac output) achievable. This results, in particular, from increased stiffness of the heart that decreases its ability to rapidly fill during diastole.

12.19 Hypertension

Hypertension is defined as a chronically increased systemic arterial pressure. Although the clinical definition of hypertension is a blood pressure above 140/90 mmHg, new guidelines suggest that interventions to lower blood pressure should be instituted at systolic pressures of 130 to 139 mmHg and diastolic pressures of 85 to 89 mmHg.

Hypertension is a serious public-health problem. Over a billion people worldwide (26% of the adult population), and 76 million (34%) in the U.S. population are estimated to suffer from this condition. Hypertension is a contributing cause to some of the leading causes of disability and death. One of the organs most affected is the heart. Because the left ventricle in a hypertensive person must chronically pump against an increased arterial pressure (afterload), it develops an adaptive increase in muscle mass called ***left ventricular hypertrophy.*** In the early phases of the disease, this hypertrophy helps maintain the heart's function as a pump. With time, however, changes in the organization and properties of myocardial cells occur, and these result in diminished contractile function and heart failure. The presence of hypertension also enhances the possible development of atherosclerosis and heart attacks, kidney damage, and ***stroke***—the rupture of a cerebral blood vessel, causing localized brain damage. Long-term data on the link between blood pressure and health show that for every 20 mmHg increase in systolic pressure and every 10 mmHg increase in diastolic pressure, the risk of heart disease and stroke doubles.

Hypertension is categorized according to its causes. Hypertension of uncertain cause is diagnosed as ***primary hypertension*** (formerly called "essential hypertension"). ***Secondary hypertension*** is the term used when there are identified causes. Primary hypertension accounts for over 90% of all cases.

By definition, the causes of primary hypertension are unknown, though a number of genetic and environmental factors are suspected to be involved. In cases in which the condition appears to be inherited, a number of genes have been implicated, including some coding for enzymes involved in the renin-angiotensin-aldosterone pathway (see Chapter 14) and some involved in the regulation of endothelial cell function and arteriolar smooth muscle contraction. Although, theoretically, hypertension could result from an increase either in cardiac output or in total peripheral resistance, it appears that in most cases of well-established primary hypertension, increased total peripheral resistance caused by reduced arteriolar radius is the most significant factor.

A number of environmental risk factors contribute to the development of primary hypertension. Recent studies show that lifestyle changes that reduce those factors result in lowered blood pressure, both in hypertensive and healthy people. Obesity and the frequently associated insulin insensitivity (discussed in Chapter 16) are risk factors, and weight loss significantly reduces blood pressure in most people. Chronic, high salt intake is also associated with hypertension, and recent research has revealed mechanisms by which even slight elevations in plasma Na^+ levels lead to chronic overstimulation of the sympathetic nervous system, constriction of arterioles, and narrowing of the lumen of arteries. These vascular changes are the hallmark in many cases of primary hypertension. Significant reduction in blood pressure occurred in experimental subjects who ate a low-salt diet in a large, well-designed study known as DASH (Dietary Approaches to Stop Hypertension). In addition to obesity and excessive salt intake, other environmental factors hypothesized to contribute to primary hypertension include smoking; excess alcohol consumption; diets low in fruits, vegetables, and whole grains; diets low in vitamin D and calcium; lack of exercise; chronic stress; excess caffeine consumption; maternal smoking; low birth weight; and not being breast-fed as an infant.

There are a number of well-characterized causes of secondary hypertension. Damage to the kidneys or their blood supply can lead to ***renal hypertension,*** in which increased renin release leads to excessive concentrations of the potent vasoconstrictor angiotensin II and inappropriately decreased urine production by the kidneys, resulting in excessive extracellular fluid volume. Some individuals are genetically predisposed to excess renal Na^+ reabsorption. These patients respond well to a low-sodium diet or to drugs called ***diuretics,*** which cause increased Na^+ and water loss in the urine (see Chapter 14). A number of endocrine disorders result in hypertension, such as syndromes involving hypersecretion of cortisol or thyroid hormone (see Chapter 11). Medications such as oral contraceptives and nonsteroidal anti-inflammatory drugs can also contribute to hypertension. Recently, a link has been established between hypertension and the abnormal nighttime breathing pattern, sleep apnea (see Chapter 13).

The major categories of drugs used to treat hypertension are summarized in **Table 12.9.** These drugs all act in ways that decrease cardiac output and/or total peripheral resistance. You will note in subsequent sections of this chapter that these same drugs are also used to treat heart failure and in both the prevention and treatment of heart attacks. One reason for this overlap is that these three diseases are causally interrelated. For example, as noted in this section, hypertension is a major risk factor for the development of heart disease. In addition, though, the drugs often have multiple cardiovascular effects, which may play different roles in the treatment of the different diseases.

12.20 Heart Failure

Heart failure (also called ***congestive heart failure***) is a collection of signs and symptoms that occur when the heart fails to pump an adequate cardiac output. This may happen for many reasons; two examples are pumping against a chronically increased arterial pressure in hypertension, and structural damage to the myocardium due to decreased coronary blood flow. It has become standard practice to separate people with heart failure into two categories: (1) those with diastolic dysfunction (problems with ventricular filling) and (2) those with systolic dysfunction (problems with ventricular ejection). Many people with heart failure, however, exhibit elements of both categories.

In ***diastolic dysfunction,*** the wall of the ventricle has reduced compliance. Its abnormal stiffness results in a reduced ability to fill adequately at normal diastolic filling pressures. The result is a reduced end-diastolic volume (even though the end-diastolic pressure in the stiff ventricle may be quite high),

TABLE 12.9 Drugs Used to Treat Hypertension
Diuretics: These drugs increase urinary excretion of sodium and water (Chapter 14). They tend to decrease cardiac output with little or no change in total peripheral resistance.
β-adrenergic receptor blockers: These drugs exert their antihypertensive effects mainly by reducing cardiac output.
Ca^{2+} channel blockers: These drugs reduce the entry of Ca^{2+} into vascular smooth muscle cells, causing them to contract less strongly and lowering total peripheral resistance. (Surprisingly, it has been found that despite their effectiveness in lowering blood pressure, at least some of these drugs may significantly increase the risk of a heart attack. Consequently, their use as therapy for hypertension is under intensive review.)
Angiotensin-converting enzyme (ACE) inhibitors: As Chapter 14 will describe, the final step in the formation of angiotensin II, a vasoconstrictor, is mediated by an enzyme called angiotensin-converting enzyme. Drugs that block this enzyme therefore reduce the concentration of angiotensin II in plasma, which causes arteriolar vasodilation, lowering total peripheral resistance. The same effect can be achieved with drugs that block the receptors for angiotensin II. A reduction in plasma angiotensin II or blockage of its receptors is also protective against the development of heart wall changes that lead to heart failure.
Drugs that antagonize one or more components of the sympathetic nervous system: The major effect of these drugs is to reduce sympathetic mediated stimulation of arteriolar smooth muscle and thereby reduce total peripheral resistance. Examples include drugs that inhibit the brain centers that mediate the sympathetic outflow to arterioles, and drugs that block α-adrenergic receptors on the arterioles.

which results in a reduced stroke volume by the Frank–Starling mechanism. In pure diastolic dysfunction, ventricular compliance is decreased but ventricular contractility is normal.

Several situations may lead to decreased ventricular compliance, but by far the most common is the existence of systemic hypertension. As noted in the previous section, hypertrophy results when the left ventricle pumps against a chronically increased arterial pressure (afterload). The structural and biochemical changes associated with this hypertrophy make the ventricle stiff and less able to expand.

In contrast to diastolic dysfunction, ***systolic dysfunction*** results from myocardial damage, like that resulting from a heart attack (discussed next). This type of dysfunction is characterized by a decrease in cardiac contractility—a lower stroke volume at any given end-diastolic volume. This is manifested as a decrease in ejection fraction and, as illustrated in **Figure 12.65**, a downward shift of the ventricular-function curve. The affected ventricle does not hypertrophy, but note that the end-diastolic volume increases.

The reduced cardiac output of heart failure, regardless of whether it is due to diastolic or systolic dysfunction, triggers the arterial baroreceptor reflexes. In this situation, these reflexes are elicited more than usual because, for unknown reasons, the afferent baroreceptors are less sensitive. In other words, the baroreceptors discharge less rapidly than normal at any given mean or pulsatile arterial pressure and the brain interprets this decreased discharge as a larger-than-usual decrease in pressure. The results of the reflexes are that (1) heart rate is increased through increased sympathetic and decreased parasympathetic activation of the heart; and (2) total peripheral resistance is increased by increased sympathetic activation of systemic arterioles, as well as by increased plasma concentrations of the two major hormonal vasoconstrictors—angiotensin II and vasopressin. The reflex increases in heart rate and total peripheral resistance are initially beneficial in restoring cardiac output and arterial pressure, just as if the changes in these parameters had been triggered by hemorrhage.

Maintained chronically throughout the period of cardiac failure, the baroreceptor reflexes also bring about fluid retention and an expansion—often massive—of the extracellular volume. This is because, as Chapter 14 describes, the neuroendocrine efferent components of the reflexes cause the kidneys to reduce their excretion of sodium and water. The retained fluid then causes expansion of the extracellular volume. Because the plasma volume is part of the extracellular fluid volume, plasma volume also increases. This in turn increases venous pressure, venous return, and end-diastolic ventricular volume, which tends to restore stroke volume toward normal by the Frank–Starling mechanism (see Figure 12.65). Thus, fluid retention is also, at least initially, an adaptive response to decreased cardiac output.

However, problems emerge as the fluid retention progresses. For one thing, when a ventricle with systolic dysfunction (as opposed to a normal ventricle) becomes very distended with blood, its force of contraction actually decreases and the situation worsens. Second, the fluid retention, with its accompanying elevation in venous pressure, causes edema—accumulation of interstitial fluid. Why does an increased venous pressure cause edema? The capillaries drain via venules into the veins; so when venous pressure increases, the capillary pressure also increases and causes increased filtration of fluid out of the capillaries into the interstitial fluid (review Figure 12.42). Thus, most of the fluid retained by the kidneys ends up as extra interstitial fluid rather than extra plasma. Swelling of the legs and feet is particularly prominent.

Most important in this regard, failure of the *left* ventricle —whether due to diastolic or systolic dysfunction—leads to ***pulmonary edema***, the accumulation of fluid in the interstitial spaces of the lung or in the air spaces themselves. This impairs pulmonary gas exchange. The reason for such accumulation is that the left ventricle fails to pump blood to the same extent as the right ventricle, so the volume of blood in all the pulmonary vessels increases. The resulting engorgement of pulmonary capillaries increases the capillary pressure above its normally very low value, causing filtration to occur at a rate faster than the lymphatics can remove the fluid. This situation usually worsens at night. During the day, because of the patient's upright posture, fluid accumulates in the legs; then the fluid is slowly absorbed back into the capillaries when the patient lies down at night, thereby expanding the plasma volume and precipitating the development of pulmonary edema.

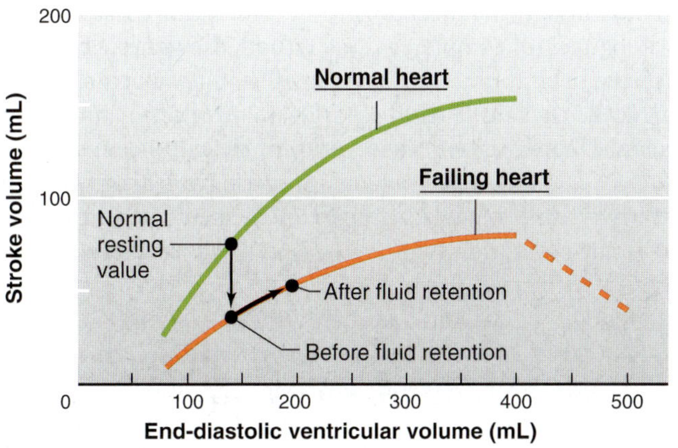

Figure 12.65 Relationship between end-diastolic ventricular volume and stroke volume in a normal heart and one with heart failure due to systolic dysfunction (decreased contractility). The normal curve was shown previously in Figure 12.24. With decreased contractility, the ventricular-function curve is displaced downward; that is, there is a lower stroke volume at any given end-diastolic volume. Fluid retention causes an increase in end-diastolic volume and restores stroke volume toward normal by the Frank–Starling mechanism. Note that this compensation occurs even though contractility—the basic defect—has not been altered by the fluid retention.

PHYSIOLOGICAL INQUIRY

- Estimate the ejection fraction of the failing heart at a typical normal end-diastolic volume.

Answer can be found at end of chapter.

TABLE 12.10	Types of Drugs Used to Treat Heart Failure

Diuretics: Drugs that increase urinary excretion of sodium and water (Chapter 14). These drugs eliminate the excessive fluid accumulation contributing to edema and/or worsening myocardial function.

Cardiac inotropic drugs: Drugs that enhance β-adrenergic receptor pathways and drugs such as ***digitalis,*** which increases ventricular contractility by increasing cytosolic Ca^{2+} concentration in the myocardial cell, can increase cardiac output in the short term. The use of these drugs is currently controversial, however, because although they clearly improve the symptoms of heart failure, they do not prolong life and, in some studies, seem to have shortened it.

Vasodilator drugs: Drugs that lower total peripheral resistance and thus the arterial blood pressure (afterload) the failing heart must pump against. Some inhibit a component of the sympathetic nervous pathway to the arterioles (α-adrenergic receptor blockers), whereas others block the formation of angiotensin II (angiotensin-converting enzyme [ACE] inhibitors, see Chapter 14). In addition, the ACE inhibitors prevent or reverse the maladaptive remodeling of the myocardium that is mediated by the increased plasma concentration of angiotensin II in heart failure.

β-adrenergic receptor blockers: Drugs that block the major adrenergic receptors in the myocardium. The mechanism by which this action improves heart failure is unknown. You may predict that such an action, by blocking sympathetically induced increases in cardiac contractility, would be counterproductive (note above that β-*agonists* are sometimes used, which is more intuitive). One hypothesis is that excess sympathetic stimulation of the heart reflexively produced by the decreased cardiac output of heart failure may cause an excessive elevation of cytosolic Ca^{2+} concentration, which would lead to cell apoptosis and necrosis; β-adrenergic receptor blockers would prevent this.

Another component of the reflex response to heart failure that is at first beneficial but ultimately becomes maladaptive is the increase in total peripheral resistance, mediated by the sympathetic neurons to arterioles and by angiotensin II and vasopressin. By chronically maintaining the arterial blood pressure the failing heart must pump against, this increased resistance makes the failing heart work harder.

One obvious treatment for heart failure is to correct, if possible, the precipitating cause (for example, hypertension). Table 12.10 lists the types of drugs most often used for treatment. Finally, although cardiac transplantation is often the treatment of choice, the paucity of donor hearts, the high costs, and the challenges of postsurgical care render it a feasible option for only a very small number of patients. Considerable research has also been directed toward the development of artificial hearts, though success has been limited to date.

12.21 Hypertrophic Cardiomyopathy

Hypertrophic cardiomyopathy is a condition that frequently leads to heart failure. It is one of the most common inherited cardiac diseases, occurring in about one out of 500 people. As the name implies, it is characterized by an increase in thickness of the heart muscle, in particular, the interventricular septum and the wall of the left ventricle. In conjunction with wall thickening, there is a disruption of the orderly array of myocytes and conducting cells within the walls. The thickening of the septum interferes with the ejection of blood through the aortic valve, particularly during exercise, which can prevent cardiac output from increasing sufficiently to meet tissue metabolic requirements. The heart itself is commonly a victim of this reduction in blood flow, and one symptom that can be an early warning sign is the associated chest pain (***angina pectoris*** or, more commonly, angina). Moreover, disruption of the conduction pathway can lead to dangerous, sometimes fatal arrhythmias. Many people with this disease have no symptoms, so it can go undetected until it has progressed to an advanced stage. For these reasons, hypertrophic cardiomyopathy is most often the cause in the rare circumstance when a young athlete suffers sudden, unexpected cardiac death. If it progresses without treatment, it can lead to heart failure, with all of the consequences discussed previously. Although the mechanisms by which this disease process develops are not completely understood, the genetic mutations that have been found to cause it involve mainly proteins of the contractile system, including myosin, troponin, and tropomyosin. Depending on the severity of the condition when it is discovered, treatments include administering drugs that prevent arrhythmias, surgical repair of the septum and valve, or heart transplantation.

12.22 Coronary Artery Disease and Heart Attacks

We have seen that the myocardium does not extract oxygen and nutrients from the blood within the atria and ventricles but depends upon its own blood supply via the coronary arteries. In ***coronary artery disease,*** changes in one or more of the coronary arteries cause insufficient blood flow (***ischemia***) to the heart. The result may be myocardial damage in the affected region, or even death of that portion of the heart—a ***myocardial infarction,*** or ***heart attack.*** Many patients with coronary artery disease experience recurrent transient episodes of inadequate coronary blood flow and angina, usually during exertion or emotional tension, before ultimately suffering a heart attack.

The symptoms of myocardial infarction include prolonged chest pain, often radiating to the left arm; nausea; vomiting; sweating; weakness; and shortness of breath. Diagnosis is made by ECG changes typical of infarction and by detection of specific cardiac muscle proteins in plasma. These proteins leak out into the blood when the muscle is damaged;

the most commonly detected are the myocardial-specific isoform of the enzyme creatine kinase, and cardiac troponin.

Approximately 1.1 million Americans have a new or recurrent heart attack each year, and over 40% of them die from it. Sudden cardiac deaths during myocardial infarction are due mainly to ***ventricular fibrillation,*** an abnormality in impulse conduction triggered by the damaged myocardial cells. This conduction pattern results in completely uncoordinated ventricular contractions that are ineffective in producing flow. (Note that ventricular fibrillation is usually fatal, whereas atrial fibrillation, as described earlier in this chapter, generally causes only minor cardiac problems.) A small fraction of individuals with ventricular fibrillation can be saved if emergency resuscitation procedures are applied immediately after the attack. This treatment is ***cardiopulmonary resuscitation*** (***CPR***), a repeated series of chest compressions sometimes accompanied by mouth-to-mouth respirations that circulate a small amount of oxygenated blood to the brain, heart, and other vital organs when the heart has stopped. CPR is then followed by definitive treatment, including ***defibrillation,*** a procedure in which electrical current is passed through the heart to try to halt the abnormal electrical activity causing the fibrillation. ***Automatic electronic defibrillators*** (***AEDs***) are now commonly found in public places. These devices make it relatively simple to render timely aid to victims of ventricular fibrillation.

The major cause of coronary artery disease is the presence of atherosclerosis in these vessels (**Figure 12.66**). ***Atherosclerosis*** is a disease of arteries characterized by a thickening of the portion of the arterial vessel wall closest to the lumen with plaques made up of (1) large numbers of cells, including smooth muscle cells, macrophages (derived from blood monocytes), and lymphocytes; (2) deposits of cholesterol and other fatty substances, both within cells and extracellularly; and (3) dense layers of connective tissue matrix. Such atherosclerotic plaques are one cause of aging-related arteriosclerosis.

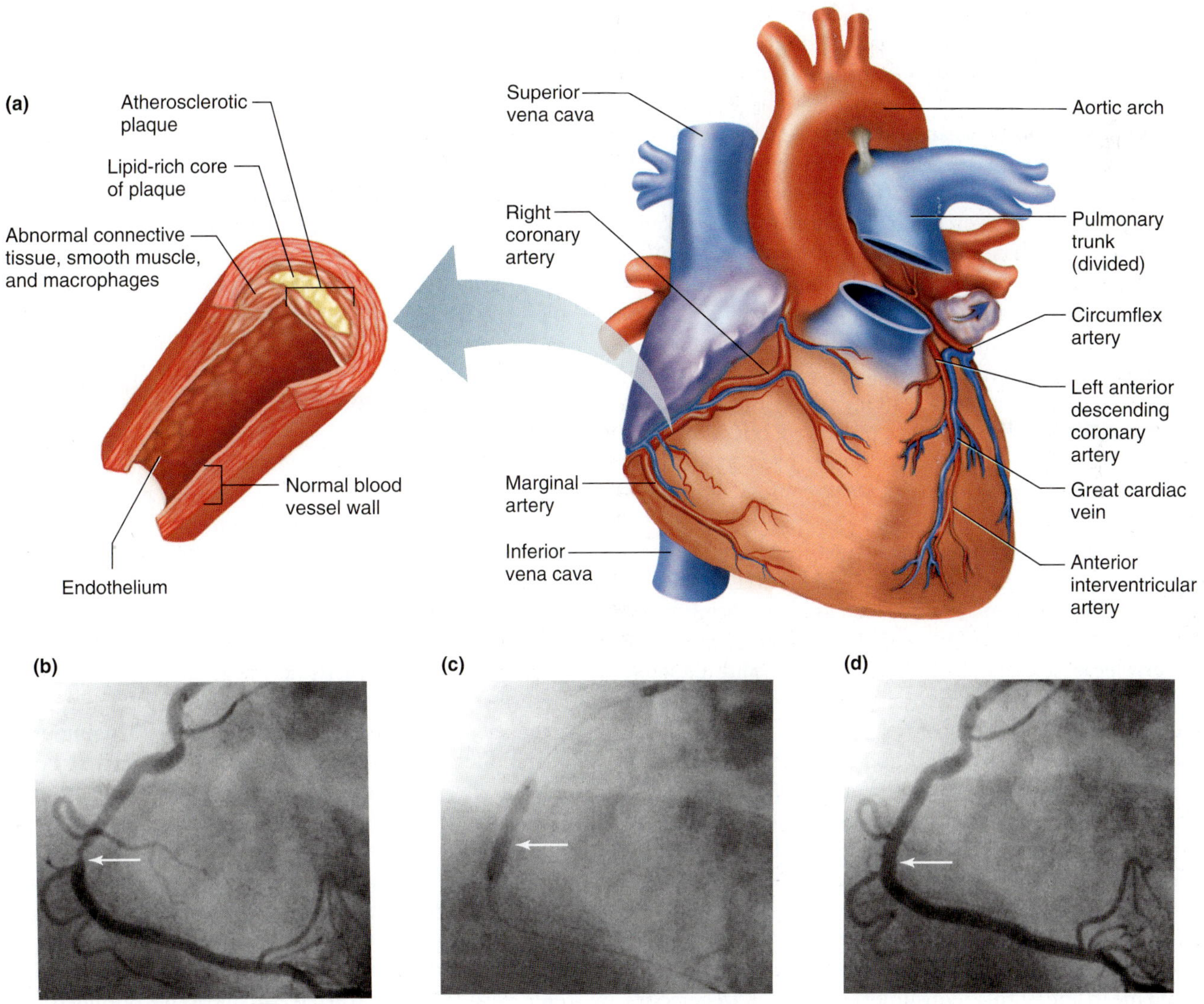

Figure 12.66 AP|R Coronary artery disease and its treatment. (a) Anterior view of the heart showing the major coronary vessels. Inset demonstrates narrowing due to atherosclerotic plaque. (b) Dye-contrast x-ray angiography performed by injecting radiopaque dye shows a significant occlusion of the right coronary artery (arrow). (c) A guide wire is used to position and inflate a dye-filled balloon in the narrow region, and a wire-mesh stent is inserted. (d) Blood flows freely through the formerly narrowed region after the procedure. Photos (b), (c), and (d) courtesy of Matthew R. Wolff, M.D.

Atherosclerosis reduces coronary blood flow by several mechanisms. The extra muscle cells and various deposits in the wall bulge into the lumen of the vessel and increase resistance to flow. Also, dysfunctional endothelial cells in the atherosclerotic area release excess vasoconstrictors (e.g., endothelin-1) and lower-than-normal amounts of vasodilators (nitric oxide and prostacyclin). These processes are progressive, sometimes leading ultimately to complete occlusion. Total occlusion is usually caused, however, by the formation of a blood clot (***coronary thrombosis***) in the narrowed atherosclerotic artery, and this triggers the heart attack.

The processes that lead to atherosclerosis are complex and still not completely understood. It is likely that the damage is initiated by agents that injure the endothelium and underlying smooth muscle, leading to an inflammatory and proliferative response that may well be protective at first but ultimately becomes excessive.

Cigarette smoking, high blood concentrations of certain types of cholesterol and the amino acid homocysteine, hypertension, diabetes, obesity, a sedentary lifestyle, and stress are all risk factors that can increase the incidence and severity of the atherosclerotic process and coronary artery disease. Prevention efforts therefore focus on eliminating or minimizing these risk factors through lifestyle changes and/or medications. In a sense, menopause can also be considered a risk factor for coronary artery disease because the incidence of heart attacks in women is very low until after menopause.

A few words about exercise are warranted here because of some potential confusion. Although it is true that a sudden burst of strenuous physical activity can sometimes trigger a heart attack, the risk is greatly reduced in individuals who perform regular physical activity. The overall risk of heart attack at any time can be reduced as much as 35% to 55% by maintaining an active rather than sedentary lifestyle. In general, the more you exercise, the better the protective effect, but any exercise is better than none. For example, even moderately paced walking three to four times a week confers significant benefit.

Regular exercise is protective against heart attacks for a variety of reasons. Among other things, it induces (1) decreased myocardial oxygen demand due to decreases in resting heart rate and blood pressure; (2) increased diameter of coronary arteries; (3) decreased severity of hypertension and diabetes, two major risk factors for atherosclerosis; (4) decreased total plasma cholesterol concentration with simultaneous increase in the plasma concentration of a "good" cholesterol-carrying lipoprotein (HDL, discussed in Chapter 16); (5) decreased tendency of blood to clot and improved ability of the body to dissolve blood clots; and (6) better control of blood glucose due to increased sensitivity to the hormone insulin (see Chapter 16).

Nutrition can also play a role in protecting against heart attacks. Reduction in the intake of saturated fat (a type abundant in red meat) and regular consumption of fruits, vegetables, whole grains, and fish may help by reducing the concentration of "bad" cholesterol (LDLs, discussed in Chapter 16) in the blood. This form of cholesterol contributes to the buildup of atherosclerotic plaques in blood vessels. Supplements like folic acid (a B vitamin; also called folate or folacin) may also be protective, in this case because folic acid helps reduce the blood concentration of the amino acid homocysteine, one of the risk factors for heart attacks. Homocysteine is an intermediary in the metabolism of methionine and cysteine. In increased amounts, it exerts several proatherosclerotic effects, including damaging the endothelium of blood vessels. Folic acid is involved in a metabolic reaction that lowers the plasma concentration of homocysteine.

Finally, there is the question of alcohol and coronary artery disease. In many studies, moderate alcohol intake—red wine, in particular—has been shown to reduce the risk of dying from a heart attack. Likely contributing to this effect is the observed increase in HDL concentration and inhibition of blood clot formation that result from low doses of alcohol. However, alcohol—particularly at higher doses—increases the chances of an early death from a variety of other diseases (cancer and cirrhosis of the liver, for example) and accidents. Because of these complex health effects and the potential to develop alcohol dependence (see Chapter 8), doctors do not recommend that patients start drinking alcohol for health benefits. For those who do drink, the recommendation is to have no more than one standard drink per day. (One standard drink is approximately 12 ounces of beer, 5 ounces of wine, or 1.5 ounces of 80-proof liquor.)

A variety of drugs can be used for the prevention and treatment of angina and coronary artery disease. For example, vasodilator drugs such as ***nitroglycerin*** (which is a vasodilator because it is converted in the body to nitric oxide) help by dilating the coronary arteries and the systemic arterioles and veins. The arteriolar effect lowers total peripheral resistance, thereby lowering arterial blood pressure and the work the heart must do to eject blood. The venous dilation, by decreasing venous pressure, reduces venous return and thereby the stretch of the ventricle and its oxygen requirement during subsequent contraction. In addition, drugs that block β-adrenergic receptors are used to reduce the arterial pressure in people with hypertension. They reduce myocardial work and cardiac output by inhibiting the effect of sympathetic neurons on heart rate and contractility. Drugs that prevent or reverse clotting within hours of its occurrence are also extremely important in the treatment (and prevention) of heart attacks. Use of these drugs, including aspirin, will be described in Section F of this chapter. Finally, a variety of drugs decrease plasma cholesterol by influencing one or more metabolic pathways for cholesterol (Chapter 16). For example, one group of drugs, sometimes referred to as "statins," interferes with a critical enzyme involved in the liver's synthesis of cholesterol.

There are several interventions for coronary artery disease after cardiac angiography (described earlier in this chapter) identifies an area of narrowing or occlusion. ***Coronary balloon angioplasty*** involves threading a catheter with a balloon at its tip into the occluded artery and then expanding the balloon (Figure 12.66c). This procedure enlarges the lumen by stretching the vessel and breaking up abnormal tissue deposits. It is generally accompanied by the placement of ***coronary stents*** in the narrowed or occluded coronary vessel (Figure 12.66d). Stents are tubes made of a stainless steel lattice that provide a scaffold within a vessel to open it and keep it open. Researchers are testing stents made of a hardened, biodegradable polymer that is absorbed after 6 months to 1 year. Another surgical treatment is ***coronary bypass,*** in which a new vessel is attached across an area of occluded coronary artery. The new vessel is often a vein taken from elsewhere in the patient's body. Despite the widespread use of these surgical interventions and their proven effectiveness in relieving the pain of angina, evidence accumulated over the past 20 years suggests that such procedures have a limited effect on long-term survival after a cardiac event or on the prevention of future events.

Atherosclerosis does not attack only the coronary vessels. Many arteries of the body are subject to this same occluding process, and wherever the atherosclerosis becomes severe, the resulting symptoms reflect the decrease in blood flow to the specific area. For example, occlusion of a cerebral artery due to atherosclerosis and its associated blood clotting can cause a stroke. (Recall that rupture of a cerebral vessel, as sometimes occurs in hypertension, is another cause of stroke.) People with atherosclerotic cerebral vessels may also suffer reversible neurological deficits known as ***transient ischemic attacks*** (***TIAs***), lasting minutes to hours, without actually experiencing a stroke at the time.

Finally, note that both myocardial infarcts and strokes due to occlusion may result when a fragment of blood clot or fatty deposit breaks off and then lodges elsewhere, completely blocking a smaller vessel. The fragment is called an ***embolus,*** and the process is ***embolism.*** See Chapter 19 for more information about embolisms.

SECTION E SUMMARY

Hemorrhage and Other Causes of Hypotension

I. The physiological responses to hemorrhage are summarized in Figures 12.52, 12.56, 12.58, and 12.59.

II. Hypotension can be caused by loss of body fluids, by cardiac malfunction, by strong emotion, and by liberation of vasodilator chemicals.

III. Shock is any situation in which blood flow to the tissues is low enough to cause damage to them.

The Upright Posture

I. In the upright posture, gravity acting upon unbroken columns of blood reduces venous return by increasing vascular pressures in the veins and capillaries in the limbs.
   a. The increased venous pressure distends the veins, causing venous pooling, and the increased capillary pressure causes increased filtration out of the capillaries.
   b. These effects are minimized by contraction of the skeletal muscles in the legs.

Exercise

I. The cardiovascular changes that occur in endurance-type exercise are illustrated in Figures 12.61, 12.62, and 12.64.

II. The changes are due to active hyperemia in the exercising skeletal muscles and heart; increased sympathetic outflow to the heart, arterioles, and veins; and decreased parasympathetic outflow to the heart.

III. The increase in cardiac output depends not only on the autonomic influences on the heart but on factors that help increase venous return.

IV. Training can increase a person's maximal oxygen consumption by increasing maximal stroke volume and thus cardiac output.

Hypertension

I. Hypertension is usually due to increased total peripheral resistance resulting from increased arteriolar vasoconstriction.

II. More than 90% of cases of hypertension are called *primary hypertension,* meaning that a specific cause of the increased arteriolar vasoconstriction is unknown. However, obesity, excessive salt intake, and a variety of other environmental factors clearly contribute to the development of hypertension.

Heart Failure

I. Heart failure can occur as a result of diastolic or systolic dysfunction; in both cases, cardiac output becomes inadequate.

II. This leads to fluid retention by the kidneys and formation of edema because of increased capillary pressure.

III. Pulmonary edema can occur when the left ventricle fails.

Hypertrophic Cardiomyopathy

I. Hypertrophic cardiomyopathy is a disease caused by genetic mutations in genes coding for cardiac contractile proteins.

II. It results in thickening of the left ventricle wall and septum, and disruption of the orderly array of myocytes and conducting cells.

III. If not successfully treated, it can result in sudden death by arrhythmia or heart failure.

Coronary Artery Disease and Heart Attacks

I. Insufficient coronary blood flow can cause damage to the heart.

II. Sudden death from a heart attack is usually due to ventricular fibrillation.

III. The major cause of reduced coronary blood flow is atherosclerosis, an occlusive disease of the arteries.

IV. People may suffer intermittent attacks of angina pectoris without actually suffering a heart attack at the time of the pain.

V. Atherosclerosis can also cause strokes and symptoms of inadequate blood flow in other areas.

VI. Coronary artery disease incidence is reduced by exercise, good nutrition, and avoiding smoking.

VII. Treatments for coronary artery disease include drugs that dilate blood vessels, reduce blood pressure, and prevent blood clotting. Balloon angioplasty and coronary bypass are surgical treatments.

SECTION E REVIEW QUESTIONS

1. Draw a flow diagram illustrating the reflex compensation for hemorrhage.
2. What happens to plasma volume and interstitial fluid volume following a hemorrhage?
3. What causes hypotension during a severe allergic response?
4. How does gravity influence effective blood volume?

5. Describe the role of the skeletal muscle pump in decreasing capillary filtration.
6. List the directional changes that occur during exercise for all relevant cardiovascular variables. What are the specific efferent mechanisms that bring about these changes?
7. What factors enhance venous return during exercise?
8. Diagram the control of autonomic outflow during exercise.
9. What is the limiting cardiovascular factor in endurance exercise?
10. What changes in cardiac function occur at rest and during exercise as a result of endurance training?
11. What is the abnormality in most cases of established hypertension? How does excess salt ingestion contribute?
12. State how fluid retention can help restore stroke volume in heart failure.
13. How does heart failure lead to edema in the pulmonary and systemic vascular beds?
14. Name the major risk factors for atherosclerosis.
15. Describe changes in lifestyle that may help prevent coronary artery disease.
16. List some ways that coronary artery disease can be treated.

SECTION E KEY TERMS

autotransfusion 415
maximal oxygen consumption ($\dot{V}_{O_2}$max) 420

SECTION E CLINICAL TERMS

angina pectoris 424
angiotensin-converting enzyme (ACE) inhibitors 422
atherosclerosis 425
automatic electronic defibrillator (AED) 425
β-adrenergic receptor blocker 424
Ca^{2+} channel blocker 422
cardiac inotropic drug 424
cardiogenic shock 417
cardiopulmonary resuscitation (CPR) 425
congestive heart failure 422
coronary artery disease 424
coronary balloon angioplasty 426
coronary bypass 427
coronary stent 426
coronary thrombosis 426
defibrillation 425
diastolic dysfunction 422
digitalis 424
diuretic 422
embolism 427
embolus 427
heart attack 424
heart failure 422
hypertension 421
hypertrophic cardiomyopathy 424
hypotension 415
hypovolemic shock 417
ischemia 424
left ventricular hypertrophy 421
low-resistance shock 417
myocardial infarction 424
nitroglycerin 426
primary hypertension 421
pulmonary edema 423
renal hypertension 422
secondary hypertension 421
shock 417
stroke 421
systolic dysfunction 423
transient ischemic attack (TIA) 427
vasodilator drug 424
vasovagal syncope 416
ventricular fibrillation 425

SECTION F Blood and Hemostasis

Blood was defined earlier as a mixture of cellular components suspended in a fluid called plasma. In this section, we will take a more detailed look at blood cells and plasma and then discuss the complex mechanisms that prevent excessive blood loss following injury.

12.23 Plasma

Plasma consists of a large number of organic and inorganic substances dissolved in water. A list of the major substances dissolved in plasma and their typical concentrations can be found inside the back cover of this book.

The **plasma proteins** constitute most of the plasma solutes, by weight. Their role in exerting an osmotic pressure that favors the absorption of extracellular fluid into capillaries was described in Section C of this chapter. They can be classified into three broad groups: the **albumins,** the **globulins,** and **fibrinogen.** The first two have many overlapping functions, which are discussed in relevant sections throughout the book. The albumins are the most abundant of the three plasma protein groups and are synthesized by the liver. Fibrinogen functions in clotting, discussed in detail in the latter part of this section. **Serum** is plasma with fibrinogen and other proteins involved in clotting removed. Cells normally do not take up plasma proteins; plasma proteins perform their functions in the plasma itself or in the interstitial fluid. In addition to proteins, plasma contains nutrients, metabolic waste products, hormones, and a variety of mineral electrolytes including Na^+, K^+, Cl^-, and others.

12.24 The Blood Cells

All blood cells are descended from a single population of cells called **pluripotent hematopoietic stem cells,** which are undifferentiated cells capable of giving rise to precursors (progenitors) of any of the different blood cells (**Figure 12.67**). When a pluripotent stem cell divides, its two daughter cells either remain pluripotent stem cells or become committed to a particular developmental pathway. The first branching yields either lymphoid stem cells, which give rise to the lymphocytes, or myeloid stem cells, the progenitors of all the other varieties. At some point, the proliferating offspring of the myeloid stem cells become committed to differentiating along only one path—for example, into erythrocytes.

Erythrocytes

The major function of erythrocytes is gas transport; they carry oxygen taken in by the lungs and carbon dioxide produced by the cells. Erythrocytes contain large amounts of the protein **hemoglobin** with which oxygen and, to a lesser extent, carbon dioxide reversibly combine. Oxygen binds to

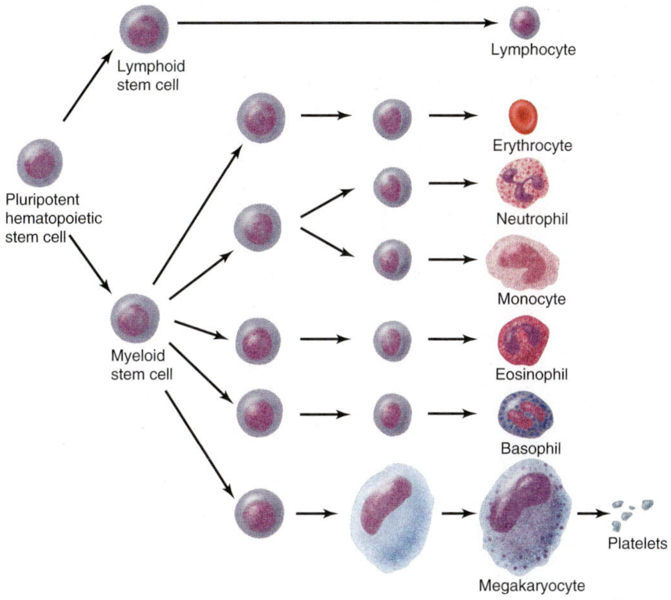

Figure 12.67 AP|R Production of blood cells by the bone marrow. For simplicity, no attempt has been made to differentiate the appearance of the various precursors. Adapted from Golde and Gasson.

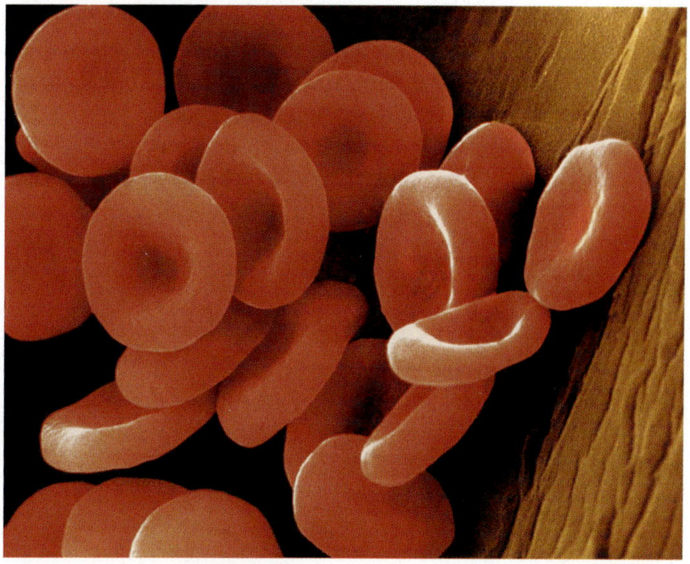

Figure 12.68 AP|R Electron micrograph of erythrocytes.

iron atoms (Fe^{2+}) in the hemoglobin molecules. The average concentration of hemoglobin is 14 g/100 mL blood in women and 15.5 g/100 mL in men. Chapter 13 further describes the structure and functions of hemoglobin.

Erythrocytes are an excellent example of the general principle of physiology that structure is a determinant of—and has coevolved with—function. They have the shape of a biconcave disk—that is, a disk thicker at the edges than in the middle, like a doughnut with a center depression on each side instead of a hole (**Figure 12.68**). This shape and their small size (7 μm in diameter) impart to the erythrocytes a high surface-area-to-volume ratio, so that oxygen and carbon dioxide can diffuse rapidly to and from the interior of the cell.

The site of erythrocyte production is the soft interior of certain bones called **bone marrow,** specifically, the red bone marrow. With differentiation, the erythrocyte precursors produce hemoglobin, but then they ultimately lose their nuclei and organelles—their machinery for protein synthesis. Young erythrocytes in the bone marrow still contain a few ribosomes, which produce a weblike (reticular) appearance when treated with special stains, an appearance that gives these young erythrocytes the name **reticulocyte.** Normally, erythrocytes lose these ribosomes about a day after leaving the bone marrow, so reticulocytes constitute only about 1% of circulating erythrocytes. In the presence of unusually rapid erythrocyte production, however, many more reticulocytes can be found in the blood, a phenomenon of clinically diagnostic usefulness.

Because erythrocytes lack nuclei and most organelles, they can neither reproduce themselves nor maintain their normal structure for very long. The average life span of an erythrocyte is approximately 120 days, which means that almost 1% of the erythrocytes are destroyed and must be replaced every day. This amounts to 250 billion cells per day! Destruction of damaged or dying erythrocytes normally occurs in the spleen and the liver. As we will later describe, most of the iron released in the process is conserved. The major breakdown product of hemoglobin is **bilirubin,** which is returned to the circulation and gives plasma its characteristic yellowish color (Chapter 15 will describe the fate of this substance).

Iron

As noted previously, iron is the element to which oxygen binds on a hemoglobin molecule within an erythrocyte. Small amounts of iron are lost from the body via the urine, feces, sweat, and cells sloughed from the skin. Women lose an additional amount via menstrual blood. In order to remain in iron balance, the amount of iron lost from the body must be replaced by ingestion of iron-containing foods. Particularly rich sources of iron are meat, liver, shellfish, egg yolk, beans, nuts, and cereals. A significant disruption of iron balance can result in either ***iron deficiency***, leading to inadequate hemoglobin production, or an excess of iron in the body (***hemochromatosis***), which results in abnormal iron deposits and damage in various organs, including the liver, heart, pituitary gland, pancreas, and joints.

The homeostatic control of iron balance resides primarily in the intestinal epithelium, which actively absorbs iron from ingested foods. Normally, only a small fraction of ingested iron is absorbed. However, this fraction is increased or decreased in a negative feedback manner, depending upon the state of the body's iron balance—the more iron in the body, the less ingested iron is absorbed (the mechanism will be described in Chapter 15).

The body has a considerable store of iron, mainly in the liver, bound up in a protein called **ferritin.** Ferritin serves as a buffer against iron deficiency. About 50% of the total body iron is in hemoglobin, 25% is in other heme-containing proteins (mainly the cytochromes) in the cells of the body, and 25% is in liver ferritin.

The recycling of iron is very efficient (**Figure 12.69**). As old erythrocytes are destroyed in the spleen (and liver), their iron is released into the plasma and bound to an iron-transport plasma protein called **transferrin.** Transferrin delivers almost all of this iron to the bone marrow to be incorporated into new erythrocytes. Recirculation of erythrocyte iron is very important because it involves 20 times more iron per day than the body absorbs and excretes.

Folic Acid and Vitamin B_{12}

Folic acid, a vitamin found in large amounts in leafy plants, yeast, and liver, is required for synthesis of the nucleotide base thymine. It is, therefore, essential for the formation of DNA and thus for normal cell division. When this vitamin is not present in adequate amounts, impairment of cell division occurs throughout the body but is most striking in rapidly proliferating cells, including erythrocyte precursors. As a result, fewer erythrocytes are produced when folic acid is deficient.

The production of normal erythrocyte numbers also requires extremely small quantities (one-millionth of a gram per day) of a cobalt-containing molecule, **vitamin B_{12}** (also called cobalamin), because this vitamin is required for the action of folic acid. Vitamin B_{12} is found only in animal products, and strictly vegetarian diets tend to be deficient in it. Also, the absorption of vitamin B_{12} from the gastrointestinal tract requires a protein called **intrinsic factor,** which is secreted by the stomach (see Chapter 15). Lack of this protein, therefore, causes vitamin B_{12} deficiency, and the resulting erythrocyte deficiency is known as ***pernicious anemia.***

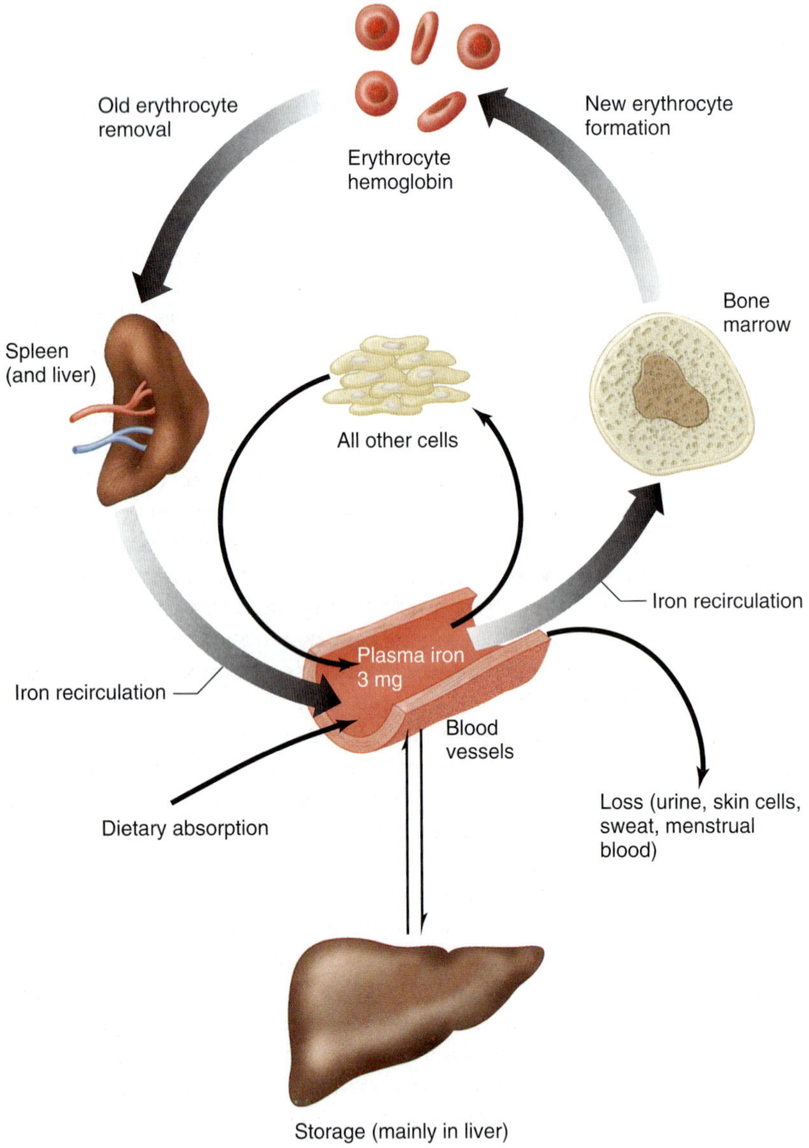

Figure 12.69 Summary of iron balance. The thickness of the arrows correlates with the amount of iron involved. In the steady state, the rate of gastrointestinal iron absorption equals the rate of iron loss via urine, skin, and menstrual flow. Adapted from Crosby.

Regulation of Erythrocyte Production

In a typical person, the total volume of circulating erythrocytes remains remarkably constant because of reflexes that regulate the bone marrow's production of these cells. In the previous section, we stated that iron, folic acid, and vitamin B_{12} must be present for normal erythrocyte production, or **erythropoiesis.** However, none of these substances constitutes the signal that regulates the production rate.

The direct control of erythropoiesis is exerted primarily by a hormone called **erythropoietin,** which is secreted into the blood mainly by a particular group of hormone-secreting connective tissue cells in the kidneys. Erythropoietin acts on the bone marrow to stimulate the proliferation of erythrocyte progenitor cells and their differentiation into mature erythrocytes.

Erythropoietin is normally secreted in small amounts that stimulate the bone marrow to produce erythrocytes at a rate adequate to replace the usual loss. The erythropoietin secretion rate is increased markedly above basal values when there is a decreased oxygen delivery to the kidneys. Situations in which this occurs include insufficient pumping of blood by the heart, lung disease, anemia (a decrease in number of erythrocytes or in hemoglobin concentration), prolonged exercise, and exposure to high altitude. As a result of the increase in erythropoietin secretion, plasma erythropoietin concentration, erythrocyte production, and the oxygen-carrying capacity of the blood all increase. Therefore, oxygen delivery to the tissues returns toward normal (**Figure 12.70**). Testosterone, the male sex hormone, also stimulates the release of erythropoietin. This accounts in part for the higher hematocrit in men than in women.

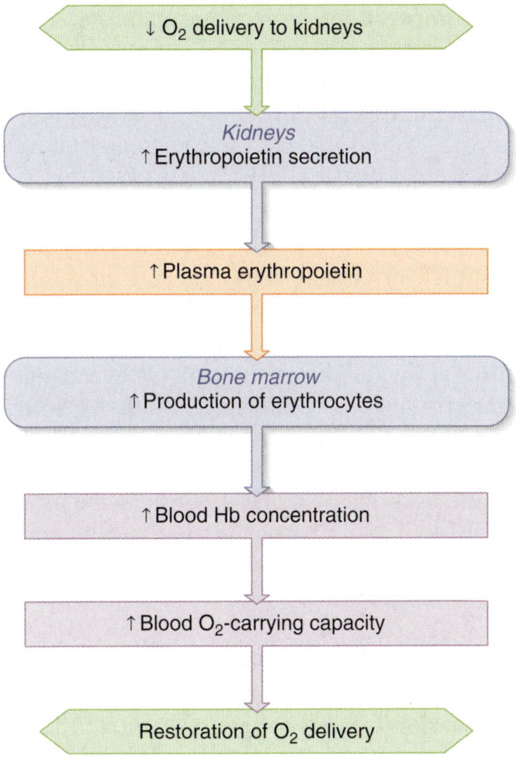

Figure 12.70 Reflex by which decreased oxygen delivery to the kidneys increases erythrocyte production via increased erythropoietin secretion.

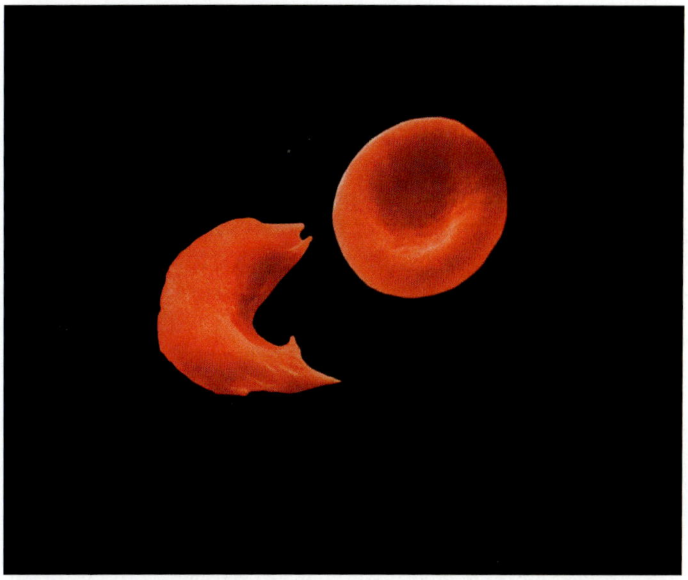

Figure 12.71 APR Digitally colorized scanning electron micrograph of red blood cells from a patient with sickle cell anemia. The cell at left assumed this sickle shape after exposure to low-oxygen conditions.

Anemia

As just described, ***anemia*** is defined as a decrease in the ability of the blood to carry oxygen due to (1) a decrease in the total number of erythrocytes, each having a normal quantity of hemoglobin; (2) a diminished concentration of hemoglobin per erythrocyte; or (3) a combination of both. Anemia has a wide variety of causes, some of which are listed in **Table 12.11.**

Sickle-cell disease (formerly called *sickle-cell anemia*) is due to a genetic mutation that alters one amino acid in the hemoglobin chain. At the low oxygen levels existing in many capillaries, the abnormal hemoglobin molecules interact with each other to form fiberlike polymers that distort the erythrocyte membrane and cause the cell to form sickle shapes or other bizarre forms (**Figure 12.71**). This causes both the blockage of capillaries, with consequent tissue damage and pain, and the destruction of the deformed erythrocytes, with consequent anemia. Sickle-cell disease is an example of a disease that is manifested fully only in people homozygous for the mutated gene (that is, they have two copies of the mutated gene, one from each parent). In heterozygotes (one mutated copy and one normal gene), people who are said to have sickle-cell trait, the normal gene codes for normal hemoglobin and the mutated gene for the abnormal hemoglobin. The erythrocytes in this case contain both types of hemoglobin, but symptoms are observed only when the oxygen level is unusually low, as at high altitude. The persistence of the sickle-cell mutation in humans is due to the fact that heterozygotes are more resistant to ***malaria,*** a blood infection caused by a protozoan parasite that is spread by mosquitoes in tropical regions. See the Chapter 2 Clinical Case Study for a case discussion of sickle-cell trait.

TABLE 12.11	Major Causes of Anemia
Dietary deficiencies of iron (***iron-deficiency anemia***), vitamin B_{12}, or folic acid	
Bone marrow failure due to toxic drugs or cancer	
Blood loss from the body (hemorrhage)	
Inadequate secretion of erythropoietin in kidney disease	
Excessive destruction of erythrocytes (for example, sickle-cell disease)	

Finally, there also exist conditions in which there are more erythrocytes than normal, a condition called ***polycythemia.*** An example, to be described in Chapter 13, is the polycythemia that occurs in high-altitude dwellers. In this case, the increased number of erythrocytes is an adaptive response because it increases the oxygen-carrying capacity of blood exposed to low oxygen levels. As discussed earlier, however, increasing the hematocrit increases the viscosity of blood. Therefore, polycythemia makes the flow of blood through blood vessels more difficult and puts a strain on the heart. Abuse of synthetic erythropoietin and the subsequent extreme polycythemia have resulted in the deaths of competitive bicyclists—one reason that such "blood doping" is banned in sports.

Leukocytes

Circulating in the blood and interspersed among various tissues are white blood cells, or leukocytes (see Figure 12.67). The leukocytes are all involved in immune defenses and include neutrophils, eosinophils, monocytes, macrophages, basophils, and lymphocytes. A brief description of their functions follows; these functions are detailed in Chapter 18.

- **Neutrophils** are phagocytes and the most abundant leukocytes. They are found in blood but leave capillaries and enter tissues during inflammation. After neutrophils engulf microbes such as bacteria by phagocytosis, the bacteria are destroyed within endocytotic vacuoles by proteases, oxidizing compounds, and antibacterial proteins called **defensins.** The production and release of neutrophils from bone marrow are greatly stimulated during the course of an infection.
- **Eosinophils** are found in the blood and in the mucosal surfaces lining the gastrointestinal, respiratory, and urinary tracts, where they fight off invasions by eukaryotic parasites. In some cases, eosinophils act by releasing toxic chemicals that kill parasites, and in other cases by phagocytosis.
- **Monocytes** are phagocytes that circulate in the blood for a short time, after which they migrate into tissues and organs and develop into macrophages.
- **Macrophages** are strategically located where they will encounter invaders, including epithelia in contact with the external environment, such as skin and the linings of respiratory and digestive tracts. Macrophages are large phagocytes capable of engulfing viruses and bacteria.
- **Basophils** are secretory cells. They secrete an anticlotting factor called heparin at the site of an infection, which helps the circulation flush out the infected site. Basophils also secrete histamine, which attracts infection-fighting cells and proteins to the site.
- **Lymphocytes** are comprised of several different types of cells that play key roles in protecting against specific pathogens, including viruses, bacteria, toxins, and cancer cells. Some lymphocytes directly kill pathogens, and others secrete antibodies into the circulation that bind to foreign molecules and begin the process of their destruction.

Platelets

The circulating platelets are colorless, nonnucleated cell fragments that contain numerous granules and are much smaller than erythrocytes. Platelets are produced when cytoplasmic portions of large bone marrow cells, termed **megakaryocytes,** pinch off and enter the circulation (see Figure 12.67). Platelet functions in blood clotting are described later in this section.

Regulation of Blood Cell Production

In children, the marrow of most bones produces blood cells. By adulthood, however, only the bones of the chest, base of the skull, spinal vertebrae, pelvis, and ends of the limb bones remain active. The bone marrow in an adult weighs almost as much as the liver, and it produces cells at an enormous rate.

Proliferation and differentiation of the various progenitor cells is stimulated, at multiple points, by a large number of protein hormones and paracrine agents collectively termed **hematopoietic growth factors (HGFs)**. Erythropoietin is one example of an HGF. Others are listed for reference in **Table 12.12.** (Nomenclature can be confusing in this area because the HGFs belong to a still larger general family of messengers called cytokines, which are described in Chapter 18.)

The physiology of the HGFs is very complex because (1) there are so many types, (2) any given HGF is often produced by a variety of cell types throughout the body, and (3) HGFs often exert other actions in addition to stimulating blood cell production. Moreover, there are many interactions of the HGFs on particular bone marrow cells and processes. For example, although erythropoietin is the major stimulator of erythropoiesis, at least 10 other HGFs cooperate in the process. Finally, in several cases, the HGFs not only stimulate differentiation and proliferation of progenitor cells but also inhibit the usual programmed death (apoptosis) of these cells.

The administration of specific HGFs is proving to be of considerable clinical importance. Examples are the use of erythropoietin in persons having a deficiency of this hormone due to kidney disease and the use of granulocyte colony-stimulating factor (G-CSF) to stimulate granulocyte production in individuals whose bone marrow has been damaged by anticancer drugs.

12.25 Hemostasis: The Prevention of Blood Loss

The stoppage of bleeding is known as **hemostasis** (do not confuse this word with *homeostasis*). Physiological hemostatic mechanisms are most effective in dealing with injuries in

TABLE 12.12 Reference Table of Major Hematopoietic Growth Factors (HGFs)

Name	Stimulates Progenitor Cells Leading To:
Erythropoietin	Erythrocytes
Colony-stimulating factors (CSFs) (example: granulocyte CSF)	Granulocytes and monocytes
Interleukins (example: interleukin 3)	Various leukocytes
Thrombopoietin	Platelets (from megakaryocytes)
Stem cell factor	Many types of blood cells

small vessels—arterioles, capillaries, and venules, which are the most common sources of bleeding in everyday life. In contrast, the body usually cannot control bleeding from a medium or large artery. Venous bleeding leads to less rapid blood loss because veins have low blood pressure. Indeed, the decrease in hydrostatic pressure induced by raising the bleeding part above the level of the heart level may stop hemorrhage from a vein. In addition, if the venous bleeding is internal, the accumulation of blood in the tissues may increase interstitial pressure enough to eliminate the pressure gradient required for continued blood loss. Accumulation of blood in the tissues can occur as a result of bleeding from any vessel type and is known as a ***hematoma.***

When a blood vessel is severed or otherwise injured, its immediate inherent response is to constrict. The mechanism is not completely understood but most likely involves changes in local vasodilator and constrictor substances released by endothelial cells and blood cells (see Figure 12.36). This short-lived response slows the flow of blood in the affected area. In addition, this constriction presses the opposed endothelial surfaces of the vessel together and this contact induces a stickiness capable of keeping them "glued" together.

Permanent closure of the vessel by constriction and contact stickiness occurs only in the very smallest vessels of the microcirculation, however, and the staunching of bleeding ultimately depends upon two other interdependent processes that occur in rapid succession: (1) formation of a platelet plug and (2) blood coagulation (clotting). The blood platelets are involved in both processes.

Formation of a Platelet Plug

The involvement of platelets in hemostasis requires their adhesion to a surface. Injury to a vessel disrupts the endothelium and exposes the underlying connective-tissue collagen fibers. Platelets adhere to collagen, largely via an intermediary called **von Willebrand factor (vWF)**, a plasma protein secreted by endothelial cells and platelets. This protein binds to exposed collagen molecules, changes its conformation, and becomes able to bind platelets. Thus, vWF forms a bridge between the damaged vessel wall and the platelets.

Binding of platelets to collagen triggers the platelets to release the contents of their secretory vesicles, which contain a variety of chemical agents. Many of these agents, including adenosine diphosphate (ADP) and serotonin, then act locally to induce multiple changes in the metabolism, shape, and surface proteins of the platelets, a process called **platelet activation.** Some of these changes cause new platelets to adhere to the old ones, a positive feedback phenomenon termed **platelet aggregation,** which rapidly creates a **platelet plug** inside the vessel.

Chemical agents in the platelets' secretory vesicles are not the only stimulators of platelet activation and aggregation. Adhesion of the platelets rapidly induces them to synthesize **thromboxane A_2,** a member of the eicosanoid family, from arachidonic acid in the platelet plasma membrane. Thromboxane A_2 is released into the extracellular fluid and acts locally to further stimulate platelet aggregation and release of their secretory vesicle contents (**Figure 12.72**).

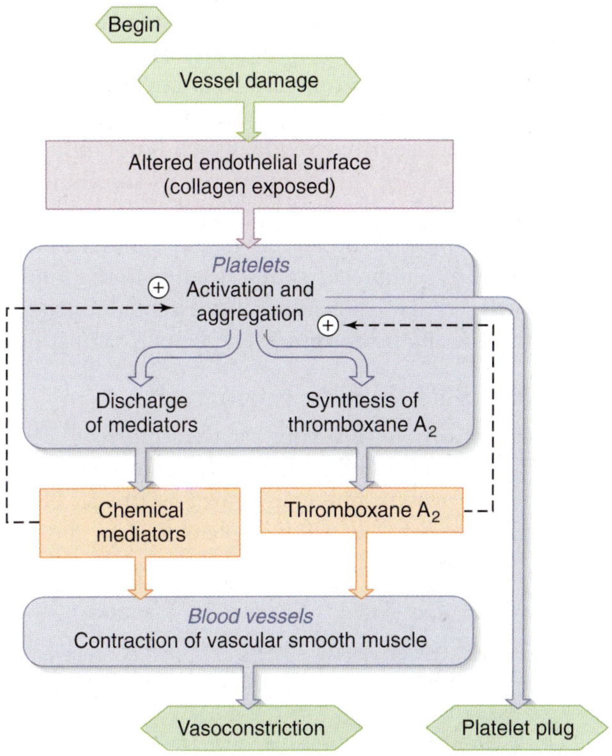

Figure 12.72 Sequence of events leading to formation of a platelet plug and vasoconstriction following damage to a blood vessel wall. Note the two positive feedbacks in the pathways.

Fibrinogen, a plasma protein whose essential role in blood clotting is described in the next section, also plays a crucial role in the platelet aggregation produced by the factors previously described. It does so by forming the bridges between aggregating platelets. The receptors (binding sites) for fibrinogen on the platelet plasma membrane become exposed and activated during platelet activation.

The platelet plug can completely seal small breaks in blood vessel walls. Its effectiveness is further enhanced by another property of platelets—contraction. Platelets contain a very high concentration of actin and myosin (see Chapter 9), which are stimulated to interact in aggregated platelets. This causes compression and strengthening of the platelet plug. (When they occur in a test tube, this contraction and compression are termed *clot retraction.*)

While the plug is being built up and compacted, the vascular smooth muscle in the damaged vessel is simultaneously being stimulated to contract (see Figure 12.72), thereby decreasing the blood flow to the area and the pressure within the damaged vessel. This vasoconstriction is the result of platelet activity, for it is mediated by thromboxane A_2 and by several chemicals contained in the platelet's secretory vesicles.

Once started, why does the platelet plug not continuously expand, spreading away from the damaged endothelium along intact endothelium in both directions? One important reason involves the ability of the adjacent undamaged endothelial cells to synthesize and release the eicosanoid known as **prostacyclin** (also termed **prostaglandin I_2 [PGI_2]**), which is a profound inhibitor of platelet aggregation. Thus, whereas platelets possess the enzymes that produce thromboxane A_2

from arachidonic acid, normal endothelial cells contain a different enzyme that converts intermediates formed from arachidonic acid not to thromboxane A_2 but to prostacyclin (**Figure 12.73**). In addition to prostacyclin, the adjacent endothelial cells also release **nitric oxide,** which is not only a vasodilator (see Section C of this chapter) but also an inhibitor of platelet adhesion, activation, and aggregation.

The platelet plug is built up very rapidly and is the primary mechanism used to seal breaks in vessel walls. In the following section, we will see that platelets are also essential for the next, more slowly occurring hemostatic event: blood coagulation.

Blood Coagulation: Clot Formation

Blood coagulation, or **clotting,** is the transformation of blood into a solid gel called a **clot** or **thrombus,** which consists mainly of a protein polymer known as **fibrin.** Clotting occurs locally around the original platelet plug and is the dominant hemostatic defense. Its function is to support and reinforce the platelet plug and to solidify blood that remains in the wound channel.

Figure 12.74 summarizes, in very simplified form, the events leading to clotting. These events, like platelet aggregation, are initiated when injury to a vessel disrupts the endothelium and permits the blood to contact the underlying tissue. This contact initiates a locally occurring cascade of chemical activations. At each step of the cascade, an inactive plasma protein, or "factor," is converted (activated) to a proteolytic enzyme, which then catalyzes the generation of the next enzyme in the sequence. Each of these activations results from the splitting of a small peptide fragment from the inactive plasma protein precursor, thereby exposing the active site of the enzyme. However, several of the plasma protein factors, following their activation, function not as enzymes but rather as cofactors for enzymes.

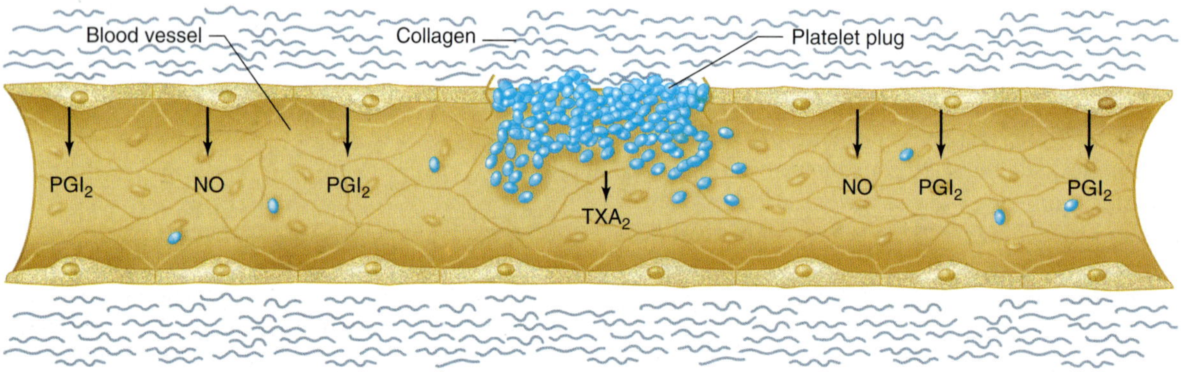

Figure 12.73 Prostacyclin (prostaglandin I_2 [PGI_2]) and nitric oxide (NO), both produced by endothelial cells, inhibit platelet aggregation and therefore prevent the spread of platelet aggregation from a damaged site. TXA_2 = Thromboxane A_2.

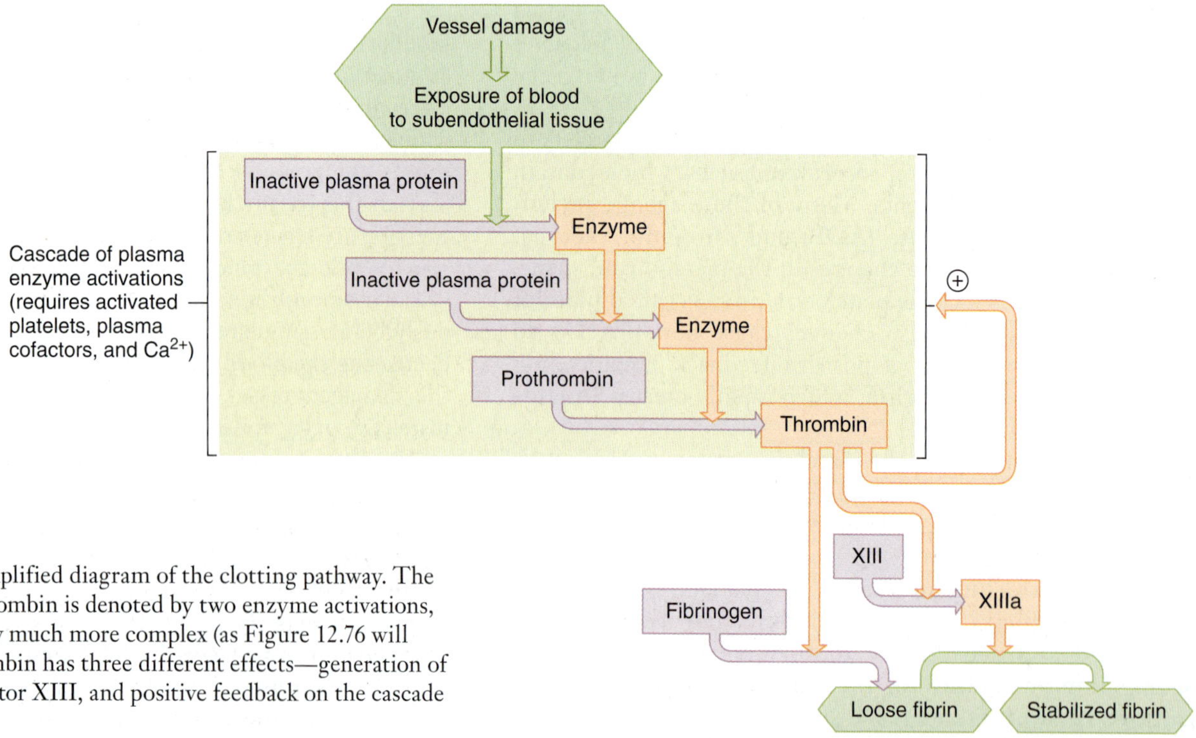

Figure 12.74 Simplified diagram of the clotting pathway. The pathway leading to thrombin is denoted by two enzyme activations, but the story is actually much more complex (as Figure 12.76 will show). Note that thrombin has three different effects—generation of fibrin, activation of factor XIII, and positive feedback on the cascade leading to itself.

For simplicity, Figure 12.74 gives no specifics about the cascade until the key point at which the plasma protein **prothrombin** is converted to the enzyme **thrombin.** Thrombin then catalyzes a reaction in which several polypeptides are split from molecules of the large, rod-shaped plasma protein fibrinogen. The fibrinogen remnants then bind to each other to form fibrin. The fibrin, initially a loose mesh of interlacing strands, is rapidly stabilized and strengthened by the enzymatically mediated formation of covalent cross-linkages. This chemical linking is catalyzed by an enzyme known as factor XIIIa, which is formed from plasma protein factor XIII in a reaction also catalyzed by thrombin.

Thus, thrombin catalyzes not only the formation of loose fibrin but also the activation of factor XIII, which stabilizes the fibrin network. However, thrombin does even more than this—it exerts a profound positive feedback effect on its own formation. It does so by activating several proteins in the cascade and also by activating platelets. Therefore, once thrombin formation has begun, reactions leading to much more thrombin generation are activated by this initial thrombin. We will make use of this crucial fact later when we describe the specifics of the cascade leading to thrombin.

In the process of clotting, many erythrocytes and other cells are trapped in the fibrin meshwork (**Figure 12.75**), but the essential component of the clot is fibrin, and clotting can occur in the absence of all cellular elements except platelets. Activated platelets are essential because several of the cascade reactions take place on the surface of the platelets. As noted earlier, platelet activation occurs early in the hemostatic response as a result of platelet adhesion to collagen, but in addition, thrombin is an important stimulator of platelet activation. The activation causes the platelets to display specific plasma membrane receptors that bind several of the clotting factors, and this permits the reactions to take place on the surface of the platelets. The activated platelets also display particular phospholipids, called **platelet factor** (**PF**), which functions as a cofactor in the steps mediated by the bound clotting factors.

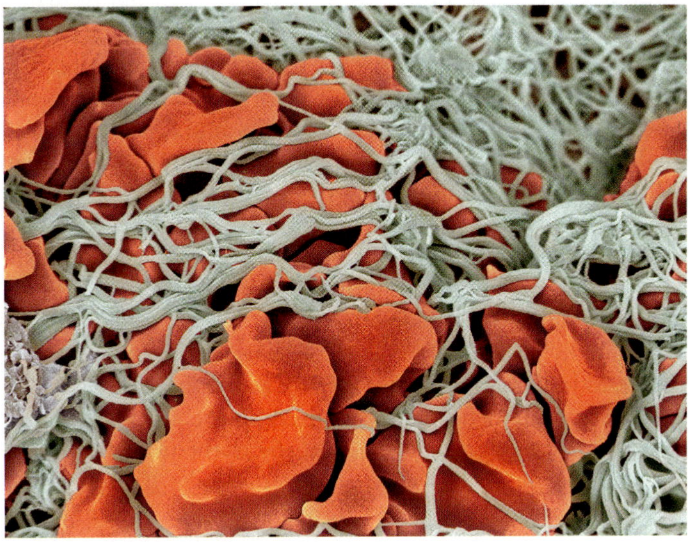

Figure 12.75 Scanning electron micrograph of erythrocytes enmeshed in fibrin.

In addition to protein factors, plasma Ca^{2+} is required at various steps in the clotting cascade. However, Ca^{2+} concentration in the plasma can never decrease enough to cause clotting defects because death would occur from muscle paralysis or cardiac arrhythmias before such low concentrations were reached.

Now we present the specifics of the early portions of the clotting cascade—those leading from vessel damage to the prothrombin–thrombin reaction. These early reactions consist of two seemingly parallel pathways that merge at the step just before the prothrombin–thrombin reaction. Under physiological conditions, however, the two pathways are not parallel but are actually activated sequentially, with thrombin serving as the link between them. There are also several points at which the two pathways interact. It will be clearer, however, if we first discuss the two pathways as though they were separate and then deal with their actual interaction. The pathways are called (1) the **intrinsic pathway,** so named because everything necessary for it is in the blood; and (2) the **extrinsic pathway,** so named because a cellular element outside the blood is needed. **Figure 12.76** will be an essential reference for this entire discussion. Also, **Table 12.13** is a reference list of the names of and synonyms for the substances in these pathways.

The first plasma protein in the intrinsic pathway (upper left of Figure 12.76) is called factor XII. It can become activated to factor XIIa when it contacts certain types of surfaces, including the collagen fibers underlying damaged endothelium. The contact activation of factor XII to XIIa is a complex process that requires the participation of several other plasma proteins not shown in Figure 12.76. Contact activation also explains why blood coagulates when it is taken from the body and put in a glass tube. This has nothing whatever to do with exposure to air but happens because the glass surface acts like collagen and induces the same activation of factor XII and aggregation of platelets as a damaged vessel surface. A silicone coating delays clotting by reducing the activating effects of the glass surface.

Factor XIIa then catalyzes the activation of factor XI to factor XIa, which activates factor IX to factor IXa. This last factor then activates factor X to factor Xa, which is the enzyme that converts prothrombin to thrombin. Note in Figure 12.76 that another plasma protein—factor VIIIa—serves as a cofactor (not an enzyme) in the factor IXa–mediated activation of factor X. The importance of factor VIII in clotting is emphasized by the fact that the disease ***hemophilia,*** characterized by excessive bleeding, is usually due to a genetic absence of this factor. (In a smaller number of cases, hemophilia is due to an absence of factor IX.)

Now we turn to the extrinsic pathway for initiating the clotting cascade (upper right of Figure 12.76). This pathway begins with a protein called **tissue factor,** which is not a plasma protein. It is located instead on the outer plasma membrane of various tissue cells, including fibroblasts and other cells in the walls of blood vessels outside the endothelium. The blood is exposed to these subendothelial cells when vessel damage disrupts the endothelial lining. Tissue factor on these cells then binds a plasma protein, factor VII, which becomes activated to factor VIIa. The complex of tissue factor and factor VIIa on the plasma membrane of the tissue cell then

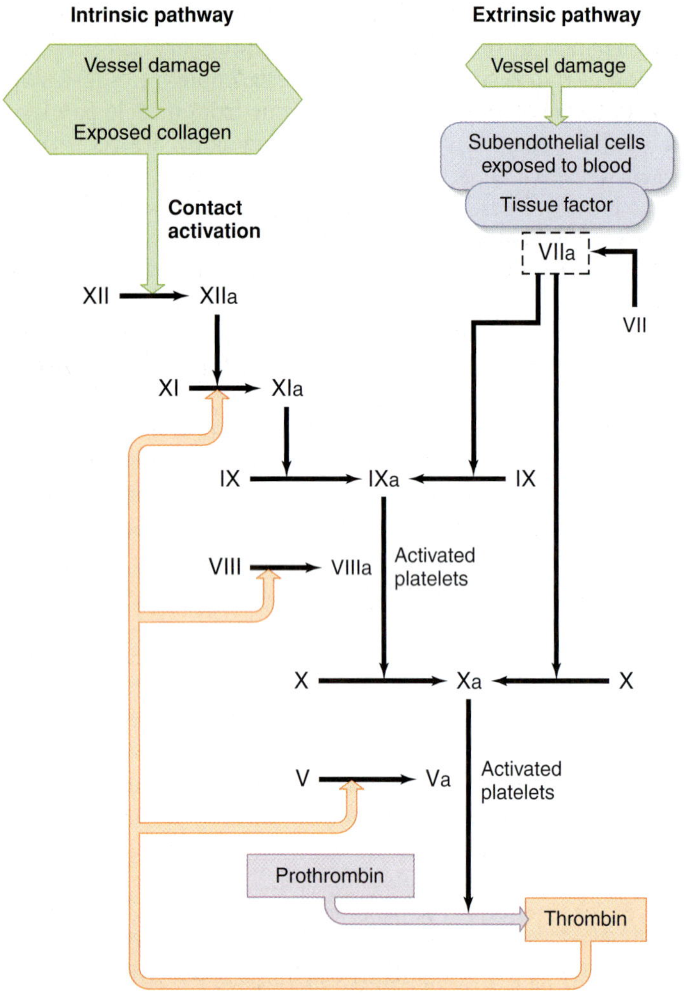

Figure 12.76 Two clotting pathways—intrinsic and extrinsic—merge and can lead to the generation of thrombin. Under most physiological conditions, however, factor XII and the contact-activation step that begins the intrinsic pathway probably play little, if any, role in clotting. Rather, clotting is initiated solely by the extrinsic pathway, as described in the text. You may think that factors IX and X were accidentally transposed in the intrinsic pathway, but this is not the case; the order of activation really is XI, IX, and X. For the sake of clarity, the roles Ca^{2+} plays in clotting are not shown.

PHYSIOLOGICAL INQUIRY

- Which would affect normal blood clotting more, a mutation that blocked the production of clotting factor XII, or one that blocked production of factor VII?

Answer can be found at end of chapter.

catalyzes the activation of factor X. In addition, it catalyzes the activation of factor IX, which can then help activate even more factor X by way of the intrinsic pathway.

In summary, clotting can theoretically be initiated either by the activation of factor XII or by the generation of the tissue factor–factor VIIa complex. The two paths merge at factor Xa, which then catalyzes the conversion of prothrombin to thrombin, which catalyzes the formation of fibrin. As shown in Figure 12.76, thrombin also contributes to the activation of (1) factors XI and VIII in the intrinsic pathway and (2) factor V, with factor Va then serving as a cofactor for factor Xa. Not shown in the figure is the fact that thrombin also activates platelets.

As stated earlier, under physiological conditions, the two pathways just described actually are activated sequentially. To understand how this works, turn again to Figure 12.76; hold your hand over the first part of the intrinsic pathway so that you can eliminate the contact activation of factor XII, and then begin the description in the next paragraph at the top of the extrinsic pathway in the figure.

The extrinsic pathway, with its tissue factor, is the usual way of initiating clotting in the body, and factor XII—the beginning of the full intrinsic pathway—normally plays little if any role (in contrast to its initiation of clotting in test tubes or within the body in several unusual situations). Thus, thrombin is initially generated only by the extrinsic pathway. The amount of thrombin is too small, however, to produce adequate, sustained coagulation. It *is* large enough, though, to trigger thrombin's positive feedback effects on the intrinsic pathway—activation of factors V, VIII, and XI and of platelets. This is all that is needed to trigger the intrinsic pathway independently of factor XII. This pathway then generates the large amounts of thrombin required for adequate coagulation. The extrinsic pathway, therefore, via its initial generation of small amounts of thrombin, provides the means for recruiting the more potent intrinsic pathway without the participation of factor XII. In essence, thrombin eliminates the need for factor XII. Moreover, thrombin not only recruits the intrinsic pathway but facilitates the prothrombin–thrombin step itself by activating factor V and platelets.

Finally, note that the liver plays several important indirect roles in clotting (**Figure 12.77**); as a result, persons with liver disease often have serious bleeding problems. First, the liver is the site of production for many of the plasma clotting factors. Second, the liver produces bile salts (Chapter 15), and these are important for normal intestinal absorption of the lipid-soluble substance **vitamin K.** The liver requires this vitamin to produce prothrombin and several other clotting factors.

TABLE 12.13 Official Designations for Clotting Factors, Along with Synonyms More Commonly Used

Factor I (fibrinogen)
Factor Ia (fibrin)
Factor II (prothrombin)
Factor IIa (thrombin)
Factor III (tissue factor, tissue thromboplastin)
Factor IV (Ca^{2+})
Factors V, VII, VIII, IX, X, XI, XII, and XIII are the inactive forms of these factors; the active forms add an "a" (e.g., factor XIIa). There is no factor VI.
Platelet factor (PF)

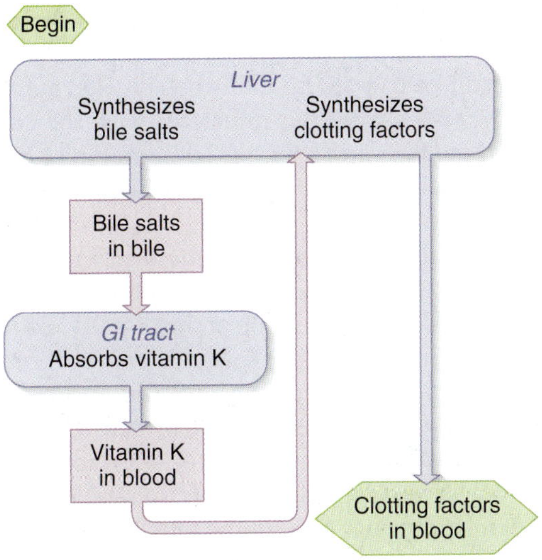

Figure 12.77 Roles of the liver in blood clotting.

PHYSIOLOGICAL INQUIRY

- How might prolonged treatment with antibiotics result in the side effect of impaired blood clotting? (*Hint:* Read about vitamin K in Chapter 15.)

Answer can be found at end of chapter.

Anticlotting Systems

Earlier, we described how the release of prostacyclin and nitric oxide by endothelial cells inhibits platelet aggregation. Because this aggregation is an essential precursor for clotting, these agents reduce the magnitude and extent of clotting. In addition, however, the body has mechanisms for limiting clot formation itself and for dissolving a clot after it has formed. The presence of mechanisms that both favor and limit blood clotting is a good example of the general principle of physiology that most physiological functions are controlled by multiple regulatory systems, often working in opposition.

Factors That Oppose Clot Formation

There are at least three different mechanisms that oppose clot formation, thereby helping to limit this process and prevent it from spreading excessively. Defects in any of these natural anticoagulant mechanisms are associated with abnormally high risk of clotting, a condition called ***hypercoagulability*** (see Chapter 19 for a case discussion of a patient with this condition).

The first anticoagulant mechanism acts during the initiation phase of clotting and utilizes the plasma protein called **tissue factor pathway inhibitor** (**TFPI**), which is secreted mainly by endothelial cells. This substance binds to tissue factor–factor VIIa complexes and inhibits the ability of these complexes to generate factor Xa. This anticoagulant mechanism is the reason that the extrinsic pathway by itself can generate only small amounts of thrombin.

The second anticoagulant mechanism is triggered by thrombin. As illustrated in **Figure 12.78**, thrombin can bind to an endothelial cell receptor known as **thrombomodulin.** This binding eliminates all of thrombin's clot-producing effects and causes the bound thrombin to bind a particular plasma protein, **protein C** (distinguish this from protein kinase C, Chapter 5). The binding to thrombin activates protein C, which, in combination with yet another plasma protein, then inactivates factors VIIIa and Va. We saw earlier that thrombin directly activates factors VIII and V when the endothelium is damaged, and now we see that it indirectly inactivates them via protein C in areas where the endothelium is intact. **Table 12.14** summarizes the effects—both stimulatory and inhibitory—of thrombin on the clotting pathways.

A third naturally occurring anticoagulant mechanism is a plasma protein called **antithrombin III,** which inactivates thrombin and several other clotting factors. The activity of antithrombin III is greatly enhanced when it binds to **heparin,** a substance present on the surface of endothelial cells. Antithrombin III prevents the spread of a clot by rapidly inactivating clotting factors that are carried away from the immediate site of the clot by the flowing blood.

The Fibrinolytic System

TFPI, protein C, and antithrombin III all function to *limit* clot formation. The system to be described now, however, dissolves a clot *after* it is formed.

A fibrin clot is not designed to last forever. It is a temporary fix until permanent repair of the vessel occurs. The **fibrinolytic** (or thrombolytic) **system** is the principal effector of clot removal. The physiology of this system (**Figure 12.79**) is analogous to that of the clotting system; it constitutes a plasma

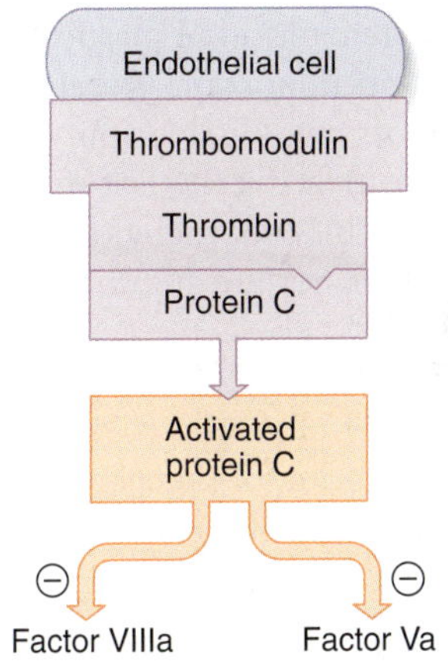

Figure 12.78 Thrombin indirectly inactivates factors VIIIa and Va via protein C. To activate protein C, thrombin must first bind to a thrombin receptor, thrombomodulin, on endothelial cells; this binding also eliminates thrombin's procoagulant effects. The ⊖ symbol indicates inactivation of factors Va and VIIIa.

TABLE 12.14	Actions of Thrombin
Procoagulant	Cleaves fibrinogen to fibrin Activates clotting factors XI, VIII, V, and XIII Stimulates platelet activation
Anticoagulant	Activates protein C, which inactivates clotting factors VIIIa and Va

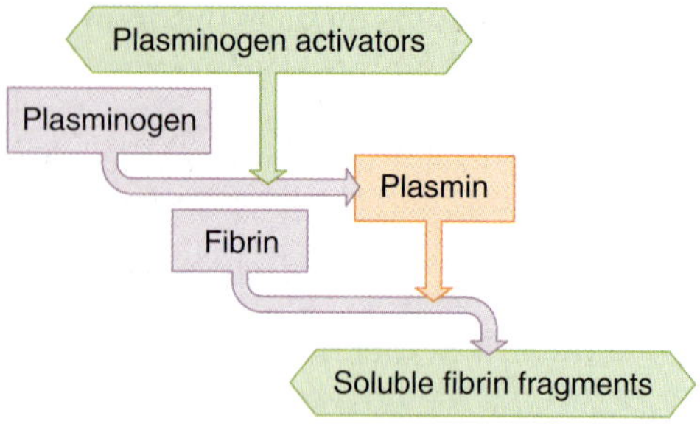

Figure 12.79 Basic fibrinolytic system. There are many different plasminogen activators and many different pathways for initiating their activity.

proenzyme, **plasminogen,** which can be activated to the active enzyme **plasmin** by protein **plasminogen activators.** Once formed, plasmin digests fibrin, thereby dissolving the clot.

The fibrinolytic system is proving to be every bit as complicated as the clotting system, with multiple types of plasminogen activators and pathways for generating them, as well as several inhibitors of these plasminogen activators. In describing how this system can be set into motion, we restrict our discussion to one example—the particular plasminogen activator known as **tissue plasminogen activator (t-PA),** which is secreted by endothelial cells. During clotting, both plasminogen and t-PA bind to fibrin and become incorporated throughout the clot. The binding of t-PA to fibrin is crucial because t-PA is a very weak enzyme in the absence of fibrin. The presence of fibrin profoundly increases the ability of t-PA to catalyze the generation of plasmin from plasminogen. Fibrin, therefore, is an important initiator of the fibrinolytic process that leads to its own dissolution.

The secretion of t-PA is the last of the various anticlotting functions exerted by endothelial cells that we have mentioned in this chapter. They are summarized in **Table 12.15**.

Anticlotting Drugs

Various drugs are used clinically to prevent or reverse clotting, and a brief description of their actions serves as a review of key clotting mechanisms. One of the most common uses of these drugs is in the prevention and treatment of myocardial infarction (heart attack), which, as described in Section E, is often the result of damage to endothelial cells. Such damage not only triggers clotting but interferes with the endothelial cells' normal *anticlotting* functions. For example, atherosclerosis interferes with the ability of endothelial cells to secrete nitric oxide.

Aspirin inhibits the cyclooxygenase enzyme in the eicosanoid pathways that generate prostaglandins and thromboxanes (see Chapter 5). Because thromboxane A_2, produced by the platelets, is important for platelet aggregation, aspirin reduces both platelet aggregation and the ensuing coagulation. Importantly, low doses of aspirin cause a steady-state decrease in *platelet* cyclooxygenase (COX) activity but not *endothelial-cell* cyclooxygenase; so the formation of prostacyclin—the prostaglandin that opposes platelet aggregation—is not impaired. (There is a reason for this difference between the responses of platelet and endothelial-cell cyclooxygenase to drugs. Platelets, once formed and released from megakaryocytes, have lost their ability to synthesize proteins. Therefore, when their COX is irreversibly blocked, thromboxane A_2 synthesis is gone for that platelet's lifetime. In contrast, the endothelial cells produce new COX molecules to replace the ones blocked by the drug.) Aspirin appears to be effective at preventing heart attacks. In addition, the administration of aspirin following a heart attack significantly reduces the incidence of sudden death and a recurrent heart attack.

A variety of drugs that interfere with platelet function by mechanisms different from those of aspirin also have great promise in the treatment or prevention of heart attacks. In particular, certain drugs block the binding of fibrinogen to platelets and thus interfere with platelet aggregation.

Drugs known collectively as ***oral anticoagulants*** interfere with clotting factors. One type interferes with the action of vitamin K, which in turn reduces the synthesis of clotting factors by the liver. Another type recently developed includes drugs that specifically inactivate factor Xa. Heparin, the naturally occurring endothelial-cell cofactor for antithrombin III, can also be administered as a drug, which then binds to endothelial cells and inhibits clotting.

TABLE 12.15 Anticlotting Roles of Endothelial Cells

Action	Result
Normally provide an intact barrier between the blood and subendothelial connective tissue	Platelet aggregation and the formation of tissue factor–factor VIIa complexes are not triggered.
Synthesize and release PGI_2 and nitric oxide	These inhibit platelet activation and aggregation.
Secrete tissue factor pathway inhibitor	This inhibits the ability of tissue factor–factor VIIa complexes to generate factor Xa.
Bind thrombin (via thrombomodulin), which then activates protein C	Active protein C inactivates clotting factors VIIIa and Va.
Display heparin molecules on the surfaces of their plasma membranes	Heparin binds antithrombin III, and this molecule then inactivates thrombin and several other clotting factors.
Secrete tissue plasminogen activator	Tissue plasminogen activator catalyzes the formation of plasmin, which dissolves clots.

In contrast to aspirin, the fibrinogen blockers, the oral anticoagulants, and heparin, all of which prevent clotting, the fifth type of drug—plasminogen activators—dissolves a clot after it is formed. The use of such drugs is termed ***thrombolytic therapy***. Intravenous administration of ***recombinant t-PA*** within a few hours after myocardial infarction significantly reduces myocardial damage and mortality. Recombinant t-PA has also been effective in reducing brain damage following a stroke caused by blood vessel occlusion. In addition, exciting new clinical studies suggest that a plasminogen activator found in vampire bat saliva may be even more effective than t-PA at protecting the brain after an ischemic stroke. Its name includes the genus and species of the animal—***Desmodus rotundus salivary plasminogen activator*** (*DSPA*).

SECTION F SUMMARY

Plasma

I. Plasma is the liquid component of blood; it contains proteins (albumins, globulins, and fibrinogen), nutrients, metabolic end products, hormones, and inorganic electrolytes.

II. Plasma proteins, synthesized by the liver, play many roles within the bloodstream, such as exerting osmotic pressure for absorption of interstitial fluid and participating in the clotting reaction.

The Blood Cells

I. The blood cells, which are suspended in plasma, include erythrocytes, leukocytes, and platelets.

II. Erythrocytes, which make up more than 99% of blood cells, contain hemoglobin, an oxygen-binding protein. Oxygen binds to the iron in hemoglobin.
   a. Erythrocytes are produced in the bone marrow and destroyed in the spleen and liver.
   b. Iron, folic acid, and vitamin B_{12} are essential for erythrocyte formation.
   c. The hormone erythropoietin, which is produced by the kidneys in response to low oxygen supply, stimulates erythrocyte differentiation and production by the bone marrow.

III. The leukocytes include neutrophils, eosinophils, basophils, monocytes, and lymphocytes.

IV. Platelets are cell fragments essential for blood clotting.

V. Blood cells are descended from stem cells in the bone marrow. Hematopoietic growth factors control their production.

Hemostasis: The Prevention of Blood Loss

I. The initial response to blood vessel damage is vasoconstriction and the sticking together of the opposed endothelial surfaces.

II. The next events are formation of a platelet plug followed by blood coagulation (clotting).

III. Platelets adhere to exposed collagen in a damaged vessel and release the contents of their secretory vesicles.
   a. These substances help cause platelet activation and aggregation.
   b. This process is also enhanced by von Willebrand factor, secreted by the endothelial cells, and by thromboxane A_2, produced by the platelets.
   c. Fibrin forms the bridges between aggregating platelets.
   d. Contractile elements in the platelets compress and strengthen the plug.

IV. The platelet plug does not spread along normal endothelium because the latter secretes prostacyclin and nitric oxide, both of which inhibit platelet aggregation.

V. Blood is transformed into a solid gel when, at the site of vessel damage, plasma fibrinogen is converted into fibrin molecules, which then bind to each other to form a mesh.

VI. This reaction is catalyzed by the enzyme thrombin, which also activates factor XIII, a plasma protein that stabilizes the fibrin meshwork.

VII. The formation of thrombin from the plasma protein prothrombin is the end result of a cascade of reactions in which an inactive plasma protein is activated and then enzymatically activates the next protein in the series.
   a. Thrombin exerts a positive feedback stimulation of the cascade by activating platelets and several clotting factors.
   b. Activated platelets, which display platelet factor and binding sites for several activated plasma factors, are essential for the cascade.

VIII. In the body, the cascade usually begins via the extrinsic clotting pathway when tissue factor forms a complex with factor VIIa. This complex activates factor X, which then catalyzes the conversion of small amounts of prothrombin to thrombin. This thrombin then recruits the intrinsic pathway by activating factor XI and factor VIII, as well as platelets, and this pathway generates large amounts of thrombin.

IX. The liver requires vitamin K for the normal production of prothrombin and other clotting factors.

X. Clotting is limited by three events:
   a. Tissue factor pathway inhibitor inhibits the tissue factor–factor VIIa complex.
   b. Protein C, activated by thrombin, inactivates factors VIIIa and Va.
   c. Antithrombin III inactivates thrombin and several other clotting factors.

XI. Clots are dissolved by the fibrinolytic system.
   a. A plasma proenzyme, plasminogen, is activated by plasminogen activators to plasmin, which digests fibrin.
   b. Tissue plasminogen activator is secreted by endothelial cells and is activated by fibrin in a clot.

SECTION F REVIEW QUESTIONS

1. Give average values for total blood volume, erythrocyte volume, plasma volume, and hematocrit.
2. What are the different classes of plasma proteins, and which are the most abundant?
3. Which solute is found in the highest concentration in plasma?
4. Summarize the production, life span, and destruction of erythrocytes.
5. What are the routes of iron gain, loss, and distribution? How is iron recycled when erythrocytes are destroyed?
6. Describe the control of erythropoietin secretion and the effect of this hormone.
7. State the relative proportions of erythrocytes and leukocytes in blood.
8. Diagram the derivation of the different blood cell types.
9. Describe the sequence of events leading to platelet activation and aggregation and the formation of a platelet plug. What helps keep this process localized?
10. Diagram the clotting pathway beginning with prothrombin.
11. What is the role of platelets in clotting?
12. List all the procoagulant effects of thrombin.
13. How is the clotting cascade initiated? How does the extrinsic pathway recruit the intrinsic pathway?

14. Describe the roles of the liver and vitamin K in clotting.
15. List three ways in which clotting is limited.
16. Diagram the fibrinolytic system.
17. How does fibrin help initiate the fibrinolytic system?
18. Which symptoms of pericarditis mimic a heart attack, and which symptoms differentiate the conditions? (See the Clinical Case Study.)

SECTION F KEY TERMS

SECTION F CLINICAL TERMS

CHAPTER 12

Clinical Case Study: Chest Pain in a 48-Year-Old Woman

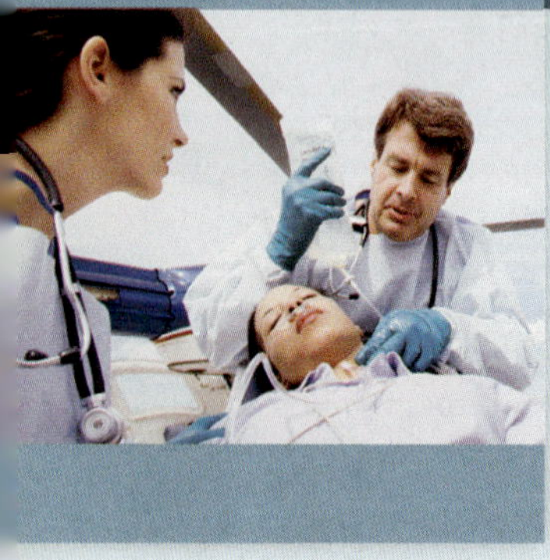

A 48-year-old woman arrived at the emergency room, complaining of chest pain. She reported being ill for about a week. At first, she just had a runny nose, cough, and sore throat. Over the past 4 days, she had developed pain in her chest and back that seemed worse with inspiration and when she was lying down. After getting into bed that evening, she had suddenly experienced sharp, stabbing pain in her chest and left shoulder, upon which she had called an ambulance.

Because the emergency room physician suspected the woman was experiencing a heart attack, an intravenous line was started, through which she was given nitroglycerin and heparin to prevent blood clot formation. Supplemental inspired oxygen was administered via a nasal tube while a history was taken and further tests were performed. Prior to this episode, she had been in good health; she reported no personal or family history of heart disease. Her heart rate was 105 beats/minute, blood pressure was 115/65 mmHg, and body temperature was 101°F (38.5°C) (normal = 98.6°F/37°C). Auscultation with a stethoscope detected rasping sounds associated with systole and diastole that obscured the normal heart sounds. A 12-lead electrocardiogram showed slight elevations of her ST segment in all of the leads except aVR and V1. A venous blood sample revealed normal hemoglobin and cardiac troponin concentrations, but the white blood cell count was mildly elevated. She was transferred to the cardiac catheterization lab for angiography, which showed minor atherosclerosis but no blocked coronary arteries. Her chest pain continued despite the nitroglycerin, and she also began to experience dizziness and a headache. When an additional measurement showed her blood pressure had decreased to 80/50 mmHg, the nitroglycerin and heparin were discontinued. What had seemed at first like a heart attack turned out to be a case of acute ***pericarditis.***

Pericarditis is an inflammation of the fibrous pericardial sac that surrounds the heart. It can be caused by viral, bacterial, or fungal infection and also by autoimmune conditions in which the body's own tissues come under immune attack (see Chapter 18). Normally, the pericardial space is extremely narrow and filled with a lubricating fluid that allows the heart to move within the thoracic cavity with a minimum of friction. In pericarditis, the membranes swell and roughen, and a large volume of fluid—either an

(continued)

(continued)

interstitial fluid exudate, blood, or pus—can build up inside the space. Friction between the roughened pericardial and epicardial membranes can produce grating or rasping sounds in concert with the heart's movements. These sounds are audible with a stethoscope and can be loud enough to make detection of the normal heart sounds difficult.

Some of the symptoms mimic those of a myocardial infarction (heart attack): chest, shoulder, or back pain; rapid heart rate; and changes in the appearance of the ST segment on an electrocardiogram. Because of the high potential for permanent cardiac damage or death from myocardial infarction, caretakers of patients with these symptoms often err on the side of immediately assuming a myocardial infarct is occurring. Nitroglycerin is given to dilate coronary arteries, and heparin or similar drugs may be given to inhibit blood clots that could occlude coronary arteries.

Information gradually emerged in this case, however, that suggested pericarditis as the correct diagnosis. Sharp chest pain that increases with inspiration (because pressure is placed on the heart when the lungs expand) and when lying down (because gravity presses the heart against the pericardial sac wall) are hallmark characteristics of pericarditis. Also, in myocardial infarction, there are changes in the ST segment only of those leads with vectors oriented through the ischemic areas; in pericarditis, ST segment changes are generally observed in most of the leads. The lack of coronary obstruction observed during angiography, combined with the failure of heparin and nitroglycerin to reduce the pain, also argued against cardiac ischemia and infarct in this case. (The decrease in this patient's blood pressure, dizziness, and headache were likely caused by a nitroglycerin-induced decrease in total peripheral resistance.) Finally, the blood concentration of cardiac troponin is generally increased beginning 8 hours after chest pain in a heart attack, but not in a patient with pericarditis.

Treatment of patients with pericarditis is directed toward pain management and addressing the cause of the inflammation. A nonsteroidal anti-inflammatory drug (see Chapter 5) or aspirin is generally prescribed; if the condition is secondary to autoimmune disease, corticosteroid treatment may also be administered (see Chapter 11). The early symptoms—elevated white blood cell count and fever in the present case—suggested the possibility of an infection, and a subsequent throat culture detected the presence of streptococcal bacteria. Therefore, in addition to pain medication, the woman was prescribed a course of antibiotics, after which she returned to good health.

Clinical term: pericarditis

See Chapter 19 for complete, integrative case studies.

CHAPTER 12 TEST QUESTIONS

Answers found in Appendix A.

1. Which of the following contains blood with the lowest oxygen content?
   a. aorta
   b. left atrium
   c. right ventricle
   d. pulmonary veins
   e. systemic arterioles
2. If other factors are equal, which of the following vessels would have the lowest resistance?
   a. length = 1 cm, radius = 1 cm
   b. length = 4 cm, radius = 1 cm
   c. length = 8 cm, radius = 1 cm
   d. length = 1 cm, radius = 2 cm
   e. length = 0.5 cm, radius = 2 cm
3. Which of the following correctly ranks pressures during isovolumetric contraction of a normal cardiac cycle?
   a. left ventricular > aortic > left atrial
   b. aortic > left atrial > left ventricular
   c. left atrial > aortic > left ventricular
   d. aortic > left ventricular > left atrial
   e. left ventricular > left atrial > aortic
4. Considered as a whole, the body's capillaries have
   a. smaller cross-sectional area than the arteries.
   b. less total blood flow than in the veins.
   c. greater total resistance than the arterioles.
   d. slower blood velocity than in the arteries.
   e. greater total blood flow than in the arteries.
5. Which of the following would *not* result in tissue edema?
   a. an increase in the concentration of plasma proteins
   b. an increase in the pore size of systemic capillaries
   c. an increase in venous pressure
   d. blockage of lymph vessels
   e. a decrease in the protein concentration of the plasma
6. Which statement comparing the systemic and pulmonary circuits is *true?*
   a. The blood flow is greater through the systemic.
   b. The blood flow is greater through the pulmonary.
   c. The absolute pressure is higher in the pulmonary.
   d. The blood flow is the same in both.
   e. The pressure gradient is the same in both.
7. What is mainly responsible for the delay between the atrial and ventricular contractions?
   a. the shallow slope of AV node pacemaker potentials
   b. slow action potential conduction velocity of AV node cells
   c. slow action potential conduction velocity along atrial muscle cell membranes
   d. slow action potential conduction in the Purkinje network of the ventricles
   e. greater parasympathetic nerve firing to the ventricles than to the atria
8. Which of the following pressures is closest to the mean arterial blood pressure in a person whose systolic blood pressure is 135 mmHg and pulse pressure is 50 mmHg?
   a. 110 mmHg c. 102 mmHg e. 85 mmHg
   b. 78 mmHg d. 152 mmHg

9. Which of the following would help restore homeostasis in the first few moments after a person's mean arterial pressure became elevated?
   a. a decrease in baroreceptor action potential frequency
   b. a decrease in action potential frequency along parasympathetic neurons to the heart
   c. an increase in action potential frequency along sympathetic neurons to the heart
   d. a decrease in action potential frequency along sympathetic neurons to arterioles
   e. an increase in total peripheral resistance
10. Which is *false* about L-type Ca^{2+} channels in cardiac ventricular muscle cells?
    a. They are open during the plateau of the action potential.
    b. They allow Ca^{2+} entry that triggers sarcoplasmic reticulum Ca^{2+} release.
    c. They are found in the T-tubule membrane.
    d. They open in response to depolarization of the membrane.
    e. They contribute to the pacemaker potential.
11. Which correctly pairs an ECG phase with the cardiac event responsible?
    a. P wave: Depolarization of the ventricles
    b. P wave: Depolarization of the AV node
    c. QRS wave: Depolarization of the ventricles
    d. QRS wave: Repolarization of the ventricles
    e. T wave: Repolarization of the atria
12. When a person engages in strenuous, prolonged exercise,
    a. blood flow to the kidneys is reduced.
    b. cardiac output is reduced.
    c. total peripheral resistance increases.
    d. systolic arterial blood pressure is reduced.
    e. blood flow to the brain is reduced.
13. Hematocrit is increased
    a. when a person has a vitamin B_{12} deficiency.
    b. by an increase in secretion of erythropoietin.
    c. when the number of white blood cells is increased.
    d. by a hemorrhage.
    e. in response to excess oxygen delivery to the kidneys.
14. The principal site of erythrocyte production is
    a. the liver.
    b. the kidneys.
    c. the bone marrow.
    d. the spleen.
    e. the lymph nodes.
15. Which is *not* part of the cascade leading to formation of a blood clot?
    a. contact between the blood and collagen found outside the blood vessels
    b. prothrombin converted to thrombin
    c. formation of a stabilized fibrin mesh
    d. activated platelets
    e. secretion of tissue plasminogen activator (t-PA) by endothelial cells

CHAPTER 12 GENERAL PRINCIPLES ASSESSMENT

Answers found in Appendix A.

1. A general principle of physiology states that *information flow between cells, tissues, and organs is an essential feature of homeostasis and allows for integration of physiological processes.* How is this principle demonstrated by the relationship between the circulatory and endocrine systems?
2. The left AV valve has only two large leaflets, while the right AV valve has three smaller leaflets. It is a general principle of physiology that *structure is a determinant of—and has coevolved with—function.* Although it is unknown why the two valves differ in structure in this way, what difference in the functional demands of the left side of the heart might explain why there is one less valve leaflet than on the right side?
3. Two of the body's important fluid compartments are those of the interstitial fluid and plasma. How does the liver's production of plasma proteins interact with those compartments to illustrate the general principle of physiology, *controlled exchange of materials occurs between compartments and across cellular membranes?*

CHAPTER 12 QUANTITATIVE AND THOUGHT QUESTIONS

Answers found at www.mhhe.com/widmaier13.

1. A person is found to have a hematocrit of 35%. Can you conclude that there is a decreased volume of erythrocytes in the blood? Explain.
2. Which would cause a greater increase in resistance to flow, a doubling of blood viscosity or a halving of tube radius?
3. If all plasma membrane Ca^{2+} channels in contractile cardiac muscle cells were blocked with a drug, what would happen to the muscle's action potentials and contraction?
4. A person with a heart rate of 40 has no P waves but normal QRS complexes on the ECG. What is the explanation?
5. A person has a left ventricular systolic pressure of 180 mmHg and an aortic systolic pressure of 110 mmHg. What is the explanation?
6. A person has a left atrial pressure of 20 mmHg and a left ventricular pressure of 5 mmHg during ventricular filling. What is the explanation?
7. A patient is taking a drug that blocks β-adrenergic receptors. What changes in cardiac function will the drug cause?
8. What is the mean arterial pressure in a person with a systolic pressure of 160 mmHg and a diastolic pressure of 100 mmHg?
9. A person is given a drug that doubles the blood flow to her kidneys but does not change the mean arterial pressure. What must the drug be doing?
10. A blood vessel removed from an experimental animal dilates when exposed to acetylcholine. After the endothelium is scraped from the lumen of the vessel, it no longer dilates in response to this mediator. Explain.
11. A person is accumulating edema throughout the body. Average capillary pressure is 25 mmHg, and lymphatic function is normal. What is the most likely cause of the edema?
12. A person's cardiac output is 7 L/min and mean arterial pressure is 140 mmHg. What is the person's total peripheral resistance?

13. The following data are obtained for an experimental animal before and after administration of a drug.

Before: Heart rate = 80 beats/min; Stroke volume = 80 mL/beat

After: Heart rate = 100 beats/min; Stroke volume = 64 mL/beat

Total peripheral resistance remains unchanged.

What has the drug done to mean arterial pressure?

14. When the nerves from all the arterial baroreceptors are cut in an experimental animal, what happens to mean arterial pressure?

15. What happens to the hematocrit within several hours after a hemorrhage?

16. If a woman's mean arterial pressure is 85 mmHg and her systolic pressure is 105 mmHg, what is her pulse pressure?

17. When a heart is transplanted into a patient, it is not possible to connect autonomic neurons from the medullary cardiovascular centers to the new heart. Will such a patient be able to increase cardiac output during exercise?

18. The P wave records the spread of depolarization of the atria on a lead I ECG as an upright wave form. Referring to the orientation of the ECG leads in Figure 12.15, what difference in the shape of the P wave might you expect when recording with lead aVR?

19. Given the following cardiac performance data,

Cardiac output (*CO*) = 5400 mL/min

Heart rate (*HR*) = 75 beats/min

End-systolic volume (*ESV*) = 60 mL

calculate the ejection fraction (*EF*).

20. Which is potentially more dangerous, a small blood clot that forms within a systemic vein, or the same thing occurring in a pulmonary vein?

CHAPTER 12 ANSWERS TO PHYSIOLOGICAL INQUIRIES

Figure 12.1 The hematocrit would be 33% because the red blood cell volume is the difference between total blood volume and plasma volume (4.5 − 3.0 = 1.5 L), and hematocrit is determined by the fraction of whole blood that is red blood cells (1.5 L/4.5 L = 0.33, or 33%).

Figure 12.3 The major change in blood flow would be an increase to certain abdominal organs, notably the stomach and small intestines. This change would provide the additional oxygen and nutrients required to meet the increased metabolic demands of digestion and absorption of the breakdown products of food. Blood flow to the brain and other organs would not be expected to change significantly, but there might be a small increase in blood flow to the skeletal muscles associated with chewing and swallowing. Consequently, the total blood flow in a resting person during and following a meal would be expected to increase.

Figure 12.5 No. The flow on side *B* would be doubled, but still less than that on side *A*. The summed wall area would be the same in both sides. The formula for circumference of a circle is $2\pi r$; so the wall circumference in side *A* would be $2 \times 3.14 \times 2 = 12.56$; for the two tubes on side *B*, it would be $(2 \times 3.14 \times 1) + (2 \times 3.14 \times 1) = 12.56$. However, the total cross section through which flow occurs would be larger in side *A* than in side *B*. The formula for cross-sectional area of a circle is πr^2, so the area of side *A* would be $3.14 \times 2^2 = 12.56$, whereas the summed area of the tubes in side *B* would be $(3.14 \times 1^2) + (3.14 \times 1^2) = 6.28$. Thus, even with two outflow tubes on side *B*, there would be more flow through side *A*

Figure 12.8 A: If this diagram included a systemic portal vessel, the order of structures in the lower box would be: aorta → arteries → arterioles → capillaries → venules → portal vessel → capillaries → venules → veins → vena cava. Examples of portal vessels include the hepatic portal vein, which carries blood from the intestines to the liver (Chapter 15), and the hypothalamo–pituitary portal vessels (Figure 11.13).

Figure 12.12 The rate of ion flux across a membrane depends on both the permeability of the membrane to the ion, and the electrochemical gradient for the ion (see Chapter 6, Section B). During the plateau of the cardiac action potential, the membrane potential is positive and closer to the Ca^{2+} equilibrium potential (which also has a positive value) than it is to the K^+ equilibrium potential (which has a negative value). Thus, Ca^{2+} has a high permeability and a low electrochemical driving force, while K^+ has a lower permeability but a higher electrochemical driving force. These factors offset each other, and the oppositely directed currents end up being nearly the same.

Figure 12.13 Purkinje cell action potentials have a depolarizing pacemaker potential, like node cells (though the slope is much more gradual), and a rapid upstroke and broad plateau, like cardiac muscle cells.

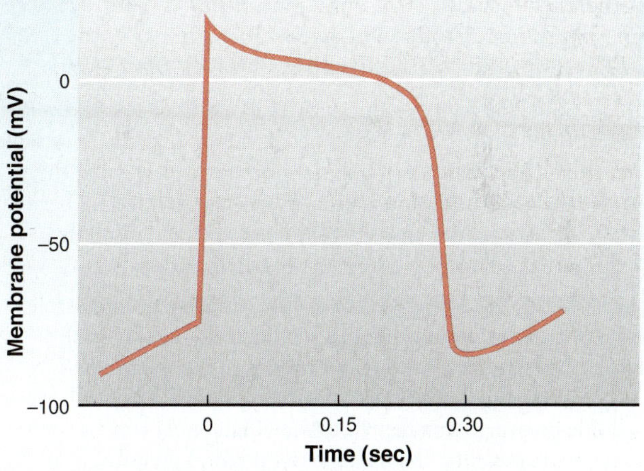

Figure 12.14 Reducing the L-type Ca^{2+} current in AV node cells would decrease the rate at which action potentials are conducted between the atria and ventricles. On the ECG tracing, this would be indicated by a longer interval between the P wave (atrial depolarization) and the QRS wave (ventricular depolarization).

Figure 12.16 A reduction in current through voltage-gated K^+ channels delays the repolarization of ventricular muscle cell action potentials. Thus, the T wave (ventricular repolarization) of the ECG wave is delayed relative to the QRS waves (ventricular depolarization). This fact gives the name to the condition "long QT syndrome."

Figure 12.20 Aortic blood would not have significantly lower-than-normal oxygen levels. Compare this figure with

Figure 12.19; the pressure in the left ventricle is higher than the right throughout the entire cardiac cycle. This pressure gradient would favor blood flow through the hole in the septum only from the left ventricle into the right. Thus, pulmonary artery blood would be higher in oxygen than normal (because blood in the left ventricle has just come from the lungs), but deoxygenated blood would not dilute the blood flowing into the aorta.

Figure 12.21 The patient most likely has a damaged semilunar valve that is stenotic and insufficient. A "whistling" murmur generally results from blood moving forward through a stenotic valve, whereas a lower-pitched "gurgling" murmur occurs when blood leaks backward through a valve that does not close properly. Systole and ejection occur between the two normal heart sounds, whereas diastole and filling occur after the second heart sound. Thus, a whistle between the heart sounds indicates a stenotic semilunar valve, and the gurgle following the second heart sound would arise from an insufficient semilunar valve. It is most likely that a single valve is both stenotic and insufficient in this case. Diagnosis could be confirmed by determining where on the chest wall the sounds were loudest and by diagnostic imaging techniques.

Figure 12.22 The delay between atrial and ventricular contractions is caused by slow propagation of the action potential through the AV node, which is a result of the relatively slow rate that the cells are depolarized by the L-type Ca^{2+} current. Parasympathetic stimulation slows AV node cell propagation further by reducing the current through L-type Ca^{2+} channels, which in turn increases the AV nodal delay.

Figure 12.25 Ejection fraction (EF) = Stroke volume (SV)/End-diastolic volume (EDV); End-systolic volume (ESV) = $EDV - SV$. Based on the graph, under control conditions, the SV is 75 mL and during sympathetic stimulation it is 110 mL. Thus: Control $ESV = 140 - 75 = 65$ mL, and $EF = 75/140 = 53.6\%$; Sympathetic $ESV = 140 - 110 = 30$ mL, and $EF = 110/140 = 78.6\%$.

Figure 12.27 Parasympathetic activity can influence stroke volume indirectly, via the effect on heart rate. If all other variables were held constant (in particular, venous return), slowing the heart rate would allow more time for the ventricles to fill between beats, and the greater end-diastolic volume would result in a larger stroke volume by the Frank–Starling mechanism.

Figure 12.31 At resting heart rate, the time spent in diastole is twice as long as that spent in systole (i.e., $\frac{1}{3}$ of the total cycle is spent near systolic pressures) and the mean pressure is approximately $\frac{1}{3}$ of the distance from diastolic pressure to systolic pressure. At a heart rate in which equal time is spent in systole and diastole, the mean arterial blood pressure would be approximately halfway between those two pressures.

Figure 12.33 If the only change from what is shown in (a) was dilation of tube 3, there would be a net decrease in the resistance to flow out of the pressure reservoir. If the rate of refilling the reservoir remains constant, then the height of fluid (hydrostatic pressure) in the reservoir would decrease to a new steady-state level. Compared to what (b) currently shows, tubes 1, 3, 4, and 5 would all have less flow because their resistance is the same but the pressure gradient would be less, whereas tube 2 would have greater flow because its diameter remained large and its resistance low. An analogous experiment is shown in Figure 12.49.

Figure 12.34 When the arterial pressure is increased, the blood flow through the arteriole will initially increase because the ΔP is higher but the resistance is unchanged (or the resistance might even be lower if the increased pressure stretches it). Within the next few minutes, however, the local oxygen concentration will increase and local metabolite concentrations will decrease, inducing vasoconstriction of the arteriole. This increases resistance, and blood flow will thus decrease toward the level it was prior to the increase in arterial pressure.

Figure 12.40 Venous blood leaving that tissue would be lower in oxygen and nutrients (like glucose) and higher in metabolic wastes (like carbon dioxide).

Figure 12.42 Injecting a liter of crystalloid to replace the lost blood would initially restore the volume (and, therefore, the capillary hydrostatic pressure), but it would dilute the plasma proteins remaining in the bloodstream. As a result, the main force opposing capillary filtration (π_c) would be reduced, causing an increase in net filtration of fluid from the capillaries into the interstitial fluid space. A plasma injection, however, restores the plasma volume as well as the plasma proteins. Thus, the Starling forces remain in balance, and more of the injected volume remains within the vasculature.

Figure 12.46 The increase in sympathetic activity and pumping of the skeletal and inspiratory muscles during vigorous exercise would increase the flow of blood out of the systemic veins and back to the heart, so the percentage of the total blood contained in the veins would decrease compared to the resting levels. At the same time, increased metabolic activity of the skeletal muscles would cause arteriolar dilation and increased blood flow (see Figure 12.34a), so the percentage of total blood in systemic arterioles and capillaries would be greater than at rest.

Figure 12.47 Ingestion of fluids supports the net filtration of fluid at capillaries by transiently elevating vascular pressure (and, therefore, P_c) and reducing the concentration of plasma proteins (and, therefore, π_c). Although reflex mechanisms described in the next section and in Chapter 14 minimize and eventually reverse changes in blood pressure and plasma osmolarity, you could expect a transient increase in interstitial fluid formation and lymph flow after ingesting extra fluids.

Table 12.6 The relative total resistance of the two circuits can be calculated using the equation, $MAP = CO \times TPR$. Rearranging, $TPR = MAP/CO$. Thus, for the systemic circuit, the total resistance $= 93/5 = 18.6$, while for the pulmonary circuit, $R = 15/5 = 3$. Relative to the total pulmonary resistance, then, the systemic resistance is $18.6/3 = 6.2$ times greater.

Figure 12.53 There is a transient reduction in pressure at the baroreceptors when you first stand up. This occurs because gravity has a significant impact on blood flow. While lying down, the effect of gravity is minimal because baroreceptors and the rest of the vasculature are basically level with the heart. Upon standing, gravity resists the return of blood from below the heart (where the majority of the vascular volume exists). This transiently reduces cardiac output and, thus, blood pressure. Section E of this chapter provides a detailed description of this phenomenon and explains how the body compensates for the effects of gravity.

Figure 12.54 Because the normal resting value is in the center of the steepest part of the curve, baroreceptor action potential frequency is maximally sensitive to small changes in mean arterial pressure in either direction, and that sensitivity can be maintained with minor upward or downward changes in the homeostatic set point.

Table 12.7 The hematocrit is the fraction of the total blood volume that is made up of erythrocytes. Thus, the normal hematocrit in this case was $2300/5000 \times 100 = 46\%$.

Immediately after the hemorrhage, it was 1840/4000 × 100 = 46%; 18 h later, it was 1840/4900 × 100 = 37%. The hemorrhage itself did not change hematocrit because erythrocytes and plasma were lost in equal proportions. However, over the next 18 h, there was a net shift of interstitial fluid into the blood plasma due to a reduction in P_c. Because this occurs faster than does the production of new red blood cells, this "autotransfusion" resulted in a dilution of the remaining erythrocytes in the bloodstream. In the days and weeks that follow, increased erythropoietin will stimulate the replacement of the lost erythrocytes, and the lost ECF volume will be replaced by ingestion and decreased urine output.

Figure 12.61 Exercising in extreme heat can result in fainting due to an inability to maintain sufficient blood flow to the brain. This occurs because maintaining homeostasis of body temperature places demands on the cardiovascular system beyond those of exercising muscles alone. Sweat glands secrete fluid from the plasma onto the skin surface to facilitate evaporative cooling, and arterioles to the skin dilate, directing blood toward the surface for radiant cooling. With reduced blood volume and large amounts of blood flowing to the skeletal muscles and skin, cardiac output may not be sufficient to maintain flow to the brain and other tissues at adequate levels.

Figure 12.65 The normal end-diastolic volume is 135 mL, and the graph shows that the stroke volume is approximately 40 mL at this volume for the failing heart. The ejection fraction would thus be approximately 40/135 = 29.6%. This is significantly lower than the normal heart (70/135 = 51.8%).

Figure 12.76 Blood clotting would be inhibited significantly more without factor VII. Normal activation of blood clotting begins with activation of factor VII, which not only initiates the extrinsic pathway but also sequentially activates the intrinsic pathway when thrombin activates factors XI, VIII, and V. This sequence would not be disrupted by the absence of factor XII. Conversely, in the absence of factor VII, the extrinsic pathway cannot be activated at all.

Figure 12.77 As described in Chapter 15, production by gut bacteria can be a significant source of vitamin K when dietary intake is low. Antibiotic treatment kills not only harmful bacteria but also the beneficial gut bacteria that produce vitamin K. It is thus possible for a prolonged course of antibiotics to cause vitamin K deficiency and thus a deficiency of clotting factor synthesis.

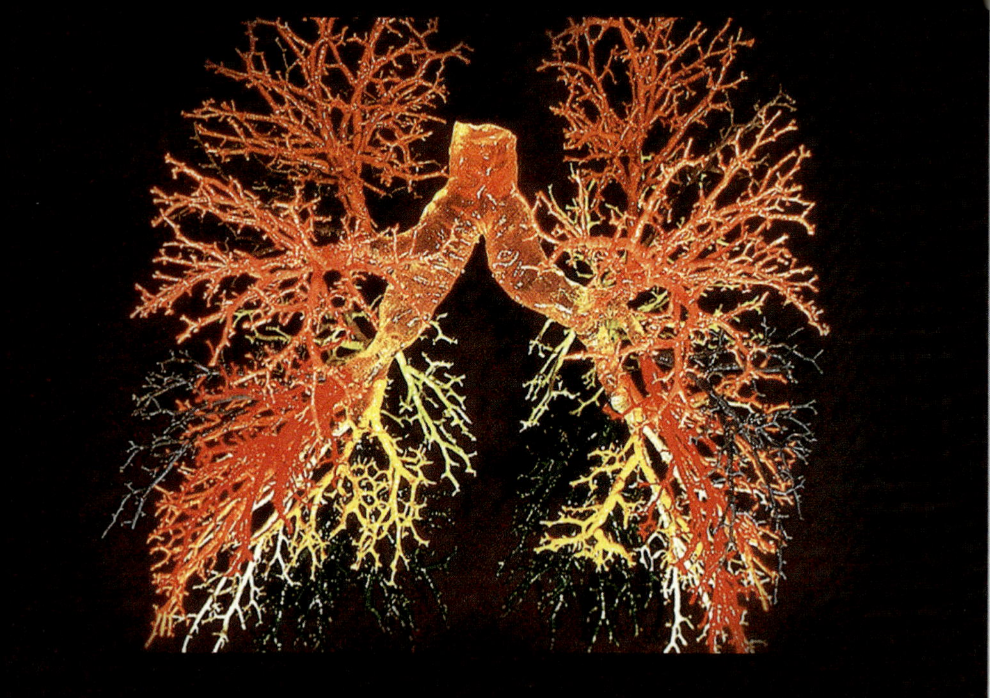

Resin cast of the pulmonary arteries and bronchi.

13 Respiratory Physiology

In the previous chapter, you learned that the major role of the cardiovascular system is to deliver nutrients and oxygen to the tissues and to remove carbon dioxide and other waste products of metabolism. In this chapter, you will learn how the respiratory system is intimately associated with the cardiovascular system and is responsible for taking up oxygen from the environment and delivering it to the blood, as well as eliminating carbon dioxide from the blood.

Respiration can have two quite different meanings: (1) utilization of oxygen in the metabolism of organic molecules by cells, often termed *internal* or *cellular respiration*, as described in Chapter 3; and (2) the exchange of oxygen and carbon dioxide between an organism and the external environment, often called *pulmonary physiology*. The adjective pulmonary refers to the lungs. The second meaning is the subject of this chapter. Human cells obtain most of their energy from chemical reactions involving oxygen. In addition, cells must be able to eliminate carbon dioxide, the major end product of oxidative metabolism. A unicellular organism can exchange oxygen and carbon dioxide directly with the external environment, but this is obviously impossible for most cells of a complex organism like a human being. Therefore, the evolution of large animals required the development of specialized structures for the entire animal to exchange oxygen and carbon dioxide with the external environment. In humans and other mammals, the **respiratory system** includes the oral and nasal cavities, the lungs, the series of tubes leading to the lungs, and the chest structures responsible for moving air into and out of the lungs during breathing.

As you read about the structure, function, and control of the respiratory system, you will encounter numerous examples of the general principles of physiology that were outlined in Chapter 1. The principle that physiological processes are governed by the laws of chemistry and physics is demonstrated when describing the binding of oxygen and carbon dioxide to hemoglobin, the handling by the blood of acid produced by metabolism, and the factors that control the inflation and deflation of the lungs. The diffusion of gases is an excellent example of the general principle of physiology that states that controlled exchange of materials occurs between compartments and across cellular membranes. You will learn how the functional units of the lung, the alveoli, are elegant examples of the general principle of physiology that structure is a determinant of—and has coevolved with—function. Finally, the central nervous system control of respiration is yet another example of how homeostasis is essential for health and survival.

13.1 Organization of the Respiratory System

There are two lungs, the right and left, each divided into lobes. The lungs consist mainly of tiny air-containing sacs called **alveoli** (singular, **alveolus**), which number approximately 300 million in an adult. The alveoli are the sites of gas exchange with the blood. The **airways** are the tubes that air flows through from the external environment to the alveoli and back.

Inspiration (inhalation) is the movement of air from the external environment through the airways into the alveoli during breathing. **Expiration** (exhalation) is movement in the opposite direction. An inspiration and expiration constitute a **respiratory cycle.** During the entire respiratory cycle, the right ventricle of the heart pumps blood through the pulmonary arteries and arterioles and into the capillaries surrounding each alveolus. In a healthy adult at rest, approximately 4 L of fresh air enters and leaves the alveoli per minute, while 5 L of blood, the cardiac output, flows through the pulmonary capillaries. During heavy exercise, the airflow can increase 20-fold, and the blood flow five- to sixfold.

The Airways and Blood Vessels

During inspiration, air passes through the nose or the mouth (or both) into the **pharynx,** a passage common to both air and food (**Figure 13.1**). The pharynx branches into two tubes: the esophagus, through which food passes to the stomach, and the **larynx,** which is part of the airways. The larynx houses the **vocal cords,** two folds of elastic tissue stretched horizontally across its lumen. The flow of air past the vocal cords causes them to vibrate, producing sounds. The nose, mouth, pharynx, and larynx are collectively termed the **upper airways.**

The larynx opens into a long tube, the **trachea,** which in turn branches into two **bronchi** (singular, **bronchus**),

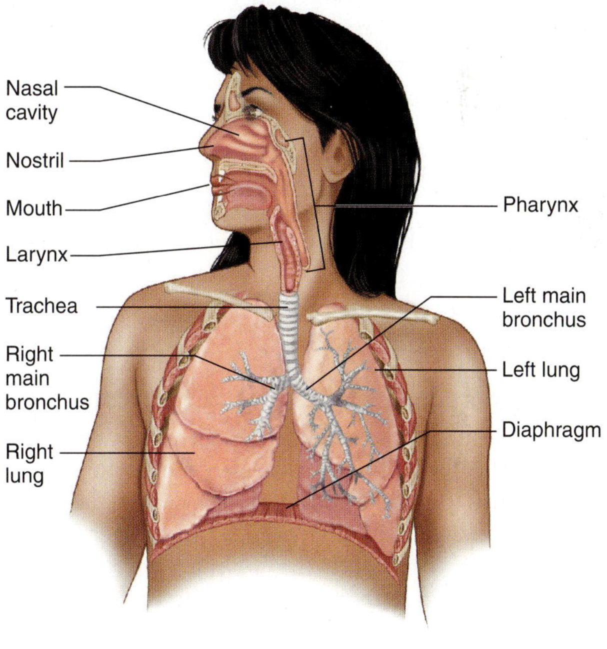

Figure 13.1 APIR Organization of the respiratory system. The ribs have been removed in front, and the lungs are shown in a way that makes visible the major airways within them. *Not shown:* The pharynx continues posteriorly to the esophagus.

one of which enters each lung. Within the lungs, there are more than 20 generations of branchings, each resulting in narrower, shorter, and more numerous tubes; their names are summarized in **Figure 13.2.** The walls of the trachea and bronchi contain rings of cartilage, which give them their cylindrical shape and support them. The first airway branches that no longer contain cartilage are termed **bronchioles,** which branch into the smaller, **terminal bronchioles.** Alveoli first begin to appear attached to the walls of the **respiratory bronchioles.** The number of alveoli increases in the alveolar ducts (see Figure 13.2), and the

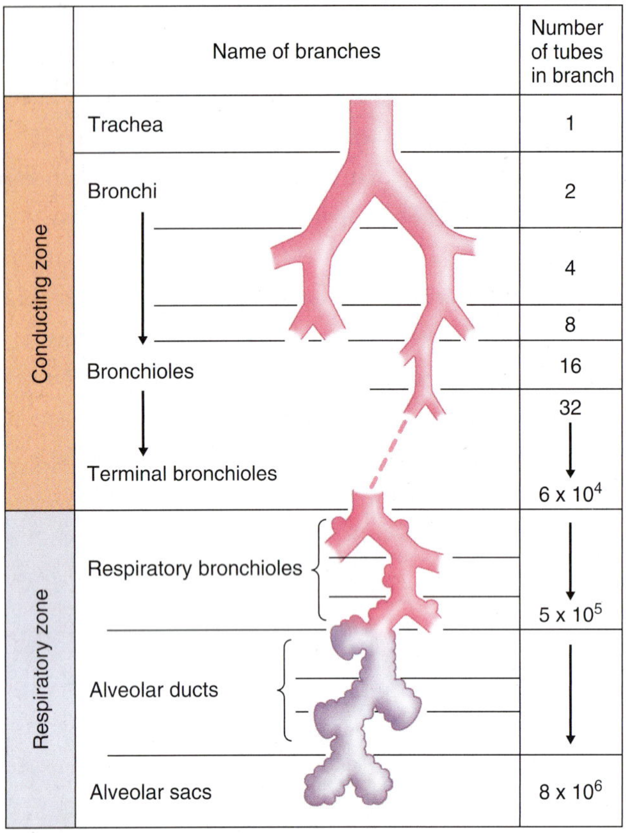

Figure 13.2 APIR Airway branching. Asymmetries in branching patterns between the right and left bronchial trees are not depicted. The diameters of the airways and alveoli are not drawn to scale.

airways then end in grapelike clusters called **alveolar sacs** that consist entirely of alveoli (**Figure 13.3**). The bronchioles are surrounded by smooth muscle, which contracts or relaxes to alter bronchiolar radius, in much the same way that the radius of small blood vessels (arterioles) is controlled, as you learned in Chapter 12.

The airways beyond the larynx can be divided into two zones. The **conducting zone** extends from the top of the trachea to the beginning of the respiratory bronchioles. This zone contains no alveoli and does not exchange gases with the blood. The **respiratory zone** extends from the respiratory bronchioles down. This zone contains alveoli and is the region where gases exchange with the blood.

The oral and nasal cavities trap airborne particles in nasal hairs and mucus. The epithelial surfaces of the airways, to the end of the respiratory bronchioles, contain cilia that constantly beat upward toward the pharynx. They also contain glands and individual epithelial cells that secrete mucus, and macrophages which can phagocytize inhaled pathogens. Particulate matter, such as dust contained in the inspired air, sticks to the mucus, which is continuously and slowly moved by the cilia to the pharynx and then swallowed. This so-called mucous escalator is important in keeping the lungs clear of particulate matter and the many bacteria that enter the body on dust particles. Ciliary activity and number can be decreased by many noxious agents, including the smoke from chronic cigarette smoking. This is why smokers often cough up mucus that the cilia would normally have cleared.

The airway epithelium also secretes a watery fluid upon which the mucus can ride freely. The production of this fluid is impaired in the disease ***cystic fibrosis*** (***CF***), the most common lethal genetic disease among Caucasians, in which the mucous layer becomes thick and dehydrated, obstructing the airways. CF is caused by an autosomal recessive mutation in an epithelial chloride channel called the **CF transmembrane conductance regulator** (**CFTR**) protein. This results in problems with salt and water movement across cell membranes, which leads to thickened secretions and a high incidence of lung infection. It is usually treated with (1) therapy to improve clearance of mucus from the lung and (2) the aggressive use of antibiotics to prevent pneumonia. Although the treatment of CF has improved over the past few decades, median life expectancy is still only about 35 years. Ultimately, lung transplantation may be required. In addition to the lungs, other organs are usually affected—particularly in the secretory components of the gastrointestinal tract (for example, the exocrine pancreas).

Constriction of bronchioles in response to irritation helps to prevent particulate matter and irritants from entering the sites of gas exchange. Another protective mechanism against infection is provided by cells called macrophages that are present in the airways and alveoli. These cells engulf and destroy inhaled particles and bacteria that have reached the alveoli. Macrophages, like the ciliated epithelium of the airways, are injured by cigarette smoke and air pollutants. The physiology of the conducting zone is summarized in **Table 13.1**.

The pulmonary blood vessels generally accompany the airways and also undergo numerous branchings. The smallest of these vessels branch into networks of capillaries that richly supply the alveoli (see Figure 13.3). As you learned in Chapter 12, the pulmonary circulation has a very low resistance to the flow of blood compared to the systemic circulation, and for this reason the pressures within all pulmonary blood vessels are low. This is an important adaptation that minimizes accumulation of fluid in the interstitial spaces of the lungs (see Figure 12.42 for a description of Starling forces and the movement of fluid across capillaries).

Site of Gas Exchange: The Alveoli

The alveoli are tiny, hollow sacs whose open ends are continuous with the lumens of the airways (**Figure 13.4a**). Typically, a single alveolar wall separates the air in two adjacent alveoli. Most of the air-facing surfaces of the wall are lined by a continuous layer, one cell thick, of flat epithelial cells termed **type I alveolar cells.** Interspersed between these cells are thicker, specialized cells termed **type II alveolar cells** (**Figure 13.4b**) that produce a detergent-like substance called surfactant.

The alveolar walls contain capillaries and a very small interstitial space, which consists of interstitial fluid and a loose meshwork of connective tissue (see Figure 13.4b). In many places, the interstitial space is absent altogether, and the basement membranes of the alveolar-surface epithelium and

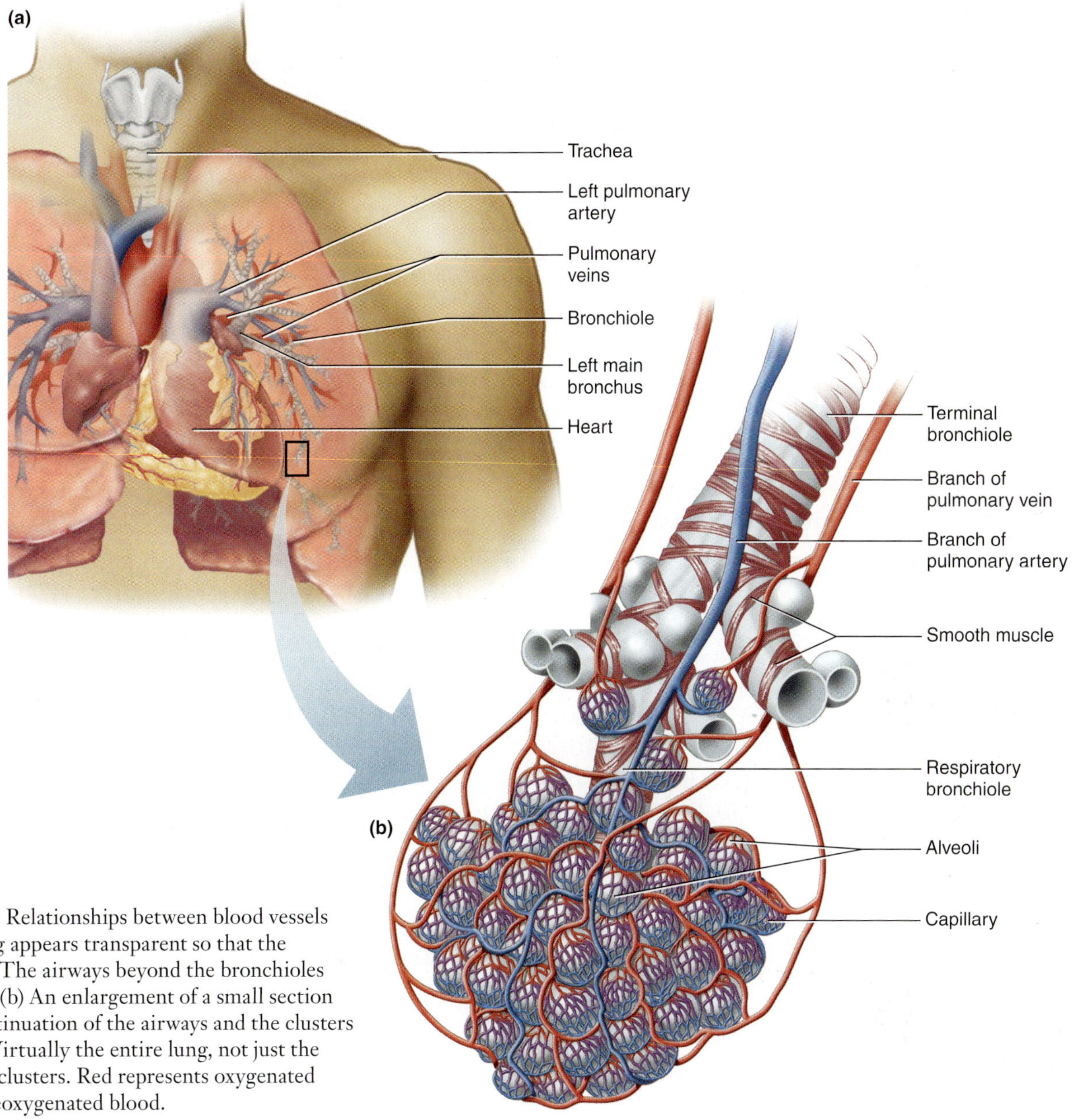

Figure 13.3 AP|R Relationships between blood vessels and airways. (a) The lung appears transparent so that the relationships are visible. The airways beyond the bronchioles are too small to be seen. (b) An enlargement of a small section of part (a) shows the continuation of the airways and the clusters of alveoli at their ends. Virtually the entire lung, not just the surface, consists of such clusters. Red represents oxygenated blood; blue represents deoxygenated blood.

the capillary-wall endothelium fuse. Thus, the blood within an alveolar-wall capillary is separated from the air within the alveolus by an extremely thin barrier (0.2 μm, compared with the 7 μm diameter of an average red blood cell). The total surface area of alveoli in contact with capillaries is roughly the size of a tennis court. This extensive area and the thinness of the barrier permit the rapid exchange of large quantities of oxygen and carbon dioxide by diffusion. These are excellent examples of two of the general principles of physiology—that physiological processes require the transfer and balance of matter (in this case, oxygen and carbon dioxide) and energy between compartments, and that structure (in this case, the thinness of the diffusion barrier and the enormous surface area for gas exchange) is a determinant of—and has coevolved with—function (the transfer of oxygen and carbon dioxide between the alveolar air and the blood in the pulmonary capillaries).

In some of the alveolar walls, pores permit the flow of air between alveoli. This route can be very important when the airway leading to an alveolus is occluded by disease, because some air can still enter the alveolus by way of the pores between it and adjacent alveoli.

TABLE 13.1	Functions of the Conducting Zone of the Airways
Provides a low-resistance pathway for airflow. Resistance is physiologically regulated by changes in contraction of bronchiolar smooth muscle and by physical forces acting upon the airways.	
Defends against microbes, toxic chemicals, and other foreign matter. Cilia, mucus, and macrophages perform this function.	
Warms and moistens the air.	
Phonates (vocal cords).	

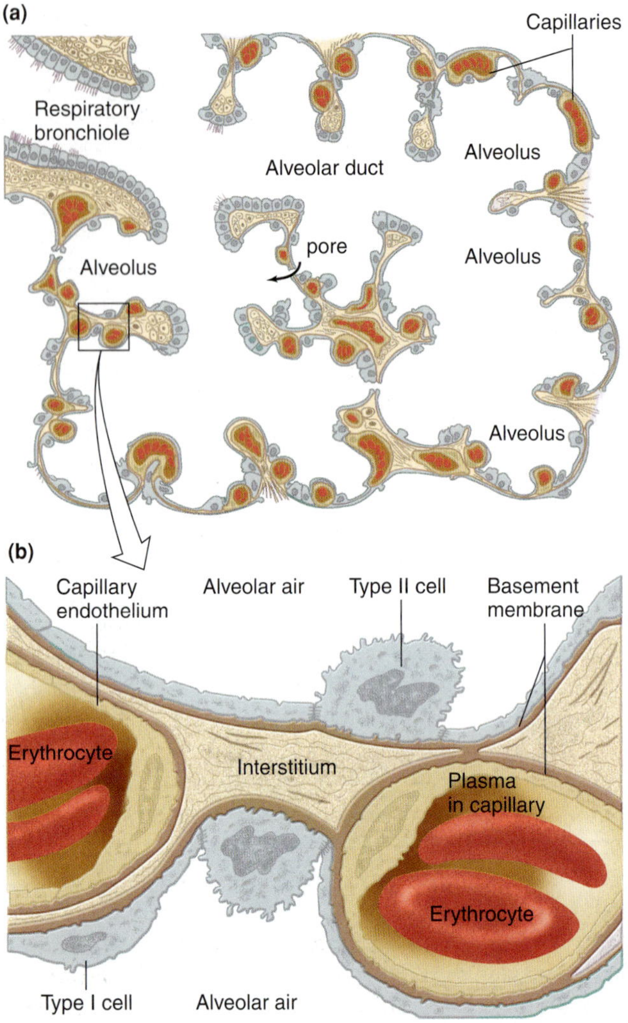

Figure 13.4 APR (a) Cross section through an area of the respiratory zone. There are 18 alveoli in this figure, only four of which are labeled. Two often share a common wall. (b) Schematic enlargement of a portion of an alveolar wall. (a) From R. O. Greep and L. Weiss, *Histology*, 3rd ed., McGraw-Hill, New York. (b) Adapted from Gong and Drage.

PHYSIOLOGICAL INQUIRY

- What consequences would result if inflammation caused a buildup of fluid in the alveoli and interstitial spaces?

Answer can be found at end of chapter.

Relation of the Lungs to the Thoracic (Chest) Wall

The lungs, like the heart, are situated in the **thorax,** the compartment of the body between the neck and abdomen. *Thorax* and *chest* are synonyms. The thorax is a closed compartment bounded at the neck by muscles and connective tissue and completely separated from the abdomen by a large, dome-shaped sheet of skeletal muscle called the **diaphragm** (see Figure 13.1). The wall of the thorax is formed by the spinal column, the ribs, the breastbone (sternum), and several groups of muscles that run between the ribs that are collectively called the **intercostal muscles.** The thoracic wall also contains large amounts of connective tissue with elastic properties.

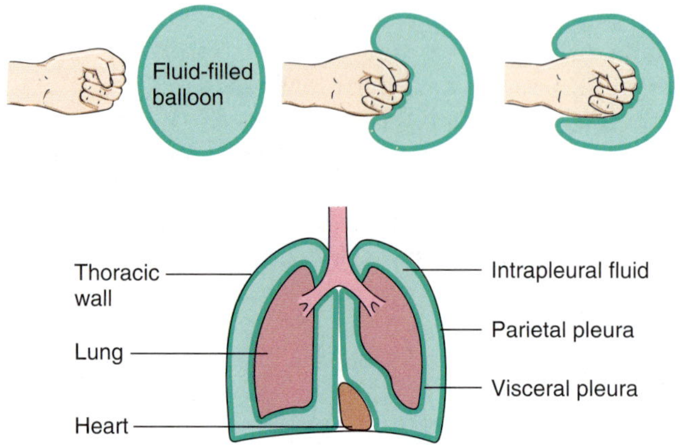

Figure 13.5 APR Relationship of lungs, pleura, and thoracic wall, shown as analogous to pushing a fist into a fluid-filled balloon. Note that there is no communication between the right and left intrapleural fluids. For purposes of illustration, the volume of intrapleural fluid is greatly exaggerated. It normally consists of an extremely thin layer of fluid between the pleural membrane lining the inner surface of the thoracic wall (the parietal pleura) and the membrane lining the outer surface of the lungs (the visceral pleura).

Each lung is surrounded by a completely closed sac, the **pleural sac,** consisting of a thin sheet of cells called **pleura.** The pleural sac of one lung is separate from that of the other lung. The relationship between a lung and its pleural sac can be visualized by imagining what happens when you push a fist into a fluid-filled balloon. The arm shown in Figure 13.5 represents the major bronchus leading to the lung, the fist is the lung, and the balloon is the pleural sac. The fist becomes coated by one surface of the balloon. In addition, the balloon is pushed back upon itself so that its opposite surfaces lie close together but are separated by a thin layer of fluid. Unlike the hand and balloon, the pleural surface coating the lung known as the **visceral pleura** is firmly attached to the lung by connective tissue. Similarly, the outer layer, called the **parietal pleura,** is attached to and lines the interior thoracic wall and diaphragm. The two layers of pleura in each sac are very close but not attached to each other. Rather, they are separated by an extremely thin layer of **intrapleural fluid,** the total volume of which is only a few milliliters. The intrapleural fluid totally surrounds the lungs and lubricates the pleural surfaces so that they can slide over each other during breathing. As we will see in the next section, changes in the hydrostatic pressure of the intrapleural fluid—the **intrapleural pressure** (P_{ip})—cause the lungs and thoracic wall to move in and out together during normal breathing.

A way to visualize the apposition of the two pleural surfaces is to put a drop of water between two glass microscope slides. The two slides can easily slide over each other but are very difficult to pull apart.

13.2 Ventilation and Lung Mechanics

This section highlights that physiological processes are dictated by the laws of chemistry and physics, one of the general principles of physiology described in Chapter 1.

Understanding the forces that control the inflation and deflation of the lung and the flow of air between the lung and the environment requires some knowledge of several fundamental physical laws. Furthermore, understanding of these forces is necessary to appreciate several pathophysiological events, such as the collapse of a lung due to an air leak into the chest cavity. We begin with an overview of these physical processes and the steps involved in respiration (**Figure 13.6**) before examining each step in detail.

Ventilation is defined as the exchange of air between the atmosphere and alveoli. Like blood, air moves by *bulk flow* from a region of high pressure to one of low pressure. Bulk flow can be described by the equation

$$F = \Delta P/R \quad (13\text{–}1)$$

Stated differently, flow (F) is proportional to the pressure difference (ΔP) between two points and inversely proportional to the resistance (R). (Notice that this equation is the same one used to describe the movement of blood through blood vessels, described in Chapter 12.) For airflow into or out of the lungs, the relevant pressures are the gas pressure in the alveoli—the **alveolar pressure (P_{alv})**—and the gas pressure at the nose and mouth, normally **atmospheric pressure (P_{atm})**, which is the pressure of the air surrounding the body:

$$F = (P_{alv} - P_{atm})/R \quad (13\text{–}2)$$

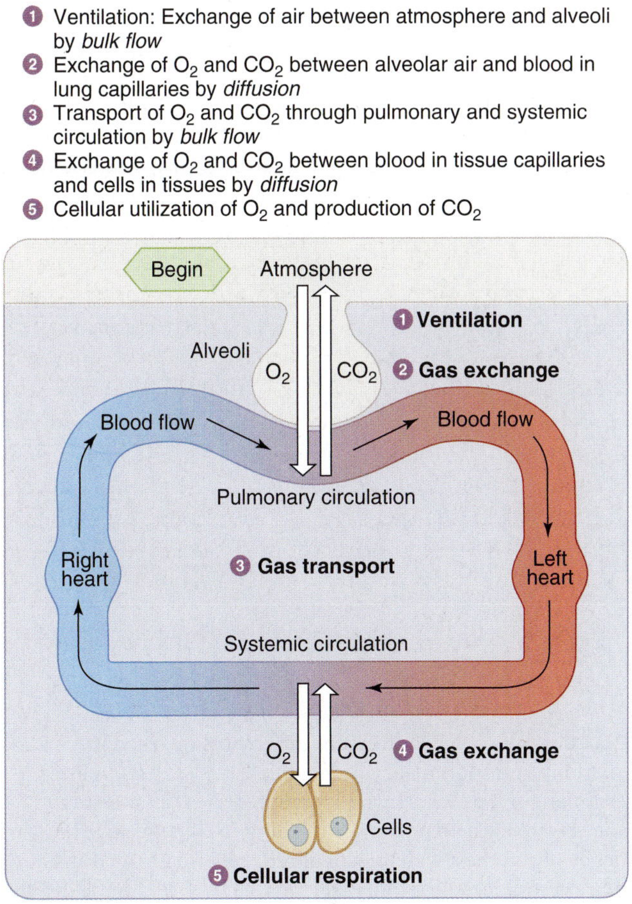

Figure 13.6 The steps of respiration.

A very important point must be made here: All pressures in the respiratory system, as in the cardiovascular system, are given *relative to atmospheric pressure*, which is 760 mmHg at sea level but which decreases in proportion to an increase in altitude. For example, the alveolar pressure between breaths is said to be 0 mmHg, which means that it is the same as atmospheric pressure at any given altitude. From equation 13–2, when there is no airflow, $F = 0$; therefore, $P_{alv} - P_{atm} = 0$, and $P_{alv} = P_{atm}$.

During ventilation, air moves into and out of the lungs because the alveolar pressure is alternately less than and greater than atmospheric pressure (**Figure 13.7**). In accordance with equation 13.2 describing airflow, a negative value reflects an inward-directed pressure gradient and a positive value indicates an outward-directed gradient. Thus, when P_{alv} is less than P_{atm}, $P_{alv} - P_{atm}$ is negative and airflow is inward (inspiration). When P_{alv} is greater than P_{atm}, $P_{alv} - P_{atm}$ is positive and airflow is outward (expiration). These alveolar pressure changes are caused, as we will see, by changes in the dimensions of the chest wall and lungs.

To understand how a change in lung dimensions causes a change in alveolar pressure, you need to learn one more basic physical principle described by **Boyle's law,** which is represented by the equation $P_1V_1 = P_2V_2$ (**Figure 13.8**). At constant temperature, the relationship between the pressure (P) exerted by a fixed number of gas molecules and the volume (V) of their container is as follows: An increase in the volume of the container decreases the pressure of the gas, whereas a decrease in the container volume increases the pressure. In other words, in a closed system, the pressure of a gas and the volume of its container are inversely proportional.

It is essential to recognize the correct sequence of events that determine the inspiration and then expiration of a breath. During inspiration and expiration, the volume of the "container"—the lungs—is made to change, and these changes then cause, by Boyle's law, the alveolar pressure changes that drive airflow into or out of the lungs. Our descriptions of ventilation must focus, therefore, on how the changes in lung dimensions are brought about.

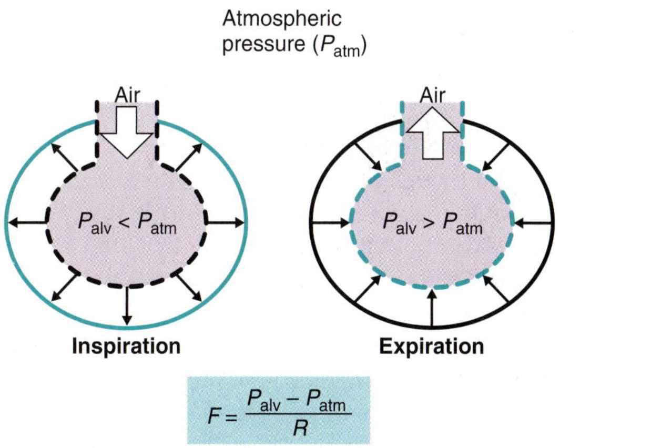

Figure 13.7 APIR Relationships required for ventilation. When the alveolar pressure (P_{alv}) is less than atmospheric pressure (P_{atm}), air enters the lungs. Flow (F) is directly proportional to the pressure difference ($P_{alv} - P_{atm}$) and inversely proportional to airway resistance (R). Black lines show lung's position at beginning of inspiration or expiration, and blue lines show position at end of inspiration or expiration.

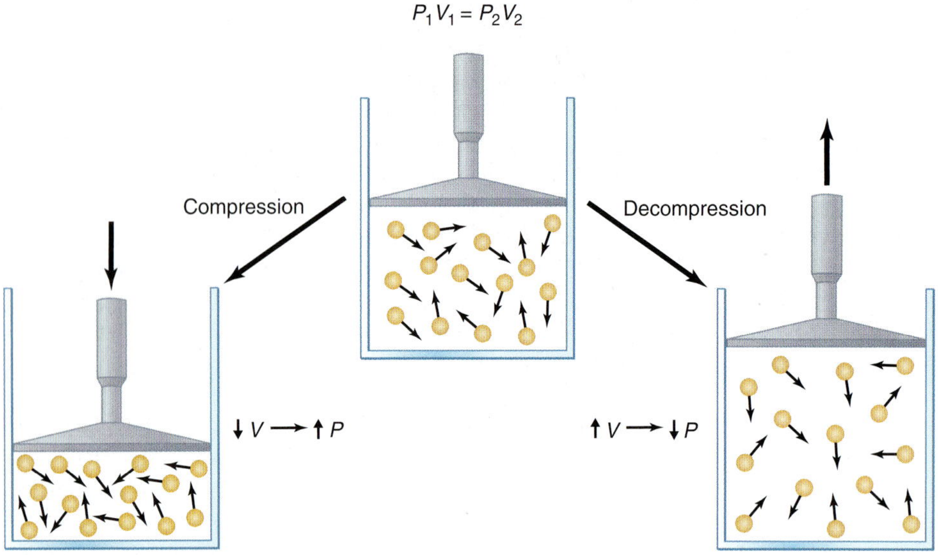

Figure 13.8 APIR Boyle's law: The pressure exerted by a constant number of gas molecules (at a constant temperature) is inversely proportional to the volume of the container. As the container is compressed, the pressure in the container increases. When the container is decompressed, the pressure inside decreases.

There are no muscles attached to the lung surface to pull the lungs open or push them shut. Rather, the lungs are passive elastic structures—like balloons—and their volume, therefore, depends on other factors. The first of these is the difference in pressure between the inside and outside of the lung, termed the **transpulmonary pressure (P_{tp})**. The second is how stretchable the lungs are, which determines how much they expand for a given change in P_{tp}. The rest of this section and the next three sections focus on transpulmonary pressure; stretchability will be discussed later in the section on lung compliance.

The pressure inside the lungs is the air pressure inside the alveoli (P_{alv}), and the pressure outside the lungs is the pressure of the intrapleural fluid surrounding the lungs (P_{ip}). Thus,

$$\text{Transpulmonary pressure} = P_{alv} - P_{ip} \quad \text{(13–3)}$$
$$P_{tp} = P_{alv} - P_{ip}$$

Compare this equation to equation 13–2 (the equation that describes airflow into or out of the lungs), as it will be essential to distinguish these equations from each other (**Figure 13.9**).

Transpulmonary pressure is the **transmural pressure** that governs the static properties of the lungs. *Transmural* means "across a wall" and, by convention, is represented by the pressure in the inside of the structure (P_{in}) minus the pressure outside the structure (P_{out}). Inflation of a balloonlike structure like the lungs requires an increase in the transmural pressure such that P_{in} increases relative to P_{out}.

Table 13.2 and Figure 13.9 show the major transmural pressures of the respiratory system. The transmural pressure acting on the lungs (P_{tp}) is $P_{alv} - P_{ip}$ and, on the chest wall, (P_{cw}) is $P_{ip} - P_{atm}$. The muscles of the chest wall contract and cause the chest wall to expand during inspiration; simultaneously, the diaphragm contracts downward, further enlarging the thoracic cavity. As the volume of the thoracic cavity expands, P_{ip} decreases. P_{tp} becomes more positive as a result and the lungs expand. As this occurs, P_{alv} becomes more negative compared to P_{atm} (due to Boyle's law), and air flows inward (inspiration, equation 13–2). Therefore, the transmural pressure across the lungs (P_{tp}) is increased to fill them with air by actively decreasing the pressure surrounding the lungs (P_{ip}) relative to the pressure inside the lungs (P_{alv}). When the respiratory muscles relax, elastic recoil of the lungs drives passive expiration back to the starting point.

How Is a Stable Balance Achieved Between Breaths?

Figure 13.10 illustrates the transmural pressures of the respiratory system at rest—that is, at the end of an unforced expiration when the respiratory muscles are relaxed and there is no airflow. By definition, if there is no airflow, P_{alv} must equal P_{atm} (see equation 13–2). Because the lungs always have air in them, the transmural pressure of the lungs (P_{tp}) must always be positive; therefore, $P_{alv} > P_{ip}$. At rest, when there is no airflow and $P_{alv} = 0$, P_{ip} must be negative, providing the force that keeps the lungs open and the chest wall in.

What are the forces that cause P_{ip} to be negative? The first, the **elastic recoil** of the lungs, is defined as the tendency of an elastic structure to oppose stretching or distortion. Even

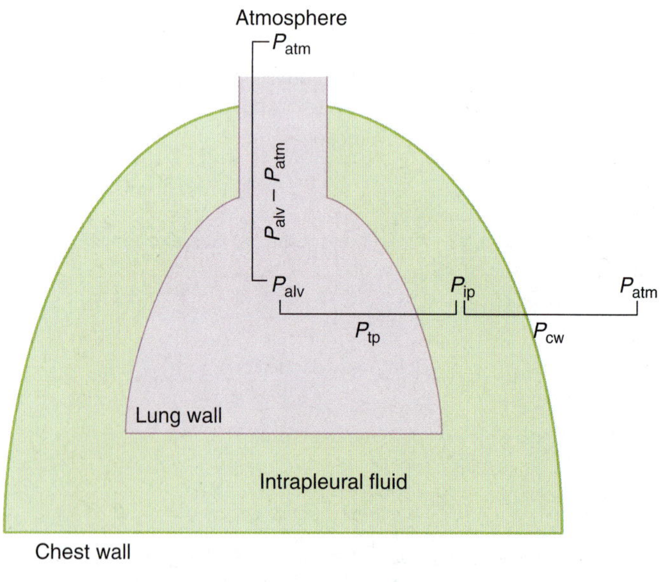

Figure 13.9 APIR Pressure differences involved in ventilation. Transpulmonary pressure ($P_{tp} = P_{alv} - P_{ip}$) is a determinant of lung size. Intrapleural pressure (P_{ip}) at rest is a balance between the tendency of the lung to collapse and the tendency of the chest wall to expand. P_{cw} represents the transmural pressure across the chest wall ($P_{ip} - P_{atm}$). $P_{alv} - P_{atm}$ is the driving pressure gradient for airflow into and out of the lungs. (The volume of intrapleural fluid is greatly exaggerated for visual clarity.)

TABLE 13.2 Two Important Transmural Pressures of the Respiratory System

Transmural Pressure	$P_{in} - P_{out}$*	Value at Rest	Explanatory Notes
Transpulmonary (P_{tp})	$P_{alv} - P_{ip}$	$0 - [-4] = 4$ mmHg	Pressure difference holding lungs open (opposes inward elastic recoil of the lung)
Chest wall (P_{cw})	$P_{ip} - P_{atm}$	$-4 - 0 = -4$ mmHg	Pressure difference holding chest wall in (opposes outward elastic recoil of the chest wall)

*P_{in} is pressure inside the structure, and P_{out} is pressure surrounding the structure.

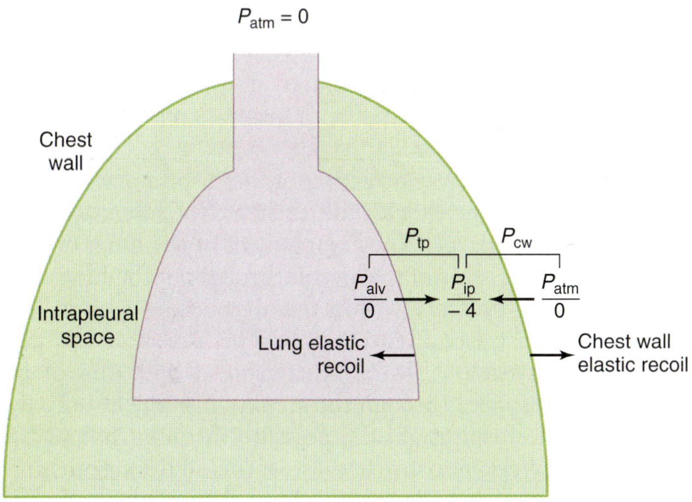

Figure 13.10 AP|R Alveolar (P_{alv}), intrapleural (P_{ip}), transpulmonary (P_{tp}), and trans-chest-wall (P_{cw}) pressures (mmHg) at the end of an unforced expiration—that is, between breaths when there is no airflow. The transpulmonary pressure ($P_{alv} - P_{ip}$) exactly opposes the elastic recoil of the lung, and the lung volume remains stable. Similarly, trans-chest-wall pressure ($P_{ip} - P_{atm}$) is balanced by the outward elastic recoil of the chest wall. Notice that the transmural pressure is the pressure inside the wall minus the pressure outside the wall. (The volume of intrapleural fluid is greatly exaggerated for clarity.)

at rest, the lungs contain air, and their natural tendency is to collapse because of elastic recoil. The lungs are held open by the positive P_{tp}, which, at rest, exactly opposes elastic recoil. The chest wall also has elastic recoil, and, at rest, its natural tendency is to expand.

At rest, all of these transmural pressures balance each other out. It is clear that the subatmospheric (negative) intrapleural pressure (P_{ip}) is the essential factor keeping the lungs partially expanded between breaths. An extremely important question is, "What is the reason for a subatmospheric ('negative') P_{ip}?"

As the lungs tend to collapse and the thoracic wall tends to expand, they move ever so slightly away from each other. This causes an infinitesimal enlargement of the fluid-filled intrapleural space between them. But fluid cannot expand the way air can, so even this tiny enlargement of the intrapleural space—so small that the pleural surfaces still remain in contact with each other—decreases the intrapleural pressure to below atmospheric pressure. In this way, the elastic recoil of both the lungs and chest wall creates the subatmospheric intrapleural pressure that keeps them from moving apart more than a very tiny amount. Again, imagine trying to pull apart two glass slides that have a drop of water between them. The fluid pressure generated between the slides will be lower than atmospheric pressure.

The importance of the transpulmonary pressure in achieving this stable balance can be seen when, during surgery or trauma, the chest wall is pierced without damaging the lung. Atmospheric air enters the intrapleural space through the wound, a phenomenon called ***pneumothorax***, and the intrapleural pressure increases from −4 mmHg to 0 mmHg. That is, P_{ip} increases from 4 mmHg lower than P_{atm} to a P_{ip} value equal to P_{atm}. The transpulmonary pressure acting to hold the lung open is thus eliminated, and the lung collapses (**Figure 13.11**).

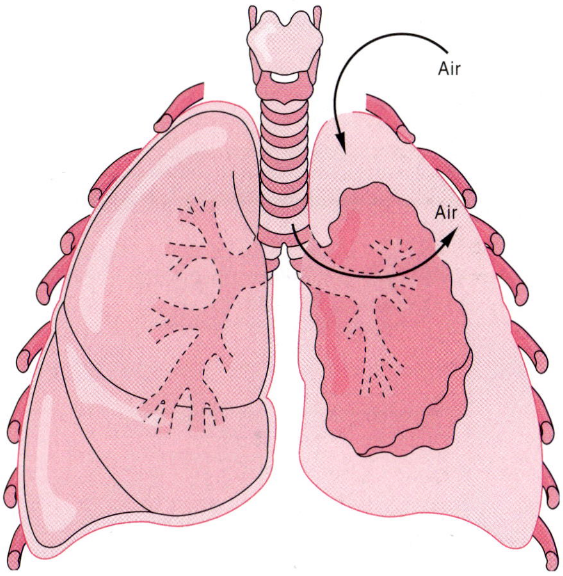

Figure 13.11 Pneumothorax. The lung collapses as air enters from the pleural cavity either from inside the lung or from the atmosphere through the thoracic wall. The combination of lung elastic recoil and surface tension causes collapse of the lung when pleural and airway pressures equalize.

PHYSIOLOGICAL INQUIRY

- How can a collapsed lung be re-expanded in a patient with a pneumothorax? (*Hint:* What changes in P_{ip} and P_{tp} would be needed to re-expand the lung?)

Answer can be found at end of chapter.

At the same time, the chest wall moves outward because its elastic recoil is also no longer opposed. Also notice in Figure 13.11 that a pneumothorax can result when a hole is made in the lung such that a significant amount of air leaks from inside the lung to the pleural space. This can occur, for example, when high airway pressure is applied during artificial ventilation of a premature infant whose lung surface tension is high and whose lungs are fragile. The thoracic cavity is divided into right and left sides by the mediastinum—the central part of the thorax containing the heart, trachea, esophagus and other structures—so a pneumothorax is often unilateral.

Inspiration

Figure 13.12 and **Figure 13.13** summarize the events that occur during normal inspiration at rest. Inspiration is initiated by the neurally induced contraction of the diaphragm and the external intercostal muscles located between the ribs (**Figure 13.14**). The diaphragm is the most important inspiratory muscle that acts during normal quiet breathing. When activation of the motor neurons within the **phrenic nerves** innervating the diaphragm causes it to contract, its dome moves downward into the abdomen, enlarging the thorax (see Figure 13.14). Simultaneously, activation of the motor neurons in the intercostal nerves to the inspiratory intercostal muscles causes them to contract, leading to an upward and outward movement of the ribs and a further increase in thoracic size. Also notice in Figure 13.14 that there are several other sets of muscles that participate in the expansion of the thoracic cavity, which become important during a maximal inspiration.

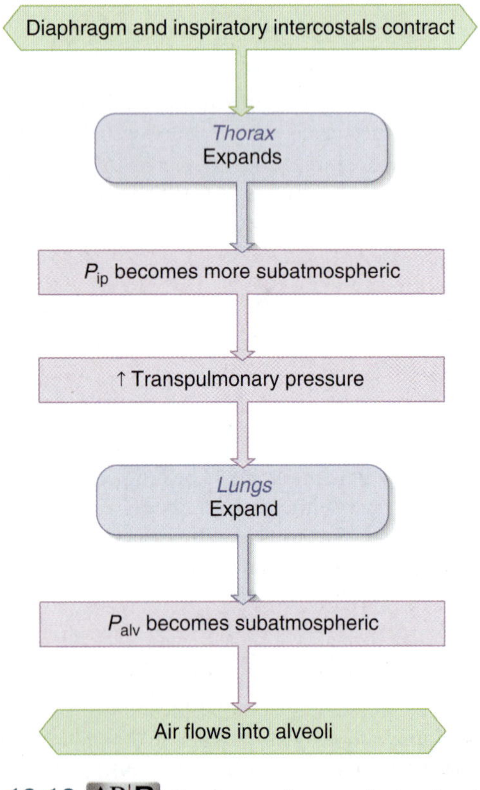

Figure 13.12 APIR Sequence of events during inspiration. Figure 13.13 illustrates these events quantitatively.

The crucial point is that contraction of the inspiratory muscles, by *actively* increasing the size of the thorax, upsets the stability set up by purely elastic forces between breaths. As the thorax enlarges, the thoracic wall moves ever so slightly farther away from the lung surface. The intrapleural fluid pressure therefore becomes even more subatmospheric than it was between breaths. This decrease in intrapleural pressure *increases* the transpulmonary pressure. Therefore, the force acting to expand the lungs—the transpulmonary pressure—is now greater than the elastic recoil exerted by the lungs at this moment, and so the lungs expand further. Note in Figure 13.13 that, by the end of inspiration, equilibrium *across the lungs* is once again established because the more inflated lungs exert a greater elastic recoil, which equals the increased transpulmonary pressure. In other words, lung volume is stable whenever transpulmonary pressure is balanced by the elastic recoil of the lungs (that is, at the end of both inspiration and expiration when there is no airflow).

Therefore, when contraction of the inspiratory muscles actively increases the thoracic dimensions, the lungs are passively forced to enlarge. The enlargement of the lungs causes an increase in the sizes of the alveoli throughout the lungs. By Boyle's law, the pressure within the alveoli decreases to less than atmospheric (see Figure 13.13). This produces the difference in pressure ($P_{alv} < P_{atm}$) that causes a bulk flow of air from the atmosphere through the airways into the alveoli. By the end of the inspiration, the pressure in the alveoli again equals atmospheric pressure because of this additional air, and airflow ceases.

Expiration

Figure 13.13 and **Figure 13.15** summarize the sequence of events that occur during expiration. At the end of inspiration, the motor neurons to the diaphragm and inspiratory intercostal muscles decrease their firing and so these muscles relax. The diaphragm and chest wall are no longer actively pulled outward by the muscle contractions, and so they start to recoil inward to their original smaller dimensions that existed between breaths. This immediately makes the intrapleural pressure less subatmospheric, thereby *decreasing* the transpulmonary pressure. Therefore, the transpulmonary pressure acting to expand the lungs is now smaller than the elastic recoil exerted by the more expanded lungs and the lungs passively recoil to their original dimension.

As the lungs become smaller, air in the alveoli becomes temporarily compressed so that, by Boyle's law, alveolar pressure exceeds atmospheric pressure (see Figure 13.13). Therefore, air flows from the alveoli through the airways out into the atmosphere. Thus, expiration at rest is passive, depending only upon the relaxation of the inspiratory muscles and the elastic recoil of the stretched lungs.

Under certain conditions, such as during exercise, expiration of larger volumes is achieved by contraction of a different set of intercostal muscles and the abdominal muscles, which *actively* decrease thoracic dimensions (see Figure 13.14). The internal intercostal muscles insert on the ribs in such a way that their contraction pulls the chest wall downward and inward, thereby decreasing thoracic volume. Contraction of

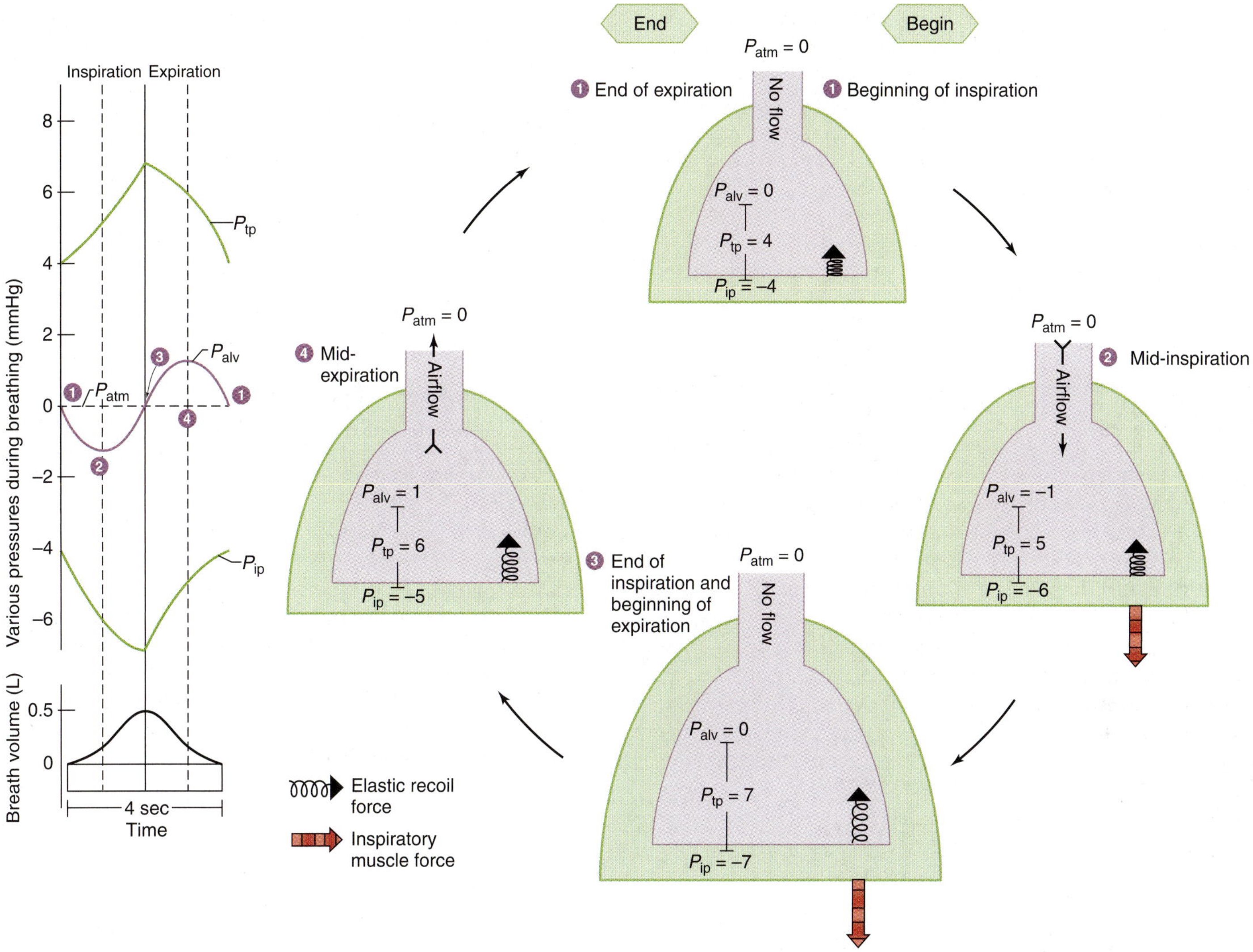

Figure 13.13 AP|R Summary of alveolar (P_{alv}), intrapleural (P_{ip}), and transpulmonary (P_{tp}) pressure changes and airflow during a typical respiratory cycle. At the end of expiration ①, P_{alv} is equal to P_{atm} and there is no airflow. At mid-inspiration ②, the chest wall is expanding, lowering P_{ip} and making P_{tp} more positive. This expands the lung, making P_{alv} negative and results in an inward airflow. At end of inspiration ③, the chest wall is no longer expanding but has yet to start passive recoil. Because lung size is not changing and the glottis is open to the atmosphere, P_{alv} is equal to P_{atm} and there is no airflow. As the respiratory muscles relax, the lungs and chest wall start to passively collapse due to elastic recoil. At mid-expiration ④, the lung is collapsing, thus compressing alveolar gas. As a result, P_{alv} is positive relative to P_{atm} and airflow is outward. The cycle starts over again at the end of expiration. Notice that throughout a typical respiratory cycle with a normal tidal volume, P_{ip} is negative relative to P_{atm}. In the graph on the left, the difference between P_{alv} and P_{ip} ($P_{alv} - P_{ip}$) at any point along the curves is equivalent to P_{tp}. For clarity, the chest-wall elastic recoil (as in Figure 13.10) is not shown.

PHYSIOLOGICAL INQUIRY

- How do the changes in P_{tp} between each step (①–④) explain whether the volume of the lung is increasing or decreasing?

Answer can be found at end of chapter.

the abdominal muscles increases intra-abdominal pressure and forces the relaxed diaphragm up into the thorax.

Lung Compliance

To repeat, the degree of lung expansion at any instant is proportional to the transpulmonary pressure, $P_{alv} - P_{ip}$. But just how much any given change in transpulmonary pressure expands the lungs depends upon the stretchability, or compliance, of the lungs. **Lung compliance (C_L)** is defined as the magnitude of the change in lung volume (ΔV_L) produced by a given change in the transpulmonary pressure:

$$C_L = \Delta V_L / \Delta P_{tp} \quad (13\text{–}4)$$

Thus, the greater the lung compliance, the easier it is to expand the lungs at any given change in transpulmonary pressure (**Figure 13.16**). Compliance can be considered the inverse of stiffness. A low lung compliance means

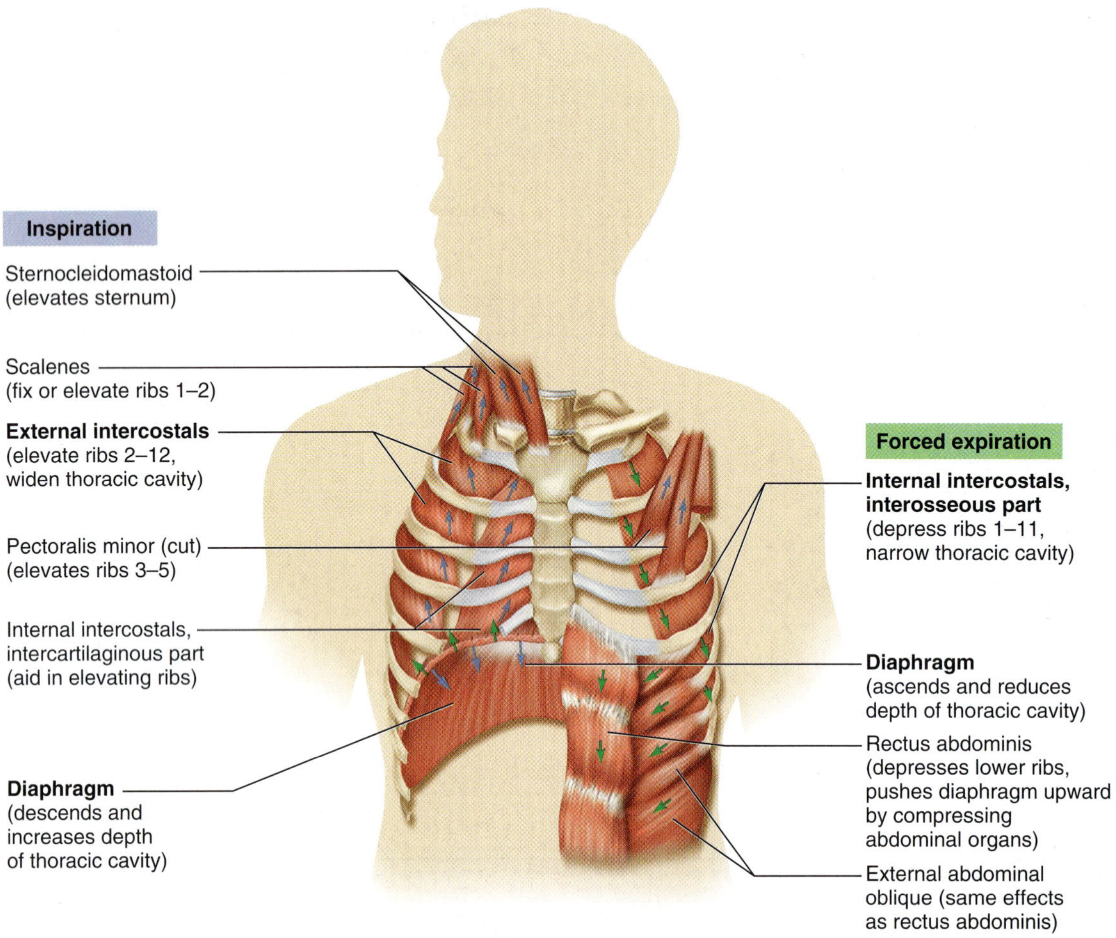

Figure 13.14 APIR The muscles of respiration. The muscles in bold are the primary muscles of respiration; the others are accessory. Blue arrows indicate muscles active during inspiration; green arrows indicate muscles active during forced expiration. Notice that the diaphragm is active during inspiration and passively moves up during a forced expiration due to pressure from the abdomen.

that a greater-than-normal transpulmonary pressure must be developed across the lung to produce a given amount of lung expansion. In other words, when lung compliance is abnormally low (increased stiffness), intrapleural pressure must be made more subatmospheric than usual during inspiration to achieve lung expansion. This requires more vigorous contractions of the diaphragm and inspiratory intercostal muscles. Thus, the less compliant the lung, the more energy is required to produce a given amount of expansion. Persons with low lung compliance due to disease tend to breathe shallowly and at a higher frequency to inspire an adequate volume of air.

Determinants of Lung Compliance

There are two major determinants of lung compliance. One is the stretchability of the lung tissues, particularly their elastic connective tissues. Thus, a thickening of the lung tissues decreases lung compliance. However, an equally if not more important determinant of lung compliance is not the elasticity of the lung tissues but the surface tension at the air–water interfaces within the alveoli.

The surface of the alveolar cells is moist, so the alveoli can be pictured as air-filled sacs lined with water. At an air–water interface, the attractive forces between the water molecules, known as **surface tension,** make the water lining like a stretched balloon that constantly tends to shrink and resists further stretching. Thus, expansion of the lung requires energy not only to stretch the connective tissue of the lung but also to overcome the surface tension of the water layer lining the alveoli.

Indeed, the surface tension of pure water is so great that were the alveoli lined with pure water, lung expansion would require exhausting muscular effort and the lungs would tend to collapse. It is extremely important, therefore, that the type II alveolar cells secrete the detergent-like substance mentioned earlier, known as **surfactant,** which markedly reduces the cohesive forces between water molecules on the alveolar surface. Therefore, surfactant lowers the surface tension, which increases lung compliance and makes it easier to expand the lungs.

Surfactant is a mixture of both lipids and proteins, but its major component is a phospholipid that inserts its hydrophilic end into the water layer lining the alveoli; its hydrophobic ends form a monomolecular layer between the air and water at the alveolar surface. The amount of surfactant tends to decrease when breaths are small and constant. A deep breath, which people normally intersperse frequently in their breathing pattern, stretches the type II cells, which stimulates the secretion of surfactant. This is why patients who have had thoracic or abdominal surgery

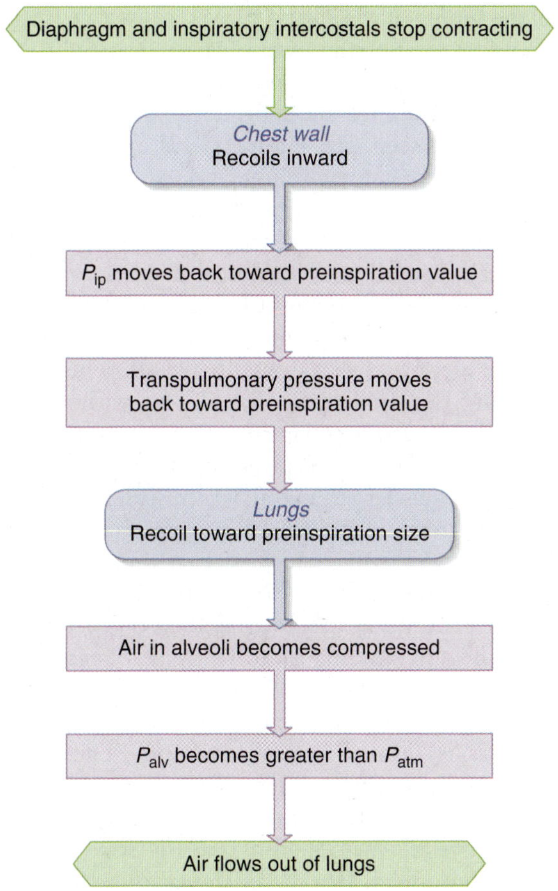

Figure 13.15 AP|R Sequence of events during expiration. Figure 13.13 illustrates these events quantitatively.

$$\text{Compliance} = \frac{\Delta \text{ Lung volume}}{\Delta (P_{alv} - P_{ip})} = \frac{\Delta V}{\Delta P_{tp}}$$

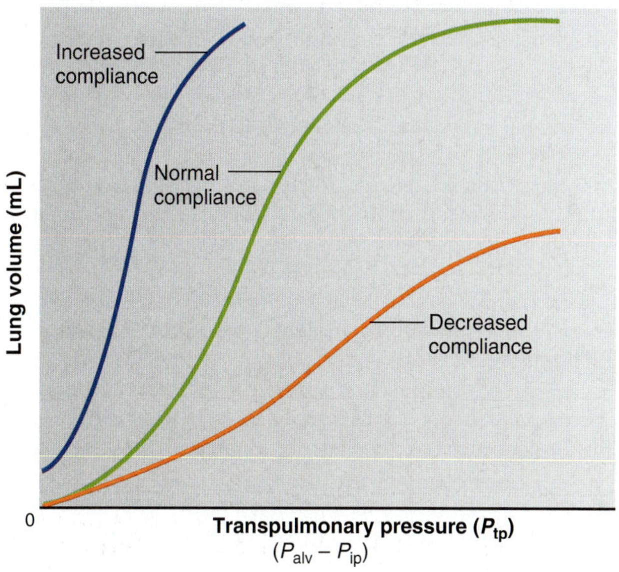

Figure 13.16 A graphic representation of lung compliance. Changes in lung volume and transpulmonary pressure are measured as a subject takes progressively larger breaths. When compliance is lower than normal (the lung is stiffer), there is a lesser increase in lung volume for any given increase in transpulmonary pressure. When compliance is increased, as in emphysema, small decreases in P_{tp} allow the lung to collapse.

PHYSIOLOGICAL INQUIRY

- Premature infants with inadequate surfactant have decreased lung compliance (respiratory distress syndrome of the newborn). If surfactant is not available to administer for therapy, what can be done to inflate the lung?

Answer can be found at end of chapter.

and are breathing shallowly because of the pain must be urged to take occasional deep breaths.

The **Law of Laplace** describes the relationship between pressure (P), surface tension (T), and the radius (r) of an alveolus, shown in **Figure 13.17**:

$$P = 2T/r \qquad (13\text{–}5)$$

As the radius inside the alveolus decreases, the pressure increases. Now imagine two alveoli next to each other sharing an alveolar duct (see Figure 13.17). The radius of alveolus a (r_a) is greater than the radius of alveolus b (r_b). If surface tension (T) were equivalent between these two alveoli, alveolus b would have a higher pressure than alveolus a by the Law of Laplace. If P_b is higher than P_a, air would flow from alveolus b into alveolus a, and alveolus b would collapse. Therefore, small alveoli would be unstable and would collapse into large alveoli. Another important property of surfactant is that it stabilizes alveoli of different sizes by altering surface tension, depending on the surface area of the alveolus. As an alveolus gets smaller, the

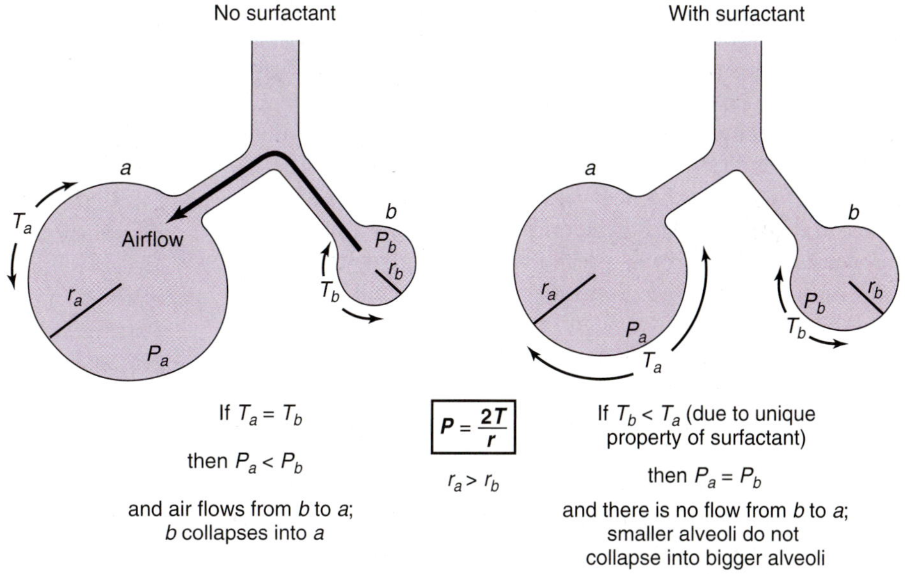

Figure 13.17 Stabilizing effect of surfactant. P is pressure inside the alveoli, T is a surface tension, and r is the radius of the alveolus. The Law of Laplace is described by the equation in the box.

TABLE 13.3	Some Important Facts About Pulmonary Surfactant
Pulmonary surfactant is a mixture of phospholipids and protein.	
It is secreted by type II alveolar cells.	
It lowers the surface tension of the water layer at the alveolar surface, which increases lung compliance, thereby making it easier for the lungs to expand.	
Its effect is greater in smaller alveoli, thus reducing the surface tension of small alveoli below that of larger alveoli. This stabilizes the alveoli.	
A deep breath increases its secretion by stretching the type II cells. Its concentration decreases when breaths are small.	
Production in the fetal lung occurs in late gestation and is stimulated by the increase in cortisol (glucocorticoid) secretion that occurs then.	

molecules of surfactant on its inside surface are less spread out, thus reducing surface tension. The reduction in surface tension helps to maintain a pressure in smaller alveoli equal to that in larger ones. This gives stability to alveoli of different sizes. **Table 13.3** summarizes some of the important aspects of pulmonary surfactant.

A striking example of what occurs when surfactant is deficient is the disease known as ***respiratory distress syndrome of the newborn.*** This is a leading cause of death in premature infants, in whom the surfactant-synthesizing cells may be too immature to function adequately. Respiratory movements in the fetus do not require surfactant because the lungs are filled with amniotic fluid, and the fetus receives oxygen from the maternal blood. Because of low lung compliance, the affected infant can inspire only by the most strenuous efforts, which may ultimately cause complete exhaustion, inability to breathe, lung collapse, and death. Before the development of newer treatments over the past 30 years, almost half of infants with this condition died. Current therapy includes assisted breathing with a mechanical ventilator and the administration of natural or synthetic surfactant given through the infant's trachea. These improved methods of treatment have markedly reduced mortality, and most infants treated adequately now survive.

Airway Resistance

As previously stated, the volume of air that flows into or out of the alveoli per unit time is directly proportional to the pressure difference between the atmosphere and alveoli and is inversely proportional to the resistance to flow of the airways (see equation 13–2). The factors that determine airway resistance are analogous to those determining vascular resistance in the circulatory system: tube length, tube radius, and interactions between moving molecules (gas molecules, in this case). As in the circulatory system, the most important factor by far is the radius of the tube—airway resistance is inversely proportional to the fourth power of the airway radii.

Airway resistance to airflow is normally so small that very small pressure differences produce large volumes of airflow. As we have seen (see Figure 13.13), the average atmosphere-to-alveoli pressure difference during a normal breath when at rest is about 1 mmHg; yet approximately 500 mL of air is moved by this tiny difference.

Physical, neural, and chemical factors affect airway radii and therefore resistance. One important physical factor is the transpulmonary pressure, which exerts a distending force on the airways, just as on the alveoli. This is a major factor keeping the smaller airways—those without cartilage to support them—from collapsing. Because transpulmonary pressure increases during inspiration (see Figure 13.13), airway radius becomes larger and airway resistance lower as the lungs expand during inspiration. The opposite occurs during expiration.

A second physical factor holding the airways open is the elastic connective-tissue fibers that link the outside of the airways to the surrounding alveolar tissue. These fibers are pulled upon as the lungs expand during inspiration; in turn, they help pull the airways open even more than between breaths. This is termed **lateral traction.** Thus, both the transpulmonary pressure and lateral traction act in the same direction, reducing airway resistance during inspiration.

Such physical factors also explain why the airways become narrower and airway resistance increases during a forced expiration. The increase in intrapleural pressure compresses the small conducting airways and decreases their radii. Therefore, because of increased airway resistance, there is a limit to how much one can increase the airflow rate during a forced expiration no matter how intense the effort. The harder one pushes, the greater the compression of the airways, further limiting expiratory airflow.

In addition to these physical factors, a variety of neuroendocrine and paracrine factors can influence airway smooth muscle and thereby airway resistance. For example, the hormone epinephrine relaxes airway smooth muscle by an effect on beta-adrenergic receptors, whereas the leukotrienes, members of the eicosanoid family produced in the lungs during inflammation, contract the muscle.

Why are we concerned with all the physical and chemical factors that *can* influence airway resistance when airway resistance is normally so low that it poses no impediment to airflow? The reason is that, under abnormal circumstances, changes in these factors may cause significant increases in airway resistance. Asthma and chronic obstructive pulmonary disease provide important examples, as we see next.

Asthma

Asthma is a disease characterized by intermittent episodes in which airway smooth muscle contracts strongly, markedly increasing airway resistance. The basic defect in asthma is chronic inflammation of the airways, the causes of which vary from person to person and include, among others, allergy, viral infections, and sensitivity to environmental factors. The underlying inflammation makes the airway smooth muscles hyperresponsive and causes them to contract strongly in response to such things as exercise (especially in cold, dry air), cigarette smoke, environmental pollutants, viruses, allergens, normally released bronchoconstrictor chemicals, and a variety of other potential triggers. In fact, the incidence of asthma is increasing in the United States, possibly due in part to environmental pollution.

The first aim of therapy for asthma is to reduce the chronic inflammation and airway hyperresponsiveness with ***anti-inflammatory drugs,*** particularly leukotriene inhibitors and inhaled glucocorticoids. The second aim is to overcome acute excessive airway smooth muscle contraction with ***bronchodilator drugs,*** which relax the airways. The latter drugs work on the airways either by relaxing airway smooth muscle or by blocking the actions of bronchoconstrictors. For example, one class of bronchodilator drugs mimics the normal action of epinephrine on beta-2 (β_2) adrenergic receptors. Another class of inhaled drugs blocks muscarinic cholinergic receptors, which have been implicated in bronchoconstriction.

Chronic Obstructive Pulmonary Disease

The term ***chronic obstructive pulmonary disease (COPD)*** refers to emphysema, chronic bronchitis, or a combination of the two. These diseases, which cause severe difficulties not only in ventilation but in oxygenation of the blood, are among the major causes of disability and death in the United States. In contrast to asthma, increased smooth muscle contraction is *not* the cause of the airway obstruction in these diseases.

Emphysema is discussed later in this chapter; suffice it to say here that the cause of obstruction in this disease is destruction and collapse of the smaller airways.

Chronic bronchitis is characterized by excessive mucus production in the bronchi and chronic inflammatory changes in the small airways. The cause of obstruction is an accumulation of mucus in the airways and thickening of the inflamed airways. The same agents that cause emphysema—smoking, for example—also cause chronic bronchitis, which is why the two diseases frequently coexist. Bronchitis may also be acute—for example, in response to viral infections such as those that cause upper respiratory infections. In such cases, the coughing and excess sputum and phlegm production associated with acute bronchitis typically resolve within 2 to 3 weeks.

Lung Volumes and Capacities

Normally, the volume of air entering the lungs during a single inspiration—the **tidal volume** (V_t)—is approximately equal to the volume leaving on the subsequent expiration. The tidal volume during normal quiet breathing—the resting tidal volume—is approximately 500 mL depending on body size. As illustrated in **Figure 13.18,** the maximal amount of air that can be increased above this value during deepest inspiration—the **inspiratory reserve volume (IRV)**—is about 3000 mL—that is, six times greater than resting tidal volume.

After expiration of a resting tidal volume, the lungs still contain a large volume of air. As described earlier, this is the resting position of the lungs and chest wall when there is no contraction of the respiratory muscles; this amount of air—the **functional residual capacity (FRC)**—averages about 2400 mL. Thus, the 500 mL of air inspired with each resting breath adds to and mixes with the much larger volume of air already in the lungs; then 500 mL of the total is expired. Through maximal active contraction of the expiratory muscles, it is possible to expire much more of the air remaining after the resting tidal volume has been expired. This additional expired volume—the **expiratory reserve volume (ERV)**—is about 1200 mL. Even after a maximal active expiration, approximately 1200 mL of air still remains in the lungs—the **residual volume (RV)**. Thus, the lungs are never completely emptied of air.

The **vital capacity (VC)** is the maximal volume of air a person can expire after a maximal inspiration. Under these conditions, the person is expiring both the resting tidal volume and the inspiratory reserve volume just inspired, plus the expiratory reserve volume (see Figure 13.18). In other words, the vital capacity is the sum of these three volumes and is an important measurement when assessing pulmonary function.

A variant on this measurement is the ***forced expiratory volume in 1 sec*** (FEV_1), in which the person takes a maximal inspiration and then exhales maximally as fast as possible. The important value is the fraction of the total "forced" vital capacity expired in 1 sec. Healthy individuals can expire approximately 80% of the vital capacity in 1 sec.

Measurement of vital capacity and FEV_1 are useful diagnostically and are known as ***pulmonary function tests.*** For example, people with ***obstructive lung diseases*** (increased airway resistance as in asthma) typically have an FEV_1 that is less than 80% of the vital capacity because it is difficult for them to expire air rapidly through the narrowed airways. In contrast to obstructive lung diseases, ***restrictive lung diseases*** are characterized by normal airway resistance but impaired respiratory movements because of abnormalities in the lung tissue, the pleura, the chest wall, or the neuromuscular machinery. Restrictive lung diseases are typically characterized by a reduced vital capacity but a normal ratio of FEV_1 to vital capacity.

Alveolar Ventilation

The total ventilation per minute—the **minute ventilation** ($\dot{V}_E$)—is equal to the tidal volume multiplied by the respiratory rate:

$$\underset{(\text{mL/min})}{\text{Minute ventilation}} = \underset{(\text{mL/breath})}{\text{Tidal volume}} \times \underset{(\text{breaths/min})}{\text{Respiratory rate}}$$

$$\dot{V}_E = V_t \cdot f \qquad (13\text{–}6)$$

For example, at rest, a typical healthy adult moves approximately 500 mL of air in and out of the lungs with each breath and takes 12 breaths each minute. The minute ventilation is therefore 500 mL/breath × 12 breaths/minute = 6000 mL of air per minute. However, because of dead space, not all this air is available for exchange with the blood, as we see next.

Dead Space

The conducting airways have a volume of about 150 mL. Exchanges of gases with the blood occur only in the alveoli and not in this 150 mL of the airways. Picture, then, what occurs during expiration of a tidal volume of 500 mL. The

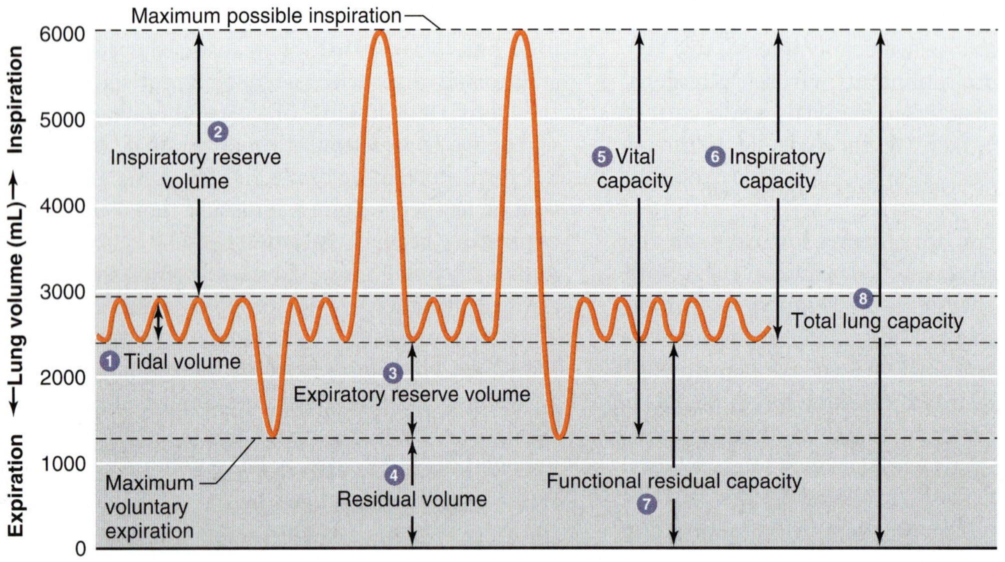

Respiratory Volumes and Capacities for an Average Young Adult Male		
Measurement	Typical Value*	Definition
Respiratory Volumes		
1 Tidal volume (TV)	500 mL	Amount of air inhaled or exhaled in one breath
2 Inspiratory reserve volume (IRV)	3000 mL	Amount of air in excess of tidal inspiration that can be inhaled with maximum effort
3 Expiratory reserve volume (ERV)	1200 mL	Amount of air in excess of tidal expiration that can be exhaled with maximum effort
4 Residual volume (RV)	1200 mL	Amount of air remaining in the lungs after maximum expiration; keeps alveoli inflated between breaths and mixes with fresh air on next inspiration
Respiratory Capacities		
5 Vital capacity (VC)	4700 mL	Amount of air that can be exhaled with maximum effort after maximum inspiration (ERV + TV + IRV); used to assess strength of thoracic muscles as well as pulmonary function
6 Inspiratory capacity (IC)	3500 mL	Maximum amount of air that can be inhaled after a normal tidal expiration (TV + IRV)
7 Functional residual capacity (FRC)	2400 mL	Amount of air remaining in the lungs after a normal tidal expiration (RV + ERV)
8 Total lung capacity (TLC)	5900 mL	Maximum amount of air the lungs can contain (RV + VC)

*Typical value at rest

Figure 13.18 Lung volumes and capacities recorded on a spirometer, an apparatus for measuring inspired and expired volumes. When the subject inspires, the pen moves up; with expiration, it moves down. The capacities are the sums of two or more lung volumes. The lung volumes are the four distinct components of total lung capacity. Note that residual volume, total lung capacity, and functional residual capacity cannot be measured with a spirometer.

500 mL of air is forced out of the alveoli and through the airways. Approximately 350 mL of this alveolar air is exhaled at the nose or mouth, but approximately 150 mL remains in the airways at the end of expiration. During the next inspiration (**Figure 13.19**), 500 mL of air flows into the alveoli, but the first 150 mL entering the alveoli is not atmospheric air but the 150 mL left behind in the airways from the last breath. Thus, only 350 mL of new atmospheric air enters the alveoli during the inspiration. The end result is that 150 mL of the 500 mL of atmospheric air entering the respiratory system during each inspiration never reaches the alveoli but is merely moved in and out of the airways. Because these airways do not permit gas exchange with the blood, the space within them is called the **anatomical dead space (V_D)**.

Thus, the volume of *fresh* air entering the alveoli during each inspiration equals the tidal volume *minus* the volume of air in the anatomical dead space. For the previous example,

Tidal volume (V_t) = 500 mL

Anatomical dead space (V_D) = 150 mL

Fresh air entering alveoli in one inspiration (V_A) =
500 mL − 150 mL = 350 mL

The total volume of fresh air entering the alveoli per minute is called the **alveolar ventilation ($\dot{V}_A$)**:

$$\underset{(\text{mL/min})}{\text{Alveolar ventilation}} = \left(\underset{(\text{mL/breath})}{\text{Tidal volume}} - \underset{(\text{mL/breath})}{\text{Dead space}}\right) \times \underset{(\text{breaths/min})}{\text{Respiratory rate}}$$

$$\dot{V}_A = (V_t - V_D) \cdot f \qquad (13\text{–}7)$$

Alveolar ventilation, rather than minute ventilation, is the more important factor in the effectiveness of gas exchange.

Figure 13.19 Effects of anatomical dead space on alveolar ventilation. Anatomical dead space is the volume of the conducting airways. Of a 500 mL tidal volume breath, 350 mL enters the airway involved in gas exchange. The remaining 150 mL remains in the conducting airways and does not participate in gas exchange.

PHYSIOLOGICAL INQUIRY

- What would be the effect of breathing through a plastic tube with a length of 20 cm and diameter of 4 cm? (*Hint:* Use the formula for the volume of a perfect cylinder.)

Answer can be found at end of chapter.

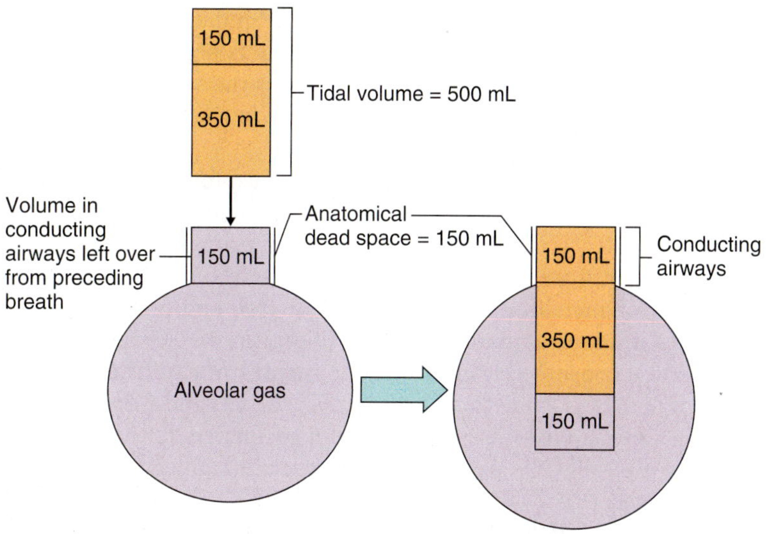

This generalization is demonstrated readily by the data in Table 13.4. In this experiment, subject A breathes rapidly and shallowly, B normally, and C slowly and deeply. Each subject has exactly the same minute ventilation; that is, each is moving the same amount of air in and out of the lungs per minute. Yet, when we subtract the anatomical-dead-space ventilation from the minute ventilation, we find marked differences in alveolar ventilation. Subject A has no alveolar ventilation and would become unconscious in several minutes, whereas C has a considerably greater alveolar ventilation than B, who is breathing normally.

Another important generalization drawn from this example is that increased *depth* of breathing is far more effective in increasing alveolar ventilation than an equivalent increase in breathing *rate*. Conversely, a decrease in depth can lead to a critical reduction in alveolar ventilation. This is because a fixed volume of each tidal volume goes to the dead space. If the tidal volume decreases, the fraction of the tidal volume going to the dead space increases until, as in subject A, it may represent the entire tidal volume. On the other hand, any increase in tidal volume goes entirely toward increasing alveolar ventilation. These concepts have important physiological implications. Most situations that produce an increase in ventilation, such as exercise, reflexively call forth a relatively greater increase in breathing depth than in breathing rate.

The anatomical dead space is not the only type of dead space. Some fresh inspired air is not used for gas exchange with the blood even though it reaches the alveoli because some alveoli may, for various reasons, have little or no blood supply. This volume of air is known as **alveolar dead space.** It is quite small in healthy persons but may be very large in persons with several kinds of lung disease. As we shall see, local mechanisms that match air and blood flows minimize the alveolar dead space. The sum of the anatomical and alveolar dead spaces is known as the **physiological dead space.** This is also known as wasted ventilation because it is air that is inspired but does not participate in gas exchange with blood flowing through the lungs.

13.3 Exchange of Gases in Alveoli and Tissues

We have now completed the discussion of the lung mechanics that produce alveolar ventilation, but this is only the first step in the respiratory process. Oxygen must move across the alveolar membranes into the pulmonary capillaries, be transported by the blood to the tissues, leave the tissue capillaries and enter the extracellular fluid, and finally cross plasma membranes to gain entry into cells. Carbon dioxide must follow a similar path, but in reverse.

In the steady state, the volume of oxygen that leaves the tissue capillaries and is consumed by the body cells per unit time is equal to the volume of oxygen added to the blood

TABLE 13.4 Effect of Breathing Patterns on Alveolar Ventilation

Subject	Tidal Volume (mL/breath)	×	Frequency (breaths/min)	=	Minute Ventilation (mL/min)	Anatomical-Dead-Space Ventilation (mL/min)	Alveolar Ventilation (mL/min)
A	150		40		6000	150 × 40 = 6000	0
B	500		12		6000	150 × 12 = 1800	4200
C	1000		6		6000	150 × 6 = 900	5100

in the lungs during the same time period. Similarly, in the steady state, the rate at which carbon dioxide is produced by the body cells and enters the systemic blood is the same as the rate at which carbon dioxide leaves the blood in the lungs and is expired.

The amount of oxygen the cells consume and the amount of carbon dioxide they produce, however, are not necessarily identical. The balance depends primarily upon which nutrients are used for energy, because the enzymatic pathways for metabolizing carbohydrates, fats, and proteins generate different amounts of CO_2. The ratio of CO_2 produced to O_2 consumed is known as the **respiratory quotient** (**RQ**). The RQ is 1 for carbohydrate, 0.7 for fat, and 0.8 for protein. On a mixed diet, the RQ is approximately 0.8; that is, 8 molecules of CO_2 are produced for every 10 molecules of O_2 consumed.

Figure 13.20 presents typical exchange values during 1 min for a person at rest with an RQ of 0.8, assuming a cellular oxygen consumption of 250 mL/min, a carbon dioxide production of 200 mL/min, an alveolar ventilation of 4000 mL/min (4 L/min), and a cardiac output of 5000 mL/min (5 L/min).

Because only 21% of the atmospheric air is oxygen, the total oxygen entering the alveoli per min in our illustration is 21% of 4000 mL, or 840 mL/min. Of this inspired oxygen, 250 mL crosses the alveoli into the pulmonary capillaries, and the rest is subsequently exhaled. Note that blood entering the lungs already contains a large quantity of oxygen, to which the new 250 mL is added. The blood then flows from the lungs to the left side of the heart and is pumped by the left ventricle through the aorta, arteries, and arterioles into the tissue capillaries, where 250 mL of oxygen leaves the blood per minute for cells to take up and utilize. Thus, the quantities of oxygen added to the blood in the lungs and removed in the tissues are the same.

The story reads in reverse for carbon dioxide. A significant amount of carbon dioxide already exists in systemic arterial blood; to this is added an additional 200 mL per minute, the amount the cells produce, as blood flows through tissue capillaries. This 200 mL leaves the blood each minute as blood flows through the lungs and is expired.

Blood pumped by the heart carries oxygen and carbon dioxide between the lungs and tissues by bulk flow, but diffusion is responsible for the net movement of these molecules between the alveoli and blood, and between the blood and the cells of the body. Understanding the mechanisms involved in these diffusional exchanges depends upon some basic chemical and physical properties of gases, which we will now discuss.

Partial Pressures of Gases

Gas molecules undergo continuous random motion. These rapidly moving molecules collide and exert a pressure, the magnitude of which is increased by anything that increases the rate of movement. The pressure a gas exerts is proportional to temperature (because heat increases the speed at which molecules move) and the concentration of the gas—that is, the number of molecules per unit volume.

As **Dalton's law** states, in a mixture of gases, the pressure each gas exerts is independent of the pressure the others exert. This is because gas molecules are normally so far apart that they do not affect each other. Each gas in a mixture behaves as

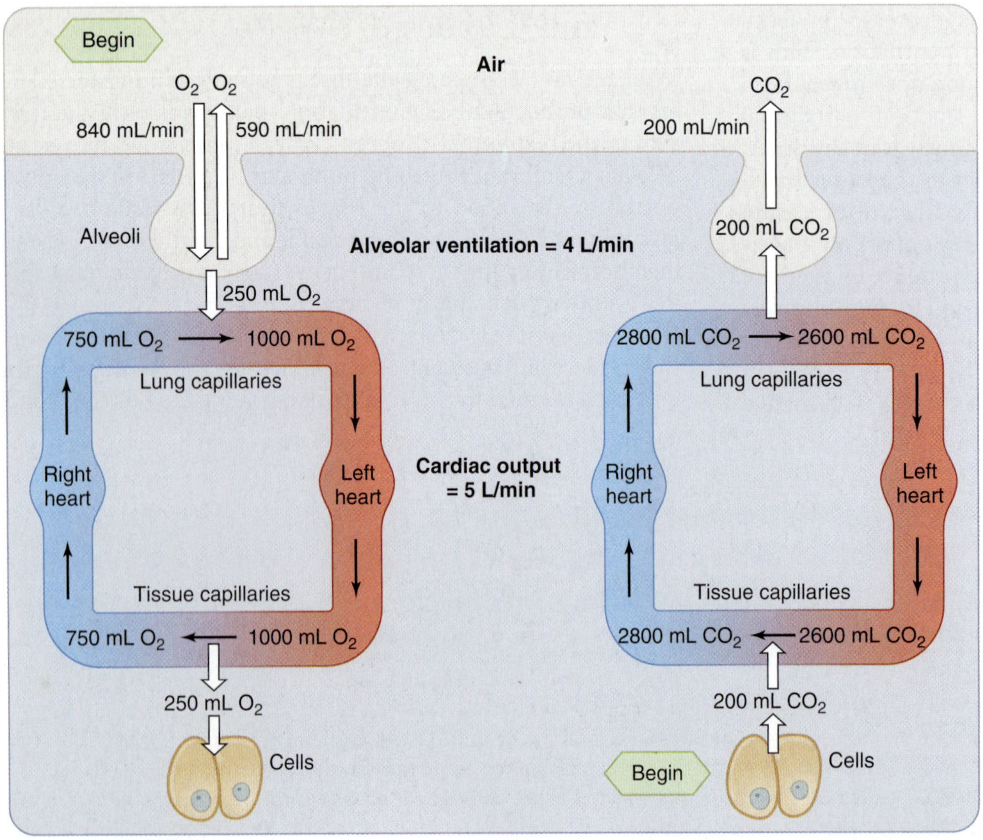

Figure 13.20 Summary of typical oxygen and carbon dioxide exchanges between atmosphere, lungs, blood, and tissues *during 1 min* in a resting individual. Note that the values in this figure for oxygen and carbon dioxide in blood are *not* the values per liter of blood but, rather, the amounts transported *per minute* in the cardiac output (5 L in this example). The volume of oxygen in 1 L of arterial blood is 200 mL O_2/L of blood—that is, 1000 mL O_2/5 L of blood.

though no other gases are present, so the total pressure of the mixture is simply the sum of the individual pressures. These individual pressures, termed **partial pressures,** are denoted by a P in front of the symbol for the gas. For example, the partial pressure of oxygen is expressed as P_{O_2}. The partial pressure of a gas is directly proportional to its concentration. Net diffusion of a gas will occur from a region where its partial pressure is high to a region where it is low. An appreciation of the importance of Dalton's law is another example of the general principle that physiological processes are dictated by the laws of chemistry and physics.

Atmospheric air consists of approximately 79% nitrogen and approximately 21% oxygen, with very small quantities of water vapor, carbon dioxide, and inert gases. The sum of the partial pressures of all these gases is called atmospheric pressure, or barometric pressure. It varies in different parts of the world as a result of local weather conditions and gravitational differences due to altitude; at sea level, it is 760 mmHg. Because the partial pressure of any gas in a mixture is the fractional concentration of that gas times the total pressure of all the gases, the P_{O_2} of atmospheric air at sea level is 0.21×760 mmHg $=$ 160 mmHg at sea level.

Diffusion of Gases in Liquids

When a liquid is exposed to air containing a particular gas, molecules of the gas will enter the liquid and dissolve in it. Another physical law, called **Henry's law,** states that the amount of gas dissolved will be directly proportional to the partial pressure of the gas with which the liquid is in equilibrium. A corollary is that, at equilibrium, the partial pressures of the gas molecules in the liquid and gaseous phases must be identical. Suppose, for example, that a closed container contains both water and gaseous oxygen. Oxygen molecules from the gas phase constantly bombard the surface of the water, some entering the water and dissolving. The number of molecules striking the surface is directly proportional to the P_{O_2} of the gas phase, so the number of molecules entering the water and dissolving in it is also directly proportional to the P_{O_2} As long as the P_{O_2} in the gas phase is higher than the P_{O_2} in the liquid, there will be a net diffusion of oxygen into the liquid. Diffusion equilibrium will be reached only when the P_{O_2} in the liquid is equal to the P_{O_2} in the gas phase, and there will then be no further net diffusion between the two phases.

Conversely, if a liquid containing a dissolved gas at high partial pressure is exposed to a lower partial pressure of that same gas in a gas phase, a net diffusion of gas molecules will occur out of the liquid into the gas phase until the partial pressures in the two phases become equal.

The exchanges *between* gas and liquid phases described in the preceding two paragraphs are precisely the phenomena occurring in the lungs between alveolar air and pulmonary capillary blood. In addition, *within* a liquid, dissolved gas molecules also diffuse from a region of higher partial pressure to a region of lower partial pressure, an effect that underlies the exchange of gases between cells, extracellular fluid, and capillary blood throughout the body.

Why must the diffusion of gases into or within liquids be presented in terms of partial pressures rather than "concentrations," the values used to deal with the diffusion of all other solutes? The reason is that the concentration of a gas in a liquid is proportional not only to the partial pressure of the gas but also to the solubility of the gas in the liquid. The more soluble the gas, the greater its concentration will be at any given partial pressure. Thus, if a liquid is exposed to two different gases having the same partial pressures, at equilibrium the *partial pressures* of the two gases will be identical in the liquid, but the *concentrations* of the gases in the liquid will differ, depending upon their solubilities in that liquid.

With these basic gas properties as the foundation, we can now discuss the diffusion of oxygen and carbon dioxide across alveolar and capillary walls and plasma membranes. The partial pressures of these gases in air and in various sites of the body for a resting person at sea level appear in **Figure 13.21.** We start our discussion with the alveolar gas pressures because their values set those of systemic arterial blood. This fact cannot be emphasized too strongly: The alveolar P_{O_2} and P_{CO_2}

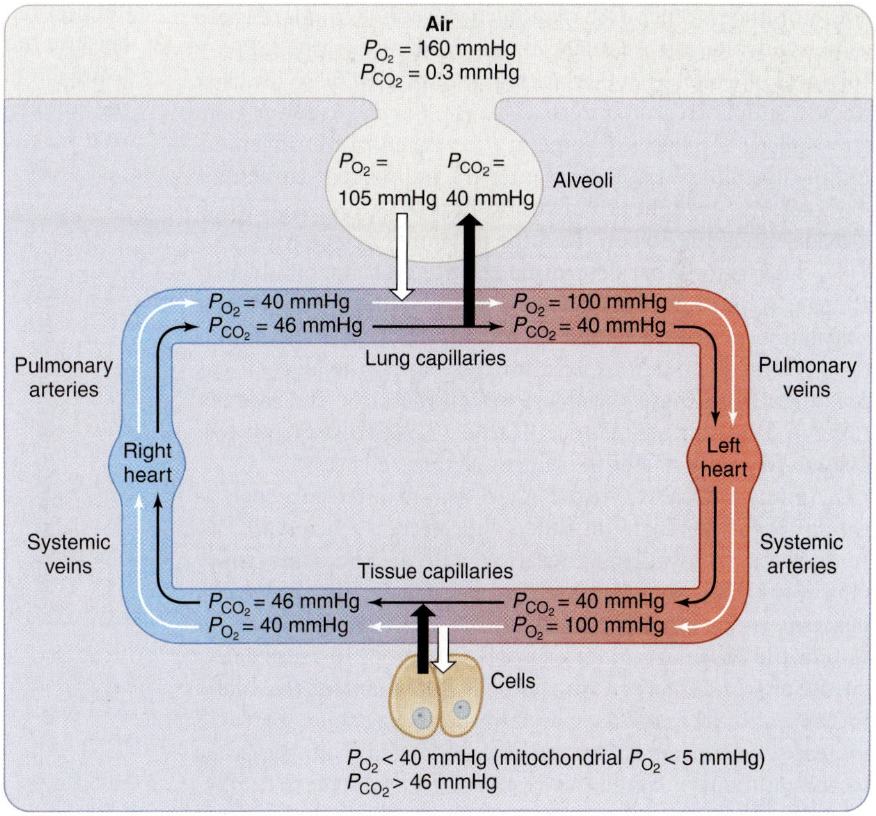

Figure 13.21 APIR Partial pressures of carbon dioxide and oxygen in inspired air at sea level and in various places in the body. The reason that the alveolar P_{O_2} and pulmonary vein P_{O_2} are not exactly the same is described later in the text. Note also that the P_{O_2} in the systemic arteries is shown as identical to that in the pulmonary veins; for reasons involving the anatomy of the blood flow through the lungs, the systemic arterial value is actually slightly less, but we have ignored this for the sake of clarity.

TABLE 13.5 Effects of Various Conditions on Alveolar Gas Pressures		
Condition	**Alveolar P_{O_2}**	**Alveolar P_{CO_2}**
Breathing air with low P_{O_2}	Decreases	No change*
↑ Alveolar ventilation and unchanged metabolism	Increases	Decreases
↓ Alveolar ventilation and unchanged metabolism	Decreases	Increases
↑ Metabolism and unchanged alveolar ventilation	Decreases	Increases
↓ Metabolism and unchanged alveolar ventilation	Increases	Decreases
Proportional increases in metabolism and alveolar ventilation	No change	No change

*Breathing air with low P_{O_2} has no direct effect on alveolar P_{CO_2}. However, as described later in the text, people in this situation will reflexively increase their ventilation, and that will lower P_{CO_2}.

determine the systemic arterial P_{O_2} and P_{CO_2}. So, what determines alveolar gas pressures?

Alveolar Gas Pressures

Typical alveolar gas pressures are P_{O_2} = 105 mmHg and P_{CO_2} = 40 mmHg. (*Note:* We do not deal with nitrogen, even though it is the most abundant gas in the alveoli, because nitrogen is biologically inert under normal conditions and does not undergo net exchange in the alveoli.) Compare these values with the gas pressures in the air being breathed: P_{O_2} = 160 mmHg and P_{CO_2} = 0.3 mmHg, the latter value so low that we will simply treat it as zero. The alveolar P_{O_2} is lower than atmospheric P_{O_2} because some of the oxygen in the air entering the alveoli leaves them to enter the pulmonary capillaries. Alveolar P_{CO_2} is higher than atmospheric P_{CO_2} because carbon dioxide enters the alveoli from the pulmonary capillaries.

The factors that determine the precise value of alveolar P_{O_2} are (1) the P_{O_2} of atmospheric air, (2) the rate of alveolar ventilation, and (3) the rate of total-body oxygen consumption. Although equations exist for calculating the alveolar gas pressures from these variables, we will describe the interactions in a qualitative manner (**Table 13.5**). To start, we will assume that only one of the factors changes at a time.

First, a decrease in the P_{O_2} of the inspired air, such as would occur at high altitude, will decrease alveolar P_{O_2}. A decrease in alveolar ventilation will do the same thing (**Figure 13.22**) because less fresh air is entering the alveoli per unit time. Finally, an increase in the oxygen consumption in the cells during, for example, strenuous physical activity, results in a decrease in the oxygen content of the blood returning to the lungs compared to the resting state. This will increase the concentration gradient of oxygen from the lungs to the pulmonary capillaries resulting in an increase in oxygen diffusion. If alveolar ventilation does not change, this will lower alveolar P_{O_2} because a larger fraction of the oxygen in the entering fresh air will leave the alveoli to enter the blood for use by the tissues. (Recall that in the steady state, the volume of oxygen entering the blood in the lungs per unit time is always equal to the volume utilized by the tissues.) This discussion has been in terms of factors that lower alveolar P_{O_2}; just reverse the direction of change of the three factors to see how to increase alveolar P_{O_2}.

The situation for alveolar P_{CO_2} is analogous, again assuming that only one factor changes at a time. There is normally essentially no carbon dioxide in inspired air and so we can ignore that factor. A decreased alveolar ventilation will decrease the amount of carbon dioxide exhaled, thereby increasing the alveolar P_{CO_2} (see Figure 13.22). Increased production of carbon dioxide will also increase the alveolar P_{CO_2} because more carbon dioxide will be diffusing into the alveoli from the blood per unit time. Recall that in the steady state, the volume of carbon dioxide entering the alveoli per unit time is always equal to the volume produced by the tissues. Just

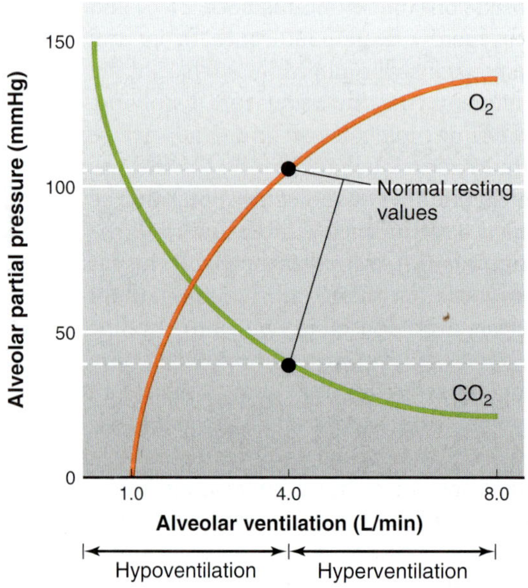

Figure 13.22 Effects of increasing or decreasing alveolar ventilation on alveolar partial pressures in a person having a constant metabolic rate (cellular oxygen consumption and carbon dioxide production). Note that alveolar P_{O_2} approaches zero when alveolar ventilation is about 1 L/min. At this point, all the oxygen entering the alveoli crosses into the blood, leaving virtually no oxygen in the alveoli.

TABLE 13.6	Normal Gas Pressure			
	Venous Blood	Arterial Blood	Alveoli	Atmosphere
P_{O_2}	40 mmHg	100 mmHg*	105 mmHg*	160 mmHg
P_{CO_2}	46 mmHg	40 mmHg	40 mmHg	0.3 mmHg

*The reason that the arterial P_{O_2} and alveolar P_{O_2} are not exactly the same is described later in this chapter.

reverse the direction of the changes to see how to decrease alveolar P_{CO_2}.

For simplicity, we assumed only one factor would change at a time, but if more than one factor changes, the effects will either add to or subtract from each other. For example, if oxygen consumption and alveolar ventilation both increase at the same time, their opposing effects on alveolar P_{O_2} will tend to cancel each other out, and alveolar P_{O_2} will not change.

This last example emphasizes that, at any particular atmospheric P_{O_2}, it is the *ratio* of oxygen consumption to alveolar ventilation that determines alveolar P_{O_2}—the higher the ratio, the lower the alveolar P_{O_2}. Similarly, alveolar P_{CO_2} is determined by the ratio of carbon dioxide production to alveolar ventilation—the higher the ratio, the higher the alveolar P_{CO_2}.

We can now define two terms that denote the adequacy of ventilation—that is, the relationship between metabolism and alveolar ventilation. These definitions are stated in terms of carbon dioxide rather than oxygen. ***Hypoventilation*** exists when there is an increase in the ratio of carbon dioxide production to alveolar ventilation. In other words, a person is hypoventilating if the alveolar ventilation cannot keep pace with the carbon dioxide production. The result is that alveolar P_{CO_2} increases above the normal value. ***Hyperventilation*** exists when there is a decrease in the ratio of carbon dioxide production to alveolar ventilation, that is, when alveolar ventilation is actually too great for the amount of carbon dioxide being produced. The result is that alveolar P_{CO_2} decreases below the normal value.

Note that "hyperventilation" is not synonymous with "increased ventilation." Hyperventilation represents increased ventilation *relative to metabolism*. Thus, for example, the increased ventilation that occurs during moderate exercise is not hyperventilation because, as we will see, the increase in production of carbon dioxide in this situation is proportional to the increased ventilation.

Gas Exchange Between Alveoli and Blood

The blood that enters the pulmonary capillaries is systemic venous blood pumped to the lungs through the pulmonary arteries. Having come from the tissues, it has a relatively high P_{CO_2} (46 mmHg in a healthy person at rest) and a relatively low P_{O_2} (40 mmHg) (see Figure 13.21 and **Table 13.6**). The differences in the partial pressures of oxygen and carbon dioxide on the two sides of the alveolar-capillary membrane result in the net diffusion of oxygen from alveoli to blood and of carbon dioxide from blood to alveoli. (For simplicity, we are ignoring the small diffusion barrier provided by the interstitial space.) As this diffusion occurs, the P_{O_2} in the pulmonary capillary blood increases and the P_{CO_2} decreases. The net diffusion of these gases ceases when the capillary partial pressures become equal to those in the alveoli.

In a healthy person, the rates at which oxygen and carbon dioxide diffuse are high enough and the blood flow through the capillaries slow enough that complete equilibrium is reached well before the blood reaches the end of the capillaries (**Figure 13.23**).

Thus, the blood that leaves the pulmonary capillaries to return to the heart and be pumped into the systemic arteries has essentially the same P_{O_2} and P_{CO_2} as alveolar air. (They are not exactly the same, for reasons given later.) Accordingly, the factors described in the previous section—atmospheric P_{O_2}, cellular oxygen consumption and carbon dioxide production, and alveolar ventilation—determine the alveolar gas pressures, which then determine the systemic arterial gas pressures.

Given that diffusion between alveoli and pulmonary capillaries normally achieves complete equilibration, the more capillaries that participate in this process, the more total

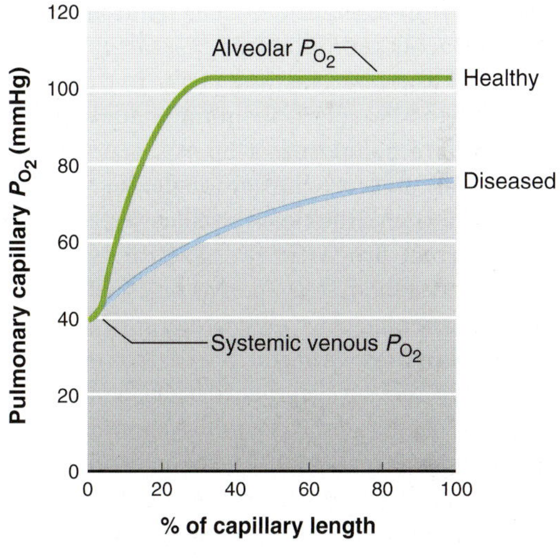

Figure 13.23 APR Equilibration of blood P_{O_2} with an alveolus with a P_{O_2} of 105 mmHg along the length of a pulmonary capillary. Note that in an abnormal alveolar-diffusion barrier (diseased), the blood is not fully oxygenated.

PHYSIOLOGICAL INQUIRY

- What is the effect of exercise on P_{O_2} at the end of a capillary in a normal region of the lung? In a region of the lung with diffusion limitation due to disease?

Answers can be found at end of chapter.

oxygen and carbon dioxide are exchanged. Many of the pulmonary capillaries at the apex (top) of each lung are normally closed at rest. During exercise, these capillaries open and receive blood, thereby enhancing gas exchange. The mechanism by which this occurs is a simple physical one; the pulmonary circulation at rest is at such a low blood pressure that the pressure in these apical capillaries is inadequate to keep them open, but the increased cardiac output of exercise increases pulmonary vascular pressures, which opens these capillaries.

The diffusion of gases between alveoli and capillaries may be impaired in a number of ways (see Figure 13.23), resulting in inadequate oxygen diffusion into the blood. For one thing, the total surface area of all of the alveoli in contact with pulmonary capillaries may be decreased. In ***pulmonary edema,*** some of the alveoli may become filled with fluid. (As described in Section C of Chapter 12, edema is the accumulation of fluid in tissues; in the alveoli, this increases the diffusion barrier for gases.) Diffusion may also be impaired if the alveolar walls become severely thickened with connective tissue (fibrotic), as, for example, in the disease called ***diffuse interstitial fibrosis.*** In this disease, fibrosis may arise from infection, autoimmune disease, hypersensitivity to inspired substances, exposure to toxic airborne chemicals, and many other causes. Typical symptoms of these types of diffusion diseases are shortness of breath and poor oxygenation of blood. Pure diffusion problems of these types are restricted to oxygen and usually do not affect the elimination of carbon dioxide, which diffuses more rapidly than oxygen.

Matching of Ventilation and Blood Flow in Alveoli

The major disease-induced cause of inadequate oxygen movement between alveoli and pulmonary capillary blood is not a problem with diffusion but, instead, is due to the mismatching of the air supply and blood supply in individual alveoli.

The lungs are composed of approximately 300 million alveoli, each capable of receiving carbon dioxide from, and supplying oxygen to, the pulmonary capillary blood. To be most efficient, the correct proportion of alveolar airflow (ventilation) and capillary blood flow (perfusion) should be available to *each* alveolus. Any mismatching is termed ***ventilation–perfusion inequality.***

The major effect of ventilation–perfusion inequality is to decrease the P_{O_2} of systemic arterial blood. Indeed, largely because of gravitational effects on ventilation and perfusion, there is enough ventilation–perfusion inequality in healthy people to decrease the arterial P_{O_2} about 5 mmHg. One effect of upright posture is to increase the filling of blood vessels at the bottom of the lung due to gravity, which contributes to a difference in blood-flow distribution in the lung. This is the major explanation of the fact, given earlier, that the P_{O_2} of blood in the pulmonary veins and systemic arteries is normally about 5 mmHg less than that of average alveolar air (see Table 13.6).

In disease states, regional changes in lung compliance, airway resistance, and vascular resistance can cause marked ventilation–perfusion inequalities. The extremes of this phenomenon are easy to visualize: (1) There may be ventilated alveoli with no blood supply at all (dead space or wasted ventilation) due to a blood clot, for example; or (2) there may be blood flowing through areas of lung that have no ventilation (this is termed a ***shunt***) due to collapsed alveoli, for example. However, the inequality need not be all-or-none to be significant.

Carbon dioxide elimination is also impaired by ventilation–perfusion inequality but not nearly to the same degree as oxygen uptake. Although the reasons for this are complex, small increases in arterial P_{CO_2} lead to increases in alveolar ventilation, which usually prevent further increases in arterial P_{CO_2}. Nevertheless, severe ventilation–perfusion inequalities in disease states can lead to an increase in arterial P_{CO_2}.

There are several local homeostatic responses within the lungs that minimize the mismatching of ventilation and blood flow and thereby maximize the efficiency of gas exchange (**Figure 13.24**). Probably the most important of these is a direct effect of low oxygen on pulmonary blood vessels. A decrease in ventilation within a group of alveoli—which might occur, for example, from a mucous plug blocking the small airways—leads to a decrease in alveolar P_{O_2} and the area around it, including the blood vessels. A decrease in P_{O_2} in these alveoli and nearby blood vessels leads to vasoconstriction, diverting blood flow away from the poorly ventilated area. This local adaptive effect, unique to the pulmonary arterial blood vessels, ensures that blood flow is directed away from diseased areas of the lung toward areas that are well ventilated. Another factor to improve the match between ventilation and perfusion can occur if there is a local decrease in blood flow within a lung region due to, for example, a small blood clot in a pulmonary arteriole. A local decrease in blood flow brings less systemic CO_2 to that area, resulting in a local decrease in P_{CO_2}. This causes local bronchoconstriction, which diverts airflow away to areas of the lung with better perfusion.

The net adaptive effects of vasoconstriction and bronchoconstriction are to (1) supply less blood flow to poorly ventilated areas, thus diverting blood flow to well-ventilated areas;

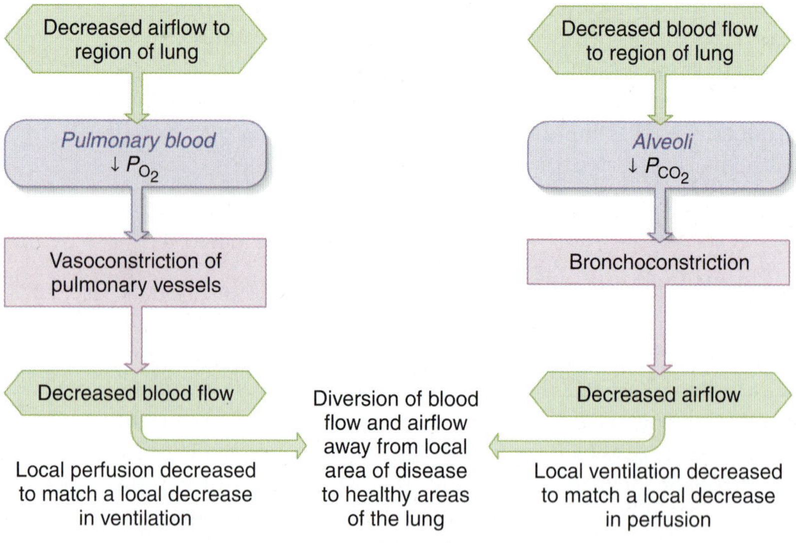

Figure 13.24 Local control of ventilation–perfusion matching.

and (2) redirect air away from diseased or damaged alveoli and toward healthy alveoli. These factors greatly improve the efficiency of pulmonary gas exchange, but they are not perfect even in the healthy lung. There is always a small mismatch of ventilation and perfusion, which, as just described, leads to the normal alveolar-arterial O_2 gradient of about 5 mmHg.

Gas Exchange Between Tissues and Blood

As the systemic arterial blood enters capillaries throughout the body, it is separated from the interstitial fluid by only the thin capillary wall, which is highly permeable to both oxygen and carbon dioxide. The interstitial fluid, in turn, is separated from the intracellular fluid by the plasma membranes of the cells, which are also quite permeable to oxygen and carbon dioxide. Metabolic reactions occurring within cells are constantly consuming oxygen and producing carbon dioxide. Therefore, as shown in Figure 13.21, intracellular P_{O_2} is lower and P_{CO_2} higher than in arterial blood. The lowest P_{O_2} of all—less than 5 mmHg—is in the mitochondria, the site of oxygen utilization. As a result, a net diffusion of oxygen occurs from blood into cells and, within the cells, into the mitochondria, and a net diffusion of carbon dioxide occurs from cells into blood. In this manner, as blood flows through systemic capillaries, its P_{O_2} decreases and its P_{CO_2} increases. This accounts for the systemic venous blood values shown in Figure 13.21 and Table 13.6.

In summary, the supply of new oxygen to the alveoli and the consumption of oxygen in the cells create P_{O_2} gradients that produce net diffusion of oxygen from alveoli to blood in the lungs and from blood to cells in the rest of the body. Conversely, the production of carbon dioxide by cells and its elimination from the alveoli via expiration create P_{CO_2} gradients that produce net diffusion of carbon dioxide from cells to blood in the rest of the body and from blood to alveoli in the lungs.

13.4 Transport of Oxygen in Blood

Table 13.7 summarizes the oxygen content of systemic arterial blood, referred to simply as arterial blood. Each liter normally contains the number of oxygen molecules equivalent to 200 mL of pure gaseous oxygen at atmospheric pressure. The oxygen is present in two forms: (1) dissolved in the plasma and erythrocyte cytosol and (2) reversibly combined with hemoglobin molecules in the erythrocytes.

TABLE 13.7 Oxygen Content of Systemic Arterial Blood at Sea Level

1 liter (L) arterial blood contains		
	3 mL	O_2 physically dissolved (1.5%)
	197 mL	O_2 bound to hemoglobin (98.5%)
Total:	200 mL	O_2
Cardiac output = 5 L/min		
O_2 carried to tissues/min = 5 L/min × 200 mL O_2/L		
= 1000 mL O_2/min		

As predicted by Henry's law, the amount of oxygen dissolved in blood is directly proportional to the P_{O_2} of the blood. Because the solubility of oxygen in water is relatively low, only 3 mL can be dissolved in 1 L of blood at the normal arterial P_{O_2} of 100 mmHg. The other 197 mL of oxygen in a liter of arterial blood—more than 98% of the oxygen content in the liter—is transported in the erythrocytes, reversibly combined with hemoglobin.

Each **hemoglobin** molecule is a protein made up of four subunits bound together. Each subunit consists of a molecular group known as **heme** and a polypeptide attached to the heme. The four polypeptides of a hemoglobin molecule are collectively called **globin.** Each of the four heme groups in a hemoglobin molecule (Figure 13.25) contains one atom of iron (Fe^{2+}), to which molecular oxygen binds. Because each iron atom can bind one molecule of oxygen, a single hemoglobin molecule can bind four oxygen molecules (see Figure 2.19). However, for simplicity, the equation for the reaction between oxygen and hemoglobin is usually written in terms of a single polypeptide–heme subunit of a hemoglobin molecule:

$$O_2 + Hb \rightleftharpoons HbO_2 \quad (13\text{–}8)$$

Therefore, hemoglobin can exist in one of two forms—**deoxyhemoglobin (Hb)** and **oxyhemoglobin (HbO_2).** In a blood sample containing many hemoglobin molecules, the fraction of all the hemoglobin in the form of oxyhemoglobin is expressed as the **percent hemoglobin saturation:**

$$\text{Percent Hb saturation} = \frac{O_2 \text{ bound to Hb}}{\text{Maximal capacity of Hb to bind } O_2} \times 100 \quad (13\text{–}9)$$

For example, if the amount of oxygen bound to hemoglobin is 40% of the maximal capacity, the sample is said to

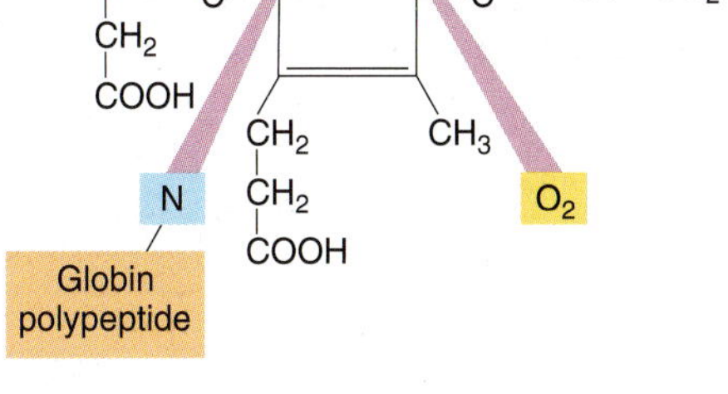

Figure 13.25 Heme in two dimensions. Oxygen binds to the iron atom (Fe^{2+}). Heme attaches to a polypeptide chain by a nitrogen atom to form one subunit of hemoglobin. Four of these subunits bind to each other to make a single hemoglobin molecule. See Figure 2.19, which shows the arrangements of polypeptide chains that make up the hemoglobin molecule.

be 40% saturated. The denominator in this equation is also termed the **oxygen-carrying capacity** of the blood.

What factors determine the percent hemoglobin saturation? By far the most important is the blood P_{O_2}. Before turning to this subject, however, it must be stressed that the *total amount* of oxygen carried by hemoglobin in the blood depends not only on the percent saturation of hemoglobin but also on how much hemoglobin is in each liter of blood. A significant decrease in hemoglobin in the blood is called ***anemia.*** For example, if a person's blood contained only half as much hemoglobin per liter as normal, then at any given percent saturation, the oxygen content of the blood would be only half as much. The most common way in which the hemoglobin content of blood is decreased is due to a low hematocrit, for example, due to chronic blood loss and to certain dietary deficiencies resulting in inadequate production of erythrocytes in the bone marrow.

What Is the Effect of P_{O_2} on Hemoglobin Saturation?

Based on equation 13–8 and the law of mass action (see Chapter 3), it is evident that increasing the blood P_{O_2} should increase the combination of oxygen with hemoglobin. The quantitative relationship between these variables is shown in **Figure 13.26**, which is called an **oxygen–hemoglobin dissociation curve.** (The term *dissociate* means "to separate," in this case, oxygen from hemoglobin; it could just as well have been called an "oxygen–hemoglobin association" curve.) The curve is sigmoid because, as stated earlier, each hemoglobin molecule contains four subunits. Each subunit can combine with one molecule of oxygen, and the reactions of the four subunits occur sequentially, with each combination facilitating the next one.

This combination of oxygen with hemoglobin is an example of cooperativity, as described in Chapter 3, and is a classic example of the general principle of physiology that understanding the laws of chemistry and physics is vital to understanding function. The explanation in this case is as follows. The globin units of deoxyhemoglobin are tightly held by electrostatic bonds in a conformation with a relatively low affinity for oxygen. The binding of oxygen to a heme molecule breaks some of these bonds between the globin subunits, leading to a conformation change that leaves the remaining oxygen-binding sites more exposed. Thus, the binding of one oxygen molecule to deoxyhemoglobin increases the affinity of the remaining sites on the same hemoglobin molecule, and so on.

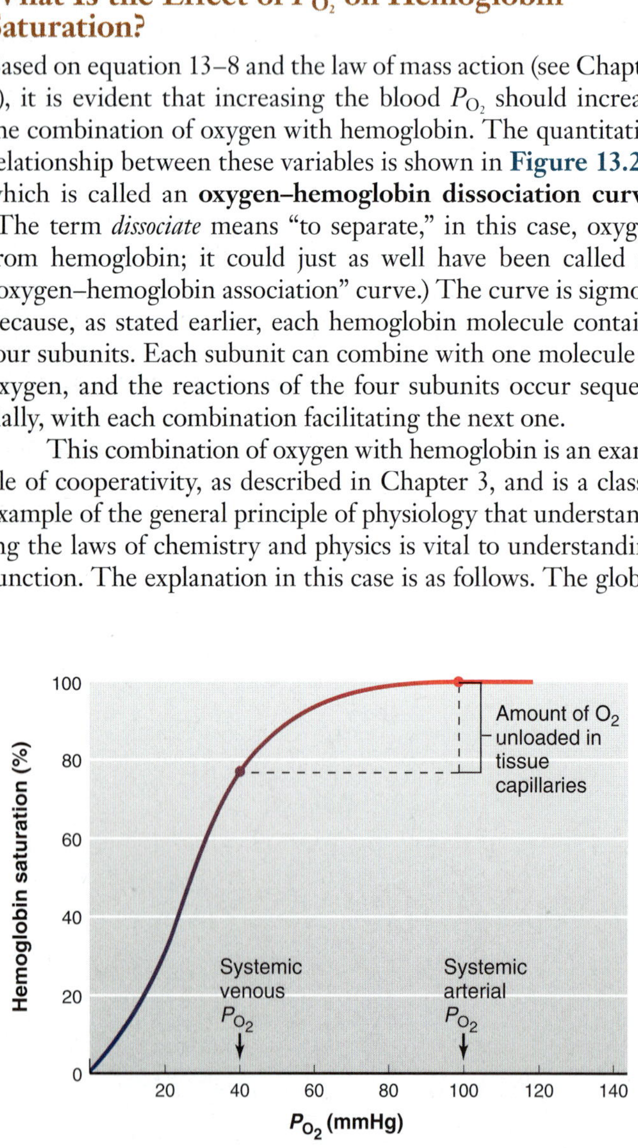

Figure 13.26 Oxygen–hemoglobin dissociation curve. This curve applies to blood at 37°C and a normal arterial H^+ concentration. At any given blood hemoglobin concentration, the *y*-axis could also have plotted oxygen content in milliliters of oxygen. At 100% saturation, the amount of hemoglobin in normal blood carries 200 mL of oxygen.

The shape of the oxygen–hemoglobin dissociation curve is extremely important in understanding oxygen exchange. The curve has a steep slope between 10 and 60 mmHg P_{O_2} and a relatively flat portion (or plateau) between 70 and 100 mmHg P_{O_2}. Thus, the extent to which oxygen combines with hemoglobin increases very rapidly as the P_{O_2} increases from 10 to 60 mmHg, so that at a P_{O_2} of 60 mmHg, approximately 90% of the total hemoglobin is combined with oxygen. From this point on, a further increase in P_{O_2} produces only a small increase in oxygen binding.

This plateau at higher P_{O_2} values has a number of important implications. In many situations, including at high altitude and with pulmonary disease, a moderate reduction occurs in alveolar and therefore arterial P_{O_2}. Even if the P_{O_2} decreased from the normal value of 100 to 60 mmHg, the total quantity of oxygen carried by hemoglobin would decrease by only 10% because hemoglobin saturation is still close to 90% at a P_{O_2} of 60 mmHg. The plateau provides an excellent safety factor so that even a significant limitation of lung function still allows almost normal oxygen saturation of hemoglobin.

The plateau also explains why, in a healthy person at sea level, increasing the alveolar (and therefore the arterial) P_{O_2} either by hyperventilating or by breathing 100% oxygen does not appreciably increase the total content of oxygen in the blood. A small additional amount dissolves; but because hemoglobin is already almost completely saturated with oxygen at the normal arterial P_{O_2} of 100 mmHg, it simply cannot pick up any more oxygen when the P_{O_2} is increased beyond this point. This applies only to healthy people at sea level. If a person initially has a low arterial P_{O_2} because of lung disease or high altitude, then there would be a great deal of deoxyhemoglobin initially present in the arterial blood. Therefore, increasing the alveolar and thereby the arterial P_{O_2} would result in significantly more oxygen transport.

The steep portion of the curve from 60 mmHg down to 20 mmHg is ideal for unloading oxygen in the tissues. That is, for a small decrease in P_{O_2} due to diffusion of oxygen from the blood to the cells, a large quantity of oxygen can be unloaded in the peripheral tissue capillary.

We now retrace our steps and reconsider the movement of oxygen across the various membranes, this time including hemoglobin in our analysis. It is essential to recognize that the oxygen bound to hemoglobin does *not* contribute directly to the P_{O_2} of the blood; only dissolved oxygen does so. Therefore, oxygen diffusion is governed only by the dissolved portion, a fact that permitted us to ignore hemoglobin in discussing transmembrane partial pressure gradients. However, the presence of hemoglobin plays a critical role in determining the *total amount* of oxygen that will diffuse, as illustrated by a simple example (**Figure 13.27**). Two solutions separated by a semipermeable membrane contain equal quantities of oxygen. The gas pressures in both solutions are equal, and no net diffusion

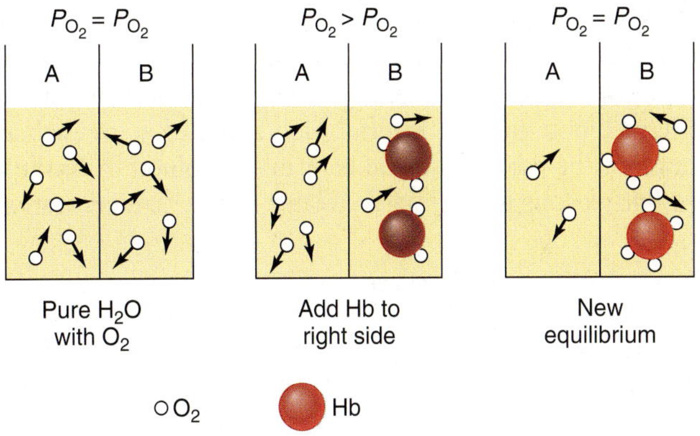

Figure 13.27 Effect of added hemoglobin on oxygen distribution between two compartments containing a fixed number of oxygen molecules and separated by a semipermeable membrane. At the new equilibrium, the P_{O_2} values are again equal to each other but lower than before the hemoglobin was added. However, the total oxygen—in other words, the oxygen dissolved plus that combined with hemoglobin—is now much higher on the right side of the membrane. Adapted from Comroe.

of oxygen occurs. Addition of hemoglobin to compartment B disturbs this equilibrium because much of the oxygen combines with hemoglobin. Despite the fact that the total *quantity* of oxygen in compartment B is still the same, the number of *dissolved* oxygen molecules has decreased. Therefore, the P_{O_2} of compartment B is less than that of A, and so there is a net diffusion of oxygen from A to B. At the new equilibrium, the oxygen pressures are once again equal, but almost all the oxygen is in compartment B and has combined with hemoglobin.

Let us now apply this analysis to capillaries of the lungs and tissues (**Figure 13.28**). The plasma and erythrocytes entering the lungs have a P_{O_2} of 40 mmHg. As we can see from Figure 13.26, hemoglobin saturation at this P_{O_2} is 75%. The alveolar P_{O_2}—105 mmHg—is higher than the blood P_{O_2} and so oxygen diffuses from the alveoli into the plasma. This increases plasma P_{O_2} and induces diffusion of oxygen into the erythrocytes, elevating erythrocyte P_{O_2} and causing increased combination of oxygen and hemoglobin. Most of the oxygen diffusing into the blood from the alveoli does not remain dissolved but combines with hemoglobin. Therefore, the blood P_{O_2} normally remains less than the alveolar P_{O_2} until hemoglobin is virtually 100% saturated. Thus, the diffusion gradient favoring oxygen movement into the blood is maintained despite the very large transfer of oxygen.

In the tissue capillaries, the process is reversed. Because the mitochondria of the cells all over the body are utilizing oxygen, the cellular P_{O_2} is less than the P_{O_2} of the surrounding interstitial fluid. Therefore, oxygen is continuously diffusing into the cells. This causes the interstitial fluid P_{O_2} to always be less than the P_{O_2} of the blood flowing through the tissue capillaries, so net diffusion of oxygen occurs from the plasma within the capillary into the interstitial fluid. As a result, plasma P_{O_2} becomes lower than erythrocyte P_{O_2}, and oxygen diffuses out of the erythrocyte into the plasma. The decrease in erythrocyte P_{O_2} causes the dissociation of oxygen from hemoglobin, thereby liberating oxygen, which then diffuses out of the erythrocyte. The net result is a transfer, purely by diffusion, of large quantities of oxygen from hemoglobin to plasma to interstitial fluid to the mitochondria of tissue cells.

In most tissues under resting conditions, hemoglobin is still 75% saturated as the blood leaves the tissue capillaries. This fact underlies an important local mechanism by which cells can obtain more oxygen whenever they increase their activity. For example, an exercising muscle consumes more oxygen, thereby lowering its tissue P_{O_2}. This increases the blood-to-tissue P_{O_2} gradient. As a result, the rate of oxygen

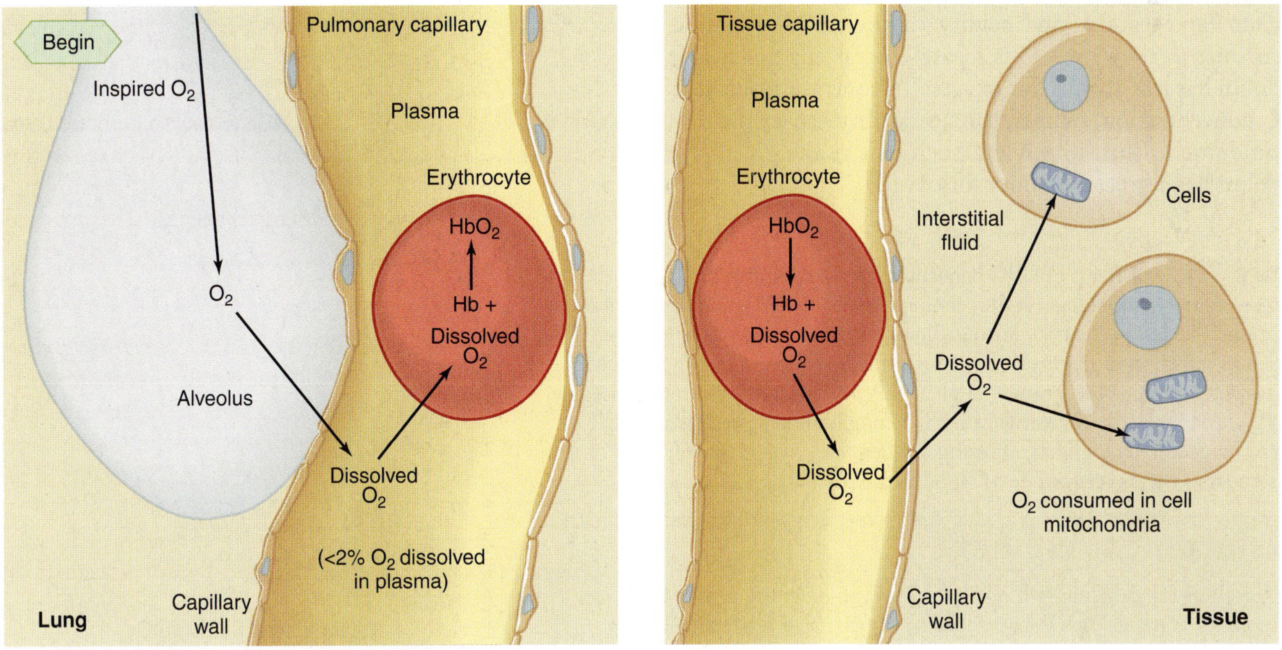

Figure 13.28 APIR Oxygen movement in the lungs and tissues. Movement of inspired air into the alveoli is by bulk flow; all movements across membranes are by diffusion.

diffusion from blood to cells increases. In turn, the resulting reduction in erythrocyte P_{O_2} causes additional dissociation of hemoglobin and oxygen. In this manner, the extraction of oxygen from blood in an exercising muscle is much greater than the usual 25%. In addition, an increased blood flow to the muscles, called active hyperemia (Chapter 12), also contributes greatly to the increased oxygen supply.

Effect of Carbon Monoxide on Oxygen Binding to Hemoglobin

Carbon monoxide is a colorless, odorless gas that is a product of the incomplete combustion of hydrocarbons, such as gasoline. It is one of the more common causes of sickness and death due to poisoning, both intentional and accidental. Its most striking pathophysiological characteristic is its extremely high affinity—210 times that of oxygen—for the oxygen-binding sites in hemoglobin. For this reason, it reduces the amount of oxygen that combines with hemoglobin in pulmonary capillaries by competing for these sites. It also exerts a second deleterious effect: It alters the hemoglobin molecule so as to shift the oxygen–hemoglobin dissociation curve to the left, thus decreasing the unloading of oxygen from hemoglobin in the tissues. As we will see later, the situation is worsened by the fact that persons suffering from carbon monoxide poisoning do not show any reflex increase in their ventilation.

Effects of CO_2 and Other Factors in the Blood and Different Isoforms on Hemoglobin Saturation

At any given P_{O_2}, a variety of other factors influence the degree of hemoglobin saturation. These include blood P_{CO_2}, H^+ concentration, temperature, the concentration of a substance produced by erythrocytes called **2,3-diphosphoglycerate (DPG)** (also known as bisphosphoglycerate [BPG]), and the presence of a special kind of hemoglobin usually only found in the fetal blood. As illustrated in **Figure 13.29**, an increase in DPG concentration, temperature, and acidity causes the dissociation curve to shift to the right. This means that at any given P_{O_2}, hemoglobin has less affinity for oxygen. In contrast, a decrease in DPG concentration, temperature, or acidity causes the dissociation curve to shift to the left, such that at any given P_{O_2}, hemoglobin has a greater affinity for oxygen.

The effects of increased P_{CO_2}, H^+ concentration, and temperature are continuously exerted on the blood in tissue capillaries, because each of these factors is greater in tissue capillary blood than in arterial blood. The P_{CO_2} is increased because of the carbon dioxide entering the blood from the tissues. For reasons to be described later, the H^+ concentration is

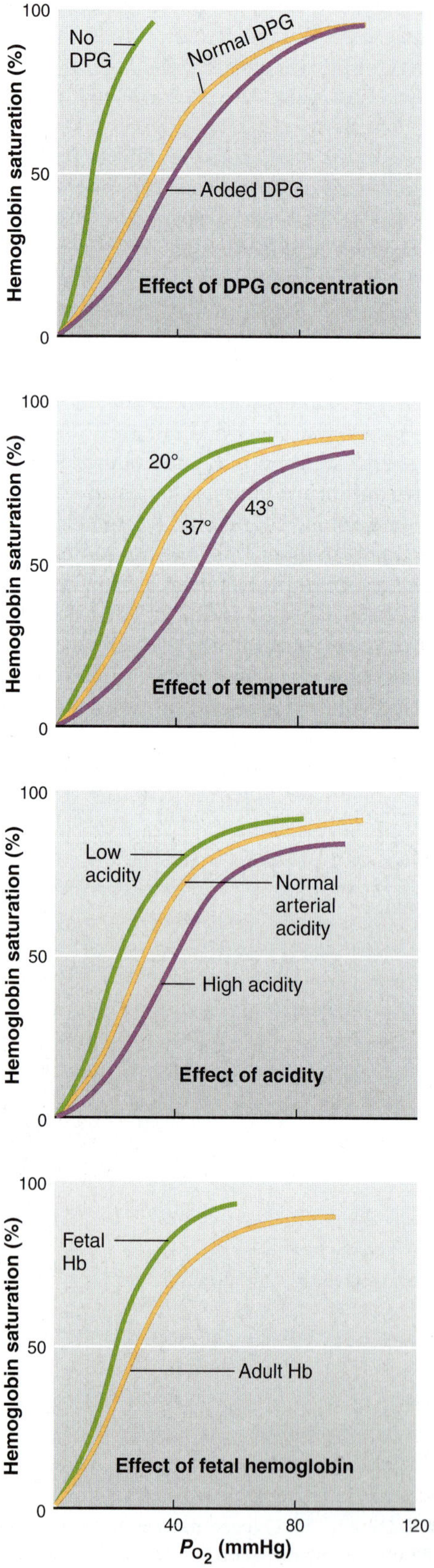

Figure 13.29 Effects of DPG concentration, temperature, acidity, and the presence of fetal hemoglobin on the relationship between P_{O_2} and hemoglobin saturation. The temperature of normal blood, of course, never diverges from 37°C as much as shown in the figure, but the principle is still the same when the changes are within the physiological range. High acidity and low acidity can be caused by high P_{CO_2} and low P_{CO_2}, respectively. Fetal hemoglobin has a higher affinity for oxygen than adult hemoglobin, allowing an adequate oxygen content from oxygen diffusion from the maternal to fetal blood in the placenta. Adapted from Comroe.

PHYSIOLOGICAL INQUIRY

- Researchers are developing blood substitutes to meet the demand for emergency transfusions. What would be the effect of artificial blood in which binding of O_2 is not altered by acidity?

Answer can be found at end of chapter.

increased because of the elevated P_{CO_2} and the release of metabolically produced acids such as lactic acid. The temperature is increased because of the heat produced by tissue metabolism. Hemoglobin exposed to this elevated blood P_{CO_2}, H^+ concentration, and temperature as it passes through the tissue capillaries has a decreased affinity for oxygen. Thus, hemoglobin gives up even more oxygen than it would have if the decreased tissue capillary P_{O_2} had been the only operating factor.

The more metabolically active a tissue is, the greater its P_{CO_2}, H^+ concentration, and temperature will be. At any given P_{O_2}, this causes hemoglobin to release more oxygen during passage through the tissue's capillaries and provides the more active cells with additional oxygen. Here, then, is another local mechanism that increases oxygen delivery to tissues with increased metabolic activity.

What is the mechanism by which these factors influence the affinity of hemoglobin for oxygen? Carbon dioxide and H^+ do so by combining with the globin portion of hemoglobin and altering the conformation of the hemoglobin molecule. Therefore, these effects are a form of allosteric modulation (Chapter 3). An elevated temperature also decreases hemoglobin's affinity for oxygen by altering its conformation.

DPG, which is produced during glycolysis, reversibly binds with hemoglobin, allosterically causing it to have a lower affinity for oxygen (see Figure 13.29). Erythrocytes have no mitochondria and, therefore, rely exclusively upon glycolysis. Consequently, erythrocytes contain large quantities of DPG, which is present in only trace amounts in cells with mitochondria. The net result is that whenever DPG levels increase, there is enhanced unloading of oxygen from hemoglobin as blood flows through the tissues. Such an increase in DPG concentration is triggered by a variety of conditions associated with inadequate oxygen supply to the tissues and helps to maintain oxygen delivery. For example, the increase in DPG is important during exposure to high altitude when the P_{O_2} of the blood is decreased because DPG increases the unloading of oxygen in the tissue capillaries.

Finally, the fetus has a unique form of hemoglobin called **fetal hemoglobin** (see Figure 13.29). Fetal hemoglobin contains subunits that are coded for by different genes than those that are expressed postnatally. These subunits alter the shape of the final protein and result in a hemoglobin molecule that has a higher affinity for oxygen than adult hemoglobin. That is, fetal hemoglobin binds considerably more oxygen than adult hemoglobin at any given P_{O_2}. This allows an increase in oxygen uptake across the placental diffusion barrier. Therefore, although fetal arterial P_{O_2} is much lower than that in the air-breathing newborn, fetal hemoglobin allows adequate oxygen uptake in the placenta to supply the developing fetus.

13.5 Transport of Carbon Dioxide in Blood

Remember that CO_2 is a waste product that has toxicity in part because it generates H^+. Large changes in H^+ concentration, if not buffered, would lead to significant changes in pH, thus altering the tertiary structure of proteins, including enzymes. In a resting person, metabolism generates about 200 mL of carbon dioxide per minute. When arterial blood flows through tissue capillaries, this volume of carbon dioxide diffuses from the tissues into the blood (**Figure 13.30a**).

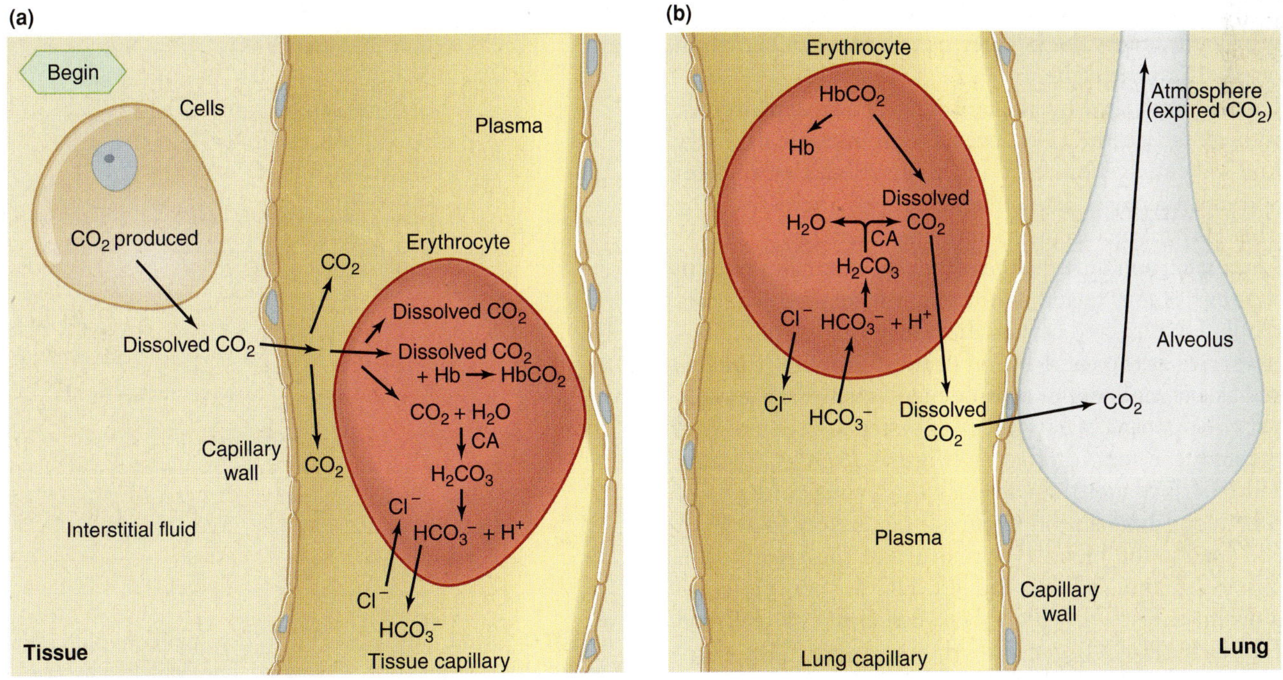

Figure 13.30 APR Summary of CO_2 movement. Expiration of CO_2 is by bulk flow, whereas all movements of CO_2 across membranes are by diffusion. Arrows reflect relative proportions of the fates of the CO_2. About two-thirds of the CO_2 entering the blood in the tissues ultimately is converted to HCO_3^- in the erythrocytes because carbonic anhydrase (CA) is located there, but most of the HCO_3^- then moves out of the erythrocytes into the plasma in exchange for Cl^- (the "chloride shift"). See Figure 13.31 for the fate of the H^+ generated in the erythrocytes.

Carbon dioxide is much more soluble in water than is oxygen, so blood carries more dissolved carbon dioxide than dissolved oxygen. Even so, only about 10% of the carbon dioxide entering the blood dissolves in the plasma and erythrocytes. In order to transport all of the CO_2 produced in the tissues to the lung, CO_2 in the blood must be carried in other forms.

Another 25% to 30% of the carbon dioxide molecules entering the blood react reversibly with the amino groups of hemoglobin to form **carbaminohemoglobin.** For simplicity, this reaction with hemoglobin is written as

$$CO_2 + Hb \rightleftharpoons HbCO_2 \quad (13\text{–}10)$$

This reaction is aided by the fact that deoxyhemoglobin, formed as blood flows through the tissue capillaries, has a greater affinity for carbon dioxide than does oxyhemoglobin.

The remaining 60% to 65% of the carbon dioxide molecules entering the blood in the tissues is converted to HCO_3^-:

$$CO_2 + H_2O \underset{}{\overset{\text{carbonic anhydrase}}{\rightleftharpoons}} \underset{\text{carbonic acid}}{H_2CO_3} \rightleftharpoons \underset{\text{bicarbonate}}{HCO_3^-} + H^+ \quad (13\text{–}11)$$

The first reaction in equation 13–11 is rate limiting and is very slow unless catalyzed in both directions by the enzyme **carbonic anhydrase.** This enzyme is present in the erythrocytes but not in the plasma; therefore, this reaction occurs mainly in the erythrocytes. In contrast, carbonic acid dissociates very rapidly into HCO_3^- and H^+ without any enzyme assistance. Once formed, most of the HCO_3^- moves out of the erythrocytes into the plasma via a transporter that exchanges one HCO_3^- for one chloride ion (this is called the "chloride shift," which maintains electroneutrality). HCO_3^- leaving the erythrocyte favors the balance of the reaction shown in equation 13–11 to the right.

The reactions shown in equation 13–11 also explain why, as mentioned earlier, the H^+ concentration in tissue capillary blood and systemic venous blood is higher than that in arterial blood and increases as metabolic activity increases. The fate of this H^+ will be discussed in the next section.

Because carbon dioxide undergoes these various fates in blood, it is customary to add up the amounts of dissolved carbon dioxide, HCO_3^-, and carbon dioxide in carbaminohemoglobin to arrive at the **total-blood carbon dioxide,** which is measured as a component of routine blood chemistry testing.

Just the opposite events occur as systemic venous blood flows through the lung capillaries (**Figure 13.30b**). Because the blood P_{CO_2} is higher than alveolar P_{CO_2}, a net diffusion of CO_2 from blood into alveoli occurs. This loss of CO_2 from the blood lowers the blood P_{CO_2} and drives the reactions in equations 13–10 and 13–11 to the left. HCO_3^- and H^+ combine to produce H_2CO_3, which then dissociates to CO_2 and H_2O. Similarly, $HbCO_2$ generates Hb and free CO_2. Normally, as fast as CO_2 is generated from HCO_3^- and H^+ and from $HbCO_2$, it diffuses into the alveoli. In this manner, the CO_2 that was delivered into the blood in the tissues is now delivered into the alveoli, from where it is eliminated during expiration.

13.6 Transport of Hydrogen Ion Between Tissues and Lungs

As blood flows through the tissues, a fraction of oxyhemoglobin loses its oxygen to become deoxyhemoglobin, while simultaneously a large quantity of carbon dioxide enters the blood and undergoes the reactions that generate HCO_3^- and H^+. What happens to this H^+?

Deoxyhemoglobin has a much greater affinity for H^+ than does oxyhemoglobin, so it binds (buffers) most of the H^+ (**Figure 13.31**). Indeed, deoxyhemoglobin can be abbreviated HbH rather than Hb to denote its binding of H^+. In effect, the reaction is

$$HbO_2 + H^+ \rightleftharpoons HbH + O_2$$

In this manner, only a small amount of the H^+ generated in the blood remains free. This explains why venous blood (pH = 7.36) is only slightly more acidic than arterial blood (pH = 7.40).

As the venous blood passes through the lungs, this reaction is reversed. Deoxyhemoglobin becomes converted to oxyhemoglobin and, in the process, releases the H^+ it picked up in the tissues. The H^+ reacts with HCO_3^- to produce carbonic acid, which, under the influence of carbonic anhydrase, dissociates to form carbon dioxide and water. The carbon dioxide diffuses into the alveoli to be expired. Normally, all the H^+ that is generated in the tissue capillaries from the reaction of carbon dioxide and water recombines with HCO_3^- to form carbon

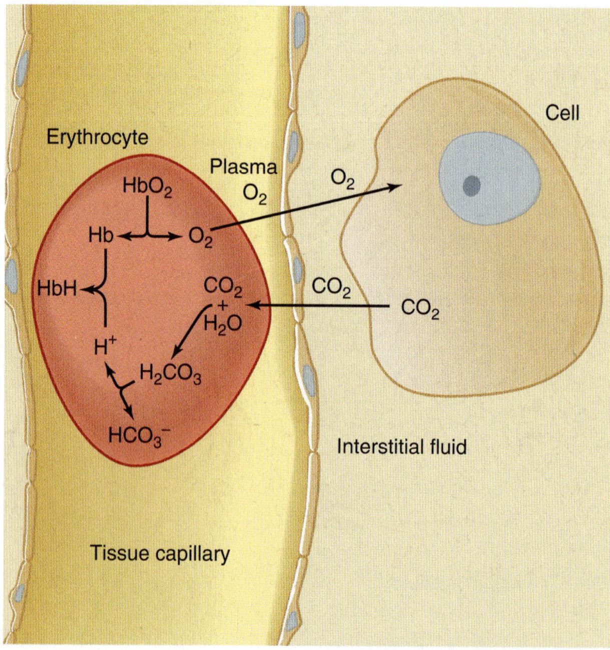

Figure 13.31 Binding of H^+ by hemoglobin as blood flows through tissue capillaries. This reaction is facilitated because deoxyhemoglobin, formed as oxygen dissociates from hemoglobin, has a greater affinity for H^+ than does oxyhemoglobin. For this reason, "Hb" and "HbH" are both abbreviations for deoxyhemoglobin. For simplicity, not shown is that H^+ binding to HbO_2 increases oxygen unloading.

TABLE 13.8 Effects of Various Factors on Hemoglobin

The affinity of hemoglobin for oxygen is decreased by

- Increased H^+ concentration
- Increased P_{CO_2}
- Increased temperature
- Increased DPG concentration

The affinity of hemoglobin for both H^+ and CO_2 is decreased by increased P_{O_2}; that is, deoxyhemoglobin has a greater affinity for H^+ and CO_2 than does oxyhemoglobin.

dioxide and water in the pulmonary capillaries. Therefore, none of this H^+ appears in the *arterial* blood.

What happens when a person is hypoventilating or has a lung disease that prevents normal elimination of carbon dioxide? Not only would arterial P_{CO_2} increase as a result, but so would arterial H^+ concentration. Increased arterial H^+ concentration due to carbon dioxide retention is termed ***respiratory acidosis.*** Conversely, hyperventilation would decrease arterial P_{CO_2} and H^+ concentration, producing ***respiratory alkalosis.***

The factors that influence the binding of CO_2 and O_2 by hemoglobin are summarized in **Table 13.8**.

Another aspect of the remarkable hemoglobin molecule is its ability to bind and transport **nitric oxide.** A present hypothesis is that as blood passes through the lungs, hemoglobin picks up and binds not only oxygen but also nitric oxide that is synthesized there, carries it to the peripheral tissues, and releases it along with oxygen. Simultaneously, via a different binding site, when nitric oxide production is increased in peripheral tissue (see Chapter 12), hemoglobin can pick up and catabolize nitric oxide. Theoretically, this cycle could play an important role in determining the peripheral concentration of nitric oxide and, thereby, the overall effect of this vasodilator agent. For example, by supplying net nitric oxide to the periphery, the process could cause additional vasodilation by systemic blood vessels. This would have effects on both local blood flow and systemic arterial blood pressure.

13.7 Control of Respiration

The control of breathing at rest, altitude, and during and after exercise has intrigued physiologists for centuries. It is a wonderful example of several general principles of physiology, including how homeostasis is essential for health and survival, and how physiological functions are controlled by multiple regulatory systems, often working in opposition.

Neural Generation of Rhythmic Breathing

The diaphragm and intercostal muscles are skeletal muscles and therefore do not contract unless motor neurons stimulate them to do so. Thus, breathing depends entirely upon cyclical respiratory muscle excitation of the diaphragm and the intercostal muscles by their motor neurons. Destruction of these neurons or a disconnection between their origin in the brain stem and the respiratory muscles results in paralysis of the respiratory muscles and death, unless some form of artificial respiration can be instituted.

Inspiration is initiated by a burst of action potentials in the spinal motor neurons to inspiratory muscles like the diaphragm. Then the action potentials cease, the inspiratory muscles relax, and expiration occurs as the elastic lungs recoil. In situations such as exercise when the contraction of expiratory muscles facilitates expiration, the neurons to these muscles, which were not active during inspiration, begin firing during expiration.

By what mechanism are impulses in the neurons innervating the respiratory muscles alternately increased and decreased? Control of this neural activity resides primarily in neurons in the medulla oblongata, the same area of the brain that contains the major cardiovascular control centers. (For the rest of this chapter, we will refer to the medulla oblongata simply as the medulla.) There are two main anatomical components of the **medullary respiratory center** (**Figure 13.32**). The neurons of the **dorsal respiratory group** (**DRG**) primarily fire during inspiration and have input to the spinal motor neurons that activate respiratory muscles involved in inspiration—the diaphragm and inspiratory intercostal muscles. The primary inspiratory muscle at rest is the diaphragm, which is innervated by the phrenic nerves. The **ventral respiratory group** (**VRG**) is the other main complex of neurons in the medullary respiratory center. The **respiratory rhythm generator** is located in the **pre-Bötzinger complex** of neurons in the upper part of the VRG. This rhythm generator appears to be composed of pacemaker cells and a complex neural network that, acting together, set the basal respiratory rate.

The VRG contains expiratory neurons that appear to be most important when large increases in ventilation are required (for example, during strenuous physical activity). During active expiration, motor neurons activated by the expiratory output from the VRG cause the expiratory muscles to contract. This helps to move air out of the lungs rather than depending only on the passive expiration that occurs during quiet breathing.

During quiet breathing, the respiratory rhythm generator activates inspiratory neurons in the VRG that depolarize the inspiratory spinal motor neurons, causing the inspiratory muscles to contract. When the inspiratory motor neurons stop firing, the inspiratory muscles relax, allowing passive expiration. During increases in breathing, the inspiratory and expiratory motor neurons and muscles are not activated at the same time but, rather, alternate in function.

The medullary inspiratory neurons receive a rich synaptic input from neurons in various areas of the pons, the part of the brainstem just above the medulla. This input fine-tunes the output of the medullary inspiratory neurons and may help terminate inspiration by inhibiting them. It is likely that an area of the lower pons called the **apneustic center** is the major source of this output, whereas an area of the upper pons called the **pneumotaxic center** modulates the activity of the apneustic center (see Figure 13.32). The pneumotaxic center, also known as the **pontine respiratory group,** helps to smooth the transition between inspiration and expiration.

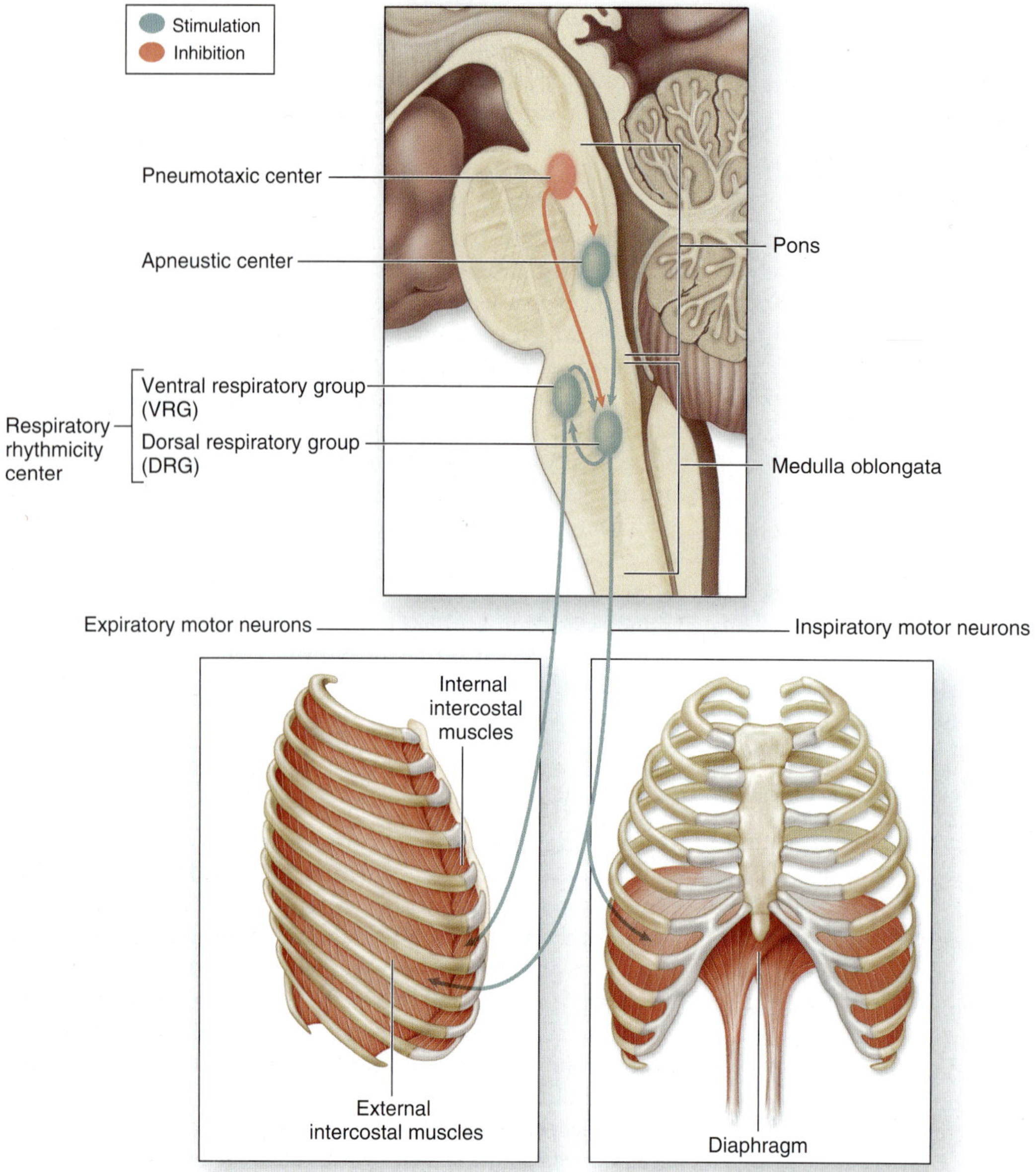

Figure 13.32 APIR A simplified depiction of the brainstem centers that control respiratory rate and depth. Inspiratory motor neurons are driven primarily by the DRG while expiratory motor neurons (active mostly during forced expiration and strenuous exercise) are driven primarily by the VRG. Note that DRG and VRG innervate each other allowing phasic inspiration and expiration. The centers in the upper pons are primarily responsible for fine-tuning respiratory control.

The respiratory nerves in the medulla and pons also receive synaptic input from higher centers of the brain such that the pattern of respiration is controlled voluntarily during speaking, diving, and even with emotions and pain.

Another cutoff signal for inspiration comes from **pulmonary stretch receptors,** which lie in the airway smooth muscle layer and are activated by a large lung inflation. Action potentials in the afferent nerve fibers from the stretch receptors travel to the brain and inhibit the activity of the medullary inspiratory neurons. This is called the **Hering–Breuer reflex.** Thus, feedback from the lungs helps to terminate inspiration by inhibiting inspiratory nerves in the DRG. However, this reflex plays a role in setting respiratory rhythm only under conditions of very large tidal volumes, as in strenuous exercise. The arterial chemoreceptors described next also have important input to the respiratory control centers such that the rate and depth of respiration can be increased when the levels of arterial oxygen decrease, or when arterial carbon dioxide or H^+ concentration increases.

A final point about the medullary inspiratory neurons is that they are quite sensitive to inhibition by drugs such as barbiturates and morphine. Death from an overdose of these drugs is often due directly to a cessation of breathing.

Control of Ventilation by P_{O_2}, P_{CO_2}, and H^+ Concentration

Respiratory rate and tidal volume are not fixed but can be increased or decreased over a wide range. For simplicity, we will describe the control of ventilation without discussing whether rate or depth makes the greater contribution to the change.

There are many inputs to the medullary inspiratory neurons, but the most important for the automatic control of ventilation at rest come from peripheral (arterial) chemoreceptors and central chemoreceptors.

The **peripheral chemoreceptors,** located high in the neck at the bifurcation of the common carotid arteries and in the thorax on the arch of the aorta (**Figure 13.33**) are called

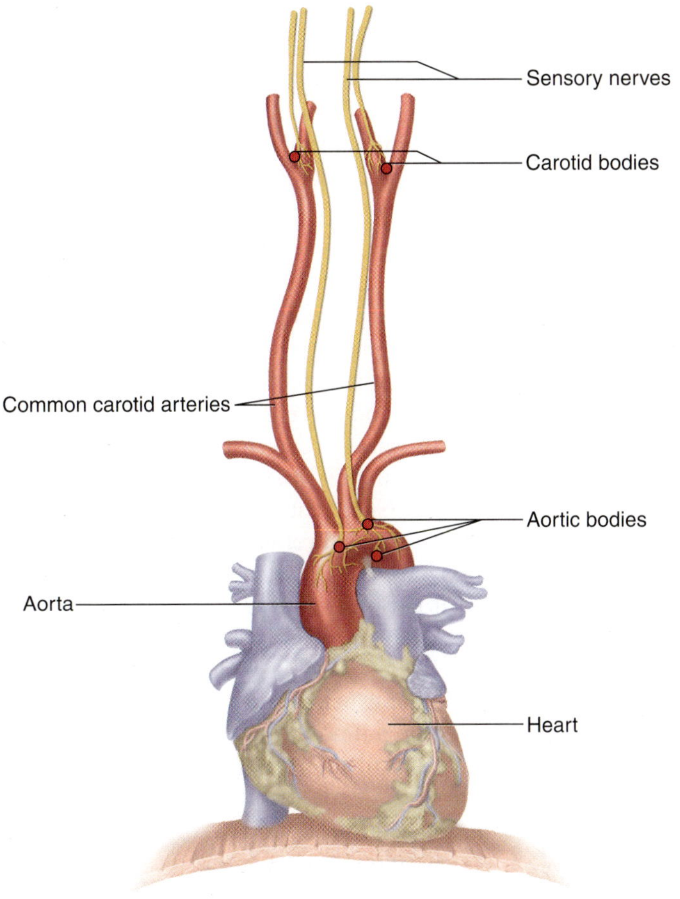

Figure 13.33 AP|R Location of the carotid and aortic bodies. Note that each carotid body is quite close to a carotid sinus, the major arterial baroreceptor (see Figure 12.53). Both right and left common carotid bifurcations contain a carotid sinus and a carotid body.

PHYSIOLOGICAL INQUIRY

- Several decades ago, removal of the carotid bodies was tried as a treatment for asthma. It was thought that it would reduce shortness of breath and airway hyperreactivity. What would be the effect of bilateral carotid body removal on someone taking a trip to the top of a mountain (an altitude of 3000 meters)? (*Hint:* Look ahead to Table 13.10.)

Answer can be found at end of chapter.

the **carotid bodies** and **aortic bodies,** respectively. In both locations, they are quite close to, but distinct from, the arterial baroreceptors and are in intimate contact with the arterial blood. The carotid bodies, in particular, are strategically located to monitor oxygen supply to the brain. The peripheral chemoreceptors are composed of specialized receptor cells stimulated mainly by a decrease in the arterial P_{O_2} and an increase in the arterial H^+ concentration (**Table 13.9**). These cells communicate synaptically with neuron terminals from which afferent nerve fibers pass to the brainstem. There they provide excitatory synaptic input to the medullary inspiratory neurons. The carotid body input is the predominant peripheral chemoreceptor involved in the control of respiration.

TABLE 13.9	Major Stimuli for the Central and Peripheral Chemoreceptors
Peripheral chemoreceptors—carotid bodies and aortic bodies—respond to changes in the arterial blood. They are stimulated by • Significantly decreased P_{O_2} (hypoxia) • Increased H^+ concentration (metabolic acidosis) • Increased P_{CO_2} (respiratory acidosis)	
Central chemoreceptors—located in the medulla oblongata—respond to changes in the *brain extracellular fluid.* They are stimulated by increased P_{CO_2} via associated changes in H^+ concentration (see equation 13–11).	

The **central chemoreceptors** are located in the medulla and, like the peripheral chemoreceptors, provide excitatory synaptic input to the medullary inspiratory neurons. They are stimulated by an increase in the H^+ concentration of the brain's extracellular fluid. As we will see later, such changes result mainly from changes in blood P_{CO_2}.

Control by P_{O_2}

Figure 13.34 illustrates an experiment in which healthy subjects breathe low-P_{O_2} gas mixtures for several minutes. The experiment is performed in a way that keeps arterial P_{CO_2} constant so that the pure effects of changing only P_{O_2} can be studied. Little increase in ventilation is observed until the oxygen concentration of the inspired air is reduced enough to lower arterial P_{O_2} to 60 mmHg. Beyond this point, any further reduction in arterial P_{O_2} causes a marked reflex increase in ventilation.

This reflex is mediated by the peripheral chemoreceptors (**Figure 13.35**). The low arterial P_{O_2} increases the rate at which the receptors discharge, resulting in an increased number of action potentials traveling up the afferent nerve fibers and stimulating the medullary inspiratory neurons. The resulting increase in ventilation provides more oxygen to the

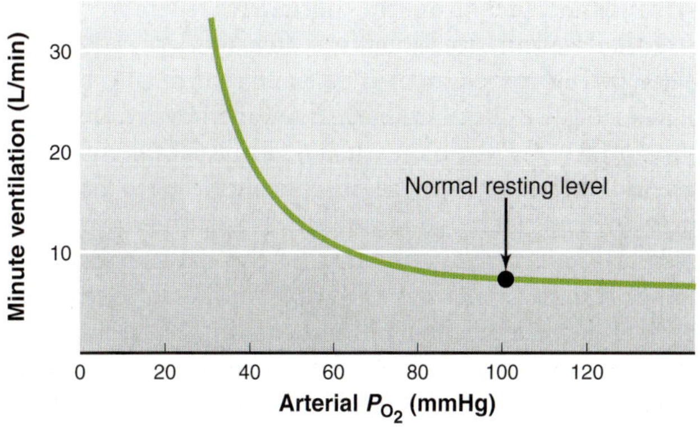

Figure 13.34 The effect on ventilation of breathing different oxygen mixtures. The arterial P_{CO_2} was maintained at 40 mmHg throughout the experiment.

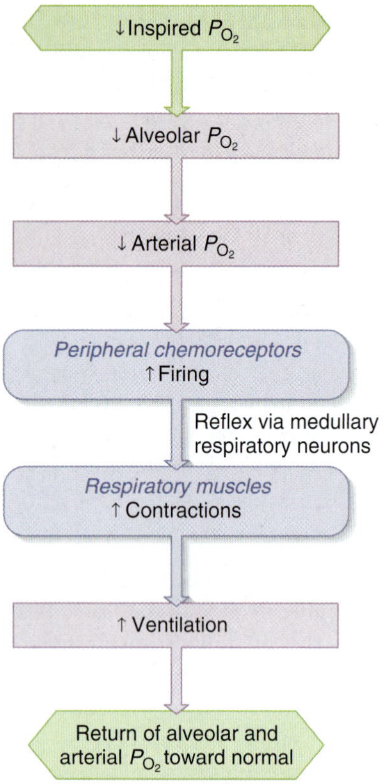

Figure 13.35 Sequence of events by which a low arterial P_{O_2} causes hyperventilation, which maintains alveolar (and, hence, arterial) P_{O_2} at a value higher than would exist if the ventilation had remained unchanged.

alveoli and minimizes the decrease in alveolar and arterial P_{O_2} produced by the low-P_{O_2} gas mixture.

It may seem surprising that we are insensitive to smaller reductions of arterial P_{O_2} but look again at the oxygen–hemoglobin dissociation curve (see Figure 13.26). Total oxygen transport by the blood is not really reduced very much until the arterial P_{O_2} falls below about 60 mmHg. Therefore, increased ventilation would not result in much more oxygen being added to the blood until that point is reached.

To reiterate, the peripheral chemoreceptors respond to decreases in arterial P_{O_2}, as occurs in lung disease or exposure to high altitude. However, the peripheral chemoreceptors are *not* stimulated in situations in which modest reductions take place in the oxygen *content* of the blood but no change occurs in arterial P_{O_2}. As stated earlier, anemia is a decrease in the amount of hemoglobin present in the blood without a decrease in arterial P_{O_2}, because the concentration of dissolved oxygen in the arterial blood is normal; that is, the P_{O_2} of arterial blood is determined primarily by the oxygen-diffusion capacity of the lung, whereas the total amount of oxygen in the blood is also dependent on the amount of hemoglobin there to carry the oxygen. Therefore, mild to moderate anemia, in which arterial P_{O_2} is usually normal, does not activate peripheral chemoreceptors and does not stimulate increased ventilation.

This same analysis holds true when oxygen content is reduced moderately by the presence of carbon monoxide, which, as described earlier, reduces the amount of oxygen combined with hemoglobin by competing for these sites. Because carbon monoxide does not affect the amount of oxygen that can dissolve in blood and does not alter the oxygen-diffusion capacity of the lung, the arterial P_{O_2} is unaltered, and no increase in peripheral chemoreceptor output or ventilation occurs.

Control by P_{CO_2}

Figure 13.36 illustrates an experiment in which subjects breathe air with variable quantities of carbon dioxide added. The presence of carbon dioxide in the inspired air causes an increase in alveolar P_{CO_2}, and therefore the diffusion gradient for CO_2 is reversed from the normal situation. This results in a net uptake of CO_2 from the alveolar air and, therefore, an increase in arterial P_{CO_2}. Note that even a very small increase in arterial P_{CO_2} causes a marked reflex increase in ventilation. Experiments like this have documented that the reflex mechanisms controlling ventilation prevent small increases in arterial P_{CO_2} to a much greater degree than they prevent equivalent decreases in arterial P_{O_2}.

Of course, we do not usually breathe bags of gas containing carbon dioxide. Some pulmonary diseases, such as emphysema, can cause the body to retain carbon dioxide, resulting in an increase in arterial P_{CO_2} that stimulates ventilation. This promotes the elimination of the carbon dioxide. Conversely, if arterial P_{CO_2} decreases below normal levels for whatever reason, this removes some of the stimulus for ventilation. This reduces ventilation and allows metabolically produced carbon dioxide to accumulate, thereby returning the P_{CO_2} to normal. In this manner, the arterial P_{CO_2} is stabilized near the normal value of 40 mmHg.

The ability of changes in arterial P_{CO_2} to control ventilation reflexively is largely due to associated changes in H^+ concentration (see equation 13–11). As summarized in

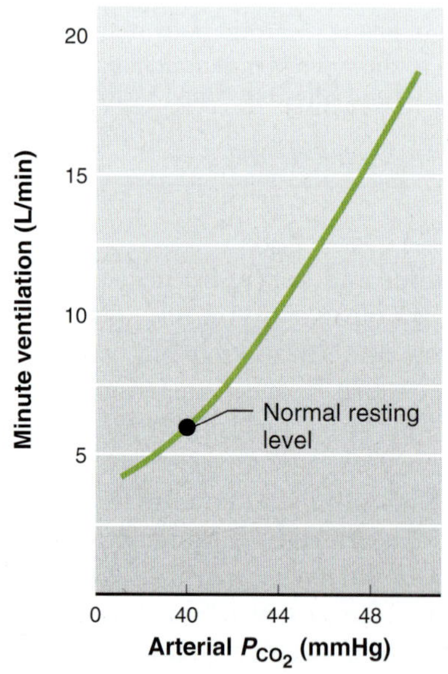

Figure 13.36 Effects on respiration of increasing arterial P_{CO_2} achieved by adding CO_2 to inspired air.

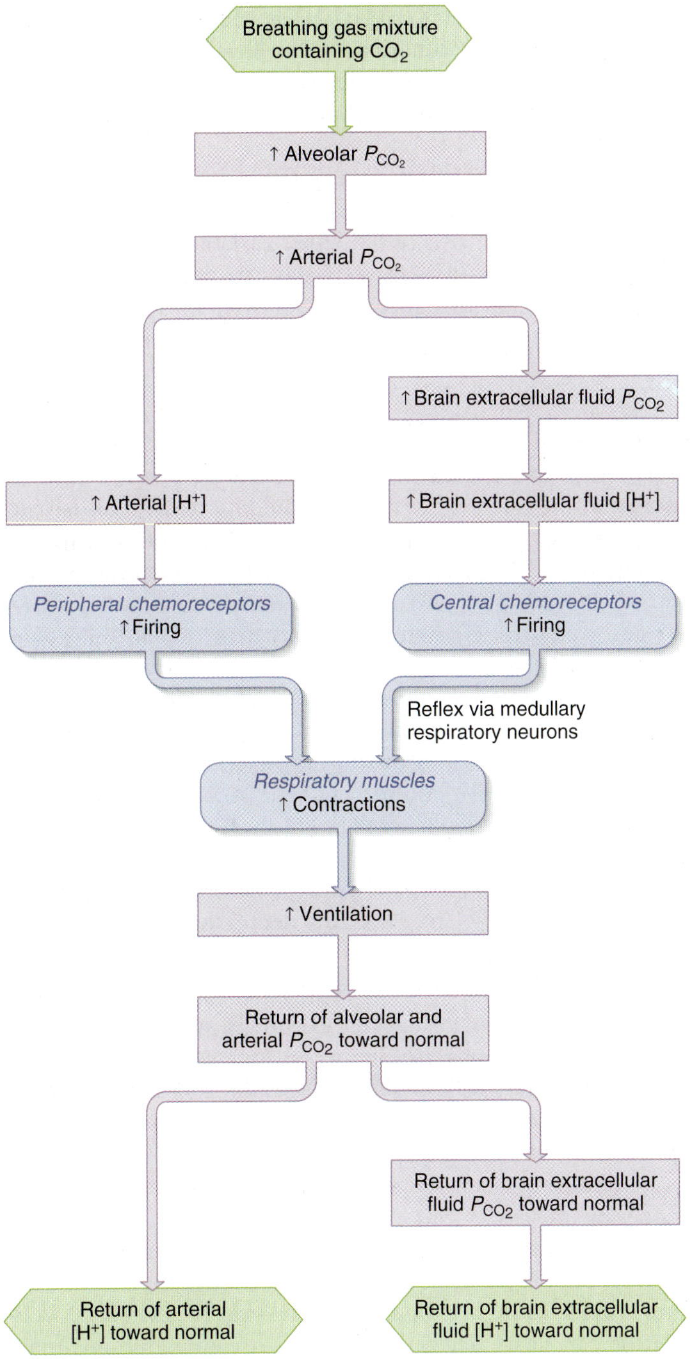

Figure 13.37 Pathways by which increased arterial P_{CO_2} stimulates ventilation. Note that the peripheral chemoreceptors are stimulated by an *increase* in H^+ concentration, whereas they are also stimulated by a *decrease* in P_{O_2} (see Figure 13.35).

Figure 13.37, both the peripheral and central chemoreceptors initiate the pathways that mediate these reflexes. The peripheral chemoreceptors are stimulated by the increased arterial H^+ concentration resulting from the increased P_{CO_2}. At the same time, because carbon dioxide diffuses rapidly across the membranes separating capillary blood and brain tissue, the increase in arterial P_{CO_2} causes a rapid increase in brain extracellular fluid P_{CO_2}. This increased P_{CO_2} increases *brain extracellular fluid* H^+ concentration, which stimulates the central chemoreceptors. Inputs from both the peripheral and central chemoreceptors stimulate the medullary inspiratory neurons to increase ventilation. The end result is a return of arterial and brain extracellular fluid P_{CO_2} and H^+ concentration toward normal. Of the two sets of receptors involved in this reflex response to elevated P_{CO_2}, the central chemoreceptors are the more important, accounting for about 70% of the increased ventilation.

It should also be noted that the effects of increased P_{CO_2} and decreased P_{O_2} not only exist as independent inputs to the medulla but potentiate each other's effects. The acute ventilatory response to combined low P_{O_2} and high P_{CO_2} is considerably greater than the sum of the individual responses.

Throughout this section, we have described the stimulatory effects of carbon dioxide on ventilation via reflex input to the medulla, but very high levels of carbon dioxide actually *inhibit* ventilation and may be lethal. This is because such concentrations of carbon dioxide act directly on the medulla to inhibit the respiratory neurons by an anesthesia-like effect, another example of a harmful effect of excess carbon dioxide. Other symptoms caused by very high blood P_{CO_2} include severe headaches, restlessness, and dulling or loss of consciousness.

Control by Changes in Arterial H^+ Concentration That Are Not Due to Changes in Carbon Dioxide

We have seen that retention or excessive elimination of carbon dioxide causes respiratory acidosis and respiratory alkalosis, respectively. There are, however, many normal and pathological situations in which a change in arterial H^+ concentration is due to some cause other than a primary change in P_{CO_2}. This is termed ***metabolic acidosis*** when H^+ concentration is increased and ***metabolic alkalosis*** when it is decreased. In such cases, the peripheral chemoreceptors play the major role in altering ventilation.

For example, the addition of lactic acid to the blood, as in strenuous exercise, causes hyperventilation almost entirely by stimulation of the peripheral chemoreceptors (**Figure 13.38** and **Figure 13.39**). The central chemoreceptors are only

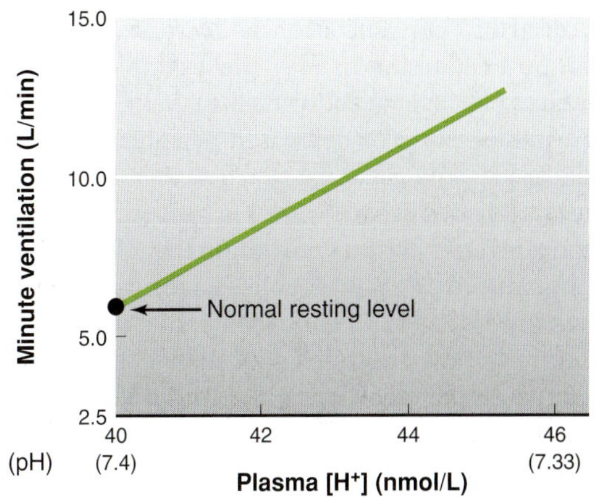

Figure 13.38 Changes in ventilation in response to an elevation of plasma H^+ concentration produced by the administration of lactic acid. Adapted from Lambertsen.

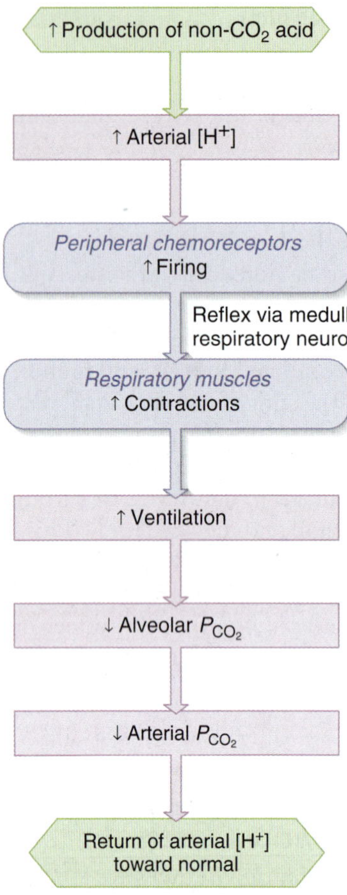

Figure 13.39 Reflexively induced hyperventilation minimizes the change in arterial H^+ concentration when acids are produced in excess in the body. Note that under such conditions, arterial P_{CO_2} is reflexively reduced below its normal value.

minimally stimulated in this case because brain H^+ concentration is increased to only a small extent, at least early on, by the H^+ generated from the lactic acid. This is because H^+ penetrates the blood–brain barrier very slowly. In contrast, as described earlier, carbon dioxide penetrates the blood–brain barrier easily and changes brain H^+ concentration.

The converse of the previous situation is also true: When arterial H^+ concentration is decreased by any means other than by a reduction in P_{CO_2} (for example, by the loss of H^+ from the stomach when vomiting), ventilation is reflexively depressed because of decreased peripheral chemoreceptor output.

The adaptive value such reflexes have in regulating arterial H^+ concentration is shown in Figure 13.39. The increased ventilation induced by a metabolic acidosis reduces arterial P_{CO_2}, which lowers arterial H^+ concentration back toward normal. Similarly, hypoventilation induced by a metabolic alkalosis results in an elevated arterial P_{CO_2} and a restoration of H^+ concentration toward normal.

Notice that when a change in arterial H^+ concentration due to some acid unrelated to carbon dioxide influences ventilation via the peripheral chemoreceptors, P_{CO_2} is displaced from normal. This is a reflex that regulates arterial H^+ concentration at the expense of changes in arterial P_{CO_2}. Maintenance of normal arterial H^+ is necessary because most enzymes of the body function best at physiological pH.

Figure 13.40 summarizes the control of ventilation by P_{O_2}, P_{CO_2}, and H^+ concentration.

Control of Ventilation During Exercise

During exercise, the alveolar ventilation may increase as much as 20-fold. On the basis of our three variables—P_{O_2}, P_{CO_2}, and H^+ concentration—it may seem easy to explain the mechanism that induces this increased ventilation. This is not the case, however, and the major stimuli to ventilation during exercise, at least moderate exercise, remain unclear.

Increased P_{CO_2} *as the Stimulus?*

It would seem logical that, as the exercising muscles produce more carbon dioxide, blood P_{CO_2} would increase. This is true, however, only for systemic *venous* blood but not for systemic *arterial* blood. Why is it that arterial P_{CO_2} does not increase during exercise? Recall two facts from the section on alveolar gas pressures: (1) Arterial P_{CO_2} is determined by alveolar P_{CO_2}, and (2) alveolar P_{CO_2} is determined by the ratio of carbon dioxide production to alveolar ventilation. During moderate exercise, the alveolar ventilation increases in exact proportion to the increased carbon dioxide production, so alveolar and therefore arterial P_{CO_2} do not change. In fact, in very strenuous exercise, the alveolar ventilation increases relatively more than carbon dioxide production. In other words, during strenuous exercise, a person may hyperventilate; thus, alveolar and systemic arterial P_{CO_2} may actually decrease (**Figure 13.41**)!

Decreased P_{O_2} *as the Stimulus?*

The story is similar for oxygen. Although systemic *venous* P_{O_2} decreases during exercise due to an increase in oxygen consumption in the tissues, alveolar P_{O_2} and, therefore, systemic *arterial* P_{O_2} usually remain unchanged (see Figure 13.41). This is because cellular oxygen consumption and alveolar ventilation increase in exact proportion to each other, at least during moderate exercise.

This is a good place to recall an important point made in Chapter 12. In healthy individuals, ventilation is not the limiting factor in strenuous exercise—cardiac output is. Ventilation can, as we have just seen, increase enough to maintain arterial P_{O_2}.

Increased H^+ *Concentration as the Stimulus?*

Because the arterial P_{CO_2} does not change during moderate exercise and decreases during strenuous exercise, there is no accumulation of excess H^+ resulting from carbon dioxide accumulation. However, during strenuous exercise, there *is* an increase in arterial H^+ concentration (see Figure 13.41) due to the generation and release of lactic acid into the blood. This change in H^+ concentration is responsible, in part, for stimulating the hyperventilation accompanying strenuous exercise.

Other Factors

A variety of other factors play some role in stimulating ventilation during exercise. These include (1) reflex input from mechanoreceptors in joints and muscles, (2) an increase in

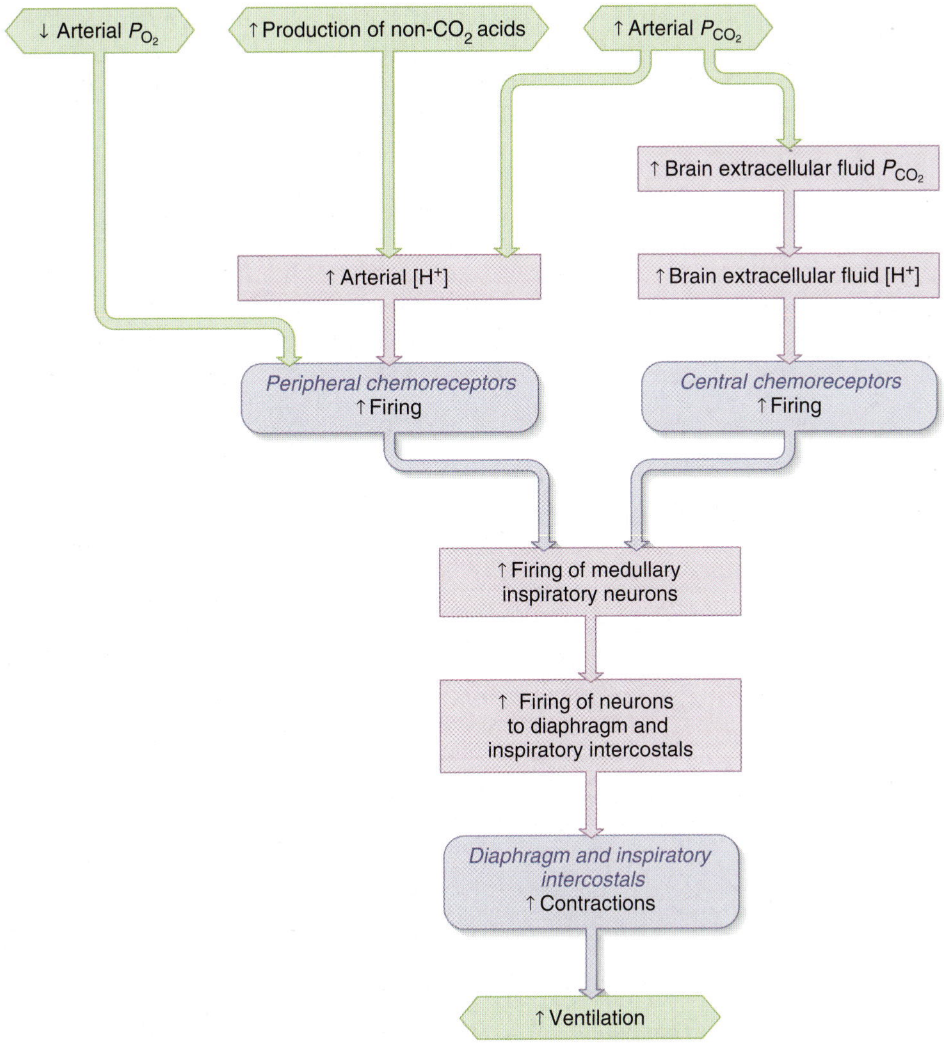

Figure 13.40 Summary of the major chemical inputs that stimulate ventilation. This is a combination of Figures 13.35, 13.37, and 13.39. When arterial P_{O_2} increases or when P_{CO_2} or H^+ concentration decreases, ventilation is reflexively decreased.

body temperature, (3) inputs to the respiratory neurons via branches from axons descending from the brain to motor neurons supplying the exercising muscles (central command), (4) an increase in the plasma epinephrine concentration, (5) an increase in the plasma potassium concentration due to movement of potassium out of the exercising muscles, and (6) a conditioned (learned) response mediated by neural input to the respiratory centers. The operation of factors (1) and (3) are most likely and can be seen in **Figure 13.42**. There is an abrupt increase—within seconds—in ventilation at the onset of exercise and an equally abrupt decrease at the end; these changes occur too rapidly to be explained by alteration of chemical constituents of the blood or by altered body temperature.

Figure 13.43 summarizes various factors that influence ventilation during exercise. The possibility that oscillatory changes in arterial P_{O_2}, P_{CO_2}, or H^+ concentration occur—despite unchanged average levels of these variables—and play some role has been proposed, but this remains unproven.

Other Ventilatory Responses

Protective Reflexes

A group of responses protect the respiratory system from irritant materials. Most familiar are the cough and the sneeze reflexes, which originate in sensory receptors located between airway epithelial cells. The receptors for the sneeze reflex are in the nose or pharynx; those for cough are in the larynx, trachea, and bronchi. When the receptors initiating a cough are stimulated, the medullary respiratory neurons reflexively cause a deep inspiration and a violent expiration. In this manner, particles and secretions are moved from smaller to larger airways and aspiration of materials into the lungs is also prevented.

Alcohol inhibits the cough reflex, which may partially explain the susceptibility of alcoholics to choking and pneumonia.

Another example of a protective reflex is the immediate cessation of respiration that is often triggered when noxious agents are inhaled. Chronic smoking may cause a loss of this reflex.

Voluntary Control of Breathing

Although we have discussed in detail the involuntary nature of most respiratory reflexes, the voluntary control of respiratory movements is important. Voluntary control is accomplished by descending pathways from the cerebral cortex to the motor neurons of the respiratory muscles. This voluntary control of respiration cannot be maintained when the involuntary stimuli, such as an elevated P_{CO_2} or H^+ concentration, become intense. An example is the inability to hold your breath for very long.

The opposite of breath holding—deliberate hyperventilation—lowers alveolar and arterial P_{CO_2} and increases P_{O_2}. Unfortunately, swimmers sometimes voluntarily hyperventilate immediately before underwater swimming to be able to hold their breath longer. We say "unfortunately" because the low P_{CO_2} may still permit breath holding at a time when the exertion is decreasing the arterial P_{O_2} to levels that can cause unconsciousness and lead to drowning.

Besides the obvious forms of voluntary control, respiration must also be controlled during such complex actions as speaking, singing, and swallowing.

Reflexes from J Receptors

In the lungs, either in the capillary walls or the interstitium, are a group of sensory receptors called **J receptors.** They are normally dormant but are stimulated by an increase in lung

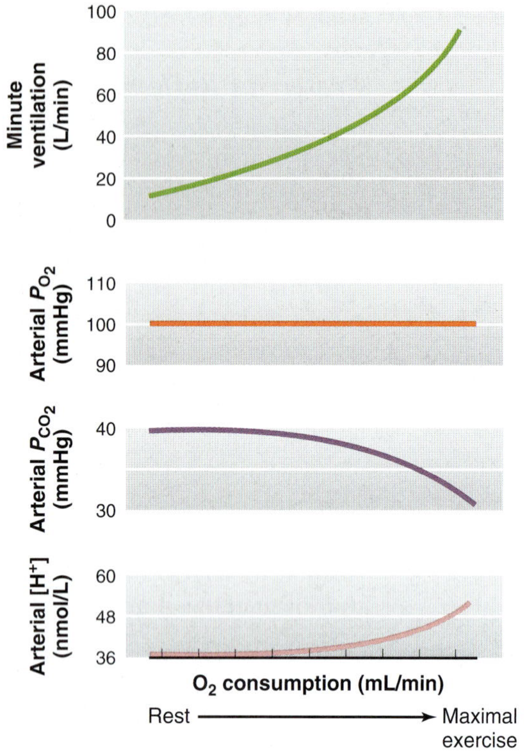

Figure 13.41 The effect of exercise on ventilation, arterial gas pressures, and H^+ concentration. All these variables remain constant during moderate exercise; any change occurs only during strenuous exercise, when the person is actually hyperventilating (decrease in P_{CO_2}). Adapted from Comroe.

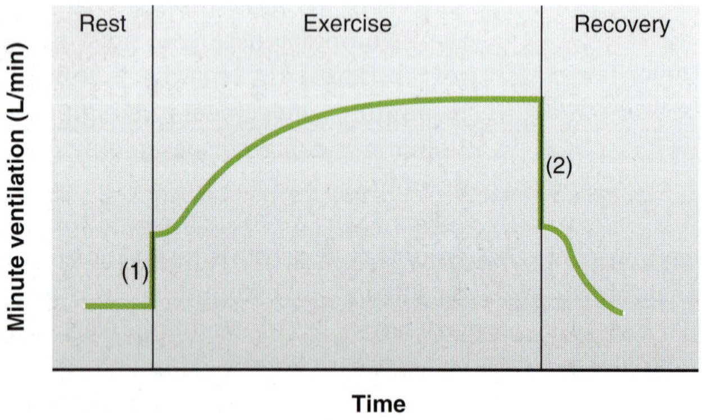

Figure 13.42 Ventilation changes during exercise. Note (1) the abrupt increase at the onset of exercise and (2) the equally abrupt but larger decrease at the end of exercise.

interstitial pressure caused by the collection of fluid in the interstitium. Such an increase occurs during the vascular congestion caused by either occlusion of a pulmonary vessel (called a ***pulmonary embolism***) or left ventricular heart failure (Chapter 12), as well as by strenuous exercise in healthy people. The main reflex effects are rapid breathing (tachypnea) and a dry cough. In addition, neural input from J receptors gives rise to sensations of pressure in the chest and ***dyspnea***—the feeling that breathing is labored or difficult.

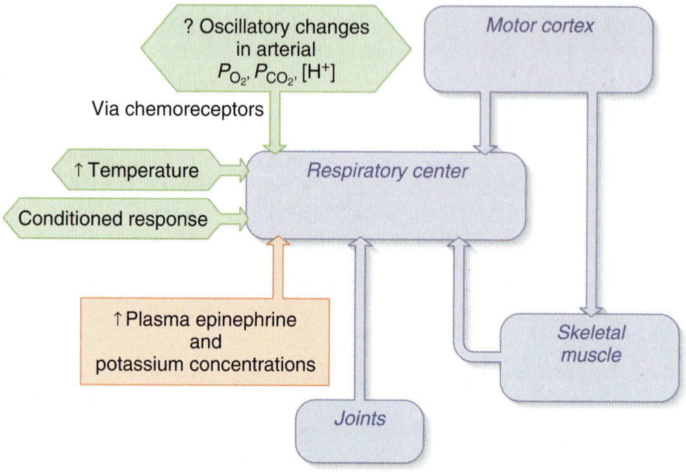

Figure 13.43 Summary of factors that stimulate ventilation during exercise. *Note:* "?" indicates a theoretical input.

PHYSIOLOGICAL INQUIRY

- The existence of chemoreceptors in the pulmonary artery has been suggested. Hypothesize a function for peripheral chemoreceptors located on and sensing the P_{O_2} and P_{CO_2} of the blood in the pulmonary artery.

Answer can be found at end of chapter.

13.8 Hypoxia

Hypoxia is defined as a deficiency of oxygen at the tissue level. There are many potential causes of hypoxia, but they can be classified into four general categories: (1) ***hypoxic hypoxia*** (also termed ***hypoxemia***), in which the arterial P_{O_2} is reduced; (2) ***anemic hypoxia*** or ***carbon monoxide hypoxia,*** in which the arterial P_{O_2} is normal but the total oxygen *content* of the blood is reduced because of inadequate numbers of erythrocytes, deficient or abnormal hemoglobin, or competition for the hemoglobin molecule by carbon monoxide; (3) ***ischemic hypoxia*** (also called *hypoperfusion hypoxia*), in which blood flow to the tissues is too low; and (4) ***histotoxic hypoxia,*** in which the quantity of oxygen reaching the tissues is normal but the cell is unable to utilize the oxygen because a toxic agent—cyanide, for example—has interfered with the cell's metabolic machinery.

Hypoxic hypoxia is a common cause of hypoxia. The primary causes of hypoxic hypoxia in disease are listed in **Table 13.10**. Exposure to the reduced P_{O_2} of high altitude also causes hypoxic hypoxia but is, of course, not a disease. The brief summaries in Table 13.10 provide a review of many of the key aspects of respiratory physiology and pathophysiology described in this chapter.

This table also emphasizes that some of the diseases that produce hypoxia also produce carbon dioxide retention and an increased arterial P_{CO_2} (***hypercapnia***). In such cases, treating only the oxygen deficit by administering oxygen may be inadequate because it does nothing about the hypercapnia. Indeed,

TABLE 13.10 Causes of a Decreased Arterial P_{O_2} (Hypoxic Hypoxia) in Disease

I. ***Hypoventilation*** may be caused by
   A. A defect anywhere along the respiratory control pathway, from the medulla through the respiratory muscles
   B. Severe thoracic cage abnormalities
   C. Major obstruction of the upper airway

The hypoxemia of hypoventilation is always accompanied by an increased arterial P_{CO_2}.

II. ***Diffusion impairment*** results from thickening of the alveolar membranes or a decrease in their surface area. In turn, it causes blood P_{O_2} and alveolar P_{O_2} to fail to equilibrate. Often, it is apparent only during exercise. Arterial P_{CO_2} is either normal because carbon dioxide diffuses more readily than oxygen or reduced if the hypoxemia reflexively stimulates ventilation.

III. A ***shunt*** is
   A. An anatomical abnormality of the cardiovascular system that causes mixed venous blood to bypass ventilated alveoli in passing from the right side of the heart to the left side
   B. An intrapulmonary defect in which mixed venous blood perfuses unventilated alveoli. Arterial P_{CO_2} generally does not increase because the effect of the shunt on arterial P_{CO_2} is counterbalanced by the increased ventilation reflexively stimulated by the hypoxemia.

IV. ***Ventilation–perfusion inequality*** is by far the most common cause of hypoxemia. It occurs in chronic obstructive lung diseases and many other lung diseases. Arterial P_{CO_2} may be normal or increased, depending upon how much ventilation is reflexively stimulated.

such therapy may be dangerous. The primary respiratory drive in such patients is the hypoxia, because for several reasons the reflex ventilatory response to an increased P_{CO_2} may be lost in chronic situations. The administration of pure oxygen may cause such patients to stop breathing; consequently, such individuals are typically treated with a mixture of air and oxygen rather than 100% oxygen.

Why Do Ventilation–Perfusion Abnormalities Affect O_2 More Than CO_2?

As described in Table 13.10, ventilation–perfusion inequalities often cause hypoxemia without associated increases in P_{CO_2}. The explanation for this resides in the fundamental difference between the transport of O_2 and the transport of CO_2 in the blood. Recall that the shape of the oxygen–hemoglobin dissociation curve is sigmoidal (see Figure 13.26). An increase in P_{O_2} above 100 mmHg does not add much oxygen to hemoglobin that is already almost 100% saturated. If poorly ventilated, diseased alveoli are perfused with blood and they will contribute blood with low oxygen to the pulmonary vein and, thus, to the general circulation. If increases in ventilation ensue in order to compensate for this, the increase in P_{O_2} in the healthy part of the lung does not add much oxygen to the blood from that region because of the minimal increase in oxygen saturation. As blood from these different areas of the lung mix in the pulmonary vein, the net result is still deoxygenated blood (hypoxemia).

The situation for CO_2, however, is very different. The CO_2 content curve is relatively linear because CO_2 is transported in the blood mainly as highly soluble HCO_3^-, which does not reach saturating levels at physiological concentrations. Therefore, although poorly ventilated areas of the lungs do cause increases in the CO_2 content of the blood entering the pulmonary vein (because CO_2 accumulates in the alveoli in those areas), a compensatory increase in ventilation *lowers* CO_2 content below normal in the blood from the well-ventilated areas of the lung. The net result, as blood mixes in the pulmonary vein in this case, is essentially normal arterial CO_2 content and P_{CO_2}. Thus, clinically significant ventilation–perfusion mismatching can lead to low arterial P_{O_2} with normal P_{CO_2}.

Emphysema

The pathophysiology of emphysema, a major cause of hypoxia, offers an instructive review of many basic principles of respiratory physiology. ***Emphysema*** is characterized by a loss of elastic tissue and the destruction of the alveolar walls leading to an increase in compliance. Furthermore, atrophy and collapse of the lower airways—those from the terminal bronchioles on down—can occur. The lungs actually self-destruct, attacked by proteolytic enzymes secreted by leukocytes in response to a variety of factors. Cigarette smoking is by far the most important of these factors; it stimulates the release of the proteolytic enzymes and destroys other enzymes that normally protect the lung against them.

As a result of alveolar-wall loss, adjacent alveoli fuse to form fewer but larger alveoli, and there is a loss of the pulmonary capillaries that were originally in the walls. The merging of alveoli, often into huge balloonlike structures, reduces the *total* surface area available for diffusion, and this impairs gas exchange. Moreover, because the destructive changes are not uniform throughout the lungs, some areas may receive large amounts of air and little blood, whereas others show just the opposite pattern. The result is marked ventilation–perfusion inequality.

In addition to problems in gas exchange, emphysema is associated with a large increase in airway resistance, which greatly increases the work of breathing and, if severe enough, may cause hypoventilation. This is why emphysema is classified, as noted earlier in this chapter, as a "chronic *obstructive* pulmonary disease." The airway obstruction in emphysema is caused by the collapse of the lower airways, particularly during expiration. To understand this, recall that two physical factors passively holding the airways open are the transpulmonary pressure and the lateral traction of connective-tissue fibers attached to the airway exteriors. Both of these factors are diminished in emphysema because of the destruction of the lung elastic tissues, so the airways collapse.

In summary, patients with emphysema suffer from decreased elastic recoil of the lungs, increased airway resistance, decreased total area available for diffusion, and ventilation–perfusion inequality. The result, particularly of the ventilation–perfusion inequality, is always some degree of hypoxia. As already explained, an increase in arterial P_{CO_2} will not occur until the disease becomes extensive and prevents increases in alveolar ventilation.

Acclimatization to High Altitude

Atmospheric pressure progressively decreases as altitude increases. Thus, at the top of Mt. Everest (approximately 29,029 ft or 8848 m), the atmospheric pressure is 253 mmHg, compared to 760 mmHg at sea level. The air is still 21% oxygen, which means that the inspired P_{O_2} is 53 mmHg (0.21 × 253 mmHg). Therefore, the alveolar and arterial P_{O_2} must decrease as persons ascend unless they breathe pure oxygen. The highest villages permanently inhabited by people are in the Andes at approximately 18,000 ft (5486 m).

The effects of oxygen deprivation vary from one individual to another, but most people who ascend rapidly to altitudes above 10,000 ft experience some degree of ***mountain sickness*** (***altitude sickness***). This disorder consists of breathlessness, headache, nausea, vomiting, insomnia, fatigue, and impairment of mental processes. Much more serious is the appearance, in some individuals, of life-threatening pulmonary edema, which is the leakage of fluid from the pulmonary capillaries into the alveolar walls and eventually the airspaces themselves. This occurs because of the development of pulmonary hypertension, as pulmonary arterioles reflexively constrict in the presence of low oxygen, as described earlier. Brain edema can also occur. Supplemental oxygen and diuretic therapy are used to treat mountain sickness; diuretics help reduce blood pressure, including in the pulmonary circulation, by promoting water loss in the urine. This reduces the amount of fluid leaving the capillaries in the lungs and brain.

Over the course of several days, the symptoms of mountain sickness usually disappear, although maximal physical capacity remains reduced. Acclimatization to high altitude is achieved by the compensatory mechanisms listed in **Table 13.11**.

TABLE 13.11 Acclimatization to the Hypoxia of High Altitude
The peripheral chemoreceptors stimulate ventilation.
Erythropoietin, a hormone secreted primarily by the kidneys, stimulates erythrocyte synthesis—resulting in increased erythrocyte and hemoglobin concentration in blood—and the oxygen-carrying capacity of blood.
DPG increases and shifts the oxygen–hemoglobin dissociation curve to the right, facilitating oxygen unloading in the tissues. However, this DPG change is not always adaptive and may be maladaptive. For example, at very high altitudes, a right shift in the curve impairs oxygen *loading* in the lungs, an effect that outweighs any benefit from facilitation of *unloading* in the tissues.
Increases in skeletal muscle capillary density (due to hypoxia-induced expression of the genes that code for angiogenic factors), number of mitochondria, and muscle myoglobin occur, all of which increase oxygen transfer.
Plasma volume can be decreased, resulting in an increased concentration of the erythrocytes and hemoglobin in the blood.

Finally, note that the responses to high altitude are essentially the same as the responses to hypoxia from any other cause. Thus, a person with severe hypoxia from lung disease may show many of the same changes—increased hematocrit, for example—as a high-altitude sojourner.

13.9 Nonrespiratory Functions of the Lungs

The lungs perform a variety of functions in addition to their roles in gas exchange and regulation of H^+ concentration. Most notable are the influences they have on the arterial concentrations of a large number of biologically active substances. Many substances (neurotransmitters and paracrine agents, for example) released locally into interstitial fluid may diffuse into capillaries and thus make their way into the systemic venous system. The lungs partially or completely remove some of these substances from the blood and thereby prevent them from reaching other locations in the body via the arteries. The cells that perform this function are the endothelial cells lining the pulmonary capillaries.

In contrast, the lungs may also produce new substances and add them to the blood. Some of these substances play local regulatory roles within the lungs, but if produced in large enough quantity, they may diffuse into the pulmonary capillaries and be carried to the rest of the body. For example, inflammatory responses (see Chapter 18) in the lung may lead, via excessive release of potent chemicals such as histamine, to alterations of systemic blood pressure or flow. In at least one case, the lungs contribute to the production of a hormone, angiotensin II, which is produced by the action of an enzyme located on endothelial cells throughout much of the body (see Chapter 14).

Finally, the lungs also act as a sieve that traps small blood clots generated in the systemic circulation, thereby preventing them from reaching the systemic arterial blood where they could occlude blood vessels in other organs.

Table 13.12 summarizes the functions of the respiratory system.

TABLE 13.12 Functions of the Respiratory System
Provides oxygen
Eliminates carbon dioxide
Regulates the blood's hydrogen ion concentration (pH) in coordination with the kidneys
Forms speech sounds (phonation)
Defends against microbes
Influences arterial concentrations of chemical messengers by removing some from pulmonary capillary blood and producing and adding others to this blood
Traps and dissolves blood clots arising from systemic veins such as those in the legs

SUMMARY

Organization of the Respiratory System

I. The respiratory system comprises the lungs, the airways leading to them, and the chest structures responsible for moving air into and out of them.
   a. The conducting zone of the airways consists of the trachea, bronchi, and terminal bronchioles.
   b. The respiratory zone of the airways consists of the alveoli, which are the sites of gas exchange, and those airways to which alveoli are attached.
   c. The alveoli are lined by type I cells and some type II cells, which produce surfactant.
   d. The lungs and interior of the thorax are covered by pleura; between the two pleural layers is an extremely thin layer of intrapleural fluid.

II. The lungs are elastic structures whose volume depends upon the pressure difference across the lungs—the transpulmonary pressure—and how stretchable the lungs are.

III. The steps involved in respiration are summarized in Figure 13.6. In the steady state, the net volumes of oxygen and carbon dioxide exchanged in the lungs per unit time are equal to the net volumes exchanged in the tissues.

Ventilation and Lung Mechanics

I. Bulk flow of air between the atmosphere and alveoli is proportional to the difference between the alveolar and atmospheric pressures and inversely proportional to the airway resistance: $F = (P_{alv} - P_{atm})/R$.

II. Between breaths at the end of an unforced expiration, $P_{atm} = P_{alv}$, no air is flowing, and the dimensions of the lungs and thoracic cage are stable as the result of opposing elastic forces. The lungs are stretched and are attempting to recoil, whereas the chest wall is compressed and attempting to move outward. This creates a subatmospheric intrapleural pressure and hence a transpulmonary pressure that opposes the forces of elastic recoil.

III. During inspiration, the contractions of the diaphragm and inspiratory intercostal muscles increase the volume of the thoracic cage.
   a. This makes intrapleural pressure more subatmospheric, increases transpulmonary pressure, and causes the lungs to expand to a greater degree than they do between breaths.
   b. This expansion initially makes alveolar pressure subatmospheric, which creates the pressure difference between the atmosphere and alveoli to drive airflow into the lungs.

IV. During expiration, the inspiratory muscles cease contracting, allowing the elastic recoil of the lungs to return them to their original between-breaths size.
   a. This initially compresses the alveolar air, raising alveolar pressure above atmospheric pressure and driving air out of the lungs.
   b. In forced expirations, the contraction of expiratory intercostal muscles and abdominal muscles actively decreases chest dimensions.

V. Lung compliance is determined by the elastic connective tissues of the lungs and the surface tension of the fluid lining the alveoli. The latter is greatly reduced—and compliance increased—by surfactant, produced by the type II cells of the alveoli. Surfactant also stabilizes alveoli by decreasing surface tension in smaller alveoli.

VI. Airway resistance determines how much air flows into the lungs at any given pressure difference between atmosphere and alveoli. The major determinants of airway resistance are the radii of the airways.

VII. The vital capacity is the sum of resting tidal volume, inspiratory reserve volume, and expiratory reserve volume. The volume expired during the first second of a forced vital capacity measurement is the FEV_1 and normally averages 80% of forced vital capacity.

VIII. Minute ventilation is the product of tidal volume and respiratory rate. Alveolar ventilation = (Tidal volume − Anatomical dead space) × Respiratory rate.

Exchange of Gases in Alveoli and Tissues

I. Exchange of gases in lungs and tissues is by diffusion as a result of differences in partial pressures. Gases diffuse from a region of higher partial pressure to one of lower partial pressure. At rest and at a respiratory quotient (RQ) of 0.8, oxygen consumption is approximately 250 mL per minute, whereas carbon dioxide production is approximately 200 mL per minute.

II. Normal alveolar gas pressure for oxygen is 105 mmHg and for carbon dioxide is 40 mmHg.
   a. At any given inspired P_{O_2}, the ratio of oxygen consumption to alveolar ventilation determines alveolar P_{O_2}—the higher the ratio, the lower the alveolar P_{O_2}.
   b. The higher the ratio of carbon dioxide production to alveolar ventilation, the higher the alveolar P_{CO_2}.

III. The average value at rest for systemic venous P_{O_2} is 40 mmHg and for P_{CO_2} is 46 mmHg.

IV. As systemic venous blood flows through the pulmonary capillaries, there is net diffusion of oxygen from alveoli to blood and of carbon dioxide from blood to alveoli. By the end of each pulmonary capillary, the blood gas pressures have become equal to those in the alveoli.

V. Inadequate gas exchange between alveoli and pulmonary capillaries may occur when the alveolar-capillary surface area is decreased, when the alveolar walls thicken, or when there are ventilation–perfusion inequalities.

VI. Significant ventilation–perfusion inequalities cause the systemic arterial P_{O_2} to be reduced. An important mechanism for opposing mismatching is that a low local P_{O_2} causes local vasoconstriction, diverting blood away from poorly ventilated areas.

VII. In the tissues, net diffusion of oxygen occurs from blood to cells and net diffusion of carbon dioxide from cells to blood.

Transport of Oxygen in Blood

I. Each liter of systemic arterial blood normally contains 200 mL of oxygen, more than 98% bound to hemoglobin and the rest dissolved.

II. The major determinant of the degree to which hemoglobin is saturated with oxygen is blood P_{O_2}.
   a. Hemoglobin is almost 100% saturated at the normal systemic arterial P_{O_2} of 100 mmHg. The fact that saturation is already more than 90% at a P_{O_2} of 60 mmHg permits relatively normal uptake of oxygen by the blood even when alveolar P_{O_2} is moderately reduced.
   b. Hemoglobin is 75% saturated at the normal systemic mixed venous P_{O_2} of 40 mmHg. Thus, only 25% of the oxygen has dissociated from hemoglobin and diffused into the tissues.

III. The affinity of hemoglobin for oxygen is decreased by an increase in P_{CO_2}, H^+ concentration, and temperature. All these conditions exist in the tissues and facilitate the dissociation of oxygen from hemoglobin.

IV. The affinity of hemoglobin for oxygen is also decreased by binding DPG, which is synthesized by the erythrocytes. DPG increases in situations associated with inadequate oxygen supply and helps maintain oxygen release in the tissues.

Transport of Carbon Dioxide in Blood

I. When carbon dioxide molecules diffuse from the tissues into the blood, 10% remain dissolved in plasma and erythrocytes, 25% to 30% combine in the erythrocytes with deoxyhemoglobin to form carbamino compounds, and 60% to 65% combine in the erythrocytes with water to form carbonic acid, which then dissociates to yield HCO_3^- and H^+. Most of the HCO_3^- then moves out of the erythrocytes into the plasma in exchange for chloride ions.

II. As venous blood flows through lung capillaries, blood P_{CO_2} decreases because of the diffusion of carbon dioxide out of the blood into the alveoli, and the reactions are reversed.

Transport of Hydrogen Ion Between Tissues and Lungs

I. Most of the H^+ generated in the erythrocytes from carbonic acid during blood passage through tissue capillaries binds to deoxyhemoglobin because deoxyhemoglobin, formed as oxygen unloads from oxyhemoglobin, has a high affinity for H^+.

II. As the blood flows through the lung capillaries, H^+ bound to deoxyhemoglobin is released and combines with HCO_3^- to yield carbon dioxide and water.

Control of Respiration

I. Breathing depends upon cyclical inspiratory muscle excitation by the nerves to the diaphragm and intercostal muscles. This neural activity is triggered by the medullary inspiratory neurons.

II. The medullary respiratory center is composed of the dorsal respiratory group, which contains inspiratory neurons, and the ventral respiratory group, where the respiratory rhythm generator is located.

III. The most important inputs to the medullary inspiratory neurons for the involuntary control of ventilation are from the peripheral chemoreceptors—the carotid and aortic bodies—and the central chemoreceptors.

IV. Ventilation is reflexively stimulated via the peripheral chemoreceptors by a decrease in arterial P_{O_2} but only when the decrease is large.

V. Ventilation is reflexively stimulated via both the peripheral and central chemoreceptors when the arterial P_{CO_2} increases even a slight amount. The stimulus for this reflex is not the increased P_{CO_2} itself but the concomitant increased H^+ concentration in arterial blood and brain extracellular fluid.

VI. Ventilation is also stimulated, mainly via the peripheral chemoreceptors, by an increase in arterial H^+ concentration resulting from causes other than an increase in P_{CO_2}. The result of this reflex is to restore H^+ concentration toward normal by lowering P_{CO_2}.

VII. Ventilation is reflexively inhibited by an increase in arterial P_{O_2} and by a decrease in arterial P_{CO_2} or H^+ concentration.

VIII. During moderate exercise, ventilation increases in exact proportion to metabolism, but the signals causing this are not known. During very strenuous exercise, ventilation increases more than metabolism.

a. The proportional increases in ventilation and metabolism during moderate exercise cause the arterial P_{O_2}, P_{CO_2}, and H^+ concentration to remain unchanged.

b. Arterial H^+ concentration increases during very strenuous exercise because of increased lactic acid production. This accounts for some of the hyperventilation that occurs.

IX. Ventilation is also controlled by reflexes originating in airway receptors and by conscious intent.

Hypoxia

I. The causes of hypoxic hypoxia are listed in Table 13.10.

II. During exposure to hypoxia, as at high altitude, oxygen supply to the tissues is maintained by the five responses listed in Table 13.11.

Nonrespiratory Functions of the Lungs

I. The lungs influence arterial blood concentrations of biologically active substances by removing some from systemic venous blood and adding others to systemic arterial blood.

II. The lungs also act as sieves that trap and dissolve small clots formed in the systemic tissues.

REVIEW QUESTIONS

1. List the functions of the respiratory system.
2. At rest, how many liters of air flow in and out of the lungs and how many liters of blood flow through the lungs per minute?
3. Describe four functions of the conducting portion of the airways.
4. Which respiration steps occur by diffusion and which by bulk flow?
5. What are normal values for intrapleural pressure, alveolar pressure, and transpulmonary pressure at the end of an unforced expiration?
6. Between breaths at the end of an unforced expiration, in what directions do the lungs and chest wall tend to move? What prevents them from doing so?
7. State typical values for oxygen consumption, carbon dioxide production, and cardiac output at rest. How much oxygen (in milliliters per liter) is present in systemic venous and systemic arterial blood?
8. Write the equation relating airflow into or out of the lungs to alveolar pressure, atmospheric pressure, and airway resistance.
9. Describe the sequence of events that cause air to move into the lungs during inspiration and out of the lungs during expiration. Diagram the changes in intrapleural pressure and alveolar pressure.
10. What factors determine lung compliance? Which is most important?
11. How does surfactant increase lung compliance? How does surfactant stabilize alveoli by preventing small alveoli from emptying into large alveoli?
12. How is airway resistance influenced by airway radii?
13. List the physical factors that alter airway resistance.
14. Contrast the causes of increased airway resistance in asthma, emphysema, and chronic bronchitis.
15. What distinguishes lung capacities, as a group, from lung volumes?
16. State the formula relating minute ventilation, tidal volume, and respiratory rate. Give representative values for each in a normal person at rest.
17. State the formula for calculating alveolar ventilation. What is an average value for alveolar ventilation?

18. The partial pressure of a gas is dependent upon what two factors?
19. State the alveolar partial pressures for oxygen and carbon dioxide in a healthy person at rest.
20. What factors determine alveolar partial pressures?
21. What is the mechanism of gas exchange between alveoli and pulmonary capillaries? In a healthy person at rest, what are the gas pressures at the end of the pulmonary capillaries relative to those in the alveoli?
22. Why does thickening of alveolar membranes impair oxygen movement but has little effect on carbon dioxide exchange?
23. What is the major result of ventilation–perfusion inequalities throughout the lungs? Describe homeostatic responses that minimize mismatching.
24. What generates the diffusion gradients for oxygen and carbon dioxide in the tissues?
25. In what two forms is oxygen carried in the blood? What are the normal quantities (in milliliters per liter) for each form in arterial blood?
26. Describe the structure of hemoglobin.
27. Draw an oxygen–hemoglobin dissociation curve. Put in the points that represent systemic venous and systemic arterial blood (ignore the rightward shift of the curve in systemic venous blood). What is the adaptive importance of the plateau? Of the steep portion?
28. Would breathing pure oxygen cause a large increase in oxygen transport by the blood in a healthy person? In a person with a low alveolar P_{O_2}?
29. Describe the effects of increased P_{CO_2}, H^+ concentration, and temperature on the oxygen–hemoglobin dissociation curve. How are these effects adaptive for oxygen unloading in the tissues?
30. Describe the effects of increased DPG on the oxygen–hemoglobin dissociation curve. What is the adaptive importance of the effect of DPG on the curve?
31. Draw figures showing the reactions carbon dioxide undergoes entering the blood in the tissue capillaries and leaving the blood in the alveoli. What fractions are contributed by dissolved carbon dioxide, HCO_3^-, and carbaminohemoglobin?
32. What happens to most of the H^+ formed in the erythrocytes from carbonic acid? What happens to blood H^+ concentration as blood flows through tissue capillaries?
33. What are the effects of P_{O_2} on carbaminohemoglobin formation and H^+ binding by hemoglobin?
34. Describe the area of the brain in which automatic control of rhythmic respirations resides.
35. Describe the function of the pulmonary stretch receptors.
36. What changes stimulate the peripheral chemoreceptors? The central chemoreceptors?
37. Why is it that moderate anemia or carbon monoxide exposure does not stimulate the peripheral chemoreceptors?
38. Is respiratory control more sensitive to small changes in arterial P_{O_2} or in arterial P_{CO_2}?
39. Describe the pathways by which increased arterial P_{CO_2} stimulates ventilation. What pathway is more important?
40. Describe the pathway by which a change in arterial H^+ concentration independent of altered carbon dioxide influences ventilation. What is the adaptive value of this reflex?
41. What happens to arterial P_{O_2}, P_{CO_2}, and H^+ concentration during moderate and strenuous exercise? List other factors that may stimulate ventilation during exercise.
42. List four general causes of hypoxic hypoxia.
43. Explain how ventilation–perfusion mismatch due to regional lung disease can cause hypoxic hypoxia but not hypercapnia.
44. Describe two general ways in which the lungs can alter the concentrations of substances other than oxygen, carbon dioxide, and H^+ in the arterial blood.
45. List two types of sleep apnea. Why does nasal CPAP prevent obstructive sleep apnea?

KEY TERMS

airway 447
alveolar dead space 461
alveolar pressure (P_{alv}) 451
alveolar ventilation ($\dot{V}_A$) 461
alveolar sac 448
alveolus (alveoli) 447
anatomical dead space (V_D) 460
aortic body 475
apneustic center 473
atmospheric pressure (P_{atm}) 451
Boyle's law 451
bronchus (bronchi) 447
bronchiole 447
carbaminohemoglobin 472
carbonic anhydrase 472
carotid body 475
central chemoreceptor 475
conducting zone 448
cystic fibrosis transmembrane conductance regulator (CFTR) 448
Dalton's law 462
deoxyhemoglobin (Hb) 467
diaphragm 450
2,3-diphosphoglycerate (DPG) 470
dorsal respiratory group (DRG) 473
elastic recoil 452
expiration 447
expiratory reserve volume (ERV) 459
fetal hemoglobin 471
functional residual capacity (FRC) 459
globin 467
heme 467
hemoglobin 467
Henry's law 463
Hering–Breuer reflex 474
inspiration 447
inspiratory reserve volume (IRV) 459
intercostal muscle 450
intrapleural fluid 450
intrapleural pressure (P_{ip}) 450
J receptor 479
larynx 447
lateral traction 458
Law of Laplace 457
lung compliance (C_L) 455
medullary respiratory center 473
minute ventilation ($\dot{V}_E$) 459
nitric oxide 473
oxygen-carrying capacity 468
oxygen–hemoglobin dissociation curve 468
oxyhemoglobin (HbO_2) 467
parietal pleura 450
partial pressure 463
percent hemoglobin saturation 467
peripheral chemoreceptor 474
pharynx 447
phrenic nerves 454
physiological dead space 461
pleura 450
pleural sac 450
pneumotaxic center 463
pontine respiratory group 473
pre-Bötzinger complex 473
pulmonary 446
pulmonary stretch receptor 474
residual volume (RV) 459
respiration 446
respiratory bronchiole 447
respiratory cycle 447
respiratory quotient (RQ) 462
respiratory rhythm generator 473
respiratory system 447
respiratory zone 448
surface tension 456
surfactant 456
terminal bronchioles 447
thorax 450
tidal volume (V_t) 459
total-blood carbon dioxide 472
trachea 447
transmural pressure 452
transpulmonary pressure (P_{tp}) 452
type I alveolar cell 448
type II alveolar cell 448
upper airways 447
ventilation 451
ventral respiratory group (VRG) 473
visceral pleura 450
vital capacity (VC) 459
vocal cord 447

CLINICAL TERMS

CHAPTER 13

Clinical Case Study: High Blood Pressure and Chronic Sleepiness in an Obese Man

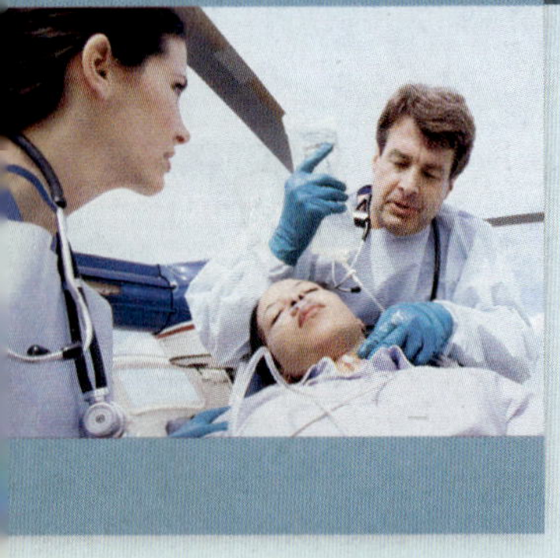

An obese man is discovered to have high blood pressure (hypertension) and is sleepy all of the time. His wife reports that he snores very loudly and often sounds like he stops breathing in his sleep. The doctor orders a sleep study, and the diagnosis of obstructive sleep apnea is made.

Sleep apnea is characterized by periodic cessation of breathing during sleep. This results in the combination of hypoxemia and hypercapnia (termed ***asphyxia***). In severe cases, this may occur more than 20 times an hour. During a sleep study, these frequent blood oxygen desaturations are documented. Sleep apnea has two general types. ***Central sleep apnea*** is primarily due to a decrease in neural output from the respiratory center in the medulla to the phrenic motor nerve to the diaphragm. ***Obstructive sleep apnea*** is caused by increased airway resistance because of narrowing or collapse of the upper airways (primarily the pharynx) during inspiration (Figure 13.44). Obstructive sleep apnea may occur in as much as 4% of the adult population with a greater frequency in elderly persons and in men. Significant snoring may be an early sign of the eventual development of obstructive sleep apnea. Obesity is clearly a contributing factor because the excess fat in the neck decreases the diameter of the upper airways. A decrease in the activity of the upper airway dilating muscles, particularly during REM sleep, also contributes to airway collapse. Finally, anatomical narrowing and increased compliance of the upper airways contributes to periodic inspiratory obstruction during sleep.

Untreated sleep apnea can have many serious consequences, including hypertension of the pulmonary arteries (pulmonary hypertension) and added strain on the right ventricle of the heart. This can lead to heart failure and abnormal heart rhythm, either of which can be fatal. The periodic arousal that occurs during these apneic episodes results in serious disruption of normal sleep patterns and can lead to sleepiness during the day (***daytime somnolence***). Increased catecholamine release during these frequent arousals can also contribute to the development of high blood pressure.

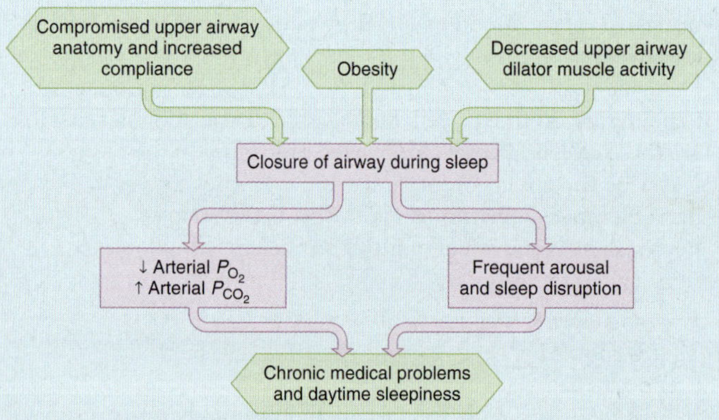

Figure 13.44 Pathogenesis of obstructive sleep apnea.

A variety of treatments exist for obstructive sleep apnea. Surgery such as laser-assisted widening of the soft palate and uvula can sometimes be of benefit. Weight loss is often quite helpful. However, the mainstay of therapy is ***continuous positive airway pressure*** (***CPAP***) (Figure 13.45). The patient wears a small mask over the nose during sleep, which is attached to a positive-pressure-generating device. By increasing airway pressure greater than P_{atm}, the collapse of the upper airways during inspiration is prevented. Although the CPAP nasal mask may seem obtrusive, many patients sleep much better with it, and many of the symptoms resolve with this treatment. Our patient was treated with CPAP during the night and also was able to lose a considerable amount of body weight. As a result, his daytime somnolence and hypertension improved over the next year.

(continued)

(continued)

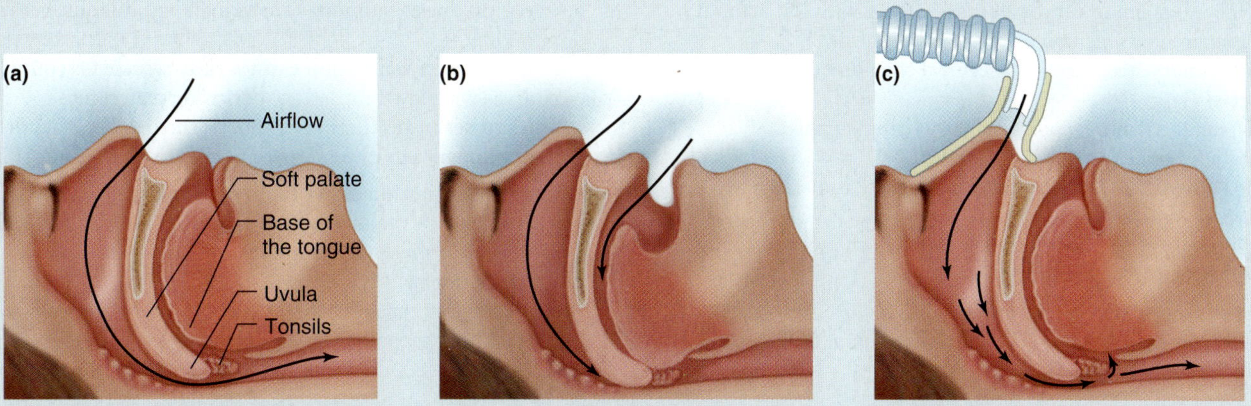

During normal sleep, air flows freely past the structures in the throat.

During sleep apnea, airflow is completely blocked.

With CPAP, a mask over the nose gently directs air into the throat to keep the air passage open.

Figure 13.45 The pathophysiology and a standard treatment of obstructive sleep apnea. (a) Normal sleep with air flowing freely past the structures of the throat during an inspiration. (b) In obstructive sleep apnea (particularly with the patient sleeping in the supine position), the soft palate, uvula, and tongue occlude the airway, greatly increasing the resistance to airflow. (c) Continuous positive airway pressure (CPAP) is applied with a nasal mask, preventing airway collapse.

Clinical terms: asphyxia, central sleep apnea, continuous positive airway pressure (CPAP), daytime somnolence, obstructive sleep apnea, sleep apnea

See Chapter 19 for complete, integrative case studies.

CHAPTER 13 TEST QUESTIONS

Answers found in Appendix A.

1. If P_{atm} = 0 mmHg and P_{alv} = −2 mmHg, then
   a. transpulmonary pressure (P_{tp}) is 2 mmHg.
   b. it is the end of the normal inspiration and there is no airflow.
   c. it is at the end of the normal expiration and there is no airflow.
   d. transpulmonary pressure (P_{tp}) is −2 mmHg.
   e. air is flowing into the lung.
2. Transpulmonary pressure (P_{tp}) increases by 3 mmHg during a normal inspiration. In subject A, 500 mL of air is inspired. In subject B, 250 mL of air is inspired for the same change in P_{tp}. Which is *true?*
   a. The compliance of the lung of subject B is less than that of subject A.
   b. The airway resistance of subject A is greater than that of subject B.
   c. The surface tension in the lung of subject B is less than that in subject A.
   d. The lung of subject A is deficient in surfactant.
   e. The compliance cannot be estimated from the data provided.
3. If alveolar ventilation is 4200 mL/min, respiratory frequency is 12 breaths per minute, and tidal volume is 500 mL, what is the anatomical-dead-space ventilation?
   a. 1800 mL/min
   b. 6000 mL/min
   c. 350 mL/min
   d. 1200 mL/min
   e. It cannot be determined from the data provided.
4. Which of the following will increase alveolar P_{O_2}?
   a. increase in metabolism and no change in alveolar ventilation
   b. breathing air with 15% oxygen at sea level
   c. increase in alveolar ventilation matched by an increase in metabolism
   d. increased alveolar ventilation with no change in metabolism
   e. carbon monoxide poisoning
5. Which of the following will cause the largest increase in systemic arterial oxygen saturation in the blood?
   a. an increase in red cell concentration (hematocrit) of 20%
   b. breathing 100% O_2 in a healthy subject at sea level
   c. an increase in arterial P_{O_2} from 40 to 60 mmHg
   d. hyperventilation in a healthy subject at sea level
   e. breathing a gas with 5% CO_2, 21% O_2, and 74% N_2 at sea level
6. In arterial blood with a P_{O_2} of 60 mmHg, which of the following situations will result in the lowest blood oxygen saturation?
   a. decreased DPG with normal body temperature and blood pH
   b. elevated body temperature, acidosis, and increased DPG
   c. decreased body temperature, alkalosis, and increased DPG
   d. normal body temperature with alkalosis
   e. elevated body temperature with alkalosis
7. Which of the following is *not* true about asthma?
   a. The basic defect is chronic airway inflammation.
   b. It is always caused by an allergy.
   c. The airway smooth muscle is hyperresponsive.
   d. It can be treated with inhaled steroid therapy.
   e. It can be treated with bronchodilator therapy.

8. Which of the following is *true?*
   a. Peripheral chemoreceptors increase firing with low arterial P_{O_2} but are not sensitive to an increase in arterial P_{CO_2}.
   b. The primary stimulus to the central chemoreceptors is low arterial P_{O_2}.
   c. Peripheral chemoreceptors increase firing during a metabolic alkalosis.
   d. The increase in ventilation during exercise is due to a decrease in arterial P_{O_2}.
   e. Peripheral and central chemoreceptors both increase firing when arterial P_{CO_2} increases.
9. Ventilation–perfusion inequalities lead to hypoxemia because
   a. the relationship between P_{CO_2} and the content of CO_2 in blood is sigmoidal.
   b. a decrease in ventilation–perfusion matching in a lung region causes pulmonary arteriolar vasodilation in that region.
   c. increases in ventilation cannot fully restore O_2 content in areas with low ventilation–perfusion matching.
   d. increases in ventilation cannot normalize P_{CO_2}.
   e. pulmonary blood vessels are not sensitive to changes in P_{O_2}.
10. After the expiration of a normal tidal volume, a subject breathes in as much air as possible. The volume of air inspired is the
    a. inspiratory reserve volume.
    b. vital capacity.
    c. inspiratory capacity.
    d. total lung capacity.
    e. functional residual capacity.

CHAPTER 13 GENERAL PRINCIPLES ASSESSMENT

Answers found in Appendix A.

1. A general principle of physiology highlighted throughout this chapter is that *physiological processes are dictated by the laws of chemistry and physics.* What are some examples of how this applies to lung mechanics and the transport of oxygen and carbon dioxide in blood?
2. How is the anatomy of the alveoli and pulmonary capillaries an example of the principle that *structure is a determinant of—and has coevolved with—function?*
3. A general principle of physiology is that *most physiological functions are controlled by multiple regulatory systems, often working in opposition.* What are some examples of factors that have opposing regulatory effects on alveolar ventilation in humans?

CHAPTER 13 QUANTITATIVE AND THOUGHT QUESTIONS

Answers found at www.mhhe.com/widmaier13.

1. At the end of a normal expiration, a person's lung volume is 2 L, his alveolar pressure is 0 mmHg, and his intrapleural pressure is −4 mmHg. He then inhales 800 mL of air. At the end of inspiration, the alveolar pressure is 0 mmHg and the intrapleural pressure is −8 mmHg. Calculate this person's lung compliance.
2. A patient is unable to produce surfactant. To inhale a normal tidal volume, will her intrapleural pressure have to be more or less subatmospheric during inspiration, relative to a healthy person?
3. A 70 kg adult patient is artificially ventilated by a machine during surgery at a rate of 20 breaths/min and a tidal volume of 250 mL/breath. Assuming a normal anatomical dead space of 150 mL, is this patient receiving an adequate alveolar ventilation?
4. Why must a person floating on the surface of the water and breathing through a snorkel increase his tidal volume and/or breathing frequency if alveolar ventilation is to remain normal?
5. A healthy person breathing room air voluntarily increases alveolar ventilation twofold and continues to do so until reaching new steady-state alveolar gas pressures for oxygen and carbon dioxide. Are the new values higher or lower than normal?
6. A person breathing room air has an alveolar P_{O_2} of 105 mmHg and an arterial P_{O_2} of 80 mmHg. Could hypoventilation due to, say, respiratory muscle weakness produce these values?
7. A person's alveolar membranes have become thickened enough to moderately decrease the rate at which gases diffuse across them at any given partial pressure differences. Will this person necessarily have a low arterial P_{O_2} at rest? During exercise?
8. A person is breathing 100% oxygen. How much will the oxygen content (in milliliters per liter of blood) of the arterial blood increase compared to when the person is breathing room air?
9. Which of the following have higher values in systemic venous blood than in systemic arterial blood: plasma P_{CO_2}, erythrocyte P_{CO_2}, plasma bicarbonate concentration, erythrocyte bicarbonate concentration, plasma hydrogen ion concentration, erythrocyte hydrogen ion concentration, erythrocyte carbamino concentration?
10. If the spinal cord were severed where it joins the brainstem, what would happen to respiration?
11. Which inspired gas mixture leads to the largest increase in minute ventilation?
    a. 10% O_2/5% CO_2
    b. 100% O_2/5% CO_2
    c. 21% O_2/5% CO_2
    d. 10% O_2/0% CO_2
    e. 0.1% CO/5% CO_2
12. Patients with severe uncontrolled type 1 diabetes mellitus produce large quantities of certain organic acids. Can you predict the ventilation pattern in these patients and whether their arterial P_{O_2} and P_{CO_2} would increase or decrease?
13. Why does an inspired O_2 of 100% increase arterial P_{O_2} much more in a patient with ventilation–perfusion mismatch than in a patient with pure anatomical shunt?

CHAPTER 13 ANSWERS TO PHYSIOLOGICAL INQUIRIES

Figure 13.4 The rate of diffusion of gases between the air and the capillaries may be decreased due to the increased resistance to diffusion (see Chapter 4 for discussion of forces affecting diffusion).

Figure 13.11 A tube is placed through the chest wall into the now enlarged pleural space. (The original hole causing the pneumothorax would need to be repaired first.) Suction is then applied to the chest tube. The negative pressure decreases P_{ip} below P_{atm} and thereby increases P_{tp}, which results in re-expansion of the lung.

Figure 13.13

	P_{alv}	P_{ip}	P_{tp} $(P_{alv} - P_{ip})$	Change in Lung Volume
1	0	–4	4	
				P_{tp} is increasing → lung volume↑
2	–1	–6	5	
				P_{tp} is increasing → lung volume↑
3	0	–7	7	
				P_{tp} is decreasing → lung volume↓
4	1	–5	6	
				P_{tp} is decreasing → lung volume↓
1	0	–4	4	

Note: The actual volume increase or decrease in mL is determined by the compliance of the lung (see Figure 13.16).

Figure 13.16 Anything that increases P_{tp} during inspiration will, theoretically, increase lung volume. This can be done with positive airway pressure generated by mechanical ventilation, which will increase P_{alv}. This approach can work but also increases the risk of pneumothorax by inducing air leaks from the lung into the intrapleural space.

Figure 13.19 The anatomical dead space would be increased by about 251 mL (or 251 cm^3). (The volume of the tube can be approximated as that of a perfect cylinder [$\pi r^2 h = 3.1416 \times 2^2 \times 20$].) This large increase in anatomical dead space would decrease alveolar ventilation (see Table 13.5), and tidal volume would have to be increased in compensation. (There would also be an increase in airway resistance, which is discussed later.)

Figure 13.23 The increase in cardiac output with exercise greatly increases pulmonary blood flow and decreases the amount of time erythrocytes are exposed to increased oxygen from the alveoli. In a normal region of the lung, there is a large safety factor such that a large increase in blood flow still allows normal oxygen uptake. However, even small increases in the rate of capillary blood flow in a diseased portion of the lung will decrease oxygen uptake due to a loss of this safety factor.

Figure 13.29 Less O_2 will be unloaded in peripheral tissue as the blood is exposed to increased P_{CO_2} and decreased pH because the oxygen–hemoglobin dissociation curve will not shift to the right as it does in real blood. Also, less O_2 will be loaded in the lungs as P_{CO_2} diffuses from blood into the alveoli because the oxygen–hemoglobin dissociation curve will not shift to the left as it normally would with removal of CO_2 and decreased acidity.

Figure 13.33 The ventilatory response to the hypoxia of altitude would be greatly diminished, and it is likely that the person would be extremely hypoxemic as a result. Carotid body removal did not help in the treatment of asthma, and this approach was abandoned.

Figure 13.43 These receptors may facilitate the increase in alveolar ventilation that occurs during exercise because pulmonary artery P_{O_2} will decrease and pulmonary artery P_{CO_2} will increase.

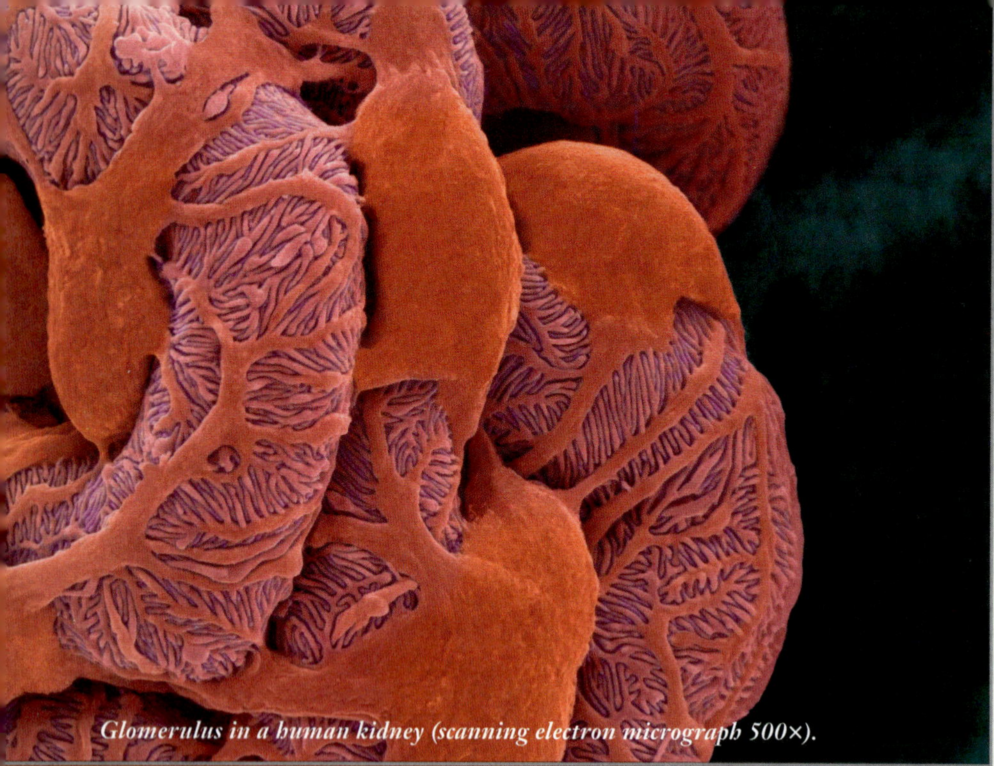

Glomerulus in a human kidney (scanning electron micrograph 500×).

14 The Kidneys and Regulation of Water and Inorganic Ions

The importance of normal electrolyte concentrations in the function of excitable tissue was explained in reference to neurons (Chapter 6) and muscle (Chapter 9) and in the homeostasis of bone in Chapter 11. You have also learned about how the maintenance of normal hydration is important in cardiovascular function in Chapter 12. Finally, Chapter 13 highlighted the importance of the respiratory system in the short-term control of acid–base balance. We now deal with the homeostatic regulation of body water volume and balance, and the inorganic ion composition of the internal environment. Furthermore, this chapter explains how the urinary system eliminates organic waste products of metabolism and, working with the respiratory system, is critical to the long-term control of acid–base balance. The kidneys play the central role in these processes.

Regulation of the total-body balance of any substance can be studied in terms of the balance concept described in Chapter 1. Theoretically, a substance can appear in the body either as a result of ingestion or synthesized as a product of metabolism. On the loss side of the balance, a substance can be excreted from the body or can be broken down by metabolism. Therefore, if the quantity of any substance in the body is to be maintained within a normal homeostatic range over a period of time, the total amounts ingested and produced must equal the total amounts excreted and broken down. Reflexes that alter excretion via the urine constitute the major mechanisms that regulate the body balances of water and many of the inorganic ions that determine the properties of the extracellular fluid. Typical values for the extracellular concentrations of these ions appeared in Table 4.1. We will first describe the general principles of kidney function, then apply this information to how the kidneys process specific substances like Na^+, H_2O, H^+, and K^+ and participate in reflexes that regulate these substances.

As you read about the structure, function, and control of the function of kidney, you will encounter numerous examples of the general principles of physiology that were outlined in Chapter 1. The homeostatic control of the excretion of metabolic wastes, as well as the ability of the kidneys to reclaim needed ions and organic molecules that would otherwise be lost in the process, is a hallmark of the general principle of physiology that homeostasis is essential for health and survival; failure of kidney function not only causes a buildup of toxic waste products in the body but can also lead to a loss of important ions and nutrients (such as glucose and amino acids) in the urine. Another general principle of physiology—that most physiological functions are controlled by multiple regulatory systems, often working in opposition—is apparent in the renal system. An example is the control of the filtration rate of the kidney. The general principle of physiology that controlled exchange of materials occurs between compartments and across cellular membranes is also integral to this chapter—as already mentioned, total-body balance of important nutrients and ions is precisely controlled by the healthy kidneys. Finally, the functional unit of the kidney—the nephron—and the blood vessels associated with it are elegant examples of the general principle of physiology that structure is a determinant of—and has coevolved with—function; form and function are inextricably intertwined.

SECTION A
Basic Principles of Renal Physiology

14.1 Renal Functions

The adjective **renal** means "pertaining to the kidneys." The kidneys process the plasma portion of blood by removing substances from it and, in a few cases, by adding substances to it. In so doing, they perform a variety of functions, as summarized in **Table 14.1**.

First, the kidneys play a central role in regulating the water concentration, inorganic ion composition, acid–base balance, and the fluid volume of the internal environment (e.g., blood volume). They do so by excreting just enough water and inorganic ions to keep the amounts of these substances in the body within a narrow homeostatic range. For example, if you increase your consumption of salt (sodium chloride), your kidneys will increase the amount of the salt excreted to match the intake. Alternatively, if there is not enough salt in the body, the kidneys will excrete very little salt.

Second, the kidneys excrete metabolic waste products into the urine as fast as they are produced. This keeps waste products, which can be toxic, from accumulating in the body. These metabolic wastes include **urea** from the catabolism of protein, **uric acid** from nucleic acids, **creatinine** from muscle creatine, the end products of hemoglobin breakdown (which give urine much of its color), and many others.

A third function of the kidneys is the urinary excretion of some foreign chemicals—such as drugs, pesticides, and food additives—and their metabolites.

TABLE 14.1	Functions of the Kidneys
I.	Regulation of water, inorganic ion balance, and acid–base balance (in cooperation with the lungs; Chapter 13)
II.	Removal of metabolic waste products from the blood and their excretion in the urine
III.	Removal of foreign chemicals from the blood and their excretion in the urine
IV.	Gluconeogenesis
V.	Production of hormones/enzymes: A. Erythropoietin, which controls erythrocyte production (Chapter 12) B. Renin, an enzyme that controls the formation of angiotensin, which influences blood pressure and sodium balance (this chapter) C. Conversion of 25-hydroxyvitamin D to 1,25-dihydroxyvitamin D, which influences calcium balance (Chapter 11)

A fourth function is gluconeogenesis. During prolonged fasting, the kidneys synthesize glucose from amino acids and other precursors and release it into the blood (see Figure 3.48).

Finally, the kidneys act as endocrine glands, releasing at least two hormones: erythropoietin (described in Chapter 12), and 1,25-dihydroxyvitamin D (described in Chapter 11). The kidneys also secrete an enzyme, renin (pronounced "REE-nin"), that is important in the control of blood pressure and sodium balance (described later in this chapter).

14.2 Structure of the Kidneys and Urinary System

The two kidneys lie in the back of the abdominal wall but not actually in the abdominal cavity. They are retroperitoneal, meaning they are just behind the peritoneum, the lining of this cavity. The urine flows from the kidneys through the **ureters** into the **bladder** and then is eliminated via the **urethra** (**Figure 14.1a**). The major structural components of the kidney are shown in cross section in **Figure 14.1b**. The indented surface of the kidney is called the **hilum,** through which courses the blood vessels perfusing (**renal artery**) and draining (**renal vein**) the kidneys. The nerves that innervate the kidney and the tube that drains urine from the kidney (the ureter) also pass through the hilum. The ureter is formed from the **calyces** (singular, **calyx**), which are funnel-shaped structures that drain urine into the ureter. Also notice that the kidney is surrounded by a protective **capsule** made of connective tissue. The kidney is divided into an outer **renal cortex** and inner **renal medulla,** described in more detail later. The connection between the tip of the medulla and the calyx is called the **papilla.**

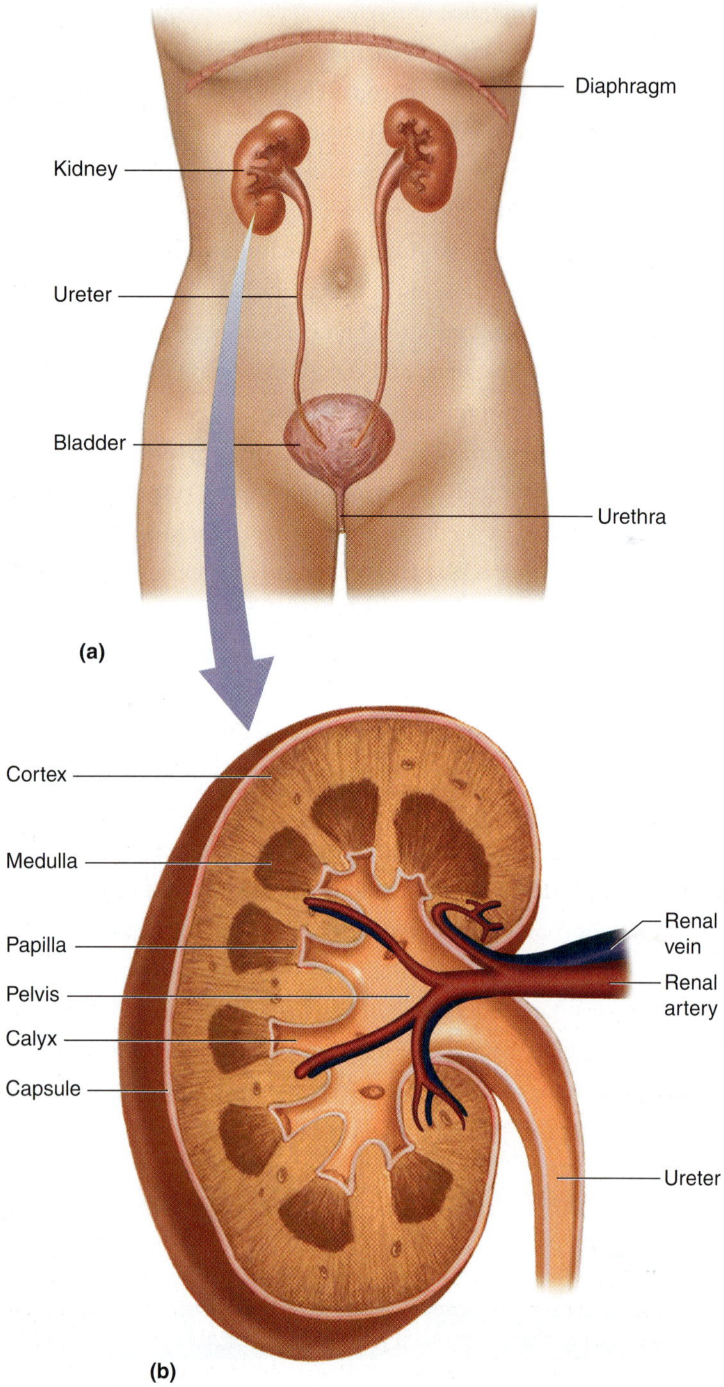

Figure 14.1 APIR (a) Urinary system in a woman. In the male, the urethra passes through the penis (Chapter 17). The diaphragm is shown for orientation. (b) Major structural components of the kidney. Kibble, 2009.

Each kidney contains approximately 1 million similar subunits called **nephrons.** Each nephron consists of (1) an initial filtering component called the **renal corpuscle** and (2) a **tubule** that extends from the renal corpuscle (**Figure 14.2a**). The renal tubule is a very narrow, hollow cylinder made up of a single layer of epithelial cells resting

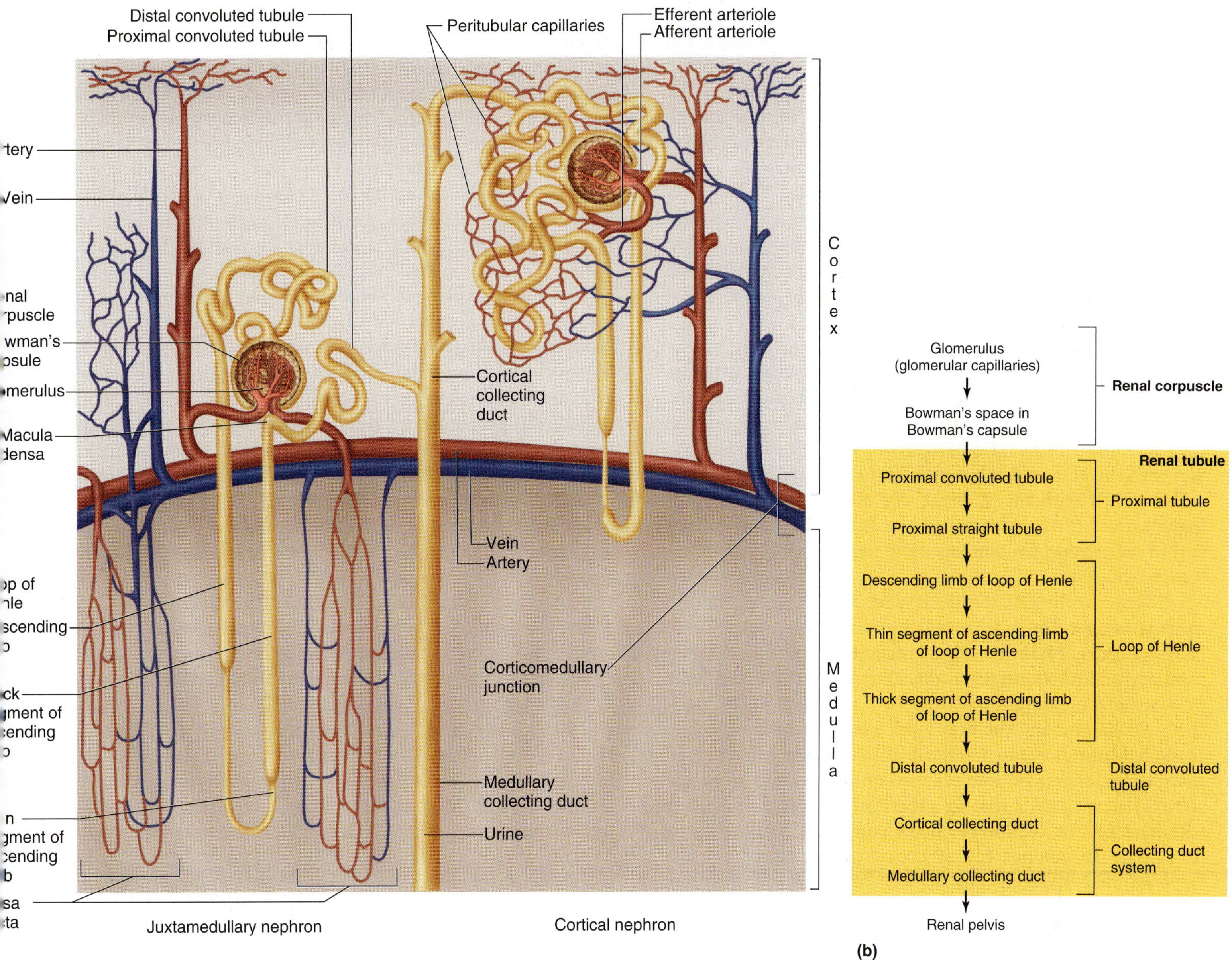

Figure 14.2 APR Basic structure of a nephron. (a) Anatomical organization. The macula densa is not a distinct segment but a plaque of cells in the ascending loop of Henle where the loop passes between the arterioles supplying its renal corpuscle of origin. The outer area of the kidney is called the cortex, and the inner is called the medulla. Two types of nephrons are shown—the juxtamedullary nephrons have long loops of Henle that penetrate deeply into the medulla, whereas the cortical nephrons have short (or no) loops of Henle. Note that the efferent arterioles of juxtamedullary nephrons give rise to long, looping vasa recta, whereas efferent arterioles of cortical nephrons give rise to peritubular capillaries. Not shown (for clarity) are the peritubular capillaries surrounding the portions of the juxtamedullary nephron's tubules located in the cortex. These peritubular capillaries arise primarily from other cortical nephrons. (b) Consecutive segments of the nephron. All segments in the yellow area are parts of the renal tubule; the terms to the right of the brackets are commonly used for several consecutive segments.

on a basement membrane. The epithelial cells differ in structure and function along the length of the tubule, and at least eight distinct segments are now recognized (**Figure 14.2b**). It is customary, however, to group two or more contiguous tubular segments when discussing function, and we will follow this practice.

The renal corpuscle forms a filtrate from blood that is free of cells, larger polypeptides, and proteins. This filtrate then leaves the renal corpuscle and enters the tubule. As it flows through the tubule, substances are added to or removed from it. Ultimately, the fluid remaining at the end of each nephron combines in the collecting ducts and exits the kidneys as urine.

Let us look first at the anatomy of the renal corpuscles—the filters. The renal corpuscle is a classic example of the general principle of physiology that structure is a determinant of function. Not only do the many capillaries in each corpuscle greatly increase the surface area for filtration of waste products from the plasma, but their structure creates an efficient sieve for the ultrafiltration of plasma. Each renal corpuscle contains a compact tuft of interconnected capillary loops called the **glomerulus** (plural, *glomeruli*), or **glomerular capillaries** (Figure 14.2 and **Figure 14.3a**). Each glomerulus is supplied with blood by an arteriole called an **afferent arteriole.** The glomerulus protrudes into a fluid-filled capsule called **Bowman's capsule.** The combination of a glomerulus and a Bowman's capsule constitutes a renal corpuscle. As blood flows through the glomerulus, about 20% of the plasma filters into Bowman's capsule. The remaining blood then leaves the glomerulus by the **efferent arteriole.**

One way of visualizing the relationships within the renal corpuscle is to imagine a loosely clenched fist—the glomerulus—punched into a balloon—the Bowman's capsule. (This is similar to the depiction of the pleural sacs around each lung in Figure 13.5). The part of Bowman's capsule in contact with the glomerulus becomes pushed inward but does not make contact with the opposite side of the capsule. Accordingly, a fluid-filled space called the **Bowman's space** exists within the capsule. Protein-free fluid filters from the glomerulus into this space.

Blood in the glomerulus is separated from the fluid in Bowman's space by a filtration barrier consisting of three layers (**Figure 14.3b, c**). These include (1) the single-celled capillary endothelium, (2) a noncellular proteinaceous layer of basement membrane (also termed *basal lamina*) between the endothelium and the next layer, and (3) the single-celled epithelial lining of Bowman's capsule. The epithelial cells in this region, called **podocytes,** are quite different from the simple flattened cells that line the rest of Bowman's capsule (the part of the "balloon" not in contact with the "fist"). They have an octopus-like structure in that they possess a large number of extensions, or foot processes. Fluid filters first across the endothelial cells, then through the basement membrane, and finally between the foot processes of the podocytes.

In addition to the capillary endothelial cells and the podocytes, **mesangial cells**—a third cell type—are modified smooth muscle cells that surround the glomerular capillary loops but are not part of the filtration pathway. Their function will be described later.

The segment of the tubule that drains Bowman's capsule is the **proximal tubule,** comprising the proximal convoluted tubule and the proximal straight tubule shown in Figure 14.2b. The next portion of the tubule is the **loop of Henle,** which is a sharp, hairpinlike loop consisting of a **descending limb** coming from the proximal tubule and an **ascending limb** leading to the next tubular segment, the **distal convoluted tubule.** Fluid flows from the distal convoluted tubule into the **collecting-duct system,** which is comprised of the **cortical collecting duct** and then the **medullary collecting duct.** The reasons for the terms *cortical* and *medullary* will be apparent shortly.

From Bowman's capsule to the collecting-duct system, each nephron is completely separate from the others. This separation ends when multiple cortical collecting ducts merge. The result of additional mergings from this point on is that the urine drains into the kidney's central cavity, the **renal pelvis,** via several hundred large medullary collecting ducts. The renal pelvis is continuous with the ureter draining that kidney (**Figure 14.4**).

There are important regional differences in the kidney (see Figures 14.1b, 14.2, and 14.4). The outer portion is the renal cortex, and the inner portion is the renal medulla. The cortex contains all the renal corpuscles. The loops of Henle extend from the cortex for varying distances down into the medulla. The medullary collecting ducts pass through the medulla on their way to the renal pelvis.

All along its length, the part of each tubule in the cortex is surrounded by capillaries called the **peritubular capillaries.** Note that we have now mentioned two sets of capillaries in the kidneys—the glomerular capillaries (glomeruli) and the peritubular capillaries. Within each nephron, the two sets of capillaries are connected to each other by an efferent arteriole, the vessel by which blood leaves the glomerulus (see Figure 14.2 and Figure 14.3a). Thus, the renal circulation is very unusual in that it includes *two* sets of arterioles and *two* sets of capillaries. After supplying the tubules with blood, the peritubular capillaries then join to form the veins by which blood leaves the kidney.

Nephrons are of two general types (see Figure 14.2a). About 15% of the nephrons are **juxtamedullary,** which means that the renal corpuscle lies in the part of the cortex closest to the cortical–medullary junction. The Henle's loops of these nephrons plunge deep into the medulla and, as we will see, are responsible for generating an osmotic gradient in the medulla responsible for the reabsorption of water. In close proximity to the juxtamedullary nephrons are long capillaries known as the **vasa recta,** which also loop deeply into the medulla and then return to the cortical–medullary junction. The majority of nephrons are **cortical,** meaning their renal corpuscles are located in the outer cortex and their Henle's loops do not penetrate deep into the medulla. In fact, some cortical nephrons do not have a Henle's loop at all; they are involved in reabsorption and secretion but do not contribute to the hypertonic medullary interstitium described later in the chapter.

One additional anatomical detail involving both the tubule and the arterioles is important. Near its end, the ascending limb of each loop of Henle passes between the afferent and efferent arterioles of that loop's own nephron (see Figure 14.2). At this point, there is a patch of cells in the wall of the ascending limb as it becomes the distal convoluted tubule called the **macula densa,** and the wall of the afferent arteriole contains secretory cells known as **juxtaglomerular (JG) cells.** The combination of macula densa and juxtaglomerular cells is known as the **juxtaglomerular apparatus (JGA)** (see Figure 14.3a and **Figure 14.5**). The juxtaglomerular cells secrete renin into the blood.

14.3 Basic Renal Processes

Urine formation begins with the filtration of plasma from the glomerular capillaries into Bowman's space. This process is termed **glomerular filtration,** and the filtrate is called

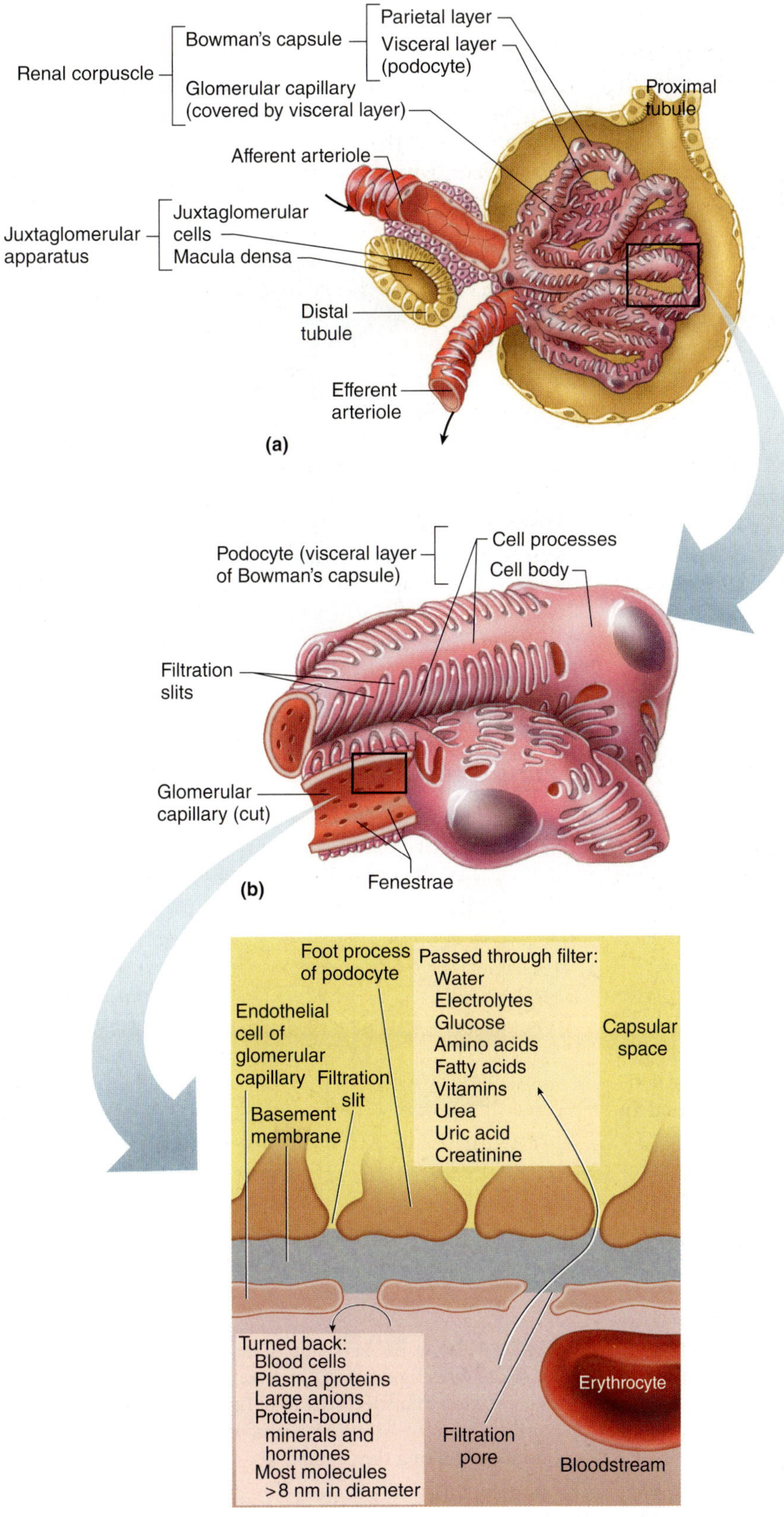

a. Blood flows into the glomerulus through the afferent arterioles and leaves the glomerulus through the efferent arterioles. The proximal tubule exits Bowman's capsule.

b. Podocytes of Bowman's capsule surround the capillaries. Filtration slits between the podocytes allow fluid to pass into Bowman's capsule. The glomerulus is composed of capillary endothelium that is fenestrated. Surrounding the endothelial cells is a basement membrane.

c. Substances in the blood are filtered through capillary pores between endothelial cells (single layer). The filtrate then passes across the basement membrane and through filtration slit between the foot processes (also called pedicels) and enters the capsular space. From here, the filtrate is transported to the lumen of the proximal convoluted tubule.

Figure 14.3 AP|R The renal corpuscle. (a) Anatomy of the renal corpuscle. (b) Inset view of podocytes and capillaries. (c) Glomerular filtration membrane.

PHYSIOLOGICAL INQUIRY

- What would happen if a significant number of glomerular capillaries were clogged, as can happen in someone with very high blood glucose concentrations for a long period of time (as can occur in untreated diabetes mellitus)?

Answer can be found at end of chapter.

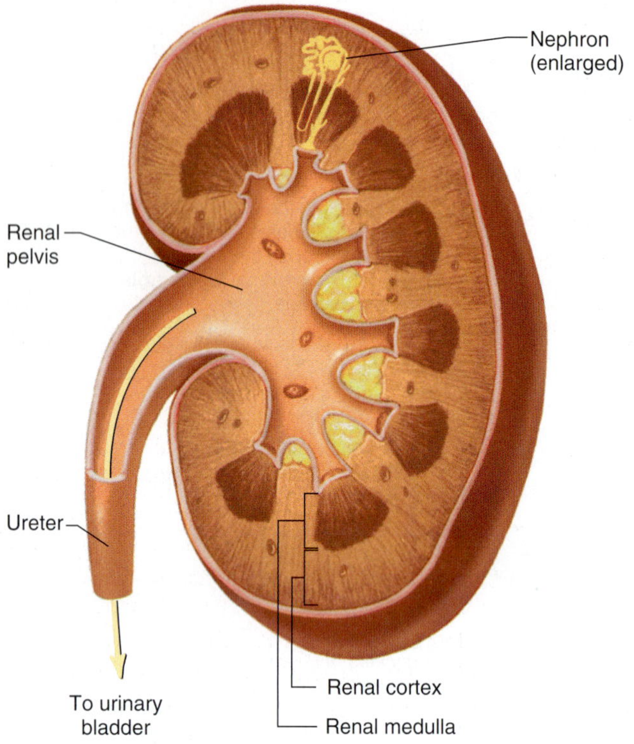

Figure 14.4 APIR Section of a human kidney. For clarity, the juxtamedullary nephron illustrated to show nephron orientation is not to scale—its outline would not be clearly visible without a microscope. The outer kidney, which contains all the renal corpuscles, is the cortex, and the inner kidney is the medulla. Note that in the medulla, the loops of Henle and the collecting ducts run parallel to each other. The medullary collecting ducts drain into the renal pelvis.

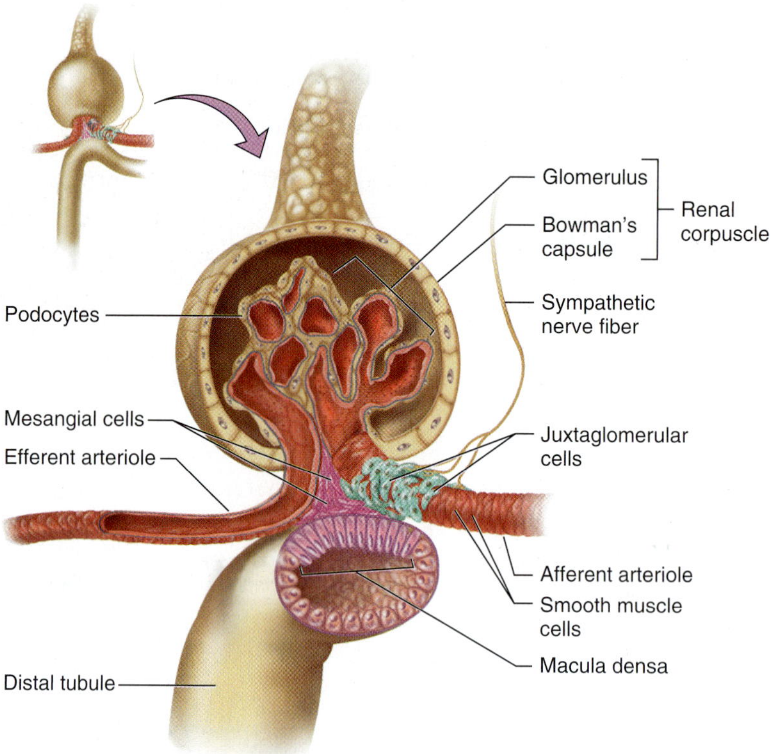

Figure 14.5 APIR The juxtaglomerular apparatus.

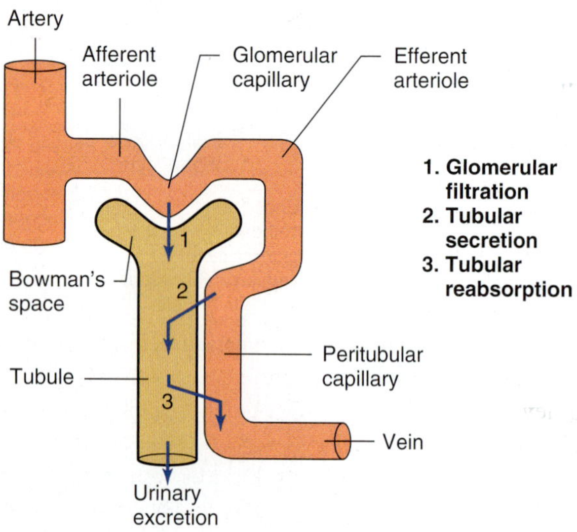

Figure 14.6 APIR The three basic components of renal function. This figure is to illustrate only the *directions* of reabsorption and secretion, not specific sites or order of occurrence. Depending on the particular substance, reabsorption and secretion can occur at various sites along the tubule.

the **glomerular filtrate.** It is cell-free and, except for larger proteins, contains all the substances in virtually the same concentrations as in plasma. This type of filtrate is also termed an *ultrafiltrate.*

During its passage through the tubules, the filtrate's composition is altered by movements of substances from the tubules to the peritubular capillaries, and vice versa (**Figure 14.6**). When the direction of movement is from tubular lumen to peritubular capillary plasma, the process is called **tubular reabsorption** or, simply, reabsorption. Movement in the opposite direction—that is, from peritubular plasma to tubular lumen—is called **tubular secretion** or, simply, secretion. Tubular secretion is also used to denote the movement of a solute from the cell interior to the lumen in the cases in which the kidney tubular cells themselves generate the substance.

To summarize, a substance can gain entry to the tubule and be excreted in the urine by glomerular filtration or tubular secretion or both. Once in the tubule, however, the substance does not have to be excreted but can be completely reabsorbed. Thus, the amount of any substance excreted in the urine is equal to the amount filtered plus the amount secreted minus the amount reabsorbed.

$$\text{Amount excreted} = \text{Amount filtered} + \text{Amount secreted} - \text{Amount reabsorbed}$$

It is important to stress that not all these processes—filtration, secretion, and reabsorption—apply to all substances. For example, important solutes like glucose are completely reabsorbed, whereas toxins are secreted and not reabsorbed.

To emphasize the general principles of renal function, **Figure 14.7** illustrates the renal handling of three hypothetical substances that might be found in blood. Approximately

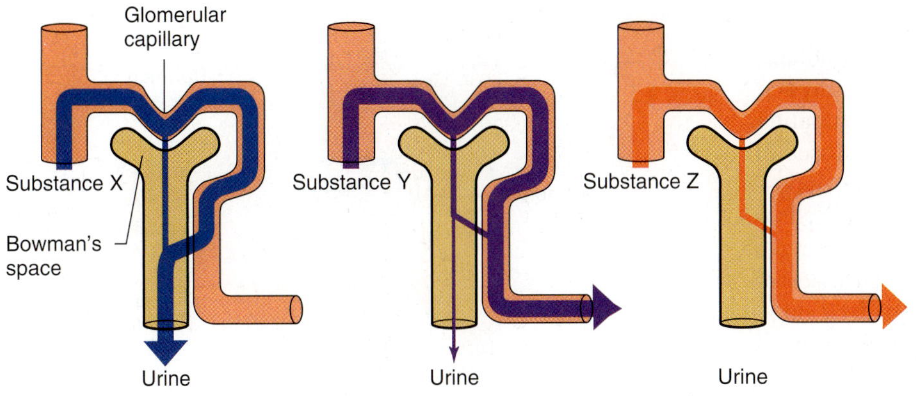

Figure 14.7 APR Renal handling of three hypothetical filtered substances X, Y, and Z. X is filtered and secreted but not reabsorbed. Y is filtered, and a fraction is then reabsorbed. Z is filtered and completely reabsorbed. The thickness of each line in this hypothetical example suggests the magnitude of the process.

20% of the plasma that enters the glomerular capillaries is filtered into Bowman's space. This filtrate, which contains X, Y, and Z in the same concentrations as in the capillary plasma, enters the proximal tubule and begins to flow through the rest of the tubule. Simultaneously, the remaining 80% of the plasma, containing X, Y, and Z, leaves the glomerular capillaries via the efferent arteriole and enters the peritubular capillaries.

Assume that the tubule can secrete 100% of the peritubular capillary substance X into the tubular lumen but cannot reabsorb X. Therefore, by the combination of filtration and tubular secretion, the plasma that originally entered the renal artery is cleared of all of its substance X, which leaves the body via the urine. Logically, this tends to be the pattern for renal handling of foreign substances that are potentially harmful to the body.

By contrast, assume that the tubule can reabsorb but not secrete Y and Z. The amount of Y reabsorption is moderate so that some of the filtered material is not reabsorbed and escapes from the body. For Z, however, the reabsorptive mechanism is so powerful that all the filtered Z is reabsorbed back into the plasma. Therefore, no Z is lost from the body. Hence, for Z, the processes of filtration and reabsorption have canceled each other out and the net result is as though Z had never entered the kidney. Again, it is logical to assume that substance Y is important to retain but requires maintenance within a homeostatic range; substance Z is presumably very important for health and is therefore completely reabsorbed.

A specific combination of filtration, tubular reabsorption, and tubular secretion applies to each substance in the plasma. The critical point is that, for many substances, the rates at which the processes proceed are subject to physiological control. By triggering changes in the rates of filtration, reabsorption, or secretion whenever the amount of a substance in the body is higher or lower than the normal limits, homeostatic mechanisms can regulate the substance's bodily balance. For example, consider what happens when a normally hydrated person drinks more water than usual. Within 1 to 2 hours, all the excess water has been excreted in the urine, partly as a result of an increase in filtration but mainly as a result of decreased tubular reabsorption of water. In this example, the kidneys are the effector organs of a homeostatic process that maintains total-body water within very narrow limits.

Although glomerular filtration, tubular reabsorption, and tubular secretion are the three basic renal processes, a fourth process—metabolism by the tubular cells—is also important for some substances. In some cases, the renal tubular cells remove substances from blood or glomerular filtrate and metabolize them, resulting in their disappearance from the body. In other cases, the cells *produce* substances and add them either to the blood or tubular fluid; the most important of these, as we will see, are ammonium ion, hydrogen ion, and HCO_3^-.

In summary, one can evaluate the normal renal processing of any given substance by asking a series of questions:

1. To what degree is the substance filterable at the renal corpuscle?
2. Is the substance reabsorbed?
3. Is the substance secreted?
4. What factors regulate the quantities filtered, reabsorbed, or secreted?
5. What are the pathways for altering renal excretion of the substance to maintain stable body balance?

Glomerular Filtration

As stated previously, the glomerular filtrate—that is, the fluid in Bowman's space—normally contains no cells but contains all plasma substances except proteins in virtually the same concentrations as in plasma. This is because glomerular filtration is a bulk-flow process in which water and all low-molecular-weight substances (including smaller polypeptides) move together. Most plasma proteins—the albumins and globulins—are excluded almost entirely from the filtrate. One reason for their exclusion is that the renal corpuscles restrict the movement of such high-molecular-weight substances. A second reason is that the filtration pathways in the corpuscular membranes are negatively charged, so they oppose the movement of these plasma proteins, most of which are negatively charged.

The only exceptions to the generalization that all nonprotein plasma substances have the same concentrations in the glomerular filtrate as in the plasma are certain low-molecular-weight substances that would otherwise be filterable but are bound to plasma proteins and therefore not filtered. For example, half the plasma calcium and virtually all of the plasma fatty acids are bound to plasma protein and so are not filtered.

Forces Involved in Filtration

Once again we return to the general principle that physiological processes are dictated by the laws of chemistry and physics; the importance of physical forces is critical to understanding the fundamental processes of homeostasis. As was discussed in Chapter 12, filtration across capillaries is determined by opposing Starling forces. To review, Starling forces are (1) the hydrostatic pressure difference across the capillary wall that favors filtration and (2) the protein concentration difference across the wall that creates an osmotic force that opposes filtration.

This also applies to the glomerular capillaries, as summarized in **Figure 14.8.** The blood pressure in the glomerular capillaries—the glomerular capillary hydrostatic pressure (P_{GC})—is a force favoring filtration. The fluid in Bowman's space exerts a hydrostatic pressure (P_{BS}) that opposes this filtration. Another opposing force is the osmotic force (π_{GC}) that results from the presence of protein in the glomerular capillary plasma. Recall that there is usually no protein in the filtrate in Bowman's space because of the unique structure of the areas of filtration in the glomerulus, so the osmotic force in Bowman's space (π_{BS}) is zero. The unequal distribution of protein causes the water concentration of the plasma to be slightly less than that of the fluid in Bowman's space, and this difference in water concentration favors fluid movement by osmosis from Bowman's space into the glomerular capillaries—that is, it opposes glomerular filtration.

Note that, in Figure 14.8, the value given for this osmotic force—29 mmHg—is slightly larger than the value—28 mmHg—for the osmotic force given in Chapter 12 for plasma in all arteries and nonrenal capillaries. The reason is that, unlike the situation elsewhere in the body, enough water filters out of the glomerular capillaries that the protein left behind in the plasma becomes more concentrated than in arterial plasma. In other capillaries, in contrast, little water filters out and the capillary protein concentration remains essentially unchanged from its value in arterial plasma. In other words, unlike the situation in other capillaries, the plasma protein concentration and, therefore, the osmotic force increase from the beginning to the end of the glomerular capillaries. The value given in Figure 14.8 for the osmotic force is the average value along the length of the capillaries.

To summarize, the **net glomerular filtration pressure** is the sum of three relevant forces:

$$\text{Net glomerular filtration pressure} = P_{GC} - P_{BS} - \pi_{GC}$$

Normally, the net filtration pressure is always positive because the glomerular capillary hydrostatic pressure (P_{GC}) is larger than the sum of the hydrostatic pressure in Bowman's space (P_{BS}) and the osmotic force opposing filtration (π_{GC}). The net glomerular filtration pressure initiates urine formation by forcing an essentially protein-free filtrate of plasma out of the glomerulus and into Bowman's space and then down the tubule into the renal pelvis.

Rate of Glomerular Filtration

The volume of fluid filtered from the glomeruli into Bowman's space per unit time is known as the **glomerular filtration rate (GFR).** GFR is determined not only by the net filtration pressure but also by the permeability of the corpuscular membranes and the surface area available for filtration. In other words, at any given net filtration pressure, the GFR will be directly proportional to the membrane permeability and the surface area. The glomerular capillaries are much more permeable to fluid than most other capillaries. Therefore, the net glomerular filtration pressure causes massive filtration of fluid into Bowman's space. In a 70 kg person, the GFR averages 180 L/day (125 mL/min)! This is much higher than the combined net filtration of 4 L/day of fluid across all the other capillaries in the body, as described in Chapter 12.

When we recall that the total volume of plasma in the cardiovascular system is approximately 3 L, it follows that the kidneys filter the entire plasma volume about 60 times a day. This opportunity to process such huge volumes of plasma enables the kidneys to regulate the constituents of the internal environment rapidly and to excrete large quantities of waste products.

GFR is not a fixed value but is subject to physiological regulation. This is achieved mainly by neural and hormonal input

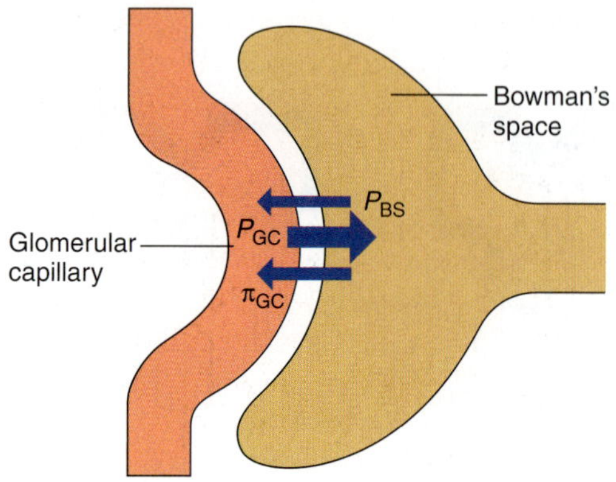

Forces	mmHg
Favoring filtration:	
Glomerular capillary blood pressure (P_{GC})	60
Opposing filtration:	
Fluid pressure in Bowman's space (P_{BS})	15
Osmotic force due to protein in plasma (π_{GC})	29
Net glomerular filtration pressure = $P_{GC} - P_{BS} - \pi_{GC}$	16

Figure 14.8 APIR Forces involved in glomerular filtration. The symbol π denotes the osmotic force due to the presence of protein in glomerular capillary plasma. (*Note:* The concentration of protein in Bowman's space is so low that π_{BS}, a force that would favor filtration, is considered zero.)

PHYSIOLOGICAL INQUIRY

- What would be the effect of an increase in plasma albumin (the most abundant plasma protein) on glomerular filtration rate (GFR)?

Answer can be found at end of chapter.

to the afferent and efferent arterioles, which causes changes in net glomerular filtration pressure (**Figure 14.9**). The glomerular capillaries are unique in that they are situated between two sets of arterioles—the afferent and efferent arterioles. Constriction of the afferent arterioles decreases hydrostatic pressure in the glomerular capillaries (P_{GC}). This is similar to arteriolar constriction in other organs and is due to a greater loss of pressure between arteries and capillaries (**Figure 14.9a**).

In contrast, efferent arteriolar constriction alone has the opposite effect on P_{GC} in that it *increases* it (**Figure 14.9b**). This occurs because the efferent arteriole lies beyond the glomerulus, so that efferent arteriolar constriction tends to "dam back" the blood in the glomerular capillaries, raising P_{GC}. Dilation of the efferent arteriole (**Figure 14.9c**) decreases P_{GC} and thus GFR, whereas dilation of the afferent arteriole increases P_{GC} and thus GFR (**Figure 14.9d**). Finally, simultaneous constriction or dilation of both sets of arterioles tends to leave P_{GC} unchanged because of the opposing effects. The control of GFR is an example of the general principle of physiology that most physiological functions are controlled by multiple regulatory systems, often working in opposition.

In addition to the neural and endocrine input to the arterioles, there is also neural and humoral input to the mesangial cells that surround the glomerular capillaries. Contraction of these cells reduces the surface area of the capillaries, which causes a decrease in GFR at any given net filtration pressure.

It is possible to measure the total amount of any nonprotein or non-protein-bound substance filtered into Bowman's space by multiplying the GFR by the plasma concentration of the substance. This amount is called the **filtered load** of the substance. For example, if the GFR is 180 L/day and plasma glucose concentration is 1 g/L, then the filtered load of glucose is 180 L/day $\times$ 1 g/L = 180 g/day.

Once the filtered load of the substance is known, it can be compared to the amount of the substance excreted. This indicates whether the substance undergoes net tubular reabsorption or net secretion. Whenever the quantity of a substance excreted in the urine is less than the filtered load, tubular reabsorption must have occurred. Conversely, if the amount excreted in the urine is greater than the filtered load, tubular secretion must have occurred.

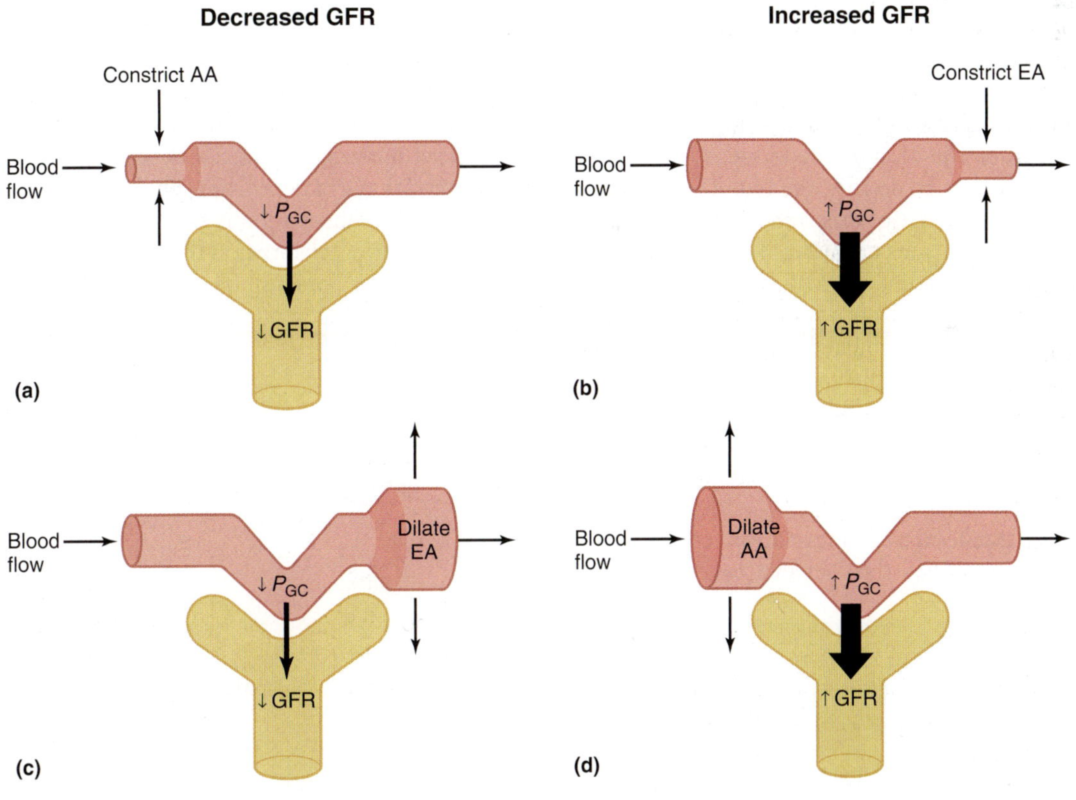

Figure 14.9 APIR Control of GFR by constriction or dilation of afferent arterioles (AA) or efferent arterioles (EA). (a) Constriction of the afferent arteriole or (c) dilation of the efferent arteriole reduces P_{GC}, thus decreasing GFR. (b) Constriction of the efferent arteriole or (d) dilation of the afferent arteriole increases P_{GC}, thus increasing GFR.

PHYSIOLOGICAL INQUIRY

- Describe the immediate consequences of a blood clot occluding the afferent arteriole or the efferent arteriole.

Answer can be found at end of chapter.

Tubular Reabsorption

Table 14.2 summarizes data for a few plasma components that undergo filtration and reabsorption. It gives an idea of the magnitude and importance of reabsorptive mechanisms. The values in this table are typical for a healthy person on an average diet. There are at least three important conclusions we can draw from this table: (1) The filtered loads are enormous, generally larger than the amounts of the substances in the body. For example, the body contains about 40 L of water, but the volume of water filtered each day is 180 L. (2) Reabsorption of waste products is relatively incomplete (as in the case of urea), so that large fractions of their filtered loads are excreted in the urine. (3) Reabsorption of most useful plasma components, such as water, inorganic ions, and organic nutrients, is relatively complete so that the amounts excreted in the urine are very small fractions of their filtered loads.

An important distinction should be made between reabsorptive processes that can be controlled physiologically and those that cannot. The reabsorption rates of most organic nutrients, such as glucose, are always very high and are not physiologically regulated. Thus, the filtered loads of these substances are normally completely reabsorbed, with none appearing in the urine. For these substances, like substance Z in Figure 14.7, it is as though the kidneys do not exist because the kidneys do not eliminate these substances from the body at all. Therefore, the kidneys do not regulate the plasma concentrations of these organic nutrients. Rather, the kidneys merely maintain whatever plasma concentrations already exist.

Recall that a major function of the kidneys is to eliminate soluble waste products. To do this, the blood is filtered in the glomeruli. One consequence of this is that substances necessary for normal body functions are filtered from the plasma into the tubular fluid. To prevent the loss of these important nonwaste products, the kidneys have powerful mechanisms to reclaim useful substances from tubular fluid while simultaneously allowing waste products to be excreted. The reabsorptive rates for water and many ions, although also very high, are under physiological control. For example, if water intake is decreased, the kidneys can increase water reabsorption to minimize water loss.

In contrast to glomerular filtration, the crucial steps in tubular reabsorption—those that achieve movement of a substance from tubular lumen to interstitial fluid—do *not* occur by bulk flow because there are inadequate pressure differences across the tubule and inadequate permeability of the tubular membranes. Instead, two other processes are involved. (1) The reabsorption of some substances from the tubular lumen is by diffusion, often across the tight junctions connecting the tubular epithelial cells (**Figure 14.10**). (2) The reabsorption of all other substances involves mediated transport, which requires the participation of transport proteins in the plasma membranes of tubular cells.

The final step in reabsorption is the movement of substances from the interstitial fluid into peritubular capillaries that occurs by a combination of diffusion and bulk flow. We will assume that this final process occurs automatically once the substance reaches the interstitial fluid.

TABLE 14.2 Average Values for Several Components That Undergo Filtration and Reabsorption

Substance	Amount Filtered per Day	Amount Excreted per Day	Percentage Reabsorbed
Water, L	180	1.8	99
Sodium, g	630	3.2	99.5
Glucose, g	180	0	100
Urea, g	54	30	44

Reabsorption by Diffusion

The reabsorption of urea by the proximal tubule provides an example of passive reabsorption by diffusion. An analysis of urea concentrations in the proximal tubule will help clarify the mechanism. Because the corpuscular membranes are freely filterable to urea, the urea concentration in the fluid within Bowman's space is the same as that in the peritubular capillary plasma and the interstitial fluid surrounding the tubule. Then, as the filtered fluid flows through the proximal tubule, water reabsorption occurs (by mechanisms to be described later). This removal of water increases the concentration of urea in the tubular fluid so it is higher than in the interstitial fluid and peritubular capillaries. Therefore, urea diffuses down this concentration gradient from tubular lumen to peritubular capillary. Urea reabsorption is thus dependent upon the reabsorption of water. Reabsorption by diffusion in this manner occurs for a variety of lipid-soluble organic substances, both naturally occurring and foreign (e.g., the pesticide DDT).

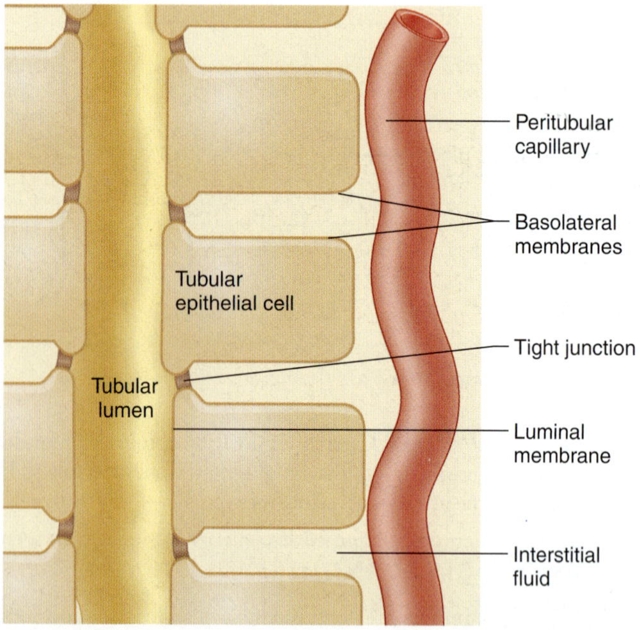

Figure 14.10 APIR Diagrammatic representation of tubular epithelium. The luminal membrane is also called the apical membrane.

Reabsorption by Mediated Transport

Figure 14.10 demonstrates that a substance reabsorbed by mediated transport must first cross the **luminal membrane** (also called the *apical membrane*) that separates the tubular lumen from the cell interior. Then, the substance diffuses through the cytosol of the cell and, finally, crosses the **basolateral membrane,** which begins at the tight junctions and constitutes the plasma membrane of the sides and base of the cell. The movement by this route is termed *transcellular* epithelial transport.

A substance does not need to be actively transported across *both* the luminal and basolateral membranes in order to be actively transported across the overall epithelium, thus moving from lumen to interstitial fluid against its electrochemical gradient. For example, Na^+ moves "downhill" (passively) into the cell across the luminal membrane either by diffusion or by facilitated diffusion and then is actively transported "uphill" out of the cell across the basolateral membrane via Na^+/K^+-ATPases in this membrane.

The reabsorption of many substances is coupled to the reabsorption of Na^+. The cotransported substance moves uphill into the cell via a secondary active cotransporter as Na^+ moves downhill into the cell via this same cotransporter. This is precisely how glucose, many amino acids, and other organic substances undergo tubular reabsorption. The reabsorption of several inorganic ions is also coupled in a variety of ways to the reabsorption of Na^+.

Many of the mediated-transport-reabsorptive systems in the renal tubule have a limit to the amounts of material they can transport per unit time known as the **transport maximum** (T_m). This is because the binding sites on the membrane transport proteins become saturated when the concentration of the transported substance increases to a certain level. An important example is the secondary active-transport proteins for glucose, located in the proximal tubule. As noted earlier, glucose does not usually appear in the urine because all of the filtered glucose is reabsorbed. This is illustrated in **Figure 14.11,** which shows the relationship between plasma glucose concentrations and the filtered load, reabsorption, and excretion of glucose. Plasma glucose concentration in a healthy person normally does not exceed 150 mg/100 mL even after the person eats a sugary meal. Notice that this level of plasma glucose is below the threshold at which glucose starts to appear in urine (***glucosuria***). Also notice that the T_m for the entire kidney is higher than the threshold for glucosuria. This is because the nephrons have a range of T_m values that, when averaged, give a T_m for the entire kidney, as shown in Figure 14.11. When plasma glucose concentration exceeds the transport maximum for a significant number of nephrons, glucose starts to appear in urine. In people with significant hyperglycemia (for example, in poorly controlled ***diabetes mellitus***), the plasma glucose concentration often exceeds the threshold value of 200 mg/100 mL, so that the filtered load exceeds the ability of the nephrons to reabsorb glucose. In other words, although the capacity of the kidneys to reabsorb glucose can be normal in diabetes mellitus, the tubules cannot reabsorb the large increase in the filtered load of glucose. As you will learn later in this chapter and in Chapter 16, the high filtered load of glucose can also lead to significant disruption of normal renal function (***diabetic nephropathy***).

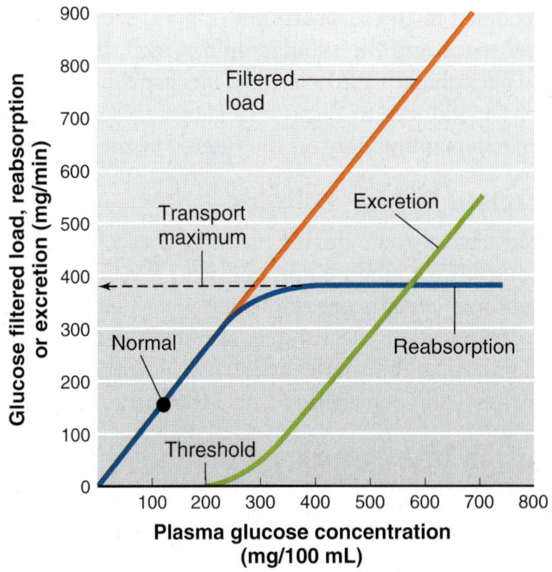

Figure 14.11 The relationship between plasma glucose concentration and the rate of glucose filtered (filtered load), reabsorbed, or excreted. The dotted line shows the transport maximum, which is the maximum rate at which glucose can be reabsorbed. Notice that as plasma glucose exceeds its threshold, glucose begins to appear in the urine.

PHYSIOLOGICAL INQUIRY

- How would you calculate the filtered load and excretion rate of glucose?

Answer can be found at end of chapter.

The pattern described for glucose is also true for a large number of other organic nutrients. For example, most amino acids and water-soluble vitamins are filtered in large amounts each day, but almost all of these filtered molecules are reabsorbed by the proximal tubule. If the plasma concentration becomes high enough, however, reabsorption of the filtered load will not be as complete and the substance will appear in larger amounts in the urine. Thus, people who ingest very large quantities of vitamin C have increased plasma concentrations of vitamin C. Eventually, the filtered load may exceed the tubular reabsorptive T_m for this substance, and any additional ingested vitamin C is excreted in the urine.

Tubular Secretion

Tubular secretion moves substances from peritubular capillaries into the tubular lumen. Like glomerular filtration, it constitutes a pathway from the blood into the tubule. Like reabsorption, secretion can occur by diffusion or by transcellular mediated transport. The most important substances secreted by the tubules are H^+ and K^+. However, a large number of normally occurring organic anions, such as choline and creatinine, are also secreted; so are many foreign chemicals such as penicillin. Active secretion of a substance requires active transport either from the blood side (the interstitial fluid) into the tubule cell (across the basolateral membrane) or out of the cell into the lumen (across the luminal membrane). As in reabsorption, tubular secretion is usually coupled to the reabsorption of Na^+. Secretion from the interstitial space into the tubular fluid, which draws substances from the peritubular capillaries, is a mechanism to increase the ability of the kidneys to dispose of substances at a higher rate rather than depending only on the filtered load.

Metabolism by the Tubules

We noted earlier that, during fasting, the cells of the renal tubules synthesize glucose and add it to the blood. They can also catabolize certain organic substances, such as peptides, taken up from either the tubular lumen or peritubular capillaries. Catabolism eliminates these substances from the body just as if they had been excreted into the urine.

Regulation of Membrane Channels and Transporters

Tubular reabsorption or secretion of many substances is under physiological control. For most of these substances, control is achieved by regulating the activity or concentrations of the membrane channel and transporter proteins involved in their transport. This regulation is achieved by hormones and paracrine or autocrine factors.

Understanding the structure, function, and regulation of renal, tubular-cell ion channels and transporters makes it possible to explain the underlying defects in some genetic diseases. For example, a genetic mutation can lead to an abnormality in the Na^+–glucose cotransporter that mediates reabsorption of glucose in the proximal tubule. This can lead to the appearance of glucose in the urine (***familial renal glucosuria***). Contrast this condition to diabetes mellitus, in which the ability to reabsorb glucose is usually normal but the filtered load of glucose exceeds the threshold for the tubules to reabsorb glucose (see Figure 14.11).

"Division of Labor" in the Tubules

To excrete waste products adequately, the GFR must be very large. This means that the filtered volume of water and the filtered loads of all the nonwaste plasma solutes are also very large. *The primary role of the proximal tubule is to reabsorb most of this filtered water and these solutes.* Furthermore, with K^+ as the one major exception, the proximal tubule is the major site of solute secretion. Henle's loop also reabsorbs relatively large quantities of the major ions and, to a lesser extent, water.

Extensive reabsorption by the proximal tubule and Henle's loop ensures that the masses of solutes and the volume of water entering the tubular segments beyond Henle's loop are relatively small. These distal segments then do the fine-tuning for most substances, determining the final amounts excreted in the urine by adjusting their rates of reabsorption and, in a few cases, secretion. It should not be surprising, therefore, that most homeostatic controls act upon the more distal segments of the tubule.

14.4 The Concept of Renal Clearance

A useful way of quantifying renal function is in terms of clearance. The renal **clearance** of any substance is the volume of plasma from which that substance is completely removed ("cleared") by the kidneys per unit time. Every substance has its own distinct clearance value, but the units are always in volume of plasma per unit of time. The basic clearance formula for any substance S is

$$\text{Clearance of } S = \frac{\text{Mass of } S \text{ excreted per unit time}}{\text{Plasma concentration of } S}$$

Thus, the clearance of a substance is a measure of the volume of plasma completely cleared of the substance per unit time. This accounts for the mass of the substance excreted in the urine.

Because the mass of S excreted per unit time is equal to the urine concentration of S multiplied by the urine volume during that time, the formula for the clearance of S becomes

$$C_S = \frac{U_S V}{P_S}$$

where

C_S = Clearance of S
U_S = Urine concentration of S
V = Urine volume per unit time
P_S = Plasma concentration of S

Let us examine some particularly interesting examples of clearance. What would be the clearance of glucose, for example, under normal conditions? Recall from Figure 14.11 that all of the glucose filtered from the plasma into the glomeruli is normally reabsorbed by the epithelial cells of the proximal tubules. Therefore, the clearance of glucose (C_{gl}) can be written as the following equation:

$$C_{gl} = \frac{(U_{gl})(V)}{(P_{gl})}$$

where the subscript "gl" indicates glucose. Because glucose is usually completely reabsorbed, its urinary concentration under normal conditions is zero (see Table 14.2). Therefore, this equation reduces to

$$C_{gl} = \frac{(0)(V)}{(P_{gl})} \text{ or } C_{gl} = 0$$

The clearance of glucose is normally zero because all of the glucose that is filtered from the plasma into the glomeruli is reabsorbed back into the blood. As shown in Figure 14.11, only when the T_m for glucose is exceeded would the clearance become a positive value, which, as described earlier, would suggest the possibility of renal disease or very high blood glucose such as in untreated diabetes mellitus.

Now imagine a substance that is freely filtered but neither reabsorbed nor secreted. In other words, such a substance is not physiologically important like glucose—nor toxic like certain compounds that are secreted—and is, therefore, "ignored" by the kidneys. The human body does not produce such compounds that perfectly fit these characteristics, but there are examples found in nature. One such compound is the polysaccharide called **inulin** (not insulin), which is present in some of the vegetables and fruits that we eat. If inulin were infused intravenously in a person, what would happen? The amount of inulin entering the nephrons from the plasma—that is, the filtered load—would be equal to the amount of inulin excreted in the urine, and none of it would be reabsorbed or secreted. Recall that the filtered load of a substance is the glomerular filtration rate (GFR) multiplied by the plasma concentration of the substance. The excreted amount of the substance is *UV*, as just described. Therefore, for the special case of inulin (subscript "in"),

$$(GFR)(P_{in}) = (U_{in})(V)$$

By rearranging this equation, we get an equation that looks like the general equation for clearance shown earlier:

$$GFR = \frac{(U_{in})(V)}{(P_{in})}$$

In other words, the GFR of a person is equal to the clearance of inulin (*UV/P*)! If it were necessary to determine the GFR of a person, for example, someone suspected of having kidney disease, a physician would only need to determine the clearance of inulin. **Figure 14.12** shows a mathematical example of the renal handling of inulin. Notice that the GFR is 7.5 L/h, which is 125 mL/min, as described earlier in this section.

The clearance of any substance handled by the kidneys in the same way as inulin—filtered, but not reabsorbed, secreted, or metabolized—would equal the GFR. Unfortunately, there are no substances normally present in the plasma that perfectly meet these criteria, and for technical reasons it is not practical to perform an inulin clearance test in clinical situations. For clinical purposes, the **creatinine clearance** (C_{Cr}) is commonly used to approximate the GFR as follows. Creatinine is a waste product released by muscle; it is filtered at the renal corpuscle but does not undergo reabsorption. It does undergo a small amount of secretion, however, so that some peritubular plasma is cleared of its creatinine by secretion. Therefore, C_{Cr} slightly overestimates the GFR but is close enough to be highly useful in most clinical situations.

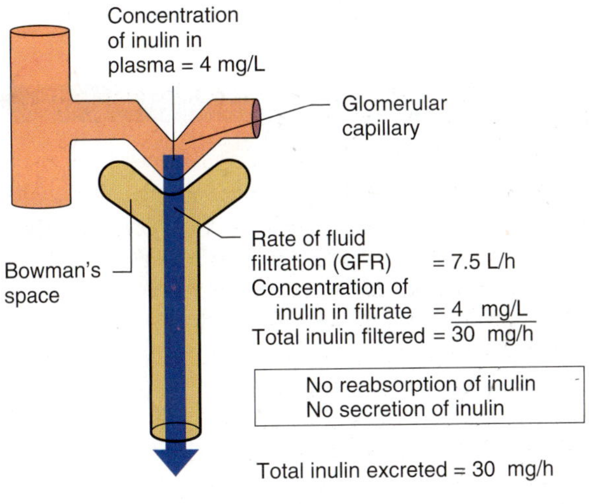

Figure 14.12 Example of renal handling of inulin, a substance that is filtered by the renal corpuscles but is neither reabsorbed nor secreted by the tubule. Therefore, the mass of inulin excreted per unit time is equal to the mass filtered during the same time period. As explained in the text, the clearance of inulin is equal to the glomerular filtration rate.

Usually, the concentration of creatinine in the blood is the only measurement necessary because it is assumed that creatinine production by the body is constant and similar between individuals. Therefore, an increase in creatinine concentration in the blood usually indicates a decrease in GFR, one of the hallmarks of kidney disease.

This leads to an important generalization. When the clearance of any substance is greater than the GFR, that substance must undergo tubular secretion. Look back at our hypothetical substance X (see Figure 14.7): X is filtered, and all the X that escapes filtration is secreted; no X is reabsorbed. Consequently, all the plasma that enters the kidney per unit time is cleared of its X. Therefore, the clearance of X is a measure of **renal plasma flow.** A substance that is handled like X is the organic anion para-aminohippurate (PAH), which is used for this purpose experimentally. (Like inulin, it must be administered intravenously.)

A similar logic leads to another important generalization. When the clearance of a filterable substance is less than the GFR, that substance must undergo some reabsorption. Performing calculations such as these provides important information about the way in which the kidneys handle a given solute. Suppose a newly developed drug is being tested for its safety and effectiveness. The dose of drug required to achieve a safe and therapeutic effect will depend at least in part on how rapidly it is cleared by the kidneys. Assume that we measure the clearance of the drug and find that it is greater than the GFR as determined by creatinine clearance. This means that the drug is secreted into the nephron tubules and a higher dose of drug than otherwise predicted may be needed to reach an optimal concentration in the blood.

14.5 Micturition

Urine flow through the ureters to the bladder is propelled by contractions of the ureter wall smooth muscle. The urine is stored in the bladder and intermittently ejected during urination, or **micturition.**

The bladder is a balloonlike chamber with walls of smooth muscle collectively termed the **detrusor muscle.** The contraction of the detrusor muscle squeezes on the urine in the bladder lumen to produce urination. That part of the detrusor muscle at the base (or "neck") of the bladder where the urethra begins functions as the **internal urethral sphincter.** Just below the internal urethral sphincter, a ring of skeletal muscle surrounds the urethra. This is the **external urethral sphincter,** the contraction of which can prevent urination even when the detrusor muscle contracts strongly.

The neural controls that influence bladder structures during the phases of filling and micturition are shown in **Figure 14.13.** While the bladder is filling, the parasympathetic input to the detrusor muscle is minimal, and, as a result, the muscle is relaxed. Because of the arrangement of the smooth muscle fibers, when the detrusor muscle is relaxed, the internal urethral sphincter is passively closed. Additionally, there is strong sympathetic input to the internal urethral sphincter and strong input by the somatic motor neurons to the external urethral sphincter. Therefore, the detrusor muscle is relaxed and both the internal and external sphincters are closed during the filling phase.

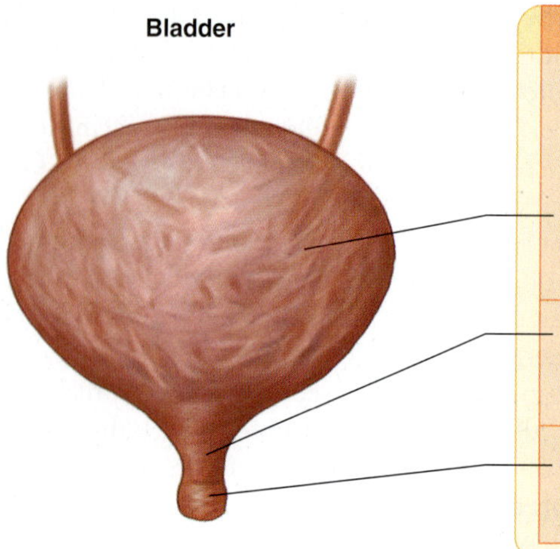

Muscle	Innervation: Type	Innervation: During filling	Innervation: During micturition
Detrusor (smooth muscle)	Parasympathetic (causes contraction)	Inhibited	Stimulated
Internal urethral sphincter (smooth muscle)	Sympathetic (causes contraction)	Stimulated	Inhibited
External urethral sphincter (skeletal muscle)	Somatic motor (causes contraction)	Stimulated	Inhibited

Figure 14.13 APIR Control of the bladder.

What happens during micturition? As the bladder fills with urine, the pressure within it increases, which stimulates stretch receptors in the bladder wall. The afferent neurons from these receptors enter the spinal cord and stimulate the parasympathetic neurons, which then cause the detrusor muscle to contract. When the detrusor muscle contracts, the change in shape of the bladder pulls open the internal urethral sphincter. Simultaneously, the afferent input from the stretch receptors reflexively inhibits the sympathetic neurons to the internal urethral sphincter, which further contributes to its opening. In addition, the afferent input also reflexively inhibits the somatic motor neurons to the external urethral sphincter, causing it to relax. Both sphincters are now open, and the contraction of the detrusor muscle can produce urination.

We have thus far described micturition as a local spinal reflex, but descending pathways from the brain can also profoundly influence this reflex, determining the ability to prevent or initiate micturition voluntarily. Loss of these descending pathways as a result of spinal cord damage eliminates the ability to voluntarily control micturition. As the bladder distends, the input from the bladder stretch receptors causes, via ascending pathways to the brain, a sense of bladder fullness and the urge to urinate. But in response to this, urination can be voluntarily prevented by activating descending pathways that stimulate both the sympathetic nerves to the internal urethral sphincter and the somatic motor nerves to the external urethral sphincter. In contrast, urination can be voluntarily initiated via the descending pathways to the appropriate neurons. Complex interactions in different areas in the brain control micturition. Briefly, there are areas in the brainstem that can both facilitate and inhibit voiding. Furthermore, an area of the midbrain can inhibit voiding, and an area of the posterior hypothalamus can facilitate voiding. Finally, strong inhibitory input from the cerebral cortex, learned during toilet training in early childhood, prevents involuntary urination.

Incontinence

Incontinence is the involuntary release of urine, which can be a disturbing problem both socially and hygienically. The most common types are ***stress incontinence*** (due to sneezing, coughing, or exercise) and ***urge incontinence*** (associated with the desire to urinate). Incontinence is more common in women and may occur one to two times per week in more than 25% of women older than 60. It is very common in older women in nursing homes and assisted-living facilities. In women, stress incontinence is usually due to a loss of urethral support provided by the anterior vagina (see Figure 17.17a). Medications (such as estrogen-replacement therapy to improve vaginal tone) can often relieve stress incontinence. Severe cases may require surgery to improve vaginal support of the bladder and urethra. The cause of urge incontinence is often unknown in individual patients. However, any irritation to the bladder or urethra (e.g., with a bacterial infection) can cause urge incontinence. Urge incontinence can be treated with drugs such as tolterodine or oxybutynin, which antagonize the effects of the parasympathetic nerves on the detrusor muscle. Because these drugs are anticholinergic, they can have side effects such as blurred vision, constipation, and increased heart rate.

SECTION A SUMMARY

Renal Functions

I. The kidneys regulate the water and ionic composition of the body, excrete waste products, excrete foreign chemicals, produce glucose during prolonged fasting, and release factors and hormones into the blood (renin, 1,25-dihydroxyvitamin D, and erythropoietin). The first three functions are accomplished by continuous processing of the plasma.

Structure of the Kidneys and Urinary System

I. Each nephron in the kidneys consists of a renal corpuscle and a tubule.
   a. Each renal corpuscle comprises a capillary tuft, termed a glomerulus, and a Bowman's capsule that the tuft protrudes into.
   b. The tubule extends from Bowman's capsule and is subdivided into the proximal tubule, loop of Henle, distal convoluted tubule, and collecting-duct system. At the level of the collecting ducts, multiple tubules join and empty into

the renal pelvis, from which urine flows through the ureters to the bladder.

c. Each glomerulus is supplied by an afferent arteriole, and an efferent arteriole leaves the glomerulus to branch into peritubular capillaries, which supply the tubule.

Basic Renal Processes

I. The three basic renal processes are glomerular filtration, tubular reabsorption, and tubular secretion. In addition, the kidneys synthesize and/or catabolize certain substances. The excretion of a substance is equal to the amount filtered plus the amount secreted minus the amount reabsorbed.

II. Urine formation begins with glomerular filtration—approximately 180 L/day—of essentially protein-free plasma into Bowman's space.
  a. Glomerular filtrate contains all plasma substances other than proteins (and substances bound to proteins) in virtually the same concentrations as in plasma.
  b. Glomerular filtration is driven by the hydrostatic pressure in the glomerular capillaries and is opposed by both the hydrostatic pressure in Bowman's space and the osmotic force due to the proteins in the glomerular capillary plasma.

III. As the filtrate moves through the tubules, certain substances are reabsorbed either by diffusion or by mediated transport.
  a. Substances to which the tubular epithelium is permeable are reabsorbed by diffusion because water reabsorption creates tubule-interstitium-concentration gradients for them.
  b. Active reabsorption of a substance requires the participation of transporters in the luminal or basolateral membrane.
  c. Tubular reabsorption rates are very high for nutrients, ions, and water, but they are lower for waste products.
  d. Many of the mediated-transport systems exhibit transport maximums. When the filtered load of a substance exceeds the transport maximum, large amounts may appear in the urine.

IV. Tubular secretion, like glomerular filtration, is a pathway for the entrance of a substance into the tubule.

The Concept of Renal Clearance

I. The clearance of any substance can be calculated by dividing the mass of the substance excreted per unit time by the plasma concentration of the substance.

II. GFR can be measured by means of the inulin clearance and estimated by means of the creatinine clearance.

Micturition

I. In the basic micturition reflex, bladder distension stimulates stretch receptors that trigger spinal reflexes; these reflexes lead to contraction of the detrusor muscle, mediated by parasympathetic neurons, and relaxation of both the internal and the external urethral sphincters, mediated by inhibition of the neurons to these muscles.

II. Voluntary control is exerted via descending pathways to the parasympathetic nerves supplying the detrusor muscle, the sympathetic nerves supplying the internal urethral sphincter, and the motor nerves supplying the external urethral sphincter.

III. Incontinence is the involuntary release of urine that occurs most commonly in elderly people (particularly women).

SECTION A REVIEW QUESTIONS

1. What are the functions of the kidneys?
2. What three hormones/factors do the kidneys secrete into the blood?
3. Fluid flows in sequence through what structures from the glomerulus to the bladder? Blood flows through what structures from the renal artery to the renal vein?
4. What are the three basic renal processes that lead to the formation of urine?
5. How does the composition of the glomerular filtrate compare with that of plasma?
6. Describe the forces that determine the magnitude of the GFR. What is a normal value of GFR?
7. Contrast the mechanisms of reabsorption for glucose and urea. Which one shows a T_m?
8. Diagram the sequence of events leading to micturition.

SECTION A KEY TERMS

afferent arteriole 494
ascending limb 494
basolateral membrane 501
bladder 492
Bowman's capsule 494
Bowman's space 494
calyx 492
capsule 492
clearance 502
collecting-duct system 494
cortical (nephron) 494
cortical collecting duct 494
creatinine 491
creatinine clearance (C_{Cr}) 503
descending limb 494
detrusor muscle 503
distal convoluted tubule 494
efferent arteriole 494
external urethral sphincter 503
filtered load 499
glomerular capillaries 494
glomerular filtrate 496
glomerular filtration 494
glomerular filtration rate (GFR) 498
glomerulus 494
hilum 492
internal urethral sphincter 503
inulin 502
juxtaglomerular apparatus (JGA) 494
juxtaglomerular (JG) cell 494
juxtamedullary (nephron) 494
loop of Henle 494
luminal membrane 501
macula densa 494
medullary collecting duct 494
mesangial cells 494
micturition 503
nephron 492
net glomerular filtration pressure 498
papilla 492
peritubular capillary 494
podocyte 494
proximal tubule 494
renal 491
renal artery 492
renal corpuscle 492
renal cortex 492
renal medulla 492
renal pelvis 494
renal plasma flow 503
renal vein 492
transport maximum (T_m) 501
tubular reabsorption 496
tubular secretion 496
tubule 492
urea 491
ureter 492
urethra 492
uric acid 491
vasa recta 494

SECTION A CLINICAL TERMS

diabetes mellitus 501
diabetic nephropathy 501
familial renal glucosuria 502
glucosuria 501
incontinence 504
stress incontinence 504
urge incontinence 504

SECTION B

Regulation of Ion and Water Balance

14.6 Total-Body Balance of Sodium and Water

Chapter 1 explained that water composes about 55% to 60% of the normal body weight, and that water is distributed throughout different compartments of the body (Figure 1.3). Since water is of such obvious importance to homeostasis, the regulation of total-body-water balance is critical to survival. This highlights two important general principles of physiology: (1) Homeostasis is essential for health and survival; and (2) controlled exchange of materials—in this case, water—occurs between compartments and across cellular membranes. **Table 14.3** summarizes total-body-water balance. These are average values that are subject to considerable normal variation. There are two sources of body water gain: (1) water produced from the oxidation of organic nutrients, and (2) water ingested in liquids and food (a rare steak is approximately 70% water). Four sites lose water to the external environment: skin, respiratory airways, gastrointestinal tract, and urinary tract. Menstrual flow constitutes a fifth potential source of water loss in women.

The loss of water by evaporation from the skin and the lining of the respiratory passageways is a continuous process. It is called **insensible water loss** because the person is unaware of its occurrence. Additional water can be made available for evaporation from the skin by the production of sweat. Normal gastrointestinal loss of water in feces is generally quite small, but it can be significant with diarrhea and vomiting.

Table 14.4 is a summary of total-body balance for sodium chloride. The excretion of Na^+ and Cl^- via the skin and gastrointestinal tract is normally small but increases markedly during severe sweating, vomiting, or diarrhea. Hemorrhage can also result in the loss of large quantities of both salt and water.

Under normal conditions, as Tables 14.3 and 14.4 show, salt and water losses equal salt and water gains, and no net change in body salt and water occurs. This matching of losses and gains is primarily the result of the regulation of urinary loss, which can be varied over an extremely wide range. For example, urinary water excretion can vary from approximately 0.4 L/day to 25 L/day, depending upon whether one is lost in the desert or drinking too much water. Similarly, some individuals ingest 20 to 25 g of sodium chloride per day, whereas a person on a low-salt diet may ingest only 0.05 g. Healthy kidneys can readily alter the excretion of salt over this range to balance loss with gain.

TABLE 14.3 Average Daily Water Gain and Loss in Adults

Intake	
In liquids	1400 mL
In food	1100 mL
Metabolically produced	350 mL
Total	**2850 mL**
Output	
Insensible loss (skin and lungs)	900 mL
Sweat	50 mL
In feces	100 mL
Urine	1800 mL
Total	**2850 mL**

14.7 Basic Renal Processes for Sodium and Water

Both Na^+ and water freely filter from the glomerular capillaries into Bowman's space because they have low molecular weights and circulate in the plasma in the free form (unbound to protein). They both undergo considerable reabsorption—normally more than 99% (see Table 14.2)—but no secretion. Most renal energy utilization is used in this enormous reabsorptive task. The bulk of Na^+ and water reabsorption (about two-thirds) occurs in the proximal tubule, but the major hormonal control of reabsorption is exerted on the distal convoluted tubules and collecting ducts.

The mechanisms of Na^+ and water reabsorption can be summarized in two generalizations: (1) Na^+ reabsorption is an active process occurring in all tubular segments except the descending limb of the loop of Henle; and (2) water reabsorption is by osmosis and is dependent upon Na^+ reabsorption.

Primary Active Na^+ Reabsorption

The essential feature underlying Na^+ reabsorption throughout the tubule is the primary active transport of Na^+ out of the cells and into the interstitial fluid, as illustrated for the proximal tubule and cortical collecting duct in **Figure 14.14.** This transport is achieved by Na^+/K^+-ATPase pumps in the basolateral membrane of the cells. The active transport of Na^+ out of the cell keeps the intracellular concentration of Na^+ low compared to the tubular lumen, so Na^+ moves "downhill" out of the tubular lumen into the tubular epithelial cells.

The mechanism of the downhill Na^+ movement across the luminal membrane into the cell varies from segment to

TABLE 14.4 Daily Sodium Chloride Intake and Loss

Intake	
Food	**8.50 g**
Output	
Sweat	0.25 g
Feces	0.25 g
Urine	8.00 g
Total	**8.50 g**

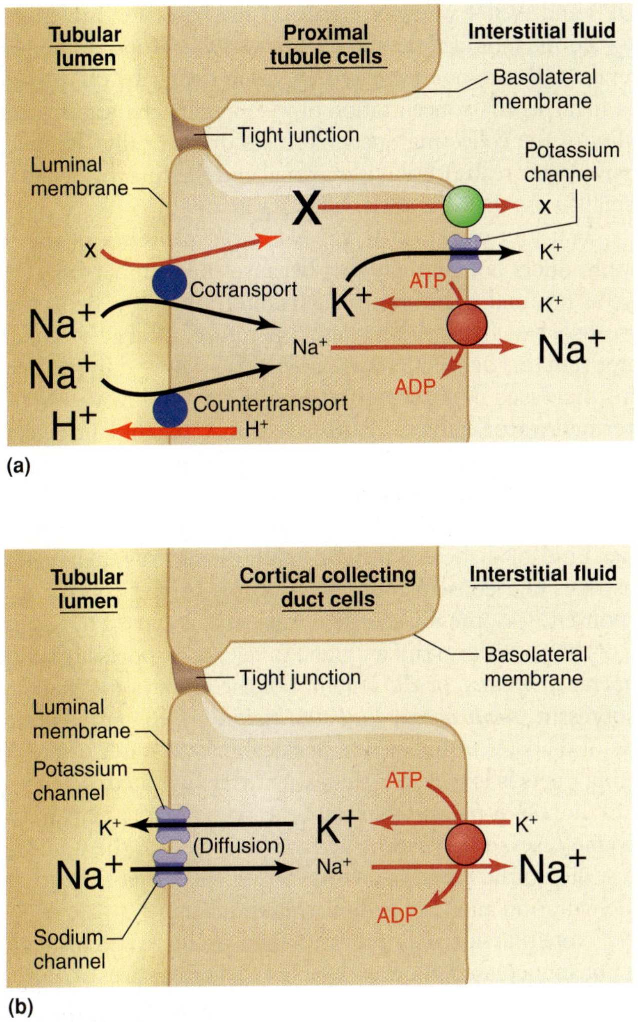

Figure 14.14 AP|R Mechanism of Na^+ reabsorption in the (a) proximal tubule and (b) cortical collecting duct. (Figure 14.15 shows the movement of the reabsorbed Na^+ from the interstitial fluid into the peritubular capillaries.) The sizes of the letters denote high and low concentrations. "X" represents organic molecules such as glucose and amino acids that are cotransported with Na^+. The fate of the K^+ that the Na^+/K^+-ATPase pumps transport is discussed in the later section dealing with renal K^+ handling.

PHYSIOLOGICAL INQUIRY

- Referring to part (b), what would be the effect of a drug that blocks the Na^+ channels in the cortical collecting duct?

Answer can be found at end of chapter.

segment of the tubule depending on which channels and/or transport proteins are present in their luminal membranes. For example, the luminal entry step in the proximal tubule cell occurs by cotransport with a variety of organic molecules, such as glucose, or by countertransport with H^+. In the latter case, H^+ moves out of the cell to the lumen as Na^+ moves into the cell (**Figure 14.14a**). Thus, in the proximal tubule, Na^+ reabsorption drives the reabsorption of the cotransported substances and secretion of H^+. In actuality, the luminal membrane of the proximal tubular cell has a brush border composed of numerous microvilli (for clarity, not shown in Figure 14.14a). This greatly increases the surface area for reabsorption. The luminal entry step for Na^+ in the cortical collecting duct occurs primarily by diffusion through Na^+ channels (**Figure 14.14b**).

The movement of Na^+ downhill from lumen into cell across the *luminal membrane* varies from one segment of the tubule to another. By contrast, the *basolateral membrane* step is the same in all Na^+-reabsorbing tubular segments—the primary active transport of Na^+ out of the cell is via Na^+/K^+-ATPase pumps in this membrane. It is this transport process that decreases intracellular Na^+ concentration and so makes possible the downhill luminal entry step.

Coupling of Water Reabsorption to Na^+ Reabsorption

As Na^+, Cl^-, and other ions are reabsorbed, water follows passively by osmosis (see Chapter 4). **Figure 14.15** summarizes this coupling of solute and water reabsorption. (1) Na^+ is transported from the tubular lumen to the interstitial fluid across the epithelial cells. Other solutes, such as glucose, amino acids, and HCO_3^-, whose reabsorption depends on Na^+ transport, also contribute to osmosis. (2) The removal of solutes from the tubular lumen decreases the local osmolarity of the tubular fluid adjacent to the cell (i.e., the local water concentration increases). At the same time, the appearance of solute in the interstitial fluid just outside the cell increases the local osmolarity (i.e., the local water concentration decreases). (3) The difference in water concentration between lumen and interstitial fluid causes net diffusion of water from the lumen across the tubular cells' plasma membranes and/or tight junctions into the interstitial fluid. (4) From there, water, Na^+, and everything else dissolved in the interstitial fluid move together by bulk flow into peritubular capillaries as the final step in reabsorption.

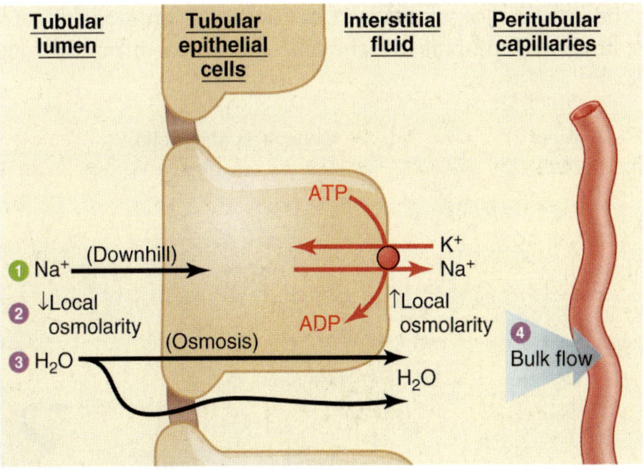

Figure 14.15 AP|R Coupling of water and Na^+ reabsorption. See text for explanation of circled numbers. The reabsorption of solutes other than Na^+—for example, glucose, amino acids, and HCO_3^-—also contributes to the difference in osmolarity between lumen and interstitial fluid, but the reabsorption of all these substances ultimately depends on direct or indirect cotransport and countertransport with Na^+ (see Figure 14.14a). Therefore, they are not shown in this figure.

Water movement across the tubular epithelium can only occur if the epithelium is permeable to water. No matter how large its concentration gradient, water cannot cross an epithelium impermeable to it. Water permeability varies from tubular segment to segment and depends largely on the presence of water channels, called **aquaporins,** in the plasma membranes. The water permeability of the proximal tubule is always very high, so this segment reabsorbs water molecules almost as rapidly as Na^+. As a result, the proximal tubule reabsorbs large amounts of Na^+ and water in the same proportions.

We will describe the water permeability of the next tubular segments—the loop of Henle and distal convoluted tubule—later. Now for the really crucial point—the water permeability of the last portions of the tubules, the cortical and medullary collecting ducts, can vary greatly due to physiological control. These are the only tubular segments in which water permeability is under such control.

The major determinant of this controlled permeability and, therefore, of passive water reabsorption in the collecting ducts is a peptide hormone secreted by the posterior pituitary gland and known as **vasopressin,** or **antidiuretic hormone** (**ADH**; see Chapter 11). Vasopressin stimulates the insertion into the luminal membrane of a particular group of aquaporin water channels made by the collecting-duct cells. More than 10 different aquaporins have been identified throughout the body, and they are identified as AQP1, AQP2, and so on. **Figure 14.16** shows the function of the aquaporin water channels in the cells of the collecting ducts of the kidney. When vasopressin from the blood enters the interstitial fluid and binds to its receptor on the basolateral membrane, the intracellular production of the second-messenger cAMP is increased. This activates the enzyme cAMP-dependent protein kinase (also called protein kinase A, or PKA), which, in turn, phosphorylates proteins that increase the rate of fusion of vesicles containing AQP2 with the luminal membrane. This leads to an increase in the number of AQP2s inserted into the luminal membrane from vesicles in the cytosol. This allows an increase in the diffusion of water down its concentration gradient across the luminal membrane into the cell. Water then diffuses through AQP3 and AQP4 water channels on the basolateral membrane into the interstitial fluid and then enters the blood. (The basolateral AQPs are not regulated by vasopressin.) In the presence of a high plasma concentration of vasopressin, the water permeability of the collecting ducts increases dramatically. Therefore, passive water reabsorption is maximal and the final urine volume is small—less than 1% of the filtered water.

Without vasopressin, the water permeability of the collecting ducts is extremely low because the number of AQP2s in the luminal membrane is minimal and very little water is reabsorbed from these sites. Therefore, a large volume of water remains behind in the tubule to be excreted in the urine. This increased urine excretion resulting from low vasopressin is termed **water diuresis. Diuresis** simply means a large urine flow from any cause. In a subsequent section, we will describe the control of vasopressin secretion.

The disease ***diabetes insipidus,*** which is distinct from the other kind of diabetes (diabetes mellitus, or "sugar diabetes"), illustrates the consequences of disorders of the control of or response to vasopressin. Diabetes insipidus is caused by the failure of the posterior pituitary gland to release vasopressin (***central diabetes insipidus***) or the inability of the kidneys to respond to vasopressin (***nephrogenic diabetes insipidus***). Regardless of the type of diabetes insipidus, the permeability to water of the collecting ducts is low even if the patient is dehydrated. A constant water diuresis is present that can be as much as 25 L/day; in such extreme cases, it may not be possible to replenish the water that is lost due to the diuresis, and the disease may lead to death due to dehydration and very high plasma osmolarity.

Note that in water diuresis, there is an increased urine flow but not an increased solute excretion. In all other cases of diuresis, termed **osmotic diuresis,** the increased urine flow is the result of a primary increase in solute excretion. For example, failure of normal Na^+ reabsorption causes both increased Na^+ excretion and increased water excretion, because, as we have seen, water reabsorption is dependent on solute reabsorption. Another example of osmotic diuresis occurs in people with uncontrolled diabetes mellitus; in this case, the glucose that escapes reabsorption

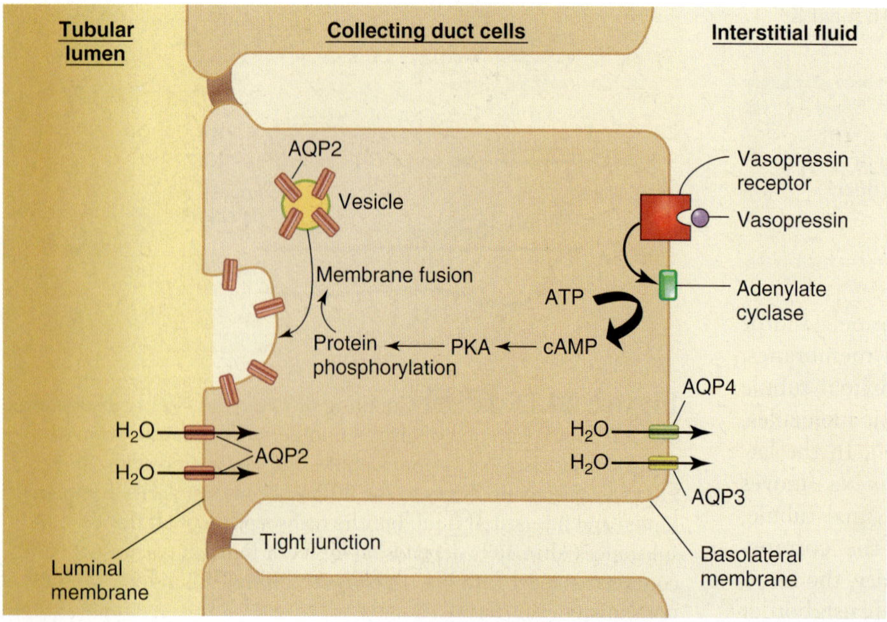

Figure 14.16 APIR The regulation and function of aquaporins (AQPs) in the medullary-collecting-duct cells to increase water reabsorption. Vasopressin binding to its receptor increases intracellular cAMP via activation of a Gs protein (not shown) and subsequent activation of adenylate cyclase. cAMP increases the activity of the enzyme protein kinase A (PKA). PKA increases the phosphorylation of specific proteins that increase the rate of the fusion of vesicles (containing AQP2) with the luminal membrane. This leads to an increase in the number of AQP2 channels in the luminal membrane. This allows increased passive diffusion of water into the cell. Water exits the cell through AQP3 and AQP4, which are not vasopressin sensitive.

because of the huge filtered load retains water in the lumen, causing it to be excreted along with the glucose.

To summarize, any loss of solute in the urine must be accompanied by water loss (osmotic diuresis), but the reverse is not true. That is, water diuresis is not necessarily accompanied by equivalent solute loss.

Urine Concentration: The Countercurrent Multiplier System

Before reading this section, you should review, by looking up in the glossary, several terms presented in Chapter 4—**hypoosmotic, isoosmotic,** and **hyperosmotic.**

In the section just concluded, we described how the kidneys produce a small volume of urine when the plasma concentration of vasopressin is high. Under these conditions, the urine is concentrated (hyperosmotic) relative to plasma. This section describes the mechanisms by which this hyperosmolarity is achieved.

The ability of the kidneys to produce hyperosmotic urine is a major determinant of the ability to survive with limited water intake. The human kidney can produce a maximal urinary concentration of 1400 mOsmol/L, almost five times the osmolarity of plasma, which is typically in the range of 285 to 300 mOsmol/L (rounded off to 300 mOsmol/L for convenience). The typical daily excretion of urea, sulfate, phosphate, other waste products, and ions amounts to approximately 600 mOsmol. Therefore, the minimal volume of urine water in which this mass of solute can be dissolved equals

$$\frac{600 \text{ mOsmol/day}}{1400 \text{ mOsmol/L}} = 0.444 \text{ L/day}$$

This volume of urine is known as the **obligatory water loss.** The loss of this minimal volume of urine contributes to dehydration when water intake is zero.

Urinary concentration takes place as tubular fluid flows through the *medullary* collecting ducts. The interstitial fluid surrounding these ducts is very hyperosmotic. In the presence of vasopressin, water diffuses out of the ducts into the interstitial fluid of the medulla and then enters the blood vessels of the medulla to be carried away.

The key question is, How does the medullary interstitial fluid become hyperosmotic? The answer involves several interrelated factors: (1) the countercurrent anatomy of the loop of Henle of juxtamedullary nephrons, (2) reabsorption of NaCl in the ascending limbs of those loops of Henle, (3) impermeability to water of those ascending limbs, (4) trapping of urea in the medulla, and (5) hairpin loops of vasa recta to minimize washout of the hyperosmotic medulla. Recall that Henle's loop forms a hairpinlike loop between the proximal tubule and the distal convoluted tubule (see Figure 14.2). The fluid entering the loop from the proximal tubule flows down the descending limb, turns the corner, and then flows up the ascending limb. The opposing flows in the two limbs are called countercurrent flows, and the entire loop functions as a **countercurrent multiplier system** to create a hyperosmotic medullary interstitial fluid.

Because the proximal tubule always reabsorbs Na^+ and water in the same proportions, the fluid entering the descending limb of the loop from the proximal tubule has the same osmolarity as plasma—300 mOsmol/L. For the moment, let us skip the descending limb because the events in it can only be understood in the context of what the *ascending* limb is doing. Along the entire length of the ascending limb, Na^+ and Cl^- are reabsorbed from the lumen into the medullary interstitial fluid (**Figure 14.17a**). In the upper (thick) portion of the ascending limb, this reabsorption is achieved by transporters that actively cotransport Na^+ and Cl^-. Such transporters are not present in the lower (thin) portion of the ascending limb, so the reabsorption there is by simple diffusion. For simplicity in the explanation of the countercurrent multiplier, we shall treat the entire ascending limb as a homogeneous structure that actively reabsorbs Na^+ and Cl^-.

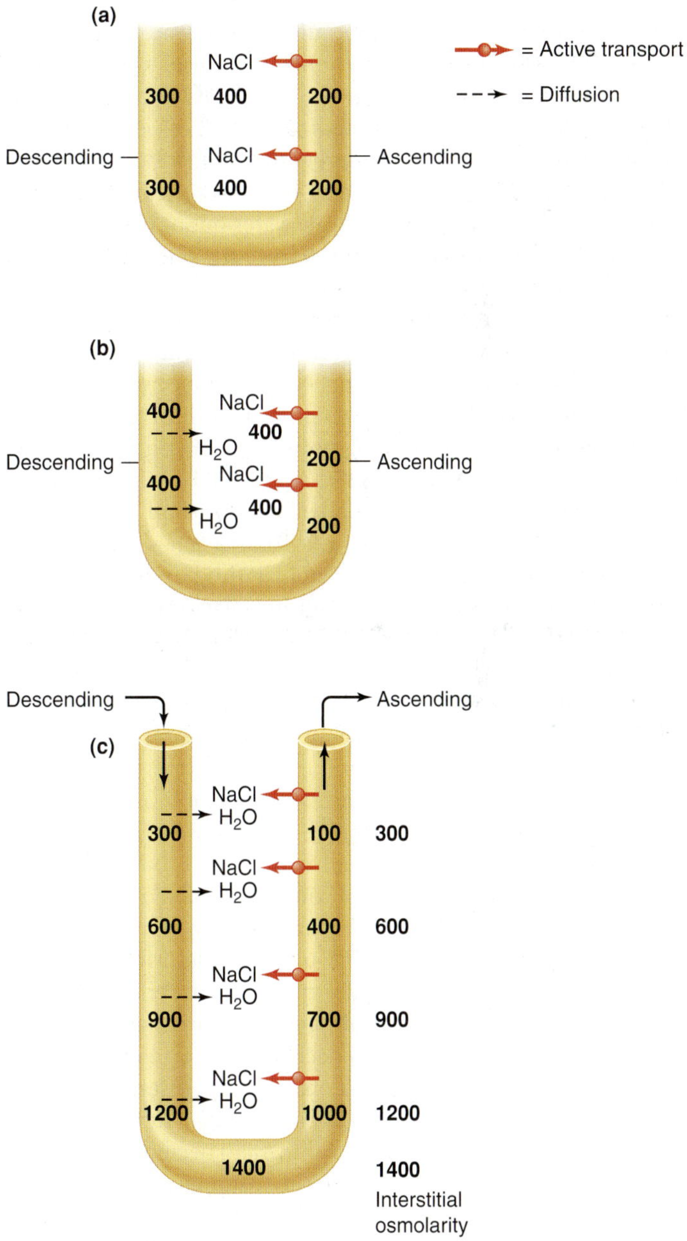

Figure 14.17 APIR Generating a hyperosmolar medullary renal interstitium. (a) NaCl active transport in ascending limbs (impermeable to H_2O). (b) Passive reabsorption of H_2O in descending limb. (c) Multiplication of osmolarity occurs with fluid flow through the tubular lumen.

Very importantly, *the ascending limb is relatively impermeable to water*, so little water follows the salt. The net result is that the interstitial fluid of the medulla becomes hyperosmotic compared to the fluid in the ascending limb because solute is reabsorbed without water.

We now return to the descending limb. This segment, in contrast to the ascending limb, does not reabsorb sodium chloride and is highly permeable to water (**Figure 14.17b**). Therefore, a net diffusion of water occurs out of the descending limb into the more concentrated interstitial fluid until the osmolarities inside this limb and in the interstitial fluid are again equal. The interstitial hyperosmolarity is maintained during this equilibration because the ascending limb continues to pump sodium chloride to maintain the concentration difference between it and the interstitial fluid.

Therefore, because of the diffusion of water, the osmolarities of the descending limb and interstitial fluid become equal, and both are higher—by 200 mOsmol/L in our example—than that of the ascending limb. This is the essence of the system: The loop countercurrent multiplier causes the interstitial fluid of the medulla to become concentrated. It is this hyperosmolarity that will draw water out of the collecting ducts and concentrate the urine. However, one more crucial feature—the "multiplication"—must be considered.

So far, we have been analyzing this system as though the flow through the loop of Henle stops while the ion pumping and water diffusion are occurring. Now, let us see what happens when we allow flow through the entire length of the descending and ascending limbs of the loop of Henle (**Figure 14.17c**). The osmolarity difference—200 mOsmol/L—that exists at each horizontal level is "multiplied" as the fluid goes deeper into the medulla. By the time the fluid reaches the bend in the loop, the osmolarity of the tubular fluid and interstitium has been multiplied to a very high osmolarity that can be as high as 1400 mOsmol/L. Keep in mind that the active sodium chloride transport mechanism in the ascending limb (coupled with low water permeability in this segment) is the essential component of the system. Without it, the countercurrent flow would have no effect on loop and medullary interstitial osmolarity, which would simply remain 300 mOsmol/L throughout.

Now we have a concentrated medullary interstitial fluid, but we must still follow the fluid within the tubules from the loop of Henle through the distal convoluted tubule and into the collecting-duct system, using **Figure 14.18** as our guide. Furthermore, urea reabsorption and trapping (described in detail later) contribute to the maximal medullary interstitial osmolarity. The countercurrent multiplier system concentrates the descending-loop fluid but then decreases the osmolarity in the ascending loop so that the fluid entering the distal convoluted tubule is actually more dilute (hypoosmotic)—100 mOsmol/L in Figure 14.18—than the plasma. The fluid becomes even more dilute during its passage through the distal convoluted tubule because this tubular segment, like the ascending loop, actively transports Na^+ and Cl^- out of the tubule but is relatively impermeable to water. This hypoosmotic fluid then enters the cortical collecting duct. Because of the significant volume reabsorption, the flow of fluid at the end of the ascending limb is much less than the flow that entered the descending limb.

As noted earlier, vasopressin increases tubular permeability to water in both the cortical and medullary collecting ducts. In contrast, vasopressin does not directly influence water reabsorption in the parts of the tubule prior to the collecting ducts. Thus, regardless of the plasma concentration of this hormone, the fluid entering the cortical collecting duct is hypoosmotic. From there on, however, vasopressin is crucial. In the presence of high concentrations of vasopressin, water reabsorption occurs by diffusion from the hypoosmotic fluid in the cortical collecting duct until the fluid in this segment becomes isoosmotic to the interstitial fluid and peritubular plasma of the cortex—that is, until it is once again at 300 mOsmol/L.

The isoosmotic tubular fluid then enters and flows through the *medullary* collecting ducts. In the presence of high plasma concentrations of vasopressin, water diffuses out of the ducts into the medullary interstitial fluid as a result of

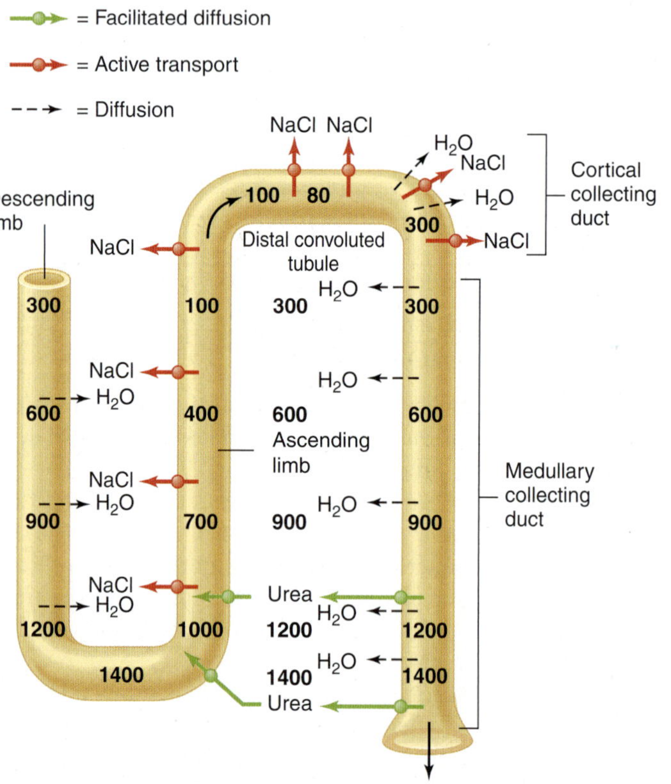

Figure 14.18 APIR Simplified depiction of the generation of an interstitial fluid osmolarity gradient by the renal countercurrent multiplier system and its role in the formation of hyperosmotic urine in the presence of vasopressin. Notice that the hyperosmotic medulla depends on NaCl reabsorption and urea trapping (described in Figure 14.20).

PHYSIOLOGICAL INQUIRY

- Certain types of lung tumors secrete one or more hormones. What would happen to plasma and urine osmolarity and urine volume in a patient with a lung tumor that secretes vasopressin?

Answer can be found at end of chapter.

the high osmolarity that the loop countercurrent multiplier system and urea trapping establish there. This water then enters the medullary capillaries and is carried out of the kidneys by the venous blood. Water reabsorption occurs all along the lengths of the medullary collecting ducts so that, in the presence of vasopressin, the fluid at the end of these ducts has essentially the same osmolarity as the interstitial fluid surrounding the bend in the loops—that is, at the bottom of the medulla. By this means, the final urine is hyperosmotic. By retaining as much water as possible, the kidneys minimize the rate at which dehydration occurs during water deprivation.

In contrast, when plasma vasopressin concentration is low, both the cortical and medullary collecting ducts are relatively impermeable to water. As a result, a large volume of hypoosmotic urine is excreted, thereby eliminating an excess of water in the body.

The Medullary Circulation

A major question arises with the countercurrent system as described previously: "Why doesn't the blood flowing through medullary capillaries eliminate the countercurrent gradient set up by the loops of Henle?" One would think that as plasma with the usual osmolarity of 300 mOsm/L enters the highly concentrated environment of the medulla, there would be massive net diffusion of Na^+ and Cl^- into the capillaries and water out of them and, thus, the interstitial gradient would be "washed away." However, the blood vessels in the medulla (vasa recta) form hairpin loops that run parallel to the loops of Henle and medullary collecting ducts. As shown in **Figure 14.19**, blood enters the top of the vessel loop at an osmolarity of 300 mOsm/L, and as the blood flows down the loop deeper and deeper into the medulla, Na^+ and Cl^- do indeed diffuse into—and water out of—the vessel. However, after the bend in the loop is reached, the blood then flows up the ascending vessel loop, where the process is almost completely reversed. Thus, the hairpin-loop structure of the vasa recta minimizes excessive loss of solute from the interstitium by *diffusion*. At the same time, both the salt and water being reabsorbed from the loops of Henle and collecting ducts are carried away in equivalent amounts by *bulk flow*, as determined by the usual capillary Starling forces. This maintains the steady-state countercurrent gradient set up by the loops of Henle. Because of NaCl and water reabsorbed from the loop of Henle and collecting ducts, the amount of blood flow leaving the vasa recta is at least twofold higher than the blood flow entering the vasa recta. Finally, the total blood flow going through all of the vasa recta is a small percentage of the total renal blood flow. This helps to minimize the washout of the hypertonic interstitium of the medulla.

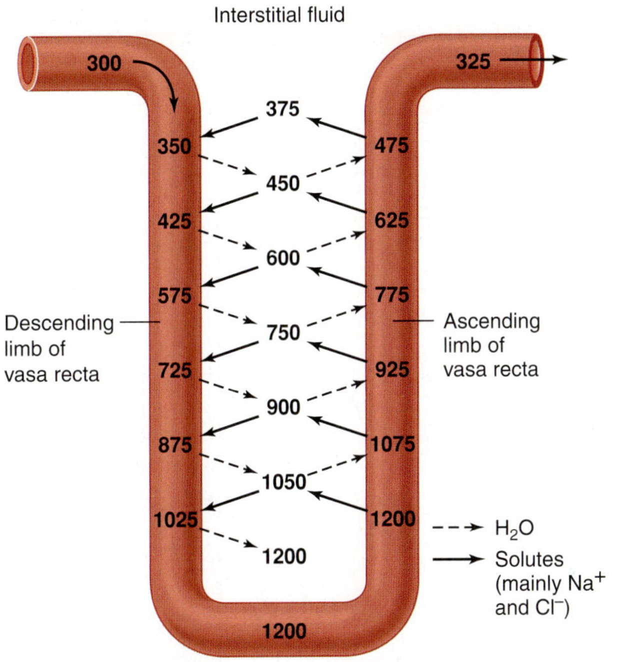

Figure 14.19 APIR Function of the vasa recta to maintain the hypertonic interstitial renal medulla. All movements of water and solutes are by diffusion. Not shown is the simultaneously occurring uptake of interstitial fluid by bulk flow.

The Recycling of Urea Helps to Establish a Hypertonic Medullary Interstitium

As was just described, the countercurrent multiplier establishes a hypertonic medullary interstitium that the vasa recta help to preserve. We already learned how the reabsorption of water in the proximal tubule mediates the reabsorption of urea by diffusion. As urea passes through the remainder of the nephron, it is reabsorbed, secreted into the tubule, and then reabsorbed again (**Figure 14.20**). This traps urea, an osmotically active molecule, in the medullary interstitium, thus increasing its osmolarity. In fact, as shown in Figure 14.18, urea contributes to the total osmolarity of the renal medulla.

Urea is freely filtered in the glomerulus. Approximately 50% of the filtered urea is reabsorbed in the proximal tubule, and the remaining 50% enters the loop of Henle. In the

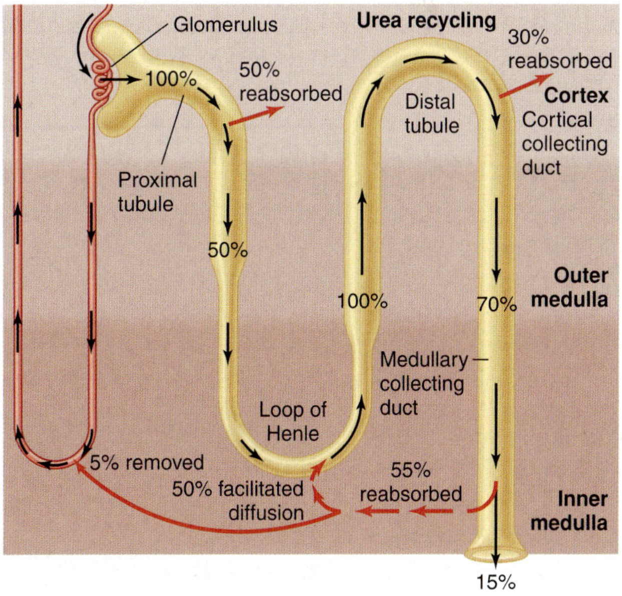

Figure 14.20 APIR Urea recycling. The recycling of urea "traps" urea in the inner medulla, which increases osmolarity and helps to establish and maintain hypertonicity.

thin descending and ascending limbs of the loop of Henle, urea that has accumulated in the medullary interstitium is secreted back into the tubular lumen by facilitated diffusion. Therefore, virtually all of the urea that was originally filtered in the glomerulus is present in the fluid that enters the distal tubule. Some of the original urea is reabsorbed from the distal tubule and cortical collecting duct. Thereafter, about half of the urea is reabsorbed from the *medullary* collecting duct, whereas only 5% diffuses into the vasa recta. The remaining amount is secreted back into the loop of Henle. Fifteen percent of the urea originally filtered remains in the collecting duct and is excreted in the urine. This recycling of urea through the medullary interstitium and minimal uptake by the vasa recta trap urea there and contribute to the high osmolarity shown in Figure 14.18. Of note is that medullary interstitial urea concentration is increased in antidiuretic states and contributes to water reabsorption. This occurs due to vasopressin, which, in addition to its effects on water permeability, also increases the permeability of the inner medullary collecting ducts to urea.

Summary of Vasopressin Control of Urine Volume and Osmolarity

This is a good place to review the reabsorption of water and the role of vasopressin in the generation of a concentrated or dilute urine. **Figure 14.21** is a convenient way to do this. First, notice that almost 75% of the volume reabsorbed in the juxtamedullary nephron is not controlled by vasopressin and occurs isosmotically in the proximal tubule. The direct effect of vasopressin in the collecting ducts participates in the development of increased osmolarity in the renal medullary interstitium. As a result, there is increased water reabsorption from the lumen in the thin descending loop of Henle with a resultant increase in tubular fluid osmolarity even though vasopressin does not have a direct effect on the loop. Note that the tubular fluid osmolarity decreases in the latter half of the loop of Henle under both conditions while there is no change in tubular fluid volume; this reflects the selective reabsorption of solutes from the tubular fluid in these water-impermeable segments of the nephron. Therefore, the ultimate determinant of the volume of urine excreted and the concentration of urine under any set of conditions is vasopressin. In the

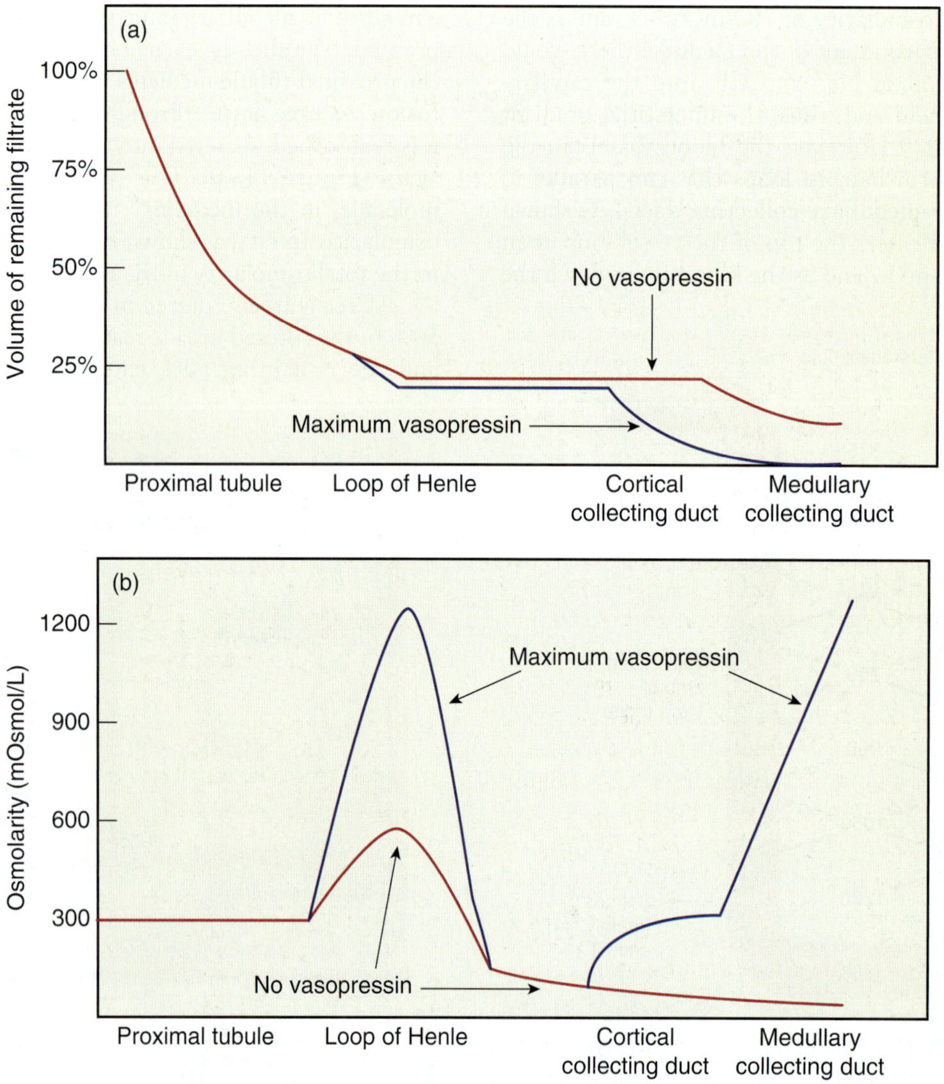

Figure 14.21 The effect of no vasopressin and maximum vasopressin concentration in the blood on (a) the volume remaining in the filtrate in the nephron as well as (b) the osmolarity of the tubular fluid along the length of the nephron.

absence of vasopressin, there is minimal water reabsorption in the collecting ducts so there is little decrease in the volume of the filtrate; this results in a diuresis and hypoosmotic urine. In the presence of maximum vasopressin during, for example, severe water restriction, most of the water is reabsorbed in the collecting ducts leading to a very small urine volume (antidiuresis) and hypertonic urine. In reality, most humans with access to water have an intermediate vasopressin concentration in the blood.

14.8 Renal Sodium Regulation

In healthy individuals, urinary Na^+ excretion increases when there is an excess of sodium in the body and decreases when there is a sodium deficit. These homeostatic responses are so precise that total-body sodium normally varies by only a few percentage points despite a wide range of sodium intakes and the occasional occurrence of large losses via the skin and gastrointestinal tract.

As we have seen, Na^+ is freely filterable from the glomerular capillaries into Bowman's space and is actively reabsorbed but not secreted. Therefore,

$$Na^+ \text{ excreted} = Na^+ \text{ filtered} - Na^+ \text{ reabsorbed}$$

The body can adjust Na^+ excretion by changing both processes on the right side of the equation. For example, when total-body sodium decreases for any reason, Na^+ excretion decreases below normal levels because Na^+ reabsorption increases.

The first issue in understanding the responses controlling Na^+ reabsorption is to determine what inputs initiate them; that is, what variables are receptors actually sensing? Surprisingly, there are no important receptors capable of detecting the total amount of sodium in the body. Rather, the responses that regulate urinary Na^+ excretion are initiated mainly by various cardiovascular baroreceptors, such as the carotid sinus, and by sensors in the kidneys that monitor the filtered load of Na^+.

As described in Chapter 12, baroreceptors respond to pressure changes within the cardiovascular system and initiate reflexes that rapidly regulate these pressures by acting on the heart, arterioles, and veins. The new information in this chapter is that *regulation of cardiovascular pressures by baroreceptors also simultaneously achieves regulation of total-body sodium.*

Na^+ is the major extracellular solute constituting, along with associated anions, approximately 90% of these solutes. Therefore, changes in total-body sodium result in similar changes in extracellular volume. Because extracellular volume comprises plasma volume and interstitial volume, plasma volume is also directly related to total-body sodium. We saw in Chapter 12 that plasma volume is an important determinant of the blood pressures in the veins, cardiac chambers, and arteries. Thus, the chain linking total-body sodium to cardiovascular pressures is completed: Low total-body sodium leads to low plasma volume, which leads to a decrease in cardiovascular pressures. These lower pressures, via baroreceptors, initiate reflexes that influence the renal arterioles and tubules so as to decrease GFR and increase Na^+ reabsorption. These latter events decrease Na^+ excretion, thereby retaining Na^+ in the body and preventing further decreases in plasma volume and cardiovascular pressures. Increases in total-body sodium have the reverse reflex effects.

To summarize, the amount of Na^+ in the body determines the extracellular fluid volume, the plasma volume component of which helps determine cardiovascular pressures, which initiate the responses that control Na^+ excretion.

Control of GFR

Figure 14.22 summarizes the major mechanisms by which an example of increased Na^+ loss elicits a decrease in GFR. The main direct cause of the reduced GFR is a reduced net glomerular filtration pressure. This occurs both as a consequence of a decreased arterial pressure in the kidneys and, more importantly,

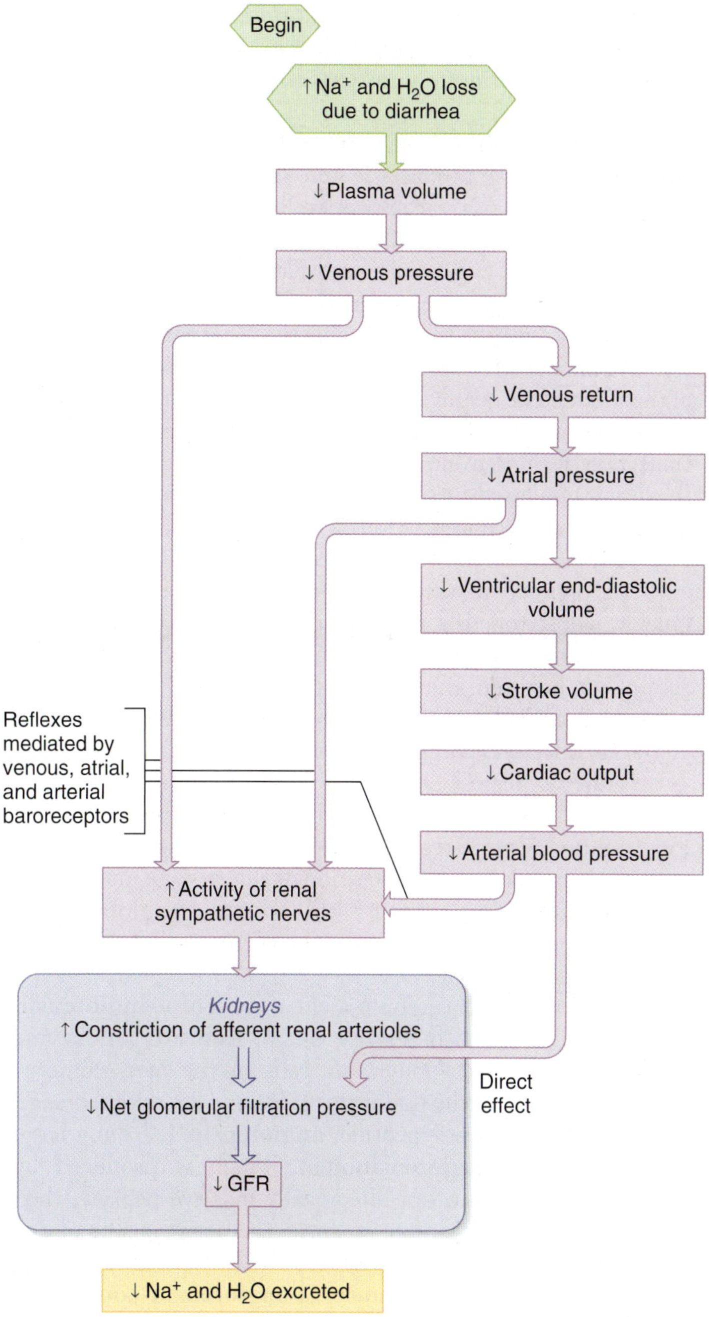

Figure 14.22 Direct and neurally mediated reflex pathways by which the GFR and, thus, Na^+ and water excretion decrease when plasma volume decreases.

as a result of reflexes acting on the renal arterioles. Note that these reflexes are the basic baroreceptor reflexes described in Chapter 12—a decrease in cardiovascular pressures causes neurally mediated reflex vasoconstriction in many areas of the body. As we will see later, the hormones angiotensin II and vasopressin also participate in this renal vasoconstrictor response.

Conversely, an increase in GFR is usually elicited by neuroendocrine inputs when an increased total-body-sodium level increases plasma volume. This increased GFR contributes to the increased renal Na^+ loss that returns extracellular volume to normal.

Control of Na^+ Reabsorption

For the long-term regulation of Na^+ excretion, the control of Na^+ reabsorption is more important than the control of GFR. The major factor determining the rate of tubular Na^+ reabsorption is the hormone aldosterone.

Aldosterone and the Renin–Angiotensin System

The adrenal cortex produces a steroid hormone, **aldosterone,** which stimulates Na^+ reabsorption by the distal convoluted tubule and the cortical collecting ducts. An action affecting these late portions of the tubule is just what one would expect for a fine-tuning input because most of the filtered Na^+ has been reabsorbed by the time the filtrate reaches the distal parts of the nephron. When aldosterone is completely absent, approximately 2% of the filtered Na^+ (equivalent to 35 g of sodium chloride per day) is not reabsorbed but excreted. In contrast, when the plasma concentration of aldosterone is high, essentially all the Na^+ reaching the distal tubule and cortical collecting ducts is reabsorbed. Normally, the plasma concentration of aldosterone and the amount of Na^+ excreted lie somewhere between these extremes.

As opposed to vasopressin, which is a peptide and acts quickly, aldosterone is a steroid and acts more slowly because it induces changes in gene expression and protein synthesis. In the case of the nephron, the proteins participate in Na^+ transport. Look again at Figure 14.14b. Aldosterone induces the synthesis of all the channels and pumps shown in the cortical collecting duct.

When a person eats a diet high in sodium, aldosterone secretion is low, whereas it is high when the person ingests a low-sodium diet or becomes sodium-depleted for some other reason. What controls the secretion of aldosterone under these circumstances? The answer is the hormone angiotensin II, which acts directly on the adrenal cortex to stimulate the secretion of aldosterone.

Angiotensin II is a component of the **renin–angiotensin system,** summarized in **Figure 14.23. Renin** is an enzyme secreted by the juxtaglomerular cells of the juxtaglomerular apparatuses in the kidneys. Once in the bloodstream, renin splits a small polypeptide, **angiotensin I,** from a large plasma protein, **angiotensinogen,** which is produced by the liver. Angiotensin I, a biologically inactive peptide, then undergoes further cleavage to form the active agent of the renin–angiotensin system, angiotensin II. This conversion is mediated by an enzyme known as **angiotensin-converting enzyme (ACE),** which is found in very high concentration on the luminal surface of capillary endothelial cells. Angiotensin II exerts many effects, but the most important are the stimulation of the secretion of aldosterone and the constriction of arterioles (described in Chapter 12). Plasma angiotensin II is high during salt depletion and low when salt intake is high. It is this change in angiotensin II that brings about the changes in aldosterone secretion.

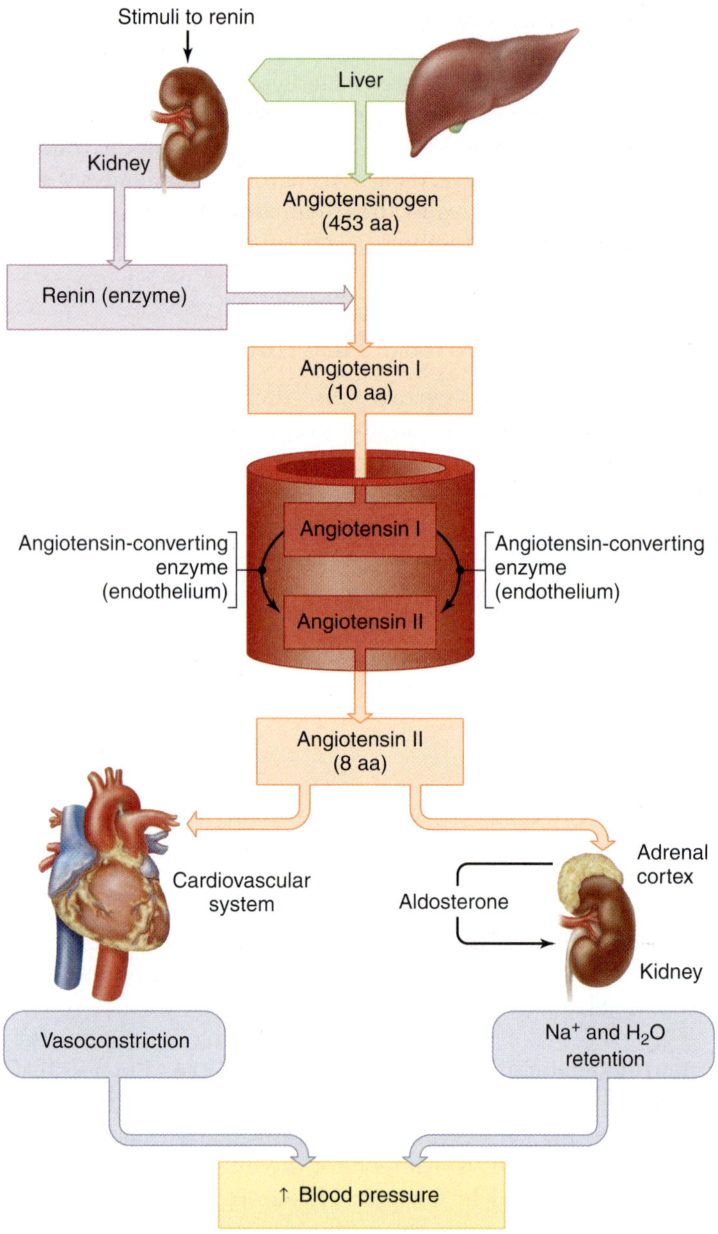

Figure 14.23 Summary of the renin–angiotensin system and the stimulation of aldosterone secretion by angiotensin II. Angiotensin-converting enzyme (ACE) is located on the surface of capillary endothelial cells. The plasma concentration of renin is the rate-limiting factor in the renin–angiotensin system; that is, it is the major determinant of the plasma concentration of angiotensin II. (aa = Amino acids)

PHYSIOLOGICAL INQUIRY

- What effect would an ACE inhibitor have on renin secretion and angiotensin II production? What effect would an angiotensin II receptor blocker (ARB) have on renin secretion and angiotensin II production? (*Hint:* Also look ahead to Figure 14.24.)

Answers can be found at end of chapter.

What causes the changes in plasma angiotensin II concentration with changes in salt balance? Angiotensinogen and angiotensin-converting enzyme are usually present in excess, so the rate-limiting factor in angiotensin II formation is the plasma renin concentration. Thus, the chain of events in salt depletion is increased renin secretion → increased plasma renin concentration → increased plasma angiotensin I concentration → increased plasma angiotensin II concentration → increased aldosterone release → increased plasma aldosterone concentration.

What are the mechanisms by which sodium depletion causes an increase in renin secretion (**Figure 14.24**)? There are at least three distinct inputs to the juxtaglomerular cells: (1) the renal sympathetic nerves, (2) intrarenal baroreceptors, and (3) the macula densa. This is an excellent example of the general principle of physiology that most physiological functions (like renin secretion) are controlled by multiple regulatory systems, often working in opposition.

The renal sympathetic nerves directly innervate the juxtaglomerular cells, and an increase in the activity of these nerves stimulates renin secretion. This makes sense because these nerves are reflexively activated via baroreceptors whenever a reduction in body sodium (and, therefore, plasma volume) decreases cardiovascular pressures (see Figure 14.22).

The other two inputs for controlling renin release—intrarenal baroreceptors and the macula densa—are contained within the kidneys and require no external neuroendocrine input (although such input can influence them). As noted earlier, the juxtaglomerular cells are located in the walls of the afferent arterioles. They are sensitive to the pressure within these arterioles and, therefore, function as **intrarenal baroreceptors.** When blood pressure in the kidneys decreases, as occurs when plasma volume is decreased, these cells are stretched less and, therefore, secrete more renin (see Figure 14.24). Thus, the juxtaglomerular cells respond simultaneously to the combined effects of sympathetic input, triggered by baroreceptors external to the kidneys, and to their own pressure sensitivity.

The other internal input to the juxtaglomerular cells is via the macula densa, which, as noted earlier, is located near the ends of the ascending loops of Henle (see Figure 14.2). The macula densa senses the amount of Na^+ in the tubular fluid flowing past it. A decreased salt delivery causes the release of paracrine factors that diffuse from the macula densa to the nearby JG cells, thereby activating them and causing the release of renin. Therefore, in an indirect way, this mechanism is sensitive to changes in sodium intake. If salt intake is low, less Na^+ is filtered and less appears at the macula densa. Conversely, a high salt intake will cause a very low rate of release of renin. If blood pressure is significantly decreased, glomerular filtration rate can decrease. This will decrease the tubular flow rate such that less Na^+ is presented to the macula densa. This input also results in increased renin release at the same time that the sympathetic nerves and intrarenal baroreceptors are doing so (see Figure 14.24).

The importance of this system is highlighted by the considerable redundancy in the control of renin secretion. Furthermore, as illustrated in Figure 14.24, the various mechanisms can all be participating at the same time.

By helping to regulate sodium balance and thereby plasma volume, the renin–angiotensin system contributes to the control of arterial blood pressure. However, this is not the only way in which it influences arterial pressure. Recall from Chapter 12 that angiotensin II is a potent constrictor of arterioles in many parts of the body and that this effect on peripheral resistance increases arterial pressure.

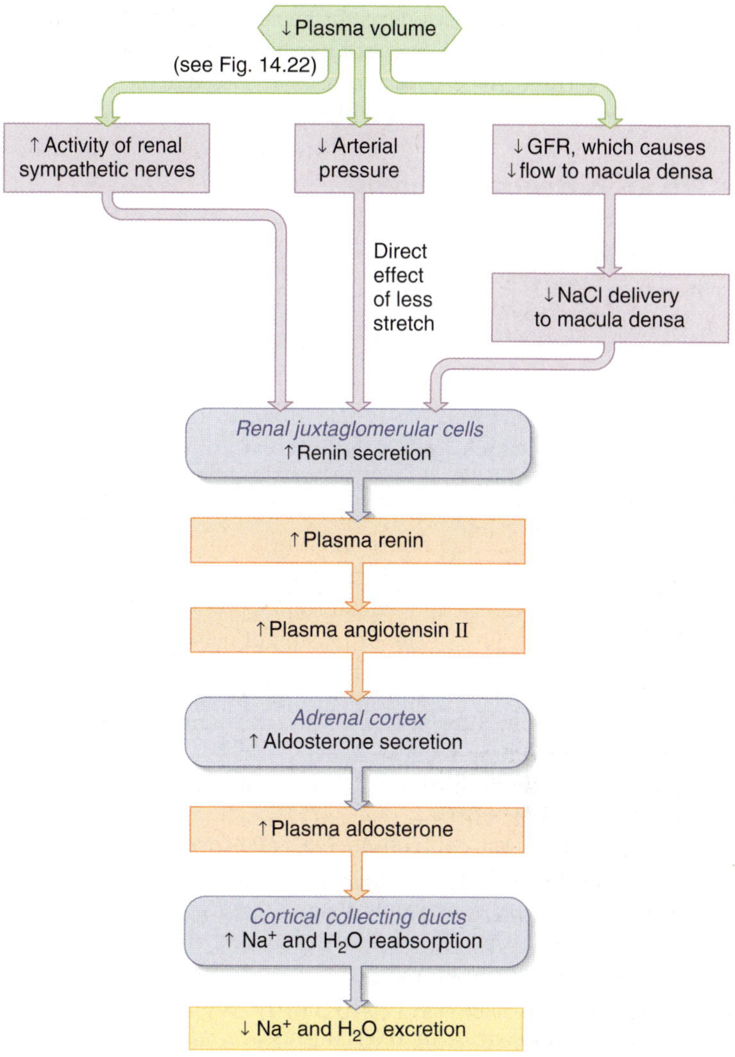

Figure 14.24 Pathways by which decreased plasma volume leads, via the renin–angiotensin system and aldosterone, to increased Na^+ reabsorption by the cortical collecting ducts and hence to decreased Na^+ excretion.

PHYSIOLOGICAL INQUIRY

- What would be the effect of denervation (removal of sympathetic neural input) of the kidneys on Na^+ and water excretion?

Answer can be found at end of chapter.

Drugs have been developed to manipulate the angiotensin II and aldosterone components of the system. ACE inhibitors, such as ***lisinopril,*** reduce angiotensin II production from angiotensin I by inhibiting angiotensin-converting enzyme. Angiotensin II receptor blockers, such as ***losartan,*** prevent angiotensin II from binding to its receptor on target tissue (e.g., vascular smooth muscle and the adrenal cortex). Finally, drugs such as ***eplerenone*** block the binding of aldosterone to its receptor in the kidney. Although these classes of drugs have different mechanisms of action, they are all effective in the treatment of hypertension. This highlights that many forms of hypertension can be attributed to the failure of the kidneys to adequately excrete Na^+ and water.

Atrial Natriuretic Peptide

Another controller is **atrial natriuretic peptide (ANP),** also known as atrial natriuretic factor (ANF) or atrial natriuretic hormone (ANH). Cells in the cardiac atria synthesize and secrete ANP. ANP acts on several tubular segments to inhibit Na^+ reabsorption. It can also act on the renal blood vessels to increase GFR, which further contributes to increased Na^+ excretion (**natriuresis**). ANP also directly inhibits aldosterone secretion, which leads to an increase in Na^+ excretion. As would be predicted, the secretion of ANP increases when there is an excess of sodium in the body, but the stimulus for this increased secretion is not alterations in Na^+ concentration. Rather, using the same logic (only in reverse) that applies to the control of renin and aldosterone secretion, ANP secretion increases because of the expansion of plasma volume that accompanies an increase in body sodium. The specific stimulus is increased atrial distension (**Figure 14.25**).

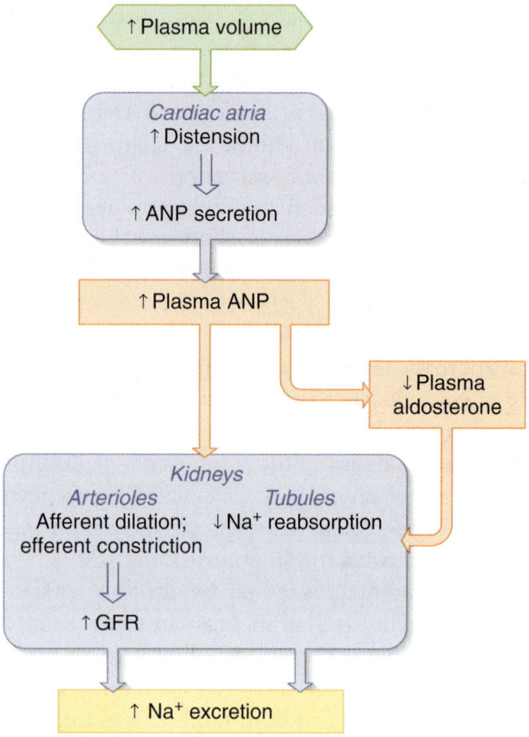

Figure 14.25 Atrial natriuretic peptide (ANP) increases Na^+ excretion.

Interaction of Blood Pressure and Renal Function

An important input controlling Na^+ reabsorption is arterial blood pressure. We have previously described how the arterial blood pressure constitutes a signal for important reflexes (involving the renin–angiotensin system and aldosterone) that influence Na^+ reabsorption. Now we are emphasizing that arterial pressure also acts locally on the tubules themselves. Specifically, an *increase* in arterial pressure *inhibits* Na^+ reabsorption and thereby increases Na^+ excretion in a process termed **pressure natriuresis.** The actual transduction mechanism of this direct effect is unknown.

Thus, an increased blood pressure reduces Na^+ reabsorption by two mechanisms: (1) It reduces the activity of the renin-angiotensin-aldosterone system, and (2) it also acts locally on the tubules. Conversely, a decreased blood pressure decreases Na^+ excretion by both stimulating the renin-angiotensin-aldosterone system and acting on the tubules to enhance Na^+ reabsorption.

Now is a good time to look back at Figure 12.57, which describes the strong, causal, reciprocal relationship between arterial blood pressure and blood volume, the result of which is that blood volume is perhaps the major long-term determinant of blood pressure. The direct effect of blood pressure on Na^+ excretion is, as Figure 12.57 shows, one of the major links in these relationships. An important hypothesis is that most people who develop hypertension do so because their kidneys, for some reason, do not excrete enough Na^+ in response to a normal arterial pressure. Consequently, at this normal pressure, some dietary sodium is retained, which causes the pressure to increase enough to produce adequate Na^+ excretion to balance sodium intake, although at an increased body sodium content. The integrated control of sodium balance is a useful example of the general principles of physiology that the functions of organ systems are coordinated with each other and that controlled exchange of materials occurs between compartments and across cellular membranes.

14.9 Renal Water Regulation

Water excretion is the difference between the volume of water filtered (the GFR) and the volume reabsorbed. Thus, the changes in GFR initiated by baroreceptor afferent input described in the previous section tend to have the same effects on water excretion as on Na^+ excretion. As is true for Na^+, however, the rate of water reabsorption is the most important factor for determining how much water is excreted. As we have seen, this is determined by vasopressin; therefore, total-body water is regulated mainly by reflexes that alter the secretion of this hormone.

As described in Chapter 11, vasopressin is produced by a discrete group of hypothalamic neurons whose axons terminate in the posterior pituitary gland, which releases vasopressin into the blood. The most important of the inputs to these neurons come from osmoreceptors and baroreceptors.

Osmoreceptor Control of Vasopressin Secretion

We have seen how changes in extracellular volume simultaneously elicit reflex changes in the excretion of *both* Na^+ and water. This is adaptive because the situations causing extracellular volume alterations are very often associated with loss or gain of both Na^+ and water in proportional amounts. In contrast, changes in total-body water with no corresponding change in total-body sodium are compensated for by altering water excretion *without altering* Na^+ *excretion.*

A crucial point in understanding how such reflexes are initiated is realizing that changes in water alone, in contrast to Na^+, have relatively little effect on extracellular volume. The reason is that water, unlike Na^+, distributes throughout all the body fluid compartments, with about two-thirds entering the intracellular compartment rather than simply staying in the extracellular compartment, as Na^+ does. Therefore, cardiovascular pressures and baroreceptors are only slightly affected by pure water gains or losses. In contrast, the major effect of water loss or gain out of proportion to Na^+ loss or gain is a change in the osmolarity of the body fluids. This is a key point because, under conditions due predominantly to water gain or loss, the sensory receptors that initiate the reflexes controlling vasopressin secretion are **osmoreceptors** in the hypothalamus. These receptors are responsive to changes in osmolarity.

As an example, imagine that you drink 2 L of water. The excess water decreases the body fluid osmolarity, which results in an inhibition of vasopressin secretion via the hypothalamic osmoreceptors (**Figure 14.26**). As a result, the water permeability of the collecting ducts decreases dramatically, water reabsorption of these segments is greatly reduced, and a large volume of hypoosmotic urine is excreted. In this manner, the excess water is eliminated and body fluid osmolarity is normalized.

At the other end of the spectrum, when the osmolarity of the body fluids increases because of water deprivation, vasopressin secretion is reflexively increased via the osmoreceptors, water reabsorption by the collecting ducts increases, and a very small volume of highly concentrated urine is excreted. By retaining relatively more water than solute, the kidneys help reduce the body fluid osmolarity back toward normal.

To summarize, regulation of body fluid osmolarity requires separation of water excretion from Na^+ excretion. That is, it requires the kidneys to excrete a urine that, relative to plasma, either contains more water than Na^+ and other solutes (water diuresis) or less water than solute (concentrated urine). This is made possible by two physiological factors: (1) osmoreceptors and (2) vasopressin-dependent water reabsorption without Na^+ reabsorption in the collecting ducts.

Baroreceptor Control of Vasopressin Secretion

The minute-to-minute control of plasma osmolarity is primarily by the osmoreceptor-mediated vasopressin secretion already described. There are, however, other important controllers of vasopressin secretion. The best understood of these is baroreceptor input to vasopressinergic neurons in the hypothalamus.

A decreased extracellular fluid volume due, for example, to diarrhea or hemorrhage, elicits an increase in aldosterone release via activation of the renin–angiotensin system. However, the decreased extracellular volume also triggers an increase in vasopressin secretion. This increased vasopressin increases the water permeability of the collecting ducts. More water is passively reabsorbed and less is excreted, so water is retained to help stabilize the extracellular volume.

This reflex is initiated by several baroreceptors in the cardiovascular system (**Figure 14.27**). The baroreceptors decrease their rate of firing when cardiovascular pressures

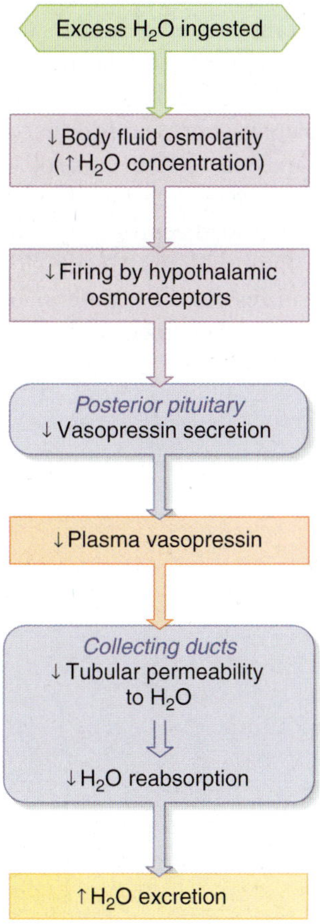

Figure 14.26 Osmoreceptor pathway that decreases vasopressin secretion and increases water excretion when excess water is ingested. The opposite events (an increase in vasopressin secretion) occur when osmolarity increases, as during water deprivation.

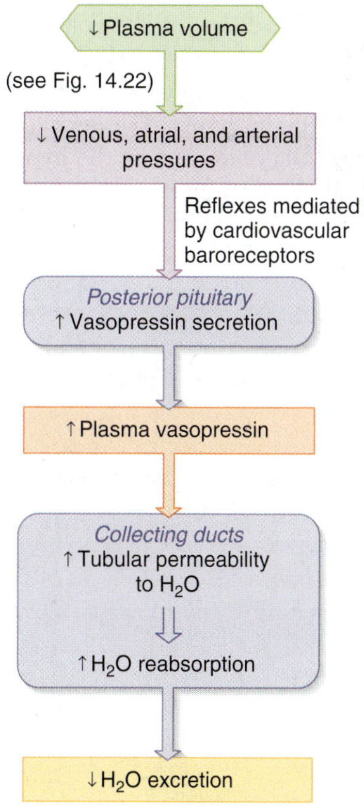

Figure 14.27 Baroreceptor pathway by which vasopressin secretion increases when plasma volume decreases. The opposite events (culminating in a decrease in vasopressin secretion) occur when plasma volume increases.

decrease, as occurs when blood volume decreases. Therefore, the baroreceptors transmit fewer impulses via afferent neurons and ascending pathways to the hypothalamus, and the result is increased vasopressin secretion. Conversely, increased cardiovascular pressures cause more firing by the baroreceptors, resulting in a decrease in vasopressin secretion. The mechanism of this inverse relationship is an inhibitory neurotransmitter released by neurons in the afferent pathway.

In addition to its effect on water excretion, vasopressin, like angiotensin II, causes widespread arteriolar constriction. This helps restore arterial blood pressure toward normal (Chapter 12).

The baroreceptor reflex for vasopressin, as just described, has a relatively high threshold—that is, there must be a sizable reduction in cardiovascular pressures to trigger it. Therefore, this reflex, compared to the osmoreceptor reflex described earlier, generally plays a lesser role under most physiological circumstances, but it can become very important in pathological states, such as hemorrhage.

Other Stimuli to Vasopressin Secretion

We have now described two afferent pathways controlling the vasopressin-secreting hypothalamic cells, one from osmoreceptors and the other from baroreceptors. To add to the complexity, the hypothalamic cells receive synaptic input from many other brain areas, so that vasopressin secretion—and, therefore, urine volume and concentration—can be altered by pain, fear, and a variety of drugs. For example, ethanol inhibits vasopressin release, and this may account for the increased urine volume produced following the ingestion of alcohol, a urine volume well in excess of the volume of the beverage consumed. Furthermore, hypoxia alters vasopressin release via afferent input from peripheral arterial chemoreceptors (see Figure 13.33) to the hypothalamus via ascending pathways from the medulla oblongata to the hypothalamus. Nausea is also a very potent stimulus of vasopressin release. The vasoconstrictor effects of vasopressin (see Chapter 12) acting on the blood vessels that perfuse the small intestines help to shift blood flow away from the gastrointestinal tract, thereby decreasing the absorption of ingested toxic substances.

14.10 A Summary Example: The Response to Sweating

Figure 14.28 shows the factors that control renal Na^+ and water excretion in response to severe sweating. You may notice the salty taste of sweat on your upper lip when you exercise. Sweat does contain Na^+ and Cl^-, in addition to water, but is actually hypoosmotic compared to the body fluids from which it is derived. Therefore, sweating causes both a decrease in extracellular volume and an increase in body fluid osmolarity. The renal retention of water and Na^+ minimizes the deviations from normal caused by the loss of water and salt in the sweat.

14.11 Thirst and Salt Appetite

Deficits of salt and water must eventually be compensated for by ingestion of these substances, because the kidneys cannot create new Na^+ or water. The kidneys can only minimize their excretion until ingestion replaces the losses.

The subjective feeling of thirst is stimulated by an increase in plasma osmolarity and by a decrease in extracellular fluid volume (**Figure 14.29**). Plasma osmolarity is the single most important stimulus under normal physiological conditions. The increase in plasma osmolarity and the decrease in extracellular fluid are precisely the same two changes that stimulate vasopressin production, and the osmoreceptors and baroreceptors that control vasopressin secretion are similar to those for thirst. The brain centers that receive input from these receptors and that mediate thirst are located in the hypothalamus, very close to those areas that synthesize vasopressin. The general principle of physiology this highlights is that information flow—in this case,

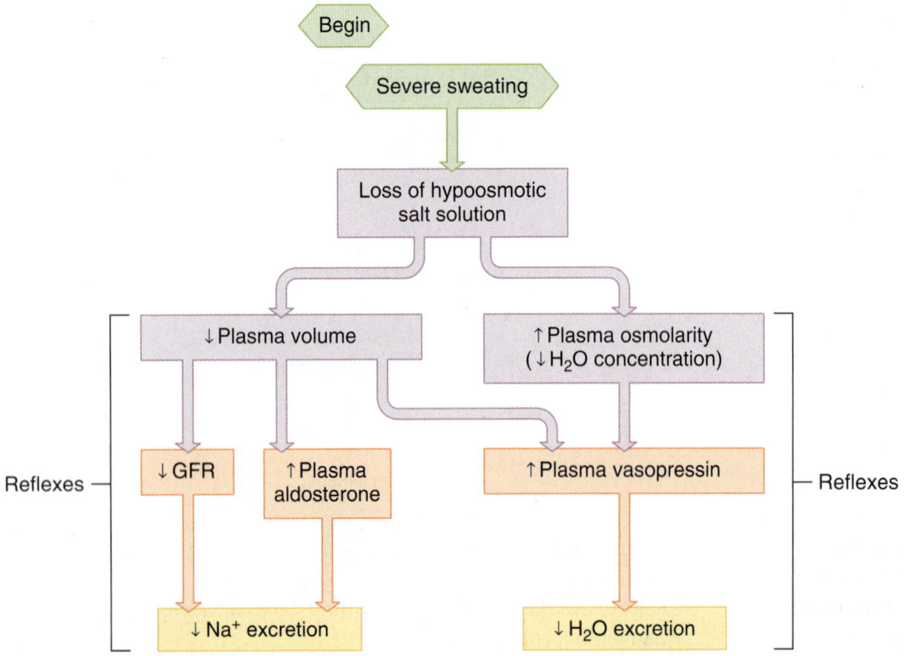

Figure 14.28 Pathways by which Na^+ and water excretion decrease in response to severe sweating. This figure is an amalgamation of Figures 14.22, 14.24, 14.27, and the reverse of Figure 14.26.

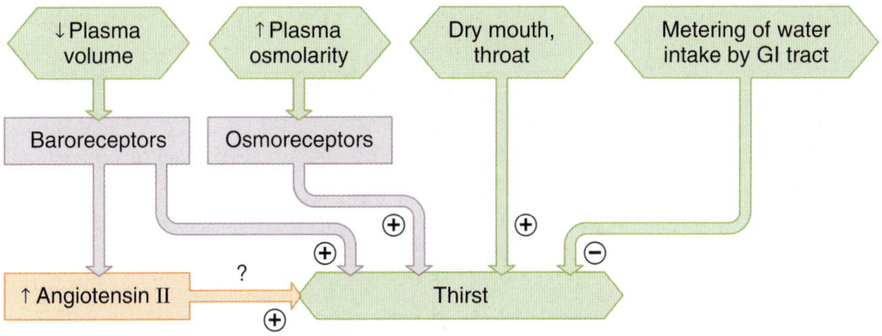

Figure 14.29 Inputs controlling thirst. The osmoreceptor input is the single most important stimulus under most physiological conditions. Psychological factors and conditioned responses are not shown. The question mark (?) indicates that evidence for the effects of angiotensin II on thirst comes primarily from experimental animals.

from the osmoreceptors to the release of vasopressin and the stimulation of thirst—is an essential feature of homeostasis and allows for the integration of physiological processes—in this case, to maintain water balance by increasing intake and minimizing loss.

There are still other pathways controlling thirst. For example, dryness of the mouth and throat causes thirst, which is relieved by merely moistening them. Some kind of "metering" of water intake by other parts of the gastrointestinal tract also occurs. For example, a thirsty person given access to water stops drinking after replacing the lost water. This occurs well before most of the water has been absorbed from the gastrointestinal tract and has a chance to eliminate the stimulatory inputs to the systemic baroreceptors and osmoreceptors. This is probably mediated by afferent sensory nerves from the mouth, throat, and gastrointestinal tract and prevents overhydration.

Salt appetite is an important part of sodium homeostasis and consists of two components, "hedonistic" appetite and "regulatory" appetite. Most mammals "like" salt and eat it whenever they can, regardless of whether they are salt-deficient. Human beings have a strong hedonistic appetite for salt, as manifested by almost universally large intakes of salt whenever it is cheap and readily available. For example, the average American consumes 10–15 g/day despite the fact that human beings can survive quite normally on less than 0.5 g/day. However, humans have relatively little regulatory salt appetite, at least until a bodily salt deficit becomes extremely large.

14.12 Potassium Regulation

K^+ is the most abundant intracellular ion. Although only 2% of total-body potassium is in the extracellular fluid, the K^+ concentration in this fluid is extremely important for the function of excitable tissues, notably, nerve and muscle. Recall from Chapter 6 that the resting membrane potentials of these tissues are directly related to the relative intracellular and extracellular K^+ concentrations. Consequently, either increases (***hyperkalemia***) or decreases (***hypokalemia***) in extracellular K^+ concentration can cause abnormal rhythms of the heart (***arrhythmias***) and abnormalities of skeletal muscle contraction and neuronal action potential conduction.

A healthy person remains in potassium balance in the steady state by daily excreting an amount of potassium in the urine equal to the amount ingested minus the amounts eliminated in feces and sweat. Like Na^+ losses, K^+ losses via sweat and the gastrointestinal tract are normally quite small, although vomiting or diarrhea can cause large quantities to be lost. The control of urinary K^+ excretion is the major mechanism regulating body potassium.

Renal Regulation of K^+

K^+ is freely filterable in the glomerulus. Normally, the tubules reabsorb most of this filtered K^+ so that very little of the filtered K^+ appears in the urine. However, the cortical collecting ducts can secrete K^+ and changes in K^+ excretion are due mainly to changes in K^+ secretion by this tubular segment (**Figure 14.30**).

During potassium depletion, when the homeostatic response is to minimize potassium loss, there is no K^+ secretion by the cortical collecting ducts. Only the small amount of filtered K^+ that escapes tubular reabsorption is excreted. With normal fluctuations in potassium intake, a variable amount of K^+ is added to the small amount filtered and not reabsorbed. This maintains total-body potassium balance.

Figure 14.14b illustrated the mechanism of K^+ secretion by the cortical collecting ducts. In this tubular segment, the K^+ pumped into the cell across the basolateral membrane by Na^+/K^+-ATPases diffuses into the tubular lumen through K^+ channels in the luminal membrane. Thus, the secretion of K^+ by the cortical collecting duct is associated with the reabsorption of Na^+ by this tubular segment. K^+ secretion does not occur in other Na^+-reabsorbing tubular segments because there are few K^+ channels in the luminal membranes of their cells. Rather, in these segments, the K^+ pumped into the cell by Na^+/K^+-ATPase simply diffuses back across the basolateral membrane through K^+ channels located there (see Figure 14.14a).

What factors influence K^+ secretion by the cortical collecting ducts to achieve homeostasis of bodily potassium?

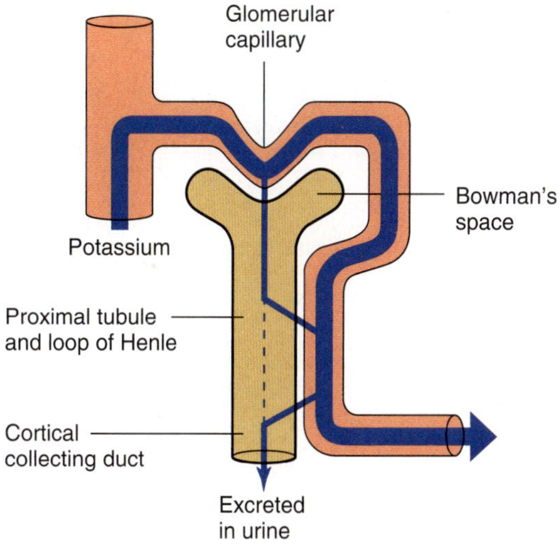

Figure 14.30 APIR Simplified model of the basic renal processing of potassium.

The single most important factor is as follows. When a high-potassium diet is ingested (**Figure 14.31**), plasma K^+ concentration increases, though very slightly, and this drives enhanced basolateral uptake via the Na^+/K^+-ATPase pumps. Thus, there is an enhanced K^+ secretion. Conversely, a low-potassium diet or a negative potassium balance, such as results from diarrhea, decreases basolateral K^+ uptake. This reduces K^+ secretion and excretion, thereby helping to reestablish potassium balance.

A second important factor linking K^+ secretion to potassium balance is the hormone aldosterone (see Figure 14.31). Besides stimulating tubular Na^+ reabsorption by the cortical collecting ducts, aldosterone simultaneously enhances K^+ secretion by this tubular segment.

The homeostatic mechanism by which an excess or deficit of potassium controls aldosterone production (see Figure 14.31) is different from the mechanism described earlier involving the renin–angiotensin system. The aldosterone-secreting cells of the adrenal cortex are sensitive to the K^+ concentration of the extracellular fluid. Thus, an increased intake of potassium leads to an increased extracellular K^+ concentration, which in turn directly stimulates the adrenal cortex to produce aldosterone. The increased plasma aldosterone concentration increases K^+ secretion and thereby eliminates the excess potassium from the body.

Conversely, a decreased extracellular K^+ concentration decreases aldosterone production and thereby reduces K^+ secretion. Less K^+ than usual is excreted in the urine, thereby helping to restore the normal extracellular concentration.

Figure 14.32 summarizes the control and major renal tubular effects of aldosterone. The fact that a single hormone regulates both Na^+ and K^+ excretion raises the question of potential conflicts between homeostasis of the two ions. For example, if a person was sodium-deficient and therefore secreting large amounts of aldosterone, the K^+-secreting effects of this hormone would tend to cause some K^+ loss even though potassium balance was normal to start with. Usually, such conflicts cause only minor imbalances because there are a variety of other counteracting controls of Na^+ and K^+ excretion.

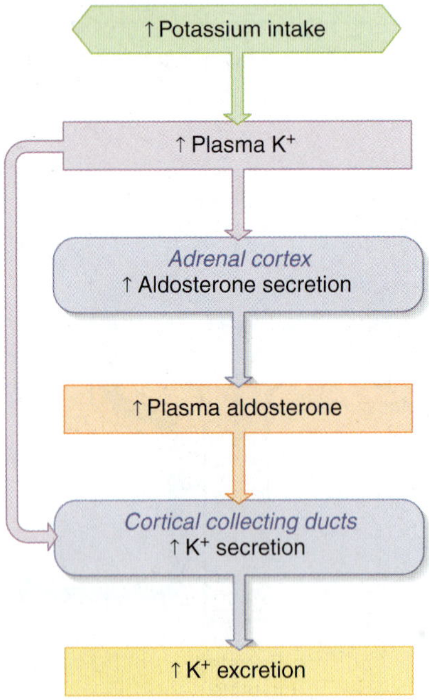

Figure 14.31 Pathways by which an increased potassium intake induces greater K^+ excretion.

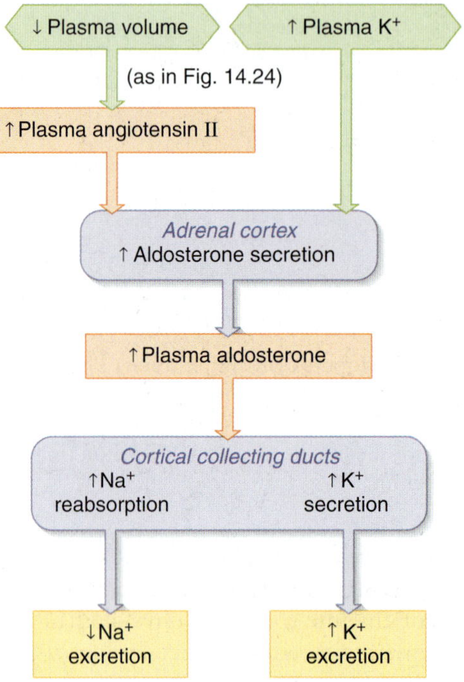

Figure 14.32 Summary of the control of aldosterone and its effects on Na^+ reabsorption and K^+ secretion.

14.13 Renal Regulation of Calcium and Phosphate Ion

Calcium and phosphate balance are controlled primarily by parathyroid hormone and $1,25(OH)_2D$, as described in detail in Chapter 11. Approximately 60% of plasma calcium is available for filtration in the kidney. The remaining plasma calcium is protein-bound or complexed with anions. Because calcium is so important in the function of every cell in the body, the kidneys have powerful mechanisms to reabsorb calcium ion from the tubular fluid. More than 60% of calcium ion reabsorption is not under hormonal control and occurs in the proximal tubule. The hormonal control of calcium ion reabsorption occurs mainly in the distal convoluted tubule and early in the cortical collecting duct. When plasma calcium is low, the secretion of parathyroid hormone (PTH) from the parathyroid glands increases. PTH stimulates the opening of calcium channels in these parts of the nephron, thereby increasing calcium ion reabsorption. As discussed in Chapter 11, another important action of PTH in the kidneys is to increase the activity of the 1-hydroxylase enzyme, thus activating 25(OH)-D to $1,25(OH)_2D$, which then goes on to increase calcium and phosphate ion absorption in the gastrointestinal tract.

About half of the plasma phosphate is ionized and is filterable. Like calcium, most of the phosphate ion that is filtered is reabsorbed in the proximal tubule. Unlike calcium ion, phosphate ion reabsorption is decreased by PTH, thereby increasing the excretion of phosphate ion. Thus, when plasma calcium is low, and PTH and calcium ion reabsorption are increased as a result, phosphate ion excretion is increased.

14.14 Summary—Division of Labor

Table 14.5 summarizes the division of labor of renal function along the renal tubule. So far, we have discussed all of these processes except the transport of acids and bases, which Section C of this chapter will cover.

14.15 Diuretics

Drugs used clinically to increase the volume of urine excreted are known as ***diuretics.*** Most act on the tubules to inhibit the reabsorption of Na^+, along with Cl^- and/or HCO_3^-, resulting in increased excretion of these ions. Because water reabsorption is dependent upon solute (particularly Na^+) reabsorption, water reabsorption is also reduced, resulting in increased water excretion.

A large variety of clinically useful diuretics are available and are classified according to the specific mechanisms by which they inhibit Na^+ reabsorption. For example, ***loop diuretics,*** such as ***furosemide,*** act on the ascending limb of the loop of Henle to inhibit the first step in Na^+ reabsorption in this segment—cotransport of Na^+ and Cl^- across the luminal membrane into the cell.

Except for one category of diuretics, called ***potassium-sparing diuretics,*** all diuretics not only increase Na^+ excretion but also cause increased K^+ excretion, which is often an unwanted side effect. The potassium-sparing diuretics inhibit Na^+ reabsorption in the cortical collecting duct, without increasing K^+ secretion there. Potassium-sparing diuretics either block the action of aldosterone (e.g., ***spironolactone*** or *eplerenone*) or block the epithelial Na^+ channel in the cortical collecting duct (e.g., ***triamterene*** or ***amiloride***). This explains why they do not cause increased K^+ excretion. ***Osmotic diuretics*** such as ***mannitol*** are filtered but not reabsorbed, thus retaining water in the urine. This is the same reason that uncontrolled diabetes mellitus and its associated glucosuria can cause excessive water loss and dehydration (see Figure 16.21).

Diuretics are among the most commonly used medications. For one thing, they are used to treat diseases characterized by renal retention of salt and water. As emphasized earlier in this chapter, the regulation of blood pressure normally produces stability of total-body-sodium mass and extracellular volume because of the close correlation between these variables. In contrast, in several types of disease, this correlation is disrupted and the reflexes that maintain blood pressure can cause renal retention of Na^+. Na^+ excretion may decrease to almost nothing despite continued sodium ingestion, leading to abnormal expansion of the extracellular fluid (***edema***). Diuretics are used to prevent or reverse this renal retention of Na^+ and water.

The most common example of this phenomenon is ***congestive heart failure*** (Chapter 12). A person with a failing heart manifests a decreased GFR and increased aldosterone secretion, both of which contribute to the virtual absence of Na^+ in the urine. The net result is extracellular volume expansion and edema. The Na^+-retaining responses are triggered by the lower cardiac output (a result of cardiac failure) and the

TABLE 14.5 Summary of "Division of Labor" in the Renal Tubules

Tubular Segment	Major Functions	Controlling Factors
Glomerulus/Bowman's capsule	Forms ultrafiltrate of plasma	Starling forces (P_{GC}, P_{BS}, π_{GC})
Proximal tubule	Bulk reabsorption of solutes and water Secretion of solutes (except K^+) and organic acids and bases	Active transport of solutes with passive water reabsorption Parathyroid hormone inhibits phosphate ion reabsorption
Loop of Henle	Establishes medullary osmotic gradient (juxtamedullary nephrons) Secretion of urea	
Descending limb	Bulk reabsorption of water	Passive water reabsorption
Ascending limb	Reabsorption of NaCl	Active transport
Distal tubule and cortical collecting ducts	Fine-tuning of the reabsorption/secretion of small quantity of solute remaining	Aldosterone stimulates Na^+ reabsorption and K^+ secretion Parathyroid hormone stimulates calcium ion reabsorption
Cortical and medullary collecting ducts	Fine-tuning of water reabsorption Reabsorption of urea	Vasopressin increases passive reabsorption of water

decrease in arterial blood pressure that results directly from this decrease in cardiac output.

Another disease in which diuretics are often used is hypertension (Chapter 12). The decrease in body sodium and water resulting from the diuretic-induced excretion of these substances brings about arteriolar dilation and a lowering of the blood pressure. The precise mechanism by which decreased body sodium causes arteriolar dilation is not known.

SECTION B SUMMARY

Total-Body Balance of Sodium and Water

I. The body gains water via ingestion and internal production, and it loses water via urine, the gastrointestinal tract, and evaporation from the skin and respiratory tract (as insensible loss and sweat).

II. The body gains Na^+ and Cl^- by ingestion and loses them via the skin (in sweat), the gastrointestinal tract, and urine.

III. For both water and Na^+, the major homeostatic control point for maintaining stable balance is renal excretion.

Basic Renal Processes for Sodium and Water

I. Na^+ is freely filterable at the glomerulus, and its reabsorption is a primary active process dependent upon Na^+/K^+-ATPase pumps in the basolateral membranes of the tubular epithelium. Na^+ is not secreted.

II. Na^+ entry into the cell from the tubular lumen is always passive. Depending on the tubular segment, it is either through channels or by cotransport or countertransport with other substances.

III. Na^+ reabsorption creates an osmotic difference across the tubule, which drives water reabsorption, largely through water channels (aquaporins).

IV. Water reabsorption is independent of the posterior pituitary gland hormone vasopressin until it reaches the collecting-duct system, where vasopressin increases water permeability. A large volume of dilute urine is produced when plasma vasopressin concentration and, hence, water reabsorption by the collecting ducts are low.

V. A small volume of concentrated urine is produced by the renal countercurrent multiplier system when plasma vasopressin concentration is high.
   a. The active transport of sodium chloride by the ascending loop of Henle causes increased osmolarity of the interstitial fluid of the medulla but a dilution of the luminal fluid.
   b. Vasopressin increases the permeability to water of the cortical collecting ducts by increasing the number of AQP2 water channels inserted into the luminal membrane. Water is reabsorbed by this segment until the luminal fluid is isoosmotic to plasma in the cortical peritubular capillaries.
   c. The luminal fluid then enters and flows through the medullary collecting ducts, and the concentrated medullary interstitium causes water to move out of these ducts, made highly permeable to water by vasopressin. The result is concentration of the collecting-duct fluid and the urine.
   d. The hairpin-loop structure of the vasa recta prevents the countercurrent gradient from being washed away.

Renal Sodium Regulation

I. Na^+ excretion is the difference between the amount of Na^+ filtered and the amount reabsorbed.

II. GFR and, hence, the filtered load of Na^+ are controlled by baroreceptor reflexes. Decreased vascular pressures cause decreased baroreceptor firing and, hence, increased sympathetic outflow to the renal arterioles, resulting in vasoconstriction and decreased GFR. These changes are generally relatively small under most physiological conditions.

III. The major control of tubular Na^+ reabsorption is the adrenal cortical hormone aldosterone, which stimulates Na^+ reabsorption in the cortical collecting ducts.

IV. The renin–angiotensin system is one of the two major controllers of aldosterone secretion. When extracellular volume decreases, renin secretion is stimulated by three inputs:
   a. Stimulation of the renal sympathetic nerves to the juxtaglomerular cells by extrarenal baroreceptor reflexes;
   b. Pressure decreases sensed by the juxtaglomerular cells, themselves acting as intrarenal baroreceptors; and
   c. A signal generated by low Na^+ or Cl^- concentration in the lumen of the macula densa.

V. Many other factors influence Na^+ reabsorption. One of these, atrial natriuretic peptide, is secreted by cells in the atria in response to atrial distension; it inhibits Na^+ reabsorption, and it also increases GFR.

VI. Arterial pressure acts locally on the renal tubules to influence Na^+ reabsorption; an increased pressure causes decreased reabsorption and, hence, increased excretion.

Renal Water Regulation

I. Water excretion is the difference between the amount of water filtered and the amount reabsorbed.

II. GFR regulation via the baroreceptor reflexes plays some role in regulating water excretion, but the major control is via vasopressin-mediated control of water reabsorption.

III. Vasopressin secretion by the posterior pituitary gland is controlled by osmoreceptors and by non-osmotic sensors such as cardiovascular baroreceptors in the hypothalamus.
   a. Via the osmoreceptors, a high body fluid osmolarity stimulates vasopressin secretion and a low osmolarity inhibits it.
   b. A low extracellular volume stimulates vasopressin secretion via the baroreceptor reflexes, and a high extracellular volume inhibits it.

A Summary Example: The Response to Sweating

I. Severe sweating can lead to a decrease in plasma volume and an increase in plasma osmolarity.

II. This will result in a decrease in GFR and an increase in aldosterone, which together decrease Na^+ excretion, and an increase in vasopressin, which decreases H_2O excretion.

III. The net result of the renal retention of Na^+ and H_2O is to minimize hypovolemia and maintain plasma osmolarity.

Thirst and Salt Appetite

I. Thirst is stimulated by a variety of inputs, including baroreceptors, osmoreceptors, and possibly angiotensin II.

II. Salt appetite is not of major regulatory importance in human beings.

Potassium Regulation

I. A person remains in potassium balance by excreting an amount of potassium in the urine equal to the amount ingested minus the amounts lost in feces and sweat.

II. K^+ is freely filterable at the renal corpuscle and undergoes both reabsorption and secretion, the latter occurring in the cortical collecting ducts and serving as the major controlled variable determining K^+ excretion.
III. When body potassium increases, extracellular potassium concentration also increases. This increase acts directly on the cortical collecting ducts to increase K^+ secretion and also stimulates aldosterone secretion. The increased plasma aldosterone then also stimulates K^+ secretion.
IV. The most common cause of hyperaldosteronism (too much aldosterone in the blood) is a noncancerous adrenal tumor (adenoma) that secretes aldosterone in the absence of stimulation from angiotensin II. Primary aldosteronism is sometimes called Conn's syndrome. The excess aldosterone causes increased renal Na^+ reabsorption and fluid retention and is a common cause of endocrine hypertension.

Renal Regulation of Calcium and Phosphate Ion

I. About half of the plasma calcium and phosphate is ionized and filterable.
II. Most calcium and phosphate ion reabsorption occurs in the proximal tubule.
III. PTH increases calcium ion absorption in the distal convoluted tubule and early cortical collecting duct. PTH decreases phosphate ion reabsorption in the proximal tubule.

Summary—Division of Labor

I. Each segment of the nephron is responsible for a different function.
II. The proximal tubule is responsible for the bulk reabsorption of solute and water.
III. The loop of Henle generates the medullary osmotic gradient that allows for the passive reabsorption of water in the collecting ducts.
IV. The distal tubules and collecting ducts are the site of most regulation (fine-tuning) of the excretion of solutes and water.

Diuretics

I. Most diuretics inhibit reabsorption of Na^+ and water, thereby enhancing the excretion of these substances. Different diuretics act on different nephron segments.

SECTION B REVIEW QUESTIONS

1. What are the sources of water gain and loss in the body? What are the sources of Na^+ gain and loss?
2. Describe the distribution of water and Na^+ between the intracellular and extracellular fluids.
3. What is the relationship between body sodium and extracellular fluid volume?
4. What is the mechanism of Na^+ reabsorption, and how is the reabsorption of other solutes coupled to it?
5. What is the mechanism of water reabsorption, and how is it coupled to Na^+ reabsorption?
6. What is the effect of vasopressin on the renal tubules, and what are the sites affected?
7. Describe the characteristics of the two limbs of the loop of Henle with regard to their transport of Na^+, Cl^-, and water.
8. Diagram the osmolarities in the two limbs of the loop of Henle, distal convoluted tubule, cortical collecting duct, cortical interstitium, medullary collecting duct, and medullary interstitium in the presence of vasopressin. What happens to the cortical and medullary collecting-duct values in the absence of vasopressin?
9. What two processes determine how much Na^+ is excreted per unit time?
10. Diagram the sequence of events in which a decrease in blood pressure leads to a decreased GFR.
11. List the sequence of events leading from increased renin secretion to increased aldosterone secretion.
12. What are the three inputs controlling renin secretion?
13. Diagram the sequence of events leading from decreased cardiovascular pressures or from an increased plasma osmolarity to an increased secretion of vasopressin.
14. What are the stimuli for thirst?
15. Which of the basic renal processes apply to potassium? Which of them is the controlled process, and which tubular segment performs it?
16. Diagram the steps leading from increased plasma potassium to increased K^+ excretion.
17. What are the two major controls of aldosterone secretion, and what are this hormone's major actions?
18. Contrast the control of calcium and phosphate ion excretion by PTH.
19. List the different types of diuretics and briefly summarize their mechanisms of action.
20. List several diseases that diuretics can be used to treat.

SECTION B KEY TERMS

aldosterone 514
angiotensin I 514
angiotensin II 514
angiotensin-converting enzyme (ACE) 514
angiotensinogen 514
antidiuretic hormone (ADH) 508
aquaporin 508
atrial natriuretic peptide (ANP) 516
countercurrent multiplier system 509
diuresis 508
hyperosmotic 509
hypoosmotic 509
insensible water loss 506
intrarenal baroreceptors 515
isoosmotic 509
natriuresis 516
obligatory water loss 509
osmoreceptor 517
osmotic diuresis 508
pressure natriuresis 516
renin 514
renin–angiotensin system 514
salt appetite 519
vasopressin 508
water diuresis 508

SECTION B CLINICAL TERMS

amiloride 521
arrhythmia 519
central diabetes insipidus 508
congestive heart failure 521
diabetes insipidus 508
diuretics 521
edema 521
eplerenone 515
furosemide 521
hyperkalemia 519
hypokalemia 519
lisinopril 515
loop diuretic 521
losartan 515
mannitol 521
nephrogenic diabetes insipidus 508
osmotic diuretics 521
potassium-sparing diuretic 521
spironolactone 521
triamterene 521

SECTION C

Hydrogen Ion Regulation

The understanding of the regulation of acid–base balance requires appreciation of a general principle of physiology that physiological processes are dictated by the laws of chemistry and physics. Metabolic reactions are highly sensitive to the H^+ concentration of the fluid in which they occur. This sensitivity is due to the influence that H^+ has on the shapes of proteins, such as enzymes, such that their function can be altered. Not surprisingly, then, the H^+ concentration of the extracellular fluid is tightly regulated. At this point, the reader might want to review the section on H^+, acidity, and pH in Chapter 2.

This regulation can be viewed in the same way as the balance of any other ion—that is, as matching gains and losses. When loss exceeds gain, the arterial plasma hydrogen ion concentration decreases and pH exceeds 7.4. This is termed ***alkalosis.*** When gain exceeds loss, the arterial plasma hydrogen ion concentration increases and the pH is less than 7.4. This is termed ***acidosis.***

14.16 Sources of Hydrogen Ion Gain or Loss

Table 14.6 summarizes the major routes for gains and losses of H^+. As described in Chapter 13, a huge quantity of CO_2—about 20,000 mmol—is generated daily as the result of oxidative metabolism. These CO_2 molecules participate in the generation of H^+ during the passage of blood through peripheral tissues via the following reactions:

$$CO_2 + H_2O \overset{\text{carbonic anhydrase}}{\rightleftharpoons} H_2CO_3 \rightleftharpoons HCO_3^- + H^+ \qquad (14\text{–}1)$$

This source does not normally constitute a net gain of H^+. This is because the H^+ generated via these reactions is reincorporated into water when the reactions are reversed during the passage of blood through the lungs (see Chapter 13). Net retention of CO_2 does occur in hypoventilation or respiratory disease and in such cases causes a net gain of H^+. Conversely, net loss of CO_2 occurs in hyperventilation, and this causes net elimination of H^+.

The body also produces both organic and inorganic acids from sources other than CO_2. These are collectively termed **nonvolatile acids.** They include phosphoric acid and sulfuric acid, generated mainly by the catabolism of proteins, as well as lactic acid and several other organic acids. Dissociation of all of these acids yields anions and H^+. Simultaneously, however, the metabolism of a variety of organic anions utilizes H^+ and produces HCO_3^-. Thus, the metabolism of "nonvolatile" solutes both generates and utilizes H^+. With the high-protein diet typical in the United States, the generation of nonvolatile acids predominates in most people, with an average net production of 40 to 80 mmol of H^+ per day.

A third potential source of the net gain or loss of H^+ in the body occurs when gastrointestinal secretions leave the body. Vomitus contains a high concentration of H^+ and so constitutes a source of net loss. In contrast, the other gastrointestinal secretions are alkaline. They contain very little H^+, but their concentration of HCO_3^- is higher than in plasma. Loss of these fluids, as in diarrhea, in essence constitutes a *gain* of H^+. Given the mass-action relationship shown in equation 14–1, *when HCO_3^- is lost from the body, it is the same as if the body had gained hydrogen ion.* This is because loss of the HCO_3^- causes the reactions shown in equation 14–1 to be driven to the right, thereby generating hydrogen ion within the body. Similarly, when the body gains HCO_3^-, it is the same as if the body had lost hydrogen ion, as the reactions of equation 14–1 are driven to the left.

Finally, the kidneys constitute the fourth source of net hydrogen ion gain or loss. That is, the kidneys can either remove H^+ from the plasma or add it.

TABLE 14.6 Sources of Hydrogen Ion Gain or Loss

Gain

- Generation of H^+ from CO_2
- Production of nonvolatile acids from the metabolism of proteins and other organic molecules
- Gain of H^+ due to loss of HCO_3^- in diarrhea or other nongastric GI fluids
- Gain of H^+ due to loss of HCO_3^- in the urine

Loss

- Utilization of H^+ in the metabolism of various organic anions
- Loss of H^+ in vomitus
- Loss of H^+ in the urine
- Hyperventilation

14.17 Buffering of Hydrogen Ion in the Body

Any substance that can reversibly bind H^+ is called a **buffer.** Most H^+ is bound by extracellular and intracellular buffers. The normal extracellular fluid pH of 7.4 corresponds to a hydrogen ion concentration of only 0.00004 mmol/L (40 nmol/L). Without buffering, the daily turnover of the 40 to 80 mmol of H^+ produced from nonvolatile acids generated in the body from metabolism would cause huge changes in body fluid hydrogen ion concentration.

The general form of buffering reactions is

$$\text{Buffer} + H^+ \rightleftharpoons \text{HBuffer} \qquad (14\text{–}2)$$

Recall the law of mass action described in Chapter 3, which governs the net direction of the reaction in equation 14–2. HBuffer is a weak acid in that it can dissociate to buffer H^+ or it can exist as the undissociated molecule (HBuffer). When H^+ concentration increases for any reason, the reaction is forced to the right and more H^+ is bound by buffer to form HBuffer. For example, when H^+ concentration is increased because of increased production of lactic acid, some of the H^+ combines with the body's buffers, so the hydrogen ion concentration does not increase as much as it otherwise would have. Conversely, when H^+ concentration decreases because of the loss of H^+ or the addition of alkali, equation 14–2 proceeds to the left and H^+ is released from HBuffer. In this manner, buffers stabilize H^+ concentration against changes in either direction.

The major extracellular buffer is the CO_2/HCO_3^- system summarized in equation 14–1. This system also plays some role in buffering within cells, but the major intracellular buffers are phosphates and proteins. An example of an intracellular protein buffer is hemoglobin, as described in Chapter 13.

This buffering does not eliminate H^+ from the body or add it to the body; it only keeps the H^+ "locked up" until balance can be restored. How balance is achieved is the subject of the rest of our description of hydrogen ion regulation.

14.18 Integration of Homeostatic Controls

The kidneys are ultimately responsible for balancing hydrogen ion gains and losses so as to maintain plasma hydrogen ion concentration within a narrow range. Thus, the kidneys normally excrete the excess H^+ from nonvolatile acids generated from metabolism—that is, all acids other than carbonic acid. An additional net gain of H^+ can occur with increased production of these nonvolatile acids, with hypoventilation or respiratory malfunction, or with the loss of alkaline gastrointestinal secretions. When this occurs, the kidneys increase the elimination of H^+ from the body to restore balance. Alternatively, if there is a net loss of H^+ from the body due to hyperventilation or vomiting, the kidneys replenish this H^+.

Although the kidneys are the ultimate hydrogen ion balancers, the respiratory system also plays a very important homeostatic role. We have pointed out that hypoventilation, respiratory malfunction, and hyperventilation can cause a hydrogen ion imbalance. Now we emphasize that when a hydrogen ion imbalance is due to a nonrespiratory cause, then ventilation is reflexively altered so as to help compensate for the imbalance. We described this phenomenon in Chapter 13 (see Figure 13.38). An increased arterial hydrogen ion concentration stimulates ventilation, which lowers arterial P_{CO_2} that, by mass action, reduces hydrogen ion concentration. Alternatively, a decreased plasma hydrogen ion concentration inhibits ventilation, thereby increasing arterial P_{CO_2} and the hydrogen ion concentration.

In this way, the respiratory system and kidneys work together. The respiratory response to altered plasma hydrogen ion concentration is very rapid (minutes) and keeps this concentration from changing too much until the more slowly responding kidneys (hours to days) can actually eliminate the imbalance. If the respiratory system is the actual cause of the hydrogen ion imbalance, then the kidneys are the sole homeostatic responder. Conversely, malfunctioning kidneys can create a hydrogen ion imbalance by eliminating too little or too much hydrogen ion from the body, and then the respiratory response is the only one in control. As you can see, therefore, the control of acid–base balance requires that the functions of organ systems be coordinated with each other—another general principle of physiology highlighted in this book.

14.19 Renal Mechanisms

The kidneys eliminate or replenish H^+ from the body by altering plasma bicarbonate concentration. The key to understanding how altering plasma bicarbonate concentration eliminates or replenishes H^+ was stated earlier. That is, the excretion of HCO_3^- in the urine increases the plasma hydrogen ion concentration just as if a hydrogen ion had been added to the plasma. Similarly, the addition of HCO_3^- to the plasma decreases the plasma hydrogen ion concentration just as if a hydrogen ion had been removed from the plasma.

Thus, when the plasma hydrogen ion concentration decreases (alkalosis) for whatever reason, the kidneys' homeostatic response is to excrete large quantities of HCO_3^-. This increases plasma hydrogen ion concentration toward normal. In contrast, when plasma hydrogen ion concentration increases (acidosis), the kidneys do not excrete HCO_3^- in the urine. Rather, kidney tubular cells produce *new* HCO_3^- and add it to the plasma. This decreases the plasma hydrogen ion concentration toward normal.

HCO_3^- Handling

HCO_3^- is completely filterable at the renal corpuscles and undergoes significant tubular reabsorption in the proximal tubule, ascending loop of Henle, and cortical collecting ducts. It can also be secreted in the collecting ducts. Therefore,

$$HCO_3^- \text{ excretion} = HCO_3^- \text{ filtered} + HCO_3^- \text{ secreted} - HCO_3^- \text{ reabsorbed}$$

For simplicity, we will ignore the secretion of HCO_3^- because it is always much less than tubular reabsorption, and we will treat HCO_3^- excretion as the difference between filtration and reabsorption.

HCO_3^- reabsorption is an active process, but it is not accomplished in the conventional manner of simply having an active pump for HCO_3^- at the luminal or basolateral membrane of the tubular cells. Instead, HCO_3^- reabsorption depends on the tubular secretion of H^+, which combines in the lumen with filtered HCO_3^-.

Figure 14.33 illustrates the sequence of events. Begin this figure inside the cell with the combination of CO_2 and H_2O to form H_2CO_3, a reaction catalyzed by the enzyme carbonic anhydrase. The H_2CO_3 immediately dissociates to yield H^+ and HCO_3^-. The HCO_3^- moves down its concentration gradient via facilitated diffusion across the basolateral membrane into interstitial fluid and then into the blood. Simultaneously, the H^+ is secreted into the lumen. Depending on the tubular segment, this secretion is achieved by some combination of primary H^+-ATPase pumps, primary H^+/K^+-ATPase pumps, and Na^+/H^+ countertransporters.

The secreted H^+, however, is not excreted. Instead, it combines in the lumen with a filtered HCO_3^- and generates CO_2 and H_2O, both of which can diffuse into the cell and be available for another cycle of hydrogen ion generation. The overall result is that the HCO_3^- filtered from the plasma at the renal corpuscle has disappeared, but its place in the plasma has been taken by the HCO_3^- that was produced inside the cell. In this manner, no net change in plasma bicarbonate concentration has occurred. It may seem inaccurate to refer to this process as

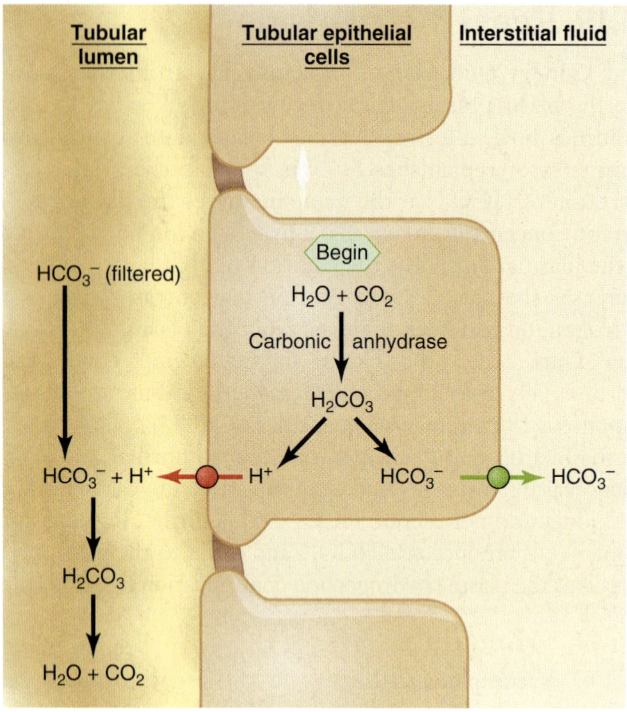

Figure 14.33 General model of the reabsorption of HCO_3^- in the proximal tubule and cortical collecting duct. Begin looking at this figure inside the cell, with the combination of CO_2 and H_2O to form H_2CO_3. As shown in the figure, active H^+-ATPase pumps are involved in the movement of H^+ out of the cell across the luminal membrane; in several tubular segments, this transport step is also mediated by Na^+/H^+ countertransporters and/or H^+/K^+-ATPase pumps.

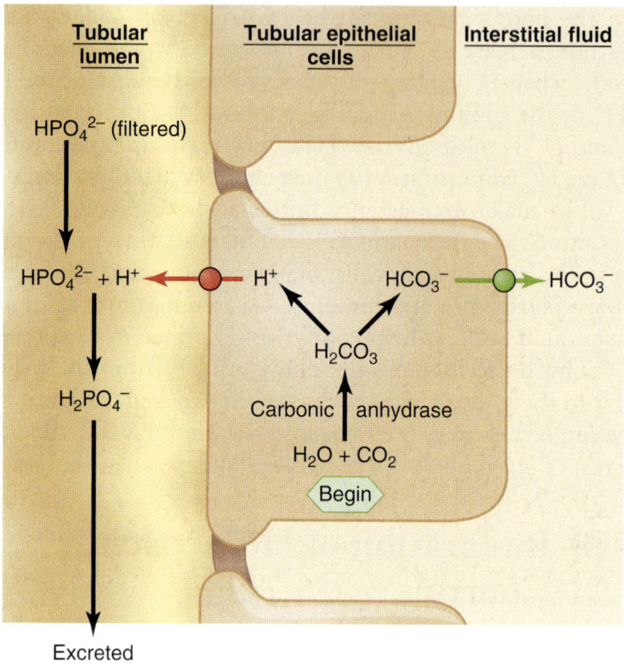

Figure 14.34 Renal contribution of new HCO_3^- to the plasma as achieved by tubular secretion of H^+. The process of intracellular H^+ and HCO_3^- generation, with H^+ moving into the lumen and HCO_3^- into the plasma, is identical to that shown in Figure 14.33. Once in the lumen of the proximal tubule, however, the H^+ combines with filtered phosphate ion ($H_2PO_4^{2-}$) rather than filtered HCO_3^- and is excreted as $H_2PO_4^-$. As described in the legend for Figure 14.33, the transport of H^+ into the lumen is accomplished not only by H^+-ATPase pumps but, in several tubular segments, by Na^+/H^+ countertransporters and/or H^+/K^+-ATPase pumps as well.

HCO_3^- "reabsorption" because the HCO_3^- that appears in the peritubular plasma is not the same HCO_3^- that was filtered. Yet, the overall result is the same as if the filtered HCO_3^- had been reabsorbed in the conventional manner like Na^+ or K^+.

Except in response to alkalosis, discussed in the next section, the kidneys normally reabsorb all filtered HCO_3^-, thereby preventing the loss of HCO_3^- in the urine.

Addition of New HCO_3^- to the Plasma

An essential concept shown in Figure 14.32 is that as long as there are still significant amounts of filtered HCO_3^- in the lumen, almost all secreted H^+ will combine with it. But what happens to any secreted H^+ once almost all the HCO_3^- has been reabsorbed and is no longer available in the lumen to combine with the H^+?

The answer, illustrated in **Figure 14.34,** is that the extra secreted H^+ combines in the lumen with a filtered nonbicarbonate buffer, the most important of which is HPO_4^{2-}. The hydrogen ion is then excreted in the urine as part of the HPO_4^{2-} ion. Now for the critical point: Note in Figure 14.34 that, under these conditions, the HCO_3^- generated within the tubular cell by the carbonic anhydrase reaction and entering the plasma constitutes a *net gain* of HCO_3^- by the plasma, not merely a replacement for filtered HCO_3^-. Therefore, when secreted hydrogen ion combines in the lumen with a buffer other than HCO_3^-, the overall effect is not merely one of HCO_3^- conservation, as in Figure 14.33, but, rather, of addition to the plasma of *new* HCO_3^-. This increases the HCO_3^- concentration of the plasma and alkalinizes it.

To repeat, significant amounts of H^+ combine with filtered nonbicarbonate buffers like HPO_4^{2-} only after the filtered HCO_3^- has virtually all been reabsorbed. The main reason is that there is such a large load of filtered HCO_3^-—25 times more than the load of filtered nonbicarbonate buffers—competing for the secreted H^+.

There is a second mechanism by which the tubules contribute new HCO_3^- to the plasma that involves not hydrogen ion secretion but, rather, the renal production and secretion of ammonium ion (NH_4^+) (**Figure 14.35**). Tubular cells, mainly those of the proximal tubule, take up glutamine from both the glomerular filtrate and peritubular plasma and metabolize it. In the process, both NH_4^+ and HCO_3^- are formed inside the cells. The NH_4^+ is actively secreted via Na^+/NH_4^+ countertransport into the lumen and excreted, while the HCO_3^- moves into the peritubular capillaries and constitutes new plasma bicarbonate.

A comparison of Figures 14.34 and 14.35 demonstrates that the overall result—renal contribution of new HCO_3^- to the plasma—is the same regardless of whether it is achieved by (1) H^+ secretion and excretion on nonbicarbonate buffers such as phosphate (see Figure 14.34) or (2) by glutamine metabolism with excretion (see Figure 14.35). It is convenient, therefore, to view the latter as representing H^+ excretion "bound" to NH_3, just as the former case constitutes H^+ excretion bound to nonbicarbonate buffers. Thus, the amount of H^+ excreted in the urine in these two forms is a measure of the amount of new HCO_3^- added to the plasma by the kidneys. Indeed, "urinary

TABLE 14.7 Renal Responses to Acidosis and Alkalosis

Responses to acidosis

- Sufficient H^+ is secreted to reabsorb all the filtered HCO_3^-.
- Still more H^+ is secreted, and this contributes new HCO_3^- to the plasma as the H^+ is excreted bound to nonbicarbonate urinary buffers such as HPO_4^{2-}.
- Tubular glutamine metabolism and ammonium excretion are enhanced, which also contributes new HCO_3^- to the plasma.

Net result: More new HCO_3^- ion than usual is added to the blood, and plasma bicarbonate is increased, thereby compensating for the acidosis. The urine is highly acidic (lowest attainable pH = 4.4).

Responses to alkalosis

- Rate of hydrogen ion secretion is inadequate to reabsorb all the filtered HCO_3^-, so significant amounts of HCO_3^- are excreted in the urine, and there is little or no excretion of H^+ on nonbicarbonate urinary buffers.
- Tubular glutamine metabolism and ammonium excretion are decreased so that little or no new HCO_3^- is contributed to the plasma from this source.

Net result: Plasma bicarbonate concentration is decreased, thereby compensating for the alkalosis. The urine is alkaline (pH > 7.4).

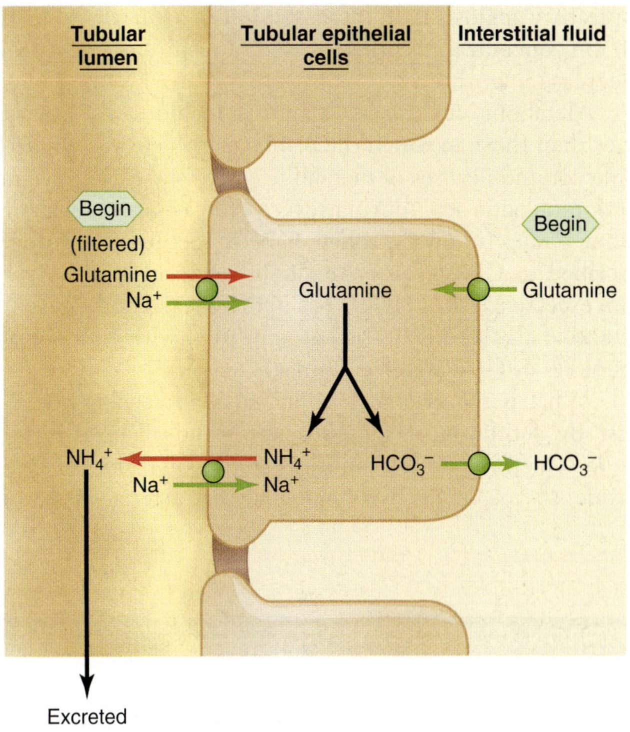

Figure 14.35 Renal contribution of new HCO_3^- to the plasma as achieved by renal metabolism of glutamine and excretion of ammonium (NH_4^+). Compare this figure to Figure 14.34. This process occurs mainly in the proximal tubule.

H^+ excretion" and "renal contribution of new HCO_3^- to the plasma" are really two sides of the same coin.

The kidneys normally contribute enough new HCO_3^- to the blood by excreting H^+ to compensate for the H^+ from nonvolatile acids generated in the body.

14.20 Classification of Acidosis and Alkalosis

The renal responses to the presence of acidosis or alkalosis are summarized in **Table 14.7.** To repeat, acidosis refers to any situation in which the hydrogen ion concentration of arterial plasma is increased above normal whereas alkalosis denotes a decrease. All such situations fit into two distinct categories (**Table 14.8**): (1) ***respiratory acidosis*** or ***alkalosis*** and (2) ***metabolic acidosis*** or ***alkalosis.***

As its name implies, respiratory acidosis results from altered alveolar ventilation. Respiratory acidosis occurs when the respiratory system fails to eliminate carbon dioxide as fast as it is produced. Respiratory alkalosis occurs when the respiratory system eliminates carbon dioxide faster than it is produced. As described earlier, the imbalance of arterial hydrogen ion concentrations in such cases is completely explainable in terms of mass action. Thus, the hallmark of

TABLE 14.8 Changes in the Arterial Concentrations of H^+, HCO_3^-, and Carbon Dioxide in Acid–Base Disorders

Primary Disorder	H^+	HCO_3^-	CO_2	Cause of HCO_3^- Change	Cause of CO_2 Change
Respiratory acidosis	↑	↑	↑	Renal compensation	Primary abnormality
Respiratory alkalosis	↓	↓	↓		
Metabolic acidosis	↑	↓	↓	Primary abnormality	Reflex ventilatory compensation
Metabolic alkalosis	↓	↑	↑		

PHYSIOLOGICAL INQUIRY

- A patient has an arterial P_{O_2} of 50 mmHg, an arterial P_{CO_2} of 60 mmHg, and an arterial pH of 7.36. Classify the acid–base disturbance and hypothesize a cause.

Answer can be found at end of chapter.

respiratory acidosis is an increase in both arterial and hydrogen ion concentration, whereas that of respiratory alkalosis is a decrease in both.

Metabolic acidosis or alkalosis includes all situations other than those in which the primary problem is respiratory. Some common causes of metabolic acidosis are excessive production of lactic acid (during severe exercise or hypoxia) or of ketone bodies (in uncontrolled diabetes mellitus or fasting, as described in Chapter 16). Metabolic acidosis can also result from excessive loss of HCO_3^-, as in diarrhea. Another cause of metabolic alkalosis is persistent vomiting, with its associated loss of H^+ as HCl from the stomach.

What is the arterial P_{CO_2} in metabolic acidosis or alkalosis? By definition, metabolic acidosis and alkalosis must be due to something other than excess retention or loss of carbon dioxide, so you might have predicted that arterial P_{CO_2} would be unchanged, but this is not the case. As emphasized earlier in this chapter, the increased hydrogen ion concentration associated with metabolic acidosis *reflexively* stimulates ventilation and decreases arterial P_{CO_2}. By mass action, this helps restore the hydrogen ion concentration toward normal. Conversely, a person with metabolic alkalosis will reflexively have ventilation inhibited. The result is an increase in arterial P_{CO_2} and, by mass action, an associated restoration of hydrogen ion concentration toward normal.

To reiterate, the plasma P_{CO_2} changes in metabolic acidosis and alkalosis are not the *cause* of the acidosis or alkalosis but the *result* of compensatory reflexive responses to nonrespiratory abnormalities. Thus, in metabolic as opposed to respiratory conditions, the arterial plasma P_{CO_2} and hydrogen ion concentration move in opposite directions, as summarized in Table 14.8.

SECTION C SUMMARY

Sources of Hydrogen Ion Gain or Loss

I. Total-body balance of H^+ is the result of both metabolic production of these ions and of net gains or losses via the respiratory system, gastrointestinal tract, and urine (Table 14.6).

II. A stable balance is achieved by regulation of urinary losses.

Buffering of Hydrogen Ion in the Body

I. Buffering is a means of minimizing changes in hydrogen ion concentration by combining these ions reversibly with anions such as HCO_3^- and intracellular proteins.

II. The major extracellular buffering system is the CO_2/HCO_3^- system, and the major intracellular buffers are proteins and phosphates.

Integration of Homeostatic Controls

I. The kidneys and the respiratory system are the homeostatic regulators of plasma hydrogen ion concentration.

II. The kidneys are the organs that achieve body hydrogen ion balance.

III. A decrease in arterial plasma hydrogen ion concentration causes reflex hypoventilation, which increases arterial and, hence, increases plasma hydrogen ion concentration toward normal. An increase in plasma hydrogen ion concentration causes reflexive hyperventilation, which decreases arterial and, hence, decreases hydrogen ion concentration toward normal.

Renal Mechanisms

I. The kidneys maintain a stable plasma hydrogen ion concentration by regulating plasma bicarbonate concentration. They can either excrete HCO_3^- or contribute new HCO_3^- to the blood.

II. HCO_3^- is reabsorbed when H^+, generated in the tubular cells by a process catalyzed by carbonic anhydrase, is secreted into the lumen and combine with filtered HCO_3^-. The secreted H^+ is not excreted in this situation.

III. In contrast, when the secreted H^+ combines in the lumen with filtered phosphate ion or other nonbicarbonate buffer, it is excreted, and the kidneys have contributed new HCO_3^- to the blood.

IV. The kidneys also contribute new HCO_3^- to the blood when they produce and excrete ammonium.

Classification of Acidosis and Alkalosis

I. Acid–base disorders are categorized as respiratory or metabolic.
   a. Respiratory acidosis is due to retention of carbon dioxide, and respiratory alkalosis is due to excessive elimination of carbon dioxide.
   b. All other causes of acidosis or alkalosis are termed *metabolic* and reflect gain or loss, respectively, of H^+ from a source other than carbon dioxide.

SECTION C REVIEW QUESTIONS

1. What are the sources of gain and loss of H^+ in the body?
2. List the body's major buffer systems.
3. Describe the role of the respiratory system in the regulation of hydrogen ion concentration.
4. How does the tubular secretion of H^+ occur, and how does it achieve HCO_3^- reabsorption?
5. How does hydrogen ion secretion contribute to the renal addition of new HCO_3^- to the blood? What determines whether secreted hydrogen ion will achieve these results or will instead cause HCO_3^- reabsorption?
6. How does the metabolism of glutamine by the tubular cells contribute new HCO_3^- to the blood and ammonium to the urine?
7. What two quantities make up "hydrogen ion excretion"? Why can this term be equated with "contribution of new HCO_3^- to the plasma"?
8. How do the kidneys respond to the presence of acidosis or alkalosis?
9. Classify the four types of acid–base disorders according to plasma hydrogen ion concentration, HCO_3^- concentration, and P_{CO_2}.
10. Explain how overuse of certain diuretics can lead to metabolic alkalosis.

SECTION C KEY TERMS

buffer 524

nonvolatile acid 524

SECTION C CLINICAL TERMS

acidosis 524

alkalosis 524

metabolic acidosis 527

metabolic alkalosis 527

respiratory acidosis 527

respiratory alkalosis 527

Clinical Case Study: Severe Kidney Disease in a Woman with Diabetes Mellitus

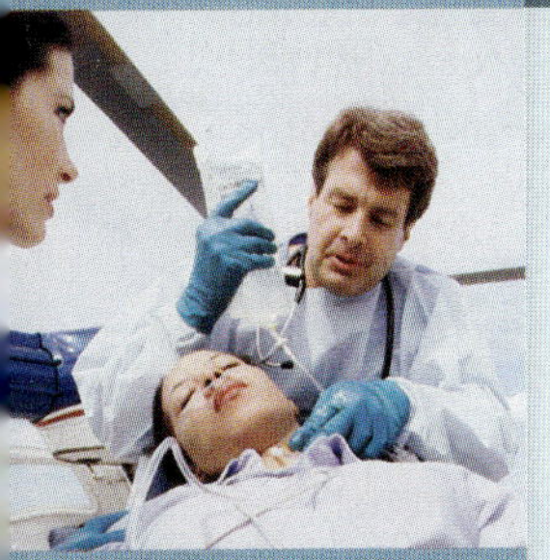

A patient with poorly controlled, long-standing type 2 diabetes mellitus has been feeling progressively weaker over the past few months. She has also been feeling generally ill and has been gaining weight although she has not changed her eating habits. During a routine visit to her family doctor, some standard blood and urine tests are ordered as an initial evaluation. In addition, her previously diagnosed mild high blood pressure has gotten significantly worse. The physician is concerned when the testing shows an increase in creatinine in her blood and a significant amount of protein in her urine. The patient is referred to a nephrologist (kidney-disease expert) who makes the diagnosis of diabetic kidney disease (diabetic nephropathy).

Many diseases affect the kidneys. Potential causes of kidney damage include congenital and inherited defects, metabolic disorders, infection, inflammation, trauma, vascular problems, and certain forms of cancer. Obstruction of the urethra or a ureter may cause injury from the buildup of pressure and may predispose the kidneys to bacterial infection. A common cause of renal failure is poorly controlled diabetes mellitus. The increase in blood glucose interferes with normal renal filtration and tubular function (see Section 14.13 of this chapter and Chapter 16), and high blood pressure common to patients with type 2 diabetes mellitus causes vascular damage in the kidney.

One of the earliest signs of a decrease in kidney function is an increase in creatinine in the blood, which was found to be the case in our patient. As described in Section 14.3 of this chapter, creatinine is a waste product of muscle metabolism that is filtered in the glomerulus and not reabsorbed. Although a small amount of creatinine is secreted in the renal tubule, creatinine clearance is a good estimate of glomerular filtration rate (GFR). Because a decrease in GFR occurs early in kidney disease, and because creatinine production is fairly constant, an increase in creatinine in the blood is a useful warning sign that creatinine clearance is decreasing and that kidney failure is occurring. Another frequent sign of kidney disease, which was also observed in our patient, is the appearance of protein in the urine. In normal kidneys, there is a tiny amount of protein in the glomerular filtrate because the filtration barrier membranes are not completely impermeable to proteins, particularly those with lower molecular weights. However, the cells of the proximal tubule completely remove this filtered protein from the tubular lumen and no protein appears in the final urine. In contrast, in diabetic nephropathy, the filtration barrier may become much more permeable to protein, and diseased proximal tubules may lose their ability to remove filtered protein from the tubular lumen. The result is that protein appears in the urine. The loss of protein in the urine leads to a decrease in the amount of protein in the blood. This results in a decrease in the osmotic force retaining fluid in the blood and subsequently the formation of edema throughout the body (see Chapter 12). In our patient, this resulted in an increase in body weight.

Although many diseases of the kidneys are self-limited and produce no permanent damage, others worsen if untreated. The symptoms of profound renal malfunction are relatively independent of the damaging agent and are collectively known as ***uremia,*** literally, "urea in the blood."

The severity of uremia depends upon how well the impaired kidneys can preserve the constancy of the internal environment. Assuming that the person continues to ingest a normal diet containing the usual quantities of nutrients and electrolytes, what problems arise? The key fact to keep in mind is that the kidney destruction markedly reduces the number of functioning nephrons. Accordingly, the many substances, particularly potentially toxic waste products that gain entry to the tubule by filtration, build up in the blood. In addition, the excretion of K^+ is impaired because there are too few nephrons capable of normal tubular secretion of this ion. The person may also develop acidosis because the reduced number of nephrons fails to add enough new HCO_3^- to the blood to compensate for the daily metabolic production of nonvolatile acids.

The remarkable fact is how large the safety factor is in renal function. In general, the kidneys are still able to perform their regulatory function quite well as long as 10% to 30% of the nephrons are functioning. This is because these remaining nephrons undergo alterations in function—filtration, reabsorption, and secretion—to compensate for the missing nephrons. For example, each remaining nephron increases its rate of K^+ secretion, so that the total amount of K^+ the kidneys excrete is maintained at normal levels. The limits of regulation are restricted, however. To use K^+ as our example again, if someone with severe renal disease were to go on a diet high in potassium, the remaining nephrons might not be able to secrete enough K^+ to prevent potassium retention.

Other problems arise in uremia because of abnormal secretion of the hormones the kidneys produce. Thus, decreased secretion of erythropoietin results in anemia (see Chapter 12). Decreased ability to form 1,25-$(OH)_2$D results in deficient absorption of calcium ion from the gastrointestinal tract, with a resulting decrease in plasma calcium, increase in PTH, and inadequate bone calcification (secondary hyperparathyroidism). Erythropoietin and 1,25-$(OH)_2$D (calcitriol) can be administered to patients with uremia to improve hematocrit and calcium balance.

In the case of the secreted enzyme renin, there is rarely too little secretion; rather, there is too much secretion by the juxtaglomerular cells of the damaged kidneys. The main reason for the increase in renin is decreased perfusion of affected nephrons (intrarenal baroreceptor). The result is increased plasma angiotensin II concentration and the development of ***renal hypertension.*** ACE inhibitors and angiotensin II receptor blockers can be used to decrease blood pressure and improve sodium and water balance. Our patient was counseled to more carefully and aggressively control her blood glucose and blood pressure with diet, exercise, and medications. She was also started on an ACE inhibitor. Unfortunately, her blood creatinine and proteinuria continued to worsen to the point of end-stage renal disease requiring hemodialysis.

Hemodialysis, Peritoneal Dialysis, and Transplantation

Failing kidneys may reach a point when they can no longer excrete water and ions at rates that maintain body balances of these substances, nor can they excrete waste products as fast as they

(continued)

(continued)

are produced. Dietary alterations can help minimize but not eliminate these problems. For example, decreasing potassium intake reduces the amount of K^+ to be excreted. The clinical techniques used to perform the kidneys' excretory functions are hemodialysis and peritoneal dialysis. The general term ***dialysis*** means to separate substances using a permeable membrane.

The artificial kidney is an apparatus that utilizes a process termed ***hemodialysis*** to remove wastes and excess substances from the blood (**Figure 14.36**). During hemodialysis, blood is pumped from one of the patient's arteries through tubing that is surrounded by special dialysis fluid. The tubing then conducts the blood back into the patient by way of a vein. The dialysis tubing is generally made of cellophane that is highly permeable to most solutes but relatively impermeable to protein and completely impermeable to blood cells—characteristics quite similar to those of capillaries. The dialysis fluid is a salt solution with ionic concentrations similar to or lower than those in normal plasma, and it contains no creatinine, urea, or other substances to be completely removed from the plasma. As blood flows through the tubing, the concentrations of nonprotein plasma solutes tend to reach diffusion equilibrium with those of the solutes in the bath fluid. For example, if the plasma K^+ concentration of the patient is above normal, K^+ diffuses out of the blood across the cellophane tubing and into the dialysis fluid. Similarly, waste products and excesses of other substances also diffuse into the dialysis fluid and thus are eliminated from the body.

Patients with acute reversible renal failure may require hemodialysis for only days or weeks. Patients like the woman in our case with chronic irreversible renal failure require treatment for the rest of their lives, however, unless they receive a kidney transplant. Such patients undergo hemodialysis several times a week.

Another way of removing excess substances from the blood is ***peritoneal dialysis,*** which uses the lining of the patient's own abdominal cavity (peritoneum) as a dialysis membrane. Fluid is injected via an indwelling plastic tube inserted through the abdominal wall into this cavity and allowed to remain there for hours, during which solutes diffuse into the fluid from the person's blood. The dialysis fluid is then removed and replaced with new fluid. This procedure can be performed several times daily by a patient who is simultaneously doing normal activities.

The long-term treatment of choice for most patients with permanent renal failure is kidney transplantation. Rejection of the transplanted kidney by the recipient's body is a potential problem, but great strides have been made in reducing the frequency of rejection (see Chapter 18). Many people who could benefit from a transplant, however, do not receive one. Currently, the major source of kidneys for transplantation is recently deceased persons. Recently, donation from a living, related donor has become more common. Because of the large safety factor, the donor can function quite normally with one kidney. In 2009, approximately 84,000 people in the United States were waiting for a kidney transplant.

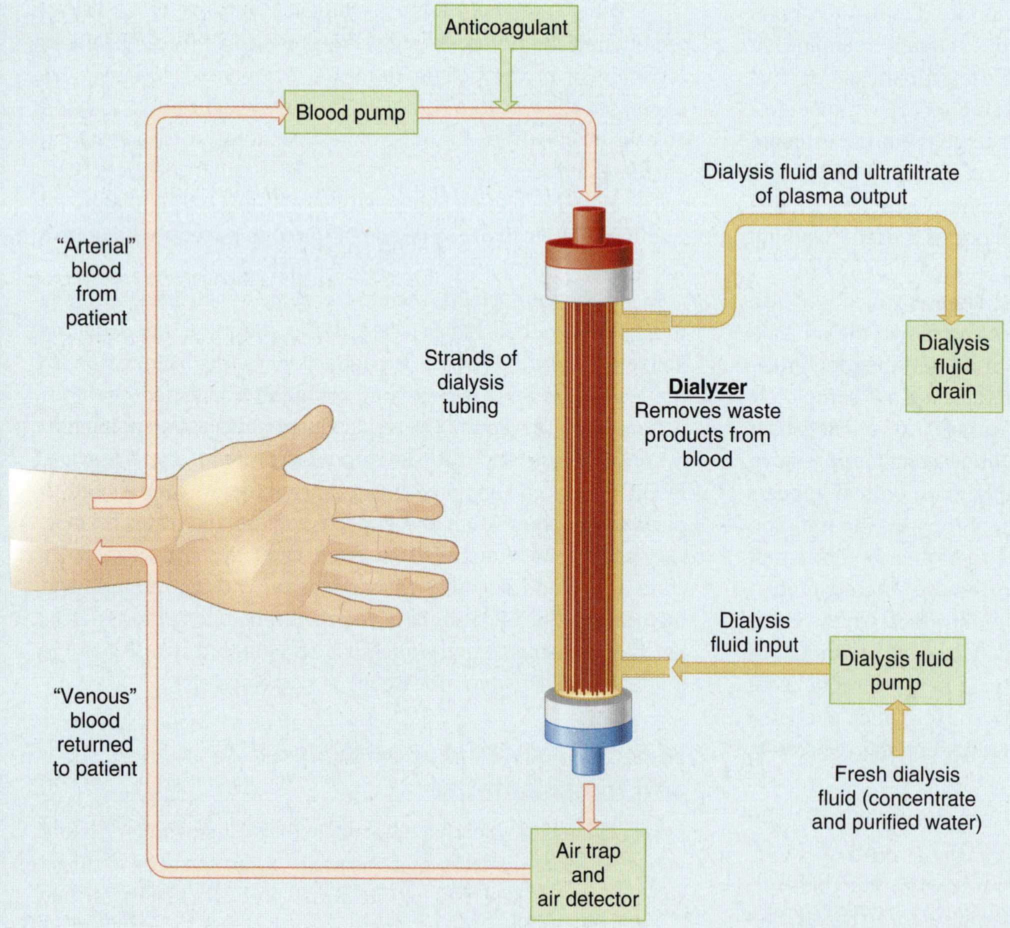

Figure 14.36 Simplified diagram of hemodialysis. Note that blood and dialysis fluid flow in opposite directions through the dialyzer (countercurrent). The blood flow can be 400 mL/min, and the dialysis fluid flow rate can be 1000 mL/min! During a 3 to 4 h dialysis session, approximately 72 to 96 L of blood and 3000 to 4000 L of dialysis fluid pass through the dialyzer. The dialyzer is composed of many strands of very thin dialysis tubing. Blood flows inside each tube, and dialysis fluid bathes the outside of the dialysis tubing. This provides a large surface area for diffusion of waste products out of the blood and into the dialysis fluid.

(continued)

(continued)

There were approximately 11,000 deceased donor and 6000 living donor kidney transplants in 2009, highlighting the shortage of transplantable kidneys. It is hoped that improved public understanding will lead to many more individuals giving permission in advance to have their kidneys and other organs used following their death. Our patient continued on hemodialysis three times a week for several years waiting for a kidney transplant. It was determined that her older brother was a compatible organ match, and he donated his kidney to our patient, allowing her to stop hemodialysis treatments. She continues to aggressively control her blood glucose and blood pressure.

Clinical terms: dialysis, hemodialysis, peritoneal dialysis, renal hypertension, uremia

See Chapter 19 for complete, integrative case studies.

CHAPTER 14 TEST QUESTIONS

Answers found in Appendix A.

1. Which of the following will lead to an increase in glomerular fluid filtration in the kidneys?
   a. an increase in the protein concentration in the plasma
   b. an increase in the fluid pressure in Bowman's space
   c. an increase in the glomerular capillary blood pressure
   d. a decrease in the glomerular capillary blood pressure
   e. constriction of the afferent arteriole
2. Which of the following is true about renal clearance?
   a. It is the amount of a substance excreted per unit time.
   b. A substance with clearance > GFR undergoes only filtration.
   c. A substance with clearance > GFR undergoes filtration and secretion.
   d. It can be calculated knowing only the filtered load of a substance and the rate of urine production.
   e. Creatinine clearance approximates renal plasma flow.
3. Which of the following will *not* lead to a diuresis?
   a. excessive sweating
   b. central diabetes insipidus
   c. nephrogenic diabetes insipidus
   d. excessive water intake
   e. uncontrolled diabetes mellitus
4. Which of the following contributes directly to the generation of a hypertonic medullary interstitium in the kidney?
   a. active Na^+ transport in the descending limb of Henle's loop
   b. active water reabsorption in the ascending limb of Henle's loop
   c. active Na^+ reabsorption in the distal convoluted tubule
   d. water reabsorption in the cortical collecting duct
   e. secretion of urea into Henle's loop
5. An increase in renin is caused by
   a. a decrease in sodium intake.
   b. a decrease in renal sympathetic nerve activity.
   c. an increase in blood pressure in the renal artery.
   d. an aldosterone-secreting adrenal tumor.
   e. essential hypertension.
6. An increase in parathyroid hormone will
   a. increase plasma 25(OH) D.
   b. decrease plasma 1,25-$(OH)_2$D.
   c. decrease calcium ion excretion.
   d. increase phosphate ion reabsorption.
   e. increase calcium ion reabsorption in the proximal tubule.
7. Which of the following is a component of the renal response to metabolic acidosis?
   a. reabsorption of H^+
   b. secretion of HCO_3^- into the tubular lumen
   c. secretion of ammonium into the tubular lumen
   d. secretion of glutamine into the interstitial fluid
   e. carbonic anhydrase-mediated production of HPO_4^{2-}
8. Which of the following is consistent with respiratory alkalosis?
   a. an increase in alveolar ventilation during mild exercise
   b. hyperventilation
   c. an increase in plasma HCO_3^-
   d. an increase in arterial CO_2
   e. urine pH < 5.0
9. Which is *true* about the difference between cortical and juxtamedullary nephrons?
   a. Most nephrons are juxtamedullary.
   b. The efferent arterioles of cortical nephrons give rise to most of the vasa recta.
   c. The afferent arterioles of the juxtamedullary nephrons give rise to most of the vasa recta.
   d. All cortical nephrons have a loop of Henle.
   e. Juxtamedullary nephrons generate a hyperosmotic medullary interstitium.
10. Which of the following is consistent with untreated chronic renal failure?
    a. proteinuria
    b. hypokalemia
    c. increased plasma 1,25-$(OH)_2$D
    d. increased plasma erythropoietin
    e. increased plasma HCO_3^-

CHAPTER 14 GENERAL PRINCIPLES ASSESSMENT

Answers found in Appendix A.

1. A general principle of physiology is that *structure is a determinant of—and has coevolved with—function.* How does the anatomy of the renal corpuscle and associated structures determine function?
2. *Physiological processes are dictated by the laws of chemistry and physics.* Give one example each of how a law of chemistry and a law of physics are important in understanding the regulation of renal function.
3. How does the control of vasopressin secretion highlight the general principle of physiology that *most physiological functions are controlled by multiple regulatory systems, often working in opposition?*

CHAPTER 14 QUANTITATIVE AND THOUGHT QUESTIONS *Answers found at www.mhhe.com/widmaier13.*

1. Substance T is present in the urine. Does this prove that it is filterable at the glomerulus?
2. Substance V is not normally present in the urine. Does this prove that it is neither filtered nor secreted?
3. The concentration of glucose in plasma is 100 mg/100 mL, and the GFR is 125 mL/min. How much glucose is filtered per minute?
4. A person is excreting abnormally large amounts of a particular amino acid. Just from the theoretical description of T_m-limited reabsorptive mechanisms in the text, list several possible causes.
5. The concentration of urea in urine is always much higher than the concentration in plasma. Does this mean that urea is secreted?
6. If a person takes a drug that blocks the reabsorption of Na^+, what will happen to the reabsorption of water, urea, Cl^-, glucose, and amino acids and to the secretion of H^+?
7. Compare the changes in GFR and renin secretion occurring in response to a moderate hemorrhage in two individuals—one taking a drug that blocks the sympathetic nerves to the kidneys and the other not taking such a drug.
8. If a person is taking a drug that completely inhibits angiotensin-converting enzyme, what will happen to aldosterone secretion when the person goes on a low-sodium diet?
9. In the steady state, what is the amount of sodium chloride excreted daily in the urine of a normal person ingesting 12 g of sodium chloride per day: (a) 12 g/day, or (b) less than 12 g/day? Explain.
10. A young woman who has suffered a head injury seems to have recovered but is thirsty all the time. What do you think might be the cause?
11. A patient has a tumor in the adrenal cortex that continuously secretes large amounts of aldosterone. What is this condition called, and what effects does this have on the total amount of sodium and potassium in her body?
12. A person is taking a drug that inhibits the tubular secretion of H^+. What effect does this drug have on the body's balance of sodium, water, and H^+?
13. How can the overuse of diuretics lead to metabolic alkalosis?

CHAPTER 14 ANSWERS TO PHYSIOLOGICAL INQUIRIES

Figure 14.3 The glomerular filtration rate would be greatly decreased. This would result in a decrease in the removal of toxic substances from the blood. As you will learn, kidney disease is a common and troubling consequence of long-term untreated diabetes mellitus.

Figure 14.8 GFR will decrease because the increase in plasma osmotic force from albumin will oppose filtration.

Figure 14.9 A blood clot occluding the afferent arteriole would decrease blood flow to that glomerulus and greatly decrease GFR in that individual glomerulus. A blood clot in the efferent arteriole would increase P_{GC} and, therefore, GFR. If this only occurred in a few glomeruli, it would not have a significant effect on renal function because of the large number of total glomeruli in the two kidneys providing a safety factor.

Figure 14.11 Filtered load = GFR × Plasma glucose concentration. Excretion rate = Urine glucose concentration × Urine flow rate.

Figure 14.14 It would decrease sodium reabsorption from the tubular fluid. This will result in an increase in urinary sodium excretion. The osmotic force of sodium will carry water with it, thus increasing urine output. Examples of such diuretics are triamterene and amiloride.

Figure 14.18 The increased vasopressin would cause maximal water reabsorption. Urine volume would be low (antidiuresis) and urine osmolarity would remain high. The continuous water reabsorption would cause a decrease in plasma sodium concentration (hyponatremia) due to dilution of sodium. Consequently, the plasma would have very low osmolarity. The decreased plasma osmolarity would not inhibit vasopressin secretion from the tumor because it is not controlled by the hypothalamic osmoreceptors. This is called the *syndrome of inappropriate antidiuretic hormone* (*SIADH*) and is one of several possible causes of hyponatremia in humans.

Figure 14.23 An ACE inhibitor will decrease angiotensin II production. The resultant increase in Na^+ and water excretion would decrease blood pressure, leading to a reflexive increase in renin secretion. An ARB would also decrease blood pressure and therefore increase renin secretion. However, with an ARB, angiotensin II would increase because angiotensin-converting-enzyme activity would be normal.

Figure 14.24 Under normal conditions, the redundant control of renin release, as indicated in this figure, as well as the participation of vasopressin (see Figure 14.27), would allow the maintenance of normal sodium and water balance even with denervated kidneys. However, during severe decreases in plasma volume, like in dehydration, the denervated kidney may not produce sufficient renin to maximally decrease Na^+ excretion.

Table 14.8 The patient has respiratory acidosis with renal compensation (hypercapnia with a normalization of arterial pH). The patient is hypoxic, which, with normal lung function, usually leads to hyperventilation and respiratory alkalosis. Therefore, the patient is likely to have chronic lung disease resulting in hypoxemia and retention of carbon dioxide (hypercapnia). We know it is chronic because the kidneys have had time to compensate for the acidosis by increasing the HCO_3^- added to the blood, thus restoring arterial pH almost to normal (see Figures 14.33 to 14.35).

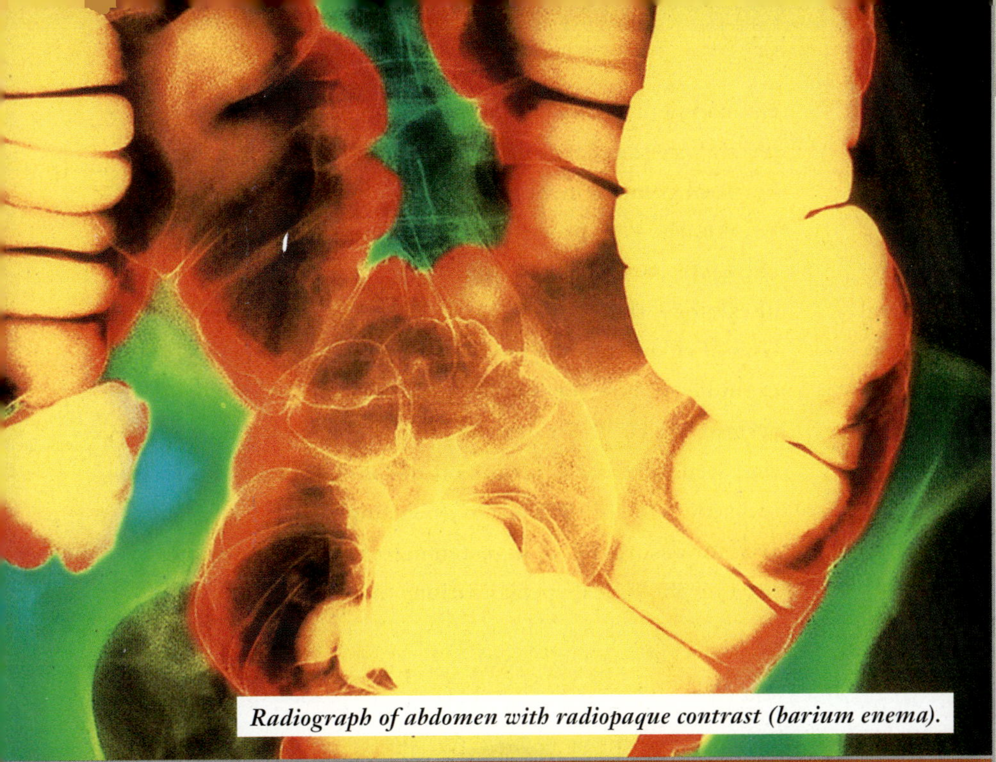

Radiograph of abdomen with radiopaque contrast (barium enema).

15 The Digestion and Absorption of Food

The digestive system is responsible for the absorption of ingested nutrients, water, minerals, and other essential factors and is central to the regulation and integration of metabolic processes throughout the body. Normal function of the digestive system is necessary for long-term whole-body homeostasis as well as normal functioning of individual organ systems. In Chapter 1, you were introduced to the concept of total-body balance where the gain of a substance in the body equals loss of that substance from the body (Figure 1.11). You will now learn several specific examples of total-body balance as they apply to the digestive system. You will also learn how the enteric nervous system, first introduced in Chapter 6, interacts with other parts of the nervous system to provide information to and from the brain, and regulates the local control of gastrointestinal function. In Chapter 14, you learned how water and electrolyte balance are achieved through the regulation of their excretion (output) by the kidneys. You will now learn about the mechanisms and integrated regulation of the absorption (input) of water, electrolytes, vitamins, and nutrients into the body.

This chapter has many examples demonstrating the general principles of physiology introduced in Chapter 1. First, the control of gastrointestinal function illustrates the general principle of physiology that information flow between cells, tissues, and organs is an essential feature of homeostasis and allows for integration of physiological processes; this is highlighted by the intimate relationship between the absorptive capacity of the gastrointestinal tract and the circulatory and lymphatic systems as pathways to deliver these nutrients to the tissues. Second, many of the functions of the gastrointestinal tract illustrate the general principle of physiology that most physiological functions are controlled by multiple regulatory systems, often working in opposition. For example, the acidity of the contents of the stomach is increased or decreased by the influence of hormones released from the gastrointestinal tract as well as paracrine factors and neuronal inputs. Third, the digestive tract regulates the transfer of materials from and to the environment, which exemplifies the general principle of physiology that controlled exchange of materials occurs between compartments and across cellular membranes. Fourth, the very process of digestion depends on basic chemistry, reflecting yet another general principle of physiology, that physiological processes are dictated by the laws of chemistry and physics. Finally, this chapter has many examples of how form follows the function of the digestive system, which illustrates the general principle of physiology that structure is a determinant of—and has coevolved with—function. One of the most vivid examples is the large surface area for absorption of ingested materials made possible by the morphological specializations of the small intestine.

15.1 Overview of the Digestive System

The **digestive system** (Figure 15.1) includes the **gastrointestinal (GI) tract,** consisting of the mouth, pharynx, esophagus, stomach, small intestine, and large intestine; and the accessory organs and tissues, consisting of the salivary glands, liver, gallbladder, and exocrine pancreas. The accessory organs are not part of the tract but secrete substances into it via connecting ducts. The GI tract is also known as the **alimentary canal.** The overall function of the digestive system is to process ingested foods into molecular forms that are then transferred, along with salts and water, to the body's internal environment, where the circulatory system can distribute them to cells. The digestive system is under the local neural control of the enteric nervous system and also of the central nervous system.

The adult gastrointestinal tract is a tube approximately 9 m (30 feet) in length, running through the body from mouth to **anus.** The lumen of the tract is continuous with the external environment, which means that its contents are technically outside the body. This fact is relevant to understanding some of the tract's properties. For example, the large intestine is colonized by billions of bacteria, most of which are harmless and even beneficial in this location. However, if the same bacteria enter the internal environment, as may happen, for example, if a portion of the large intestine is perforated, they may cause a severe infection (see Chapter 19).

Most food enters the gastrointestinal tract as large particles containing macromolecules, such as proteins and polysaccharides, which are unable to cross the intestinal epithelium. Before ingested food can be absorbed, therefore, it must be dissolved and broken down into small molecules. (Small nutrients such as vitamins and minerals do not need to be broken down and can cross the epithelium intact.) This dissolving and breaking-down process is called **digestion** and is accomplished by the action of hydrochloric acid in the stomach, bile from the liver, and a variety of digestive enzymes released by the system's exocrine glands. Each of these substances is released into the lumen of the GI tract through the process of **secretion.** In addition, some digestive enzymes are located on the luminal membranes of the intestinal epithelium. The molecules produced by digestion, along with water and small nutrients that do not require digestion, then move from the lumen of the

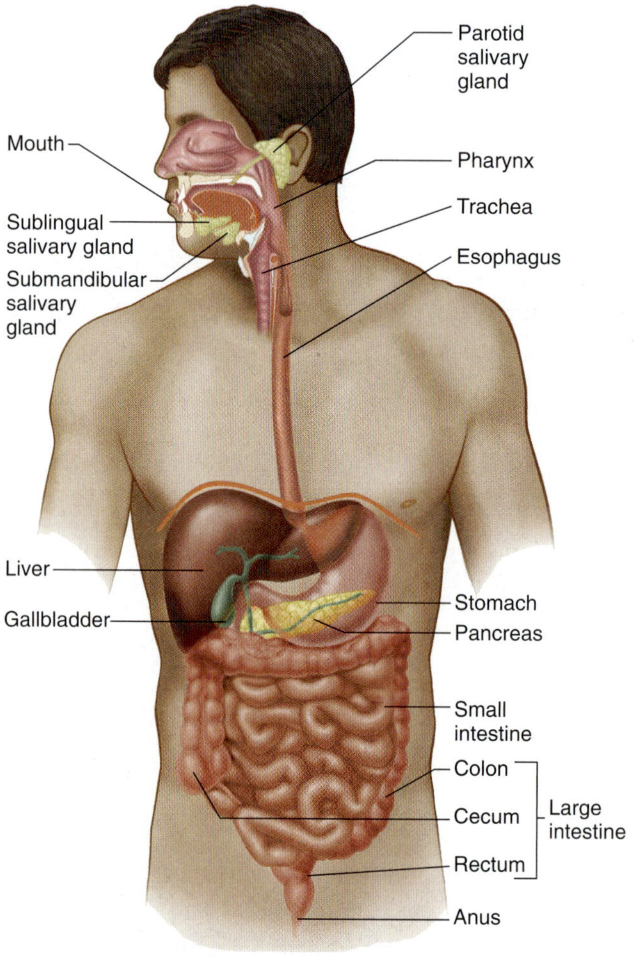

Figure 15.1 APIR Anatomy of the digestive system. The liver overlies the gallbladder and a portion of the stomach, and the stomach overlies part of the pancreas. See Table 15.1 for the functions of the organs of the digestive system.

gastrointestinal tract across a layer of epithelial cells and enter the blood or lymph. This process is called **absorption.**

While digestion, secretion, and absorption are taking place, contractions of smooth muscles in the gastrointestinal tract wall serve two functions: They mix the luminal contents with the various secretions, and they move the contents through the tract from mouth to anus. These contractions are referred to as the **motility** of the gastrointestinal tract. In some cases, muscular movements travel in a wave-like fashion in one direction along the length of a part of the tract, a process called **peristalsis.** The functions of the digestive system can be described in terms of these four major processes—digestion, secretion, absorption, and motility (**Figure 15.2**)—and the mechanisms controlling them.

Within fairly wide limits, the digestive system will absorb as much of any particular substance that is ingested, with a few important exceptions (to be described later). Therefore, the digestive system does not regulate the total amount of nutrients absorbed or their concentrations in the internal environment. The plasma concentration and distribution of the absorbed nutrients throughout the body are primarily controlled by hormones from a number of endocrine glands (see Chapters 11 and 16) and by the kidneys (see Chapter 14).

Small amounts of certain metabolic end products are excreted via the gastrointestinal tract, primarily by way of the bile. This represents a minor function of the GI tract in healthy individuals—**elimination.** In fact, the lungs and kidneys are usually responsible for the elimination of most of the body's waste products. The material known as **feces** leaves the system at the end of the gastrointestinal tract. Feces consist almost entirely of bacteria and ingested material that was neither digested nor absorbed, that is, material that was never actually absorbed into the internal environment.

15.2 Structure of the Gastrointestinal Tract Wall

From the mid-esophagus to the anus, the wall of the gastrointestinal tract has the general structure illustrated in **Figure 15.3**. Most of the luminal (inside) surface is highly convoluted, a feature that greatly increases the surface area available for absorption. From the stomach on, this surface is covered by a single layer of epithelial cells linked together along the edges of their luminal surfaces by tight junctions. Included in this epithelial layer are exocrine cells that secrete mucus into the lumen of the tract and endocrine cells that release hormones into the blood. Invaginations of the epithelium into the underlying tissue form exocrine glands that secrete acid, enzymes, water, ions, and mucus into the lumen.

Just below the epithelium is the **lamina propria,** which is a layer of loose connective tissue through which pass small blood vessels, nerve fibers, and lymphatic vessels. (Some of these structures do not appear in Figure 15.3 but are in Figure 15.4.) The lamina propria is separated from underlying tissues by the **muscularis mucosa,** which is a thin layer of smooth muscle that may be involved in the movement of villi, described subsequently. The combination of these three layers—the epithelium, lamina propria, and muscularis mucosa—is called the **mucosa** (see Figure 15.3).

Beneath the mucosa is the **submucosa,** which is a second connective-tissue layer. This layer also contains a network of neurons, the **submucosal plexus,** and blood and lymphatic vessels whose branches penetrate into both the overlying mucosa and the underlying layers of smooth muscle called the **muscularis externa.** Contractions of these muscles provide the forces for moving and mixing the gastrointestinal contents. Except for the stomach, which has three layers, the

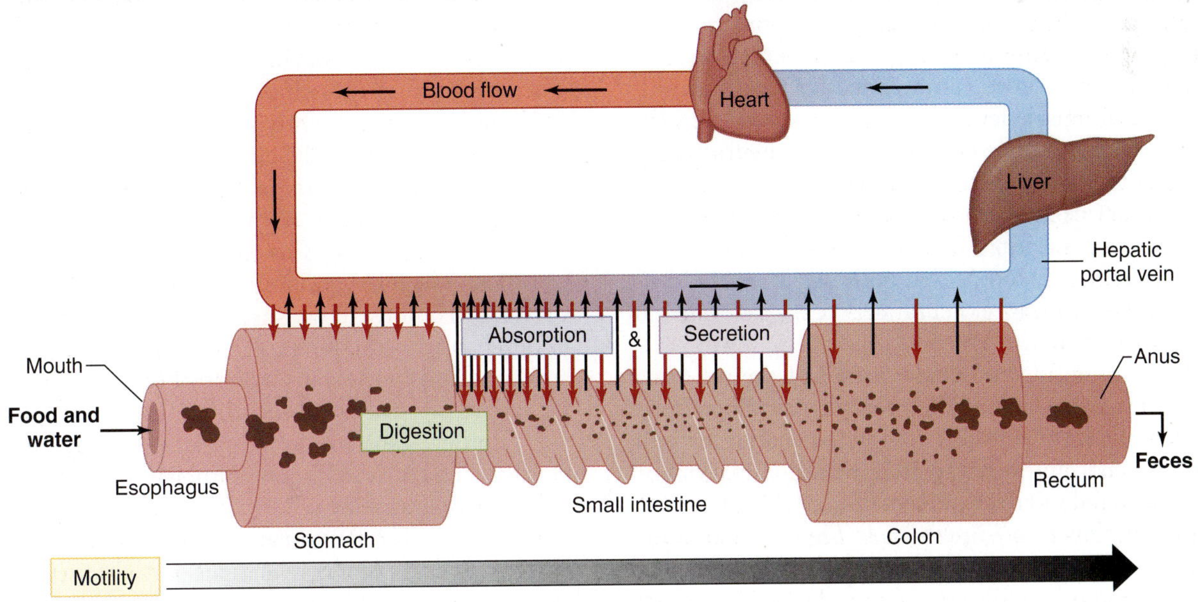

Figure 15.2 AP|R Four major processes the gastrointestinal tract carries out: digestion, secretion, absorption, and motility. Outward-pointing (black) arrows indicate absorption of the products of digestion, water, minerals, and vitamins into the blood. Inward-pointing (red) arrows represent the secretion of ions, enzymes, and bile salts into the GI tract. The length and density of the arrows indicate the relative importance of each segment of the tract; the small intestine is where most absorption and secretion occurs. The feces represent a fifth function of the GI tract: elimination. The wavy configuration of the small intestine represents muscular contractions (motility) throughout the tract.

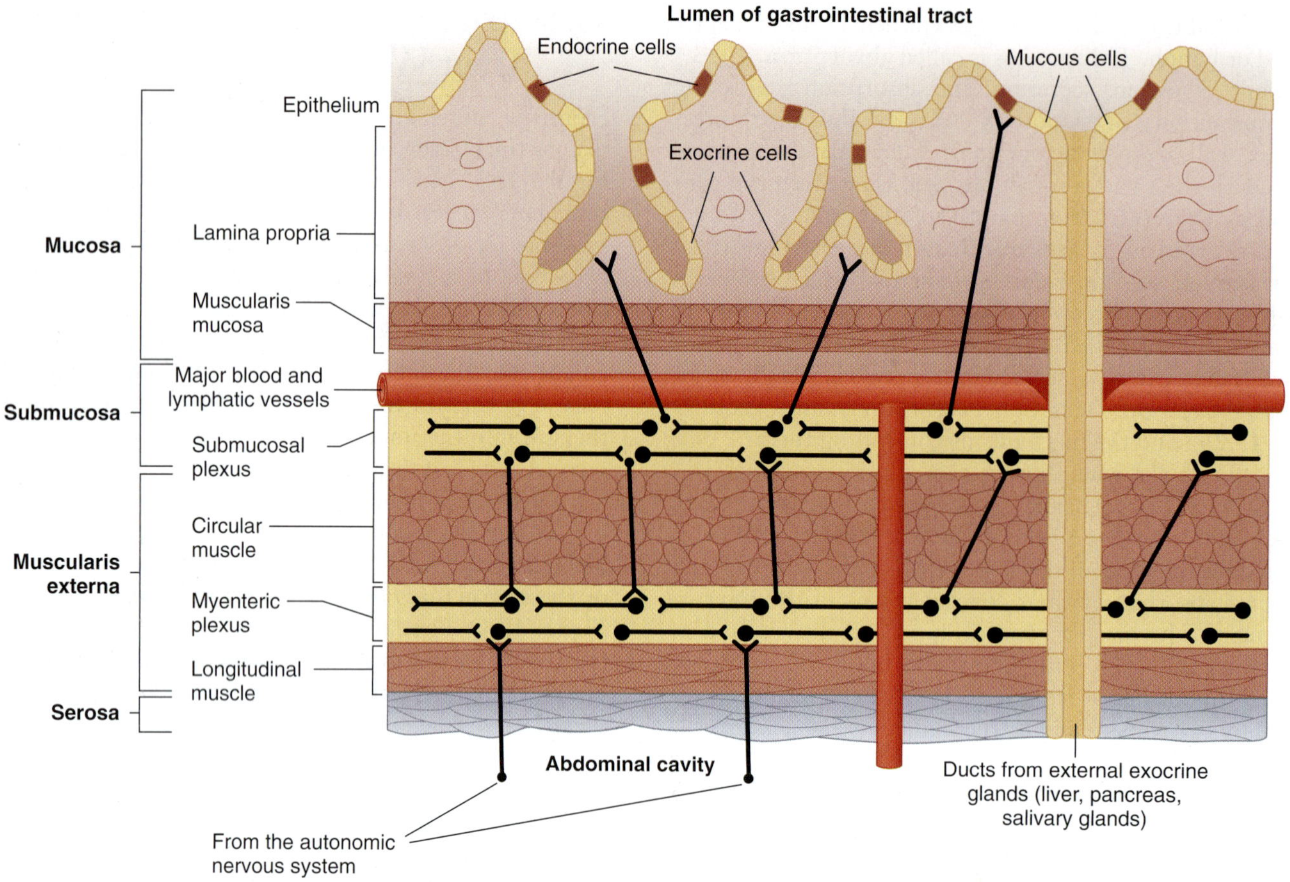

Figure 15.3 APIR Structure of the gastrointestinal wall in longitudinal section. Not shown are the smaller blood vessels and lymphatics and neural terminations on muscles.

muscularis externa has two layers: (1) a relatively thick inner layer of **circular muscle,** whose fibers are oriented in a circular pattern around the tube so that contraction produces a narrowing of the lumen; and (2) a thinner outer layer of **longitudinal muscle,** whose contraction shortens the tube. Between these two muscle layers is a second network of neurons known as the **myenteric plexus.** There are neurons projecting from the submucosal plexus to the single layer of cells on the luminal surface as well as to the myenteric plexus. The myenteric plexus is innervated by nerves from the autonomic nervous system and has neurons that project to the submucosal plexus. This complex, local neural network is described in detail later in this chapter.

Finally, surrounding the outer surface of the tube is a thin layer of connective tissue called the **serosa.** Thin sheets of connective tissue connect the serosa to the abdominal wall and support the gastrointestinal tract in the abdominal cavity.

The macro- and microscopic structure of the wall of the small intestine is shown in **Figure 15.4**. The **circular folds** (mucosa and submucosa) are covered with fingerlike projections called **villi** (singular, **villus;** see Figure 15.4). The surface of each villus is covered with a layer of epithelial cells whose surface membranes form small projections called **microvilli** (singular, **microvillus;** also known collectively as the **brush border**) (**Figure 15.5**). Interspersed between these absorptive epithelial cells with microvilli are **goblet cells** that secrete mucus that lubricates the wall of the small intestine. The combination of circular folds, villi, and microvilli increases the small intestine's surface area about 600-fold over that of a flat-surfaced tube having the same length and diameter. The human small intestine's total surface area is about 250 to 300 square meters, roughly the area of a tennis court. This is a dramatic example of the general principle of physiology that structure is a determinant of function; in this case, the greatly increased surface area of the small intestine maximizes its absorptive capacity. Just as the folding of the cerebral cortex provides a much larger number of neurons in the cranium (see Chapter 6) and the large surface area of the alveoli enhances gas exchange in the lungs (see Chapter 13), the large surface area provided by the morphology of the small intestine allows for the highly efficient absorption of nutrients.

Epithelial surfaces in the gastrointestinal tract are continuously being replaced by new epithelial cells. In the small intestine, new cells arise by cell division from cells at the base of the villi. These cells differentiate as they migrate to the top of the villus, replacing older cells that die and are discharged into the intestinal lumen. These dead cells release their intracellular enzymes into the lumen, which then contribute to the digestive process. About 17 billion epithelial cells are replaced each day, and the entire epithelium of the small intestine is replaced approximately every 5 days. It is because of this rapid cell turnover that the lining of the intestinal tract is so susceptible to

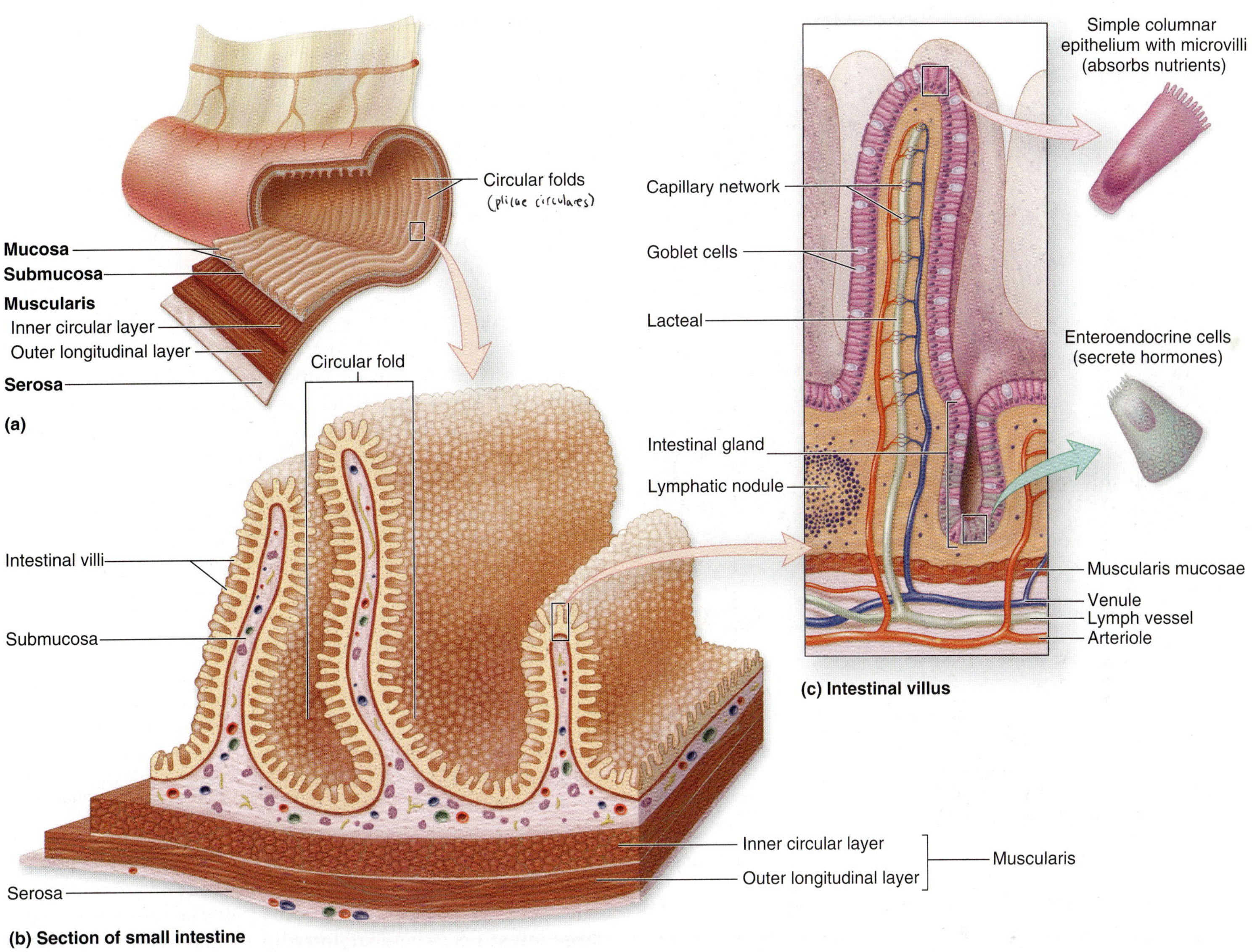

Figure 15.4 AP|R Microscopic structure of the small-intestine wall demonstrates increased surface area. (a) Circular folds formed from the mucosa and submucosa increase surface area. (b) Surface area further increased by villi formed from mucosa. (c) Structure of the villus—epithelial microvilli further increase surface area.

damage by treatments that inhibit cell division, such as anticancer drugs and radiation therapy. Also at the base of the villi are **enteroendocrine cells** that secrete hormones that, as you will learn, control a wide variety of gastrointestinal functions, including motility and exocrine pancreatic secretions.

The center of each intestinal villus is occupied by both a single, blind-ended lymphatic vessel—a **lacteal**—and a capillary network (see Figure 15.4). As we will see, most of the fat absorbed in the small intestine enters the lacteals. Material absorbed by the lacteals reaches the general circulation by eventually emptying from the lymphatic system into large veins through a structure called the **thoracic duct.**

Other absorbed nutrients enter the blood capillaries. The venous drainage from the small intestine—as well as from the large intestine, pancreas, and portions of the stomach—does not empty directly into the vena cava but passes first, via the **hepatic portal vein,** to the liver. (The term **hepatic** refers to the liver.) There it flows through a second capillary network before leaving the liver to return to the heart. Because of this portal circulation, material that is absorbed into the intestinal capillaries, in contrast to the lacteals, can be processed by the liver before entering the general circulation. This is important because the liver contains enzymes that can metabolize (detoxify) harmful compounds that may have been ingested, thereby preventing them from entering the circulation. The relationship between the lymphatic system, the circulatory system, and the absorptive surface of the GI tract shown in Figures 15.3 and 15.4 emphasizes the general principle of physiology that there is coordination between the function of different organ systems. One must understand the distribution of blood flow to the GI tract and lymphatic drainage from the GI tract to appreciate its huge absorptive and secretory capacity.

The gastrointestinal tract also has a variety of immune functions, allowing it to produce antibodies and fight

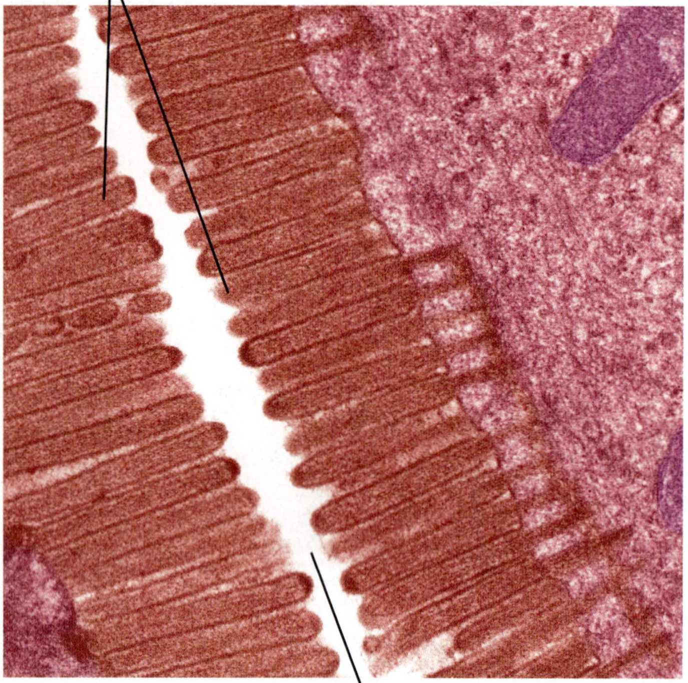

Figure 15.5 AP|R Microvilli on the surface of intestinal epithelial cells.

PHYSIOLOGICAL INQUIRY

- Do you recall learning about a brush border in any other body structure? (*Hint:* Refer back to Chapter 14.)

Answer can be found at end of chapter.

infectious organisms that are not destroyed by the acidity of the stomach. For example, the small intestine has regions of immune tissue called **Peyer's patches** that contain immune cells; these cells secrete factors (e.g., cytokines; see Chapter 18) that alter intestinal motility and kill microorganisms.

15.3 General Functions of the Gastrointestinal and Accessory Organs

Using **Table 15.1** as a guide, this section briefly surveys the gastrointestinal functions that will be described in detail later in this chapter. Digestion begins with chewing in the **mouth** where large pieces of food are broken up into smaller particles that we can swallow. **Saliva,** secreted by three pairs of exocrine **salivary glands** located in the head (see Figure 15.1), drains into the mouth through a series of short ducts. Saliva, which contains mucus, moistens and lubricates the food particles before swallowing. It also contains the enzyme **amylase,** which partially digests polysaccharides (complex sugars) described later. A third function of saliva is to dissolve some of the food molecules. Only in the dissolved state can these molecules react with chemoreceptors in the mouth, giving rise to the sensation of taste (see Chapter 7). Finally, saliva has antibacterial properties. See **Table 15.2** for the major functions of saliva.

The next segments of the tract, the **pharynx** and **esophagus,** do not contribute to digestion but provide the pathway for ingested materials to reach the stomach. The muscles in the walls of these segments control swallowing.

The **stomach** is a saclike organ located between the esophagus and the small intestine. Its functions are to store, dissolve, and partially digest the macromolecules in food and to regulate the rate at which the contents of the stomach empty into the small intestine. The acidic environment in the **gastric** (adjective for "stomach") lumen alters the ionization of polar molecules, leading to denaturation of protein (see Chapter 2). This exposes more sites for digestive enzymes to break down the proteins, and disrupts the extracellular network of connective-tissue proteins that form the structural framework of the tissues in food. Polysaccharides and fat are major food components that are not dissolved to a significant extent by acid. The low pH also kills most of the bacteria that enter along with food. This process is not completely effective, and some bacteria survive to colonize and multiply in the gastrointestinal tract, particularly the large intestine.

The digestive actions of the stomach reduce food particles to a solution known as **chyme,** which contains molecular fragments of proteins and polysaccharides; droplets of fat; and salt, water, and various other small molecules ingested in the food. Virtually none of these molecules, except water, can cross the epithelium of the gastric wall, and thus little absorption of organic nutrients occurs in the stomach.

Most absorption and digestion occur in the next section of the tract, the **small intestine,** a tube about 2.4 cm in diameter and 3 m in length, which leads from the stomach to the **large intestine.** (The small intestine is almost twice as long if removed from the abdomen because the muscular wall loses its tone.) Hydrolytic enzymes in the small intestine break down molecules of intact or partially digested carbohydrates, fats, proteins, and nucleic acids into monosaccharides, fatty acids, amino acids, and nucleotides. Some of these enzymes are on the luminal surface of the intestinal lining cells, whereas others are secreted by the pancreas and enter the intestinal lumen. The products of digestion are absorbed across the epithelial cells and enter the blood and/or lymph. Vitamins, minerals, and water, which do not require enzymatic digestion, are also absorbed in the small intestine.

The small intestine is divided into three segments: An initial short segment, the **duodenum,** is followed by the **jejunum** and then by the longest segment, the **ileum.** Normally, most of the chyme entering from the stomach is digested and absorbed in the first quarter of the small intestine in the duodenum and jejunum. Therefore, the small intestine has a very large reserve for the absorption of most nutrients; removal of portions of the small intestine as a treatment for disease does not necessarily result in nutritional deficiencies, depending on which part of the intestine is removed.

Two major organs—the pancreas and liver—secrete substances that flow via ducts into the duodenum. The **pancreas,** an elongated gland located behind the stomach, has both

TABLE 15.1 Functions of the Gastrointestinal Organs

Organ	Exocrine Secretions	Functions Related to Digestion and Absorption
Mouth and pharynx		Chewing begins; initiation of swallowing reflex
Salivary glands	Salt and water	Moisten and dissolve food
	Mucus	Lubrication
	Amylase	Polysaccharide-digesting enzyme
Esophagus		Move food to stomach by peristaltic waves
	Mucus	Lubrication
Stomach		Store, mix, dissolve, and continue digestion of food; regulate emptying of dissolved food into small intestine
	HCl	Solubilization of food particles; kill microbes; activation of pepsinogen to pepsin
	Pepsin	Begin the process of protein digestion in the stomach
	Mucus	Lubricate and protect epithelial surface
Pancreas		Secretion of enzymes and bicarbonate; also has nondigestive endocrine functions
	Enzymes	Digest carbohydrates, fats, proteins, and nucleic acids
	Bicarbonate	Neutralize HCl entering small intestine from stomach
Liver		Secretion of bile
	Bile salts	Solubilize water-insoluble fats
	Bicarbonate	Neutralize HCl entering small intestine from stomach
	Organic waste products and trace metals	Elimination in feces
Gallbladder		Store and concentrate bile between meals
Small intestine		Digestion and absorption of most substances; mixing and propulsion of contents
	Enzymes	Digestion of macromolecules
	Salt and water	Maintain fluidity of luminal contents
	Mucus	Lubrication and protection
Large intestine		Storage and concentration of undigested matter; absorption of salt and water; mixing and propulsion of contents; defecation
	Mucus	Lubrication

endocrine (see Chapter 16) and exocrine functions, but only the latter are directly involved in gastrointestinal function and are described in this chapter. The exocrine portion of the pancreas secretes digestive enzymes and a fluid rich in HCO_3^-. The high acidity of the chyme coming from the stomach would inactivate the pancreatic enzymes in the small intestine if the acid were not neutralized by the HCO_3^- in the pancreatic fluid.

TABLE 15.2 Major Functions of Saliva

Moistens and lubricates food
Initiates small amount of digestion of polysaccharides by amylase (described in detail later)
Dissolves a small amount of food (which facilitates taste)
Kills bacteria

The **liver**, a large organ located in the upper-right portion of the abdomen, has a variety of functions, which are described in various chapters. We will be concerned in this chapter primarily with the liver's exocrine functions that are directly related to the secretion of **bile.**

Bile contains HCO_3^-, cholesterol, phospholipids, bile pigments, a number of organic wastes, and—most important—a group of substances collectively termed **bile salts.** The HCO_3^-, like that from the pancreas, helps neutralize acid from the stomach, whereas the bile salts, as we shall see, solubilize dietary fat. These fats would otherwise be insoluble in water, and their solubilization increases the rates at which they are digested and absorbed.

Bile is secreted by the liver into small ducts that join to form the common hepatic duct. Between meals, secreted bile is stored in the **gallbladder,** a small sac underneath the liver that branches from the common hepatic duct. The gallbladder concentrates the organic molecules in bile by absorbing some salts and water. During a meal, the smooth muscles in the gallbladder wall contract, causing a concentrated bile solution to be injected into the duodenum via the **common bile duct** (**Figure 15.6**), an extension of the common hepatic duct.

In the small intestine, monosaccharides and amino acids are absorbed by specific transporter-mediated processes in the plasma membranes of the intestinal epithelial cells, whereas fatty acids enter these cells primarily by diffusion. Most mineral ions are actively absorbed by transporters, and water diffuses passively down osmotic gradients.

The motility of the small intestine, brought about by the smooth muscles in its walls, (1) mixes the luminal contents with the various secretions, (2) brings the contents into contact with the epithelial surface where absorption takes place, and (3) slowly advances the luminal material toward the large intestine, the next segment of the alimentary canal. Because most substances are absorbed in the small intestine, only a small amount of water, salts, and undigested material passes on to the large intestine. The large intestine temporarily stores the undigested material (some of which is metabolized by bacteria) and concentrates it by absorbing salts and water. Contractions of the **rectum,** the final segment of the large intestine, and relaxation of associated sphincter muscles expel the feces in a process called **defecation.**

The average American adult consumes about 500–800 g of food and 1200 mL of water per day, but this is only a fraction of the material entering the lumen of the gastrointestinal tract. An additional 7000 mL of fluid from salivary glands, gastric glands, pancreas, liver, and intestinal glands is secreted into the tract each day (**Figure 15.7**). Of the approximately 8 L of fluid entering the tract, 99% is absorbed; only about 100 mL is normally lost in the feces. This small amount of fluid loss represents only 4% of the total fluids lost from the body each day. Most fluid loss is via the kidneys and respiratory system. Almost all the salts in the secreted fluids are also reabsorbed into the blood. Moreover, the secreted digestive enzymes are themselves digested, and the resulting amino acids are absorbed into the blood.

Finally, a critical component in the control of gastrointestinal functions is the role of the central nervous system. The CNS receives information from the GI tract (afferent input) and has a vital influence on GI function (efferent output).

This completes our brief overview of some of the general functions of the organs of the digestive system. Because its major tasks are digestion and absorption, we begin our more detailed description with these processes. Subsequent sections of the chapter will then describe, organ by organ, regulation of the secretions and motility that produce the optimal conditions for digestion and absorption.

15.4 Digestion and Absorption

This section describes how ingested nutrients are broken down (digested) and taken up (absorbed) in the GI tract. The process of absorption illustrates the general principle of physiology that controlled exchange of materials occurs between compartments (in this case, from the lumen of the GI tract to the blood and lymph) and across cellular membranes (of the cells lining the GI tract).

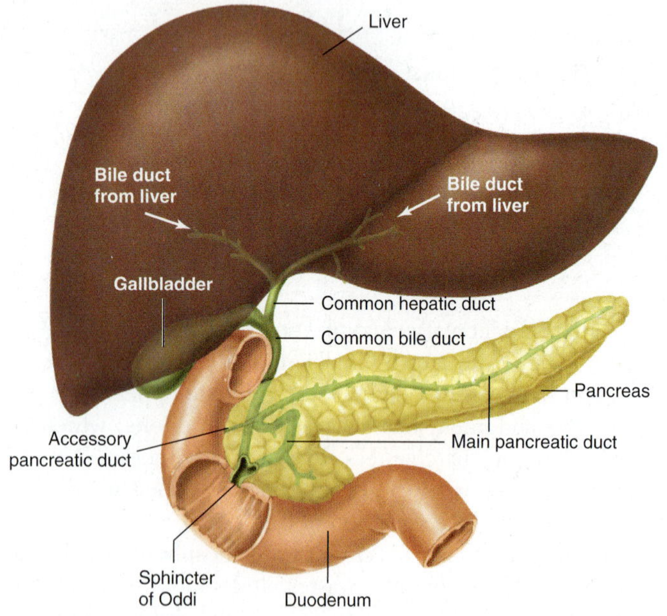

Figure 15.6 AP|R Bile ducts from the liver converge to form the common hepatic duct, from which branches the duct leading to the gallbladder. Beyond this branch, the common hepatic duct becomes the common bile duct. The common bile duct and the main pancreatic duct converge and empty their contents into the duodenum at the sphincter of Oddi. Some people have an accessory pancreatic duct.

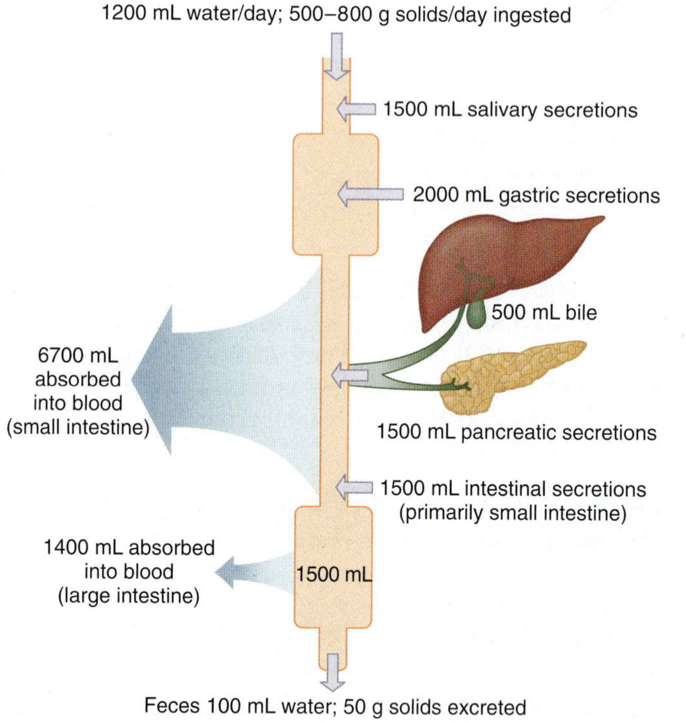

Figure 15.7 Average amounts of solids and fluid ingested, secreted, absorbed, and excreted from the gastrointestinal tract daily.

Carbohydrate

The average daily intake of carbohydrates is about 250 to 300 g per day in a typical American diet. This represents about half the average daily intake of calories. About two-thirds of this carbohydrate is the plant polysaccharide starch, and most of the remainder consists of the disaccharides sucrose (table sugar) and lactose (milk sugar) (**Table 15.3**). Only small amounts of monosaccharides are normally present in the diet. Cellulose and certain other complex polysaccharides found in vegetable matter—referred to as **fiber**—are not broken down by the enzymes in the small intestine and pass on to the large intestine, where they are partially metabolized by bacteria.

The digestion of starch by salivary amylase begins in the mouth but accounts for only a small fraction of total starch digestion. It continues very briefly in the upper part of the stomach before gastric acid inactivates the amylase. Most (~95% or more) starch digestion is completed in the small intestine by pancreatic amylase (**Figure 15.8**). The products of both salivary and pancreatic amylase are the disaccharide maltose and a mixture of short, branched chains of glucose molecules. These products, along with ingested sucrose and lactose, are broken down into monosaccharides—glucose, galactose, and fructose—by enzymes located on the luminal membranes of the small-intestine epithelial cells (brush border). These monosaccharides are then transported across the intestinal epithelium into the blood. Fructose enters the epithelial cells by facilitated diffusion via a glucose transporter (GLUT), whereas glucose and galactose undergo secondary active transport coupled to Na^+ via the sodium–glucose cotransporter (SGLT). These monosaccharides then leave the epithelial cells and enter the interstitial fluid by way of facilitated diffusion via GLUT proteins in the basolateral membranes of the epithelial cells. From there, the monosaccharides diffuse into the blood through capillary pores. Most ingested carbohydrates are digested and absorbed within the first 20% of the small intestine.

Protein

A healthy adult requires only 40 to 50 g of protein per day to supply essential amino acids and replace the nitrogen contained in amino acids that are converted to urea. A typical American diet contains about 60 to 90 g of protein per day. This represents about one-sixth of the average daily caloric intake. In addition, a large amount of protein, in the form of enzymes and mucus, is secreted into the gastrointestinal tract or enters it via the disintegration of epithelial cells. Regardless of the source, most of the protein in the lumen is broken down into dipeptides, tripeptides, and amino acids, all of which are absorbed by the small intestine.

TABLE 15.3 Carbohydrates in Food

Class	Examples	Composed Of:
Polysaccharides	Starch	Glucose
	Cellulose	Glucose
	Glycogen	Glucose
Disaccharides	Sucrose	Glucose–fructose
	Lactose	Glucose–galactose
	Maltose	Glucose–glucose
Monosaccharides	Glucose	
	Fructose	
	Galactose	

Proteins are first partially broken down to peptide fragments in the stomach by **pepsin** that, as you will learn, is produced from a precursor **pepsinogen.** Further breakdown is completed in the small intestine by **trypsin** and **chymotrypsin,** the major proteases secreted by the pancreas. These fragments can be absorbed or are further digested to free amino acids by **carboxypeptidases** from the pancreas and **aminopeptidases,** located on the luminal membranes of the small-intestine

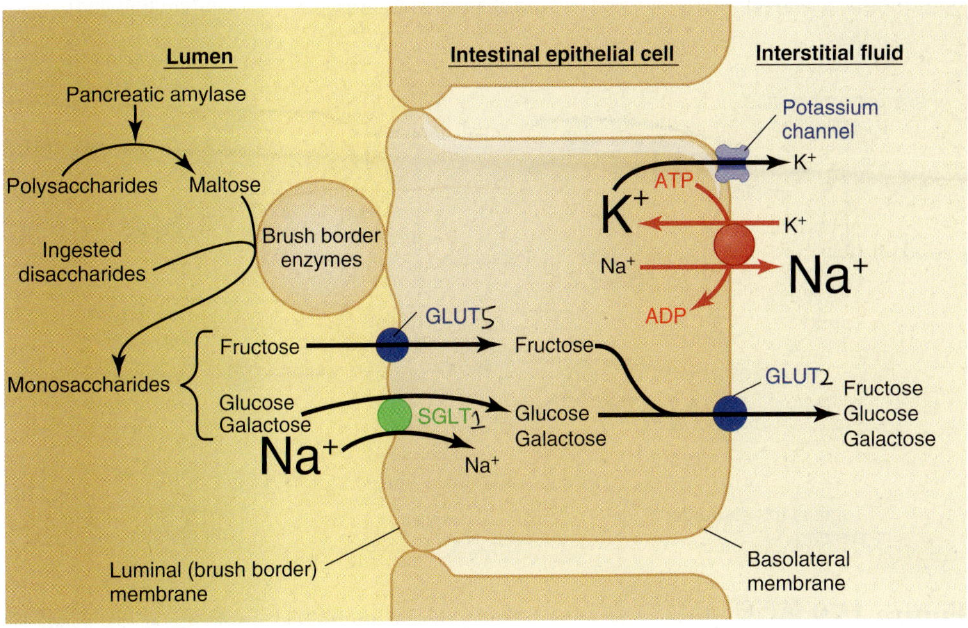

Figure 15.8 APIR Carbohydrate digestion and sugar absorption in the small intestine. Starches (polysaccharides) and ingested small sugars (disaccharides) are metabolized to simple sugars (monosaccharides) by enzymes from the pancreas and on the luminal membrane (brush border). Fructose is absorbed into the cell by facilitated diffusion via a glucose transporter (GLUT). Glucose and galactose are absorbed into the cell by cotransport with Na^+ via sodium–glucose cotransporters (SGLTs). Sugars are then absorbed across the basolateral membrane into the interstitial fluid by facilitated diffusion (GLUTs) and diffuse into the blood. The energy required for absorption is provided primarily by Na^+/K^+-ATPase pumps on the basolateral membrane. Also, remember that carbohydrate digestion begins in the mouth by salivary amylase. The wavy shape of the luminal membrane represents the brush border shown in Figure 15.5.

epithelial cells (**Figure 15.9**). These last two enzymes split off amino acids from the carboxyl and amino ends of peptide chains, respectively. At least 20 different peptidases are located on the luminal membrane of the epithelial cells, with various specificities for the peptide bonds they attack.

Most of the products of protein digestion are absorbed as short chains of two or three amino acids by a secondary active transport coupled to the H^+ gradient (see Figure 15.9). The absorption of small peptides contrasts with carbohydrate absorption, in which molecules larger than monosaccharides are not absorbed. Free amino acids, by contrast, enter the epithelial cells by secondary active transport coupled to Na^+. There are many different amino acid transporters that are specific for the different amino acids, but only one transporter is shown in Figure 15.9 for simplicity. Within the cytosol of the epithelial cell, the dipeptides and tripeptides are hydrolyzed to amino acids; these, along with free amino acids that entered the cells, then leave the cell and enter the interstitial fluid through facilitated-diffusion transporters in the basolateral membranes. As with carbohydrates, protein digestion and absorption are largely completed in the upper portion of the small intestine.

Very small amounts of intact proteins are able to cross the intestinal epithelium and gain access to the interstitial fluid. They do so by a combination of endocytosis and exocytosis. The absorptive capacity for intact proteins is much greater in infants than in adults, and antibodies (proteins involved in the immunologic defense system of the body) secreted into the mother's milk can be absorbed by the infant, providing some immunity until the infant begins to produce his or her own antibodies.

Fat

The average daily intake of lipids is 70 to 100 g per day in a typical American diet, most of this in the form of fat (triglycerides). This represents about one-third of the average daily caloric intake. Triglyceride digestion occurs to a limited extent in the mouth and stomach, but it predominantly occurs in the small intestine. The major digestive enzyme in this process is pancreatic **lipase,** which catalyzes the splitting of bonds linking fatty acids to the first and third carbon atoms of glycerol, producing two free fatty acids and a monoglyceride as products:

$$\text{Triglyceride} \xrightarrow{\text{lipase}} \text{Monoglyceride} + 2 \text{ Fatty acids}$$

The lipids in the ingested foods are insoluble in water and aggregate into large lipid droplets in the upper portion of the stomach. This is like a mixture of oil and vinegar after shaking. Because pancreatic lipase is a water-soluble enzyme, its digestive action in the small intestine can take place only at the *surface* of a lipid droplet. Therefore, if most of the ingested fat remained in large lipid droplets, the rate of triglyceride digestion would be very slow because of the small surface-area-to-volume ratio of these big fat droplets. The rate of digestion is, however, substantially increased by division of the large lipid droplets into many very small droplets, each about 1 mm in diameter, thereby increasing their surface area and accessibility to lipase action. This process is known as **emulsification,** and the resulting suspension of small lipid droplets is an emulsion.

The emulsification of fat requires (1) mechanical disruption of the large lipid droplets into smaller droplets, and (2) an emulsifying agent, which acts to prevent the smaller droplets from reaggregating back into large droplets. The mechanical disruption is provided by the motility of the gastrointestinal tract, occurring in the lower portion of the stomach and in the small intestine, which grinds and mixes the luminal contents. Phospholipids in food, along with phospholipids and bile salts secreted in the bile, provide the emulsifying agents. Phospholipids are amphipathic molecules (see Chapter 2) consisting of two nonpolar fatty acid chains attached to glycerol,

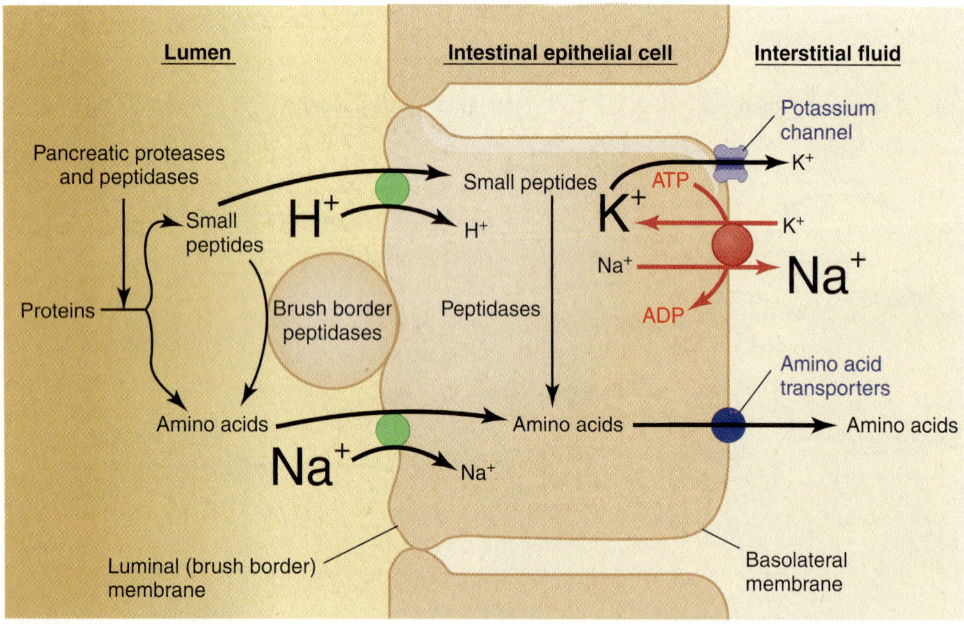

Figure 15.9 APIR Protein digestion and peptide and amino acid absorption in the small intestine. Proteins and peptides are digested in the lumen of the intestine to small peptides and amino acids. Small peptides can be absorbed by cotransport with H^+ into the cytosol where they are catabolized to amino acids by peptidases. Small peptides in the lumen are also catabolized to amino acids by peptidases located on the luminal (brush border) membrane. Amino acids are absorbed into the cytosol by cotransport with Na^+. Amino acids then cross the basolateral membrane by facilitated diffusion via many different specific amino acid transporters (only one is shown in the figure for clarity). Amino acids then diffuse into the blood from the interstitial fluid through capillary pores. The energy for these processes is provided primarily by Na^+/K^+-ATPase pumps on the basolateral membrane. Also remember that protein digestion begins in the acidic environment of the stomach. The wavy shape of the luminal membrane represents the brush border shown in Figure 15.5.

with a charged phosphate group located on glycerol's third carbon. Bile salts are formed from cholesterol in the liver and are also amphipathic (**Figure 15.10**). The nonpolar portions of the phospholipids and bile salts associate with the nonpolar interior of the lipid droplets, leaving the polar portions exposed at the water surface. There, they repel other lipid droplets that are similarly coated with these emulsifying agents, thereby preventing their reaggregation into larger fat droplets (**Figure 15.11**).

The coating of the lipid droplets with these emulsifying agents, however, impairs the accessibility of the water-soluble lipase to its lipid substrate. To overcome this problem, the pancreas secretes a protein known as **colipase,** which is amphipathic and lodges on the lipid droplet surface. Colipase binds the lipase enzyme, holding it on the surface of the lipid droplet.

Although emulsification speeds up digestion, absorption of the water-insoluble products of the lipase reaction would still be very slow if it were not for a second action of the bile salts, the formation of **micelles,** which are similar in structure to emulsion droplets but much smaller—4 to 7 nm in diameter. Micelles consist of bile salts, fatty acids, monoglycerides, and phospholipids all clustered together with the polar ends of each molecule oriented toward the micelle's surface and the nonpolar portions forming the micelle's core (**Figure 15.12**). Also included in the core of the micelle are small amounts of fat-soluble vitamins and cholesterol.

How do micelles increase absorption? Although fatty acids and monoglycerides have an extremely low solubility in water, a few molecules do exist in solution and are free to diffuse across the lipid portion of the luminal plasma membranes of the epithelial cells lining the small intestine. Micelles, containing the products of fat digestion, are in equilibrium with the small concentration of fat-digestion products that are free

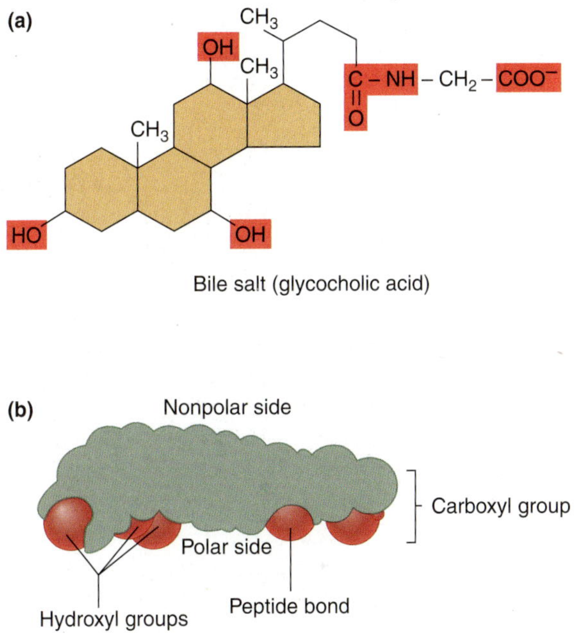

Figure 15.10 Structure of bile salts. (a) Chemical formula of glycocholic acid, one of several bile salts secreted by the liver (polar groups in color). Note the similarity to the structure of steroids (see Figure 11.4). (b) Three-dimensional structure of a bile salt, showing its polar and nonpolar surfaces.

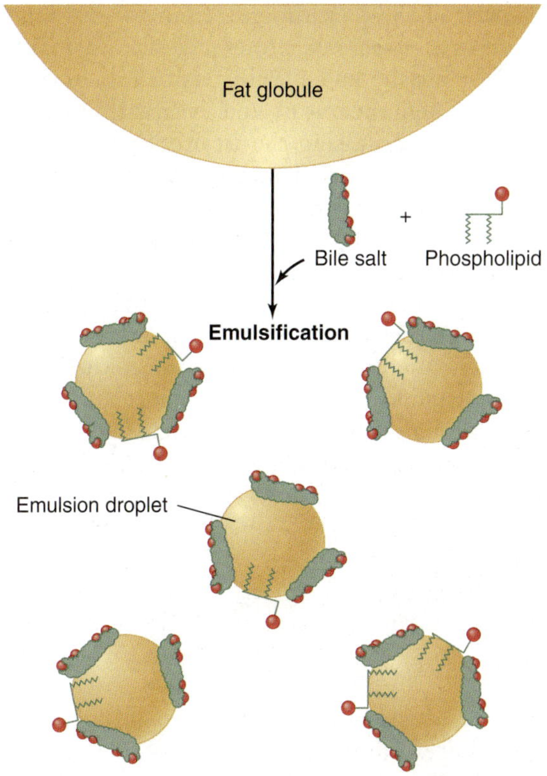

Figure 15.11 Emulsification of fat by bile salts and phospholipids. Note that the nonpolar sides (green) of bile salts and phospholipids are oriented toward fat, whereas the polar sides (red) of these compounds are oriented outward.

in solution. Thus, micelles are continuously breaking down and reforming. As the concentrations of free lipids decrease because of their diffusion into epithelial cells, more lipids are released into the free phase from micelles as they begin to break down (see Figure 15.12). Meanwhile, the process of digestion, which is still ongoing, provides additional small lipids that replenish the micelles. Micelles, therefore, provide a means of keeping most of the insoluble fat-digestion products in small, soluble aggregates, while at the same time replenishing the small amount of products in solution that are free to diffuse into the intestinal epithelium. Note that it is not the micelle that is absorbed but, rather, the individual lipid molecules released from the micelle. You can think of micelles as a "holding station" for small, nonsoluble lipids, releasing their contents slowly to prevent the lipids from coming out of solution while permitting digestion to continue unabated.

Although fatty acids and monoglycerides enter epithelial cells from the intestinal lumen, triglycerides are released on the other side of the cell into the interstitial fluid. In other words, during their passage through the epithelial cells, fatty acids and monoglycerides are resynthesized into triglycerides. This occurs in the smooth endoplasmic reticulum, where the enzymes for triglyceride synthesis are located. This process decreases the concentration of cytosolic free fatty acids and monoglycerides and thereby maintains a diffusion gradient for these molecules into the cell from the intestinal lumen. The resynthesized fat aggregates into small droplets coated with amphipathic proteins that perform an emulsifying function similar to that of bile salts.

The exit of these fat droplets from the cell follows the same pathway as a secreted protein. Vesicles containing the droplet pinch off the endoplasmic reticulum, are processed through the Golgi apparatus, and eventually fuse with the plasma membrane, releasing the fat droplet into the interstitial fluid. These 1-micron-diameter, extracellular fat droplets are known as **chylomicrons.** Chylomicrons contain not only triglycerides but other lipids (including phospholipids, cholesterol, and fat-soluble vitamins) that have been absorbed by the same process that led to fatty acid and monoglyceride movement into the epithelial cells of the small intestine.

The chylomicrons released from the epithelial cells pass into lacteals—lymphatic vessels in the intestinal villi—rather than into the blood capillaries. The chylomicrons cannot enter the blood capillaries because the basement membrane (an extracellular glycoprotein layer) at the outer surface of the capillary provides a barrier to the diffusion of large chylomicrons. In contrast, the lacteals have large pores between their endothelial cells that allow the chylomicrons to pass into the lymph. The lymph from the small intestine, as from everywhere else in the body, eventually empties into systemic veins. In Chapter 16, we describe how the lipids in the circulating blood chylomicrons are made available to the cells of the body.

Figure 15.13 summarizes the pathway fat takes in moving from the intestinal lumen into the lymphatic system.

Vitamins

The fat-soluble vitamins—A, D, E, and K—follow the pathway for fat absorption described in the previous section. They are solubilized in micelles; thus, any interference with the secretion of bile or the action of bile salts in the intestine decreases the absorption of the fat-soluble vitamins, a pathological condition called ***malabsorption.*** Malabsorption syndromes can lead

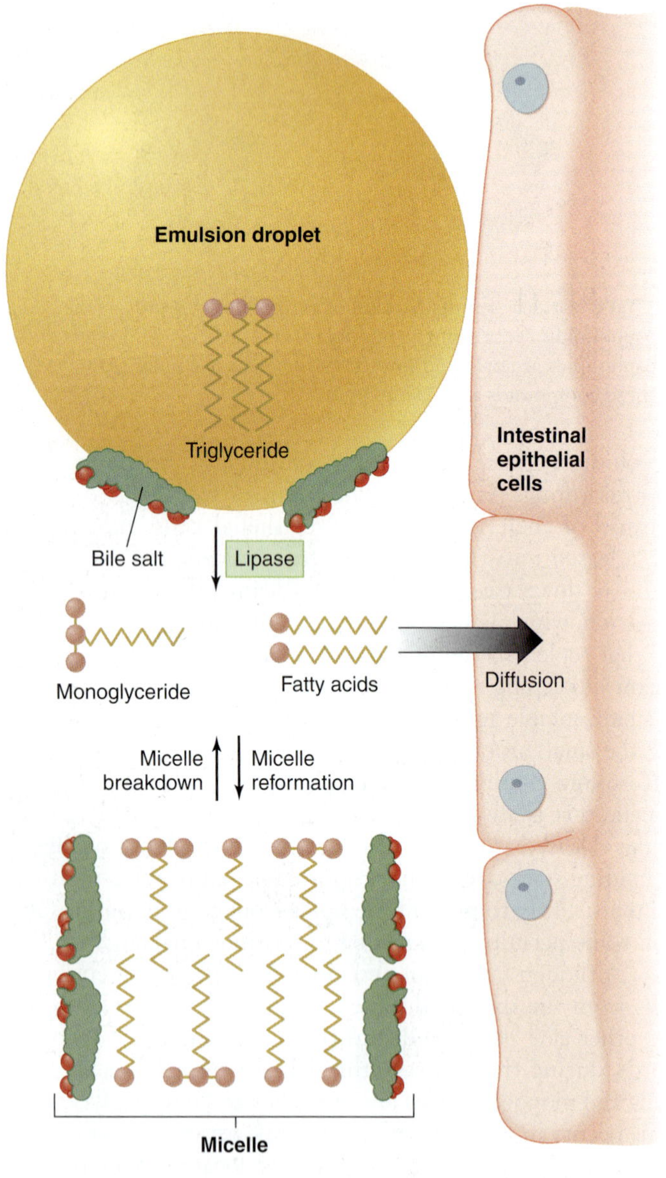

Figure 15.12 The products of fat digestion by lipase are held in solution in the micellar state, combined with bile salts and phospholipids. For simplicity, the phospholipids and colipase (see text) are not shown and the size of the micelle is greatly exaggerated. Note that micelles and free fatty acids are in equilibrium so that as fatty acids are absorbed, more can be released from the micelles.

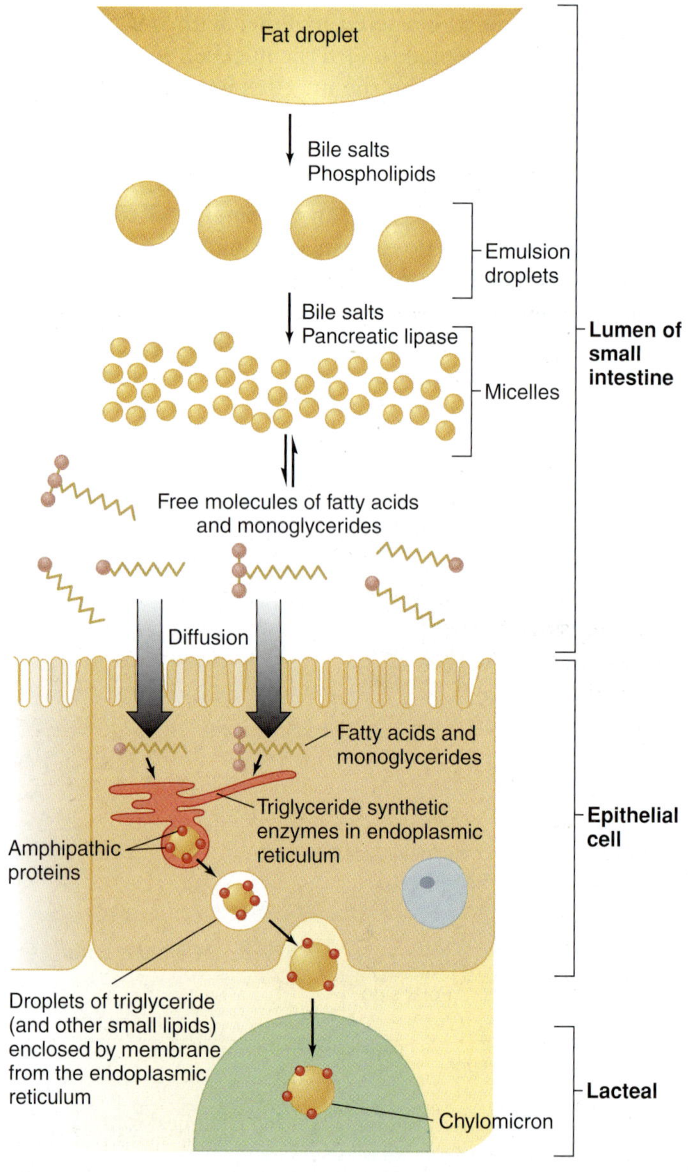

Figure 15.13 Summary of fat absorption across the epithelial cells of the small intestine.

to deficiency of fat-soluble vitamins. For example, ***nontropical sprue,*** also known as ***celiac disease*** or ***gluten-sensitive enteropathy,*** is due to an autoimmune-mediated loss of intestinal surface area due to sensitivity to the wheat proteins collectively known as **gluten.** The loss of intestinal brush border surface area can lead to decreased absorption of many nutrients, which in turn may result in a variety of health consequences. For example, it is often associated with vitamin D malabsorption, which ultimately results in a decrease in calcium ion absorption in the GI tract (see Chapter 11).

With one exception, water-soluble vitamins are absorbed by diffusion or mediated transport. The exception, vitamin B_{12} (cyanocobalamin), is a very large, charged molecule. To be absorbed, vitamin B_{12} must first bind to a protein known as **intrinsic factor,** which is secreted by the acid-secreting cells in the stomach. Intrinsic factor with bound vitamin B_{12} then binds to specific sites on the epithelial cells in the lower portion of the ileum, where vitamin B_{12} is absorbed by endocytosis. As described in Chapter 12, vitamin B_{12} is required for erythrocyte formation, and deficiencies result in ***pernicious anemia.*** This form of anemia may occur when the stomach either has been removed (for example, to treat ulcers or gastric cancer) or fails to secrete intrinsic factor (often due to autoimmune destruction of acid-producing cells). Because the absorption of vitamin B_{12} occurs in the lower part of the ileum, removal or dysfunction of this segment due to disease can also result in pernicious anemia. Although healthy individuals can absorb oral vitamin B_{12}, it is not very effective in patients with pernicious anemia because of the absence of intrinsic factor. Therefore, the treatment of pernicious anemia usually requires injections of vitamin B_{12}.

Water and Minerals

Water is the most abundant substance in chyme. Approximately 8000 mL of ingested and secreted water enters the small intestine each day, but only 1500 mL passes on to the large intestine because 80% of the fluid is absorbed in the small intestine. Small amounts of water are absorbed in the stomach, but the stomach has a much smaller surface area available for diffusion and lacks the solute-absorbing mechanisms that create the osmotic gradients necessary for net water absorption. The epithelial membranes of the small intestine are very permeable to water, and net water diffusion occurs across the epithelium whenever a water concentration difference is established by the active absorption of solutes. The mechanisms coupling solute and water absorption by epithelial cells were described in Chapter 4.

Na^+ accounts for much of the actively transported solute because it constitutes the most abundant solute in chyme. Na^+ absorption is a primary active process—using the Na^+/K^+-ATPase pumps as described in Chapter 4—and is similar to that for renal tubular Na^+ and water reabsorption (Chapter 14). Cl^- and HCO_3^- are absorbed with the Na^+ and contribute another large fraction of the absorbed solute.

Other minerals present in smaller concentrations, such as potassium, magnesium, and calcium ions, are also absorbed, as are trace elements such as iron, zinc, and iodide. Consideration of the transport processes associated with each of these is beyond the scope of this book, and we shall briefly consider as an example the absorption of only one—iron. Calcium ion absorption and its regulation were described in Chapter 11.

Iron

Iron is necessary for normal health because it is the O_2-binding component of hemoglobin, and it is also a key component of many enzymes. Only about 10% of ingested iron is absorbed into the blood each day. Iron ions are actively transported into intestinal epithelial cells, where most of them are incorporated into **ferritin,** the protein–iron complex that functions as an intracellular iron store (see Chapter 12). The absorbed iron that does not bind to ferritin is released on the blood side, where it circulates throughout the body bound to the plasma protein transferrin. Most of the iron bound to ferritin in the epithelial cells is released back into the intestinal lumen when the cells at the tips of the villi disintegrate, and the iron is then excreted in the feces.

Iron absorption depends on the body's iron content. When body stores are ample, the increased concentration of free iron in the plasma and intestinal epithelial cells leads to an increased transcription of the gene encoding the ferritin protein and, as a consequence, an increased synthesis of ferritin. This results in the increased binding of iron in the intestinal epithelial cells and a reduction in the amount of iron released into the blood. When body stores of iron decrease (for example, after a loss of blood), the production of intestinal ferritin decreases. This leads to a decrease in the amount of iron bound to ferritin, thereby increasing the unbound iron released into the blood.

Once iron has entered the blood, the body has very little means of excreting it, so it accumulates in tissues. Although the control mechanisms for iron absorption tend to maintain the iron content of the body at a fairly constant level, a very large ingestion of iron can overwhelm them, leading to an increased deposition of iron in tissues and producing toxic effects such as changes in skin pigmentation, diabetes mellitus, liver and heart failure, and decreased testicular function. This condition is termed ***hemochromatosis.*** Some people have genetically defective control mechanisms and therefore develop hemochromatosis even when iron ingestion is normal. They can be treated with frequent blood withdrawal (***phlebotomy***), which removes iron contained in red blood cells (hemoglobin) from the body.

Iron absorption also depends on the types of food ingested because it binds to many negatively charged ions in food, which can retard its absorption. For example, iron in ingested liver is much more absorbable than iron in egg yolk because the latter contains phosphates that bind the iron to form an insoluble and unabsorbable complex.

The absorption of iron is typical of that of most trace metals in several respects: (1) Cellular storage proteins and plasma carrier proteins are involved; and (2) the control of absorption, rather than urinary excretion, is the major mechanism for the homeostatic control of the body's content of the trace metal.

15.5 How Are Gastrointestinal Processes Regulated?

Unlike control systems that regulate variables in the internal environment, the control mechanisms of the gastrointestinal system regulate conditions in the lumen of the tract. With few exceptions, like those just discussed for iron and other trace metals, these control mechanisms are governed by the volume and composition of the luminal contents rather than by the nutritional state of the body.

Basic Principles

Gastrointestinal reflexes are initiated by a relatively small number of luminal stimuli: (1) distension of the wall by the volume of the luminal contents; (2) chyme osmolarity (total solute concentration); (3) chyme acidity; and (4) chyme concentrations of specific digestion products like monosaccharides, fatty acids, peptides, and amino acids. These stimuli act on mechanoreceptors, osmoreceptors, and chemoreceptors located in the wall of the tract and trigger reflexes that influence the effectors—the muscle layers in the wall of the tract and the exocrine glands that secrete substances into its lumen.

Neural Regulation

The gastrointestinal tract has its own local nervous system, a division of the autonomic nervous system known as the **enteric nervous system.** The cells in this system form two networks or plexuses of neurons, the myenteric plexus and the submucosal plexus (see Figure 15.3). These neurons either synapse with other neurons within a given plexus or end near smooth muscles, glands, and epithelial cells. Many axons leave the myenteric plexus and synapse with neurons in the submucosal plexus, and vice versa, so that neural activity in one plexus influences the activity in the other. Moreover, stimulation at one point in the plexus can lead to impulses that are conducted both up and down the tract. For example, stimuli in the upper part of the small intestine may affect smooth muscle and gland activity in the stomach as well as in the lower part of the intestinal tract. In general, the myenteric plexus influences smooth muscle activity whereas the submucosal plexus influences secretory activity.

The enteric nervous system contains adrenergic and cholinergic neurons as well as neurons that release other neurotransmitters, such as nitric oxide, several neuropeptides, and ATP.

The effectors mentioned earlier—muscle cells and exocrine glands—are supplied by neurons that are part of the enteric nervous system. This permits neural reflexes that are completely within the tract—that is, independent of the CNS. In addition, nerve fibers from both the sympathetic and parasympathetic branches of the autonomic nervous system enter the intestinal tract and synapse with neurons in both plexuses. Via these pathways, the CNS can influence the motility and secretory activity of the gastrointestinal tract.

Thus, two types of neural-reflex arcs exist (**Figure 15.14**): (1) **short reflexes** from receptors through the nerve plexuses to effector cells; and (2) **long reflexes** from receptors in the tract to the CNS by way of afferent nerves, and back to the nerve plexuses and effector cells by way of autonomic nerve fibers.

Finally, it should be noted that not all neural reflexes are initiated by signals *within* the tract. Hunger, the sight or smell of food, and the emotional state of an individual can have significant effects on the gastrointestinal tract, effects that are mediated by the CNS via autonomic neurons.

Hormonal Regulation

The hormones that control the gastrointestinal system are secreted mainly by endocrine cells scattered throughout the epithelium of the stomach and small intestine. That is, these cells

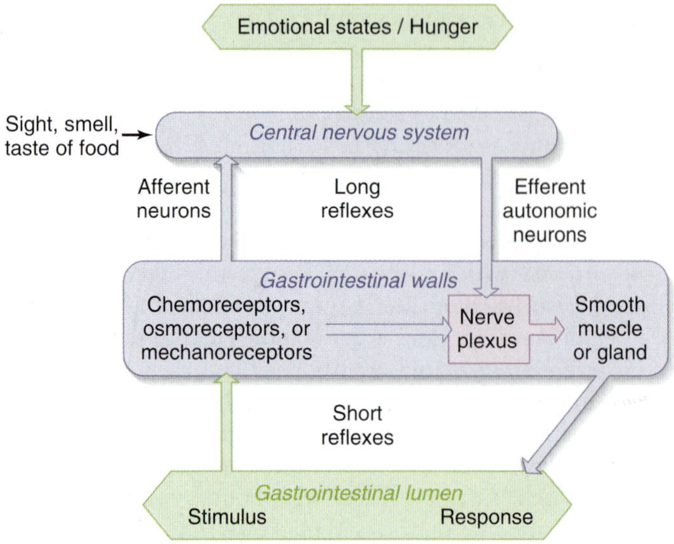

Figure 15.14 APIR Long and short neural-reflex pathways activated by stimuli in the gastrointestinal tract. The long reflexes utilize neurons that link the central nervous system to the gastrointestinal tract. Chemoreceptors are stimulated by chemicals, osmoreceptors are sensitive to changes in osmolarity (salt concentration), and mechanoreceptors respond to distension of the gastrointestinal wall.

are not clustered into discrete organs like the thyroid or adrenal glands. One surface of each endocrine cell is exposed to the lumen of the gastrointestinal tract. At this surface, various chemical substances in the chyme stimulate the cell to release its hormones from the opposite side of the cell into the blood. The gastrointestinal hormones reach their target cells via the circulation.

The four best-understood gastrointestinal hormones are **secretin, cholecystokinin (CCK), gastrin,** and **glucose-dependent insulinotropic peptide (GIP). Table 15.4** summarizes the characteristics of these GI hormones and not only serves as a reference for future discussions but also illustrates the following generalizations: (1) Each hormone participates in a feedback control system that regulates some aspect of the GI luminal environment, and (2) most GI hormones affect more than one type of target cell.

These two generalizations can be illustrated by CCK. The presence of fatty acids and amino acids in the small intestine triggers CCK secretion from cells in the small intestine into the blood. Circulating CCK then stimulates the pancreas to increase the secretion of digestive enzymes and causes the sphincter of Oddi to relax. CCK also causes the gallbladder to contract, delivering to the intestine the bile salts required for micelle formation. As fatty acids and amino acids are absorbed, their concentrations in the lumen decrease, removing the signal for CCK release.

In many cases, a single effector cell contains receptors for more than one hormone, as well as receptors for neurotransmitters and paracrine agents. The result is a variety of inputs that can affect the cell's response. One such event is the phenomenon known as **potentiation,** which is exemplified by the interaction between secretin and CCK. Secretin strongly stimulates pancreatic HCO_3^- secretion, whereas CCK is a weak stimulus of HCO_3^- secretion. Both hormones together, however, stimulate pancreatic HCO_3^- secretion more strongly

TABLE 15.4 Properties of Gastrointestinal Hormones

	Gastrin	CCK	Secretin	GIP
Chemical class	Peptide	Peptide	Peptide	Peptide
Site of production	Antrum of stomach	Small intestine	Small intestine	Small intestine
Stimuli for hormone release	Amino acids, peptides in stomach; parasympathetic nerves	Amino acids, fatty acids in small intestine	Acid in small intestine	Glucose, fat in small intestine
Factors inhibiting hormone release	Acid in stomach; somatostatin			
		Target Organ Responses		
Stomach				
Acid secretion	Stimulates	Inhibits	Inhibits	
Motility	Stimulates	Inhibits	Inhibits	
Pancreas				
HCO_3^- secretion		Potentiates secretin's actions	Stimulates	
Enzyme secretion		Stimulates	Potentiates CCK's actions	
Insulin secretion				Stimulates
Liver (bile ducts)				
HCO_3^- secretion		Potentiates secretin's actions	Stimulates	
Gallbladder				
Contraction		Stimulates		
Sphincter of Oddi		Relaxes		
Small intestine				
Motility	Stimulates ileum			
Large intestine	Stimulates mass movement			

PHYSIOLOGICAL INQUIRY

- Gastrinomas are tumors of the GI tract that secrete gastrin, leading to very high plasma concentrations. What might be some of the effects of a gastrinoma?

Answer can be found at end of chapter.

than would be predicted by the sum of their individual stimulatory effects. This is because CCK amplifies the response to secretin. One of the consequences of potentiation is that small changes in the plasma concentration of one gastrointestinal hormone can have large effects on the actions of other gastrointestinal hormones. In addition to their stimulation (or, in some cases, inhibition) of effector cell functions, the gastrointestinal hormones also have trophic (growth-promoting) effects on various tissues, including the gastric and intestinal mucosa and the exocrine portions of the pancreas. Finally, many additional GI hormones have been described, some of which are involved in the control of blood glucose by serving as a feedforward signal from the GI tract to the endocrine pancreas (see Chapter 16).

Phases of Gastrointestinal Control

The neural and hormonal control of the gastrointestinal system is, in large part, divisible into three phases—cephalic, gastric, and intestinal—according to where the stimulus is perceived.

The **cephalic** (from a Greek word for "head") **phase** is initiated when sensory receptors in the head are stimulated by sight, smell, taste, and chewing. Various emotional states can also initiate this phase. The efferent pathways for these reflexes are primarily mediated by parasympathetic fibers carried in the vagus nerves. These fibers activate neurons in the gastrointestinal nerve plexuses, which in turn affect secretory and contractile activity.

Four stimuli in the stomach initiate the reflexes that constitute the **gastric phase** of regulation: distension, acidity, amino acids, and peptides formed during the digestion of ingested protein. The responses to these stimuli are mediated by short and long neural reflexes and by release of the hormone gastrin.

Finally, the **intestinal phase** is initiated by stimuli in the intestinal tract: distension, acidity, osmolarity, and various digestive products. The intestinal phase is mediated by both short and long neural reflexes and by the gastrointestinal hormones secretin, CCK, and GIP, all of which are secreted by endocrine cells in the small intestine.

We reemphasize that each of these phases is named for the site at which the various stimuli initiate the reflex and not for the sites of effector activity. Each phase is characterized by efferent output to virtually all organs in the gastrointestinal tract. Also, these phases do not occur in temporal sequence except at the very beginning of a meal. Rather, during ingestion and the much longer absorptive period, reflexes characteristic of all three phases may be occurring simultaneously.

Keeping in mind the neural and hormonal mechanisms available for regulating gastrointestinal activity, we can now examine the specific contractile and secretory processes that occur in each segment of the gastrointestinal system.

Mouth, Pharynx, and Esophagus

Chewing

Chewing is controlled by the somatic nerves to the skeletal muscles of the mouth and jaw. In addition to the voluntary control of these muscles, rhythmic chewing motions are reflexively activated by the pressure of food against the gums, hard palate at the roof of the mouth, and tongue. Activation of these mechanoreceptors leads to reflexive inhibition of the muscles holding the jaw closed. The resulting relaxation of the jaw reduces the pressure on the various mechanoreceptors, leading to a new cycle of contraction and relaxation.

Chewing prolongs the subjective pleasure of taste. Chewing also breaks up food particles, creating a bolus that is easier to swallow and, possibly, digest. Attempting to swallow a large particle of food can lead to choking if the particle lodges over the trachea, blocking the entry of air into the lungs.

Saliva

There are three pairs of salivary glands—the parotid, sublingual, and submandibular glands (see Figure 15.1). The secretion of saliva is controlled by both sympathetic and parasympathetic neurons. Unlike their antagonistic activity in most organs, both systems stimulate salivary secretion, with the parasympathetic neurons producing the greater response. There is no hormonal regulation of salivary secretion. In the absence of ingested material, a low rate of salivary secretion keeps the mouth moist. The smell or sight of food induces a cephalic phase of salivary secretion. This reflex can be conditioned to other cues, a phenomenon made famous by Pavlov. Salivary secretion can increase markedly in response to a meal. This reflex response is initiated by chemoreceptors (acidic fruit juices are particularly strong stimuli) and pressure receptors in the walls of the mouth and on the tongue.

Increased saliva secretion is accomplished by a large increase in blood flow to the salivary glands, which is mediated primarily by an increase in parasympathetic neural activity. The volume of saliva secreted per gram of tissue is the largest secretion of any of the body's exocrine glands.

Sjögren's syndrome is a fascinating immune disorder in which many different exocrine glands are rendered nonfunctional by the infiltration of white blood cells and immune complexes. The loss of salivary gland function, which frequently occurs, can be treated by taking frequent sips of water and with oral fluoride treatment to prevent tooth decay. In addition, these patients—mostly women—can have an impaired sense of taste, difficulty chewing, and even ulcers (holes) in the mucosa of the mouth.

Swallowing

Swallowing is a complex reflex initiated when pressure receptors in the walls of the pharynx are stimulated by food or drink forced into the rear of the mouth by the tongue (**Figure 15.15a**). These receptors send afferent impulses to the **swallowing center** in the medulla oblongata of the brainstem. This center then elicits swallowing via efferent fibers to the muscles in the pharynx and esophagus as well as to the respiratory muscles.

As the ingested material moves into the pharynx, the soft palate elevates and lodges against the back wall of the pharynx, preventing food from entering the nasal cavity (**Figure 15.15b**). Impulses from the swallowing center inhibit respiration, raise the larynx, and close the **glottis** (the area around the vocal cords and the space between them), keeping food from moving into the trachea. As the tongue forces the food farther back into the pharynx, the food tilts a flap of tissue, the **epiglottis,** backward to cover the closed glottis (**Figure 15.15c**). This prevents **aspiration** of food, a potentially dangerous situation in which food travels down the trachea and can cause choking, or regurgitated stomach contents are allowed into the lungs causing damage.

The next stage of swallowing occurs in the esophagus (**Figure 15.15d**), the tube that passes through the thoracic cavity, penetrates the diaphragm (which separates the thoracic cavity from the abdominal cavity), and joins the stomach a few centimeters below the diaphragm. Skeletal muscle surrounds the upper third of the esophagus, and smooth muscle surrounds the lower two-thirds.

As described in Chapter 13, the pressure in the thoracic cavity is negative relative to atmospheric pressure, and this subatmospheric pressure is transmitted across the thin wall of the intrathoracic portion of the esophagus to the lumen. In contrast, the luminal pressure in the pharynx at the opening to the esophagus is equal to atmospheric pressure, and the pressure at the opposite end of the esophagus in the stomach is slightly greater than atmospheric pressure. Therefore, pressure differences could tend to force both air (from above) and gastric contents (from below) into the esophagus. This does not occur, however, because both ends of the esophagus are normally closed by the contraction of **sphincter** muscles. A ring of skeletal muscle surrounds the esophagus just below the pharynx and forms the **upper esophageal sphincter** (see Figure 15.15), whereas the smooth muscle in the last portion of the esophagus forms the **lower esophageal sphincter** (**Figure 15.16**).

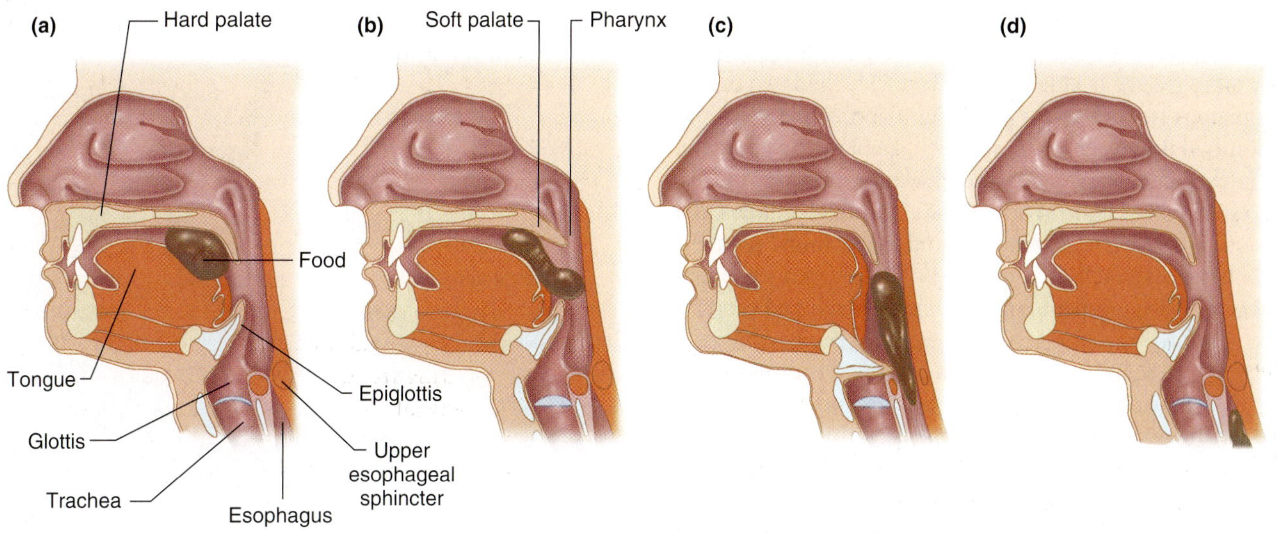

Figure 15.15 AP|R Movements of food through the pharynx and upper esophagus during swallowing. (a) The tongue pushes the food bolus to the back of the pharynx. (b) The soft palate elevates to prevent food from entering the nasal passages. (c) The epiglottis covers the glottis to prevent food or liquid from entering the trachea (aspiration), and the upper esophageal sphincter relaxes. (d) Food descends into the esophagus.

PHYSIOLOGICAL INQUIRY

- Referring to parts (b) and (c), what are some of the consequences of aspiration?

Answer can be found at end of chapter.

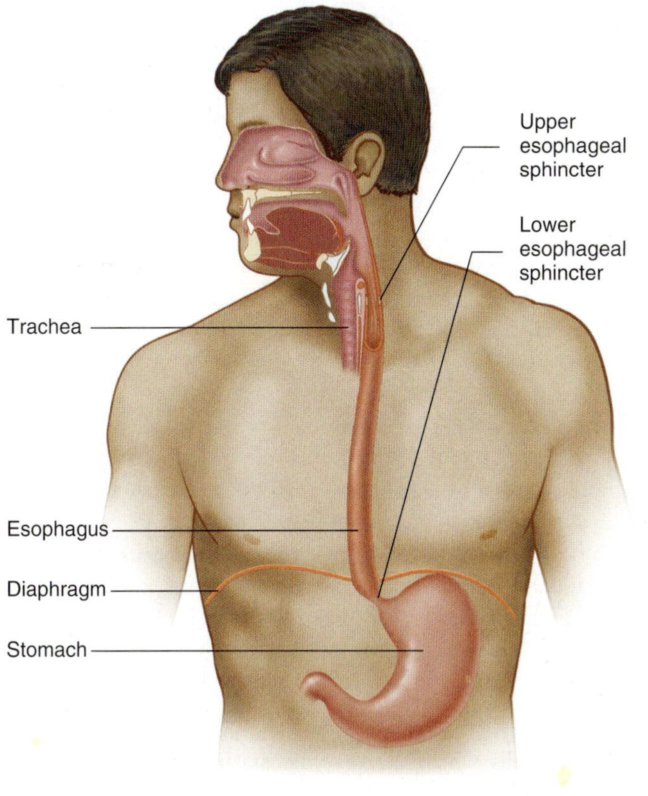

Figure 15.16 AP|R Location of upper and lower esophageal sphincters.

The esophageal phase of swallowing begins with relaxation of the upper esophageal sphincter. Immediately after the food has passed, the sphincter closes, the glottis opens, and breathing resumes. Once in the esophagus, the food moves toward the stomach by a progressive wave of muscle contractions that proceeds along the esophagus, compressing the lumen and forcing the food ahead. Such waves of contraction in the muscle layers surrounding a tube are known as **peristaltic waves.** One esophageal peristaltic wave takes about 9 seconds to reach the stomach. Swallowing can occur even when a person is upside down or in zero gravity (outer space) because it is not primarily gravity but the peristaltic wave that moves the food to the stomach.

The lower esophageal sphincter opens and remains relaxed throughout the period of swallowing, allowing the arriving food to enter the stomach. After the food passes, the sphincter closes, resealing the junction between the esophagus and the stomach.

The act of swallowing is a neural and muscular reflex coordinated by a group of brainstem nuclei collectively called the swallowing center. Both skeletal and smooth muscles are involved, so the swallowing center must direct efferent activity in both somatic nerves (to skeletal muscle) and autonomic nerves (to smooth muscle). Simultaneously, afferent fibers from receptors in the esophageal wall send information to the swallowing center; this can alter the efferent activity. For example, if a large food bolus does not reach the stomach during the initial peristaltic wave, the maintained distension of the esophagus by the bolus activates receptors that initiate reflexes, causing repeated waves of peristaltic activity (**secondary peristalsis**).

The ability of the lower esophageal sphincter to maintain a barrier between the stomach and the esophagus when swallowing is not taking place is aided by the fact that the last portion of the esophagus lies below the diaphragm and is subject to the same abdominal pressures as the stomach. In other words, if the pressure in the abdominal cavity increases, for example, during cycles of respiration or contraction of the abdominal muscles, the pressures on both the gastric contents and the terminal segment of the esophagus are increased together. This prevents the formation of a pressure gradient between the stomach and esophagus that could force the stomach's contents into the esophagus.

During pregnancy, the growth of the fetus not only increases the pressure on the abdominal contents but also can push the terminal segment of the esophagus through the diaphragm into the thoracic cavity. The sphincter is therefore no longer assisted by changes in abdominal pressure. Consequently, during the last half of pregnancy, increased abdominal pressure tends to force some of the gastric contents up into the esophagus (***gastroesophageal reflux***). The **hydrochloric acid** from the stomach irritates the esophageal walls, producing pain known as ***heartburn*** (because the pain appears to be located in the area of the heart). Heartburn often subsides in the last weeks of pregnancy prior to delivery, as the uterus descends lower into the pelvis, decreasing the pressure on the stomach.

Gastroesophageal reflux and the pain of heartburn also occur in the absence of pregnancy. Some people have less efficient lower esophageal sphincters, resulting in repeated episodes of gastric contents refluxing into the esophagus. In extreme cases, ulceration, scarring, obstruction, or perforations (holes) of the lower esophagus may occur. Gastroesophageal reflux can also occur after a large meal, which can sufficiently increase the pressure in the stomach to force acid into the esophagus. It can also cause coughing and irritation of the larynx in the absence of any esophageal symptoms, and it has even been implicated in the onset of asthmatic symptoms in susceptible individuals.

The lower esophageal sphincter undergoes brief periods of relaxation not only during a swallow but also in the absence of a swallow. During these periods of relaxation, small amounts of the acid contents from the stomach normally reflux into the esophagus. The acid in the esophagus triggers a secondary peristaltic wave and also stimulates increased salivary secretion, which helps to neutralize the acid and clear it from the esophagus.

Stomach

The epithelial layer lining the stomach invaginates into the mucosa, forming many tubular glands. Glands in the thin-walled upper portions of the **body** of the stomach (**Figure 15.17**) secrete mucus, hydrochloric acid, and the enzyme precursor pepsinogen. The uppermost part of the body of the stomach is called the **fundus** and is functionally part of the body. The lower portion of the stomach, the **antrum,** has a much thicker layer of smooth muscle and is responsible for mixing and grinding the stomach contents. The glands in this region secrete little acid but contain the endocrine cells that secrete the hormone gastrin.

The cells at the opening of the glands secrete mucus (**Figure 15.18**). Lining the walls of the glands are **parietal cells** (also known as oxyntic cells), which secrete acid and intrinsic

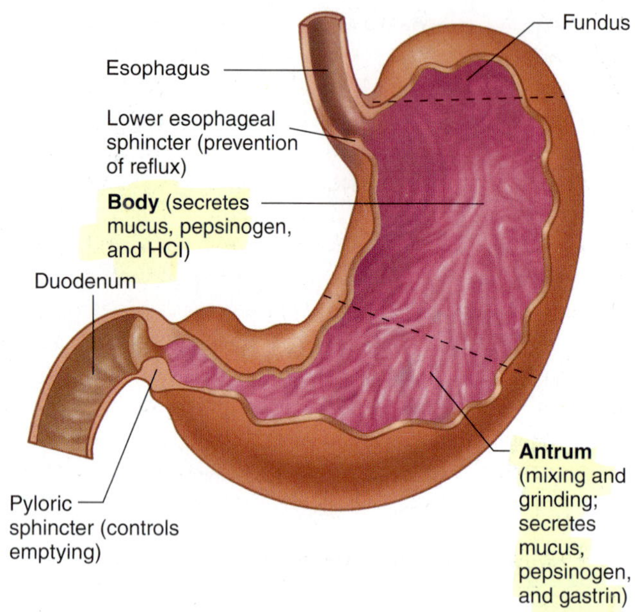

Figure 15.17 APIR The two regions of the stomach: body and antrum. The fundus is the uppermost portion of the body of the stomach and is functionally considered part of the body.

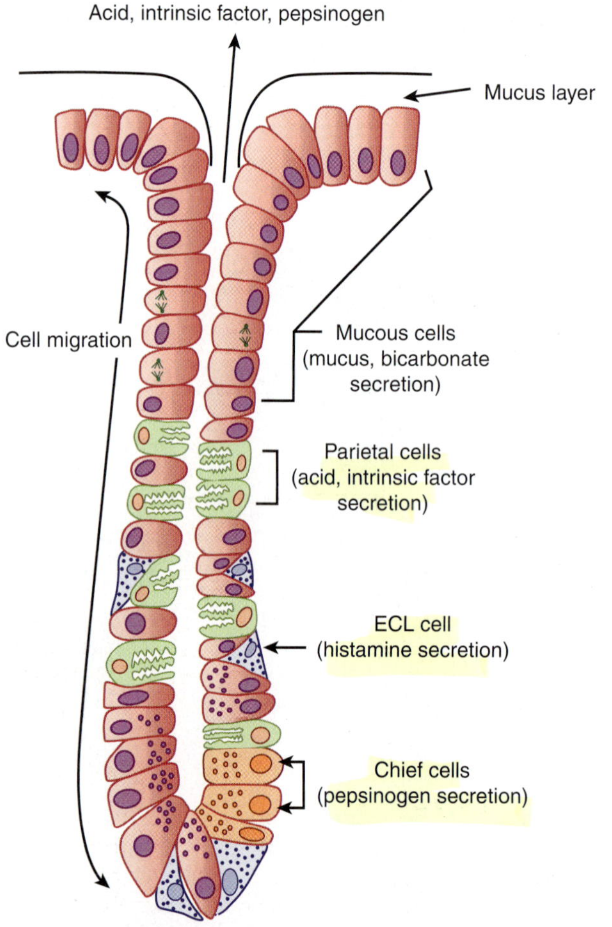

Figure 15.18 APIR A gastric gland in the stomach. Not shown are D cells, which release somatostatin and are located primarily in and around the glands in the antral region. The unique invaginations of the luminal membranes of parietal cells are called canaliculi and greatly increase the surface area for secretion.

factor, and **chief cells,** which secrete pepsinogen. The unique invaginations of the luminal membrane of parietal cells shown in Figure 15.18 are called **canaliculi** (singular, **canaliculus**); these increase the surface area of the parietal cells thereby maximizing secretion into the lumen of the stomach. This again illustrates the general principle of physiology that structure (increased surface area) is a determinant of function (efficient secretion). Thus, each of the three major exocrine secretions of the stomach—mucus, acid, and pepsinogen—is secreted by a different cell type. The gastric glands in the antrum also contain enteroendocrine cells, which secrete gastrin. In addition, **enterochromaffin-like (ECL) cells,** which release the paracrine agent histamine, and endocrine cells called D cells, which secrete the peptide **somatostatin,** are scattered throughout the tubular glands or in surrounding tissue; both of these substances play roles in regulating acid secretion by the stomach.

HCl Production and Secretion

The stomach secretes about 2 L of hydrochloric acid per day. The concentration of H^+ in the lumen of the stomach may reach >150 mM, which is 1 to 3 million times greater than the concentration in the blood. This requires an efficient production mechanism to generate large numbers of hydrogen ions. The origin of the hydrogen ions is CO_2 in the parietal cell. Recall from Chapter 13 that the enzyme carbonic anhydrase catalyzes the reaction between CO_2 with water to produce carbonic acid, which dissociates to H^+ and HCO_3^-. Primary H^+/K^+-ATPases in the luminal membrane of the parietal cells pump these hydrogen ions into the lumen of the stomach (**Figure 15.19**). This primary active transporter also pumps K^+ into the cell, which then leaks back into the lumen through K^+ channels. As H^+ is secreted into the lumen, HCO_3^- is secreted on the opposite side of the cell into the blood in exchange for Cl^-. Removal of the end products of this reaction enhance the forward rate of the reaction by the law of mass action (see Chapter 3). In this way, production and secretion of H^+ are coupled.

Increased acid secretion, stimulated by factors described in the next paragraph, results from the transfer of H^+/K^+-ATPase proteins from the membranes of intracellular vesicles to the plasma membrane by fusion of these vesicles with the membrane, thereby increasing the number of pump proteins in the plasma membrane. This process is analogous to that described in Chapter 14 for the transfer of water channels (aquaporins) to the plasma membrane of kidney collecting-duct cells in response to ADH.

Four chemical messengers regulate the insertion of H^+/K^+-ATPases into the plasma membrane and therefore acid secretion: gastrin (a gastric hormone), acetylcholine (ACh, a neurotransmitter), histamine, and somatostatin (two paracrine agents). Parietal cell membranes contain receptors for all four of these molecules (**Figure 15.20**). Somatostatin inhibits acid secretion, whereas the other three stimulate secretion. This illustrates the general principle of physiology that most physiological functions—in this case, the secretion of H^+ into the stomach lumen—are controlled by multiple regulatory systems, often working in opposition.

These chemical messengers not only act directly on the parietal cells but also influence each other's secretion. For example, histamine markedly potentiates the response to the other two stimuli, gastrin and ACh. As we will discuss later

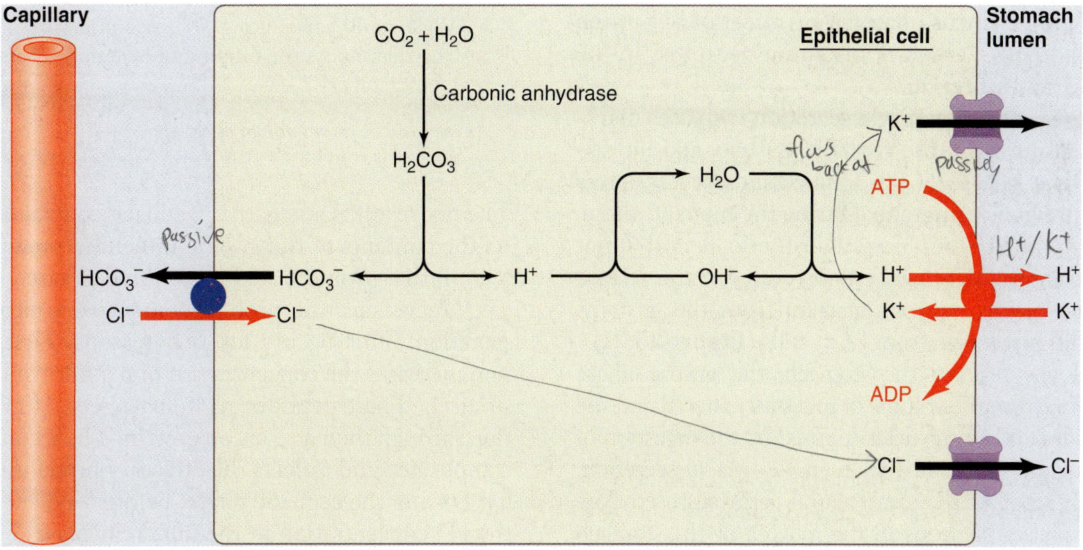

Figure 15.19 APIR Secretion of hydrochloric acid by parietal cells. The H^+ secreted into the lumen by primary active transport is derived from the breakdown of water molecules, leaving hydroxyl ion (OH^-) behind. This OH^- is neutralized by combination with other H^+ generated by the reaction between carbon dioxide and water, a reaction catalyzed by the enzyme carbonic anhydrase, which is present in high concentrations in parietal cells. The HCO_3^- formed by this reaction is transported out of the parietal cell on the blood side in exchange for Cl^-.

PHYSIOLOGICAL INQUIRY

- Why doesn't the high concentration of H^+ in the stomach lumen destroy the lining of the stomach wall?

Answer can be found at end of chapter.

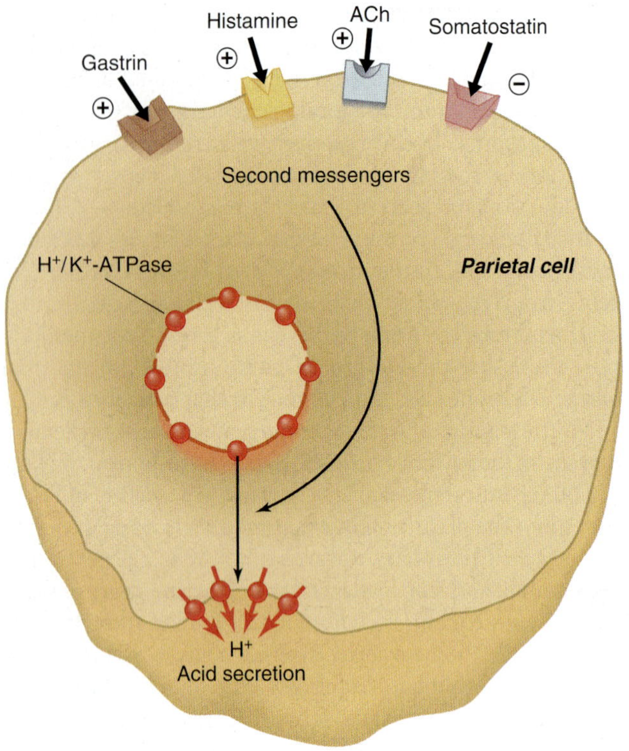

Figure 15.20 APIR The four neurohumoral inputs to parietal cells that regulate acid secretion by generating second messengers. These second messengers control the transfer of the H^+/K^+-ATPase pumps in cytoplasmic vesicle membranes to the plasma membrane. Not shown are the effects of peptides and amino acids on acid secretion.

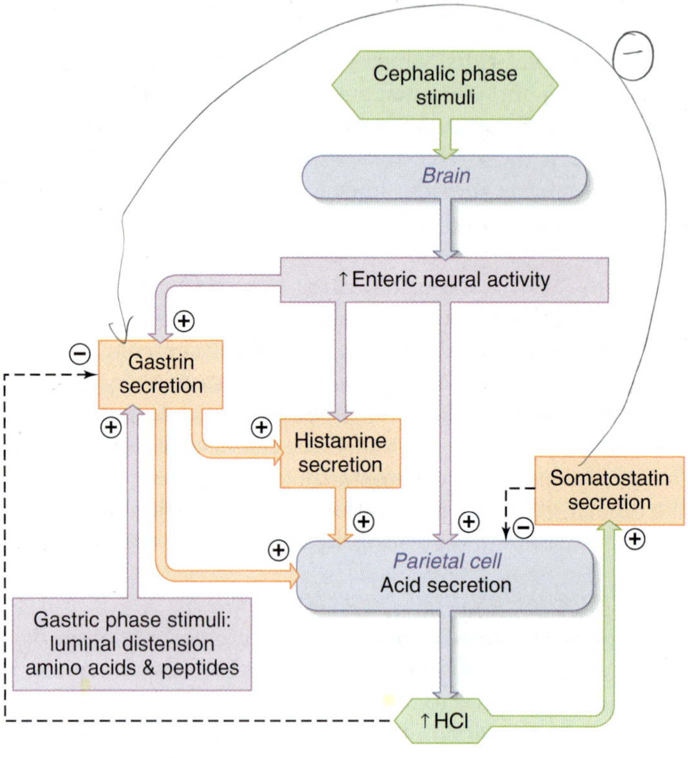

Figure 15.21 APIR Cephalic and gastric phases controlling acid secretion by the stomach. The dashed line and ⊖ indicate that an increase in acidity inhibits the secretion of gastrin and that somatostatin inhibits the release of HCl. HCl inhibition of gastrin and somatostatin inhibition of HCl are negative feedback loops limiting overproduction of HCl.

when considering ulcers, this potentiating effect of histamine is the reason that drugs that block histamine receptors in the stomach suppress acid secretion.

During a meal, the rate of acid secretion increases markedly as stimuli arising from the cephalic, gastric, and intestinal phases alter the release of the four chemical messengers described in the previous paragraph. During the cephalic phase, increased activity of efferent parasympathetic neural input to the stomach's enteric nervous system results in the release of ACh from the plexus neurons, gastrin from the gastrin-releasing cells, and histamine from ECL cells (**Figure 15.21**).

Once food has reached the stomach, the gastric phase stimuli—distension from the volume of ingested material and the presence of peptides and amino acids released by the digestion of luminal proteins—produce a further increase in acid secretion. These stimuli use some of the same neural pathways used during the cephalic phase. Neurons in the mucosa of the stomach respond to these luminal stimuli and send action potentials to the cells of the enteric nervous system, which in turn can relay signals to the gastrin-releasing cells, histamine-releasing cells, and parietal cells. In addition, peptides and amino acids can act directly on the gastrin-releasing endocrine cells to promote gastrin secretion.

The concentration of acid in the gastric lumen is itself an important determinant of the rate of acid secretion because H^+ (acid) directly inhibits gastrin secretion. It also stimulates the release of somatostatin from endocrine cells in the gastric wall. Somatostatin then acts on the parietal cells to inhibit acid secretion; it also inhibits the release of gastrin and histamine.

PHYSIOLOGICAL INQUIRY

- What would happen to gastrin secretion in a patient taking a drug that blocks the binding of histamine to its receptor on the parietal cell?

Answer can be found at end of chapter.

The net result is a negative feedback control of acid secretion. As the contents of the gastric lumen become more acidic, the stimuli that promote acid secretion decrease.

Increasing the protein content of a meal increases acid secretion. This occurs for two reasons. First, protein ingestion increases the concentration of peptides in the lumen of the stomach. These peptides, as we have seen, stimulate acid secretion through their actions on gastrin. The second reason is more complicated and reflects the effects of proteins on luminal acidity. During the cephalic phase, before food enters the stomach, the H^+ concentration in the lumen increases because there are few buffers present to bind any secreted H^+. Thereafter, the rate of acid secretion soon decreases because high acidity reflexively inhibits acid secretion (see Figure 15.21). The protein in food is an excellent buffer, however, so as it enters the stomach, the H^+ concentration decreases as H^+ binds to proteins and begins to denature them. This decrease in acidity removes the inhibition of acid secretion. The more protein in a meal, the greater the buffering of acid and the more acid secreted.

We now come to the intestinal phase that controls acid secretion—the phase in which stimuli in the early portion of the small intestine influence acid secretion by the stomach.

High acidity in the duodenum triggers reflexes that inhibit gastric acid secretion. This inhibition is beneficial because the digestive activity of enzymes and bile salts in the small intestine is strongly inhibited by acidic solutions. This reflex limits gastric acid production when the H^+ concentration in the duodenum increases due to the entry of chyme from the stomach.

Acid, distension, hypertonic solutions, solutions containing amino acids, and fatty acids in the small intestine reflexively inhibit gastric acid secretion. The extent to which acid secretion is inhibited during the intestinal phase varies, depending upon the amounts of these substances in the intestine; the net result is the same, however—balancing the secretory activity of the stomach with the digestive and absorptive capacities of the small intestine.

The inhibition of gastric acid secretion during the intestinal phase is mediated by short and long neural reflexes and by hormones that inhibit acid secretion by influencing the four signals that directly control acid secretion: ACh, gastrin, histamine, and somatostatin. The hormones released by the intestinal tract that reflexively inhibit gastric activity are collectively called **enterogastrones** and include secretin and CCK.

Table 15.5 summarizes the control of acid secretion.

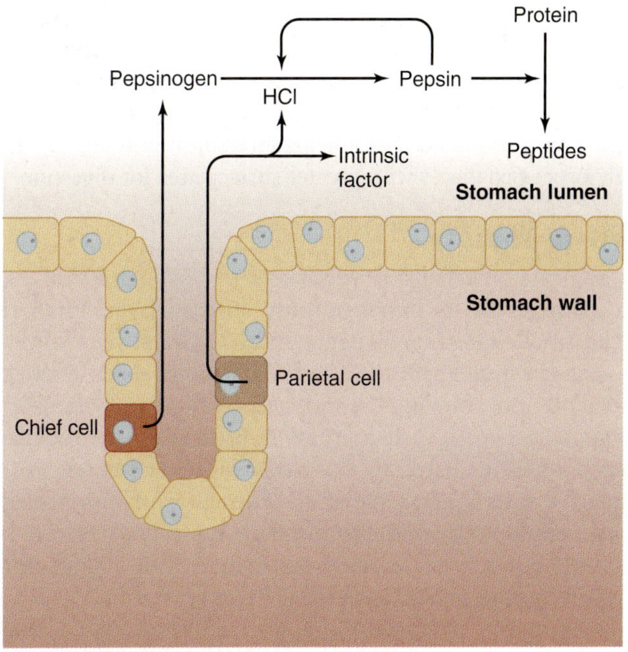

Figure 15.22 APIR Conversion of pepsinogen to pepsin in the lumen of the stomach. An increase in HCl acidifies the stomach contents. High acidity (low pH) maximizes pepsin cleavage from pepsinogen. The pepsin thus formed also catalyzes its own production by acting on additional molecules of pepsinogen. The parietal cells also secrete intrinsic factor, which is needed to absorb vitamin B_{12} in the small intestine.

Pepsin Secretion

Pepsin is secreted by chief cells in the form of an inactive precursor called pepsinogen (Figure 15.22). Exposure to low pH in the lumen of the stomach activates a very rapid, autocatalytic process in which pepsin is produced from pepsinogen.

The synthesis and secretion of pepsinogen, followed by its intraluminal activation to pepsin, provide an example of a process that occurs with many other secreted proteolytic enzymes in the gastrointestinal tract. These enzymes are synthesized and stored intracellularly in inactive forms, collectively referred to as **zymogens.** Consequently, zymogens do not act on proteins inside the cells that produce them; this protects the cell from proteolytic damage.

Pepsin is active only in the presence of a high H^+ concentration (low pH). It is irreversibly inactivated when it enters the small intestine, where the HCO_3^- secreted into the small intestine neutralizes the H^+. The primary pathway for stimulating pepsinogen secretion is input to the chief cells from the enteric nervous system. During the cephalic, gastric, and intestinal phases, most of the factors that stimulate or inhibit acid secretion exert the same effect on pepsinogen secretion. Thus, pepsinogen secretion parallels acid secretion.

Pepsin is not essential for protein digestion because in its absence, as occurs in some pathological conditions, protein can

TABLE 15.5 Control of HCl Secretion During a Meal

Stimuli	Pathways	Result
Cephalic phase Sight Smell Taste Chewing	Parasympathetic nerves to enteric nervous system	↑HCl secretion
Gastric contents (gastric phase) Distension ↑Peptides ↓H^+ concentration	Long and short neural reflexes and direct stimulation of gastrin secretion	↑HCl secretion
Intestinal contents (intestinal phase) Distension ↑H^+ concentration ↑Osmolarity ↑Nutrient concentrations	Long and short neural reflexes; secretin, CCK, and other duodenal hormones	↓HCl secretion

be completely digested by enzymes in the small intestine. However, pepsin accelerates protein digestion and normally accounts for about 20% of total protein digestion. It is also important in the digestion of collagen contained in the connective-tissue matrix of meat. This is useful because it helps shred meat into smaller, more easily processed pieces with greater surface area for digestion.

Gastric Motility

An empty stomach has a volume of only about 50 mL, and the diameter of its lumen is only slightly larger than that of the small intestine. When a meal is swallowed, however, the smooth muscles in the fundus and body relax before the arrival of food, allowing the stomach's volume to increase to as much as 1.5 L with little increase in pressure. This **receptive relaxation** is mediated by the parasympathetic nerves to the stomach's enteric nerve plexuses, with coordination provided by afferent input from the stomach via the vagus nerve and by the swallowing center in the brain. Nitric oxide and serotonin released by enteric neurons mediate this relaxation.

As in the esophagus, the stomach produces peristaltic waves in response to the arriving food. Each wave begins in the body of the stomach and produces only a ripple as it proceeds toward the antrum; this contraction is too weak to produce much mixing of the luminal contents with acid and pepsin. As the wave approaches the larger mass of wall muscle surrounding the antrum, however, it produces a more powerful contraction, which both mixes the luminal contents and *closes* the **pyloric sphincter,** a ring of smooth muscle and connective tissue between the antrum and the duodenum (**Figure 15.23**). The pyloric sphincter muscles contract upon arrival of a peristaltic wave. As a consequence of the sphincter closing, only a small amount of chyme is expelled into the duodenum with each wave. Most of the antral contents are forced backward toward the body of the stomach. This backward motion of chyme, called **retropulsion,** generates strong shear forces that helps to disperse the food particles and improve mixing of the chyme. Recall that the lower esophageal sphincter prevents this retrograde movement of stomach contents from entering the esophagus.

What is responsible for producing gastric peristaltic waves? Their rhythm (three per minute) is generated by pacemaker cells in the longitudinal smooth muscle layer. These smooth muscle cells undergo spontaneous depolarization–repolarization cycles (slow waves) known as the **basic electrical rhythm** of the stomach. These slow waves are conducted through gap junctions along the stomach's longitudinal muscle layer and also induce similar slow waves in the overlying circular muscle layer. In the absence of neural or hormonal input, however, these depolarizations are too small to cause significant contractions. Excitatory neurotransmitters and hormones act upon the smooth muscle to further depolarize the membrane, thereby bringing it closer to threshold. Action potentials may be generated at the peak of the slow-wave cycle if threshold is reached (**Figure 15.24**), causing larger contractions. The number of spikes fired with each wave determines the strength of the muscle contraction. Therefore, whereas the frequency of contraction is determined by the intrinsic basic electrical rhythm and remains essentially constant, the force of contraction—and, consequently, the amount of gastric emptying per contraction—is determined reflexively by neural and hormonal input to the antral smooth muscle.

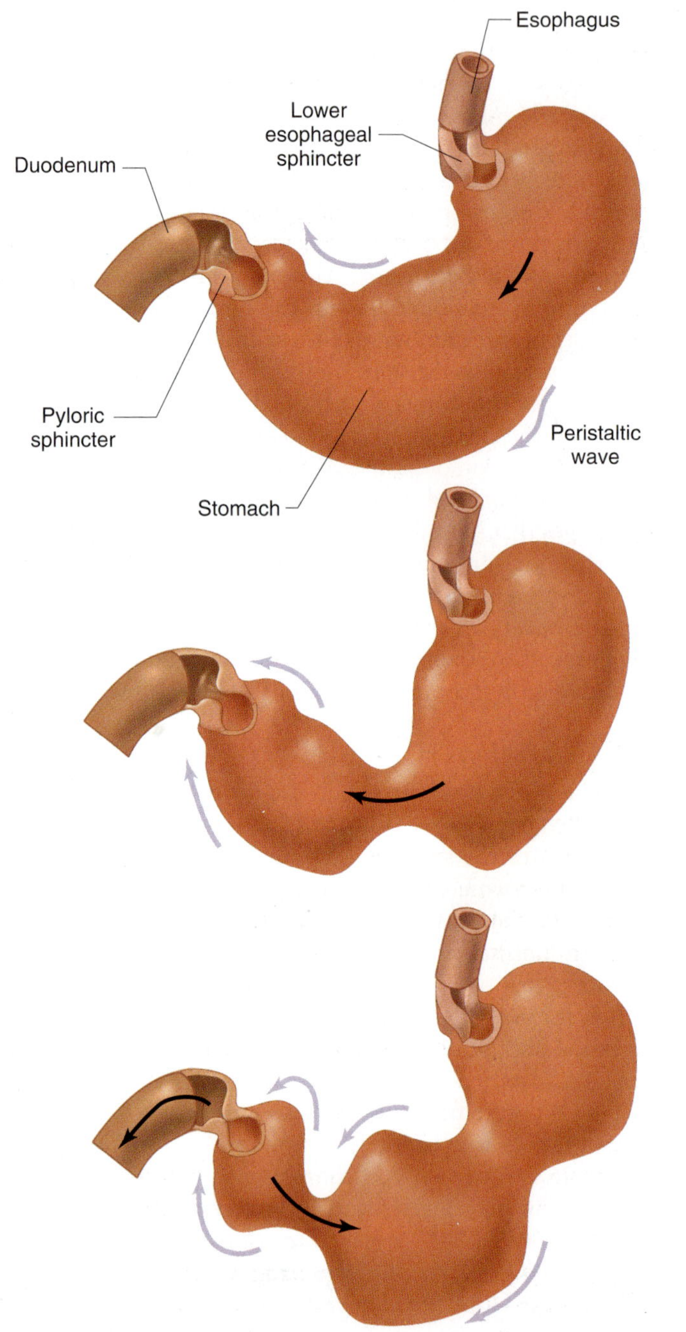

Figure 15.23 APIR Peristaltic waves passing over the stomach force a small amount of luminal material into the duodenum. Black arrows indicate movement of luminal material; purple arrows indicate movement of the peristaltic wave in the stomach wall.

The initiation of these reflexes depends upon the contents of both the stomach and small intestine. All the factors previously discussed that regulate acid secretion (see Table 15.5) can also alter gastric motility. For example, gastrin in sufficiently high concentrations increases the force of antral smooth muscle contractions. Distension of the stomach also increases the force of antral contractions through long and short reflexes triggered by mechanoreceptors in the stomach wall. Therefore, after a

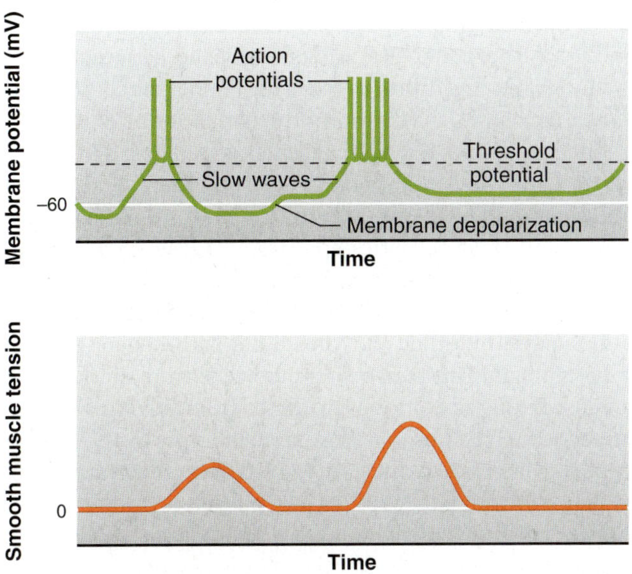

Figure 15.24 Slow-wave oscillations in the membrane potential of gastric smooth muscle fibers trigger bursts of action potentials when threshold potential is reached at the wave peak. Membrane depolarization brings the slow wave closer to threshold, increasing the action potential frequency and thus the force of smooth muscle contraction.

large meal, the force of initial stomach contractions is greater, which results in a greater emptying per contraction.

In contrast, gastric emptying is inhibited by distension of the duodenum or the presence of fat, high acidity (low pH), or hypertonic solutions in the lumen of the duodenum (**Figure 15.25**). These are the same factors that inhibit acid and pepsin secretion in the stomach. Fat is the most potent of these chemical stimuli. This prevents overfilling of the duodenum. The rate of gastric emptying has significant clinical implications particularly when considering what food type is eaten with oral medications. A meal rich in fat content tends to slow oral drug absorption due to a delay of the drug entering the small intestine through the pyloric sphincter.

Autonomic nerve fibers to the stomach can be activated by the CNS independently of the reflexes originating in the stomach and duodenum and can influence gastric motility. An increase in parasympathetic activity increases gastric motility, whereas an increase in sympathetic activity decreases motility. Via these pathways, pain and emotions can alter motility; however, different people show different gastrointestinal responses to apparently similar emotional states. As we have seen, a hypertonic solution in the duodenum is one of the stimuli inhibiting gastric emptying. This reflex prevents the fluid in the duodenum from becoming too hypertonic. It does so by slowing the rate of entry of chyme and thereby the delivery of large molecules that can rapidly be broken down into many small molecules by enzymes in the small intestine.

Once the contents of the stomach have emptied over a period of several hours, the peristaltic waves cease and the empty stomach is mostly quiescent. During this time, however, there are brief intervals of peristaltic activity that we will describe along with the events controlling intestinal motility.

Pancreatic Secretions

The exocrine portion of the pancreas secretes HCO_3^- and a number of digestive enzymes into ducts that converge into the pancreatic duct, which joins the common bile duct from the liver just before it enters the duodenum (see Figure 15.6). The enzymes are secreted by gland cells at the pancreatic end of the duct system, whereas HCO_3^- is secreted by the epithelial cells lining the ducts (**Figure 15.26**).

The pancreatic duct cells secrete HCO_3^- (produced from CO_2 and water) into the duct lumen via an apical membrane Cl^-/HCO_3^- exchanger, while the H^+ produced is exchanged for extracellular Na^+ on the basolateral side of the cell (**Figure 15.27**). The H^+ enters the pancreatic capillaries to eventually meet up in portal vein blood with the HCO_3^- produced by the stomach during the generation of luminal H^+ (see Figure 15.19). As with most transport systems, the energy for secretion of HCO_3^- is ultimately provided by Na^+/K^+-ATPase pumps on the basolateral membrane. Cl^- normally does not accumulate within the cell because these ions are recycled into the lumen through the **cystic fibrosis transmembrane conductance regulator (CFTR)** that you learned about in

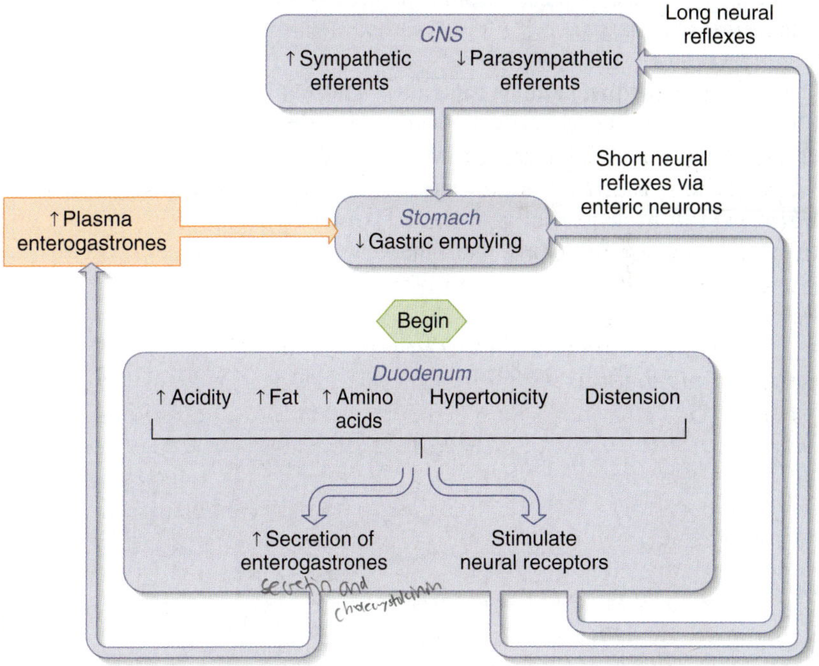

Figure 15.25 AP|R Intestinal phase pathways inhibiting gastric emptying.

PHYSIOLOGICAL INQUIRY

- What might occur if a patient whose stomach has been removed eats a large meal?

Answer can be found at end of chapter.

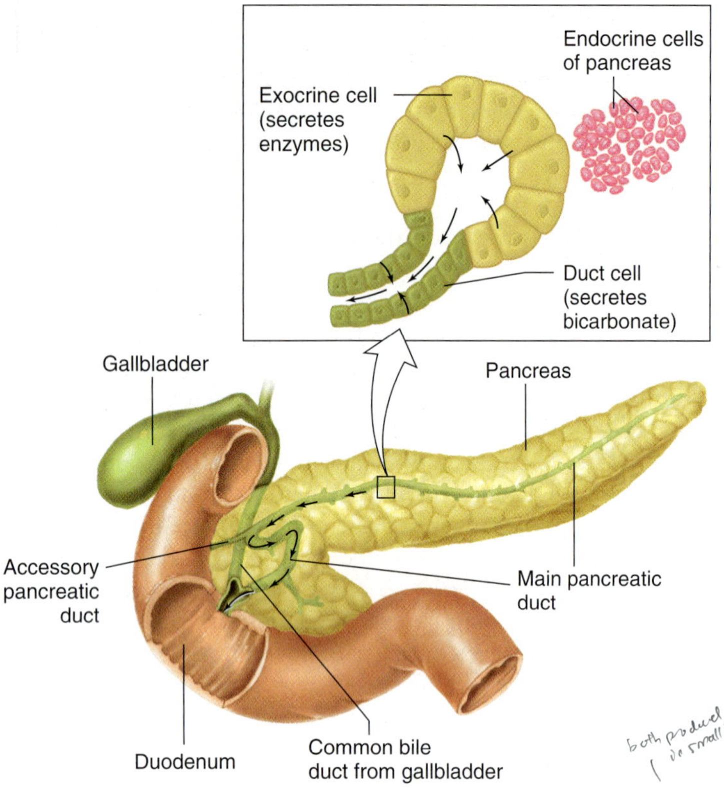

Figure 15.26 AP|R Structure of the pancreas. The exocrine portion secretes enzymes and HCO_3^- into the pancreatic ducts. The endocrine portion secretes insulin, glucagon, and other hormones into the blood.

Chapter 13. Via a paracellular route, Na^+ and water move into the ducts due to the electrochemical gradient established by chloride movement through the CFTR. This dependence on Cl^- explains why mutations in the CFTR that cause ***cystic fibrosis*** result in decreased pancreatic HCO_3^- secretion. Furthermore, the lack of normal water movement into the lumen leads to a thickening of pancreatic secretions; this can lead to clogging of the pancreatic ducts and pancreatic damage. In fact, the cystic and fibrotic (scarring) appearance of the diseased pancreas was the origin of the name of this disease.

The enzymes the pancreas secretes digest fat, polysaccharides, proteins, and nucleic acids to fatty acids, sugars, amino acids, and nucleotides, respectively. A partial list of these enzymes and their activities appears in **Table 15.6.** The proteolytic enzymes are secreted in inactive forms (zymogens), as described for pepsinogen in the stomach, and then activated in the duodenum by other enzymes. Like pepsinogen, the secretion of zymogens protects pancreatic cells from autodigestion. A key step in this activation is mediated by **enterokinase,** which is embedded in the luminal plasma membranes of the intestinal epithelial cells. Enterokinase is a proteolytic enzyme that splits off a peptide from pancreatic **trypsinogen,** forming the active enzyme trypsin. Trypsin is also a proteolytic enzyme; once activated, it activates the other pancreatic zymogens by splitting off peptide fragments (**Figure 15.28**). This activating function is in addition to the role of trypsin in digesting ingested protein. The nonproteolytic enzymes secreted by the pancreas (e.g., amylase and lipase) are released in fully active form.

Pancreatic secretion increases during a meal, mainly as a result of stimulation by the hormones secretin and CCK (see Table 15.4). Secretin is the primary stimulant for HCO_3^- secretion, whereas CCK mainly stimulates enzyme secretion.

Because the function of pancreatic HCO_3^- is to neutralize acid entering the duodenum from the stomach, it is appropriate that the major stimulus for secretin release is increased acidity in the duodenum (**Figure 15.29**). In analogous fashion, CCK stimulates the secretion of digestive enzymes, including those for fat and protein digestion, so it is appropriate that the stimuli for its release are fatty acids and amino acids in the duodenum (**Figure 15.30**). Luminal acid and fatty acids also act on afferent nerve endings in the intestinal wall, initiating reflexes that act on the pancreas to increase both enzyme and

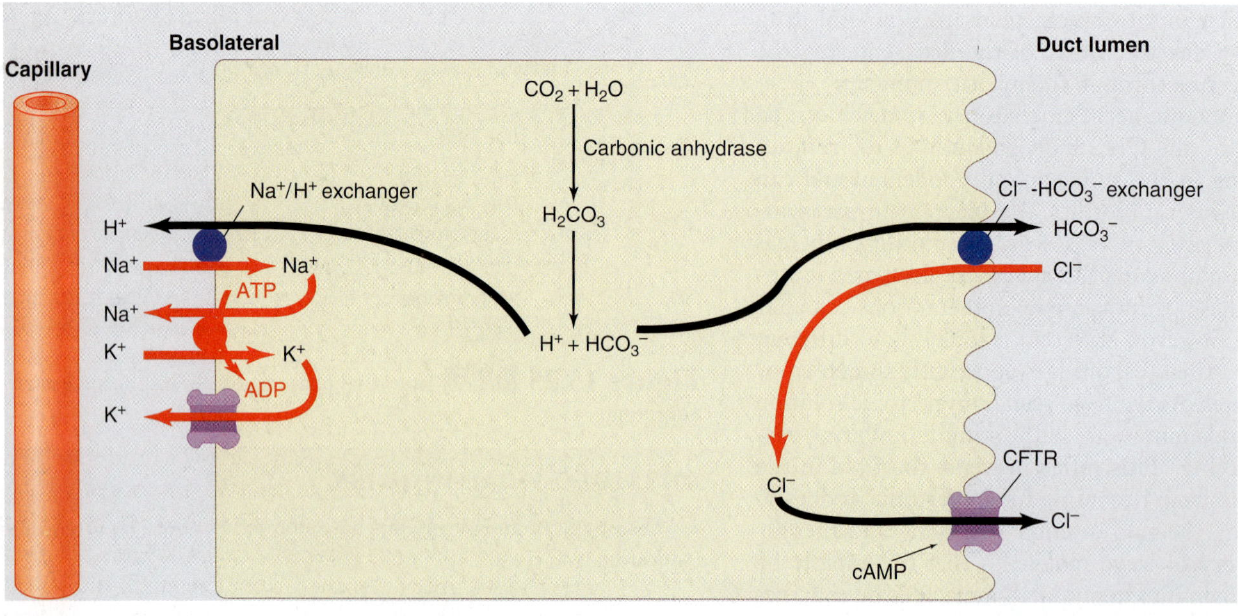

Figure 15.27 Ion-transport pathways in pancreatic duct cells. (CFTR = Cystic fibrosis transmembrane conductance regulator)

TABLE 15.6 Pancreatic Enzymes		
Enzyme	**Substrate**	**Action**
Trypsin, chymotrypsin, elastase	Proteins	Break peptide bonds in proteins to form peptide fragments
Carboxypeptidase	Proteins	Splits off terminal amino acid from carboxyl end of protein
Lipase	Fats	Splits off two fatty acids from triglycerides, forming free fatty acids and monoglycerides
Amylase	Polysaccharides	Splits polysaccharides into glucose and maltose
Ribonuclease, deoxyribonuclease	Nucleic acids	Split nucleic acids into free mononucleotides

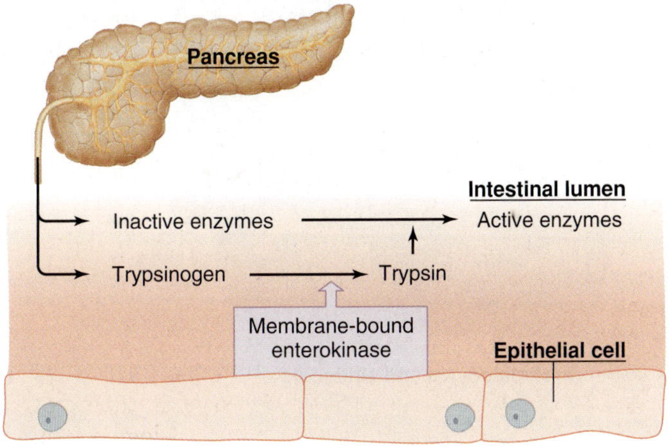

Figure 15.28 Activation of pancreatic enzyme precursors in the small intestine.

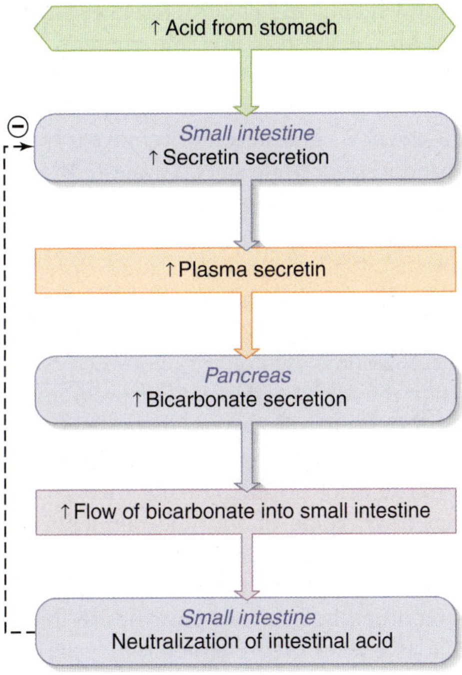

Figure 15.29 Hormonal regulation of pancreatic HCO_3^- secretion. Dashed line and ⊖ indicate that neutralization of intestinal acid (↑pH) turns off secretin secretion (negative feedback).

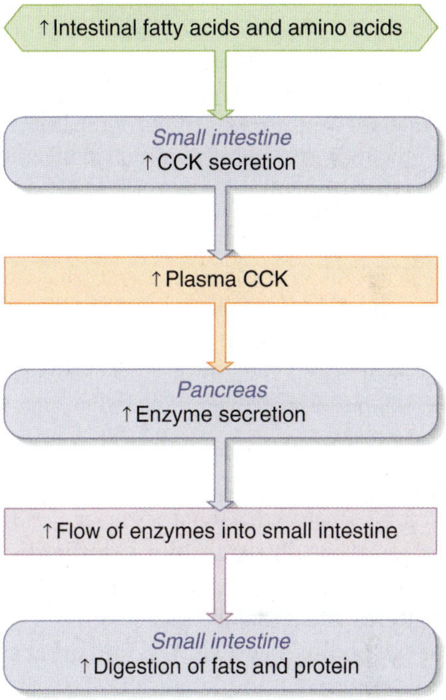

Figure 15.30 Hormonal regulation of pancreatic enzyme secretion.

HCO_3^- secretion. In these ways, the organic nutrients in the small intestine initiate neural and endocrine reflexes that control the secretions involved in their own digestion.

Although most of the pancreatic exocrine secretions are controlled by stimuli arising from the intestinal phase of digestion, cephalic and gastric stimuli also play a role by way of the parasympathetic nerves to the pancreas. Thus, the taste of food or the distension of the stomach by food will lead to increased pancreatic secretion.

Bile Secretion

The functional unit of the liver is the **hepatic lobule** (**Figure 15.31**). Within the lobule, the **portal triad** is composed of branches of the bile duct, the hepatic and portal veins, and the hepatic artery (which brings oxygenated blood to the liver). Substances absorbed from the small intestine wind up in the hepatic sinusoid either to reach the vena cava via the central vein or are taken up by the **hepatocytes** (liver cells) in

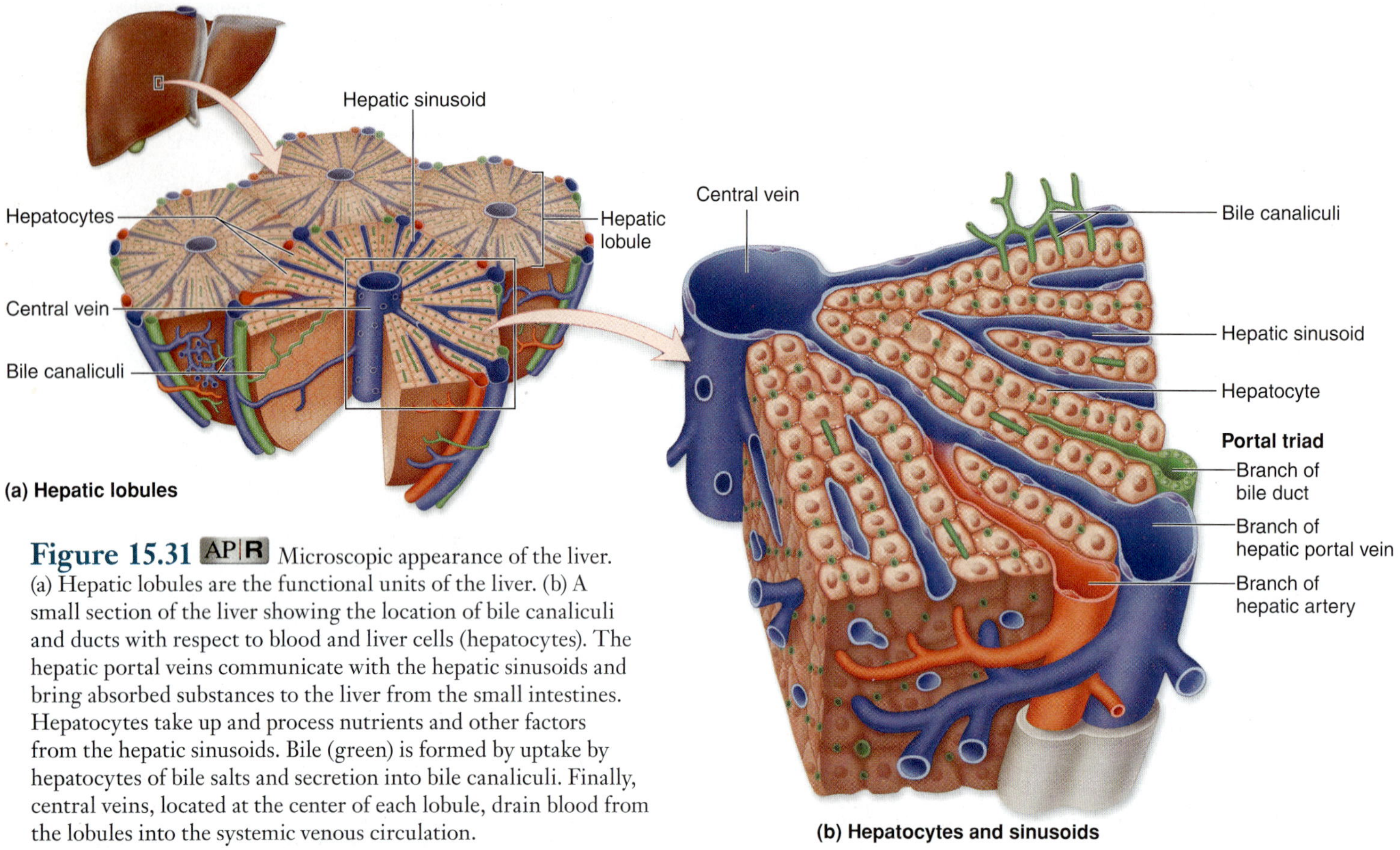

Figure 15.31 AP|R Microscopic appearance of the liver. (a) Hepatic lobules are the functional units of the liver. (b) A small section of the liver showing the location of bile canaliculi and ducts with respect to blood and liver cells (hepatocytes). The hepatic portal veins communicate with the hepatic sinusoids and bring absorbed substances to the liver from the small intestines. Hepatocytes take up and process nutrients and other factors from the hepatic sinusoids. Bile (green) is formed by uptake by hepatocytes of bile salts and secretion into bile canaliculi. Finally, central veins, located at the center of each lobule, drain blood from the lobules into the systemic venous circulation.

which they can be modified. Hepatocytes can rid the body of substances by secretion into the **bile canaliculi,** which converge to form the common hepatic bile duct (see Figure 15.6).

Bile contains six major ingredients: (1) bile salts, (2) lecithin (a phospholipid), (3) HCO_3^- and other salts, (4) cholesterol, (5) bile pigments and small amounts of other metabolic end products, and (6) trace metals. Bile salts and lecithin are synthesized in the liver and, as we have seen, help solubilize fat in the small intestine. HCO_3^- neutralizes acid in the duodenum, and the last three ingredients represent substances extracted from the blood by the liver and excreted via the bile.

The most important digestive components of bile are the bile salts. During the digestion of a fatty meal, most of the bile salts entering the intestinal tract via the bile are absorbed by specific Na^+-coupled transporters in the ileum (the last segment of the small intestine). The absorbed bile salts are returned via the portal vein to the liver, where they are once again secreted into the bile. Uptake of bile salts from portal blood into hepatocytes is driven by secondary active transport coupled to Na^+. This recycling pathway from the liver to the intestine and back to the liver is known as the **enterohepatic circulation** (**Figure 15.32**). A small amount (5%) of the bile salts escapes this recycling and is lost in the feces, but the liver synthesizes new bile salts from cholesterol to replace it. During the digestion of a meal, the entire bile salt content of the body may be recycled several times via the enterohepatic circulation.

In addition to synthesizing bile salts from cholesterol, the liver also secretes cholesterol extracted from the blood into the bile. Bile secretion, followed by excretion of cholesterol in the feces, is one of the mechanisms for maintaining cholesterol homeostasis in the blood (see Chapter 16) and is also the process by which some cholesterol-lowering drugs work. Dietary fiber also sequesters bile and thereby lowers plasma cholesterol. This occurs because the sequestered bile salts escape the enterohepatic circulation. Therefore, the liver must either synthesize new cholesterol, or remove it from the blood, or both to produce more bile salts. Cholesterol is insoluble in water, and its solubility in bile is achieved by its incorporation into micelles (whereas in blood, cholesterol is incorporated into lipoproteins). Gallstones, consisting of precipitated cholesterol, will be discussed at the end of this chapter.

Bile pigments are substances formed from the heme portion of hemoglobin when old or damaged erythrocytes are broken down in the spleen and liver. The predominant bile pigment is **bilirubin,** which is extracted from the blood by liver cells and actively secreted into the bile. Bilirubin is yellow and contributes to the color of bile. During their passage through the intestinal tract, some of the bile pigments are absorbed into the blood and are eventually excreted in the urine, giving urine its yellow color. After entering the intestinal tract, some bilirubin is modified by bacterial enzymes to form the brown pigments that give feces their characteristic color.

The components of bile are secreted by two different cell types. The bile salts, cholesterol, lecithin, and bile pigments are secreted by hepatocytes, whereas most of the HCO_3^--rich solution is secreted by the epithelial cells lining the bile ducts.

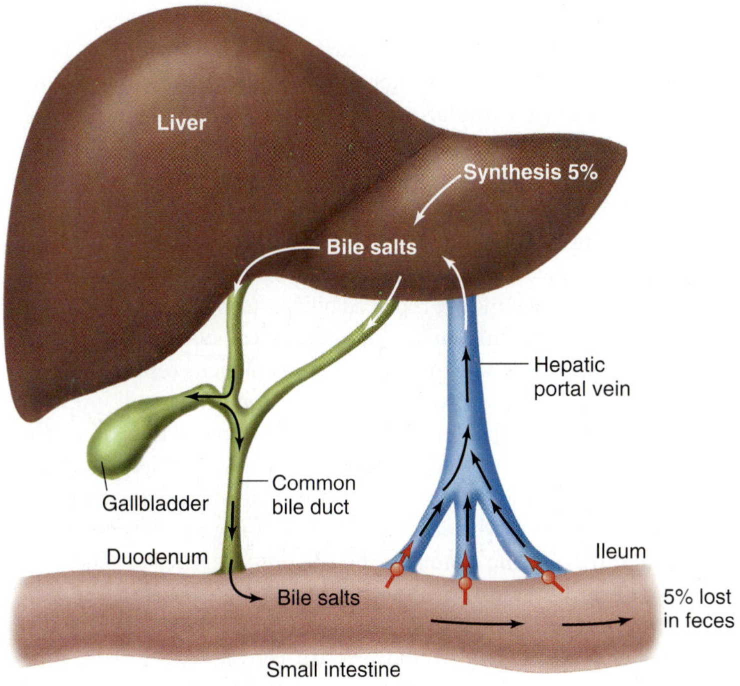

Figure 15.32 APIR Enterohepatic circulation of bile salts. Bile salts are secreted into bile (green) and enter the duodenum through the common bile duct. Bile salts are reabsorbed from the intestinal lumen into hepatic portal blood (red arrows). The liver (hepatocytes) reclaims bile salts from hepatic portal blood. The hepatic portal vein drains blood from the entire intestine, not just the ileum as shown here for simplicity.

PHYSIOLOGICAL INQUIRY

- In addition to the hepatic portal vein, can you name another portal-vein system and explain the meaning of the term *portal?*

Answer can be found at end of chapter.

Secretion of the HCO_3^--rich solution by the bile ducts, just like the secretion by the pancreas, is stimulated by secretin in response to the presence of acid in the duodenum.

Although bile secretion is greatest during and just after a meal, the liver is always secreting some bile. Surrounding the common bile duct at the point where it enters the duodenum is a ring of smooth muscle known as the **sphincter of Oddi.** When this sphincter is closed, the dilute bile secreted by the liver is shunted into the gallbladder. Here, the organic components of bile become concentrated as some NaCl and water are absorbed into the blood.

Shortly after the beginning of a fatty meal, the sphincter of Oddi relaxes and the gallbladder contracts, discharging concentrated bile into the duodenum. The signal for gallbladder contraction and sphincter relaxation is the intestinal hormone CCK—appropriately so, because, as we have seen, the presence of fat in the duodenum is a major stimulus for this hormone's release. It is from this ability to cause contraction of the gallbladder that cholecystokinin received its name: *chole,* "bile"; *cysto,* "bladder"; and *kinin,* "to move." **Figure 15.33** summarizes the factors controlling the entry of bile into the small intestine.

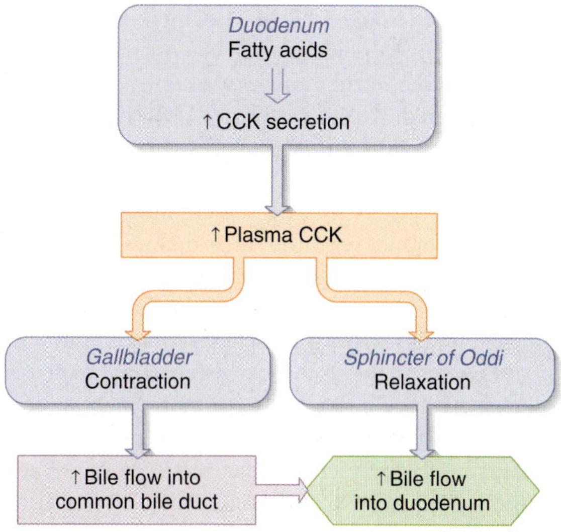

Figure 15.33 Regulation of bile entry into the small intestine.

Small Intestine

Secretion

Approximately 1500 mL of fluid is secreted by the walls of the small intestine from the blood into the lumen each day. One of the causes of water movement (secretion) into the lumen is that the intestinal epithelium at the base of the villi secretes a number of mineral ions—notably, Na^+, Cl^-, and HCO_3^-—into the lumen, and water follows by osmosis. These secretions, along with mucus, lubricate the surface of the intestinal tract and help protect the epithelial cells from excessive damage by the digestive enzymes in the lumen. Some damage to these cells still occurs, however, and the intestinal epithelium has one of the highest cell-renewal rates of any tissue in the body.

As stated earlier, water movement into the lumen also occurs when the chyme entering the small intestine from the stomach is hypertonic because of a high concentration of solutes in the meal and because digestion breaks down large molecules into many more small molecules. This hypertonicity causes the osmotic movement of water from the isotonic plasma into the intestinal lumen.

Absorption

Normally, virtually all of the fluid secreted by the small intestine is absorbed back into the blood. In addition, a much larger volume of fluid, which includes salivary, gastric, hepatic, and pancreatic secretions, as well as ingested water, is simultaneously absorbed from the intestinal lumen into the blood. Thus, overall there is a large net absorption of water from the small intestine. Absorption is achieved by the transport of ions, primarily via Na^+ and nutrient cotransport (see Figures 15.8 and 15.9) from the intestinal lumen into the blood, with water following by osmosis.

Motility

In contrast to the peristaltic waves that sweep over the stomach, the most common motion in the small intestine during digestion of a meal is a stationary contraction and relaxation of intestinal segments, with little apparent net movement toward the large intestine (**Figure 15.34**). Each contracting segment is only a few centimeters long, and the contraction lasts a few seconds. The chyme in the lumen of a contracting segment is forced both up and down the intestine. This rhythmic contraction and relaxation of the intestine, known as **segmentation,** produces a continuous division and subdivision of the intestinal contents, thoroughly mixing the chyme in the lumen and bringing it into contact with the intestinal wall.

These segmenting movements are initiated by electrical activity generated by pacemaker cells (the **interstitial cells of Cajal**) in the circular smooth muscle layer (see Figure 15.4). As with the slow waves in the stomach, this intestinal basic electrical rhythm produces oscillations in the smooth muscle membrane potential. If threshold is reached, action potentials are triggered that increase muscle contraction. The frequency of segmentation is set by the frequency of the intestinal basic electrical rhythm; unlike the stomach, however, which normally has a single rhythm (three per minute), the intestinal rhythm varies along the length of the intestine, each successive region having a slightly lower frequency than the one above. For example, segmentation in the duodenum occurs at a frequency of about 12 contractions/min, whereas in the last portion of the ileum the rate is only 9 contractions/min. Segmentation produces, therefore, a slow migration of the intestinal contents toward the large intestine because more chyme is forced downward, on average, than upward.

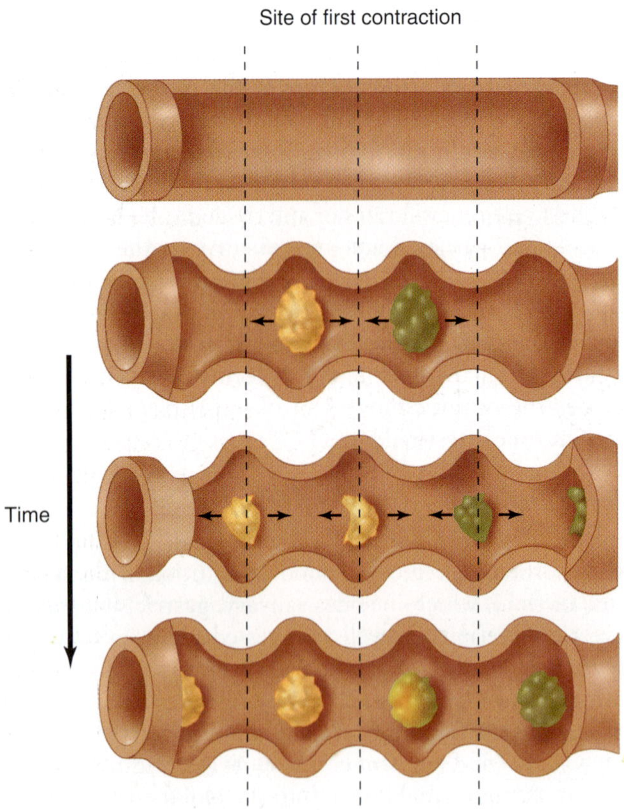

Figure 15.34 Segmentation contractions in a portion of the small intestine in which segments of the intestines contract and relax in a rhythmic pattern but do *not* undergo peristalsis. This is the rhythm encountered during a meal. Dotted lines are reference points to show the site of the first contraction in time (starting at the top). As contractions occur at the next site, the chyme is divided and pushed back and forth, mixing the luminal contents.

The intensity of segmentation can be altered by hormones, the enteric nervous system, and autonomic nerves; parasympathetic activity increases the force of contraction, and sympathetic stimulation decreases it. Thus, cephalic phase stimuli, as well as emotional states, can alter intestinal motility. As is true for the stomach, these inputs produce changes in the force of smooth muscle contraction but do not significantly change the frequencies of the basic electrical rhythms.

After most of a meal has been absorbed, the segmenting contractions cease and are replaced by a pattern of peristaltic activity known as the **migrating myoelectrical complex (MMC)**. Beginning in the lower portion of the stomach, repeated waves of peristaltic activity travel about 2 feet along the small intestine and then die out. The next MMC starts slightly farther down the small intestine so that peristaltic activity slowly migrates down the small intestine, taking about 2 h to reach the large intestine. By the time the MMC reaches the end of the ileum, new waves are beginning in the stomach, and the process repeats.

The MMC moves any undigested material still remaining in the small intestine into the large intestine and also prevents bacteria from remaining in the small intestine long enough to grow and multiply excessively. In diseases characterized by an aberrant MMC, bacterial overgrowth in the small intestine can become a major problem. Upon the arrival of a meal in the stomach, the MMC rapidly ceases in the intestine and is replaced by segmentation.

An increase in the plasma concentration of the intestinal hormone **motilin** is thought to initiate the MMC. Feeding inhibits the release of motilin; motilin stimulates MMCs via both the enteric and autonomic nervous systems.

The contractile activity in various regions of the small intestine can be altered by reflexes initiated at different points along the gastrointestinal tract. For example, segmentation intensity in the ileum increases during periods of gastric emptying; this is known as the **gastroileal reflex.** Large distensions of the intestine, injury to the intestinal wall, and various bacterial infections in the intestine lead to a complete cessation of motility, the **intestino-intestinal reflex.**

As much as 500 mL of air may be swallowed during a meal. Most of this air travels no farther than the esophagus, from which it is eventually expelled by belching. Some of the air reaches the stomach, however, and is passed on to the intestines, where its percolation through the chyme as the intestinal contents mix produces gurgling sounds that can be quite loud.

Large Intestine

Anatomy and Function

The large intestine is a tube about 6.5 cm (2.5 inches) in diameter and about 1.5 m (5 feet) long. Although the large intestine has a greater diameter than the small intestine, its epithelial surface area is far smaller because the large intestine is shorter than the small intestine, its surface is not convoluted, and its mucosa lacks villi found in the small intestine (see Figure 15.4). The first portion of the large intestine is the **cecum.** A sphincter between the ileum and the cecum is called the **ileocecal valve** (or **sphincter**) and is composed primarily of circular smooth muscle innervated by sympathetic nerves. The circular muscle contracts with distension of the colon and limits the movement of colonic contents backward into the ileum. This prevents bacteria from the large intestine from colonizing the final part of the small intestine. The **appendix** is a small, fingerlike projection that extends from the cecum and may participate in immune function but is not essential (**Figure 15.35**). The **colon** consists of three relatively straight segments—the ascending, transverse, and descending portions. The terminal portion of the descending colon is S-shaped, forming the sigmoid colon, which empties into a relatively straight segment of the large intestine, the rectum, which ends at the anus.

The primary function of the large intestine is to store and concentrate fecal material before defecation. The secretions of the large intestine are scanty, lack digestive enzymes, and consist mostly of mucus and fluid containing HCO_3^- and K^+.

About 1500 mL of chyme enters the large intestine from the small intestine each day. This material is derived largely from the secretions of the lower small intestine because most of the ingested food is absorbed before reaching the large intestine. Fluid absorption by the large intestine normally accounts for only a small fraction of the fluid absorbed by the gastrointestinal tract each day.

The primary absorptive process in the large intestine is the active transport of Na^+ from lumen to extracellular fluid, with the accompanying osmotic absorption of water. If fecal material remains in the large intestine for a long time, almost all the water is absorbed, leaving behind hard fecal pellets. There is normally a net movement of K^+ from blood into the large intestine lumen. Severe depletion of total-body potassium can result when large volumes of fluid are excreted in the feces. There is also a net movement of HCO_3^- into the lumen coupled to Cl^- absorption from the lumen, and loss of this HCO_3^- (a base) in patients with prolonged diarrhea can cause metabolic acidosis (see Chapter 14).

The large intestine also absorbs some of the products formed by the bacteria colonizing this region. It is now recognized that the colonic bacteria make a vital metabolic contribution to health. Undigested polysaccharides (fiber) are converted to short-chain fatty acids by bacteria in the large intestine and absorbed by passive diffusion as well as actively via specific short-chain fatty acid transporters. This route of absorption can represent a significant source of ingested calories and can be even more in obesity. The HCO_3^- secreted by the large intestine helps to neutralize the increased acidity resulting from the formation of these fatty acids. These bacteria also produce small amounts of vitamins, especially vitamin K, for absorption into the blood. Although this source of vitamins generally provides only a small part of the normal daily requirement, it may make a significant contribution when dietary vitamin intake is low. An individual who depends on absorption of nutrients and vitamins formed by bacteria in the large intestine can have adverse health consequences if treated with antibiotics that inhibit other species of bacteria in addition to the disease-causing bacteria.

Other bacterial products include gas (**flatus**), which is a mixture of nitrogen and carbon dioxide, with small amounts of the gases hydrogen, methane, and hydrogen sulfide. Bacterial fermentation of undigested polysaccharides produces these gases in the colon (except for nitrogen, which is derived from swallowed air) at the rate of about 400 to 700 mL/day. Certain foods (beans, for example) contain large amounts of carbohydrates that cannot be digested by intestinal enzymes but are readily metabolized by bacteria in the large intestine, producing large amounts of gas.

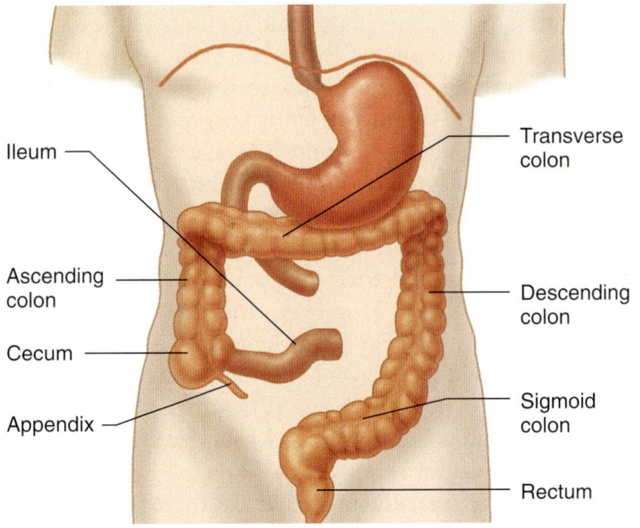

Figure 15.35 APIR The segments of the large intestine. (A portion of the ileum is shown to indicate where the large intestine connects with the small intestine.)

Motility and Defecation

Contractions of the circular smooth muscle in the large intestine produce a segmentation motion with a rhythm considerably slower (one every 30 min) than that in the small intestine. Because of the slow propulsion of the large-intestine contents, material entering the large intestine from the small intestine remains for about 18 to 24 h. This provides time for bacteria to grow and multiply. Three to four times a day, generally following a meal, a wave of intense contraction known as a **mass movement** spreads rapidly over the transverse segment of the large intestine toward the rectum. The large intestine is innervated by parasympathetic and sympathetic nerves. Parasympathetic input increases segmental contractions, whereas sympathetic input decreases colonic contractions.

The anus, the exit from the rectum, is normally closed by the **internal anal sphincter,** composed of smooth muscle, and the **external anal sphincter,** composed of skeletal muscle under voluntary control. The sudden distension of the walls of the rectum produced by the mass movement of fecal material into it initiates the neurally mediated **defecation reflex.** The conscious urge to defecate, mediated by mechanoreceptors, accompanies distension of the rectum. The reflex response consists of a contraction of the rectum and relaxation of the internal anal sphincter but *contraction* of the external anal sphincter (initially) and increased motility in the sigmoid colon. Eventually, a pressure is reached in the rectum that triggers reflex *relaxation* of the external anal sphincter, allowing the feces to be expelled.

Via descending pathways to somatic nerves to the external anal sphincter, however, brain centers can override the reflex signals that eventually would relax the sphincter, thereby keeping the external sphincter closed and allowing a person to delay defecation. In this case, the prolonged distension of the rectum initiates a reverse movement, driving the rectal contents back into the sigmoid colon. The urge to defecate then subsides until the next mass movement again propels more feces into the rectum, increasing its volume and again initiating the defecation reflex. Voluntary control of the external anal sphincter is learned during childhood. Spinal cord damage can lead to a loss of voluntary control over defecation.

Defecation is normally assisted by a deep breath, followed by closure of the glottis and contraction of the abdominal and thoracic muscles, producing an increase in abdominal pressure that is transmitted to the contents of the large intestine and rectum. This maneuver (termed the Valsalva maneuver) also causes an increase in intrathoracic pressure, which leads to a transient increase in blood pressure followed by a decrease in pressure as the venous return to the heart is decreased. The cardiovascular changes resulting from excessive strain during defecation may in rare instances precipitate a stroke or heart attack, especially in constipated elderly people with cardiovascular disease.

15.6 Pathophysiology of the Gastrointestinal Tract

Because the end result of gastrointestinal function is the absorption of nutrients, salts, and water, most malfunctions of this organ system affect either the nutritional state of the body or its salt and water content. The following are a few common examples of disordered gastrointestinal function.

Ulcers

Considering the high concentration of acid and pepsin secreted by the stomach, it is natural to wonder why the stomach does not digest itself. Several factors protect the walls of the stomach from being digested. (1) The surface of the mucosa is lined with cells that secrete slightly alkaline mucus that forms a thin layer over the luminal surface. Both the protein content of mucus and its alkalinity neutralize H^+ in the immediate area of the epithelium. In this way, mucus forms a chemical barrier between the highly acidic contents of the lumen and the cell surface. (2) The tight junctions between the epithelial cells lining the stomach restrict the diffusion of H^+ into the underlying tissues. (3) Damaged epithelial cells are replaced every few days by new cells arising by the division of cells within the gastric pits.

At times, these protective mechanisms can prove inadequate, and erosion (***ulcers***) of the gastric surface can develop. Ulcers can occur not only in the stomach but also in the lower part of the esophagus and in the duodenum. Indeed, duodenal ulcers are about 10 times more frequent than gastric ulcers, affecting about 10% of the U.S. population. Damage to blood vessels in the tissues underlying the ulcer may cause bleeding into the gastrointestinal lumen (**Figure 15.36**). On occasion, the ulcer may penetrate the entire wall, resulting in leakage of the luminal contents into the abdominal cavity. A device used to diagnose gastric and duodenal ulcers is the ***endoscope*** (see Figure 15.36). This uses either fiber-optic or video technology to directly visualize the gastric and duodenal mucosa. Furthermore, the endoscopist can apply local treatments and take samples of tissue (***biopsy***) during upper endoscopy. Similar devices can be used to visualize the colon (flexible ***sigmoidoscopy*** or ***colonoscopy***).

Ulcer formation involves breaking the mucosal barrier and exposing the underlying tissue to the corrosive action of acid and pepsin, but it is not always clear what produces the initial damage to the barrier. Although acid is essential for ulcer formation, it is not necessarily the primary factor; many patients with ulcers have normal or even subnormal rates of acid secretion.

Many factors, including genetic susceptibility, drugs, alcohol, bile salts, and an excessive secretion of acid and pepsin, may contribute to ulcer formation. The major factor, however, is the presence of a bacterium, *Helicobacter pylori*, that is present in the stomachs of a majority of patients with ulcers or ***gastritis*** (inflammation of the stomach walls). Suppression of these bacteria with antibiotics usually helps heal the damaged mucosa.

Once an ulcer has formed, the inhibition of acid secretion can remove the constant irritation and allow the ulcer to heal. Two classes of drugs are potent inhibitors of acid secretion. One class of inhibitors acts by blocking a specific class of histamine receptors (H_2) found on parietal cells, which stimulate acid secretion. An example of an H_2 receptor antagonist is ***cimetidine***. The second class of drugs directly inhibits the H^+/K^+-ATPase pump in parietal cells. Examples of these so-called proton-pump inhibitors are ***omeprazole*** and ***lansoprazole***. Although both classes of drugs are effective in healing ulcers, the ulcers tend to recur if the *Helicobacter pylori* bacteria are not removed.

Despite popular notions, the role of stress in producing ulcers remains unclear. Once the ulcer has been formed, however, emotional stress can aggravate it by increasing acid secretion and also decreasing appetite and food intake.

Vomiting

Vomiting is the forceful expulsion of the contents of the stomach and upper intestinal tract through the mouth. Like swallowing, vomiting is a complex reflex coordinated by a region in the brainstem medulla oblongata, in this case known as the **vomiting center.** Neural input to this center from receptors in many different regions of the body can initiate the vomiting reflex. For example, excessive distension of the stomach or small intestine, various substances acting upon chemoreceptors in the intestinal wall or in the brain, increased pressure within the skull, rotating movements of the head (motion sickness), intense pain, and tactile stimuli applied to the back of the throat can all initiate vomiting. The **area postrema** in the brain, which is outside the blood–brain barrier, is sensitive to toxins in the blood and can initiate vomiting. There are many chemicals (***emetics***) that can stimulate vomiting via receptors in the stomach, duodenum, or brain.

What is the adaptive value of this reflex? Obviously, the removal of ingested toxic substances before they can be absorbed is beneficial. Moreover, the nausea that usually accompanies vomiting may have the adaptive value of conditioning the individual to avoid the future ingestion of foods containing such toxic substances. Why other types of stimuli, such as those producing motion sickness, have become linked to the vomiting center is not clear.

Vomiting is usually preceded by increased salivation, sweating, increased heart rate, pallor, and nausea. The events leading to vomiting begin with a deep breath, closure of the glottis, and elevation of the soft palate. The abdominal muscles then contract, thereby increasing the abdominal pressure,

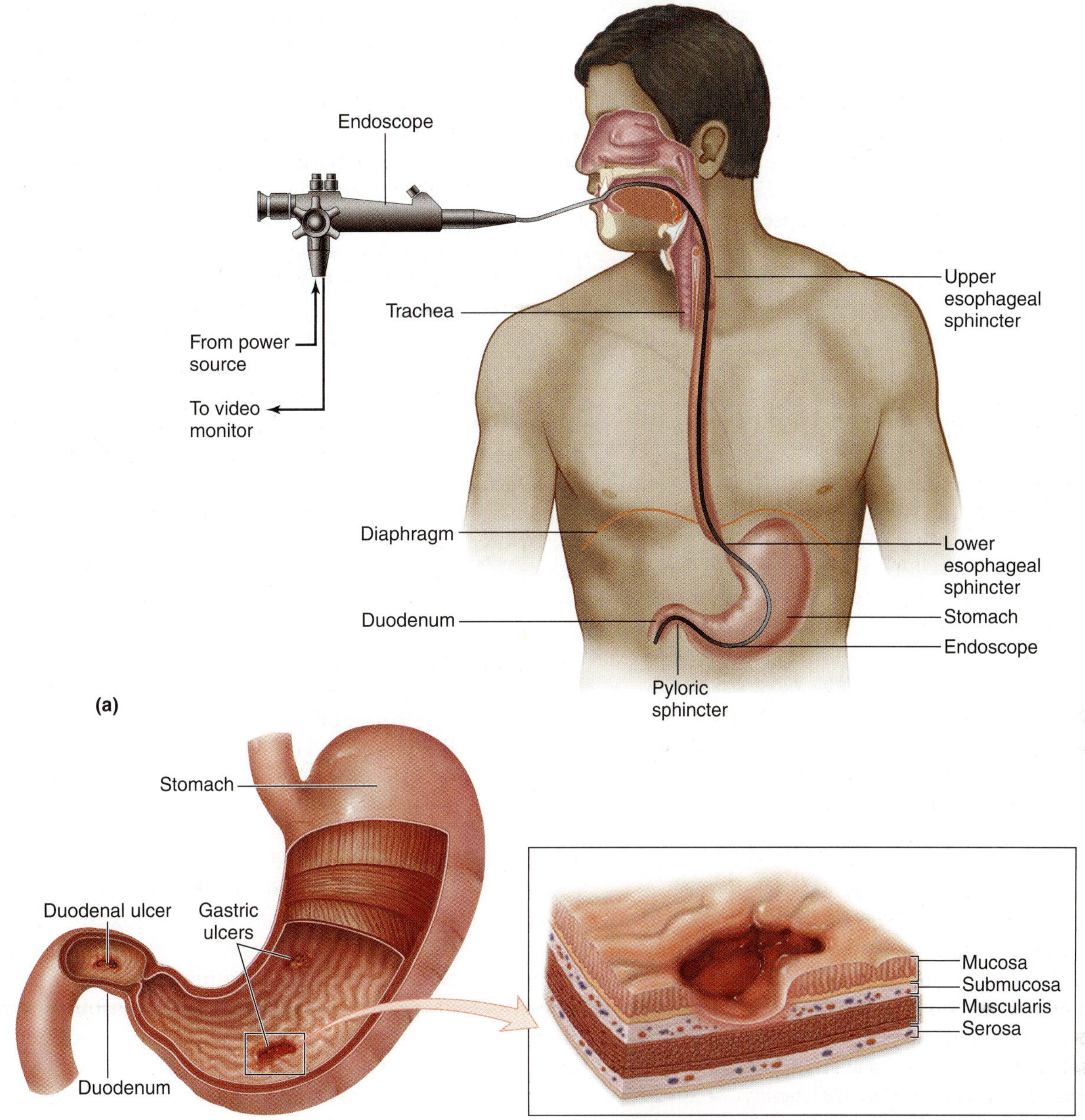

(b) Common locations of gastric and duodenal ulcers

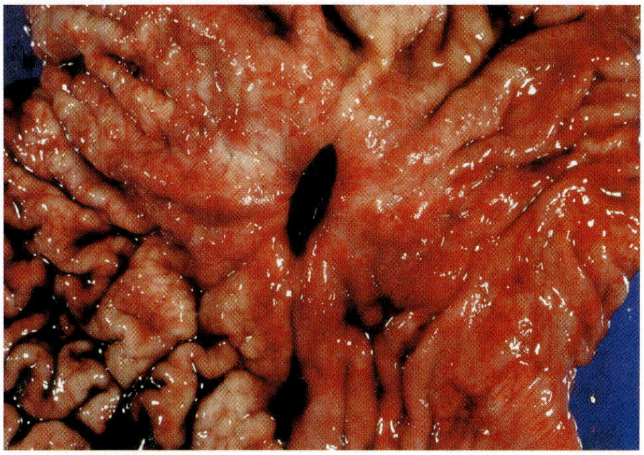

(c) Perforated gastric ulcer

Figure 15.36 APIR (a) Video endoscopy of the upper GI tract. The physician passes the endoscope through the mouth (or nose) down the esophagus, through the stomach, and into the duodenum. A light source at the tip of the endoscope illuminates the mucosa. The tip also has a miniature video chip, which transmits images up the endoscope to a video recorder. Local treatments can be applied and small tissue samples (biopsies) can be taken with the endoscope. Earlier versions of this device used fiber-optic technology. (b) and (c) Illustration and photo of the typical location and appearance of gastric and duodenal ulcers.

which is transmitted to the stomach's contents. The lower esophageal sphincter relaxes, and the high abdominal pressure forces the contents of the stomach into the esophagus. This initial sequence of events, which can occur repeatedly without expulsion via the mouth, is known as ***retching.*** Vomiting occurs when the abdominal contractions become so strong that the increased intrathoracic pressure forces the contents of the esophagus through the upper esophageal sphincter.

Vomiting is also accompanied by strong contractions in the upper portion of the small intestine—contractions that tend to force some of the intestinal contents back into the stomach for expulsion. Thus, some bile may be present in the vomitus.

Excessive vomiting can lead to large losses of the water and salts that normally would be absorbed in the small intestine. This can result in severe dehydration, upset the body's salt balance, and produce circulatory problems due to a decrease in plasma volume. The loss of acid from vomiting results in metabolic alkalosis (see Chapter 14). A variety of antiemetic drugs can suppress vomiting.

Gallstones

As described earlier, bile contains not only bile salts but also cholesterol and phospholipids, which are water-insoluble and are maintained in soluble form in the bile as micelles. When the concentration of cholesterol in the bile becomes high in relation to the concentrations of phospholipid and bile salts, cholesterol crystallizes out of solution, forming ***gallstones.*** This can occur if the liver secretes excessive amounts of cholesterol or if the cholesterol becomes overly concentrated in the gallbladder as a result of salt and water absorption. Although cholesterol gallstones are the most frequently encountered gallstones in the Western world, the precipitation of bile pigments can also occasionally be responsible for gallstone formation.

If a gallstone is small, it may pass through the common bile duct into the intestine with no complications. A larger stone may become lodged in the opening of the gallbladder, causing painful contractile spasms of the smooth muscle. A more serious complication arises when a gallstone lodges in the common bile duct, thereby preventing bile from entering the intestine. A large decrease in bile can decrease fat digestion and absorption. Furthermore, impaired absorption of the fat-soluble vitamins A, D, K, and E can occur, leading to, for example, clotting problems (vitamin K deficiency) and calcium malabsorption (due to vitamin D deficiency). The fat that is not absorbed enters the large intestine and eventually appears in the feces (a condition known as ***steatorrhea***). Furthermore, bacteria in the large intestine convert some of this fat into fatty acid derivatives that alter salt and water movements, leading to a net flow of fluid into the large intestine. The results are diarrhea and fluid and nutrient loss.

Because the duct from the pancreas joins the common bile duct just before it enters the duodenum, a gallstone that becomes lodged at this point prevents both bile and pancreatic secretions from entering the intestine. This results in failure to both neutralize acid and adequately digest most organic nutrients, not just fat. The end results are severe nutritional deficiencies.

The buildup of very high pressure in a blocked common bile duct is transmitted back to the liver and interferes with the further secretion of bile. As a result, bilirubin, which is normally secreted into the bile by uptake from the blood in the liver, accumulates in the blood and diffuses into tissues, producing a yellowish coloration of the skin and eyes known as ***jaundice.***

At birth, the liver's capacity to secrete bilirubin is not fully developed. During the first few days of life, this may result in ***hemolytic jaundice of the newborn,*** which normally clears spontaneously. Excessive accumulation of bilirubin during the neonatal period, as occurs, for example, with hemolytic disease of the newborn (see Chapter 18), carries a risk of bilirubin-induced neurological damage during a critical phase in the development of the nervous system.

Although surgery may be necessary to remove an inflamed gallbladder (***cholecystectomy***) or stones from an obstructed duct, newer techniques use drugs to dissolve gallstones. Patients who have had a cholecystectomy still make bile and transport it to the small intestine via the bile duct. Therefore, fat digestion and absorption can be maintained, but bile secretion and fat intake in the diet are no longer coupled. Thus, large, fatty meals are difficult to digest because of the absence of a large pool of bile normally released from the gallbladder in response to CCK. A diet low in fat content is usually advisable.

Lactose Intolerance

Lactose is the major carbohydrate in milk. It cannot be absorbed directly but must first be digested into its components, glucose and galactose, which are readily absorbed by active transport. Lactose is digested by the enzyme **lactase,** which is embedded in the luminal plasma membranes of intestinal epithelial cells. Lactase is usually present at birth and allows the nursing infant to digest the lactose in breast milk. Because the only dietary source of lactose is from milk and milk products, all mammals—including most humans—lose the ability to digest this disaccharide around the time of weaning. With the exception of people descended from a few regions of the world—notably, those of Northern Europe and parts of central Africa, the vast majority of people undergo a decline in lactase production beginning at about 2 years of age. This leads to ***lactose intolerance***—the inability to completely digest lactose such that its concentration increases in the small intestine. Current hypotheses for why certain populations of people retained the ability to express lactase relate to a mutation in the regulatory region of the lactase gene that occurred around the time certain groups of neolithic humans domesticated cattle as a food source.

Because the absorption of water requires prior absorption of solute to provide an osmotic gradient, the unabsorbed lactose in persons with lactose intolerance prevents some of the water from being absorbed. This lactose-containing fluid is passed on to the large intestine, where bacteria digest the lactose. They then metabolize the released monosaccharides, producing large quantities of gas (which distends the colon, producing pain) and short-chain fatty acids, which cause fluid movement into the lumen of the large intestine, producing diarrhea. The response to ingestion of milk or dairy products by adults whose lactase levels have diminished varies from mild discomfort to severely dehydrating diarrhea, according to the volume of milk and dairy products ingested and the amount of lactase present in the intestine. The person can avoid these symptoms by either drinking milk in which the lactose has been predigested with added lactase enzyme or taking pills containing lactase along with the milk.

Constipation and Diarrhea

Many people have a mistaken belief that, unless they have a bowel movement every day, the absorption of "toxic" substances from fecal material in the large intestine will somehow poison them. Attempts to identify such toxic agents in the blood following prolonged periods of fecal retention have been unsuccessful, and there appears to be no physiological necessity for having bowel movements at frequent intervals. This reinforces a point made earlier in this chapter that the contribution of the GI tract to the elimination of waste products is usually small compared to the lungs and kidneys. Whatever maintains a person in a comfortable state is physiologically adequate, whether this means a bowel movement after every meal, once a day, or only once a week.

On the other hand, some symptoms—headache, loss of appetite, nausea, and abdominal distension—may arise when defecation has not occurred for several days or even weeks, depending on the individual. These *symptoms* of ***constipation*** are caused not by toxins but by distension of the rectum. The longer that fecal material remains in the large intestine, the more water is absorbed and the harder and drier the feces become, making defecation more difficult and sometimes painful.

Decreased motility of the large intestine is the primary factor causing constipation. This often occurs in elderly people, or it may result from damage to the colon's enteric nervous system or from emotional stress.

One of the factors increasing motility in the large intestine—and thus opposing the development of constipation—is distension. As noted earlier, dietary fiber (cellulose and other complex polysaccharides) is not digested by the enzymes in the small intestine and is passed on to the large intestine, where its bulk produces distension and thereby increases motility. Bran, most fruits, and vegetables are examples of foods that have a relatively high fiber content.

Laxatives, agents that increase the frequency or ease of defecation, act through a variety of mechanisms. Fiber provides a natural laxative. Some laxatives, such as mineral oil, simply lubricate the feces, making defecation easier and less painful. Others contain magnesium and aluminum salts, which are poorly absorbed and therefore lead to water retention in the intestinal tract. Still others, such as castor oil, stimulate the motility of the colon and inhibit ion transport across the wall, resulting in decreased water absorption.

Excessive use of laxatives in an attempt to maintain a preconceived notion of regularity leads to a decreased responsiveness of the large intestine to normal defecation-promoting signals. In such cases, a long period without defecation may occur following cessation of laxative intake, appearing to confirm the necessity of taking laxatives to promote regularity.

Diarrhea is characterized by large, frequent, watery stools. Diarrhea can result from decreased fluid absorption, increased fluid secretion, or both. The increased motility that accompanies diarrhea probably does not cause most cases of diarrhea (by decreasing the time available for fluid absorption) but, rather, results from the distension produced by increased luminal fluid.

A number of bacterial, protozoan, and viral diseases of the intestinal tract cause secretory diarrhea. ***Cholera,*** which is endemic in many parts of the world, is caused by a bacterium that releases a toxin that stimulates the production of cyclic AMP in the secretory cells at the base of the intestinal villi. This leads to an increased frequency in the opening of the Cl^- channels in the luminal membrane and, hence, increased secretion of Cl^-. An accompanying osmotic flow of water into the intestinal lumen occurs, resulting in massive diarrhea that can be life threatening due to dehydration and decreased blood volume that leads to circulatory shock. The salt and water lost by this severe form of diarrhea can be balanced by ingesting a simple solution containing salt and glucose. The active absorption of these solutes is accompanied by absorption of water, which replaces the fluid lost by diarrhea. ***Traveler's diarrhea,*** produced by several species of bacteria, produces a secretory diarrhea by the same mechanism as the cholera bacterium but is usually less severe.

In addition to decreased blood volume due to salt and water loss, other consequences of severe diarrhea are potassium depletion and metabolic acidosis (see Chapter 14) resulting from the excessive fecal loss of K^+ and HCO_3^-, respectively.

SUMMARY

Overview of the Digestive System

I. The digestive system transfers digested organic nutrients, minerals, and water from the external environment to the internal environment. The four major processes used to accomplish this function are digestion, secretion, absorption, and motility.
   a. The system functions to maximize the absorption of most nutrients, not to regulate the amount absorbed.
   b. The system does not play a major role in the removal of waste products from the internal environment; therefore, elimination is usually not listed as a major function compared to the lungs and kidneys.

Structure of the Gastrointestinal Tract Wall

I. Figure 15.3 diagrams the structure of the wall of the gastrointestinal tract.
   a. The area available for absorption in the small intestine is greatly increased by the folding of the intestinal wall and by the presence of villi and microvilli on the surface of the epithelial cells.
   b. The epithelial cells lining the intestinal tract are continuously replaced by new cells arising from cell division at the base of the villi.
   c. The venous blood from the small intestine, containing absorbed nutrients other than fat, passes to the liver via the hepatic portal vein before returning to the heart. Fat is absorbed into the lymphatic vessels (lacteals) in each villus.

General Functions of the Gastrointestinal and Accessory Organs

I. Table 15.1 summarizes the names and functions of the gastrointestinal organs.

II. Each day, the gastrointestinal tract secretes about six times more fluid into the lumen than is ingested. Only 1% of this fluid is excreted in the feces.

Digestion and Absorption

I. Starch is digested by amylases secreted by the salivary glands and pancreas. The resulting products, as well as ingested disaccharides, are digested to monosaccharides by enzymes in the luminal membranes of epithelial cells in the small intestine.
   a. Most monosaccharides are then absorbed by secondary active transport.
   b. Some polysaccharides, such as cellulose, cannot be digested and pass to the large intestine, where bacteria metabolize them.

II. Proteins are broken down into small peptides and amino acids, which are absorbed by secondary active transport in the small intestine.
   a. The breakdown of proteins to peptides is catalyzed by pepsin in the stomach and by the pancreatic enzymes trypsin and chymotrypsin in the small intestine.
   b. Peptides are broken down into amino acids by pancreatic carboxypeptidase and intestinal aminopeptidase.
   c. Small peptides consisting of two to three amino acids can be actively absorbed into epithelial cells and then broken down to amino acids, which are released into the blood.

III. The digestion and absorption of fat by the small intestine require mechanisms that solubilize the fat and its digestion products.
   a. Large fat globules leaving the stomach are emulsified in the small intestine by bile salts and phospholipids secreted by the liver.
   b. Lipase from the pancreas digests fat at the surface of the emulsion droplets, forming fatty acids and monoglycerides.
   c. These water-insoluble products of lipase action, when combined with bile salts, form micelles, which are in equilibrium with the free molecules.
   d. Free fatty acids and monoglycerides diffuse across the luminal membranes of epithelial cells, where they are enzymatically recombined to form triglycerides, which are released as chylomicrons from the blood side of the cell by exocytosis.
   e. The released chylomicrons enter lacteals in the intestinal villi and pass by way of the lymphatic system and the thoracic duct to the venous blood returning to the heart.

IV. Fat-soluble vitamins are absorbed by the same pathway used for fat absorption. Most water-soluble vitamins are absorbed in the small intestine by diffusion or mediated transport. Vitamin B_{12} is absorbed in the ileum by endocytosis after combining with intrinsic factor secreted into the lumen by parietal cells in the stomach.

V. Water is absorbed from the small intestine by osmosis following the active absorption of solutes, primarily sodium chloride.

How Are Gastrointestinal Processes Regulated?

I. Most gastrointestinal reflexes are initiated by luminal stimuli: distension, osmolarity, acidity, and digestion products.
   a. Neural reflexes are mediated by short reflexes in the enteric nervous system and by long reflexes involving afferent and efferent neurons to and from the CNS.
   b. Endocrine cells scattered throughout the epithelium of the stomach secrete gastrin; and cells in the small intestine secrete secretin, CCK, and GIP. Table 15.4 lists the properties of these hormones.
   c. The three phases of gastrointestinal regulation—cephalic, gastric, and intestinal—are each named for the location of the stimulus that initiates the response.

II. Chewing breaks up food into particles suitable for swallowing, but it is not essential for the eventual digestion and absorption of food.

III. Salivary secretion is stimulated by food in the mouth acting reflexively via chemoreceptors and pressure receptors and by sensory stimuli (e.g., sight or smell of food). Both sympathetic stimulation and parasympathetic stimulation increase salivary secretion.

IV. Food moved into the pharynx by the tongue initiates swallowing, which is coordinated by the swallowing center in the brainstem medulla oblongata.
   a. Food is prevented from entering the trachea by inhibition of respiration and by closure of the glottis.
   b. The upper esophageal sphincter relaxes as food is moved into the esophagus, and then the sphincter closes.
   c. Food is moved through the esophagus toward the stomach by peristaltic waves. The lower esophageal sphincter remains open throughout swallowing.
   d. If food does not reach the stomach with the first peristaltic wave, distension of the esophagus initiates secondary peristalsis.

V. Table 15.5 summarizes the factors controlling acid secretion by parietal cells in the stomach.

VI. Pepsinogen, secreted by the gastric chief cells in response to most of the same reflexes that control acid secretion, is converted to the active proteolytic enzyme pepsin in the stomach's lumen, primarily by acid.

VII. Peristaltic waves sweeping over the stomach become stronger in the antrum, where most mixing occurs. With each wave, only a small portion of the stomach's contents is expelled into the small intestine through the pyloric sphincter.
   a. Cycles of membrane depolarization, the basic electrical rhythm generated by gastric smooth muscle, determine gastric peristaltic wave frequency. Contraction strength can be altered by neural and hormonal changes in membrane potential, which is imposed on the basic electrical rhythm.
   b. Distension of the stomach increases the force of contractions and the rate of emptying. Distension of the small intestine and fat, acid, or hypertonic solutions in the intestinal lumen inhibit gastric contractions.

VIII. The exocrine portion of the pancreas secretes digestive enzymes and HCO_3^-, all of which reach the duodenum through the pancreatic duct.
   a. The HCO_3^- neutralizes acid entering the small intestine from the stomach.
   b. Most of the proteolytic enzymes, including trypsin, are secreted by the pancreas in inactive forms. Trypsin is activated by enterokinase located on the membranes of the small-intestine cells; trypsin then activates other inactive pancreatic enzymes.
   c. The hormone secretin, released from the small intestine in response to increased luminal acidity, stimulates pancreatic HCO_3^- secretion. The small intestine releases CCK in response to the products of fat and protein digestion. CCK then stimulates pancreatic enzyme secretion.
   d. Parasympathetic stimulation increases pancreatic secretion.

IX. The liver secretes bile, the major ingredients of which are bile salts, cholesterol, lecithin, HCO_3^-, bile pigments, and trace metals.
   a. Bile salts undergo continuous enterohepatic recirculation during a meal. The liver synthesizes new bile salts to replace those lost in the feces.
   b. The greater the bile salt concentration in the hepatic portal blood, the greater the rate of bile secretion.
   c. Bilirubin, the major bile pigment, is a breakdown product of hemoglobin and is absorbed from the blood by the liver and secreted into the bile.
   d. Secretin stimulates HCO_3^- secretion by the cells lining the bile ducts in the liver.
   e. Bile is concentrated in the gallbladder by the absorption of NaCl and water.
   f. Following a meal, the release of CCK from the small intestine causes the gallbladder to contract and the sphincter of Oddi to relax, thereby injecting concentrated bile into the intestine.

X. In the small intestine, the digestion of polysaccharides and proteins increases the osmolarity of the luminal contents, producing water flow into the lumen.

XI. Na^+, Cl^-, HCO_3^-, and water are secreted by the small intestine. However, most of these secreted substances, as well as those entering the small intestine from other sources, are absorbed back into the blood.

XII. Intestinal motility is coordinated by the enteric nervous system and modified by long and short reflexes and hormones.
   a. During and shortly after a meal, the intestinal contents are mixed by segmenting movements of the intestinal wall.
   b. After most of the food has been digested and absorbed, the migrating myoelectrical complex (MMC), which moves the undigested material into the large intestine by a migrating segment of peristaltic waves, replaces segmentation.

XIII. The primary function of the large intestine is to store and concentrate fecal matter before defecation.
   a. Water is absorbed from the large intestine secondary to the active absorption of Na^+, leading to the concentration of fecal matter.
   b. Flatus is produced by bacterial fermentation of undigested polysaccharides.
   c. Three to four times a day, mass movements in the colon move its contents into the rectum.
   d. Distension of the rectum initiates defecation, which is assisted by a forced expiration against a closed glottis.
   e. Defecation can be voluntarily controlled through somatic nerves to the skeletal muscles of the external anal sphincter.

Pathophysiology of the Gastrointestinal Tract

I. The factors that normally prevent breakdown of the mucosal barrier and formation of ulcers are secretion of an alkaline mucus, tight junctions between epithelial cells, and rapid replacement of epithelial cells.
   a. The bacterium *Helicobacter pylori* is a major cause of damage to the mucosal barrier, leading to ulcers.
   b. Drugs that block histamine receptors or inhibit the H^+/K^+-ATPase pump inhibit acid secretion and promote ulcer healing.

II. Vomiting is coordinated by the vomiting center in the brainstem medulla oblongata. Contractions of abdominal muscles force the contents of the stomach into the esophagus (retching); if the contractions are strong enough, they force the contents of the esophagus through the upper esophageal sphincter into the mouth (vomiting).

III. Precipitation of cholesterol or, less often, bile pigments in the gallbladder forms gallstones, which can block the exit of the gallbladder or common bile duct. In the latter case, the failure of bile salts to reach the intestine causes decreased fat digestion and absorption; the accumulation of bile pigments in the blood and tissues causes jaundice.

IV. Lactase activity, which is present at birth, undergoes a genetically determined decrease during childhood in many individuals. In the absence of lactase, lactose cannot be digested, and its presence in the small intestine can cause diarrhea and increased flatus production when milk products are ingested.

V. Constipation is primarily the result of decreased colonic motility. The symptoms of constipation are produced by overdistension of the rectum, not by the absorption of toxic bacterial products.

VI. Diarrhea can be caused by decreased fluid absorption, increased fluid secretion, or both.

REVIEW QUESTIONS

1. List the four processes that accomplish the functions of the digestive system.
2. List the primary functions performed by each of the organs in the digestive system.
3. Approximately how much fluid is secreted into the gastrointestinal tract each day compared with the amount of food and drink ingested? How much of this appears in the feces?
4. What structures are responsible for the large surface area of the small intestine?
5. Where does the venous blood go after leaving the small intestine?
6. Identify the enzymes involved in carbohydrate digestion and the mechanism of carbohydrate absorption in the small intestine.
7. List three ways in which proteins or their digestion products can be absorbed from the small intestine.
8. Describe the process of fat emulsification.
9. What is the role of micelles in fat absorption?
10. Describe the movement of fat-digestion products from the intestinal lumen to a lacteal.
11. How does the absorption of fat-soluble vitamins differ from that of water-soluble vitamins?
12. Specify two conditions that may lead to failure to absorb vitamin B_{12}.
13. How are salts and water absorbed in the small intestine?
14. Describe the role of ferritin in the absorption of iron.
15. List the four types of stimuli that initiate most gastrointestinal reflexes.
16. Describe the location of the enteric nervous system and its role in both short and long reflexes.
17. Name the four best-understood gastrointestinal hormones and state their major functions.
18. Describe the neural reflexes leading to increased salivary secretion.
19. Describe the sequence of events that occur during swallowing.
20. List the cephalic, gastric, and intestinal phase stimuli that stimulate or inhibit acid secretion by the stomach.
21. Describe the function of gastrin and the factors controlling its secretion.

22. By what mechanism is pepsinogen converted to pepsin in the stomach?
23. Describe the factors that control gastric emptying.
24. Describe the mechanisms controlling pancreatic secretion of HCO_3^- and enzymes.
25. How are pancreatic proteolytic enzymes activated in the small intestine?
26. List the major constituents of bile.
27. Describe the recycling of bile salts by the enterohepatic circulation.
28. What determines the rate of bile secretion by the liver?
29. Describe the effects of secretin and CCK on the bile ducts and gallbladder.
30. What causes water to move from the blood to the lumen of the duodenum following gastric emptying?
31. Describe the type of intestinal motility found during and shortly after a meal and the type found several hours after a meal.
32. Describe the production of flatus by the large intestine.
33. Describe the factors that initiate and control defecation.
34. Why is the stomach's wall normally not digested by the acid and digestive enzymes in the lumen?
35. Describe the process of vomiting.
36. What are the consequences of blocking the common bile duct with a gallstone?
37. What are the consequences of the failure to digest lactose in the small intestine?
38. Contrast the factors that cause constipation with those that produce diarrhea.
39. Describe the two main types of inflammatory bowel disease.

KEY TERMS

absorption 535
alimentary canal 534
aminopeptidase 541
amylase 538
antrum 550
anus 534
appendix 561
area postrema 562
aspiration 548
basic electrical rhythm 554
bile 539
bile canaliculi 558
bile pigment 558
bile salt 539
bilirubin 558
body (of stomach) 550
brush border 536
canaliculus (parietal cell) 551
carboxypeptidase 541
cecum 560
cephalic phase 547
chief cell 551
cholecystokinin (CCK) 546
chylomicron 544
chyme 538
chymotrypsin 541
circular fold 536
circular muscle 536
colipase 543
colon 561
common bile duct 540
cystic fibrosis transmembrane conductance regulator (CFTR) 555
defecation 540
defecation reflex 561
digestion 534
digestive system 534
duodenum 538
elimination 535
emulsification 542
enteric nervous system 546
enterochromaffin-like (ECL) cell 551
enteroendocrine cell 537
enterogastrone 553
enterohepatic circulation 558
enterokinase 556
epiglottis 548
esophagus 538
external anal sphincter 561
feces 535
ferritin 545
fiber 541
flatus 561
fundus 550
gallbladder 540
gastric 538
gastric phase 548
gastrin 546
gastroileal reflex 560
gastrointestinal (GI) tract 534
glottis 548
glucose-dependent insulinotropic peptide (GIP) 546
gluten 545
goblet cells 536
hepatic 537
hepatic lobules 557
hepatic portal vein 537
hepatocyte 557
hydrochloric acid 550
ileocecal valve (sphincter) 560
ileum 538
internal anal sphincter 561
interstitial cells of Cajal 560
intestinal phase 548
intestino-intestinal reflex 560
intrinsic factor 545
jejunum 538
lactase 564
lacteal 537
lamina propria 535
large intestine 538
lipase 542
liver 539
longitudinal muscle 536
long reflex 546
lower esophageal sphincter 548
mass movement 561
micelle 543
microvilli 536
migrating myoelectrical complex (MMC) 560
motilin 560
motility 535
mouth 538
mucosa 535
muscularis externa 535
muscularis mucosa 535
myenteric plexus 536
pancreas 538
parietal cell 550
pepsin 541
pepsinogen 541
peristalsis 535
peristaltic waves 549
Peyer's patches 538
pharynx 538
portal triad 557
potentiation 546
pyloric sphincter 554
receptive relaxation 554
rectum 540
retropulsion 554
saliva 538
salivary gland 538
secondary peristalsis 549
secretin 546
secretion 534
segmentation 560
serosa 536
short reflex 546
small intestine 538
somatostatin 551
sphincter 548
sphincter of Oddi 559
stomach 538
submucosa 535
submucosal plexus 535
swallowing center 548
thoracic duct 537
trypsin 541
trypsinogen 556
upper esophageal sphincter 548
villi 536
vomiting center 562
zymogen 553

CLINICAL TERMS

biopsy 562
cholecystectomy 564
cholera 565
cimetidine 562
colonoscopy 562
constipation 565
cystic fibrosis 556
diarrhea 565
emetics 562
endoscope 562
gallstones 564
gastritis 562
gastroesophageal reflux 550
heartburn 550
hemochromatosis 545
hemolytic jaundice of the newborn 564
jaundice 564
lactose intolerance 564
lansoprazole 562
laxatives 565
malabsorption 544
nontropical sprue (celiac disease; gluten-sensitive enteropathy) 545
omeprazole 562
pernicious anemia 545
phlebotomy 545
retching 563
sigmoidoscopy 562
Sjögren's syndrome 548
steatorrhea 564
traveler's diarrhea 565
ulcers 562

Clinical Case Study: A College Student with Weight Loss, Cramps, Diarrhea, and Chills

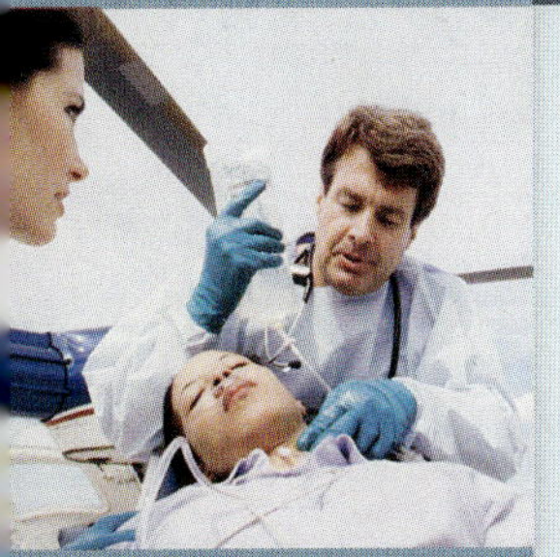

A 19-year-old college student has noticed some lower-right-quadrant abdominal cramping followed by diarrhea, particularly a few hours after eating popcorn, salads with a lot of lettuce, and uncooked vegetables. Over the semester, the cramps and diarrhea have gotten progressively worse and he has started to have fevers and chills. Despite eating a normal caloric intake, he has noticed some weight loss. He finally goes to the student health clinic, and the nurse practitioner refers him to a gastroenterologist (a physician specializing in diseases of the digestive system). After ruling out acute appendicitis, the physician orders a radiological test called a GI series with small-bowel follow-through. In these tests, the patient drinks a liquid containing barium (which is radiopaque) and then x-ray images are taken of the small and large intestine as the barium moves through the gastrointestinal tract (**Figure 15.37**). ***Strictures*** (narrowing) and other abnormalities of the intestines due to inflammation of the mucosa are readily observed with this test and were visible in the terminal ileum of our patient. Based on his symptoms and the result of the barium test, a diagnosis of inflammatory bowel disease (IBD)—specifically, Crohn's disease—was made.

The general term ***inflammatory bowel disease*** comprises two related diseases—***Crohn's disease*** and ***ulcerative colitis***. Both diseases involve chronic inflammation of the bowel. Crohn's disease can occur anywhere along the GI tract from the mouth to the anus, although it is most common near the end of the ileum, as in our patient. Colitis is confined to the colon. The incidence of IBD in the United States is 7 to 11 per 100,000 people and is most common in Caucasian people, particularly those of Ashkenazi Jewish descent. The most common ages of onset for IBD are in the late teens to early 20s and then again in people older than 60.

Although the precise cause or causes of IBD are not certain, it seems that it occurs as a combination of environmental and genetic factors. There appears to be a genetic predisposition for an abnormal response of the bowel mucosa to infection and the presence of normal luminal bacteria. Therefore, IBD appears to result from inappropriate immune and tissue-repair responses to essentially normal microorganisms in the intestinal lumen.

Active Crohn's disease shows inflammation and thickening of the bowel wall such that the lumen can become narrowed to the point at which it may even become blocked or obstructed, which can be very painful. The abdominal pain is often aggravated by eating meals rich in fiber (like uncooked vegetables and popcorn)—this roughage physically irritates the inflamed bowel. The part of the small intestine at the end of the ileum is the most common site of Crohn's disease, so the first symptoms experienced by patients with this disease are often pain in the lower-right abdomen and diarrhea. Because the disease is often accompanied by fever due to the immune response and pain in the lower-right quadrant of the abdomen, the initial symptoms can be mistaken for acute appendicitis (see Chapter 19). Because of its obstructive nature due to luminal narrowing, the abdominal pain in Crohn's disease can be temporarily relieved by defecation.

Ulcerative colitis is caused by disruption of the normal mucosa with the presence of bleeding, edema, and ulcerations (losses of tissue due to inflammation). When ulcerative colitis is most extreme, the bowel wall can get so thin and the loss of tissue so great that perforations all the way through the bowel wall can occur. The main symptoms of ulcerative colitis are diarrhea, rectal bleeding, and abdominal cramps.

The current initial treatment of IBD is the use of 5-aminosalicylate drugs, such as ***sulfasalazine,*** which appear to have both antibacterial and anti-inflammatory effects, and this is what our patient was treated with. However, he was advised by his physician that if the symptoms became more severe, additional drug therapy might be required. He was also advised to alter his diet to decrease the amount of roughage. Often, in more severe cases, the use of glucocorticoids as anti-inflammatory drugs can be very useful, although their overuse has significant risks such as loss of bone mass. It is often helpful to make adjustments in the diet to allow the inflamed bowel time to heal. Finally, new drug therapy using immunosuppressive medicines such as ***tacrolimus*** and ***cyclosporine*** show promise. When IBD becomes sufficiently severe and not responsive to drug therapy, surgery is sometimes necessary to remove the diseased bowel.

Clinical terms: Crohn's disease, cyclosporine, inflammatory bowel disease, stricture, sulfasalazine, tacrolimus, ulcerative colitis

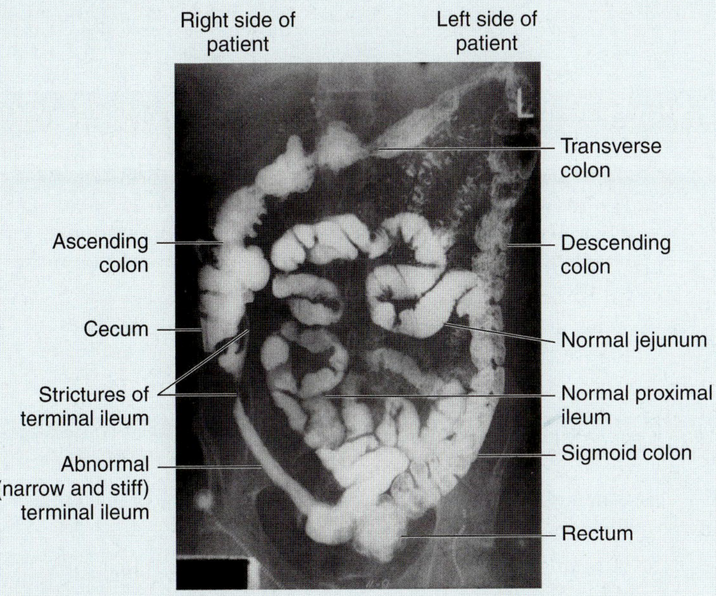

Figure 15.37 Radiograph (x-ray image) of the abdomen with barium contrast in the lumen of the small and large intestine. Notice the severe narrowing (strictures) of the terminal ileum in the lower-right quadrant of the patient, which is characteristic of Crohn's disease. This narrowing of the lumen is due to the inflammation and swelling of the mucosa. A segment of ileum below the strictures is also abnormal—it lacks the normal convolutions of the small intestine because of the inflammation of the mucosa. Figure courtesy of David Olson, M.D., Aurora St. Luke's Medical Center.

See Chapter 19 for complete, integrative case studies.

CHAPTER 15 TEST QUESTIONS

Answers found in Appendix A.

1–4: Match the gastrointestinal hormone (a–d) with its description (1–4).

Hormone:

a. gastrin
b. CCK
c. secretin
d. GIP

Description:

1. It is stimulated by the presence of acid in the small intestine and stimulates HCO_3^- release from the pancreas and bile ducts.
2. It is stimulated by glucose and fat in the small intestine and increases insulin and amplifies the insulin responses to glucose.
3. It is inhibited by acid in the stomach and stimulates acid secretion from the stomach.
4. It is stimulated by amino acids and fatty acids in the small intestine and stimulates pancreatic enzyme secretion.
5. Which of the following is *true* about pepsin?
   a. Most pepsin is released directly from chief cells.
   b. Pepsin is most active at high pH.
   c. Pepsin is essential for protein digestion.
   d. Pepsin accelerates protein digestion.
   e. Pepsin accelerates fat digestion.
6. Micelles increase the absorption of fat by
   a. binding the lipase enzyme and holding it on the surface of the lipid emulsion droplet.
   b. keeping the insoluble products of fat digestion in small aggregates.
   c. promoting direct absorption across the intestinal epithelium.
   d. metabolizing triglyceride to monoglyceride.
   e. facilitating absorption into the lacteals.
7. Which of the following inhibit/inhibits gastric HCl secretion during a meal?
   a. stimulation of the parasympathetic nerves to the enteric nervous system
   b. the sight and smell of food
   c. distension of the duodenum
   d. presence of peptides in the stomach
   e. distension of the stomach
8. Which component/components of bile is/are not primarily secreted by hepatocytes?
   a. HCO_3^-
   b. bile salts
   c. cholesterol
   d. lecithin
   e. bilirubin
9. Which of the following is *true* about segmentation in the small intestine?
   a. It is a type of peristalsis.
   b. It moves chyme only from the duodenum to the ileum.
   c. Its frequency is the same in each intestinal segment.
   d. It is unaffected by cephalic phase stimuli.
   e. It produces a slow migration of chyme to the large intestine.
10. Which of the following is the primary absorptive process in the large intestine?
    a. active transport of Na^+ from the lumen to the blood
    b. absorption of water
    c. active transport of potassium from the lumen to the blood
    d. active absorption of HCO_3^- into the blood
    e. active secretion of Cl^- from the blood

CHAPTER 15 GENERAL PRINCIPLES ASSESSMENT

Answers found in Appendix A.

1. A general principle of physiology is that *structure is a determinant of—and has coevolved with—function.* One example highlighted in this chapter is the large surface area provided by the villous and microvillous structure of the cells lining the small intestine (Figures 15.4 and 15.5). How does the anatomy of the hepatic lobule shown in Figure 15.31 provide another example of increased surface area to maximize function?
2. Another general principle of physiology states that *physiological processes are dictated by the laws of chemistry and physics.* Give at least two examples of how this principle is important in understanding the processes of absorption and secretion in the GI tract.
3. What general principle of physiology is demonstrated by Figure 15.14?

CHAPTER 15 QUANTITATIVE AND THOUGHT QUESTIONS

Answers found at www.mhhe.com/widmaier13.

1. If the salivary glands were unable to secrete amylase, what effect would this have on starch digestion?
2. Whole milk or a fatty snack consumed before the ingestion of alcohol decreases the rate of intoxication. By what mechanism may fat be acting to produce this effect?
3. A patient brought to a hospital after a period of prolonged vomiting has an elevated heart rate, decreased blood pressure, and below-normal blood K^+ and acidity. Explain these symptoms in terms of the consequences of excessive vomiting.
4. Can fat be digested and absorbed in the absence of bile salts? Explain.
5. How might damage to the lower portion of the spinal cord affect defecation?
6. One of the older but no longer used procedures in the treatment of ulcers is abdominal vagotomy, surgical cutting of the vagus (parasympathetic) nerves to the stomach. By what mechanism might this procedure help ulcers to heal and decrease the incidence of new ulcers?

CHAPTER 15 ANSWERS TO PHYSIOLOGICAL INQUIRIES

Figure 15.5 A brush border is also found along the luminal surface of the proximal tubules of the renal nephrons. Like the intestinal brush border, that of the proximal tubules is an adaptation that increases surface area and allows for increased transport of solutes across the epithelium.

Table 15.4 The most common finding is an abnormally high production of gastric (hydrochloric) acid due to gastrin stimulation of the parietal cell of the stomach (see Figure 15.21). This high acidity can cause injury to the duodenum because the pancreas cannot produce sufficient quantities of HCO_3^- to neutralize it (see Figure 15.29). The low pH in the duodenum can also inactivate pancreatic enzymes (see Figure 15.30), which can ultimately lead to diarrhea due to unabsorbed nutrients and increased fat in the stool. The spectrum of findings in a patient with a gastrinoma is called the Zollinger–Ellison syndrome.

Figure 15.15 Aspiration of food during swallowing can lead to occlusion (blockage) of the airways, which can result in a disruption of oxygen delivery and carbon dioxide removal from the pulmonary system. Aspiration of stomach contents can lead to severe lung damage primarily due to the low pH of the material.

Figure 15.19 Mucus secreted by the cells in the gastric gland (see Figure 15.18) creates a protective coating and traps HCO_3^-. This gastric mucosal barrier protects the stomach from the luminal acidity.

Figure 15.21 A decrease in histamine action would result in a decrease in acid secretion and an increase in the pH of the material in the lumen of the stomach. This would decrease the H^+-induced inhibition of gastrin secretion; consequently, gastrin secretion would increase. Because a large part of the effect of gastrin on acid secretion is by stimulating histamine release, as shown in Figure 15.21, the parietal cell acid secretion would still be decreased. This is why histamine-receptor blockers (called H2 blockers) are effective in increasing stomach pH and alleviating the symptoms of gastroesophageal reflux (heartburn) described earlier in this chapter.

Figure 15.25. A person whose stomach has been removed because of disease (e.g., cancer) must eat more frequent small meals instead of the usual three large meals per day. A large meal in the absence of the controlled emptying by the stomach could rapidly enter the intestine, producing a hypertonic solution. This hypertonic solution could cause enough water to flow (by osmosis) into the intestine from the blood to lower the blood volume and produce circulatory complications. The large distension of the intestine by the entering fluid can also trigger vomiting in such individuals. All of these symptoms produced by the rapid entry of large quantities of ingested material into the small intestine are known as the dumping syndrome. You already learned earlier in this chapter that the lack of intrinsic factor from parietal cells can lead to pernicious anemia.

Figure 15.32 A portal vein carries blood from one capillary bed to another capillary bed (rather than from capillaries to venules as described in Chapter 12). The hypothalamo–pituitary portal veins carry hypophysiotropic hormones from the capillaries of the median eminence to the anterior pituitary gland where they stimulate or inhibit the release of pituitary gland hormones (see Chapter 11).

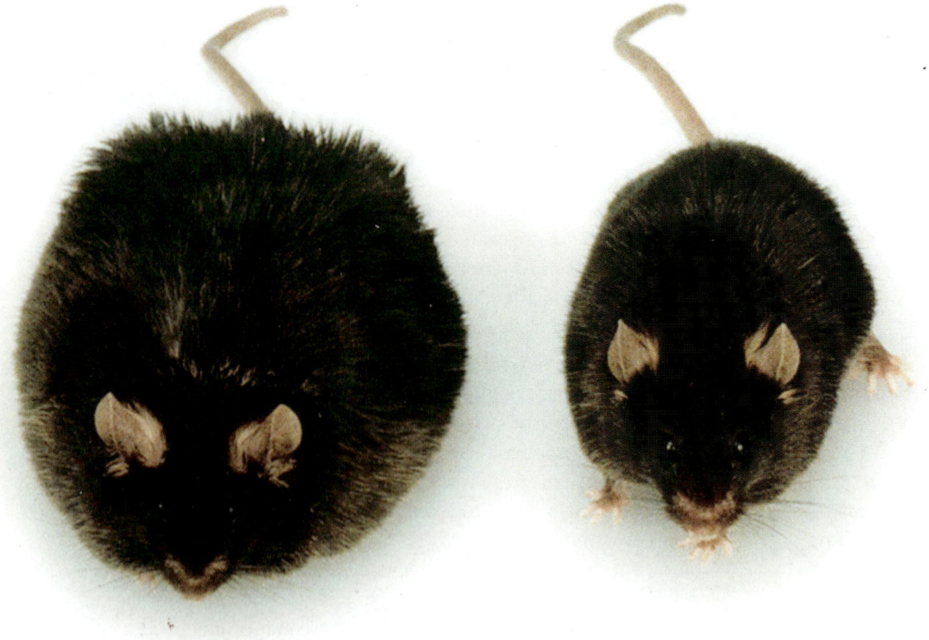

Genetically obese mouse and normal mouse.

16 Regulation of Organic Metabolism and Energy Balance

SECTION A

Control and Integration of Carbohydrate, Protein, and Fat Metabolism

SECTION B

Regulation of Total-Body Energy Balance and Temperature

Chapter 3 introduced the concepts of energy and organic metabolism at the level of the cell. This chapter deals with two topics that are concerned in one way or another with those same concepts—but for the entire body. First, this chapter describes how the metabolic pathways for carbohydrate, fat, and protein are integrated and controlled so as to provide continuous sources of energy to the various tissues and organs, even during periods of fasting. Next, the factors that determine total-body energy balance and the regulation of body temperature are described.

In Section A, you will learn how the control of metabolism is a good example of the general principle of physiology that most physiological functions are controlled by multiple regulatory systems, often working in opposition. This will be particularly evident by the opposing effects of the primary regulatory hormone insulin and the counterregulatory hormones cortisol, growth hormone, glucagon, and epinephrine on the balance of glucose and other energy sources in the blood. The control of metabolism and energy balance also illustrates the general principles of physiology that homeostasis is essential for health and survival and that physiological processes require the transfer and balance of matter and energy. In Section B, energy balance and homeostasis are again general themes. This section will also illustrate how physiological processes are dictated by the laws of chemistry and physics, particularly in relation to heat transfer between the body and the environment.

SECTION A

Control and Integration of Carbohydrate, Protein, and Fat Metabolism

16.1 Events of the Absorptive and Postabsorptive States

The regular availability of food is a very recent event in the history of humankind and, indeed, is still not universal. It is not surprising, therefore, that mechanisms have evolved for survival during alternating periods of food availability and fasting. The two functional states or periods the body undergoes in providing energy for cellular activities are the **absorptive state,** during which ingested nutrients enter the blood from the gastrointestinal tract, and the **postabsorptive state,** during which the gastrointestinal tract is empty of nutrients and the body's own stores must supply energy. Because an average meal requires approximately 4 h for complete absorption, our usual three-meal-a-day pattern places us in the postabsorptive state during the late morning, again in the late afternoon, and during most of the night. We will refer to more than 24 h without eating as fasting.

During the absorptive state, some of the ingested nutrients provide the energy requirements of the body and the remainder is added to the body's energy stores to be called upon during the next postabsorptive state. Total-body energy stores are adequate for the average person to withstand a fast of many weeks, provided water is available.

Absorptive State

The events of the absorptive state are summarized in **Figure 16.1.** A typical meal contains all three of the major energy-supplying food groups—carbohydrates, fats, and proteins—with carbohydrates constituting most of a typical meal's energy content (calories). Recall from Chapter 15 that carbohydrates and proteins are absorbed primarily as monosaccharides and amino acids, respectively, into the blood leaving the gastrointestinal tract. The blood then drains directly into the liver by way of the hepatic portal vein. This allows the liver to alter the nutrient composition of the blood before it returns to the heart to be pumped to the rest of the body. This mechanism likely evolved as a means of inactivating toxins that were inadvertently ingested with a meal; liver cells express numerous enzymes capable of chemically altering and rendering harmless a wide range of potentially toxic compounds. In contrast to monosaccharides and amino acids, fat is absorbed into the *lymph* in chylomicrons, which are too large to enter capillaries. The lymph then drains into the

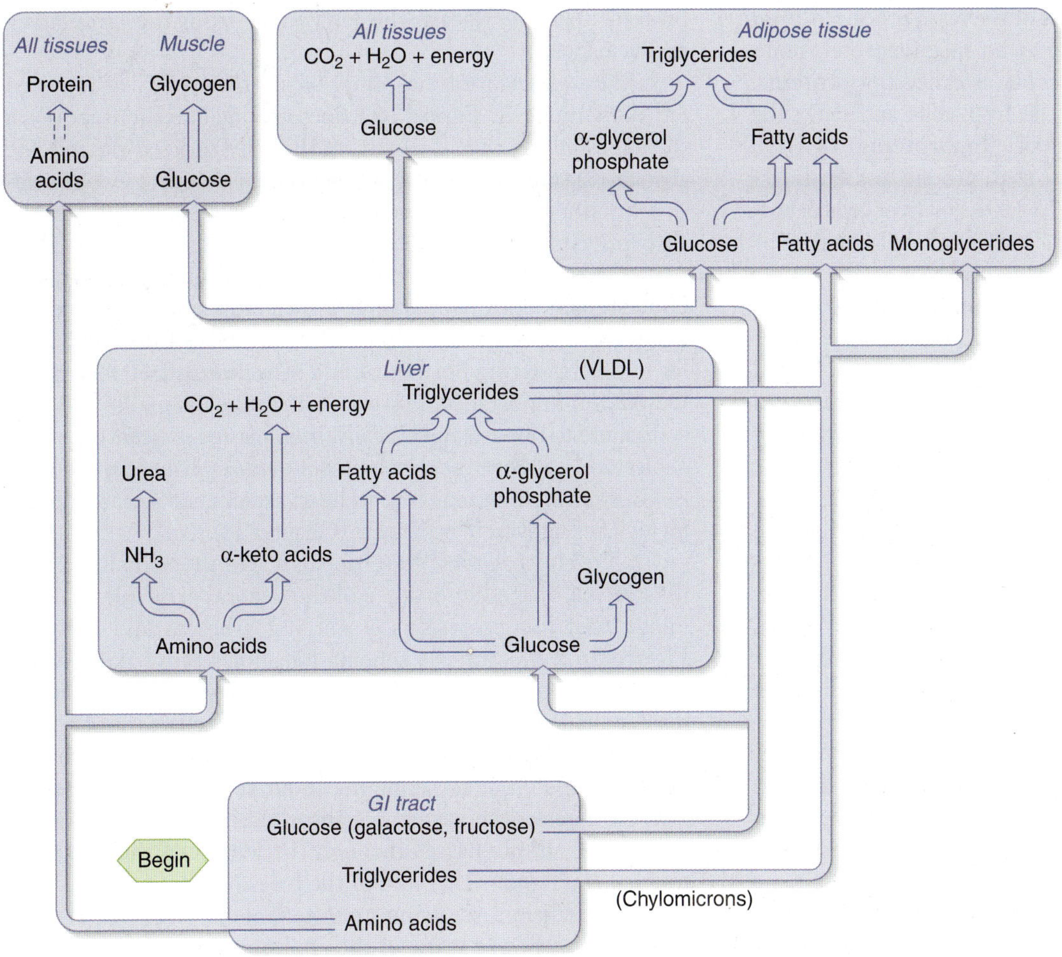

Figure 16.1 Major metabolic pathways of the absorptive state. The arrow from amino acids to protein is dashed to denote the fact that excess amino acids are not stored as protein (see text). All arrows between boxes denote transport of the substance via the blood (VLDL = very-low-density lipoproteins; Energy = ATP).

PHYSIOLOGICAL INQUIRY

- Would eating a diet that is low in fat content ensure that a person could not gain fat mass?

Answer can be found at end of chapter.

systemic venous system. Consequently, the liver cannot first modify absorbed fat before it reaches other tissues.

Absorbed Carbohydrate

Some of the carbohydrate absorbed from the gastrointestinal tract is galactose and fructose. Because these sugars are either converted to glucose by the liver or enter essentially the same metabolic pathways as glucose, we will for simplicity refer to absorbed carbohydrates as glucose.

Glucose is the body's major energy source during the absorptive state. Much of the absorbed glucose enters cells and is catabolized to carbon dioxide and water, in the process releasing energy that is used for ATP formation (as described in Chapter 3). Skeletal muscle makes up the majority of body mass, so it is the major consumer of glucose, even at rest. Skeletal muscle not only catabolizes glucose during the absorptive phase but also converts some of the glucose to the polysaccharide glycogen, which is then stored in the muscle for future use.

Adipose-tissue cells (adipocytes) also catabolize glucose for energy, but the most important fate of glucose in adipocytes during the absorptive phase is its transformation to fat (triglycerides). Glucose is the precursor of both α-glycerol phosphate and fatty acids, and these molecules are then linked together to form triglycerides, which are stored in the cell.

Another large fraction of the absorbed glucose enters liver cells. This is a very important point: During the absorptive period, there is net *uptake* of glucose by the liver. It is either stored as glycogen, as in skeletal muscle, or transformed to α-glycerol phosphate and fatty acids, which are then used to synthesize triglycerides, as in adipose tissue. Most of the fat synthesized from glucose in the liver is packaged along with specific proteins into molecular aggregates of lipids and proteins called **lipoproteins.** These aggregates are secreted by the liver cells and enter the blood. They are called **very-low-density lipoproteins (VLDLs)** because they contain much more fat than protein and fat is less dense than protein. The synthesis of VLDLs by liver cells occurs by processes similar to those for the synthesis of chylomicrons by intestinal mucosal cells, as Chapter 15 described.

Because of their large size, VLDLs in the blood do not readily penetrate capillary walls. Instead, their triglycerides are hydrolyzed mainly to monoglycerides (glycerol linked to one fatty acid) and fatty acids by the enzyme **lipoprotein lipase.** This enzyme is located on the blood-facing surface of capillary endothelial cells, especially those in adipose tissue. In adipose-tissue capillaries, the fatty acids generated by the action of lipoprotein lipase diffuse from the capillaries into the adipocytes. There, they combine with α-glycerol phosphate, supplied by glucose metabolites, to form triglycerides once again. As a result, most of the fatty acids in the VLDL triglycerides originally synthesized from glucose by the *liver* end up being stored in triglyceride in *adipose tissue.* Some of the monoglycerides formed in the blood by the action of lipoprotein lipase in adipose-tissue capillaries are also taken up by adipocytes, where enzymes can reattach fatty acids to the two available carbon atoms of the monoglyceride and thereby form a triglyceride. In addition, some of the monoglycerides travel via the blood to the liver, where they are metabolized.

To summarize, the major fates of glucose during the absorptive phase are (1) utilization for energy, (2) storage as glycogen in liver and skeletal muscle, and (3) storage as fat in adipose tissue.

Absorbed Lipids

As described in Chapter 15, many of the absorbed lipids are packaged into chylomicrons that enter the lymph and, from there, the circulation. The processing of the triglycerides in chylomicrons in plasma is similar to that just described for VLDLs produced by the liver. The fatty acids of plasma chylomicrons are released, mainly within adipose-tissue capillaries, by the action of endothelial lipoprotein lipase. The released fatty acids then diffuse into adipocytes and combine with α-glycerol phosphate, synthesized in the adipocytes from glucose metabolites, to form triglycerides.

The importance of glucose for triglyceride synthesis in adipocytes cannot be overemphasized. Adipocytes do not have the enzyme required for phosphorylation of glycerol, so α-glycerol phosphate can be formed in these cells only from glucose metabolites (refer back to Figure 3.41 to see how these metabolites are produced) and not from glycerol or any other fat metabolites.

In contrast to α-glycerol phosphate, there are three major sources of the fatty acids found in adipose-tissue triglyceride: (1) glucose that enters adipose tissue and is broken down to provide building blocks for the synthesis of fatty acids; (2) glucose that is used in the liver to form VLDL triglycerides, which are transported in the blood and taken up by the adipose tissue; and (3) ingested triglycerides transported in the blood in chylomicrons and taken up by adipose tissue. As we have seen, sources (2) and (3) require the action of lipoprotein lipase to release the fatty acids from the circulating triglycerides.

This description has emphasized the *storage* of ingested fat. For simplicity, Figure 16.1 does not include the fraction of the ingested fat that is not stored but is oxidized during the absorptive state by various organs to provide energy. The relative amounts of carbohydrate and fat used for energy during the absorptive period depend largely on the content of the meal.

One very important absorbed lipid found in chylomicrons—**cholesterol**—does not serve as a metabolic energy source but instead is a component of plasma membranes and a precursor for bile salts, steroid hormones, and other specialized molecules. Despite its importance, however, cholesterol in excess can also contribute to disease. Specifically, high plasma concentrations of cholesterol enhance the development of ***atherosclerosis***, the arterial thickening that may lead to heart attacks, strokes, and other forms of cardiovascular damage (Chapter 12).

The control of cholesterol balance in the body is a classic illustration of the importance of the general principle of physiology that homeostasis is essential for health and survival. **Figure 16.2** illustrates a schema for cholesterol balance. The two sources of cholesterol are dietary cholesterol and cholesterol synthesized within the body. Dietary cholesterol comes from animal sources, egg yolk being by far the richest in this lipid (a single large egg contains about 185 mg of cholesterol). Not all ingested cholesterol is absorbed into the blood, however; some simply passes through the length of the gastrointestinal tract and is excreted in the feces.

In addition to using ingested cholesterol, almost all cells can synthesize some of the cholesterol required for their

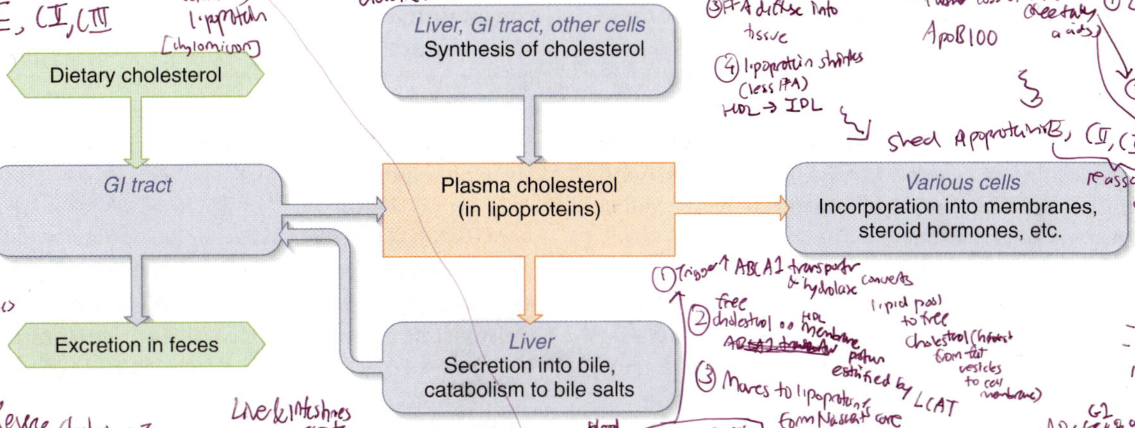

Figure 16.2 Cholesterol balance. Most of the cholesterol that is converted to bile salts, stored in the gallbladder, and secreted into the intestine gets recycled back to the liver. Changes in dietary cholesterol can modify plasma cholesterol concentration, but not usually dramatically. Cholesterol synthesis by the liver is up-regulated when dietary cholesterol is decreased, and vice versa.

own plasma membranes, but most cannot do so in adequate amounts and depend upon receiving cholesterol from the blood. This is also true of the endocrine cells that produce steroid hormones from cholesterol. Consequently, most cells *remove* cholesterol from the blood. In contrast, the liver and small intestine can produce large amounts of cholesterol, most of which *enters* the blood.

Now we look at the other side of cholesterol balance—the pathways, all involving the liver, for net cholesterol loss from the body. First, some plasma cholesterol is taken up by liver cells and secreted into the bile, which carries it to the gallbladder and from there to the lumen of the small intestine. Here, it is treated much like ingested cholesterol, some being absorbed back into the blood and the remainder excreted in the feces. Second, much of the cholesterol taken up by the liver cells is metabolized into bile salts (Chapter 15). After their production by the liver, these bile salts, like secreted cholesterol, eventually flow through the bile duct into the small intestine. (As described in Chapter 15, many of these bile salts are then reclaimed by absorption back into the blood across the epithelium of the distal small intestine.)

The liver is clearly the major organ that controls cholesterol homeostasis, for the liver can add newly synthesized cholesterol to the blood and it can remove cholesterol from the blood, secreting it into the bile or metabolizing it to bile salts. The homeostatic control mechanisms that keep plasma cholesterol concentrations within a normal range operate on all of these hepatic processes, but the single most important response involves cholesterol synthesis. The liver's synthesis of cholesterol is inhibited whenever dietary—and, therefore, plasma—cholesterol is increased. This is because cholesterol inhibits the enzyme HMG-CoA reductase, which is critical for cholesterol synthesis by the liver.

Thus, as soon as the plasma cholesterol concentration increases because of cholesterol ingestion, hepatic synthesis of cholesterol is inhibited and the plasma concentration of cholesterol remains close to its original value. Conversely, when dietary cholesterol is reduced and plasma cholesterol decreases, hepatic synthesis is stimulated (released from inhibition). This increased synthesis opposes any further decrease in plasma cholesterol. The sensitivity of this negative feedback control of cholesterol synthesis differs greatly from person to person, but it is the major reason why, for most people, it is difficult to decrease plasma cholesterol concentration very much by altering only dietary cholesterol.

So far, the maintenance of plasma cholesterol concentration within a homeostatic range has been emphasized. However, environmental and physiological factors can significantly alter plasma cholesterol concentrations. Perhaps the most important of these factors are the quantity and type of dietary fatty acids. Ingesting saturated fatty acids, which are the dominant fatty acids of animal fat (particularly high in red meats, most cheeses, and whole milk), increases plasma cholesterol. In contrast, eating either polyunsaturated fatty acids (the predominant plant fatty acids) or monounsaturated fatty acids, such as those in olive or peanut oil, decreases plasma cholesterol. The various fatty acids exert their effects on plasma cholesterol concentration by altering cholesterol synthesis, excretion, and metabolism to bile salts.

A variety of drugs now in common use are also capable of decreasing plasma cholesterol by influencing one or more of the metabolic pathways for cholesterol—for example, inhibiting HMG-CoA reductase—or by interfering with intestinal absorption of bile salts.

The story is more complicated than this, however, because not all plasma cholesterol has the same function or significance for disease. Like most other lipids, cholesterol circulates in the plasma as part of various lipoprotein complexes. These include chylomicrons, VLDLs, **low-density lipoproteins (LDLs)**, and **high-density lipoproteins (HDLs)**, each distinguished by their ratio of fat to protein. LDLs are the main cholesterol carriers, and they *deliver* cholesterol to cells throughout the body. LDLs bind to plasma membrane receptors specific for a protein component of the LDLs and are then taken up by the cells by endocytosis. In contrast to LDLs, HDLs *remove* excess cholesterol from blood and tissue, including the cholesterol-loaded cells of atherosclerotic plaques. They then deliver this cholesterol to the liver, which secretes it into the bile or converts it to bile salts. Along with LDLs, HDLs also deliver cholesterol to steroid-producing endocrine cells. Uptake of the HDLs by the liver and these endocrine cells is facilitated by the presence in their plasma membranes of large numbers of receptors specific for HDLs, which bind to the receptors and then are taken into the cells.

LDL cholesterol is often designated "bad" cholesterol because a high plasma concentration can be associated with increased deposition of cholesterol in arterial walls and a higher incidence of heart attacks. (The designation "bad" should not obscure the fact that LDL cholesterol is essential for supplying cells with the cholesterol they require to synthesize cell membranes and, in the case of the gonads and adrenal glands, steroid hormones.) Using the same criteria, HDL cholesterol has been designated "good" cholesterol.

The best single indicator of the likelihood of developing atherosclerotic disease is not necessarily total plasma cholesterol concentration but rather the ratio of plasma LDL cholesterol to plasma HDL cholesterol—the lower the ratio, the lower the risk. Cigarette smoking, a known risk factor for heart attacks, decreases plasma HDL, whereas weight reduction (in overweight persons) and regular exercise usually increase it. Estrogen not only decreases LDL but increases HDL, which explains, in part, why the incidence of coronary artery disease in premenopausal women is lower than in men. After menopause, the cholesterol values and coronary artery disease rates in women not on estrogen-replacement therapy become similar to those in men.

Finally, a variety of disorders of cholesterol metabolism have been identified. In ***familial hypercholesterolemia***, for example, LDL receptors are decreased in number or are nonfunctional. Consequently, LDL accumulates in the blood to very high concentrations. If untreated, this disease may result in atherosclerosis and heart disease at unusually young ages.

Absorbed Amino Acids

Some amino acids are absorbed into liver cells and used to synthesize a variety of proteins, including liver enzymes and plasma proteins, or they are converted to carbohydrate-like intermediates known as **α-keto acids** by removal of the amino group. This process is called deamination. The amino groups are used to synthesize urea in the liver, which enters the blood and is excreted by the kidneys. The α-keto acids can enter the Krebs (tricarboxylic acid) cycle (see Chapter 3, Figure 3.44) and be catabolized to provide energy for the liver cells. They can also be converted to fatty acids, thereby participating in fat synthesis by the liver.

Most ingested amino acids are not taken up by the liver cells but instead enter other cells (see Figure 16.1), where they may be used to synthesize proteins. All cells require a constant supply of amino acids for protein synthesis and participate in protein metabolism.

Protein synthesis is represented by a dashed arrow in Figure 16.1 to call attention to an important fact: There is a net synthesis of protein during the absorptive period, but this basically just replaces the proteins catabolized during the postabsorptive state. In other words, excess amino acids are not stored as protein in the sense that glucose is stored as glycogen or that both glucose and fat are stored as fat. Rather, ingested amino acids in excess of those required to maintain a stable rate of protein turnover are converted to carbohydrate or fat. Therefore, eating large amounts of protein does not in itself cause increases in total-body protein. Increased daily consumption of protein does, however, provide the amino acids required to support the high rates of protein synthesis occurring in growing children or in adults who increase muscle mass by engaging in weight-bearing exercises.

Table 16.1 summarizes nutrient metabolism during the absorptive period.

Postabsorptive State

As the absorptive state ends, net synthesis of glycogen, fat, and protein ceases and net catabolism of all these substances begins. The events of the postabsorptive state are summarized in **Figure 16.3**. The overall significance of these events can be understood in terms of the essential problem during the postabsorptive state: No glucose is being absorbed from the gastrointestinal tract, yet the plasma glucose concentration must be maintained because the central nervous system normally utilizes only glucose for energy. If the plasma glucose concentration decreases too much, alterations of neural activity occur, ranging from subtle impairment of mental function to seizures, coma, and even death.

Like cholesterol, the control of glucose balance is another classic example of the general principle of physiology that homeostasis is essential for health and survival. The events that maintain plasma glucose concentration fall into two categories: (1) reactions that provide sources of blood glucose; and (2) cellular utilization of fat for energy, thereby "sparing" glucose.

Sources of Blood Glucose

The sources of blood glucose during the postabsorptive state are as follows (see Figure 16.3):

1. **Glycogenolysis,** the hydrolysis of glycogen stores to monomers of glucose 6-phosphate, occurs in the liver and skeletal muscle. In the liver, glucose 6-phosphate is enzymatically converted to glucose, which then enters the blood. Hepatic glycogenolysis begins within seconds of an appropriate stimulus, such as sympathetic nervous system activation. As a result, it is the first line of defense in maintaining the plasma glucose concentration within a homeostatic range. The amount of glucose available from this source, however, can supply the body's requirements for only several hours before hepatic glycogen is nearly depleted.

TABLE 16.1 Summary of Nutrient Metabolism During the Absorptive State
Energy is provided primarily by absorbed carbohydrate in a typical meal.
There is net uptake of glucose by the liver.
Some carbohydrate is stored as glycogen in liver and muscle, but most carbohydrates and fats in excess of that used for energy are stored as fat in adipose tissue.
There is some synthesis of body proteins, but some of the amino acids in dietary protein are used for energy or converted to fat.

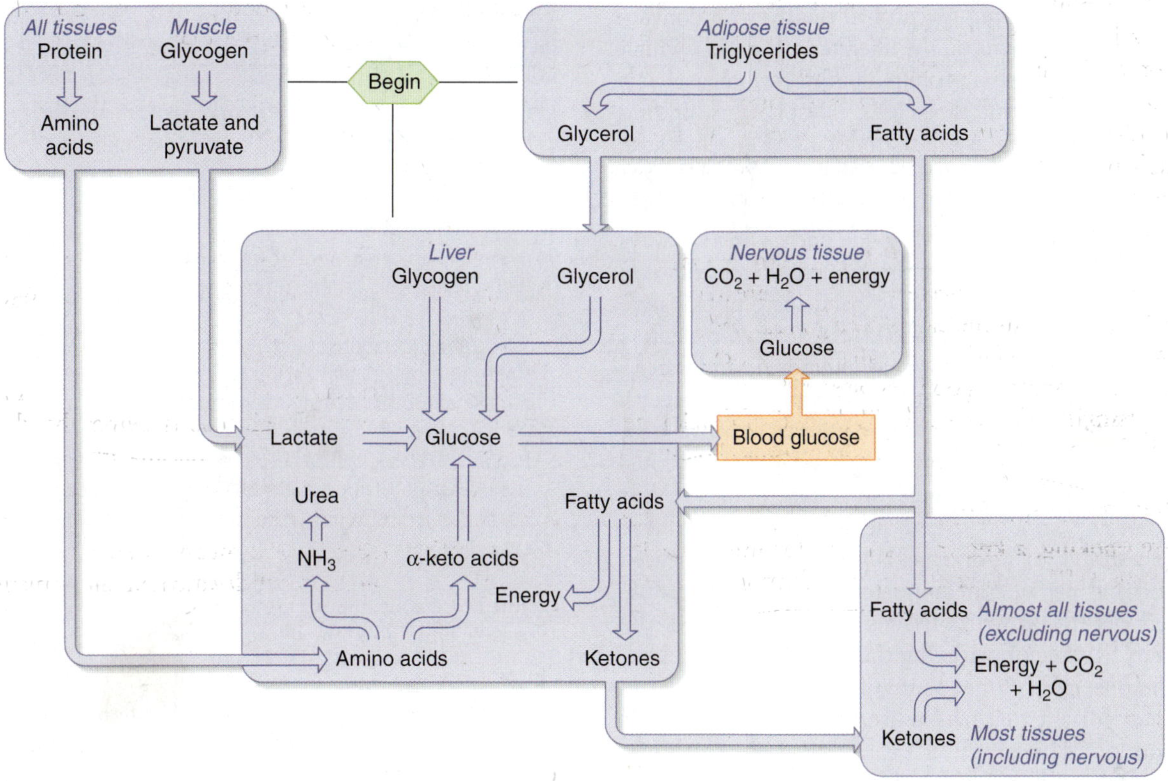

Figure 16.3 Major metabolic pathways of the postabsorptive state. The central focus is regulation of the blood glucose concentration. All arrows between boxes denote transport of the substance via the blood.

Glycogenolysis also occurs in skeletal muscle, which contains approximately the same amount of glycogen as the liver. Unlike the liver, however, muscle cells lack the enzyme necessary to form glucose from the glucose 6-phosphate formed during glycogenolysis; therefore, muscle glycogen is not a source of blood glucose. Instead, the glucose 6-phosphate undergoes glycolysis within muscle to yield ATP, pyruvate, and lactate. The ATP and pyruvate are used directly by the muscle cell. Some of the lactate, however, enters the blood, circulates to the liver, and is converted into glucose, which can then leave the liver cells to enter the blood. Thus, muscle glycogen contributes to the blood glucose indirectly via the liver's processing of lactate.

2. The catabolism of triglycerides in adipose tissue yields glycerol and fatty acids, a process termed **lipolysis.** The glycerol and fatty acids then enter the blood by diffusion. The glycerol reaching the liver is enzymatically converted through a series of steps to glucose. Thus, an important source of glucose during the postabsorptive state is the glycerol released when adipose-tissue triglyceride is broken down.
3. A few hours into the postabsorptive state, protein becomes another source of blood glucose. Large quantities of protein in muscle and other tissues can be catabolized without serious cellular malfunction. There are, of course, limits to this process, and continued protein loss during a prolonged fast ultimately means disruption of cell function, sickness, and death. Before this point is reached, however, protein breakdown can supply large quantities of amino acids. These amino acids enter the blood and are taken up by the liver, where some can be converted via the α-keto acid pathway to glucose. This glucose is then released into the blood.

Synthesis of glucose from such precursors as amino acids and glycerol is known as **gluconeogenesis**—that is, "creation of new glucose." During a 24 h fast, gluconeogenesis provides approximately 180 g of glucose. Although historically this process was considered to be almost entirely carried out by the liver with a small contribution by the kidneys, recent evidence strongly suggests that the kidneys contribute much more substantially to gluconeogenesis than previously believed.

Glucose Sparing (Fat Utilization)

The approximately 180 g of glucose per day produced by gluconeogenesis in the liver (and kidneys) during fasting supplies 720 kcal of energy. As described later in this chapter, typical total energy expenditure for an average adult is 1500 to 3000 kcal/day. Therefore, gluconeogenesis cannot supply all the energy demands of the body. An adjustment must therefore take place during the transition from the absorptive to the postabsorptive state. Most organs and tissues, other than those of the nervous system, significantly decrease their glucose catabolism and increase their fat utilization, the latter becoming the major energy source. This metabolic adjustment, known as **glucose sparing,** "spares" the glucose produced by the liver for use by the nervous system.

The essential step in this adjustment is lipolysis, the catabolism of adipose-tissue triglyceride, which liberates glycerol and fatty acids into the blood. We described lipolysis earlier in terms of its importance in providing glycerol to the liver for conversion to glucose. Now, we focus on the liberated fatty acids, which circulate bound to the plasma protein albumin, which acts as a carrier for these hydrophobic molecules. (Despite this binding to protein, they are known as free fatty acids [FFAs] because they are "free" of their attachment to glycerol.) The circulating FFAs are taken up and metabolized by almost all tissues, *excluding the nervous system.* They provide energy in two ways (see Chapter 3 for details): (1) They first undergo beta oxidation to yield hydrogen atoms (that go on to participate in oxidative phosphorylation) and acetyl CoA, and (2) the acetyl CoA enters the Krebs cycle and is catabolized to carbon dioxide and water.

The liver is unique, however, in that most of the acetyl CoA it forms from fatty acids during the postabsorptive state does not enter the Krebs cycle but is processed into three compounds collectively called **ketones,** or ketone bodies. (*Note:* Ketones are not the same as α-keto acids, which, as we have seen, are metabolites of amino acids.) Ketones are released into the blood and provide an important energy source during prolonged fasting for many tissues, *including* those of the nervous system, capable of oxidizing them via the Krebs cycle. One of the ketones is acetone, some of which is exhaled and accounts in part for the distinctive breath odor of individuals undergoing prolonged fasting.

The net result of fatty acid and ketone utilization during fasting is the provision of energy for the body while at the same time sparing glucose for the brain and nervous system. Moreover, as just emphasized, the brain can use ketones for an energy source, and it does so increasingly as ketones build up in the blood during the first few days of a fast. The survival value of this phenomenon is significant; when the brain decreases its glucose requirement by utilizing ketones, much less protein breakdown is required to supply amino acids for gluconeogenesis. Consequently, the ability to withstand a long fast without serious tissue damage is enhanced.

Table 16.2 summarizes the events of the postabsorptive state. The combined effects of glycogenolysis, gluconeogenesis, and the switch to fat utilization are so efficient that, after several days of complete fasting, the plasma glucose concentration is decreased by only a few percentage points. After 1 month, it is decreased by only 25% (although in very thin persons, this happens much sooner).

16.2 Endocrine and Neural Control of the Absorptive and Postabsorptive States

We now turn to the endocrine and neural factors that control and integrate these metabolic pathways. We will focus primarily on the following questions, summarized in **Figure 16.4**: (1) What controls net anabolism of protein, glycogen, and triglyceride in the absorptive phase, and net catabolism in the postabsorptive phase? (2) What induces the cells to utilize primarily glucose for energy during the absorptive phase but fat during the postabsorptive phase? (3) What stimulates net glucose uptake by the liver during the absorptive phase but gluconeogenesis and glucose release during the postabsorptive phase?

TABLE 16.2 Summary of Nutrient Metabolism During the Postabsorptive State
Glycogen, fat, and protein syntheses are curtailed, and net breakdown occurs.
Glucose is formed in the liver both from the glycogen stored there and by gluconeogenesis from blood-borne lactate, pyruvate, glycerol, and amino acids. The kidneys also perform gluconeogenesis during a prolonged fast.
The glucose produced in the liver (and kidneys) is released into the blood, but its utilization for energy is greatly decreased in muscle and other nonneural tissues.
Lipolysis releases adipose-tissue fatty acids into the blood, and the oxidation of these fatty acids by most cells and of ketones produced from them by the liver provides most of the body's energy supply.
The brain continues to use glucose but also starts using ketones as they build up in the blood.

The most important controls of these transitions from feasting to fasting, and vice versa, are two pancreatic hormones—**insulin** and **glucagon.** Also playing a role are the hormones epinephrine and cortisol from the adrenal glands, growth hormone from the anterior pituitary gland, and the sympathetic nerves to the liver and adipose tissue.

Insulin and glucagon are peptide hormones secreted by the **islets of Langerhans** (or, simply, pancreatic islets), clusters of endocrine cells in the pancreas. There are several distinct types of islet cells, each of which secretes a different hormone. The **beta cells** (or B cells) are the source of insulin, and the **alpha cells** (or A cells) are the source of glucagon. There are other molecules secreted by still other islet cells, but the functions of these other molecules in humans are less well established.

Insulin

Insulin is the most important controller of organic metabolism. Its secretion—and, therefore, its plasma concentration—is increased during the absorptive state and decreased during the postabsorptive state.

The metabolic effects of insulin are exerted mainly on muscle cells (both cardiac and skeletal), adipocytes, and hepatocytes. **Figure 16.5** summarizes the most important responses of these target cells. Compare the top portion of this figure to Figure 16.1 and to the left panel of Figure 16.4, and you will see that the responses to an increase in insulin are the same as the events of the absorptive-state pattern. Conversely, the effects of a decrease in plasma insulin are the same as the events of the postabsorptive pattern in Figure 16.3 and the right panel of Figure 16.4. The reason for these correspondences is that an increased plasma concentration of insulin is the major cause of the absorptive-state events, and a decreased plasma concentration of insulin is the major cause of the postabsorptive events.

Like all peptide hormones, insulin induces its effects by binding to specific receptors on the plasma membranes of its

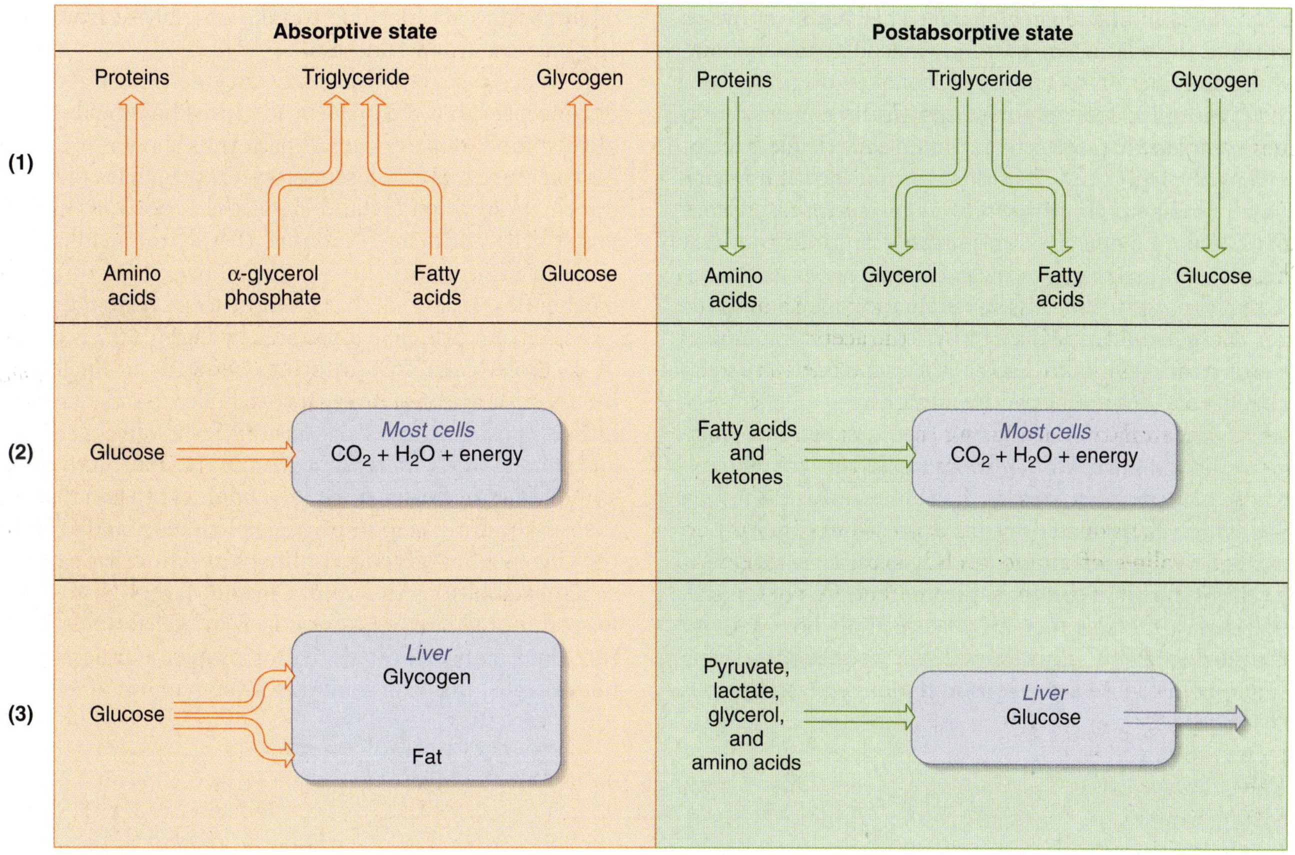

Figure 16.4 Summary of critical points in transition from the absorptive state to the postabsorptive state. The term *absorptive state* could be replaced with *actions of insulin*, and the term *postabsorptive state* with *results of decreased insulin*. The numbers at the left margin refer to discussion questions in the text.

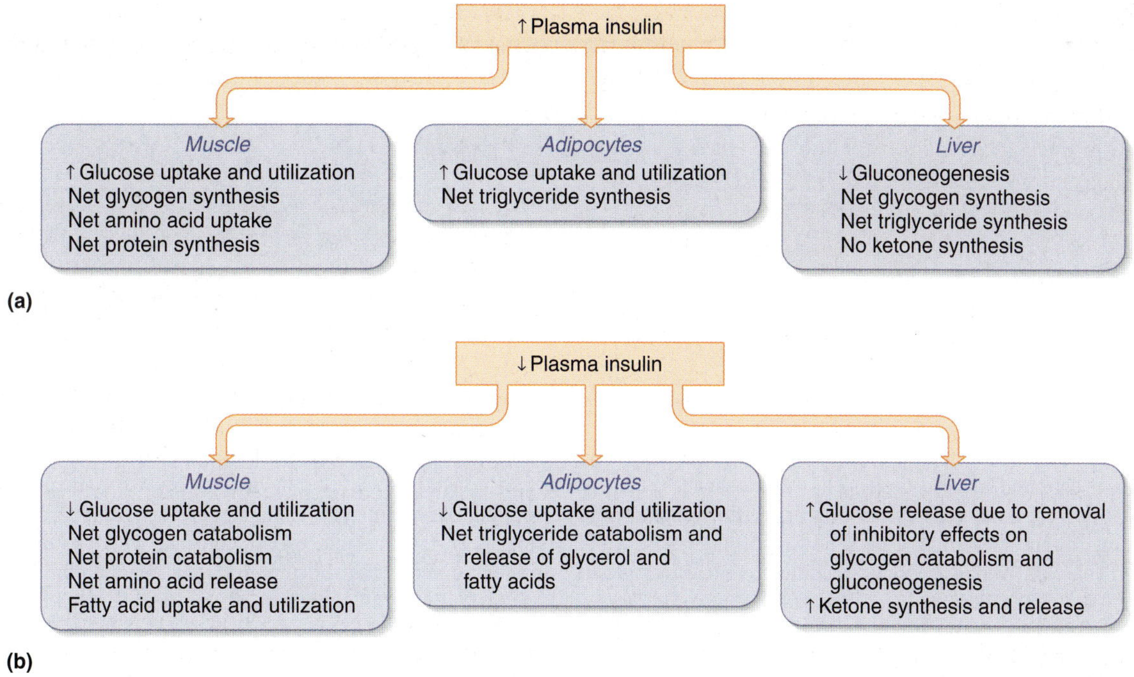

Figure 16.5 Summary of overall target-cell responses to (a) an increase or (b) a decrease in the plasma concentration of insulin. The responses in (a) are virtually identical to the absorptive-state events of Figure 16.1 and the left panel of Figure 16.4; the responses in (b) are virtually identical to the postabsorptive-state events of Figure 16.3 and the right panel of Figure 16.4.

target cells. This binding triggers signal transduction pathways that influence the plasma membrane transport proteins and intracellular enzymes of the target cell. For example, in skeletal muscle cells and adipocytes, an increased insulin concentration stimulates cytoplasmic vesicles that contain a particular type of glucose transporter (GLUT-4) in their membrane to fuse with the plasma membrane (**Figure 16.6**). The increased number of plasma membrane glucose transporters resulting from this fusion results in a greater rate of glucose diffusion from the extracellular fluid into the cells by facilitated diffusion. This illustrates the general principle of physiology that controlled exchange of materials (in this case, glucose) occurs between compartments and across cellular membranes.

Recall from Chapter 4 that glucose enters most body cells by facilitated diffusion. Multiple subtypes of glucose transporters mediate this process, however, and the subtype GLUT-4, which is regulated by insulin, is found mainly in skeletal muscle cells and adipocytes. Of great significance is that the cells of the brain express a different subtype of GLUT, one that has very high affinity for glucose and whose activity is *not* insulin-dependent. This ensures that even if the plasma insulin concentration is very low, as in prolonged fasting, cells of the brain can continue to take up glucose from the blood and maintain their function.

A description of the many enzymes whose activities and/or concentrations are influenced by insulin is beyond the scope of this book, but the overall pattern is shown in **Figure 16.7** for reference and to illustrate several principles. The essential information to understand about the actions of insulin is the target cells' ultimate responses, that is, the material summarized in Figure 16.5. Figure 16.7 shows some of the specific biochemical reactions that underlie these responses.

A major principle illustrated by Figure 16.7 is that, in each of its target cells, insulin brings about its ultimate responses by multiple actions. Take, for example, its effects on skeletal muscle cells. In these cells, insulin favors glycogen formation and storage by (1) increasing glucose transport into the cell, (2) stimulating the key enzyme (**glycogen synthase**) that catalyzes the rate-limiting step in glycogen synthesis, and (3) inhibiting the key enzyme (**glycogen phosphorylase**) that catalyzes glycogen catabolism. As a result, insulin favors glucose transformation to and storage as glycogen in skeletal muscle through three mechanisms. Similarly, for protein synthesis in skeletal muscle cells, insulin (1) increases the number of active plasma

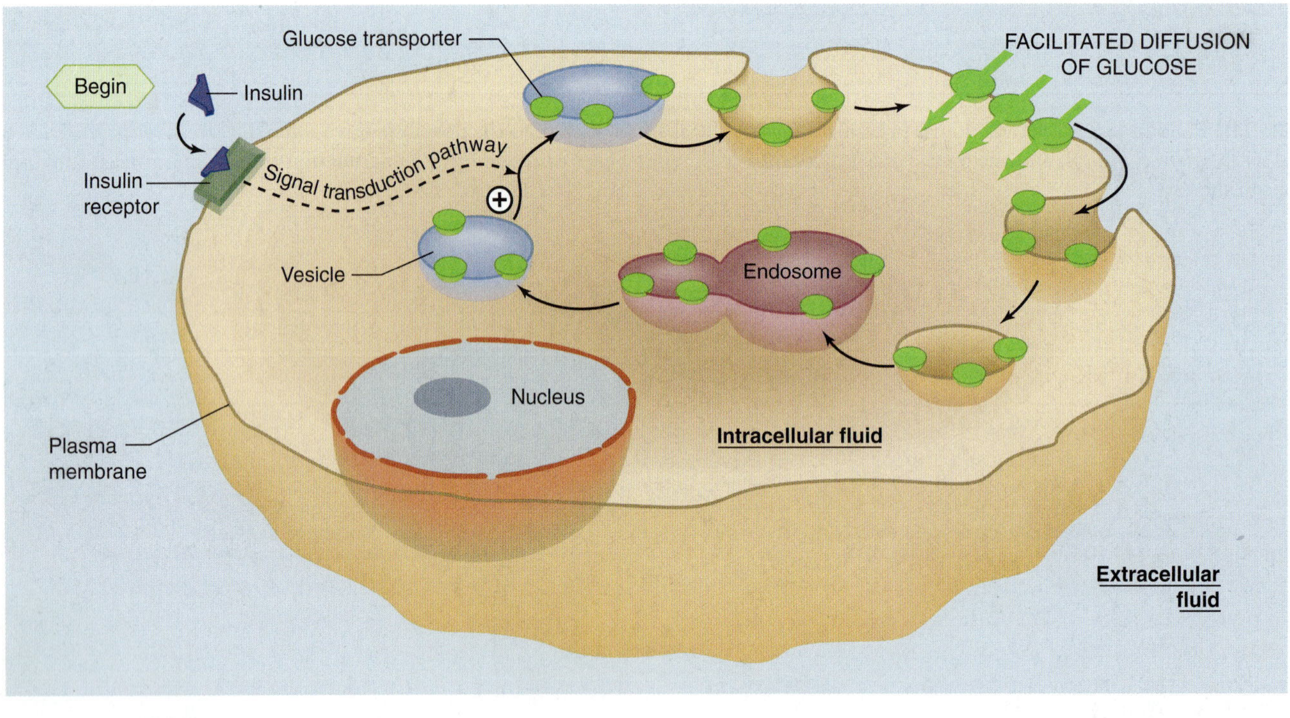

Figure 16.6 APIR Stimulation by insulin of the translocation of glucose transporters from cytoplasmic vesicles to the plasma membrane in skeletal muscle cells and adipose-tissue cells. Note that these transporters are constantly recycled by endocytosis from the plasma membrane back through endosomes into vesicles. As long as insulin concentration is elevated, the entire cycle continues and the number of transporters in the plasma membrane stays high. This is how insulin decreases the plasma concentration of glucose. In contrast, when insulin concentration decreases, the cycle is broken, the vesicles accumulate in the cytoplasm, and the number of transporters in the plasma membrane decreases. Thus, without insulin, the plasma glucose concentration would increase, because glucose transport from plasma to cells would be decreased.

PHYSIOLOGICAL INQUIRY

- What advantage is there to having insulin-dependent glucose transporters already synthesized and prepackaged in a cell, even before it is stimulated by insulin?

Answer can be found at end of chapter.

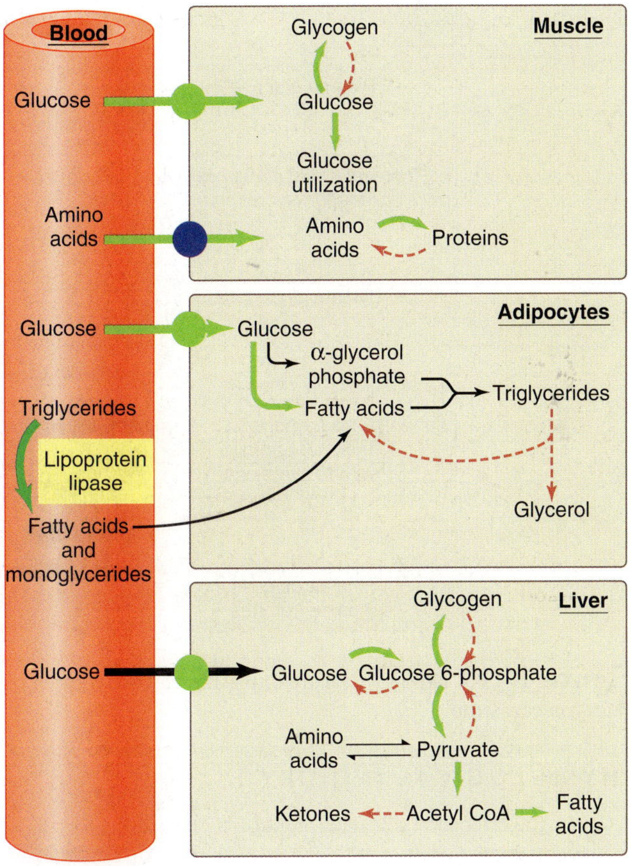

Figure 16.7 Illustration of the key biochemical events that underlie the responses of target cells to insulin as summarized in Figure 16.5. Each green arrow denotes a process stimulated by insulin, whereas a dashed red arrow denotes inhibition by insulin. Except for the effects on the transport proteins for glucose and amino acids, all other effects are exerted on insulin-sensitive enzymes. The bowed arrows denote pathways whose reversibility is mediated by different enzymes; such enzymes are commonly the ones influenced by insulin and other hormones. The black arrows are processes that are not *directly* affected by insulin but are enhanced in the presence of increased insulin as the result of mass action.

membrane transporters for amino acids, thereby increasing amino acid transport into the cells; (2) stimulates the ribosomal enzymes that mediate the synthesis of protein from these amino acids; and (3) inhibits the enzymes that mediate protein catabolism.

Control of Insulin Secretion

The major controlling factor for insulin secretion is the plasma glucose concentration. An increase in plasma glucose concentration, as occurs after a meal, acts on the beta cells of the islets of Langerhans to stimulate insulin secretion, whereas a decrease in plasma glucose removes the stimulus for insulin secretion. The feedback nature of this system is shown in **Figure 16.8**; following a meal, the increase in plasma glucose concentration stimulates insulin secretion. The insulin stimulates the entry of glucose into muscle and adipose tissue, as well as net uptake rather than net output of glucose by the liver. These effects eventually decrease the blood concentration of glucose to its premeal level, thereby removing the stimulus for insulin secretion and causing it to return to its previous level. This is a classic example of a homeostatic process regulated by negative feedback.

In addition to plasma glucose concentration, several other factors control insulin secretion (**Figure 16.9**). For example, increased amino acid concentrations stimulate insulin secretion. This is another negative feedback control; amino acid concentrations increase in the blood after ingestion of a protein-containing meal, and the increased plasma insulin stimulates the uptake of these amino acids by muscle and other cells, thereby lowering their concentrations.

There are also important hormonal controls over insulin secretion. For example, a family of hormones known as **incretins**—secreted by endocrine cells in the gastrointestinal tract in response to eating—amplifies the insulin response to glucose. The major incretins include glucagon-like peptide 1 (GLP-1) and glucose-dependent insulinotropic peptide (GIP). The actions of incretins provide a feedforward component to glucose regulation during the ingestion of a meal. Consequently, insulin secretion increases more than it would if plasma glucose were the only controller, thereby minimizing the absorptive peak in plasma glucose concentration. This mechanism minimizes the likelihood of large increases in plasma glucose after a meal, which among other things could

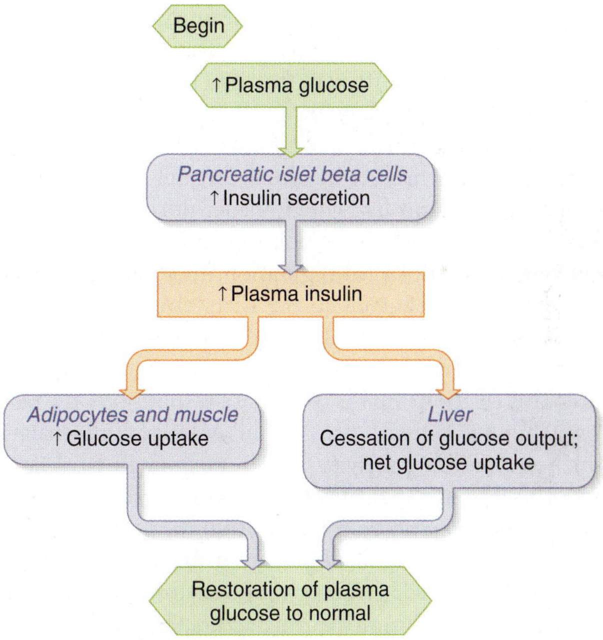

Figure 16.8 AP|R Nature of plasma glucose control over insulin secretion. As glucose concentration increases in plasma (e.g., after a meal containing carbohydrate), insulin secretion is rapidly stimulated. The increase in insulin stimulates glucose transport from extracellular fluid into cells, thus decreasing plasma glucose concentrations. Insulin also acts to inhibit hepatic glucose output.

PHYSIOLOGICAL INQUIRY

- Notice that the brain is not listed as being insulin-sensitive. Why is that advantageous?

Answer can be found at end of chapter.

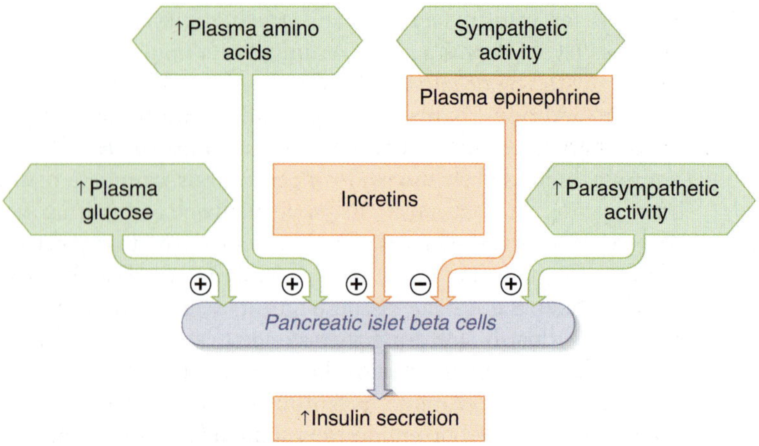

Figure 16.9 APIR Major controls of insulin secretion. The ⊕ and ⊖ symbols represent stimulatory and inhibitory actions, respectively. Incretins are gastrointestinal hormones that act as feedforward signals to the pancreas.

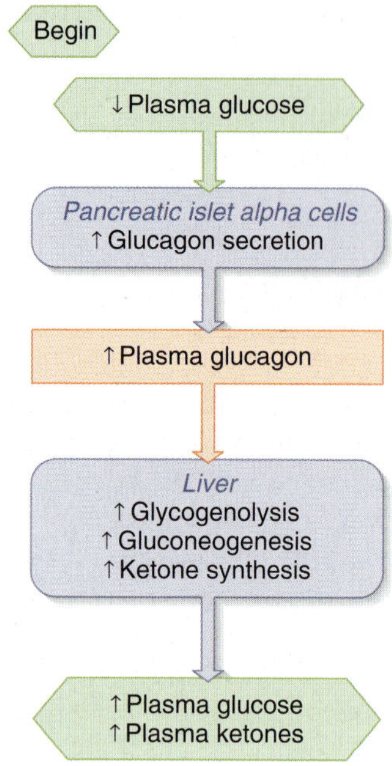

Figure 16.10 APIR Nature of plasma glucose control over glucagon secretion.

PHYSIOLOGICAL INQUIRY

- Given the effects of glucagon on plasma glucose concentrations, what effect do you think fight-or-flight (stress) reactions would have on the circulating level of glucagon?

Answer can be found at end of chapter.

exceed the capacity of the kidneys to completely reabsorb all of the glucose that appears in the filtrate in the renal nephrons. An analog of GLP-1 is currently used for the treatment of type 2 diabetes mellitus, in which the pancreas often produces insufficient insulin and the body's cells are less responsive to insulin. Injection of this analog before a meal may increase a person's circulating insulin concentration sufficiently to compensate for the decreased sensitivity of cells to insulin. The clinical features of the different forms of diabetes mellitus will be covered later in this chapter.

Finally, input of the autonomic neurons to the islets of Langerhans also influences insulin secretion. Activation of the parasympathetic neurons, which occurs during the ingestion of a meal, stimulates the secretion of insulin and constitutes a second type of feedforward regulation. In contrast, activation of the sympathetic neurons to the islets or an increase in the plasma concentration of epinephrine (the hormone secreted by the adrenal medulla) inhibits insulin secretion. The significance of this relationship for the body's response to low plasma glucose (hypoglycemia), stress, and exercise—all situations in which sympathetic activity is increased—will be described later in this chapter, but all of these are situations where an increase in plasma glucose concentration would be beneficial.

In summary, insulin plays the primary role in controlling the metabolic adjustments required for feasting or fasting. Other hormonal and neural factors, however, also play significant roles. They all oppose the action of insulin in one way or another and are known as **glucose-counterregulatory controls.** As described next, the most important of these are glucagon, epinephrine, sympathetic nerves, cortisol, and growth hormone.

Glucagon

As mentioned earlier, glucagon is the peptide hormone produced by the alpha cells of the pancreatic islets. The major physiological effects of glucagon occur within the liver and oppose those of insulin (**Figure 16.10**). Thus, glucagon (1) stimulates glycogenolysis, (2) stimulates gluconeogenesis, and (3) stimulates the synthesis of ketones. The overall results are to increase the plasma concentrations of glucose and ketones, which are important for the postabsorptive state, and to prevent hypoglycemia. The effects, if any, of glucagon on adipocyte function in humans are still unresolved.

The major stimulus for glucagon secretion is a decrease in the circulating concentration of glucose (which in turn causes a decrease in plasma insulin). The adaptive value of such a reflex is clear; a decreased plasma glucose concentration induces an increase in the secretion of glucagon into the blood, which, by its effects on metabolism, serves to restore normal blood glucose concentration by glycogenolysis and gluconeogenesis. At the same time, glucagon supplies ketones for utilization by the brain. Conversely, an increased plasma glucose concentration inhibits the secretion of glucagon, thereby helping to return the plasma glucose concentration toward normal. As a result, during the postabsorptive state, there is an increase in the glucagon/insulin ratio in the plasma, and this accounts almost entirely for the transition from the absorptive to the postabsorptive state.

The secretion of glucagon, like that of insulin, is controlled not only by the plasma concentration of glucose and other nutrients but also by neural and hormonal inputs to the islets. For example, the sympathetic nerves to the islets stimulate glucagon secretion—just the opposite of their effect on insulin secretion. The dual and opposite actions of glucagon and insulin on glucose homeostasis clearly illustrate the general principle of physiology that most physiological functions are controlled by multiple regulatory systems, often working in opposition.

Epinephrine and Sympathetic Nerves to Liver and Adipose Tissue

As noted earlier, epinephrine and the sympathetic nerves to the pancreatic islets inhibit insulin secretion and stimulate glucagon secretion. In addition, epinephrine also affects nutrient metabolism directly (**Figure 16.11**). Its major direct effects include stimulation of (1) glycogenolysis in both the liver and skeletal muscle, (2) gluconeogenesis in the liver, and (3) lipolysis in adipocytes. Activation of the sympathetic nerves to the liver and adipose tissue elicits the same responses from these organs as does circulating epinephrine.

In adipocytes, epinephrine stimulates the activity of an enzyme called **hormone-sensitive lipase (HSL)**. Once activated, HSL works along with other enzymes to catalyze the breakdown of triglycerides to free fatty acids and glycerol. Both are then released into the blood, where they serve directly as an energy source (fatty acids) or as a gluconeogenic precursor (glycerol). Not surprisingly, insulin inhibits the activity of HSL during the absorptive state, because it would not be beneficial to break down stored fat when the blood is receiving nutrients from ingested food. Thus, enhanced sympathetic nervous system activity exerts effects on organic metabolism—specifically, increased plasma concentrations of glucose, glycerol, and fatty acids—that are opposite those of insulin.

As might be predicted from these effects, low blood sugar leads to increases in both epinephrine secretion and sympathetic nerve activity to the liver and adipose tissue. This is the same stimulus that leads to increased glucagon secretion, although the receptors and pathways are totally different. When the plasma glucose concentration decreases, glucose-sensitive cells in the central nervous system (and, possibly, the liver) initiate the reflexes that lead to increased activity in the sympathetic pathways to the adrenal medulla, liver, and adipose tissue. The adaptive value of the response is the same as that for the glucagon response to hypoglycemia; blood glucose returns toward normal, and fatty acids are supplied for cell utilization.

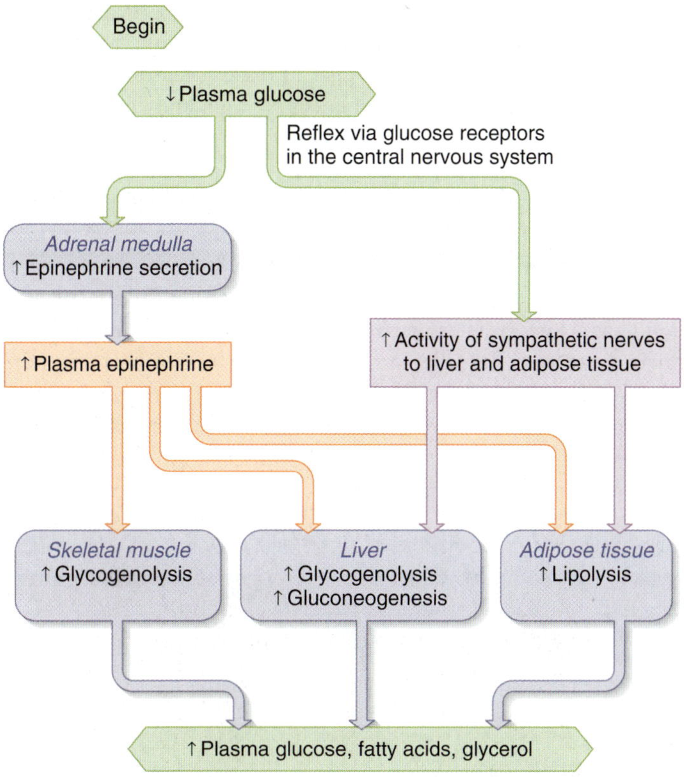

Figure 16.11 APIR Participation of the sympathetic nervous system in the response to a low plasma glucose concentration (hypoglycemia). Glycogenolysis in skeletal muscle contributes to restoring plasma glucose by releasing lactate, which is converted to glucose in the liver and released into the blood. Recall also from Figure 16.9 and the text that the sympathetic nervous system inhibits insulin and stimulates glucagon secretion, which further contributes to the increased plasma energy sources.

Cortisol

Cortisol, the major glucocorticoid produced by the adrenal cortex, plays an essential permissive role in the adjustments to fasting. We have described how fasting is associated with the stimulation of both gluconeogenesis and lipolysis; however, neither of these critical metabolic transformations occurs to the usual degree in a person deficient in cortisol. In other words, the plasma cortisol level does not need to increase much during fasting, but the presence of cortisol in the blood maintains the concentrations of the key liver and adipose-tissue enzymes required for gluconeogenesis and lipolysis—for example, HSL. Therefore, in response to fasting, people with a cortisol deficiency can develop hypoglycemia significant enough to interfere with cellular function. Moreover, cortisol can play more than a permissive role when its plasma concentration does increase, as it does during stress. At high concentrations, cortisol elicits many metabolic events ordinarily associated with fasting (**Table 16.3**). In fact, cortisol actually decreases the sensitivity of muscle and adipose cells to insulin, which helps to maintain plasma glucose concentration during fasting, thereby providing a regular source of energy for the brain. Clearly, here is another hormone that, in addition to glucagon and epinephrine, can exert actions opposite those of insulin. Indeed, people with pathologically high plasma concentrations of cortisol or who are given synthetic glucocorticoids for medical reasons can develop symptoms similar to those seen in individuals, such as those with type 2 diabetes mellitus, whose cells do not respond adequately to insulin.

TABLE 16.3 Effects of Cortisol on Organic Metabolism

I. Basal concentrations are permissive for stimulation of gluconeogenesis and lipolysis in the postabsorptive state.

II. Increased plasma concentrations cause
   A. Increased protein catabolism
   B. Increased gluconeogenesis
   C. Decreased glucose uptake by muscle cells and adipose-tissue cells
   D. Increased triglyceride breakdown

Net result: Increased plasma concentrations of amino acids, glucose, and free fatty acids

Growth Hormone

The primary physiological effects of growth hormone are to stimulate both growth and protein synthesis (by means of its effects on insulin-like growth factor 1; see Chapter 11). Compared to these effects, those it exerts on carbohydrate and lipid metabolism are less significant. Nonetheless, as is true for cortisol, either deficiency or excess of growth hormone does produce significant abnormalities in lipid and carbohydrate metabolism. Growth hormone's effects on these nutrients, in contrast to those on protein metabolism, are similar to those of cortisol and opposite those of insulin. Growth hormone (1) increases the responsiveness of adipocytes to lipolytic stimuli, (2) stimulates gluconeogenesis by the liver, and (3) reduces the ability of insulin to stimulate glucose uptake by muscle and adipose tissue. These three effects are often termed growth hormone's "anti-insulin effects." Because of these effects, some of the symptoms observed in people with acromegaly (excess growth hormone production; see the Chapter 11 Clinical Case Study) are similar to those observed in people with insulin resistance due to type 2 diabetes mellitus.

A summary of the hormonal control of metabolism is given in **Table 16.4**.

Hypoglycemia

Hypoglycemia is broadly defined as an abnormally low plasma glucose concentration. The plasma glucose concentration can decrease to very low values, usually during the postabsorptive state, in persons with several types of disorders. ***Fasting hypoglycemia*** and the relatively uncommon disorders responsible for it can be understood in terms of the regulation of blood glucose concentration. They include (1) an excess of insulin due to an insulin-producing tumor, drugs that stimulate insulin secretion, or taking too much insulin (if the person is diabetic); and (2) a defect in one or more glucose-counterregulatory controls, for example, inadequate glycogenolysis and/or gluconeogenesis due to liver disease or cortisol deficiency.

Fasting hypoglycemia causes many symptoms. Some—increased heart rate, trembling, nervousness, sweating, and anxiety—are accounted for by activation of the sympathetic nervous system caused reflexively by the hypoglycemia. Other symptoms, such as headache, confusion, dizziness, loss of coordination, and slurred speech, are direct consequences of too little glucose reaching the brain. More serious brain effects, including convulsions and coma, can occur if the plasma glucose concentration decreases sufficiently.

16.3 Energy Homeostasis in Exercise and Stress

During exercise, large quantities of fuels must be mobilized to provide the energy required for muscle contraction. These include plasma glucose and fatty acids as well as the muscle's own glycogen.

The additional plasma glucose used during exercise is supplied by the liver, both by breakdown of its glycogen stores and by gluconeogenesis. Glycerol is made available to the liver by a large increase in adipose-tissue lipolysis due to activation of HSL, with a resultant release of glycerol and fatty acids into the blood; the fatty acids serve as an additional energy source for the exercising muscle.

What happens to plasma glucose concentration during exercise? It changes very little in short-term, mild-to-moderate exercise and may even increase slightly with strenuous, short-term activity due to the counterregulatory actions of hormones. However, during prolonged exercise (**Figure 16.12**)—more than about 90 min—plasma glucose concentration does decrease but usually by less than 25%. Clearly, glucose output by the liver increases approximately in proportion to increased glucose utilization during exercise, at least until the later stages of prolonged exercise when it begins to lag somewhat.

The metabolic profile of an exercising person—increases in hepatic glucose production, triglyceride breakdown, and fatty acid utilization—is similar to a fasting person, and the endocrine controls are also the same. Exercise is characterized by a decrease in insulin secretion and an increase in glucagon secretion (see Figure 16.12), and the changes in the plasma concentrations of these two hormones are the major controls during exercise. In addition, activity of the sympathetic nervous system increases (including secretion of epinephrine) and cortisol and growth hormone secretion both increase as well.

What triggers increased glucagon secretion and decreased insulin secretion during exercise? One signal, at least during

TABLE 16.4 Summary of Glucose-Counterregulatory Controls*

	Glucagon	Epinephrine	Cortisol	Growth Hormone
Glycogenolysis	✓	✓		
Gluconeogenesis	✓	✓	✓	✓
Lipolysis		✓	✓	✓
Inhibition of glucose uptake by muscle cells and adipose tissue cells			✓	✓

*A ✓ indicates that the hormone stimulates the process; no ✓ indicates that the hormone has no major physiological effect on the process. Epinephrine stimulates glycogenolysis in both liver and skeletal muscle, whereas glucagon does so only in liver.

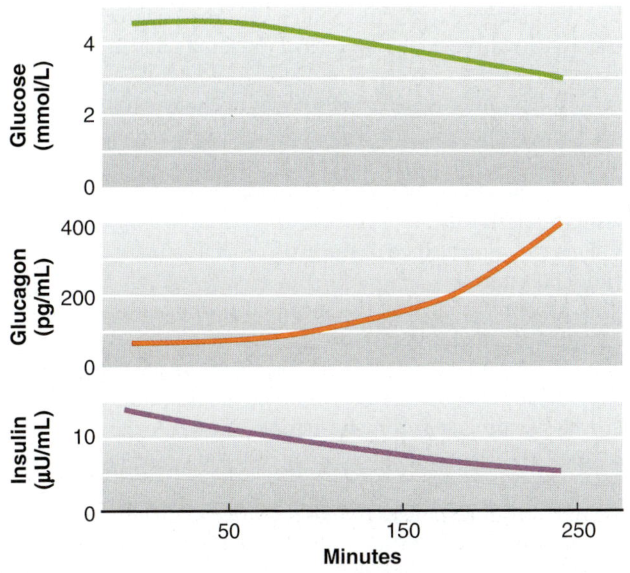

Figure 16.12 Plasma concentrations of glucose, glucagon, and insulin during prolonged (240 min) moderate exercise at a fixed intensity (pg/mL = Picograms per milliliter; μU/mL = Microunits per milliliter). Adapted from Felig and Wahren.

prolonged exercise, is the modest decrease in plasma glucose that occurs (see Figure 16.12). This is the same signal that controls the secretion of these hormones in fasting. Other inputs at all intensities of exercise include increased circulating epinephrine and increased activity of the sympathetic neurons supplying the pancreatic islets. Thus, the increased sympathetic nervous system activity characteristic of exercise not only contributes directly to energy mobilization by acting on the liver and adipose tissue but contributes indirectly by inhibiting the secretion of insulin and stimulating that of glucagon. This sympathetic output is not triggered by changes in plasma glucose concentration but is mediated by the central nervous system as part of the neural response to exercise.

One component of the response to exercise is quite different from the response to fasting; in exercise, glucose uptake and utilization by the muscles are increased, whereas during fasting they are markedly decreased. How is it that, during exercise, the movement of glucose via facilitated diffusion into skeletal muscle can remain high in the presence of decreased plasma insulin and increased plasma concentrations of cortisol and growth hormone, all of which decrease glucose uptake by skeletal muscle? By an as-yet-unidentified mechanism, muscle contraction causes migration of an intracellular store of glucose transporters to the plasma membrane and an increase in synthesis of the transporters. For this reason, even though exercising muscles require more glucose than do muscles at rest, less insulin is required to induce glucose transport into muscle cells.

Exercise and the postabsorptive state are not the only situations characterized by the endocrine profile of decreased insulin and increased glucagon, sympathetic activity, cortisol, and growth hormone. This profile also occurs in response to a variety of nonspecific stresses, both physical and emotional. The adaptive value of these endocrine responses to stress is that the resulting metabolic shifts prepare the body for exercise ("fight or flight") in the face of real or threatened injury. In addition, the amino acids liberated by the catabolism of body protein stores because of decreased insulin and increased cortisol not only provide energy via gluconeogenesis but also constitute a potential source of amino acids for tissue repair should injury occur.

Chronic, intense exercise can also be stressful for the human body. In such cases, certain nonessential functions shut down so that nutrients can be directed primarily to muscle. One of these nonessential functions is reproduction. Consequently, adolescents engaged in rigorous daily training regimens, such as Olympic-caliber gymnasts, may show delayed puberty. Similarly, women who perform chronic, intense exercise may become temporarily infertile, a condition known as ***exercise-induced amenorrhea*** (the lack of regular menstrual cycles—see Chapter 17). This condition occurs in a variety of occupations that combine weight loss and strenuous exercise, such as may occur in professional ballerinas. Whether exercise-induced infertility occurs in men is uncertain, but most evidence suggests it does not.

SECTION A SUMMARY

Events of the Absorptive and Postabsorptive States

I. During absorption, energy is provided primarily by absorbed carbohydrate. Net synthesis of glycogen, triglyceride, and protein occurs.
   a. Some absorbed carbohydrate not used for energy is converted to glycogen, mainly in the liver and skeletal muscle, but most is converted in liver and adipocytes to α-glycerol phosphate and fatty acids, which then combine to form triglycerides. The liver releases its triglycerides in very-low-density lipoproteins, the fatty acids of which are picked up by adipocytes.
   b. The fatty acids of some absorbed triglycerides are used for energy, but most are rebuilt into fat in adipose tissue.
   c. Plasma cholesterol is a precursor for the synthesis of plasma membranes, bile salts, and steroid hormones.
   d. Cholesterol synthesis by the liver is controlled so as to homeostatically regulate plasma cholesterol concentration; it varies inversely with ingested cholesterol.
   e. The liver also secretes cholesterol into the bile and converts it to bile salts.
   f. Plasma cholesterol is carried mainly by low-density lipoproteins, which deliver it to cells; high-density lipoproteins carry cholesterol from cells to the liver and steroid-producing cells. The LDL/HDL ratio correlates with the incidence of coronary heart disease.
   g. Some absorbed amino acids are converted to proteins, but excess amino acids are converted to carbohydrate and fat.
   h. There is a net uptake of glucose by the liver.

II. In the postabsorptive state, blood glucose level is maintained by a combination of glucose production by the liver and a switch from glucose utilization to fatty acid and ketone utilization by most tissues.
   a. Synthesis of glycogen, fat, and protein is curtailed, and net breakdown of these molecules occurs.
   b. The liver forms glucose by glycogenolysis of its own glycogen and by gluconeogenesis from lactate and pyruvate (from the breakdown of muscle glycogen), glycerol (from adipose-tissue lipolysis), and amino acids (from protein catabolism).

c. Glycolysis is decreased, and most of the body's energy supply comes from the oxidation of fatty acids released by adipose-tissue lipolysis and of ketones produced from fatty acids by the liver.
d. The brain continues to use glucose but also starts using ketones as they build up in the blood.

Endocrine and Neural Control of the Absorptive and Postabsorptive States

I. The major hormones secreted by the pancreatic islets of Langerhans are insulin by the beta cells and glucagon by the alpha cells.
II. Insulin is the most important hormone controlling metabolism.
  a. In muscle, it stimulates glucose uptake, glycolysis, and net synthesis of glycogen and protein. In adipose tissue, it stimulates glucose uptake and net synthesis of triglyceride. In liver, it inhibits gluconeogenesis and glucose release and stimulates the net synthesis of glycogen and triglycerides.
  b. The major stimulus for insulin secretion is an increased plasma glucose concentration, but secretion is also influenced by many other factors, which are summarized in Figure 16.9.
III. Glucagon, epinephrine, cortisol, and growth hormone all exert effects on carbohydrate and lipid metabolism that are opposite, in one way or another, to those of insulin. They increase plasma concentrations of glucose, glycerol, and fatty acids.
  a. Glucagon's physiological actions are on the liver, where glucagon stimulates glycogenolysis, gluconeogenesis, and ketone synthesis.
  b. The major stimulus for glucagon secretion is hypoglycemia, but secretion is also stimulated by other inputs, including the sympathetic nerves to the islets.
  c. Epinephrine released from the adrenal medulla in response to hypoglycemia stimulates glycogenolysis in the liver and muscle, gluconeogenesis in the liver, and lipolysis in adipocytes. The sympathetic nerves to liver and adipose tissue exert effects similar to those of epinephrine.
  d. Cortisol is permissive for gluconeogenesis and lipolysis; in higher concentrations, it stimulates gluconeogenesis and blocks glucose uptake. These last two effects are also exerted by growth hormone.
IV. Hypoglycemia is defined as an abnormally low glucose concentration in the blood. Symptoms of hypoglycemia are similar to those of sympathetic nervous system activation. However, severe hypoglycemia can lead to brain dysfunction and even death if untreated.

Energy Homeostasis in Exercise and Stress

I. During exercise, the muscles use as their energy sources plasma glucose, plasma fatty acids, and their own glycogen.
  a. Glucose is provided by the liver, and fatty acids are provided by adipose-tissue lipolysis.
  b. The changes in plasma insulin, glucagon, and epinephrine are similar to those that occur during the postabsorptive state and are mediated mainly by the sympathetic nervous system.
II. Stress causes hormonal changes similar to those caused by exercise.

SECTION A REVIEW QUESTIONS

1. Using a diagram, summarize the events of the absorptive period.
2. In what two organs does major glycogen storage occur?
3. How do the liver and adipose tissue metabolize glucose during the absorptive period?
4. How does adipose tissue metabolize absorbed triglyceride, and what are the three major sources of the fatty acids in adipose-tissue triglyceride?
5. Using a diagram, describe the sources of cholesterol gain and loss. Include the roles the liver plays in cholesterol metabolism, and describe the controls over these processes.
6. What are the effects of saturated and unsaturated fatty acids on plasma cholesterol?
7. What is the significance of the ratio of LDL cholesterol to HDL cholesterol?
8. What happens to most of the absorbed amino acids when a high-protein meal is ingested?
9. Using a diagram, summarize the events of the postabsorptive state; include the four sources of blood glucose and the pathways leading to ketone formation.
10. Distinguish between the roles of glycerol and free fatty acids during fasting.
11. List the overall responses of muscle, adipose tissue, and liver to insulin. What effects occur when the plasma insulin concentration decreases?
12. Describe several inputs controlling insulin secretion and the physiological significance of each.
13. List the effects of glucagon on the liver and their consequences.
14. Discuss two inputs controlling glucagon secretion and the physiological significance of each.
15. List the metabolic effects of epinephrine and the sympathetic nerves to the liver and adipose tissue, and state the net results of each.
16. Describe the permissive effects of cortisol and the effects that occur when plasma cortisol concentration increases.
17. List the effects of growth hormone on carbohydrate and lipid metabolism.
18. Which hormones stimulate gluconeogenesis? Glycogenolysis in the liver? Lipolysis in adipose tissue? Which hormone or hormones inhibit glucose uptake into cells?
19. Describe how plasma glucose, insulin, glucagon, and epinephrine concentrations change during exercise and stress. What causes the changes in the concentrations of the hormones?

SECTION A KEY TERMS

absorptive state 573
alpha cell 578
α-keto acid 576
beta cell 578
cholesterol 574
glucagon 578
gluconeogenesis 577
glucose-counterregulatory control 582
glucose sparing 577
glycogenolysis 576
glycogen phosphorylase 580
glycogen synthase 580
high-density lipoprotein (HDL) 575
hormone-sensitive lipase (HSL) 583
hypoglycemia 584
incretins 581
insulin 578
islets of Langerhans 578
ketone 578
lipolysis 577
lipoprotein 574
lipoprotein lipase 574
low-density lipoprotein (LDL) 575
postabsorptive state 573
very-low-density lipoprotein (VLDL) 574

SECTION A CLINICAL TERMS

atherosclerosis 574
exercise-induced amenorrhea 585
familial hypercholesterolemia 576
fasting hypoglycemia 584

SECTION B

Regulation of Total-Body Energy Balance and Temperature

16.4 General Principles of Energy Expenditure

The breakdown of organic molecules liberates the energy locked in their chemical bonds. Cells use this energy to perform the various forms of biological work, such as muscle contraction, active transport, and molecular synthesis. These processes illustrate the general principle of physiology that physiological processes are dictated by the laws of chemistry and physics. The first law of thermodynamics states that energy can be neither created nor destroyed but can be converted from one form to another. Therefore, internal energy liberated (ΔE) during breakdown of an organic molecule can either appear as heat (H) or be used to perform work (W).

$$\Delta E = H + W$$

During metabolism, about 60% of the energy released from organic molecules appears immediately as heat, and the rest is used for work. The energy used for work must first be incorporated into molecules of ATP. The subsequent breakdown of ATP serves as the immediate energy source for the work. The body is incapable of converting heat to work, but the heat released in its chemical reactions helps to maintain body temperature.

Biological work can be divided into two general categories: (1) **external work**—the movement of external objects by contracting skeletal muscles; and (2) **internal work**—all other forms of work, including skeletal muscle activity not used in moving external objects. As just stated, much of the energy liberated from nutrient catabolism appears immediately as heat. What may not be obvious is that internal work, too, is ultimately transformed to heat except during periods of growth. For example, internal work is performed during cardiac contraction, but this energy appears ultimately as heat generated by the friction of blood flow through the blood vessels.

Thus, the total energy liberated when cells catabolize organic nutrients may be transformed into body heat, can be used to do external work, or can be stored in the body in the form of organic molecules. The **total energy expenditure** of the body is therefore given by the equation

$$\text{Total energy expenditure} = \text{Internal heat produced} + \text{External work performed} + \text{Energy stored}$$

Metabolic Rate

The basic metric unit of energy is the joule. When quantifying the energy of metabolism, however, another unit is used, called the **calorie** (equal to 4.184 joules). One calorie is the amount of heat required to raise the temperature of one gram of water from 14.5°C to 15.5°C. Because the amount of energy stored in food is quite high relative to a calorie, a more convenient expression of energy in this context is the **kilocalorie (kcal),** which is equal to 1000 calories. (In the field of nutrition, the terms "Calorie" with a capital *C* and "kilocalorie" are synonyms; they are both 1000 "calories," with a small *c*.) Total energy expenditure per unit time is called the **metabolic rate.**

Because many factors cause the metabolic rate to vary (**Table 16.5**), the most common method for evaluating it specifies certain standardized conditions and measures what is known as the **basal metabolic rate** (**BMR**). In the basal condition, the subject is at rest in a room at a comfortable temperature and has not eaten for at least 12 h (i.e., is in the postabsorptive state). These conditions are arbitrarily designated "basal," even though the metabolic rate during sleep may be lower than the

TABLE 16.5 Some Factors Affecting the Metabolic Rate

Sleep (↓ during sleep)	
Age (↓ with increasing age)	
Gender (women less than men at any given size)	
Fasting (BMR decreases, which conserves energy stores)	
Height, weight, and body surface area	The presence of, or an increase in, any of these factors causes an increase in metabolic rate
Growth	
Pregnancy, menstruation, lactation	
Infection or other disease	
Body temperature	
Recent ingestion of food	
Muscular activity	
Emotional stress	
Environmental temperature	
Circulating concentrations of various hormones, especially epinephrine, thyroid hormone, and leptin	

BMR. The BMR is sometimes called the "metabolic cost of living," and most of the energy involved is expended by the heart, muscle, liver, kidneys, and brain. For the following discussion, the term *BMR* can be applied to metabolic rate only when the specified conditions are met. The next sections describe several of the important determinants of BMR and metabolic rate.

Thyroid Hormones

The thyroid hormones (T_3 and T_4) are the single most important determinant of BMR regardless of body size, age, or gender. T_3 and T_4 increase the oxygen consumption and heat production of most body tissues, a notable exception being the brain. This ability to increase BMR is known as a **calorigenic effect.**

Long-term excessive T_3 and T_4, as in people with hyperthyroidism (see Chapter 11 and the first case study in Chapter 19), induce a host of effects secondary to the calorigenic effect. For example, the increased metabolic demands markedly increase hunger and food intake. The greater intake often remains inadequate to meet metabolic demands. The resulting net catabolism of protein and fat stores leads to loss of body weight. Of importance is the fact that the more metabolically active a particular cell is, the greater are its requirements for vitamins, which serve as cofactors for many enzymes and for ATP production. Therefore, even with increased dietary intake, the onset of hyperthyroidism may result in symptoms of vitamin deficiency. Also, the greater heat production activates heat-dissipating mechanisms, such as skin vasodilation and sweating, and the person feels intolerant to warm environments. In contrast, the hypothyroid person may experience cold intolerance.

Epinephrine

Epinephrine is another hormone that exerts a calorigenic effect. This effect may be related to its stimulation of glycogen and triglyceride catabolism, as ATP hydrolysis and energy liberation occur during both the breakdown and subsequent resynthesis of these molecules. As a result, when epinephrine secretion by the adrenal medulla is stimulated, the metabolic rate increases.

Diet-Induced Thermogenesis

The ingestion of food increases the metabolic rate by 10% to 20% for a few hours after eating. This effect is known as **diet-induced thermogenesis.** Ingested protein produces the greatest effect, and carbohydrate and fat produce less. Most of the increased heat production is caused by the processing of the absorbed nutrients by the liver, the energy expended by the gastrointestinal tract in digestion and absorption, and the storage of energy in adipose and other tissue. Because of the contribution of diet-induced thermogenesis, a BMR measurement would have to be performed in the postabsorptive state. As we will see, *prolonged* alterations in food intake (either increased or decreased total calories) also have significant effects on metabolic rate.

Muscle Activity

The factor that can increase metabolic rate the most is altered skeletal muscle activity. Even minimal increases in muscle contraction significantly increase metabolic rate, and strenuous exercise may increase energy expenditure several-fold (**Figure 16.13**). Therefore, depending on the degree of physical activity, total energy expenditure may vary for a healthy young adult from a value of approximately 1500 kcal/24 h (for a sedentary individual) to more than 7000 kcal/24 h (for someone who is extremely active). Changes in muscle activity also account in part for the changes in metabolic rate that occur during sleep (decreased muscle contraction) and during exposure to a low environmental temperature (increased muscle contraction due to shivering).

Approximate Energy Expenditure During Different Types of Activity for a 70 kg (154 lb) Person

Form of Activity		Energy kcal/h
Sitting at rest	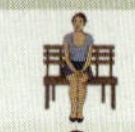	100
Walking on level ground at 4.3 km/h (2.6 mi/h)	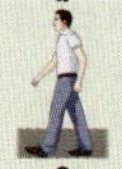	200
Walking on 3% grade at 4.3 km/h (2.6 mi/h)	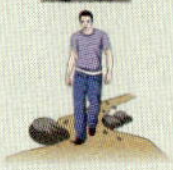	360
Weight lifting *(light workout)*	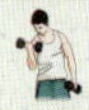	220
Bicycling on level ground at 9 km/h (5.3 mi/h)	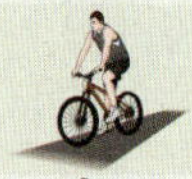	300
Shoveling snow	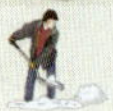	480
Jogging at 9 km/h (5.3 mi/h)	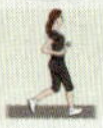	570
Rowing at 20 strokes/ min	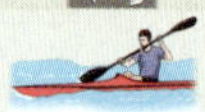	830

Figure 16.13 Rates of energy expenditure for a variety of common activities.

16.5 Regulation of Total-Body Energy Stores

Under normal conditions, for body weight to remain stable, the total energy expenditure (metabolic rate) of the body must equal the total energy intake. We have already identified the ultimate forms of energy expenditure: internal heat production, external work, and net molecular synthesis (energy storage). The source of input is the energy contained in ingested food. Therefore,

$$\text{Energy from food intake} = \text{Internal heat produced} + \text{External work} + \text{Energy stored}$$

This equation includes no term for loss of energy from the body via excretion of nutrients because normally only negligible losses occur via the urine, feces, and sloughed hair and skin. In certain diseases, however, the most important being diabetes mellitus, urinary losses of organic molecules may be quite large and would have to be included in the equation.

Rearranging the equation to focus on energy storage gives

$$\text{Energy stored} = \text{Energy from food intake} - (\text{Internal heat produced} + \text{External work})$$

Consequently, whenever energy intake differs from the sum of internal heat produced and external work, changes in energy storage occur; that is, the total-body energy content increases or decreases. Normally, energy storage is mainly in the form of fat in adipose tissue.

It is worth emphasizing at this point that "body weight" and "total-body energy content" are not synonymous. Body weight is determined not only by the amount of fat, carbohydrate, and protein in the body but also by the amounts of water, bone, and other minerals. For example, an individual can lose body weight quickly as the result of sweating or an excessive increase in urinary output. It is also possible to gain large amounts of weight as a result of water retention, as occurs, for example, during heart failure. Moreover, even focusing only on the nutrients, a constant body weight does not mean that total-body energy content is constant. The reason is that 1 g of fat contains 9 kcal, whereas 1 g of either carbohydrate or protein contains 4 kcal. Aging, for example, is usually associated with a gain of fat and a loss of protein; the result is that even though the person's body weight may stay constant, the total-body energy content has increased. Apart from these qualifications, however, in the remainder of this chapter, changes in body weight are equated with changes in total-body energy content and, more specifically, changes in body fat stores.

Body weight in adults is usually regulated around a stable set point. Theoretically, this regulation can be achieved by reflexively adjusting caloric intake and/or energy expenditure in response to changes in body weight. It was once assumed that regulation of caloric intake was the only important adjustment, and the next section will describe this process. However, it is now clear that energy expenditure can also be adjusted in response to changes in body weight.

A typical demonstration of this process in human beings follows. Total daily energy expenditure was measured in nonobese subjects at their usual body weight and again after they either lost 10% of their body weight by underfeeding or gained 10% by overfeeding. At their new body weight, the overfed subjects manifested a large (15%) increase in both resting and nonresting energy expenditure, and the underfed subjects showed a similar decrease. These changes in energy expenditure were much greater than could be accounted for simply by the altered metabolic mass of the body or having to move a larger or smaller body.

The generalization that emerges is that a dietary-induced change in total-body energy stores triggers, in negative feedback fashion, an alteration in energy expenditure that opposes the gain or loss of energy stores. This phenomenon helps explain why some dieters lose about 5 to 10 pounds fairly easily and then become stuck at a plateau.

Control of Food Intake

The control of food intake can be analyzed in the same way as any other biological control system. As the previous section emphasized, the variable being maintained in this system is total-body energy content or, more specifically, total fat stores. An essential component of such a control system is the peptide hormone **leptin,** synthesized by adipocytes and released from the cells in proportion to the amount of fat they contain. This hormone acts on the hypothalamus to cause a decrease in food intake, in part by inhibiting the release of **neuropeptide Y,** a hypothalamic neurotransmitter that stimulates appetite. Leptin also increases BMR and, therefore, plays an important role in the changes in energy expenditure that occur in response to overfeeding or underfeeding, as described in the previous section. Thus, as illustrated in **Figure 16.14**, leptin functions in a negative feedback system to maintain a stable total-body energy content by signaling to the brain how much fat is stored.

It should be emphasized that leptin is important for *long-term* matching of caloric intake to energy expenditure. In addition, it is thought that various other signals act on the hypothalamus (and other brain areas) over short periods of time to regulate individual meal length and frequency (**Figure 16.15**). These **satiety signals** (factors that decrease appetite) cause the person to cease feeling hungry and set the time period before hunger returns. For example, the rate of insulin-dependent glucose utilization by certain areas of the hypothalamus increases during eating, and this probably constitutes a satiety signal. Insulin, which increases during food absorption, also acts as a direct satiety signal. Diet-induced thermogenesis tends to increase body temperature slightly, which acts as yet another satiety signal. Finally, some satiety signals are initiated by the presence of food within the gastrointestinal tract. These include neural signals triggered by stimulation of both stretch receptors and chemoreceptors in the stomach and duodenum, as well as by certain of the hormones (cholecystokinin, for example) released from the stomach and duodenum during eating.

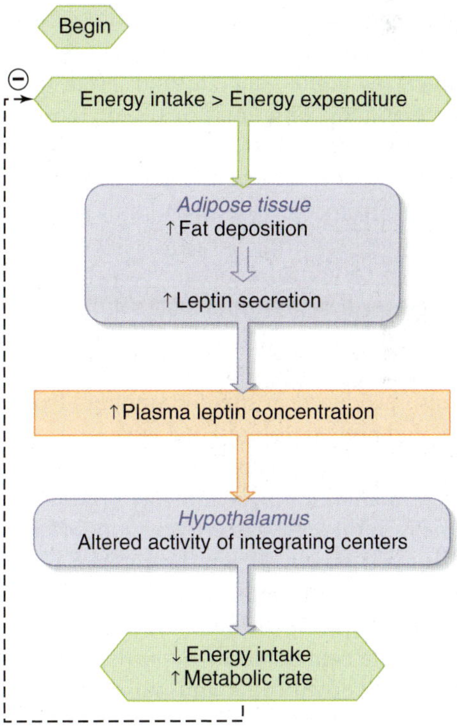

Figure 16.14 Postulated role of leptin in the control of total-body energy stores. Note that the direction of the arrows within the boxes would be reversed if energy (food) intake were less than energy expenditure.

PHYSIOLOGICAL INQUIRY

- Under what circumstances might the appetite-suppressing action of leptin be counterproductive?

Answer can be found at end of chapter.

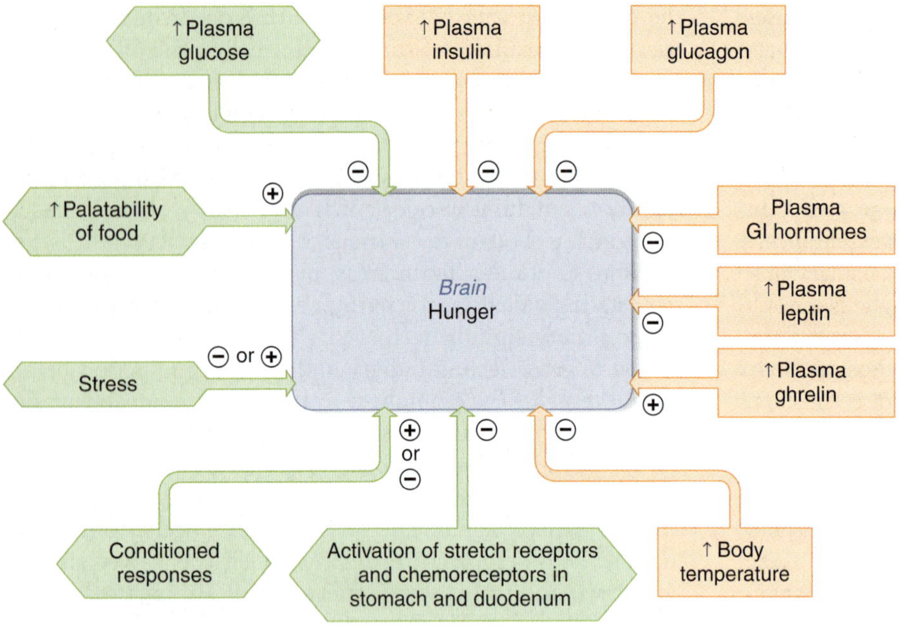

Figure 16.15 Short-term inputs controlling appetite and, consequently, food intake. The ⊖ symbols denote hunger suppression, and the ⊕ symbols denote hunger stimulation.

PHYSIOLOGICAL INQUIRY

- As shown, stretch receptors in the gut after a meal can suppress hunger. Would drinking a large glass of water before a meal be an effective means of dieting?

Answer can be found at end of chapter.

Although we have focused on leptin and other factors as satiety signals, it is important to realize that a primary function of leptin is to increase metabolic rate. If a person is subjected to starvation, his or her adipocytes begin to shrink, as catabolic hormones mobilize triglycerides from adipocytes. This decrease in size causes a proportional reduction in leptin secretion from the shrinking cells. The decrease in leptin concentration removes the signal that normally inhibits appetite and speeds up metabolism. The result is that a loss of fat mass leads to a decrease in leptin and, thereby, a decrease in BMR and an increase in appetite. This may be the true evolutionary significance of leptin, namely that its disappearance from the blood results in a decreased BMR, thereby prolonging life during periods of starvation.

In addition to leptin, another recently discovered hormone appears to be an important regulator of appetite. **Ghrelin** (GREH-lin) is a 28-amino-acid peptide synthesized and released primarily from endocrine cells in the stomach. Ghrelin is also produced in smaller amounts from other gastrointestinal and nongastrointestinal tissues.

Ghrelin has several major functions that have been identified in experimental animals and that appear to be true in humans. One is to increase growth *h*ormone *rel*ease—the derivation of the word *ghrelin*—from the anterior pituitary gland. The major function of ghrelin pertinent to this chapter is to increase hunger by stimulating NPY and other neuropeptides in the feeding centers in the hypothalamus. Ghrelin also decreases the breakdown of fat and increases gastric motility and acid production. It makes sense, then, that the major stimuli to ghrelin are fasting and a low-calorie diet.

Ghrelin, therefore, participates in several feedback loops. Fasting or a low-calorie diet leads to an increase in ghrelin. This stimulates hunger and, if food is available, food intake. The food intake subsequently decreases ghrelin, possibly through stomach distention, caloric absorption, or some other mechanism.

Overweight and Obesity

The clinical definition of ***overweight*** is a functional one, a state in which an increased amount of fat in the body results in a significant impairment of health from a variety of diseases or disorders—notably, hypertension, atherosclerosis, heart disease, diabetes, and sleep apnea. ***Obesity*** denotes a particularly large accumulation of fat—that is, extreme overweight. The difficulty has been establishing at what point fat accumulation begins to constitute a health risk. This is evaluated by epidemiologic studies that correlate disease rates with some measure of the amount of fat in the body. Currently, the preferred simple method for assessing the latter is not the body weight but the **body mass index (BMI)**, which is calculated by dividing the weight (in kilograms) by the square of the height (in meters). For example, a 70 kg person with a height of 180 cm would have a BMI of 21.6 kg/m^2 (70/1.8^2).

Current National Institutes of Health guidelines categorize BMIs of greater than 25 kg/m^2 as overweight (i.e., as having some increased health risk because of excess fat) and those greater than 30 kg/m^2 as obese, with a significantly increased health risk. According to these criteria, more than half of U.S. women and men age 20 and older are now considered to be overweight and one-quarter or more to be clinically obese! Even more troubling is that the incidence of childhood overweight and obesity is increasing in the United States and other countries. These guidelines, however, are controversial. First, the epidemiologic studies do not always agree as to where along the continuum of BMIs between 25 and 30 kg/m^2 health risks begin to significantly increase. Second, even granting increased risk above a BMI of 25 kg/m^2, the studies do not always account for confounding factors associated with being overweight or even obese, particularly a sedentary lifestyle. Instead, the increased health risk may be at least partly due to lack of physical activity, not body fat, per se.

To add to the complexity, there is growing evidence that not just total fat but where the fat is located has important consequences. Specifically, people with mostly abdominal fat are at greater risk for developing serious conditions such as diabetes and cardiovascular diseases than people whose fat is mainly in the lower body on the buttocks and thighs. There is currently no agreement as to the explanation of this phenomenon, but there are important differences in the physiology of adipose-tissue cells in these regions. For example, adipose-tissue cells in the abdomen are much more adept at breaking down fat stores and releasing the products into the blood.

What is known about the underlying causes of obesity? Identical twins who have been separated soon after birth and raised in different households manifest strikingly similar body weights and incidences of obesity as adults. Twin studies, therefore, indicate that genetic factors play an important role in obesity. It has been postulated that natural selection favored the evolution in our ancestors of so-called **thrifty genes,** which boosted the ability to store fat from each feast in order to sustain people through the next fast. Given today's relative abundance of high-fat foods in many countries, such an adaptation is now a liability. Despite the importance of genetic factors, psychological, cultural, and social factors can also play a significant role. For example, the increasing incidence of obesity in the United States and other industrialized nations during the past 40 years cannot be explained by changes in our genes.

Much recent research has focused on possible abnormalities in the leptin system as a cause of obesity. In one strain of mice (shown in the chapter-opening photo), the gene that codes for leptin is mutated so that adipose-tissue cells produce an abnormal, inactive leptin, resulting in hereditary obesity. The same is *not* true, however, for the vast majority of obese people. The leptin secreted by these people is normal, and leptin concentrations in the blood are increased, not decreased. This observation indicates that leptin secretion is not at fault in these people. Consequently, such people are leptin-resistant in much the same way that people with type 2 diabetes mellitus are insulin-resistant. Moreover, there are multiple genes that interact with one another and with environmental factors to influence a person's susceptibility to weight gain.

The methods and goals of treating obesity are now undergoing extensive rethinking. An increase in body fat must be due to an excess of energy intake over energy expenditure, and low-calorie diets have long been the mainstay of therapy. However, it is now clear that such diets alone have limited effectiveness in obese people; over 90% regain all or most of the lost weight within 5 years. Another important reason for the ineffectiveness of such diets is that, as described earlier, the person's metabolic rate decreases as leptin concentration decreases, sometimes decreasing low enough to prevent further weight loss on as little as 1000 calories a day. Because of this, many obese people continue to gain weight or remain in stable energy balance on a caloric intake equal to or less than the amount consumed by people of normal weight. These persons must either have less physical activity than normal or have lower basal metabolic rates. Finally, at least half of obese people—those who are more than 20% overweight—who try to diet down to desirable weights suffer medically, physically, and psychologically. This is what would be expected if the body were "trying" to maintain body weight (more specifically, fat stores) at the higher set point.

Such studies, taken together, indicate that crash diets are not an effective long-term method for controlling weight. Instead, caloric intake should be set at a level that can be maintained for the rest of one's life. Such an intake in an overweight person should lead to a slow, steady weight loss of no more than 1 pound per week until the body weight stabilizes at a new, lower level. The most important precept is that any program of weight loss should include increased physical activity. The exercise itself uses calories, but more importantly, it partially offsets the tendency, described earlier, for the metabolic rate to decrease during long-term caloric restriction and weight loss. Also, the combination of exercise and caloric restriction may cause the person to lose more fat and less protein than with caloric restriction alone, although some recent studies suggest this may not always be true.

Let us calculate how rapidly a person can expect to lose weight on a reducing diet (assuming, for simplicity, no change in energy expenditure). Suppose a person whose steady-state metabolic rate per 24 h is 2000 kcal goes on a 1000 kcal/day diet. How much of the person's own body fat will be required to supply this additional 1000 kcal/day? Because fat contains 9 kcal/g,

$$\frac{1000 \text{ kcal/day}}{9 \text{ kcal/g}} = 111 \text{ g/day, or } 777 \text{ g/week}$$

Approximately another 77 g of water is lost from the adipose tissue along with this fat (adipose tissue is 10% water), so that the grand total for 1 week's loss equals 854 g, or 1.8 pounds. Therefore, even on this severe diet, the person can reasonably expect to lose approximately this amount of weight per week, assuming no decrease in metabolic rate occurs.

Eating Disorders: Anorexia Nervosa and Bulimia Nervosa

Two of the major eating disorders are found primarily in adolescent girls and young women. The typical person with ***anorexia nervosa*** becomes pathologically obsessed with her weight and body image. She may decrease her food intake so severely that she may die of starvation. There are many other abnormalities associated with anorexia nervosa—cessation of menstrual periods, low blood pressure, low body temperature, and altered secretion of many hormones, including increased concentrations of ghrelin. It is likely that these are simply the results of starvation, although it is possible that some represent signs, along with the eating disturbances, of primary hypothalamic malfunction.

Bulimia nervosa, usually called simply *bulimia,* is a disorder characterized by recurrent episodes of binge eating. It is usually associated with regular self-induced vomiting and use of laxatives or diuretics, as well as strict dieting, fasting, or vigorous exercise to lose weight or to prevent weight gain. Like individuals with anorexia nervosa, those with bulimia manifest a persistent heightened concern with body weight, although they generally remain within 10% of their ideal weight. This disorder too, is accompanied by a variety of physiological abnormalities, but it is unknown in some cases whether they are causal or secondary.

In addition to anorexia and bulimia, rare lesions or tumors within the hypothalamic centers that normally regulate appetite can result in overfeeding or underfeeding.

What Should We Eat?

In recent years, more and more dietary factors have been associated with the cause or prevention of many diseases or disorders, including not only coronary artery disease but hypertension, cancer, birth defects, osteoporosis, and others. These associations come mainly from animal studies, epidemiologic studies on people, and basic research concerning potential mechanisms. Some of these findings may be difficult to interpret or may be conflicting. One of the most commonly used sets of dietary recommendations, issued by the National Research Council, is presented in **Table 16.6**.

TABLE 16.6	Summary of National Research Council Dietary Recommendations
Reduce fat intake to 30% or less of total calories; most fat consumed should be mono- or polyunsaturated fats. Reduce saturated fatty acid intake to less than 10% of calories and intake of cholesterol to less than 300 mg daily.	
Every day eat five or more servings of a combination of vegetables and fruits, especially green and yellow vegetables and citrus fruits. Also, increase complex carbohydrates by eating six or more daily servings of a combination of whole-grain breads, cereals, and legumes.	
Maintain protein intake at moderate levels (approximately 0.8 g/kg body mass).	
Balance food intake and physical activity to maintain appropriate body weight.	
Alcohol consumption is not recommended. For those who drink alcoholic beverages, limit consumption to the equivalent of 1 ounce of pure alcohol in a single day.	
Limit total daily intake of sodium to 2.3 g or less.	
Maintain adequate calcium intake.	
Avoid taking dietary supplements in excess of the RDA (Recommended Dietary Allowance) in any one day.	
Maintain an optimal intake of fluoride, particularly during the years of primary and secondary tooth formation and growth. Most bottled water does not contain fluoride.	

16.6 Regulation of Body Temperature

In the preceding discussion, it was emphasized that energy expenditure is linked to our ability to maintain a stable, homeostatic body temperature. In this section, we discuss the mechanisms by which the body gains or loses heat in a variety of healthy or pathological settings.

Humans are **endotherms,** meaning that they generate their own internal body heat and do not rely on the energy of sunlight to warm the body. Moreover, humans maintain their body temperatures within very narrow limits despite wide fluctuations in ambient temperature and are, therefore, also known as **homeotherms.** The relatively stable body temperature frees biochemical reactions from fluctuating with the external temperature. However, the maintenance of a warm body temperature (approximately 37°C in healthy persons) imposes a requirement for precise regulatory mechanisms because large elevations of temperature cause nerve malfunction and protein denaturation. Some people suffer convulsions at a body temperature of 41°C (106°F), and 43°C is considered to be the absolute limit for survival.

A few important generalizations about normal human body temperature should be stressed at the outset. (1) Oral temperature averages about 0.5°C less than rectal, which is generally used as an estimate of internal temperature (also known as **core body temperature**). Not all regions of the body, therefore, have the same temperature. (2) Internal temperature is not constant; although it does not vary much, it does change slightly in

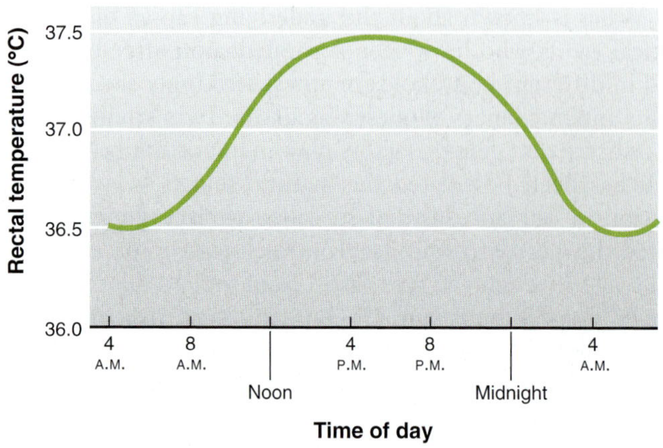

Figure 16.16 Circadian changes in core (measured as rectal) body temperature in a typical person. This figure does not take into account daily minor swings in temperature due to such things as exercise, eating, and menstrual cycle; nor are the absolute values on the *y*-axis representative of all individuals. Adapted from Scales et al.

response to activity patterns and changes in external temperature. Moreover, there is a characteristic circadian fluctuation of about 1°C (**Figure 16.16**), with temperature being lowest during the night and highest during the day. (3) An added variation in women is a higher temperature during the second half of the menstrual cycle due to the effects of the hormone progesterone.

Temperature regulation can be studied by our usual balance methods. The total heat content gained or lost by the body is determined by the net difference between heat gain (from the environment and produced in the body) and heat loss. Maintaining a stable body temperature means that, in the steady state, heat gain must equal heat loss.

Mechanisms of Heat Loss or Gain

The surface of the body can lose heat to the external environment by radiation, conduction, convection, and the evaporation of water (**Figure 16.17**). Before defining each of these processes, however, it must be emphasized that radiation, conduction, and convection can, under certain circumstances, lead to heat *gain* instead of loss.

Radiation is the process by which the surfaces of all objects constantly emit heat in the form of electromagnetic waves. It is a principle of physics that the rate of heat emission is determined by the temperature of the radiating surface. As a result, if the body surface is warmer than the various surfaces in the environment, net heat is lost from the body, the rate being directly dependent upon the temperature difference between the surfaces. Conversely, the body gains heat by absorbing electromagnetic energy emitted by the sun.

Conduction is the loss or gain of heat by transfer of thermal energy during collisions between adjacent molecules. In essence, heat is "conducted" from molecule to molecule. The body surface loses or gains heat by conduction through direct contact with cooler or warmer substances, including the air or water. Not all substances, however, conduct heat equally. Water is a better conductor of heat than is air; therefore, more heat is lost from the body in water than in air of similar temperature.

Convection is the process whereby conductive heat loss or gain is aided by movement of the air or water next to the body. For example, air next to the body is heated by conduction.

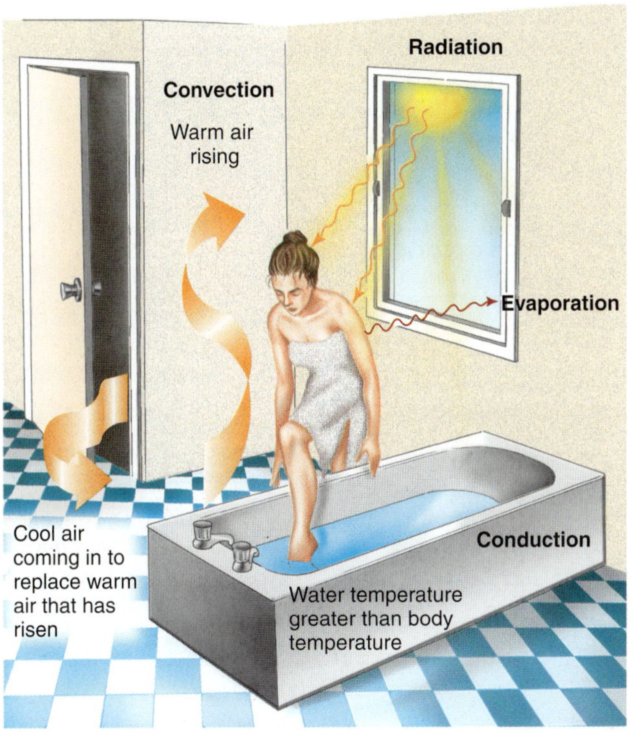

Figure 16.17 Mechanisms of heat transfer.

PHYSIOLOGICAL INQUIRY

- Evaporation is an important mechanism for eliminating heat, particularly on a hot day or when exercising. What are some of the negative consequences of this mechanism of heat loss?

Answer can be found at end of chapter.

Because warm air is less dense than cool air, the heated air around the body surface rises, thereby carrying away the heat just taken from the body. The air that moves away is replaced by cooler air, which in turn follows the same pattern. Convection is always occurring because warm air is less dense and therefore rises, but it can be greatly facilitated by external forces such as wind or fans. Consequently, convection aids conductive heat exchange by continuously maintaining a supply of cool air. Therefore, in the rest of this chapter, the term *conduction* will also imply convection.

Evaporation of water from the skin and membranes lining the respiratory tract is the other major process causing loss of body heat. A very large amount of energy—600 kcal/L—is required to transform water from the liquid to the gaseous state. As a result, whenever water vaporizes from the body's surface, the heat required to drive the process is conducted from the surface, thereby cooling it.

Temperature-Regulating Reflexes

Temperature regulation offers a classic example of a homeostatic control system, as described in Chapter 1. The balance between heat production (gain) and heat loss is continuously being disturbed, either by changes in metabolic rate (exercise being the most powerful influence) or by changes in the external environment such as air temperature. The resulting changes in body temperature are detected by thermoreceptors. These receptors initiate reflexes that change the output of various effectors so that heat production and/or loss are modified and body temperature is restored toward normal.

Figure 16.18 summarizes the components of these reflexes. There are two locations of thermoreceptors, one in the skin (**peripheral thermoreceptors**) and the other (**central thermoreceptors**) in deep body structures, including abdominal organs and thermoreceptive neurons in the hypothalamus. Because it is the core body temperature—not the skin temperature—that is maintained in a narrow homeostatic range, the central thermoreceptors provide the essential negative feedback component of the reflexes. The peripheral thermoreceptors provide feedforward information, as described in Chapter 1, and also account for the ability to identify a hot or cold area of the skin.

The hypothalamus serves as the primary overall integrator of the reflexes, but other brain centers also exert some control over specific components of the reflexes. Output from the hypothalamus and the other brain areas to the effectors is via (1) sympathetic nerves to the sweat glands, skin arterioles, and the adrenal medulla; and (2) motor neurons to the skeletal muscles.

Control of Heat Production

Changes in muscle activity constitute the major control of heat production for temperature regulation. The first muscle change in response to a decrease in core body temperature is a gradual and general increase in skeletal muscle contraction. This may lead to shivering, which consists of oscillating, rhythmic muscle contractions and relaxations occurring at a rapid rate. During shivering, the efferent motor nerves to the skeletal muscles are influenced by descending pathways under the primary control of the hypothalamus. Because almost no external work is performed by shivering, most of the energy liberated by the metabolic machinery appears as internal heat, a process known as **shivering thermogenesis.** People also use their muscles for voluntary heat-producing activities such as foot stamping and hand rubbing.

The opposite muscle reactions occur in response to heat. Basal muscle contraction is reflexively decreased, and voluntary movement is also diminished. These attempts to decrease heat production are limited, however, because basal muscle contraction is quite low to start with and because any increased core temperature produced by the heat acts *directly* on cells to increase metabolic rate. In other words, an increase in cellular temperature directly accelerates the rate at which all of its chemical reactions occur. This is due to the increased thermal motion of dissolved molecules, making it more likely that they will encounter each other. The result is that ATP is expended at a higher rate because ATP participates in many of a cell's chemical reactions. This, in turn, results in a compensatory increase in ATP production from cellular energy stores, which also generates heat as a by-product of metabolism. Thus, increasing cellular temperature can itself result in the production of additional heat through increased metabolism.

Muscle contraction is not the only process controlled in temperature-regulating reflexes. In many experimental mammals, chronic cold exposure induces an increase in metabolic rate (and therefore heat production) that is not due to increased muscle activity and is termed **nonshivering thermogenesis.** Its causes are an increased adrenal secretion of epinephrine, increased thyroid hormone secretion, and increased sympathetic activity to

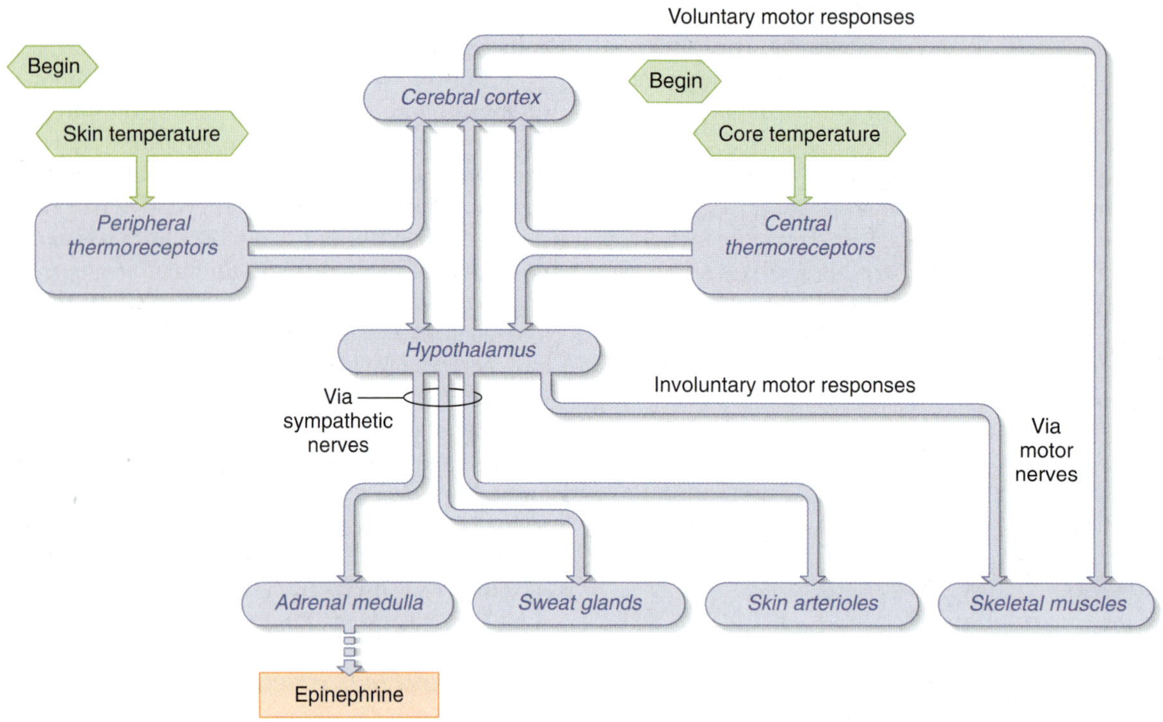

Figure 16.18 Summary of temperature-regulating mechanisms beginning with peripheral thermoreceptors and central thermoreceptors. The dashed arrow from the adrenal medulla indicates that this hormonal pathway is of minor importance in adult human beings. The solid arrows denote neural pathways. The hypothalamus influences sympathetic nerves via descending pathways.

a special type of adipose tissue called brown fat, or **brown adipose tissue.** This type of adipose tissue is stimulated by thyroid hormone, epinephrine, and the sympathetic nervous system; it contains large amounts of a class of proteins called uncoupling proteins. These proteins uncouple oxidation from phosphorylation (Chapter 3) and, in effect, make metabolism less efficient (less ATP is generated). The major product of this inefficient metabolism is heat, which then contributes to maintaining body temperature. Brown adipose tissue is present in infant humans. Nonshivering thermogenesis does occur in infants, therefore, whose shivering mechanism is not yet fully developed.

Control of Heat Loss by Radiation and Conduction

For purposes of temperature control, the body may be thought of as a central core surrounded by a shell consisting of skin and subcutaneous tissue. The temperature of the central core is regulated at approximately 37°C, but the temperature of the outer surface of the skin changes considerably.

If the skin and its underlying tissue were a perfect insulator, no heat would ever be lost from the core. The temperature of the outer skin surface would equal the environmental temperature, and net conduction would be zero. The skin is not a perfect insulator, however, so the temperature of its outer surface generally is somewhere between that of the external environment and that of the core. Instead of acting as an insulator, the skin functions as a variable regulator of heat exchange. Its effectiveness in this capacity is subject to physiological control by a change in blood flow. The more blood reaching the skin from the core, the more closely the skin's temperature approaches that of the core. In effect, the blood vessels can carry heat to the skin surface to be lost to the external environment. These vessels are controlled largely by vasoconstrictor sympathetic nerves, which are reflexively stimulated in response to cold and inhibited in response to heat. There is also a population of sympathetic neurons to the skin whose neurotransmitters cause active vasodilation. Certain areas of skin participate much more than others in all these vasomotor responses, and so skin temperatures vary with location.

Finally, the three *behavioral* mechanisms for altering heat loss by radiation and conduction are changes in surface area, changes in clothing, and choice of surroundings. Curling up into a ball, hunching the shoulders, and similar maneuvers in response to cold reduce the surface area exposed to the environment, thereby decreasing heat loss by radiation and conduction. In human beings, clothing is also an important component of temperature regulation, substituting for the insulating effects of feathers in birds and fur in other mammals. The outer surface of the clothes forms the true "exterior" of the body surface. The skin loses heat directly to the air space trapped by the clothes, which in turn pick up heat from the inner air layer and transfer it to the external environment. The insulating ability of clothing is determined primarily by the thickness of the trapped air layer. The third behavioral mechanism for altering heat loss is to seek out warmer or colder surroundings, for example, by moving from a shady spot into the sunlight.

Control of Heat Loss by Evaporation

Even in the absence of sweating, there is loss of water by diffusion through the skin, which is not completely waterproof. A similar amount is lost from the respiratory lining during expiration. These two losses are known as **insensible water loss** and amount to approximately 600 mL/day in human beings. Evaporation of this water can account for a significant fraction of total heat loss. In contrast to this passive water loss, sweating requires the active secretion of fluid by **sweat glands** and its extrusion into ducts that carry it to the skin surface.

Production of sweat is stimulated by sympathetic nerves to the glands. Sweat is a dilute solution containing sodium chloride as its major solute. Sweating rates of over 4 L/h have been reported; the evaporation of 4 L of water would eliminate almost 2400 kcal of heat from the body!

Sweat must evaporate in order to exert its cooling effect. The most important factor determining evaporation rate is the water vapor concentration of the air—that is, the relative humidity. The discomfort suffered on humid days is due to the failure of evaporation; the sweat glands continue to secrete, but the sweat simply remains on the skin or drips off.

Integration of Effector Mechanisms

By altering heat loss, changes in skin blood flow alone can regulate body temperature over a range of environmental temperatures known as the **thermoneutral zone.** In humans, the thermoneutral zone is approximately 25°C to 30°C or 75°F to 86°F for a nude individual. At temperatures lower than this, even maximal vasoconstriction of blood vessels in the skin cannot prevent heat loss from exceeding heat gain and the body must increase its heat production to maintain temperature. At environmental temperatures above the thermoneutral zone, even maximal vasodilation cannot eliminate heat as fast as it is produced, and another heat-loss mechanism—sweating—therefore comes strongly into play. At environmental temperatures above that of the body, heat is actually added to the body by radiation and conduction. Under such conditions, evaporation is the sole mechanism for heat loss. A person's ability to tolerate such temperatures is determined by the humidity and by his or her maximal sweating rate. For example, when the air is completely dry, a person can tolerate an environmental temperature of 130°C (225°F) for 20 min or longer, whereas very humid air at 46°C (115°F) is bearable for only a few minutes.

Temperature Acclimatization

Changes in the onset, volume, and composition of sweat determine the ability to adapt to chronic high temperatures. A person newly arrived in a hot environment has poor ability to do work; body temperature increases, and severe weakness may occur. After several days, there is a great improvement in work tolerance, with much less increase in body temperature, and the person is said to have acclimatized to the heat. Body temperature does not increase as much because sweating begins sooner and the volume of sweat produced is greater.

There is also an important change in the composition of the sweat, namely, a significant reduction in its salt concentration. This adaptation, which minimizes the loss of sodium ions from the body via sweat, is due to increased secretion of the adrenal cortex hormone aldosterone. The sweat-gland secretory cells produce a solution with a sodium ion concentration similar to that of plasma, but some of the sodium ions are absorbed back into the blood as the secretion flows along the sweat-gland ducts toward the skin surface. Aldosterone stimulates this absorption in a manner identical to its stimulation of sodium ion reabsorption in the renal tubules.

Cold acclimatization has been much less studied than heat acclimatization because of the difficulty of subjecting people to total-body cold stress over long enough periods to produce acclimatization. Moreover, people who live in cold climates generally dress very warmly and so would not develop acclimatization to the cold.

16.7 Fever and Hyperthermia

Fever is an increase in body temperature due to a resetting of the "thermostat" in the hypothalamus. A person with a fever still regulates body temperature in response to heat or cold but at a higher set point. The most common cause of fever is infection, but physical trauma and tissue damage can also induce fever.

The onset of fever during infection is often gradual, but it is most striking when it occurs rapidly in the form of a chill. In such cases, the temperature setting of the brain thermostat is suddenly increased. Because of this, the person feels cold, even though his or her actual body temperature may be normal. As a result, the typical actions that are used to increase body temperature, such as vasoconstriction and shivering, occur. The person may also curl up and put on blankets. This combination of decreased heat loss and increased heat production serves to drive body temperature up to the new set point, where it stabilizes. It will continue to be regulated at this new value until the thermostat is reset to normal and the fever "breaks." The person then feels hot, throws off the covers, and manifests profound vasodilation and sweating.

What is the basis for the thermostat resetting? Chemical messengers collectively termed **endogenous pyrogen** (**EP**) are released from macrophages (as well as other cell types) in the presence of infection or other fever-producing stimuli. The next steps vary depending on the precise stimulus for the release of EP. As illustrated in **Figure 16.19**, in some cases, EP probably circulates in the blood to act upon the thermoreceptors in the hypothalamus (and perhaps other brain areas), altering their input to the integrating centers. In other cases, EP may be produced by macrophage-like cells in the liver and stimulate neural receptors there that give rise to afferent neural input to the hypothalamic thermoreceptors. In both cases, the immediate cause of the resetting is a local synthesis and release of prostaglandins within the hypothalamus. ***Aspirin*** reduces fever by inhibiting this prostaglandin synthesis.

The term *EP* was coined at a time when the identity of the chemical messenger(s) was not known. At least three peptides, interleukin 1-beta (IL-1β), interleukin 6 (IL-6), and tumor necrosis factor-alpha (TNFα), are now known to function as EPs. In addition to their effects on temperature, these peptides have many other effects (described in Chapter 18) that enhance resistance to infection and promote the healing of damaged tissue.

One would expect fever, which is such a consistent feature of infection, to play some important protective role. Most evidence suggests that this is the case. For example, increased body temperature stimulates a large number of the body's defensive responses to infection, including the proliferation and activity of pathogen-fighting white blood cells. The likelihood that fever is a beneficial response raises important questions about the use of aspirin and other drugs to suppress fever during infection. It must be emphasized that these questions apply to the usual modest fevers. There is no question that an extremely high fever can be harmful—particularly in its effects on the central nervous system—and must be vigorously opposed with drugs and other forms of therapy.

Fever, then, is an increased body temperature caused by an elevation of the thermal set point. When body temperature is

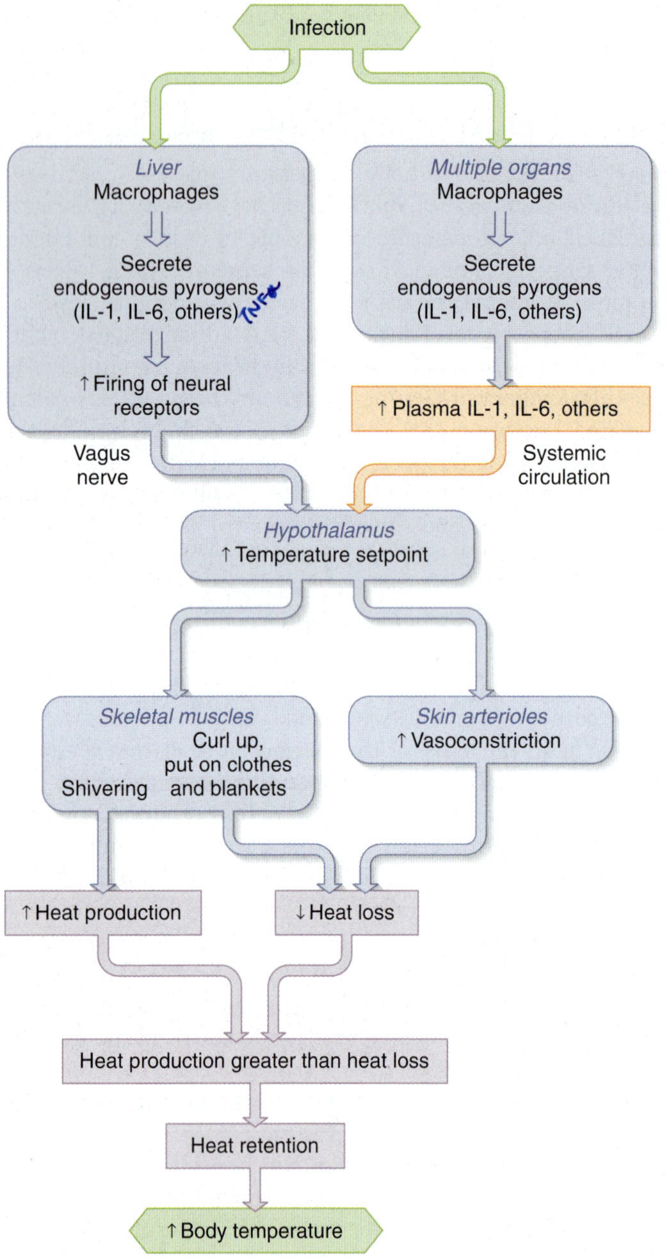

Figure 16.19 Pathway by which infection causes fever (IL-1 = Interleukin 1; IL-6 = Interleukin 6). The effector responses serve to *increase* body temperature during an infection.

elevated for any other reason beyond a narrow normal range but without a change in the temperature set point, it is termed ***hyperthermia.*** The most common cause of hyperthermia in a typical person is exercise; the increase in body temperature above set point is due to the internal heat generated by the exercising muscles.

As shown in **Figure 16.20**, heat production increases immediately during the initial stage of exercise and exceeds heat loss, causing heat storage in the body and an increase in the core temperature. This increase in core temperature triggers reflexes, via the central thermoreceptors, that cause increased heat loss. As skin blood flow and sweating increase, the discrepancy between heat production and heat loss starts to diminish but does not disappear. Therefore, core temperature continues to increase. Ultimately, core temperature will be high enough to drive (via the central thermoreceptors) the

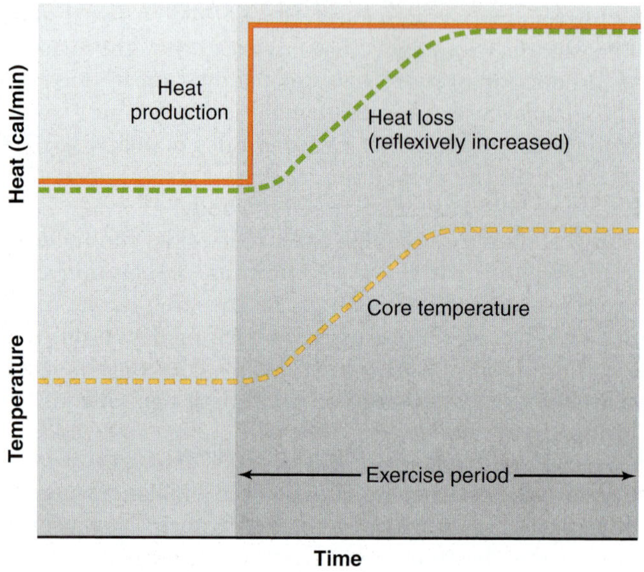

Figure 16.20 Thermal changes during exercise. Heat loss is reflexively increased. When heat loss once again equals heat production, core temperature stabilizes.

heat-loss reflexes at a rate such that heat loss once again equals heat production. At this point, core temperature stabilizes at this elevated value despite continued exercise. In some situations, hyperthermia may lead to life-threatening consequences.

Heat exhaustion is a state of collapse, often taking the form of fainting, due to hypotension brought on by depletion of plasma volume secondary to sweating and extreme dilation of skin blood vessels. Recall from Chapter 12 that blood pressure, cardiac output, and total peripheral resistance are related according to the equation $MAP = CO \times TPR$. Thus, decreases in both cardiac output (due to the decreased plasma volume) and peripheral resistance (due to the vasodilation) contribute to the hypotension. Heat exhaustion occurs as a direct consequence of the activity of heat-loss mechanisms. Because these mechanisms have been so active, the body temperature is only modestly elevated. In a sense, heat exhaustion is a safety valve that, by forcing a cessation of work in a hot environment when heat-loss mechanisms are overtaxed, prevents the larger increase in body temperature that would cause the far more serious condition of heatstroke.

In contrast to heat exhaustion, ***heatstroke*** represents a complete breakdown in heat-regulating systems so that body temperature keeps increasing. It is an extremely dangerous situation characterized by collapse, delirium, seizures, or prolonged unconsciousness—all due to greatly increased body temperature. It almost always occurs in association with exposure to or overexertion in hot and humid environments. In some individuals, particularly elderly persons, heatstroke may appear with no apparent prior period of severe sweating (refer back to the Chapter 1 Clinical Case Study for an example), but in most cases, it comes on as the end stage of prolonged untreated heat exhaustion. Exactly what triggers the transition to heatstroke is not clear, although impaired circulation to the brain due to dehydration is one factor. The striking finding, however, is that even in the face of a rapidly increasing body temperature, the person fails to sweat. Heatstroke is a positive feedback situation in which the increasing body temperature directly stimulates metabolism, that is, heat production, which further increases body temperature. For both heat exhaustion and heatstroke, the remedy is external cooling, fluid replacement, and cessation of activity.

SECTION B SUMMARY

General Principles of Energy Expenditure

I. The energy liberated during a chemical reaction appears either as heat or work.

II. Total energy expenditure = Heat produced + External work done + Energy stored

III. Metabolic rate is influenced by the many factors summarized in Table 16.5.

IV. Metabolic rate is increased by the thyroid hormones and epinephrine.

Regulation of Total-Body Energy Stores

I. Energy storage as fat can be positive when the metabolic rate is less than, or negative when the metabolic rate is greater than, the energy content of ingested food.
   a. Energy storage is regulated mainly by reflexive adjustment of food intake.
   b. In addition, the metabolic rate increases or decreases to some extent when food intake is chronically increased or decreased, respectively.

II. Food intake is controlled by leptin, which is secreted by adipose-tissue cells, and a variety of satiety factors, as summarized in Figures 16.14 and 16.15.

III. Being overweight or obese, the result of an imbalance between food intake and metabolic rate, increases the risk of many diseases.

Regulation of Body Temperature

I. Core body temperature shows a circadian rhythm, with temperature highest during the day and lowest at night.

II. The body exchanges heat with the external environment by radiation, conduction, convection, and evaporation of water from the body surface.

III. The hypothalamus and other brain areas contain the integrating centers for temperature-regulating reflexes, and both peripheral and central thermoreceptors participate in these reflexes.

IV. Body temperature is regulated by altering heat production and/or heat loss so as to change total-body heat content.
   a. Heat production is altered by increasing muscle tone, shivering, and voluntary activity.
   b. Heat loss by radiation, conduction, and convection depends on the temperature difference between the skin surface and the environment.
   c. In response to cold, skin temperature is decreased by decreasing skin blood flow through reflexive stimulation of the sympathetic nerves to the skin. In response to heat, skin temperature is increased by inhibiting these nerves.
   d. Behavioral responses, such as putting on more clothes, also influence heat loss.
   e. Evaporation of water occurs all the time as insensible loss from the skin and respiratory lining. Additional water for evaporation is supplied by sweat, stimulated by the sympathetic nerves to the sweat glands.
   f. Increased heat production is essential for temperature regulation at environmental temperatures below the thermoneutral zone, and sweating is essential at temperatures above this zone.

V. Temperature acclimatization to heat is achieved by an earlier onset of sweating, an increased volume of sweat, and a decreased salt concentration of the sweat.

Fever and Hyperthermia

I. Fever is due to a resetting of the temperature set point so that heat production is increased and heat loss is decreased in order to increase body temperature to the new set point and keep it there. The stimulus is endogenous pyrogen, in the form of interleukin 1 and other peptides.

II. The hyperthermia of exercise is due to the increased heat produced by the muscles, and it is partially offset by skin vasodilation.

III. Extreme increases in body temperature can result in heat exhaustion or heatstroke. In heat exhaustion, blood pressure decreases due to vasodilation. In heatstroke, the normal thermoregulatory mechanisms fail; thus, heatstroke can be fatal.

SECTION B REVIEW QUESTIONS

1. State the formula relating total energy expenditure, heat produced, external work, and energy storage.
2. What two hormones alter the basal metabolic rate?
3. State the equation for total-body energy balance. Describe the three possible states of balance with regard to energy storage.
4. What happens to the basal metabolic rate after a person has either lost or gained weight?
5. List several satiety signals; where do satiety signals act?
6. List three beneficial effects of exercise in a weight-loss program.
7. Compare and contrast the four mechanisms for heat loss.
8. Describe the control of skin blood vessels during exposure to cold or heat.
9. With a diagram, summarize the reflexive responses to heat or cold. What are the dominant mechanisms for temperature regulation in the thermoneutral zone and in temperatures below and above this range?
10. What changes are exhibited by a heat-acclimatized person?
11. Summarize the sequence of events leading to a fever; contrast this to the sequence leading to hyperthermia during exercise.

SECTION B KEY TERMS

basal metabolic rate (BMR) 587
body mass index (BMI) 590
brown adipose tissue 594
calorie 587
calorigenic effect 588
central thermoreceptor 593
conduction 592
convection 592
core body temperature 592
endogenous pyrogen (EP) 595
endotherm 592
evaporation 593
external work 587
diet-induced thermogenesis 588
ghrelin 590
homeotherm 592
insensible water loss 594
internal work 587
kilocalorie (kcal) 587
leptin 589
metabolic rate 587
neuropeptide Y 589
nonshivering thermogenesis 593
peripheral thermoreceptor 593
radiation 592
satiety signal 589
shivering thermogenesis 593
sweat gland 595
thermoneutral zone 595
thrifty gene 591
total energy expenditure 587

SECTION B CLINICAL TERMS

anorexia nervosa 591
aspirin 595
bulimia nervosa 591
fever 595
heat exhaustion 596
heatstroke 596
hyperthermia 596
obesity 590
overweight 590

CHAPTER 16

Clinical Case Study: An Overweight Man with Tingling, Thirst, and Blurred Vision

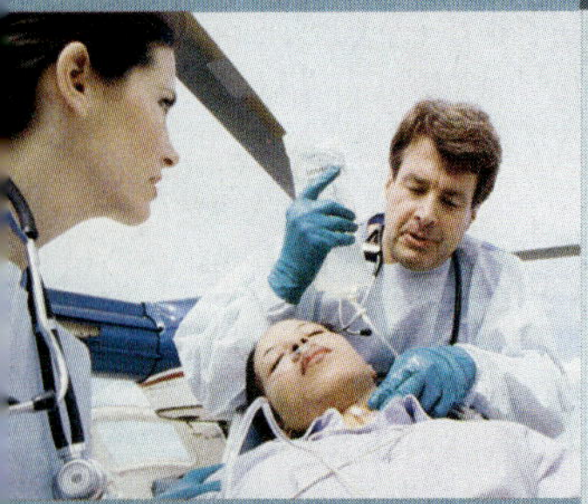

A 46-year-old man visited an ophthalmologist because of recent episodes of blurry vision. In addition to examining the man's eyes, the ophthalmologist took a medical history and assessed the patient's overall health. The patient was 6 feet tall and weighed 265 pounds (BMI equal to 36 kg/m^2). He had recently been experiencing "tingling" sensations in his hands and feet and was sleeping poorly because he was waking up several times during the night with a full bladder. He had also taken to carrying bottled water with him wherever he went, because he often felt very thirsty. He reported that he worked as a taxicab driver and rarely if ever had occasion to engage in much physical activity or exercise. The patient attributed the tingling sensations to "sitting in one position all day" and was convinced that his eye problems were the natural result of aging. Examination of the eyes, however, revealed a greatly weakened accommodation reflex in both eyes (see Chapter 7). These signs and symptoms suggested to the ophthalmologist that the patient might have ***diabetes mellitus,*** and he therefore referred the patient to a physician at the diabetes unit of his local hospital.

The physician at the hospital performed a series of tests to confirm the diagnosis of diabetes mellitus. First, the fasting plasma glucose concentration was determined on two separate days. After an overnight fast, blood was drawn and the concentration of glucose in the plasma was determined. Normal values are generally below 100 mg/dL, but the two values determined for this patient were 156 and 144 mg/dL. Consequently, a second test called an *oral glucose tolerance test* was performed. In this test, the patient fasts overnight and then drinks a solution of 75 grams of glucose dissolved in water. Two hours later, blood is drawn and again the plasma glucose concentration is determined. In healthy individuals, the plasma glucose concentration will be below 140 mg/dL by this time, because their circulating insulin will have responded to the increase in glucose and will be in the process of restoring glucose to normal. In two separate tests, however, the glucose concentrations were 215 and 236 mg/dL; these results suggested that the patient's pancreas failed to secrete sufficient insulin in response to the glucose challenge, or that the sensitivity of his cells to insulin was decreased, or both. Finally, a third test was performed to determine what percentage of the patient's hemoglobin was glycosylated. Hemoglobin is found in red blood cells, which have a lifetime of 2 to 4 months. When glucose concentrations are above normal, certain proteins including hemoglobin become bound to glucose (that is, they become glycosylated); once bound, the glucose molecules remain on hemoglobin for the lifetime of the cell. The longer the duration of the elevation in plasma glucose, the greater the percentage of glycosylated hemoglobin, abbreviated HbA1c. Therefore, this test is a measure of the average glucose values in the blood over the previous few months. Normal values are between 4% and 6%, but in our patient, HbA1c was 6.9%. Together, these tests confirmed the diagnosis of diabetes mellitus.

Diabetes mellitus can be due to a deficiency of insulin and/or to a decreased responsiveness to insulin. Diabetes mellitus is therefore classified into two distinct diseases depending on the cause. In ***type 1 diabetes mellitus*** (***T1DM***), formerly called *insulin-dependent diabetes mellitus* or *juvenile diabetes,* insulin is completely or almost completely absent from the islets of Langerhans and the plasma. Therefore, therapy with insulin is essential. In ***type 2 diabetes mellitus*** (***T2DM***), formerly called *non-insulin-dependent diabetes mellitus* or *adult-onset diabetes mellitus,* insulin is present in plasma but cellular sensitivity to insulin is less than normal (***insulin resistance***). In many patients with T2DM, the response of the pancreatic beta cells to glucose is also impaired. Therefore, therapy may involve some combination of drugs that increase cellular sensitivity to insulin, increase insulin secretion from beta cells, or decrease hepatic glucose production; or the therapy may involve insulin administration itself.

T1DM is less common, affecting approximately 5% of diabetic patients in the United States. T1DM is due to the total or near-total autoimmune destruction of the pancreatic beta cells by the body's white blood cells. As you will learn in Chapter 18, an autoimmune disease is one in which the body's immune cells attack and destroy normal, healthy tissue. The triggering events for this autoimmune response are not yet fully established. Treatment of T1DM involves the administration of insulin by injection, because insulin administered orally would be destroyed by gastrointestinal enzymes.

Because of insulin deficiency, *untreated* patients with T1DM always have increased glucose concentrations in their blood. The increase in plasma glucose occurs because (1) glucose fails to enter insulin's target cells normally, and (2) the liver continuously makes glucose by glycogenolysis and gluconeogenesis and secretes the glucose into the blood. Recall also that insulin normally suppresses lipolysis and ketone formation. Consequently, another result of the insulin deficiency is pronounced lipolysis with subsequent elevation of plasma glycerol and fatty acids. Many of the fatty acids are then converted by the liver into ketones, which are released into the blood.

If extreme, these metabolic changes culminate in the acute life-threatening emergency called ***diabetic ketoacidosis*** (**Figure 16.21**). Some of the problems are due to the effects that extremely elevated plasma glucose concentration produces on renal function. Chapter 14 pointed out that a typical person does not excrete glucose because all glucose filtered at the renal glomeruli is reabsorbed by the tubules. However, the elevated plasma glucose of diabetes mellitus increases the filtered load of glucose beyond the maximum tubular reabsorptive capacity and, therefore, large amounts of glucose are excreted. For the same reasons, large amounts of ketones may also appear in the urine. These urinary losses deplete the body of nutrients and lead to weight loss. Far worse, however, is the fact that these unreabsorbed solutes cause an osmotic diuresis—increased urinary excretion of sodium ions and water, which can lead, by the sequence of events shown in Figure 16.21, to hypotension, brain damage, and death. It should be noted, however, that apart from this extreme example, diabetics are more often prone to hypertension, not hypotension (due to several causes, including vascular and kidney damage).

The other serious abnormality in diabetic ketoacidosis is the increased plasma hydrogen ion concentration caused by the accumulation of ketones. As described in Chapter 3, ketones are four-carbon breakdown products of fatty acids. Two ketones,

(continued)

(continued)

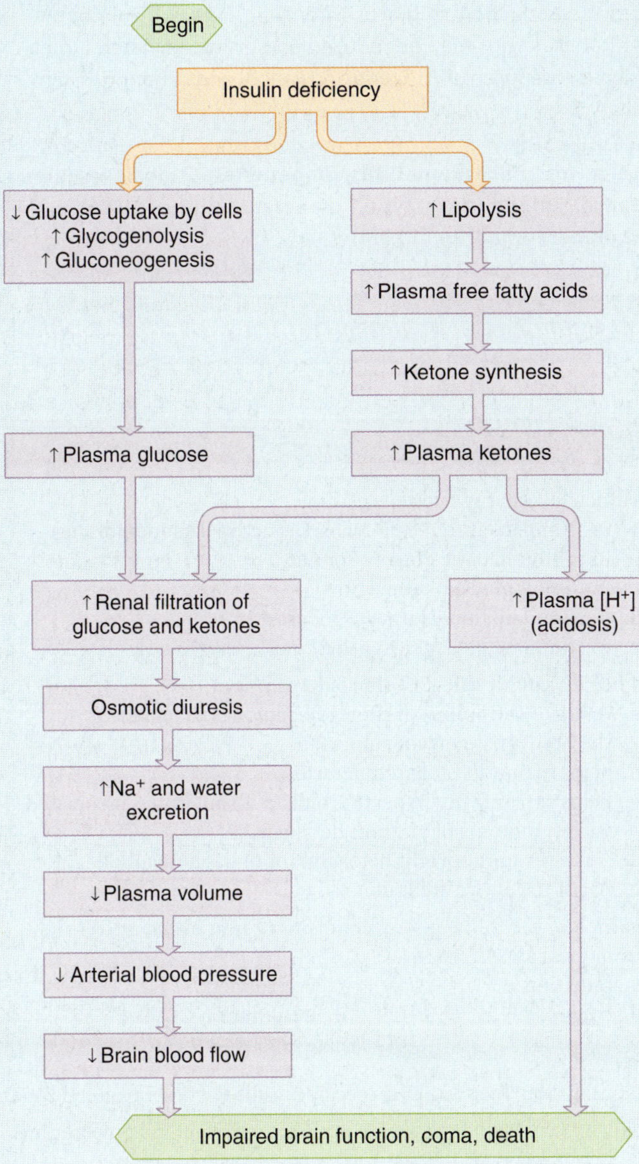

Figure 16.21 Diabetic ketoacidosis. Events caused by severe untreated insulin deficiency in type 1 diabetes mellitus.

known as hydroxybutyric acid and acetoacetic acid, are acidic at the pH of blood. This increased hydrogen ion concentration causes brain dysfunction that can contribute to coma and death.

Diabetic ketoacidosis occurs primarily in patients with *untreated* T1DM, that is, those with almost total inability to secrete insulin. However, more than 90% of diabetic patients are in the T2DM category and usually do not develop metabolic derangements severe enough to develop diabetic ketoacidosis. T2DM is a syndrome mainly of overweight adults, typically starting in middle life. However, T2DM is *not* an age-dependent syndrome. As the incidence of childhood obesity has soared in the United States, so too has the incidence of T2DM in children and adolescents. Given the earlier mention of progressive weight loss in T1DM as a symptom of diabetes, why is it that most people with T2DM are overweight? One reason is that people with T2DM, in contrast to those with T1DM, do not excrete enough glucose in the urine to cause weight loss. Moreover, in T2DM, it is the excessive weight gain that is the *cause* of the diabetes.

Several factors combine to cause T2DM. One major problem is target-cell hyporesponsiveness to insulin, termed insulin resistance. Obesity accounts for much of the insulin resistance in T2DM, although a minority of people develop T2DM without obesity for reasons that are unknown. Obesity in any person—diabetic or not—usually induces some degree of insulin resistance, particularly in muscle and adipose-tissue cells. One hypothesis is that the excess adipose tissue overproduces messengers—perhaps inflammatory cytokines—that cause downregulation of insulin-responsive glucose transporters or in some other way blocks insulin's actions. Another hypothesis is that excess fat deposition in non-adipose tissue (for example, in muscle) causes a decrease in insulin sensitivity.

As stated earlier, many people with T2DM not only have insulin resistance but also have a defect in the ability of their beta cells to secrete insulin adequately in response to an increase in the concentration of plasma glucose. In other words, although insulin resistance is the primary factor inducing hyperglycemia in T2DM, an as-yet-unidentified defect in beta-cell function prevents these cells from responding maximally to the hyperglycemia. It is currently thought that the mediators of decreased insulin sensitivity described earlier may also interfere with a normal insulin secretory response to hyperglycemia.

The most effective therapy for obese persons with T2DM is weight reduction. An exercise program is also very important because insulin sensitivity is increased by frequent endurance-type exercise, independent of changes in body weight. This occurs, at least in part, because exercise causes a substantial increase in the total number of plasma membrane glucose transporters in skeletal muscle cells. Because a program of weight reduction, exercise, and dietary modification typically requires some time before it becomes effective, T2DM patients are usually also given orally active drugs that lower plasma glucose concentration by a variety of mechanisms. A recently approved synthetic incretin and another class of drugs called ***sulfonylureas*** lower plasma glucose concentration by acting on the beta cells to stimulate insulin secretion. Other drugs increase cellular sensitivity to insulin or decrease hepatic gluconeogenesis. Finally, in some cases, the use of high doses of insulin itself is warranted in T2DM.

Unfortunately, people with either form of diabetes mellitus tend to develop a variety of chronic abnormalities, including atherosclerosis, hypertension, kidney failure, blood vessel and nerve disease, susceptibility to infection, and blindness. Chronically increased plasma glucose concentration contributes to most of these abnormalities either by causing the intracellular accumulation of certain glucose metabolites that exert harmful effects on cells when present in high concentrations or by linking glucose to proteins, thereby altering their function. In our subject, the high glucose concentrations led to an accumulation of glucose metabolites in the lenses, causing them to swell due to osmosis; this, in turn, reduced the ability of his eyes to accurately focus light on the retina. He also had signs of nerve damage evidenced by the tingling sensations in his hands and feet. In many cases, symptoms such as his diminish or even disappear within days to months of receiving therapy. Nonetheless, over the long term, the aforementioned problems may still arise.

(continued)

(continued)

Our patient was counseled to begin a program of brisk walking for 30 minutes a day, at least five times a week, with the goal of increasing the duration and intensity of the exercise over the course of several months. He was also referred to a nutritionist, who advised him on a weight-loss program that involved a reduction in total daily saturated fat and calorie intake and increased consumption of fruits and vegetables. In addition, he was started immediately on two drugs, one that increases secretion of insulin from the pancreas and one that suppresses production of glucose from the liver. With time, the need for these drugs may be reduced and even eliminated if diet and exercise are successful in reducing weight and restoring insulin sensitivity.

Clinical terms: diabetes mellitus, diabetic ketoacidosis, insulin resistance, sulfonylureas, type 1 diabetes mellitus (T1DM), type 2 diabetes mellitus (T2DM)

See Chapter 19 for complete, integrative case studies.

CHAPTER 16 TEST QUESTIONS

Answers found in Appendix A.

1. Which is *incorrect?*
   a. Fatty acids can be converted into glucose in the liver.
   b. Glucose can be converted into fatty acids in adipose cells.
   c. Certain amino acids can be converted into glucose by the liver.
   d. Triglycerides are absorbed from the GI tract in the form of chylomicrons.
   e. The absorptive state is characterized by ingested nutrients entering the blood from the GI tract.
2. During the postabsorptive state, epinephrine stimulates breakdown of adipose triglycerides by
   a. inhibiting lipoprotein lipase.
   b. stimulating hormone-sensitive lipase.
   c. increasing production of glycogen.
   d. inhibiting hormone-sensitive lipase.
   e. promoting increased adipose ketone production.
3. Which is true of strenuous, prolonged exercise?
   a. It results in an increase in plasma glucagon concentration.
   b. It results in an increase in plasma insulin concentration.
   c. Plasma glucose concentration does not change.
   d. Skeletal muscle uptake of glucose is inhibited.
   e. Plasma concentrations of cortisol and growth hormone both decrease.
4. Untreated type 1 diabetes mellitus is characterized by
   a. decreased sensitivity of adipose and skeletal muscle cells to insulin.
   b. higher-than-normal plasma insulin concentration.
   c. loss of body fluid due to increased urine production.
   d. age-dependent onset (only occurs in adults).
   e. obesity.
5. Which is *not* a function of insulin?
   a. to stimulate amino acid transport across cell membranes
   b. to inhibit hepatic glucose output
   c. to inhibit glucagon secretion
   d. to stimulate lipolysis in adipocytes
   e. to stimulate glycogen synthase in skeletal muscle
6. The calorigenic effect of thyroid hormones
   a. refers to the ability of thyroid hormones to increase the body's oxygen consumption.
   b. helps maintain body temperature.
   c. helps explain why hyperthyroidism is sometimes associated with symptoms of vitamin deficiencies.
   d. is the most important determinant of basal metabolic rate.
   e. All of the above are true.
7. Which of the following mechanisms of heat exchange results from local air currents?
   a. radiation
   b. convection
   c. conduction
   d. evaporation

True or False

8. Nonshivering thermogenesis occurs outside the thermoneutral zone.
9. Skin and core temperature are both kept constant in homeotherms.
10. Leptin inhibits and ghrelin stimulates appetite.
11. Actively contracting skeletal muscles require more insulin than they do at rest.
12. Body mass index is calculated as height in meters divided by weight in kilograms.
13. In conduction, heat moves from a surface of higher temperature to one of lower temperature.
14. Skin blood vessels constrict in response to elevated core body temperature.
15. Evaporative cooling is most efficient in dry weather.

CHAPTER 16 GENERAL PRINCIPLES ASSESSMENT

Answers found in Appendix A.

1. A general principle of physiology is that *most physiological functions are controlled by multiple regulatory systems, often working in opposition.* How is this principle illustrated by the pancreatic control of glucose homeostasis? (*Note:* Compare Figures 16.5, 16.8, and 16.10 for help.)
2. This same principle also applies to the control of appetite. Give at least five examples of factors that regulate appetite in humans, including some that stimulate and some that inhibit appetite.
3. Body temperature homeostasis is critical for maintenance of healthy cells, tissues, and organs. Using Figure 16.17 as your guide, explain how the control of body temperature reflects the general principle of physiology that *physiological processes are dictated by the laws of chemistry and physics.*

CHAPTER 16 QUANTITATIVE AND THOUGHT QUESTIONS *Answers found at www.mhhe.com/widmaier13.*

1. What happens to the triglyceride concentrations in the plasma and in adipose tissue after administration of a drug that blocks the action of lipoprotein lipase?
2. A person has a defect in the ability of her small intestine to reabsorb bile salts. What effect will this have on her plasma cholesterol concentration?
3. A well-trained athlete is found to have a moderately elevated plasma total cholesterol concentration. What additional measurements would you advise this person to have taken in order to gain a better understanding of the importance of the elevated cholesterol?
4. A resting, unstressed person has increased plasma concentrations of free fatty acids, glycerol, amino acids, and ketones. What situations might be responsible and what additional plasma measurement would distinguish among them?
5. A healthy volunteer is given an injection of insulin. The plasma concentrations of which hormones increase as a result?
6. If the sympathetic preganglionic fibers to the adrenal medulla were cut in an animal, would this eliminate the sympathetically mediated component of increased gluconeogenesis and lipolysis during exercise? Explain.
7. What are the sources of heat loss for a person immersed up to the neck in a 40°C bath?
8. Lizards regulate their body temperatures primarily through behavioral means. Can you predict what they do when they are infected with bacteria?

CHAPTER 16 ANSWERS TO PHYSIOLOGICAL INQUIRIES

Figure 16.1 Eating a diet that is low in fat content does not mean that a person cannot gain additional adipose mass, because as shown in this figure, glucose and amino acids can be converted into fat in the liver. From there, the fat is transported and deposited in adipose tissue. A diet that is low in fat but rich in sugar, for example, could still result in an increase in fat mass in the body.

Figure 16.6 Having the transporters already synthesized and packaged into intracellular vesicle membranes means that glucose transport can be tightly and quickly coupled with changes in glucose concentrations in the blood. This protects the body against the harmful effects of excess blood glucose concentrations and also prevents urinary loss of glucose by keeping the rate of glucose filtration below the maximum rate at which the kidney can reabsorb it. This tight coupling could not occur if the transporters were required to be synthesized each time a cell was stimulated by insulin.

Figure 16.8 The brain is absolutely necessary for immediate survival and can maintain glucose uptake from the plasma in the fasted state when insulin concentrations are very low.

Figure 16.10 Fight-or-flight reactions result in an increase in sympathetic nerve activity. These neurons release norepinephrine from their axon terminals (see Chapter 6), which stimulates glucagon release from the pancreas. Glucagon then contributes to the increase in energy sources such as glucose in the blood, which facilitates fight-or-flight reactions.

Figure 16.14 The body's normal response to leptin is to decrease appetite and increase metabolic rate. This would not be adaptive during times when it is important to increase body energy (fat) stores. An example of such a situation is pregnancy, when gaining weight in the form of increased fat mass is important for providing energy to the growing fetus. In nature, another example is the requirement of hibernating animals to store large amounts of fat prior to hibernation. In these cases, the effects of leptin are decreased or ignored by the brain.

Figure 16.15 In the short term, drinking water before a meal may decrease appetite by stretching the stomach, and this may contribute to eating a smaller meal. However, as described in Chapter 15, water is quickly absorbed by the GI tract and provides no calories; thus, hunger will soon return once the meal is over.

Figure 16.17 The amount of fluid in the body decreases as water evaporates from the surface of the skin. This fluid must be replaced by drinking or the body will become dehydrated. In addition, sweat is salty (as you may have noticed by the salt residue remaining on hats or clothing once the sweat has dried). This means that the body's salt content also needs to be restored. This is a good example of how maintaining homeostasis for one variable (body temperature) may result in disruption of homeostasis for other variables (water and salt).

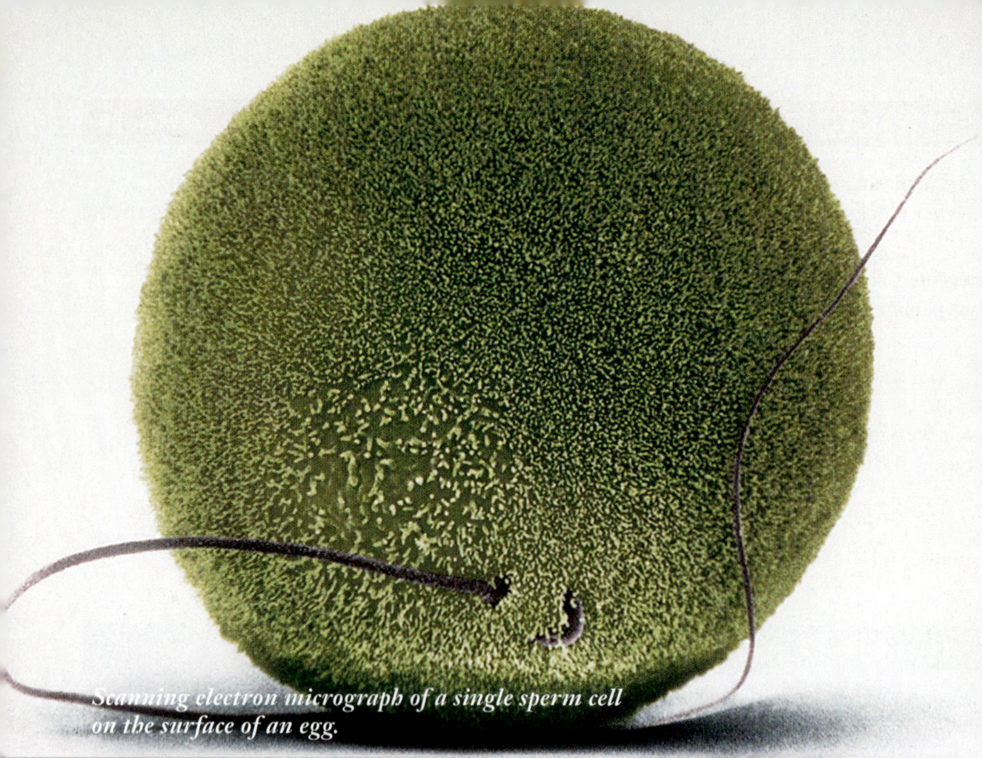

Scanning electron micrograph of a single sperm cell on the surface of an egg.

17 Reproduction

Reproduction is the process by which a species is perpetuated. As opposed to most of the physiological processes you have learned about in this book, reproduction is one of the few that is not necessary for the survival of an individual. However, normal reproductive function is essential for the production of healthy offspring and, therefore, for *survival of the species*. Sexual reproduction and the merging of parental chromosomes provide the biological variation of individuals that is necessary for adaptation of the species to our changing environment.

Reproduction includes the processes by which the male gamete (the sperm) and the female gamete (the ovum) develop, grow, and unite to produce a new and unique combination of genes in a new organism. This new entity, the zygote, develops into an embryo and then a fetus within the maternal uterus. The gametes are produced by gonads—the testes in the male and the ovaries in the female. Reproduction also includes the process by which a fetus is born. Over the course of a lifetime, reproductive functions also include sexual maturation (puberty), as well as pregnancy and lactation in women.

The gonads produce hormones that influence development of the offspring into male or female phenotypes. The gonadal hormones are controlled by and influence the secretion of hormones from the hypothalamus and the anterior pituitary gland. Together with the nervous system, these hormones regulate the cyclical activities of female reproduction, including the menstrual cycle, and provide a striking example of the general principle of physiology that most physiological processes are controlled by multiple regulatory systems, often working in opposition. The process of gamete maturation requires communication and feedback between the gonads, anterior pituitary gland, and brain, demonstrating the importance of two related general principles of physiology, namely, that information flow between cells, tissues, and organs is an essential feature of homeostasis and allows for integration of physiological processes; and that the functions of organ systems are coordinated with each other.

SECTION A

Gametogenesis, Sex Determination, and Sex Differentiation; General Principles of Reproductive Endocrinology

The primary reproductive organs are known as the **gonads:** the **testes** (singular, **testis**) in the male and the **ovaries** (singular, **ovary**) in the female. In both sexes, the gonads serve dual functions. The first of these is **gametogenesis,** which is the production of the reproductive cells, or **gametes.** These are **spermatozoa** (singular, **spermatozoan,** usually shortened to **sperm**) in males and **ova** (singular, **ovum**) in females. Secondly, the gonads secrete steroid hormones, often termed **sex hormones** or **gonadal steroids.** The major sex hormones are **androgens** (including **testosterone** and **dihydrotestosterone [DHT]**), **estrogens** (primarily **estradiol**), and **progesterone.** Both sexes have each of these hormones, but androgens predominate in males and estrogens and progesterone predominate in females.

17.1 Gametogenesis

The process of gametogenesis is depicted in **Figure 17.1.** At any point in gametogenesis, the developing gametes are called **germ cells.** The first stage in gametogenesis is proliferation of the primordial (undifferentiated) germ cells by mitosis. With the exception of the gametes, the DNA of each nucleated human cell is contained in 23 pairs of chromosomes, giving a total of 46. The two corresponding chromosomes in each pair are said to be homologous to each other, with one coming from each parent. In **mitosis,** the 46 chromosomes of the dividing cell are replicated. The cell then divides into two new cells called daughter cells. Each of the two daughter cells resulting from the division receives a full set of 46 chromosomes identical to those of the original cell. Thus, each daughter cell receives identical genetic information during mitosis.

In this manner, mitosis of primordial germ cells, each containing 46 chromosomes, provides a supply of identical germ cells for the next stages. The timing of mitosis in germ cells differs greatly in females and males. In the male, some mitosis occurs in the embryonic testes to generate the population of **primary spermatocytes** present at birth, but mitosis really begins in earnest in the male at puberty and usually continues throughout life. In the female, mitosis of germ cells in the ovary occurs primarily during fetal development, generating **primary oocytes.** The second stage of gametogenesis is **meiosis,** in which each resulting gamete receives only 23 chromosomes from a 46-chromosome germ cell, one chromosome from each homologous pair. Meiosis consists of two cell divisions in succession (see Figure 17.1). The events preceding the first meiotic division are identical to those preceding a *mitotic*

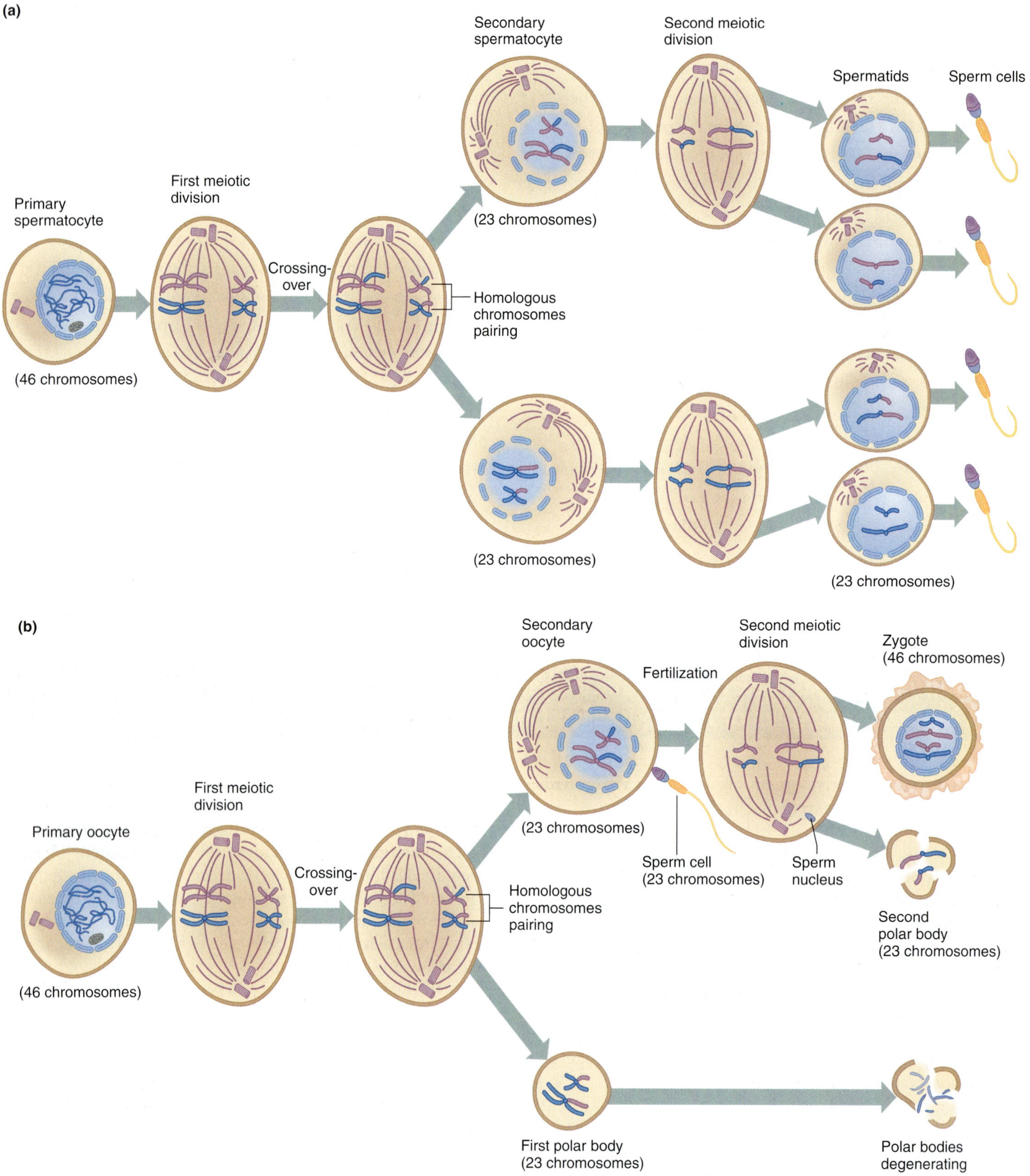

Figure 17.1 AP|R An overview of gametogenesis in (a) the testes and (b) the ovary. Only four chromosomes (two sets) are shown for clarity instead of the normal 46 in humans. Chromosomes from one parent are purple, and those from the other parent are blue. The size of the cells can vary quite dramatically in ova development.

division. During the interphase period, which precedes a mitotic division, chromosomal DNA is replicated. Thus, after DNA replication, an interphase cell has 46 chromosomes, but each chromosome consists of two identical strands of DNA, called sister chromatids, which are joined together by a centromere.

As the first meiotic division begins, homologous chromosomes, each consisting of two identical sister chromatids, come together and line up adjacent to each other. Thus, 23 pairs of homologous chromosomes (called **bivalents**) are formed. The sister chromatids of each chromosome condense into thick, rodlike structures. Then within each homologous pair, corresponding segments of homologous chromosomes align closely. This allows two nonsister chromatids to undergo an exchange of sites of breakage in a process called **crossing-over** (see Figure 17.1). Thus, crossing-over results in the recombination of genes on homologous chromosomes. Recombination is one of the most significant features of sexual reproduction that creates genetic diversity.

Following crossing-over, the homologous chromosomes line up in the center of the cell. The orientation of each pair on the equator is random, meaning that sometimes the maternal portion points to a particular pole of the cell and sometimes the paternal portion does so. The cell then divides (the first meiotic division), with the maternal chromatids of any particular pair going to one of the two cells resulting from the division and the paternal chromatids going to the other. The results of the first meiotic division are the **secondary spermatocytes** in males and the **secondary oocyte** in females. Note in Figure 17.1 that, in females, one of the two cells arising from the first meiotic division is the **first polar body** that has no function. Because of the random orientation of the homologous pairs at the equator, it is extremely unlikely that all 23 maternal chromatids will end up in one cell and all 23 paternal chromatids in the other. Over 8 million (2^{23}) different combinations of maternal and paternal chromosomes can result during this first meiotic division.

The second meiotic division occurs without any further replication of DNA. The sister chromatids—both of which were originally either maternal or paternal—of each chromosome separate and move apart into the new daughter cells. The daughter cells resulting from the second meiotic division, therefore, contain 23 one-chromatid chromosomes. Although the concept is the same, the timing of the second meiotic division is different in males and females. In males, this occurs continuously after puberty with the production of **spermatids** and ultimately mature sperm cells described in detail in the next section. In females, the second meiotic division does not occur until after fertilization of a secondary oocyte by a sperm. This results in production of the **zygote,** which contains 46 chromosomes—23 from the oocyte (maternal) and 23 from the sperm (paternal)—and the **second polar body,** which, like the first polar body, has no function.

To summarize, gametogenesis produces daughter cells having only 23 chromosomes, and two events during the first meiotic division contribute to the enormous genetic variability of the daughter cells: (1) crossing-over and (2) the random distribution of maternal and paternal chromatid pairs between the two daughter cells.

17.2 Sex Determination

The complete genetic composition of an individual is known as the **genotype.** Genetic inheritance sets the gender of the individual, or **sex determination,** which is established at the moment of fertilization. Gender is determined by genetic inheritance of two chromosomes called the **sex chromosomes.** The larger of the sex chromosomes is called the **X chromosome** and the smaller, the **Y chromosome.** Males possess one X and one Y, whereas females have two X chromosomes. Therefore, the key difference in genotype between males and females arises from this difference in one chromosome. As you will learn in the next section, the presence of the Y chromosome leads to the development of the male gonads—the testes; the absence of the Y chromosome leads to the development the female gonads—the ovaries.

The ovum can contribute only an X chromosome, whereas half of the sperm produced during meiosis are X and half are Y. When the sperm and the egg join, 50% should have XX and 50% XY. Interestingly, however, sex ratios at birth are not exactly 1:1; rather, there tends to be a slight preponderance of male births, possibly due to functional differences in sperm carrying the X versus Y chromosome.

An easy method exists for determining whether a person's cells contain two X chromosomes, the typical female pattern. When two X chromosomes are present, only one is functional; the nonfunctional X chromosome condenses to form a nuclear mass called the **sex chromatin,** or **Barr body,** which is readily observable with a light microscope. Scrapings from the cheek mucosa or white blood cells are convenient sources of cells to be examined. The single X chromosome in male cells rarely condenses to form sex chromatin.

A more exacting technique for determining sex chromosome composition employs tissue culture visualization of all the chromosomes—a **karyotype.** This technique can be used to identify a group of genetic sex abnormalities characterized by such unusual chromosomal combinations such as XXX, XXY, and XO (the O denotes the absence of a second sex chromosome). The end result of such combinations is usually the failure of normal anatomical and functional sexual development. The karyotype is also used to evaluate many other chromosomal abnormalities such as the characteristic trisomy 21 of Down syndrome described later in this chapter.

17.3 Sex Differentiation

The multiple processes involved in the development of the reproductive system in the fetus are collectively called **sex differentiation.** It is not surprising that people with atypical chromosomal combinations can manifest atypical sex differentiation. However, careful study has also revealed individuals with normal chromosomal combinations but abnormal sexual appearance and function (**phenotype**). In these people, sex differentiation has been atypical, and their gender phenotype may not correspond with the presence of XX or XY chromosomes.

It will be important to bear in mind during the following description one essential generalization: The genes directly determine only whether the individual will have testes or ovaries. The rest of sex differentiation depends upon the presence or absence of substances produced by the genetically determined gonads, in particular, the testes.

Differentiation of the Gonads

The male and female gonads derive embryologically from the same site—an area called the urogenital (or gonadal) ridge. Until the sixth week of uterine life, primordial gonads are undifferentiated (see Figure 17.2). In the genetic male, the testes begin to develop during the seventh week. A gene on the Y chromosome (the ***SRY* gene,** for *s*ex-determining *r*egion of the *Y* chromosome) is expressed at this time in the urogenital ridge cells and triggers this development. In the absence of a Y chromosome and, consequently, the *SRY* gene, testes do not develop. Instead, ovaries begin to develop in the same area.

By what mechanism does the *SRY* gene induce the formation of the testes? This gene codes for a protein, SRY, which sets into motion a sequence of gene activations ultimately leading to the formation of testes from the various embryonic cells in the urogenital ridge.

Differentiation of Internal and External Genitalia

The internal duct system and external genitalia of the fetus are capable of developing into either sexual phenotype (**Figure 17.2** and **Figure 17.3**). Before the functioning of the fetal gonads, the undifferentiated reproductive tract includes a double genital duct system, comprised of the **Wolffian ducts** and **Müllerian ducts,** and a common opening to the outside for the genital ducts and urinary system. Usually, most of the reproductive tract develops from only one of these duct systems. In the male, the Wolffian ducts persist and the Müllerian ducts regress, whereas in the female, the opposite happens. The external genitalia in the two genders and the outer part of the vagina do not develop from these duct systems, however, but from other structures at the body surface.

Which of the two duct systems and types of external genitalia develops depends on the presence or absence of fetal testes. These testes secrete testosterone and a protein hormone called **Müllerian-inhibiting substance (MIS)** (see Figure 17.2). SRY protein induces the expression of the gene for MIS; MIS then causes the degeneration of the Müllerian duct system. Simultaneously, testosterone causes the Wolffian ducts to differentiate into the epididymis, vas deferens, ejaculatory duct, and seminal vesicles. Externally and somewhat later, under the influence primarily of dihydrotestosterone (DHT) produced from testosterone in target tissue, a penis forms and the tissue near it fuses to form the scrotum (see Figure 17.3). The testes will ultimately descend into the scrotum, stimulated to do so by testosterone. Failure of the testes to descend is called ***cryptorchidism*** and is common in infants with decreased androgen secretion. Because sperm production requires about 2°C lower temperature than normal core body temperature, sperm production is usually decreased in cryptorchidism. Treatments include hormone therapy and surgical approaches to move the testes into the scrotum.

In contrast, the female fetus, not having testes (because of the absence of the *SRY* gene), does not secrete testosterone and MIS. In the absence of MIS, the Müllerian system does not degenerate but rather develops into fallopian tubes and a uterus (see Figure 17.2). In the absence of testosterone, the Wolffian ducts degenerate and a vagina and female external genitalia develop from the structures at the body surface (see Figure 17.3). Ovaries, though present in the female fetus, do not play a role in these developmental processes. In other words, female fetal development will occur automatically unless stopped from doing so by the presence of factors released from functioning testes. The events in sex determination and sex differentiation in males and females are summarized in **Figure 17.4**.

There are various conditions in which normal sex differentiation does not occur. For example, in ***androgen insensitivity syndrome*** (also called ***testicular feminization***), the genotype is XY and testes are present but the phenotype (external genitalia and vagina) is female. It is caused by a mutation in the androgen-receptor gene that renders the receptor incapable of normal binding to testosterone. Under the influence of SRY protein, the fetal testes differentiate as usual and they secrete both MIS and testosterone. MIS causes the Müllerian ducts to regress, but the inability of the Wolffian ducts to respond to testosterone also causes them to regress, and so no duct system develops. The tissues that develop into external genitalia are also unresponsive to androgen, so female external genitalia and a vagina develop. The testes do not descend, and they are usually removed when the diagnosis is made. The syndrome is usually not detected until menstrual cycles fail to begin at puberty.

Whereas androgen insensitivity syndrome is caused by a failure of the developing fetus to respond to fetal androgens, ***congenital adrenal hyperplasia*** is caused by the production of too much androgen in the fetus. Rather than the androgen coming from the fetal testes, it is caused by adrenal androgen overproduction due to a partial defect in the ability of the fetal adrenal gland to synthesize cortisol. This is almost always due to a mutation in the gene for an enzyme in the cortisol synthetic pathway (**Figure 17.5**) leading to a partial decrease in the activity of the enzyme. The resultant decrease in cortisol in the fetal blood leads to an increase in the secretion of ACTH from the fetal pituitary gland due to a loss of glucocorticoid negative feedback. The increase in fetal plasma ACTH stimulates the fetal adrenal cortex to try to make more cortisol to overcome the partial enzyme dysfunction. Remember, however, that the adrenal cortex can synthesize androgens from the same precursor as cortisol (see Figure 11.5). ACTH stimulation results in an increase in androgen production because the precursors cannot be efficiently converted to cortisol. This increase in fetal androgen production results in ***virilization*** of an XX fetus (masculinized external genitalia). If untreated in the fetus, the XX baby is usually born with ***ambiguous genitalia***—it is not obvious whether the baby is a phenotypic boy or girl. These babies require treatment with cortisol replacement.

Sexual Differentiation of the Brain

With regard to sexual behavior, differences in the brain may form during fetal and neonatal development. For example, genetic female monkeys treated with testosterone during their late fetal life manifest evidence of masculine sex behavior as adults, such as mounting. In this regard, a potentially important difference in human brain anatomy has been reported; the size of a particular nucleus (neuronal cluster) in the hypothalamus is

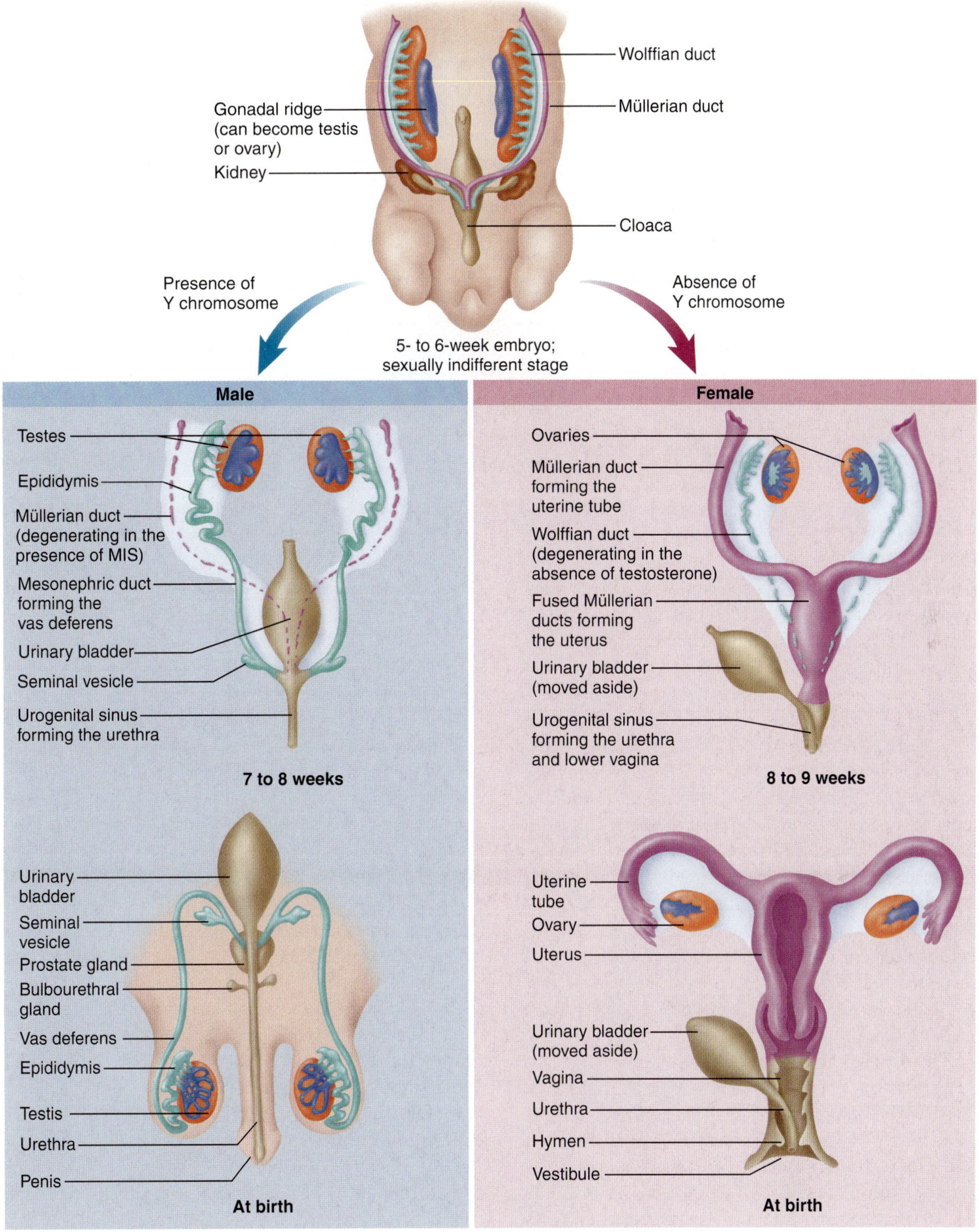

Figure 17.2 Embryonic sex differentiation of the male and female internal reproductive tracts. The testes develop in the presence of the Y chromosome (due to the expression of SRY protein), whereas the ovaries develop in the absence of the Y chromosome (due to the absence of SRY protein). In males, the testes secrete testosterone, which stimulates the maturation of the Wolffian duct into the vas deferens and associated structures, and Müllerian-inhibiting substance (MIS), which induces the degeneration of the Müllerian ducts and associated structures. At birth, the testes have descended into the scrotum. In the female, the absence of testosterone allows the Wolffian ducts to degenerate and the absence of MIS allows the Müllerian ducts to develop into the uterine (fallopian) tubes and the uterus.

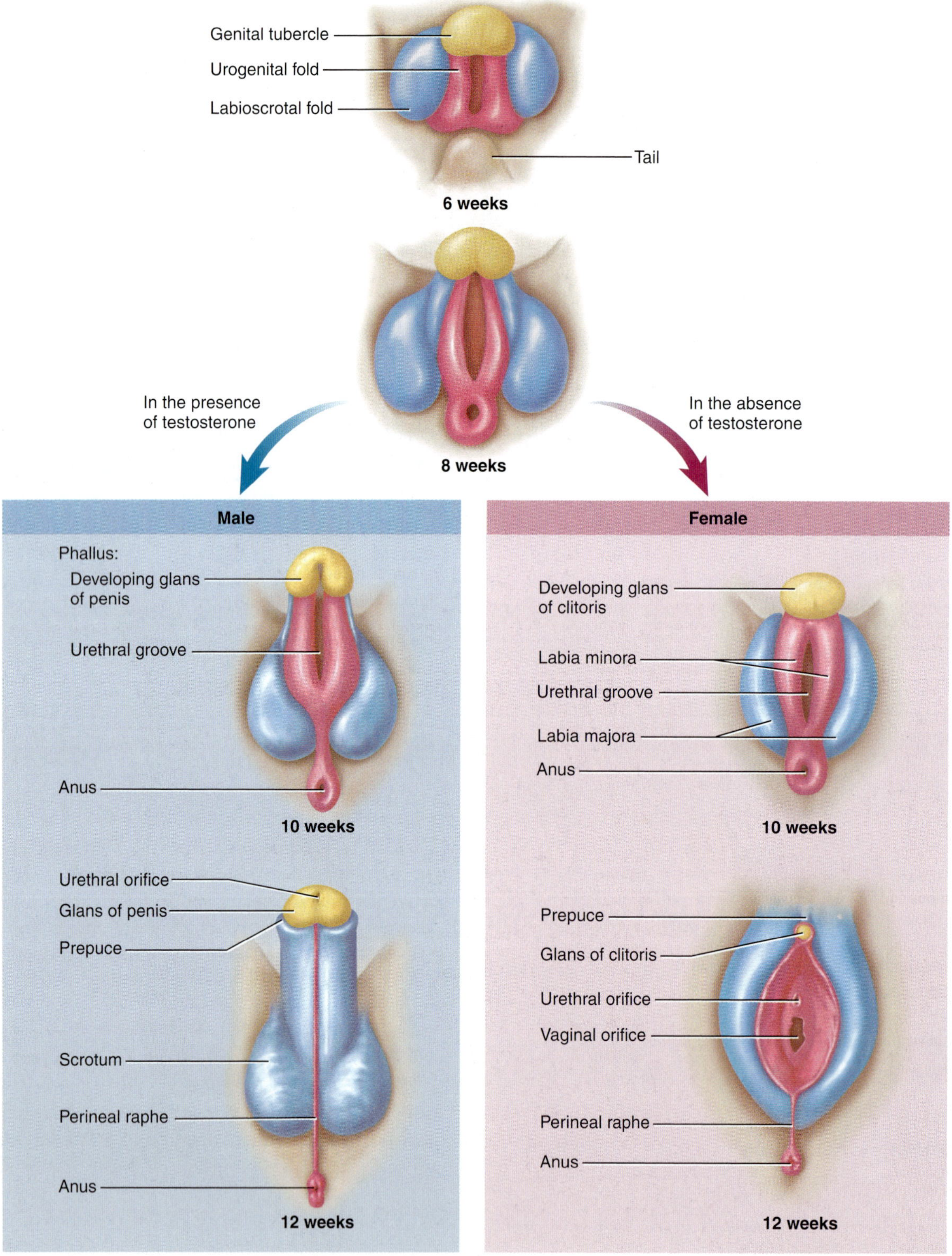

Figure 17.3 Development of the external genitalia in males and females. The major signal for sex differentiation of the external genitalia is the presence of testosterone in the male (produced by the testes shown in Figure 17.2) and its local conversion to dihydrotestosterone (DHT) in target tissue. By about 6 weeks of development, the three primordial structures of the embryo that will become the male or female external genitalia are the genital tubercle, the urogenital fold, and the labioscrotal fold. Sexual differentiation becomes apparent at 10 weeks of fetal life and is unmistakable by 12 weeks of fetal life. The female phenotype develops in the absence of testosterone and DHT. Matching colors identify homologous structures in the male and female.

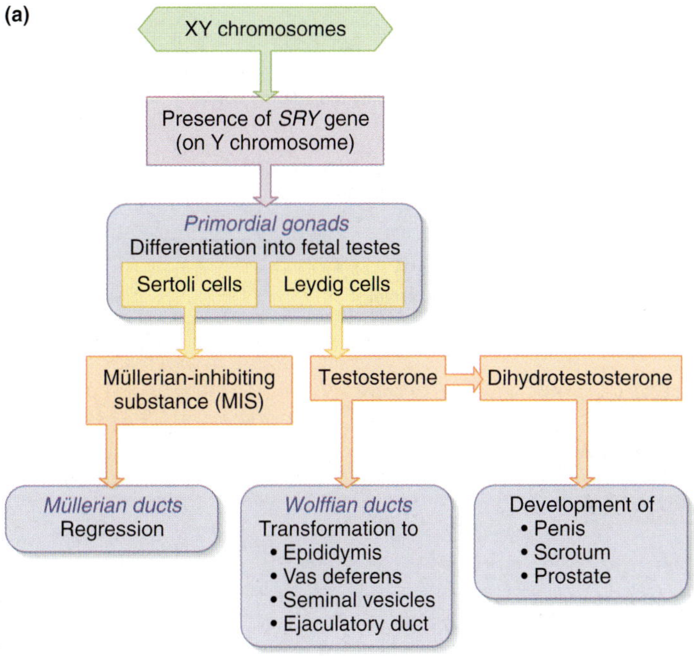

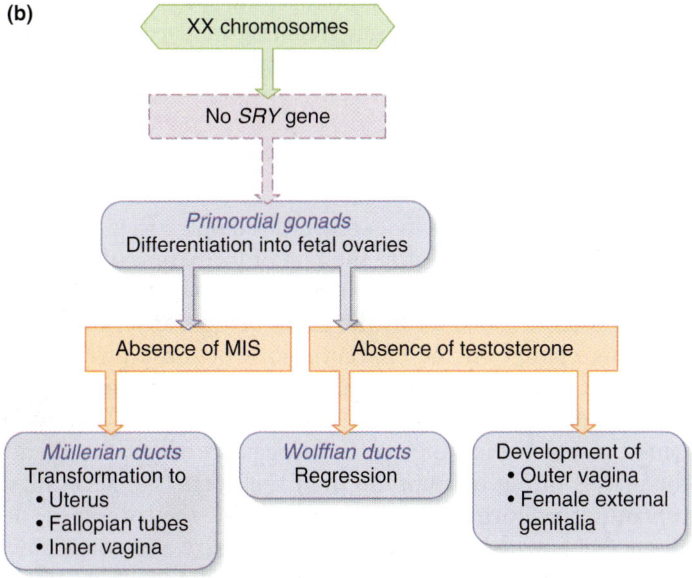

Figure 17.4 Summary of sex differentiation. (a) Male. (b) Female. The *SRY* gene codes for the SRY protein. Conversion of testosterone to dihydrotestosterone occurs primarily in target tissue. The Sertoli and Leydig cells in the testes will be described in Section C.

PHYSIOLOGICAL INQUIRY

- Referring to part (a), 5-α-reductase inhibitors, which block the conversion of testosterone to dihydrotestosterone (DHT) in target tissue, are used to treat some men with benign swelling of their prostate glands. (The prostate gland cells contain 5-α-reductase and are target tissues of locally produced DHT.) Examples of these drugs are finasteride and dutasteride. Why are pregnant women instructed not to take or even handle these drugs? (*Hint:* Some drugs can cross the placenta and enter the circulatory system of the fetus.)

Answer can be found at end of chapter.

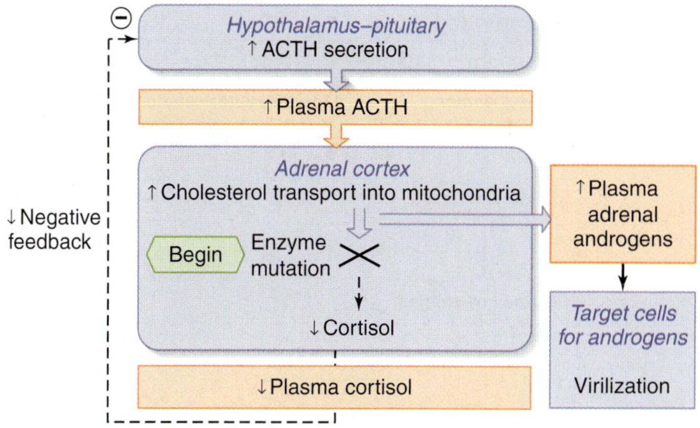

Figure 17.5 Mechanism of virilization in female fetuses with congenital adrenal hyperplasia. An enzyme defect (usually partial) in the steroidogenic pathway leads to decreased production of cortisol and a shift of precursors into the adrenal androgen pathway. Because cortisol negative feedback is decreased, ACTH release from the fetal pituitary gland increases. Although cortisol can eventually be normalized, it is at the expense of ACTH-stimulated adrenal hypertrophy and excess fetal adrenal androgen production.

significantly larger in men. There is also an increase in gonadal steroid secretion in the first year of postnatal life that contributes to the sexual differentiation of the brain. Sex-linked differences in appearance or form within a species are called **sexual dimorphisms.**

17.4 General Principles of Reproductive Endocrinology

This is a good place to review the synthesis of gonadal steroid hormones introduced in Chapter 11 (**Figure 17.6**). These steroidogenic pathways are excellent examples of how the understanding of physiological control is aided by an appreciation of fundamental chemical principles. Each step in this synthetic pathway is catalyzed by enzymes encoded by specific genes. Mutations in these enzymes can lead to atypical gonadal steroid synthesis and secretion and can have profound consequences on sexual development and function. As in the adrenal gland, steroid synthesis starts with cholesterol (see Figures 11.5 and 11.7). Testosterone belongs to a group of steroid hormones that have similar masculinizing actions and are collectively called androgens. In the male, most of the circulating testosterone is synthesized in the testes. Other circulating androgens are produced by the adrenal cortex, but they are much less potent than testosterone and are unable to maintain male reproductive function if testosterone secretion is inadequate. Furthermore, these adrenal androgens are also secreted by women. Some adrenal androgens, like dehydroepiandrosterone (DHEA) and androstenedione, are sold as dietary supplements and touted as miracle drugs with limited data showing effectiveness. Finally, some testosterone is converted to the more potent androgen dihydrotestosterone in target tissue by the action of the enzyme **5-α-reductase.**

Estrogens are a class of steroid hormones secreted in large amounts by the ovaries and placenta. There are three

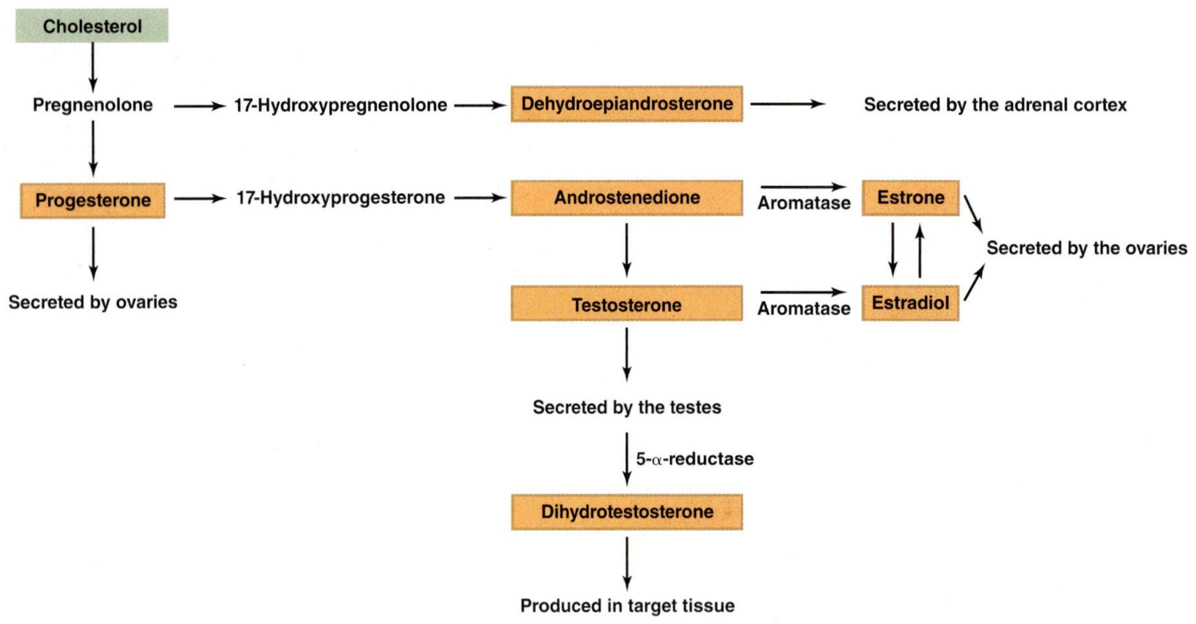

Figure 17.6 Synthesis of androgens in the testes and adrenal gland, and progesterone and estrogens in the ovaries. As in the adrenal cortex (see Figure 11.5), cholesterol is the precursor of steroid hormone synthesis. Progesterone and the estrogens (estrone and estradiol) are the main secretory products of the ovaries depending on the time in the menstrual cycle (see Figure 17.22). The adrenal cortex produces weak androgens in men and women. The primary gonadal steroid produced by the testes is testosterone, which can be activated to the more potent dihydrotestosterone (DHT) in target tissue. *Note:* Men can also produce some estrogen from testosterone by peripheral conversion due to the action of aromatase in some target tissue (particular adipocytes). For the basic chemical structure of some of these steroid hormones, see Figure 11.4.

major estrogens in humans. As noted earlier, estradiol is the predominant estrogen in the plasma. It is produced by the ovary and placenta and is often used synonymously with the generic term estrogen. **Estrone** is also produced by the ovary and placenta. **Estriol** is found primarily in pregnant women in whom it is produced by the placenta. In all cases, estrogens are produced from androgens by the enzyme **aromatase** (see Figure 17.6). Because plasma concentrations of the different estrogens vary widely depending on the circumstances, and because they have similar actions in the female, we will refer to them throughout this chapter as *estrogen.*

As mentioned earlier, estrogens are not unique to females, nor are androgens to males. Estrogen in the blood in males is derived from the release of small amounts by the testes and from the conversion of androgens to estrogen by the aromatase enzyme in some nongonadal tissues (notably, adipose tissue). Conversely, in females, small amounts of androgens are secreted by the ovaries and larger amounts by the adrenal cortex. Some of these androgens are then converted to estrogen in nongonadal tissues, just as in men, and released into the blood.

Progesterone in females is a major secretory product of the ovary at specific times of the menstrual cycle, as well as of the placenta during pregnancy (see Figure 17.6). Progesterone is also an intermediate in the synthetic pathways for adrenal steroids, estrogens, and androgens.

As described in Chapters 5 and 11, all steroid hormones act in the same general way. They bind to intracellular receptors, and the hormone–receptor complex then binds to DNA in the nucleus to alter the rate of formation of particular mRNAs. The result is a change in the rates of synthesis of the proteins coded for by the genes being transcribed. The resulting change in the concentrations of these proteins in the target cells accounts for the responses to the hormone.

As described earlier, the development of the duct systems through which the sperm or eggs are transported and the glands lining or emptying into the ducts (the **accessory reproductive organs**) is controlled by the presence or absence of gonadal hormones. The breasts are also considered accessory reproductive organs; their development is under the influence of ovarian hormones. The development of the **secondary sexual characteristics,** comprising the many external differences between males and females, is also under the influence of gonadal steroids. Examples are hair distribution, body shape, and average adult height. The secondary sexual characteristics are not directly involved in reproduction.

Reproductive function is largely controlled by a chain of hormones (**Figure 17.7**). The first hormone in the chain is **gonadotropin-releasing hormone** (**GnRH**). As described in Chapter 11, GnRH is one of the hypophysiotropic hormones involved in the control of anterior pituitary gland function. It is secreted by neuroendocrine cells in the hypothalamus, and it reaches the anterior pituitary gland via the hypothalamo–pituitary portal blood vessels. In the anterior pituitary gland, GnRH stimulates the release of the pituitary **gonadotropins—follicle-stimulating hormone**

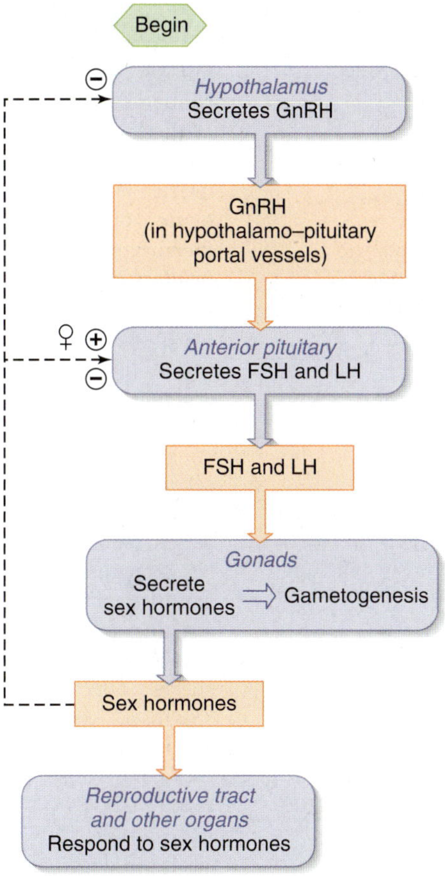

Figure 17.7 APIR General pattern of reproduction control in both males and females. GnRH, like all hypothalamic–hypophysiotropic hormones, reaches the anterior pituitary gland via the hypothalamo–hypophyseal portal vessels. The arrow within the box marked "gonads" denotes the fact that the sex hormones act locally as paracrine agents to influence the gametes. ⊖ indicates negative feedback inhibition. ♀⊕ indicates estrogen stimulation of FSH and LH in the middle of the menstrual cycle in women (positive feedback).

PHYSIOLOGICAL INQUIRY

- What would be the short- and long-term effects of removal of one of the two gonads in an adult?

Answer can be found at end of chapter.

(**FSH**) and **luteinizing hormone** (**LH**), which in turn stimulate gonadal function. The brain is, therefore, the primary regulator of reproduction.

The cell bodies of the GnRH neurons receive input from throughout the brain as well as from hormones in the blood. This is why certain stressors, emotions, and trauma to the central nervous system can inhibit reproductive function. It has recently been discovered that neurons in discrete areas of the hypothalamus synapse on GnRH neurons and release a peptide called **kisspeptin** that is intimately involved in the activation of GnRH neurons. Secretion of GnRH is triggered by action potentials in GnRH-producing hypothalamic neuroendocrine cells. These action potentials occur periodically in brief bursts, with virtually no secretion in between. The pulsatile pattern of GnRH secretion is important because the cells of the anterior pituitary gland that secrete the gonadotropins lose sensitivity to GnRH if the concentration of this hormone remains constantly elevated. This phenomenon is exploited by the administration of synthetic analogs of GnRH to men with androgen-sensitive prostate cancer and to women with estrogen-sensitive breast cancer. Although one may think that administration of a GnRH analog would stimulate FSH and LH, the constant nonpulsatile overstimulation actually decreases FSH and LH and results in a decrease in gonadal steroid secretion.

LH and FSH were named for their effects in the female, but their molecular structures are the same in both sexes. The two hormones act upon the gonads, the result being (1) the maturation of sperm or ova and (2) stimulation of sex hormone secretion. In turn, the sex hormones exert many effects on all portions of the reproductive system, including the gonads from which they come and other parts of the body as well. In addition, the gonadal steroids exert feedback effects on the secretion of GnRH, FSH, and LH. It is currently thought that gonadal steroids exert negative feedback effects on GnRH both directly and through inhibition of kisspeptin neuron cell bodies in the hypothalamus that have input to the GnRH neurons. Gonadal protein hormones such as **inhibin** also exert feedback effects on the anterior pituitary gland.

Each link in this hormonal chain is essential. A decrease in function of the hypothalamus or the anterior pituitary gland can result in failure of gonadal steroid secretion and gametogenesis just as if the gonads themselves were diseased.

As a result of changes in the amount and pattern of hormone secretions, reproductive function changes markedly during a person's lifetime and may be divided into the stages summarized in **Table 17.1**.

TABLE 17.1	Stages in the Control of Reproductive Function
During the initial stage, which begins during fetal life and ends in the first year of life (infancy), GnRH, the gonadotropins, and gonadal sex hormones are secreted at relatively high levels.	
From infancy to puberty, the secretion rates of these hormones are very low and reproductive function is quiescent.	
Beginning at puberty, hormonal secretion rates increase markedly, showing large cyclical variations in women during the menstrual cycle. This ushers in the period of active reproduction.	
Finally, reproductive function diminishes later in life, largely because the gonads become less responsive to the gonadotropins. The ability to reproduce ceases entirely in women.	

SECTION A SUMMARY

Gametogenesis

I. The first stage of gametogenesis is mitosis of primordial germ cells.

II. This is followed by meiosis, which is a sequence of two cell divisions resulting in each gamete receiving 23 chromosomes.

III. Crossing-over and random distribution of maternal and paternal chromatids to the daughter cells during meiosis cause genetic variability in the gametes.

Sex Determination

I. Gender is determined by the two sex chromosomes; males are XY, and females are XX.

Sex Differentiation

I. A gene on the Y chromosome is responsible for the development of testes. In the absence of a Y chromosome, testes do not develop and ovaries do instead.

II. When functioning male gonads are present, they secrete testosterone and MIS, so a male reproductive tract and external genitalia develop. In the absence of testes, the female system develops.

III. A sexually dimorphic brain region exists in humans and certain experimental animals that may be linked with male-type or female-type sexual behavior.

General Principles of Reproductive Endocrinology

I. The gonads have a dual function—gametogenesis and secretion of sex hormones.

II. The male gonads are the testes, which produce sperm and secrete the steroid hormone testosterone.

III. The female gonads are the ovaries, which produce ova and secrete the steroid hormones estrogen and progesterone.

IV. Gonadal function is controlled by the gonadotropins (FSH and LH) from the pituitary gland whose release is controlled by gonadotropin-releasing hormone (GnRH) from the hypothalamus.

SECTION A REVIEW QUESTIONS

1. Describe the stages of gametogenesis and how meiosis results in genetic variability.
2. State the genetic difference between males and females and a method for identifying genetic sex.
3. Describe the sequence of events, the timing, and the control of the development of the gonads and the internal and external genitalia.
4. Explain how administration of glucocorticoids to a pregnant woman would treat congenital adrenal hyperplasia in her fetus.

SECTION A KEY TERMS

accessory reproductive organ 612
androgen 605
aromatase 612
Barr body 607
bivalent 607
crossing-over 607
dihydrotestosterone (DHT) 605
estradiol 605
estriol 612
estrogen 605
estrone 612
first polar body 607
5-α-reductase 611
follicle-stimulating hormone (FSH) 612
gamete 605
gametogenesis 605
genotype 607
germ cell 605
gonad 605
gonadal steroid 605
gonadotropin 612
gonadotropin-releasing hormone (GnRH) 612
inhibin 613
karyotype 607
kisspeptin 613
luteinizing hormone (LH) 613
meiosis 605
mitosis 605
Müllerian duct 608
Müllerian-inhibiting substance (MIS) 608
ovary 605
ovum 605
phenotype 607
primary oocyte 605
primary spermatocyte 605
progesterone 605
second polar body 607
secondary oocyte 607
secondary sexual characteristic 612
secondary spermatocyte 607
sex chromatin 607
sex chromosome 607
sex determination 607
sex differentiation 607
sex hormone 605
sexual dimorphism 611
sperm 605
spermatid 607
spermatozoan 605
SRY gene 608
testis 605
testosterone 605
Wolffian duct 608
X chromosome 607
Y chromosome 607
zygote 607

SECTION A CLINICAL TERMS

ambiguous genitalia 608
androgen insensitivity syndrome 608
congenital adrenal hyperplasia 608
cryptorchidism 608
testicular feminization 608
virilization 608

SECTION B
Male Reproductive Physiology

17.5 Anatomy

The male reproductive system includes the two testes, the system of ducts that store and transport sperm to the exterior, the glands that empty into these ducts, and the penis. The duct system, glands, and penis constitute the male accessory reproductive organs.

The testes are suspended outside the abdomen in the **scrotum,** which is an outpouching of the abdominal wall and is divided internally into two sacs, one for each testis. During early fetal development, the testes are located in the abdomen; but during later **gestation** (usually in the seventh month of pregnancy), they usually descend into the scrotum (see Figure 17.2). This descent is essential for normal sperm

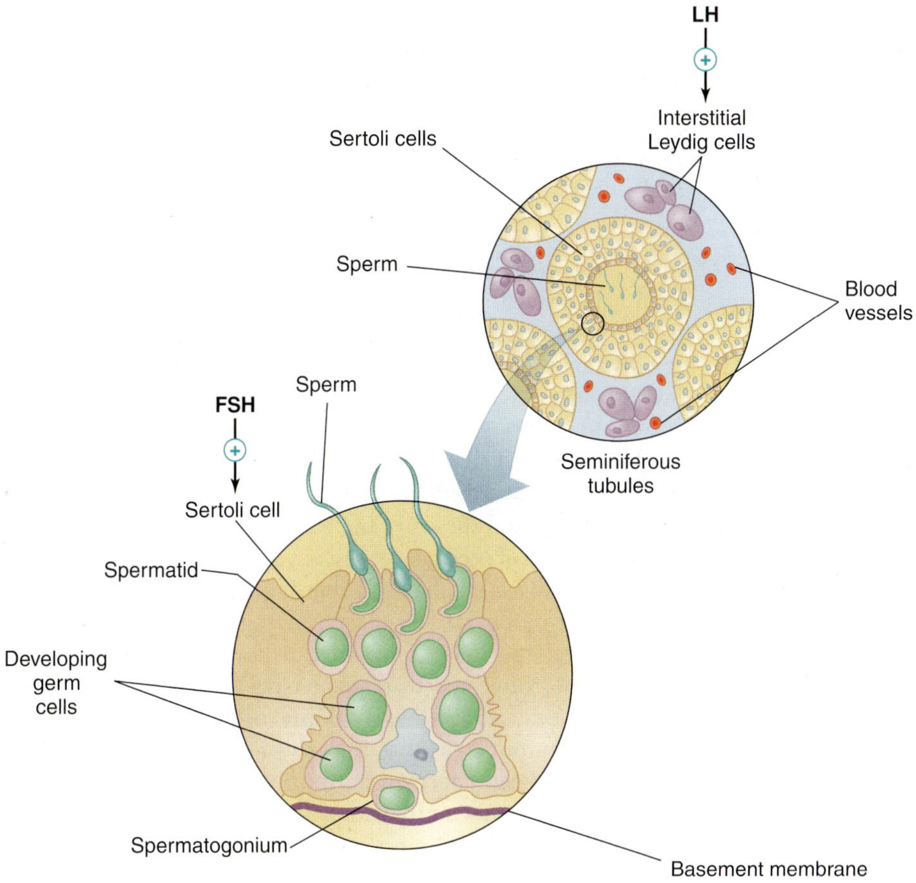

Figure 17.8 APR Cross section of an area of testis. The Sertoli cells (stimulated by FSH to increase spermatogenesis and produce inhibin) are in the seminiferous tubules, the sites of sperm production. The tubules are separated from each other by interstitial space (colored light blue) that contains Leydig cells (stimulated by LH to produce testosterone) and blood vessels.

production during adulthood, because sperm formation requires a temperature approximately 2°C lower than normal internal body temperature. Cooling is achieved by air circulating around the scrotum and by a heat-exchange mechanism in the blood vessels supplying the testes. In contrast to spermatogenesis, testosterone secretion can usually occur normally at internal body temperature, so failure of testes descent usually does not impair testosterone secretion.

The sites of **spermatogenesis** (sperm formation) in the testes are the many tiny, convoluted **seminiferous tubules** (Figure 17.8). The combined length of these tubes is 250 m (the length of over 2.5 football fields). Each seminiferous tubule is bounded by a basement membrane. In the center of each tubule is a fluid-filled lumen containing the mature sperm cells, called spermatozoa. The tubular wall is composed of developing germ cells and their supporting cells called **Sertoli cells.**

The **Leydig cells,** or interstitial cells, which lie in small, connective-tissue spaces between the tubules, are the cells that synthesize and release testosterone. Thus, the sperm-producing and testosterone-producing functions of the testes are carried out by different structures—the seminiferous tubules and Leydig cells, respectively.

The seminiferous tubules from different areas of a testis converge to form a network of interconnected tubes, the **rete testis** (Figure 17.9). Small ducts called efferent ductules leave the rete testis, pierce the fibrous covering of the testis, and empty into a single duct within a structure called the **epididymis** (plural, *epididymides*). The epididymis is loosely attached to the outside of the testis. The duct of the epididymis is so convoluted that, when straightened out at dissection, it measures 6 m. The epididymis draining each testis leads to a **vas deferens** (plural, *vasa deferentia*), a large, thick-walled tube

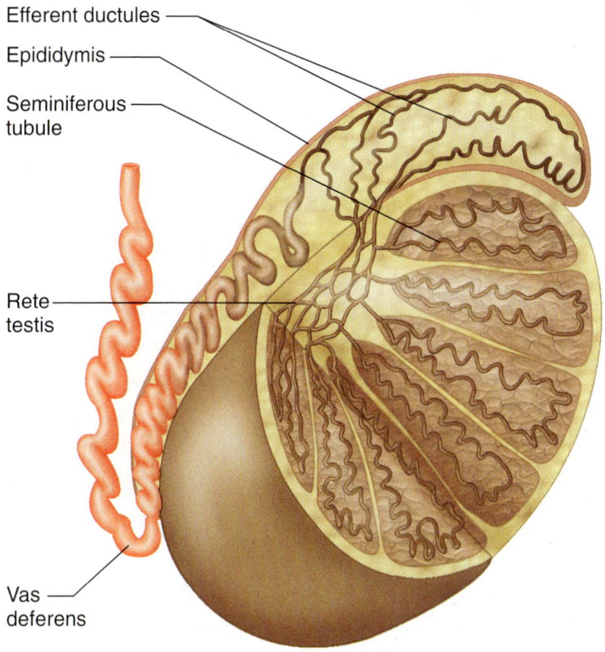

Figure 17.9 APR Section of a testis. The upper portion of the testis has been removed to show its interior.

lined with smooth muscle. Not shown in Figure 17.9 is that the vas deferens and the blood vessels and nerves supplying the testis are bound together in the **spermatic cord,** which passes to the testis through a slitlike passage, the inguinal canal, in the abdominal wall.

After entering the abdomen, the two vasa deferentia—one from each testis—continue to behind the urinary bladder base (**Figure 17.10**). The ducts from two large glands, the **seminal vesicles,** which lie behind the bladder, join the two vasa deferentia to form the two **ejaculatory ducts.** The ejaculatory ducts then enter the **prostate gland** and join the urethra, coming from the bladder. The prostate gland is a single walnut-sized structure below the bladder and surrounding the upper part of the urethra, into which it secretes fluid through hundreds of tiny openings in the side of the urethra. The urethra emerges from the prostate gland and enters the penis. The paired **bulbourethral glands,** lying below the prostate, drain into the urethra just after it leaves the prostate.

The prostate gland and seminal vesicles secrete most of the fluid in which ejaculated sperm are suspended. This fluid plus the sperm cells constitute **semen,** the sperm contributing a small percentage of the total volume. The glandular secretions contain a large number of different chemical substances, including (1) nutrients, (2) buffers for protecting the sperm against the acidic vaginal secretions and residual acidic urine in the male urethra, (3) chemicals (particularly from the seminal vesicles) that increase sperm motility, and (4) prostaglandins. The function of the prostaglandins, which are produced by the seminal vesicles, is still not clear. The bulbourethral glands contribute a small volume of lubricating mucoid secretions.

In addition to providing a route for sperm from the seminiferous tubules to the exterior, several of the duct system segments perform additional functions to be described in the section on sperm transport.

17.6 Spermatogenesis

The various stages of spermatogenesis were introduced in Figure 17.1 and are summarized in **Figure 17.11**. The undifferentiated germ cells, called spermatogonia (singular, **spermatogonium**), begin to divide mitotically at puberty. The daughter cells of this first division then divide again and again for a specified number of division cycles so that a clone of spermatogonia is produced from each stem cell spermatogonium. Some differentiation occurs in addition to cell division. The cells that result from the final mitotic division and differentiation in the series are called primary spermatocytes, and these are the cells that will undergo the first meiotic division of spermatogenesis.

It should be emphasized that if all the cells in the clone produced by each stem cell spermatogonium followed this pathway, the spermatogonia would disappear—that is, they would all be converted to primary spermatocytes. This does not occur because, at an early point, one of the cells of each clone "drops out" of the mitosis–differentiation cycle to remain a stem cell spermatogonium that will later enter into its own full sequence of divisions. One cell of the clone it produces will do likewise, and so on. Therefore, the supply of undifferentiated spermatogonia does not decrease.

Each primary spermatocyte increases markedly in size and undergoes the first meiotic division (see Figure 17.11) to form two secondary spermatocytes, each of which contains

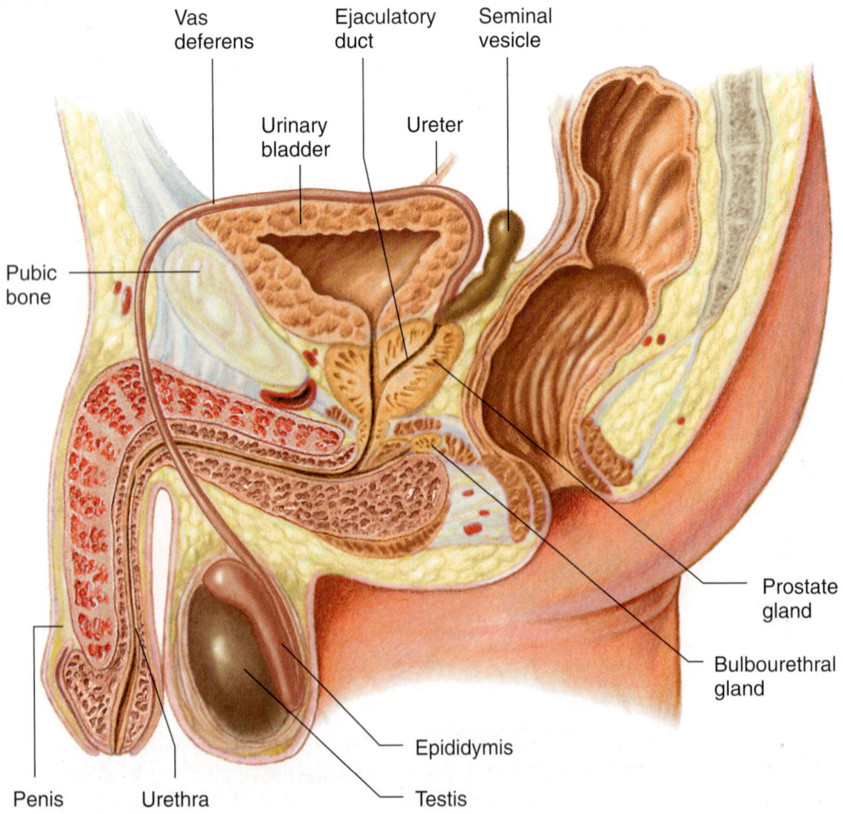

Figure 17.10 AP|R Anatomical organization of the male reproductive tract. This figure shows the testis, epididymis, vas deferens, ejaculatory duct, seminal vesicle, and bulbourethral gland on only one side of the body, but they are all paired structures. The urinary bladder and a ureter are shown for orientation but are not part of the reproductive tract. Once the ejaculatory ducts join the urethra in the prostate, the urinary and reproductive tracts have merged.

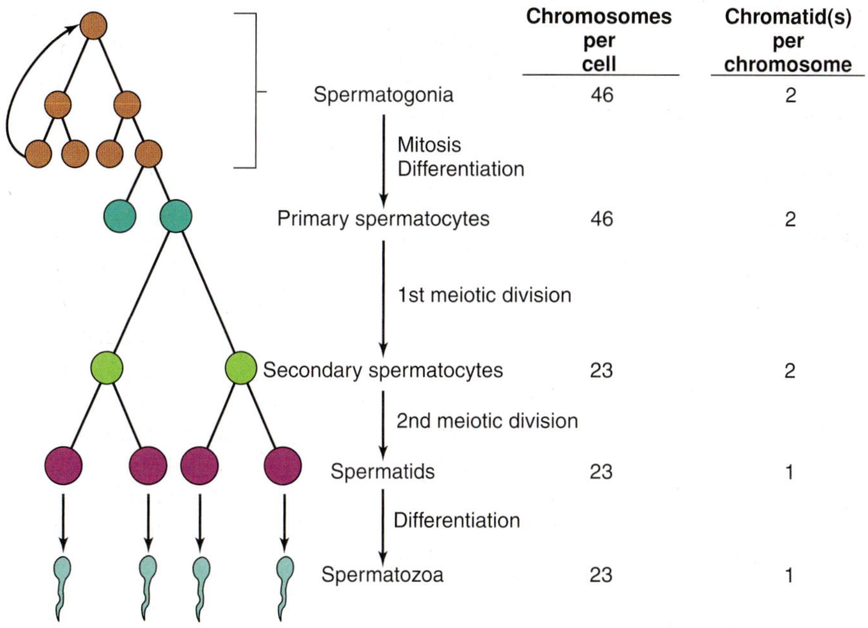

Figure 17.11 APIR Summary of spermatogenesis, which begins at puberty. Each spermatogonium yields, by mitosis, a clone of spermatogonia; for simplicity, the figure shows only two such cycles, with a third mitotic cycle generating two primary spermatocytes. The arrow from one of the spermatogonia back to a stem cell spermatogonium denotes the fact that one cell of the clone does not go on to generate primary spermatocytes but reverts to an undifferentiated spermatogonium that gives rise to a new clone. Each primary spermatocyte produces four spermatozoa.

23 two-chromatid chromosomes. Each secondary spermatocyte undergoes the second meiotic division (see Figure 17.1) to form spermatids. Thus, each primary spermatocyte, containing 46 two-chromatid chromosomes, produces four spermatids, each containing 23 one-chromatid chromosomes.

The final phase of spermatogenesis is the differentiation of the spermatids into spermatozoa (sperm). This process involves extensive cell remodeling, including elongation, but no further cell divisions. The head of a sperm cell (**Figure 17.12**) consists almost entirely of the nucleus, which contains the genetic information (DNA). The tip of the nucleus is covered by the **acrosome,** a protein-filled vesicle containing several enzymes that play an important role in fertilization. Most of the tail is a flagellum—a group of contractile filaments that produce whiplike movements capable of propelling the sperm at a velocity of 1 to 4 mm per min. Mitochondria form the midpiece of the sperm and provide the energy for movement.

The entire process of spermatogenesis, from primary spermatocyte to sperm, takes approximately 64 days. The typical human male manufactures approximately 30 million sperm per day.

Thus far, spermatogenesis has been described without regard to its orientation within the seminiferous tubules or the participation of Sertoli cells, the second type of cell in the seminiferous tubules, with which the developing germ cells are closely associated. Each seminiferous tubule is bounded by a basement membrane. Each Sertoli cell extends from the basement membrane all the way to the lumen in the center of the tubule and is joined to adjacent Sertoli cells by means of tight junctions (**Figure 17.13**). Thus, the Sertoli cells form an unbroken ring around the outer circumference of the seminiferous tubule. The tight junctions divide the tubule into two compartments—a basal compartment, between the basement membrane and the tight junctions, and a central compartment, beginning at the tight junctions and including the lumen.

The ring of interconnected Sertoli cells forms the **Sertoli cell barrier** (blood–testes barrier), which prevents the movement of many chemicals from the blood into the lumen of the seminiferous tubule and helps retain luminal fluid. This ensures proper conditions for germ cell development and differentiation in the tubules. The arrangement of Sertoli cells also permits different stages of spermatogenesis to take place in different compartments and, therefore, in different environments.

Mitotic cell divisions and differentiation of spermatogonia to yield primary spermatocytes take place entirely in the basal compartment. The primary spermatocytes then move through the tight junctions of the Sertoli cells (which open in front of them while at the same time forming new tight junctions behind them) to gain entry into the central compartment. In this central compartment, the meiotic divisions of spermatogenesis occur, and the spermatids differentiate into sperm while contained in recesses formed by invaginations of the Sertoli cell plasma membranes. When sperm formation is

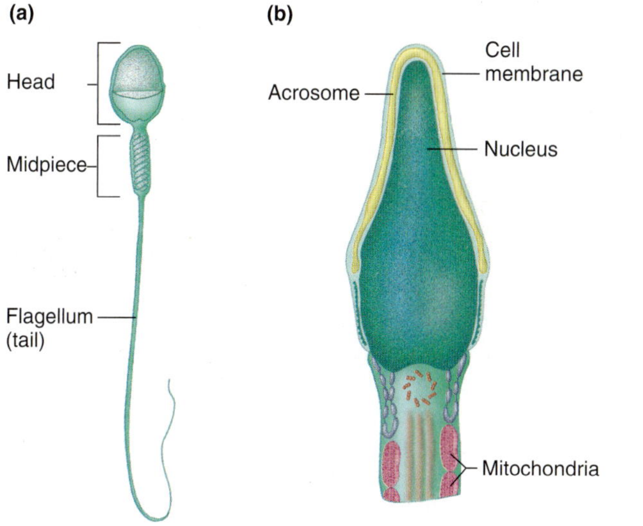

Figure 17.12 APIR (a) Diagram of a human mature sperm. (b) A close-up of the head drawn from a different angle. The acrosome contains enzymes required for fertilization of the ovum.

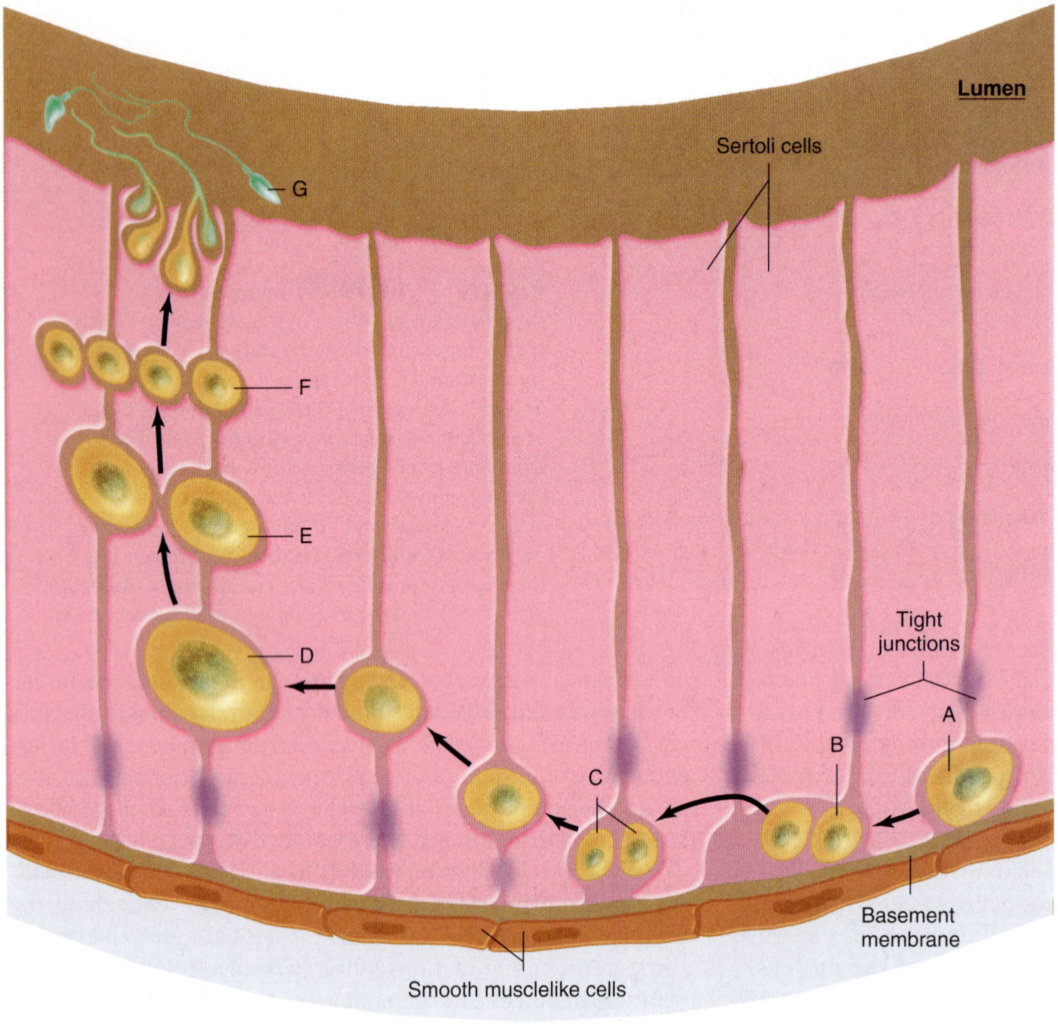

Figure 17.13 APIR Relation of the Sertoli cells and germ cells. The Sertoli cells form a ring (barrier) around the entire tubule. For convenience of presentation, the various stages of spermatogenesis are shown as though the germ cells move down a line of adjacent Sertoli cells; in reality, all stages beginning with any given spermatogonium take place between the same two Sertoli cells. Spermatogonia (A and B) are found only in the basal compartment (between the tight junctions of the Sertoli cells and the basement membrane of the tubule). After several mitotic cycles (A to B), the spermatogonia (B) give rise to primary spermatocytes (C). Each of the latter crosses a tight junction, enlarges (D), and divides into two secondary spermatocytes (E), which divide into spermatids (F), which in turn differentiate into spermatozoa (G). This last step involves loss of cytoplasm by the spermatids. Adapted from Tung.

complete, the cytoplasm of the Sertoli cell around the sperm retracts and the sperm are released into the lumen to be bathed by the luminal fluid.

Sertoli cells serve as the route by which nutrients reach developing germ cells, and they also secrete most of the fluid found in the tubule lumen. This fluid contains **androgen-binding protein** (**ABP**), which binds the testosterone secreted by the Leydig cells and crosses the Sertoli cell barrier to enter the tubule. This protein maintains a high concentration of total testosterone in the lumen of the tubule. The dissociation of free testosterone from ABP continuously bathes the developing spermatocytes and Sertoli cells in testosterone.

Sertoli cells do more than influence environment of the germ cells. In response to FSH from the anterior pituitary gland and to local testosterone produced in the Leydig cell, Sertoli cells secrete a variety of chemical messengers. These function as paracrine agents to stimulate proliferation and differentiation of the germ cells.

In addition, the Sertoli cells secrete the protein hormone inhibin, which acts as a negative feedback controller of FSH, and paracrine agents that affect Leydig cell function. The many functions of Sertoli cells, several of which remain to be described later in this chapter, are summarized in **Table 17.2**.

TABLE 17.2 Functions of Sertoli Cells
Provide Sertoli cell barrier to chemicals in the plasma
Nourish developing sperm
Secrete luminal fluid, including androgen-binding protein
Respond to stimulation by testosterone and FSH to secrete paracrine agents that stimulate sperm proliferation and differentiation
Secrete the protein hormone inhibin, which inhibits FSH secretion from the pituitary gland
Secrete paracrine agents that influence the function of Leydig cells
Phagocytize defective sperm
Secrete Müllerian-inhibiting substance (MIS), which causes the primordial female duct system to regress during embryonic life

17.7 Transport of Sperm

From the seminiferous tubules, the sperm pass through the rete testis and efferent ducts into the epididymis and from there to the vas deferens. The vas deferens and the portion of the epididymis closest to it serve as a storage reservoir for sperm until **ejaculation,** the discharge of semen from the penis.

Movement of the sperm as far as the epididymis results from the pressure that the Sertoli cells create by continuously secreting fluid into the seminiferous tubules. The sperm themselves are normally nonmotile at this time.

During passage through the epididymis, the concentration of the sperm increases dramatically due to fluid absorption from the lumen of the epididymis. Therefore, as the sperm pass from the end of the epididymis into the vas deferens, they are a densely packed mass whose transport is no longer facilitated by fluid movement. Instead, peristaltic contractions of the smooth muscle in the epididymis and vas deferens cause the sperm to move.

The absence of a large quantity of fluid accounts for the fact that ***vasectomy,*** the surgical tying off and removal of a segment of each vas deferens as a method of male contraception, does not cause the accumulation of much fluid behind the tie-off point. The sperm, which are still produced after vasectomy, do build up, however, and eventually break down, with their chemical components absorbed into the bloodstream. Vasectomy does not affect testosterone secretion because it does not alter the function of the Leydig cells. The next step in sperm transport is ejaculation.

Erection

The penis consists almost entirely of three cylindrical, vascular compartments running its entire length. Normally, the small arteries supplying the vascular compartments are constricted so that the compartments contain little blood and the penis is flaccid. During sexual excitation, the small arteries dilate, blood flow increases, the three vascular compartments become engorged with blood at high pressure, and the penis becomes rigid (**erection**). The vascular dilation is initiated by neural input to the small arteries of the penis. As the vascular compartments expand, the veins emptying them are passively compressed, further increasing the local pressure, thus contributing to the engorgement while blood flow remains elevated. This entire process occurs rapidly with complete erection sometimes taking only 5 to 10 seconds.

What are the neural inputs to the small arteries of the penis? At rest, the dominant input is from sympathetic neurons that release norepinephrine, which causes the arterial smooth muscle to contract. During erection, this sympathetic input is inhibited. Much more important is the activation of nonadrenergic, noncholinergic autonomic neurons to the arteries (**Figure 17.14**). These neurons and associated endothelial cells release **nitric oxide,** which relaxes the arterial smooth muscle.

Which receptors and afferent pathways initiate these reflexes? The primary stimulus comes from mechanoreceptors in the genital region, particularly in the head of the penis. The afferent fibers carrying the impulses synapse in the lower spinal cord on interneurons that control the efferent outflow.

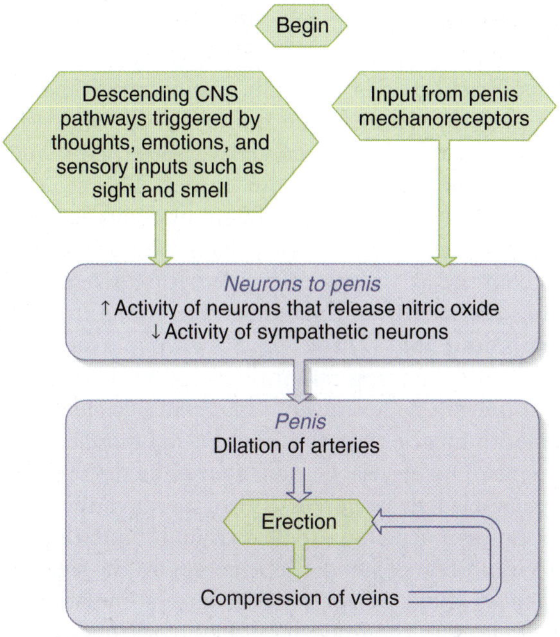

Figure 17.14 Reflex pathways for erection. Nitric oxide, a vasodilator, is the most important neurotransmitter to the arteries in this reflex.

It must be stressed, however, that higher brain centers, via descending pathways, may also exert profound stimulatory or inhibitory effects upon the autonomic neurons to the small arteries of the penis. Thus, mechanical stimuli from areas other than the penis, as well as thoughts, emotions, sights, and odors, can induce erection in the complete absence of penile stimulation (or prevent erection even though stimulation is present).

Erectile dysfunction (also called *impotence*) is the consistent inability to achieve or sustain an erection of sufficient rigidity for sexual intercourse and is a common problem. Although it can be mild to moderate in degree, complete erectile dysfunction is present in as many as 10% of adult American males between the ages of 40 and 70. During this period of life, its rate almost doubles. The organic causes are multiple and include damage to or malfunction of the efferent nerves or descending pathways, endocrine disorders, various therapeutic and "recreational" drugs (e.g., alcohol), and certain diseases, particularly diabetes mellitus. Erectile dysfunction can also be due to psychological factors (such as depression), which are mediated by the brain and the descending pathways.

There are now a group of orally active ***cGMP-phosphodiesterase type 5*** (PDE5) ***inhibitors*** including sildenafil (*Viagra*), vardenafil (*Levitra*), and tadalafil (*Cialis*) that greatly improve the ability of many men with erectile dysfunction to achieve and maintain an erection. The most important event leading to erection is the dilation of penile arteries by nitric oxide, released from autonomic neurons. Nitric oxide stimulates the enzyme guanylyl cyclase, which catalyzes the formation of cyclic GMP (cGMP), as described in Chapter 5. This second messenger then continues the signal transduction pathway leading to the relaxation of the arterial smooth muscle. The sequence of events is terminated by an enzyme-dependent breakdown of cGMP. PDE5 inhibitors block the action of this enzyme and thereby permit a higher concentration of cGMP to exist.

Ejaculation

As stated earlier, ejaculation is the discharge of semen from the penis. Ejaculation is primarily a spinal reflex mediated by afferent pathways from penile mechanoreceptors. When the level of stimulation is high enough, a patterned sequence of discharge of the efferent neurons ensues. This sequence can be divided into two phases: (1) The smooth muscles of the epididymis, vas deferens, ejaculatory ducts, prostate, and seminal vesicles contract as a result of sympathetic nerve stimulation, emptying the sperm and glandular secretions into the urethra (**emission**); and (2) the semen, with an average volume of 3 mL and containing 300 million sperm, is then expelled from the urethra by a series of rapid contractions of the urethral smooth muscle as well as the skeletal muscle at the base of the penis. During ejaculation, the sphincter at the base of the urinary bladder is closed so that sperm cannot enter the bladder, nor can urine be expelled from it. Note that erection involves inhibition of sympathetic nerves (to the small arteries of the penis), whereas ejaculation involves stimulation of sympathetic nerves (to the smooth muscles of the duct system).

The rhythmic muscular contractions that occur during ejaculation are associated with intense pleasure and many systemic physiological changes, collectively termed an **orgasm.** Marked skeletal muscle contractions occur throughout the body, and there is a transient increase in heart rate and blood pressure.

Once ejaculation has occurred, there is a latent period during which a second erection is not possible. The latent period is quite variable but may last from minutes to hours.

17.8 Hormonal Control of Male Reproductive Functions

Control of the Testes

Figure 17.15 summarizes the control of the testes. In a normal adult man, the GnRH-secreting neuroendocrine cells in the hypothalamus fire a brief burst of action potentials approximately every 90 min, secreting GnRH at these times. The GnRH reaching the anterior pituitary gland via the hypothalamo–hypophyseal portal vessels during each periodic pulse triggers the release of both LH and FSH from the same cell type, although not necessarily in equal amounts. Thus, plasma concentrations of FSH and LH also show pulsatility—rapid increases followed by slow decreases over the next 90 min or so as the hormones are slowly removed from the plasma.

There is a clear separation of the actions of FSH and LH within the testes (see Figure 17.15). FSH acts primarily on the Sertoli cells to stimulate the secretion of paracrine agents required for spermatogenesis. LH, by contrast, acts primarily on the Leydig cells to stimulate testosterone secretion. In addition to its many important systemic effects as a hormone, the testosterone secreted by the Leydig cells also acts locally, in a paracrine manner, by diffusing from the interstitial spaces into the seminiferous tubules. Testosterone enters Sertoli cells, where it facilitates spermatogenesis. Thus, despite the absence of a *direct* effect on cells in the seminiferous tubules, LH exerts an essential *indirect* effect because the testosterone secretion stimulated by LH is required for spermatogenesis.

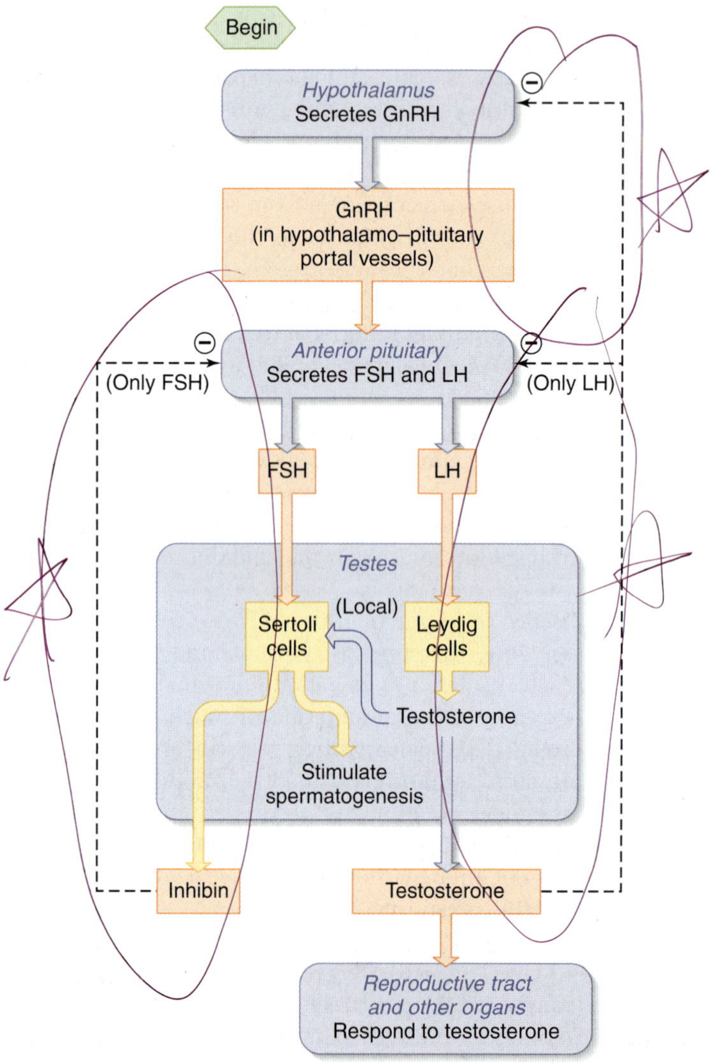

Figure 17.15 APIR Summary of hormonal control of male reproductive function. Note that FSH acts only on the Sertoli cells, whereas LH acts primarily on the Leydig cells. The secretion of FSH is inhibited mainly by inhibin, a protein hormone secreted by the Sertoli cells, and the secretion of LH is inhibited mainly by testosterone, the steroid hormone secreted by the Leydig cells. Testosterone, acting locally on Sertoli cells, stimulates spermatogenesis, whereas FSH stimulates inhibin release from Sertoli cells.

PHYSIOLOGICAL INQUIRY

- Men with decreased anterior pituitary gland function often have decreased sperm production as well as low testosterone concentrations. Would you expect the administration of testosterone alone to restore sperm production to normal?

Answer can be found at end of chapter.

The last components of the hypothalamo–hypophyseal control of male reproduction that remain to be discussed are the negative feedback effects exerted by testicular hormones. Even though FSH and LH are produced by the same cell type, their secretion rates can be altered to different degrees by negative feedback inputs.

Testosterone inhibits LH secretion in two ways (see Figure 17.15): (1) It acts on the hypothalamus to decrease the amplitude of GnRH bursts, which results in a decrease in the secretion of gonadotropins; and (2) it acts directly on the anterior pituitary gland to decrease the LH response to any given amount of GnRH.

How do the testes reduce FSH secretion? The major inhibitory signal, exerted directly on the anterior pituitary gland, is the protein hormone inhibin secreted by the Sertoli cells (see Figure 17.15). This is a logical completion of a negative feedback loop such that FSH stimulates Sertoli cells to increase both spermatogenesis and inhibin production, and inhibin decreases FSH release.

Despite all these complexities, the total amounts of GnRH, LH, FSH, testosterone, and inhibin secreted and of sperm produced do not change dramatically from day to day in the adult male. This is completely different from the large cyclical variations of activity so characteristic of female reproductive processes.

Testosterone

In addition to its essential paracrine action within the testes on spermatogenesis and its negative feedback effects on the hypothalamus and anterior pituitary gland, testosterone exerts many other effects, as summarized in **Table 17.3**.

In Chapter 11, we mentioned that some hormones undergo transformation in their target cells in order to be more effective. This is true of testosterone in many (but not all) of its target cells. In some cells, like in the adult prostate, after its entry into the cytoplasm, testosterone is converted to dihydrotestosterone (DHT), which is more potent than testosterone (see Figure 17.6). This conversion is catalyzed by the enzyme 5-α-reductase, which is expressed in several androgen target tissues. In certain other target cells (e.g., the brain), testosterone is transformed not to dihydrotestosterone but to estradiol, which is the active hormone in these cells. The enzyme aromatase catalyzes this conversion. In the latter case, the "male" sex hormone is converted to the "female" sex hormone to be active in the male. The fact that, depending on the target cells, testosterone may act as testosterone, or be converted to dihydrotestosterone or estradiol, has important pathophysiological implications because some men lack 5-α-reductase or aromatase in some tissues. Therefore, they will exhibit certain signs of testosterone deficiency but not others. For example, an XY fetus with 5-α-reductase deficiency will have normal differentiation of male reproductive duct structures (an effect of testosterone, per se) but will not have normal development of external male genitalia, which requires DHT.

TABLE 17.3 Effects of Testosterone in the Male
Required for initiation and maintenance of spermatogenesis (acts via Sertoli cells)
Decreases GnRH secretion via an action on the hypothalamus
Inhibits LH secretion via a direct action on the anterior pituitary gland
Induces differentiation of male accessory reproductive organs and maintains their function
Induces male secondary sex characteristics; opposes action of estrogen on breast growth
Stimulates protein anabolism, bone growth, and cessation of bone growth
Required for sex drive and may enhance aggressive behavior
Stimulates erythropoietin secretion by the kidneys

Therapy for ***prostate cancer*** makes use of these facts: Prostate cancer cells are stimulated by dihydrotestosterone, so the cancer can be treated with inhibitors of 5-α-reductase. Furthermore, ***male pattern baldness*** may also be treated with 5-α-reductase inhibitors because DHT tends to promote hair loss from the scalp.

Accessory Reproductive Organs

The fetal differentiation and later growth and function of the entire male duct system, glands, and penis all depend upon testosterone (see Figures 17.2 and 17.3). Following the loss of testicular function and decrease in testosterone production, the accessory reproductive organs decrease in size, the glands significantly reduce their secretion rates, and the smooth muscle activity of the ducts is diminished. Sex drive (**libido**), erection, and ejaculation are usually impaired. These defects lessen with the administration of testosterone. This would also occur with ***castration*** (removal of the gonads), which may be done to treat testicular cancer, for example.

17.9 Puberty

Puberty is the period during which the reproductive organs mature and reproduction becomes possible. In males, this usually occurs between 12 and 16 years of age. Some of the first signs of puberty are due not to gonadal steroids but to increased secretion of adrenal androgens, probably under the stimulation of adrenocorticotropic hormone (ACTH). These androgens cause the very early development of pubic and axillary (armpit) hair, as well as the early stages of the pubertal growth spurt in concert with growth hormone and insulin-like growth factor I (see Chapter 11). All other developments in puberty, however, reflect increased activity of the hypothalamo–pituitary–gonadal axis.

The amplitude and pulse frequency of GnRH secretion increase at puberty, probably stimulated by input from kisspeptin neurons in the hypothalamus. This causes increased secretion of pituitary gonadotropins, which stimulate the seminiferous tubules and testosterone secretion. Testosterone, in addition to its critical role in spermatogenesis, induces the pubertal changes that occur in the accessory reproductive organs, secondary sex characteristics, and sex drive. The mechanism of the brain change that results in increased GnRH secretion at puberty remains unknown. One important event is that the brain becomes less sensitive to the negative feedback effects of gonadal hormones at the time of puberty.

Secondary Sex Characteristics and Growth

Virtually all the male secondary sex characteristics are dependent on testosterone and its metabolite, DHT. For example, a male lacking normal testicular secretion of testosterone before puberty has minimal facial, axillary, or pubic hair. Other androgen-dependent secondary sexual characteristics are deepening of the voice resulting from the growth of the larynx, thick secretion of the skin oil glands (often causing acne), and the masculine pattern of fat distribution. Androgens also stimulate bone growth, mostly through the stimulation of growth hormone secretion. Ultimately, however, androgens terminate bone growth by causing closure of the bones' epiphyseal plates. Androgens are "anabolic steroids" in that they exert a direct stimulatory effect on protein synthesis in muscle. Finally, androgens stimulate the secretion of the hormone erythropoietin by the kidneys; this is a major reason why men have a higher hematocrit than women.

Behavior

Androgens are essential in males for the development of sex drive at puberty, and they play an important role in maintaining sex drive (libido) in the adult male. Whether androgens influence other human behaviors in addition to sexual behavior is not certain. However, there is no doubt that androgen-dependent behavioral differences based on gender do exist in other mammals. For example, aggression is clearly greater in males and is androgen-dependent.

Anabolic Steroid Use

The abuse of synthetic androgens (anabolic steroids) is a major public health problem, particularly in younger athletes. Although there are positive effects on muscle mass and athletic performance, the negative effects—such as overstimulation of prostate tissue and increase in aggressiveness—are of significant concern. Ironically, the increase in muscle mass and other masculine characteristics in men belies the fact that negative feedback has decreased LH. This results in a decrease in endogenous testosterone and FSH secretion, reducing the stimulation of spermatogenesis in Sertoli cells. This actually induces a decrease in testicular size and low sperm count (infertility) as described in the next section. In fact, administration of low doses of anabolic steroids is being tested as a potential male birth control pill.

17.10 Hypogonadism

A decrease in testosterone release from the testes—***hypogonadism***—can be caused by a wide variety of disorders. In general, they can be classified into testicular failure (primary hypogonadism) or a failure to supply the testes with appropriate gonadotrophic stimulus (secondary hypogonadism). The loss of normal testicular androgen production before puberty can lead to a failure to develop secondary sex characteristics such as deepening of the voice, pubic and axillary hair, and increased libido, as well as a failure to develop normal sperm production.

A relatively common genetic cause of primary hypogonadism is ***Klinefelter's syndrome.*** The most common cause of this disorder, occurring in 1 in 500 male births, is an extra X chromosome (XXY) caused by meiotic nondisjunction. Nondisjunction is the failure of a pair of chromosomes to separate during meiosis, such that two chromosome pairs go to one daughter cell and the other daughter cell fails to receive either chromosome. The classic form of Klinefelter's syndrome is caused by the failure of the two sex chromosomes to separate during the first meiotic division in gametogenesis (see Figure 17.1). The extra X chromosome can come from either the egg or the sperm. That is, if nondisjunction occurs in the ovary leading to an XX ovum, an XXY genotype will result if fertilized by a Y sperm. If nondisjunction occurs in the testis leading to an XY sperm, an XXY genotype will result if that sperm fertilizes a normal (single X) ovum.

Male children with the XXY genotype appear normal before puberty. However, after puberty, the testes remain small and poorly developed, with insufficient Leydig and Sertoli cell function. The abnormal Leydig cell function results in decreased concentrations of plasma and testicular testosterone; this, in turn, leads to abnormal development of the seminiferous tubules and therefore decreased sperm production. Normal secondary sex characteristics do not appear, and breast size increases (***gynecomastia***) (**Figure 17.16**). Men with this set of characteristics have relatively high gonadotropin concentrations (LH and FSH) due to loss of androgen and inhibin negative feedback. Men with Klinefelter's syndrome can be treated with androgen-replacement therapy to increase libido and decrease breast size.

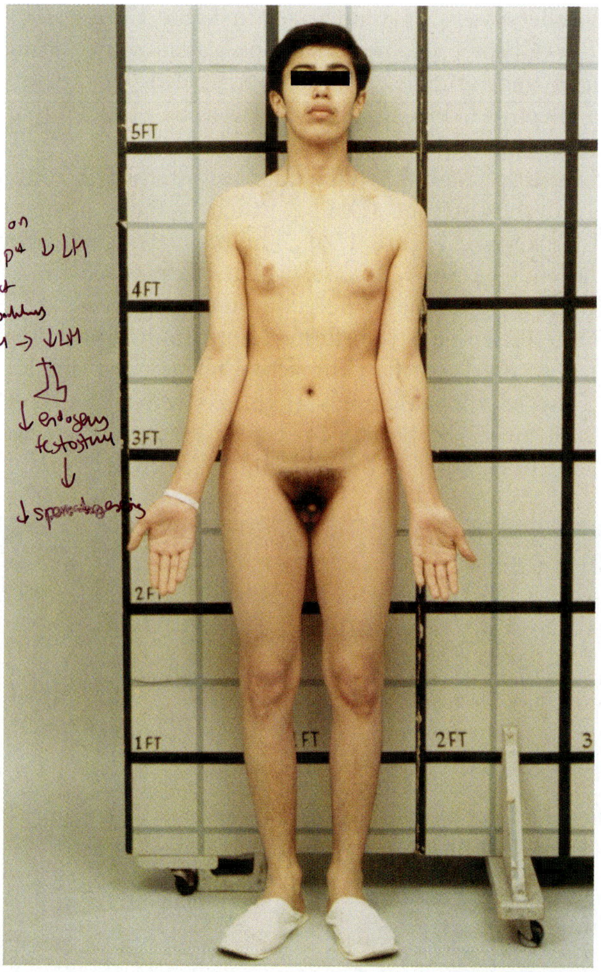

Figure 17.16 Klinefelter's syndrome in a 20-year-old man. Note relatively increased lower/upper body segment ratio, gynecomastia, small penis, and sparse body hair with a female pubic hair pattern. Courtesy of Glenn D. Braunstein, M.D.

↑ Prolactin → ↓ GnRH

Hypogonadism in men can also be caused by a decrease in LH and FSH secretion (secondary hypogonadism). Although there are many causes of the loss of function of pituitary gland cells that secrete LH and FSH, ***hyperprolactinemia*** (increased prolactin in the blood) is one of the most common. Although prolactin probably has only minor effects in men under normal conditions, the pituitary gland still has cells (lactotrophs) that secrete prolactin. Pituitary gland tumors arising from prolactin-secreting cells can develop and secrete too much prolactin. One of the effects of increased prolactin concentrations in the blood is to inhibit LH and FSH secretion from the anterior pituitary gland. (This occurs in men and women.) Hyperprolactinemia is discussed in more detail at the end of this chapter. Another cause of secondary hypogonadism is the total loss of anterior pituitary gland function, called ***hypopituitarism*** or panhypopituitarism. There are many causes of hypopituitarism, including head trauma, infection, and inflammation of the pituitary gland. When all anterior pituitary gland function is decreased or absent, male patients need to be treated with testosterone. In addition, male and female patients are treated with cortisol because of low ACTH, and with thyroid hormone because of low TSH. Children and some adults are also treated with growth hormone injections. In most circumstances, posterior pituitary gland function remains intact so that vasopressin does not need to be administered to avoid diabetes insipidus (see Chapter 14, Section B).

17.11 Andropause

Changes in the male reproductive system with aging are less drastic than those in women (described later in this chapter). Once testosterone and pituitary gland gonadotropin secretions are initiated at puberty, they continue, at least to some extent, throughout adult life. There is a steady decrease, however, in testosterone secretion, beginning at about 40 years of age, which apparently reflects slow deterioration of testicular function and failure of the gonads to respond to the pituitary gland gonadotropins. Along with the decreasing testosterone concentrations in the blood, libido decreases and sperm become less motile. Despite these events, many elderly men continue to be fertile. With aging, some men manifest increased emotional problems, such as depression, and this is sometimes referred to as the ***andropause*** (***male climacteric***). It is not clear, however, what role hormonal changes play in this phenomenon.

SECTION B SUMMARY

Anatomy

I. The male gonads, the testes, produce sperm in the seminiferous tubules and secrete testosterone from the Leydig cells.

Spermatogenesis

I. The meiotic divisions of spermatogenesis result in sperm containing 23 chromosomes, compared to the original 46 of the spermatogonia.

II. The developing germ cells are intimately associated with the Sertoli cells, which perform many functions, as summarized in Table 17.2.

Transport of Sperm

I. From the seminiferous tubules, the sperm pass into the epididymis, where they are concentrated and become mature.

II. The epididymis and vas deferens store the sperm, and the seminal vesicles and prostate secrete most of the semen.

III. Erection of the penis occurs because of vascular engorgement accomplished by relaxation of the small arteries and passive occlusion of the veins.

IV. Ejaculation includes emission—emptying of semen into the urethra—followed by expulsion of the semen from the urethra.

Hormonal Control of Male Reproductive Functions

I. Pulses of hypothalamic GnRH stimulate the anterior pituitary gland to secrete FSH and LH, which then act on the testes: FSH on the Sertoli cells to stimulate spermatogenesis and inhibin secretion, and LH on the Leydig cells to stimulate testosterone secretion.

II. Testosterone, acting locally on the Sertoli cells, is essential for maintaining spermatogenesis.

III. Testosterone exerts a negative feedback inhibition on both the hypothalamus and the anterior pituitary gland to reduce mainly LH secretion. Inhibin exerts a negative feedback inhibition on FSH secretion.

IV. Testosterone maintains the accessory reproductive organs and male secondary sex characteristics and stimulates the growth of muscle and bone. In many of its target cells, it must first undergo transformation to dihydrotestosterone or to estrogen.

Puberty

I. A change in brain function at the onset of puberty results in increases in the hypothalamo–pituitary–gonadal axis (because of increases in GnRH).

II. The first sign of puberty is the appearance of pubic and axillary hair.

Hypogonadism

I. Male hypogonadism is a decrease in testicular function. Klinefelter's syndrome (usually XXY genotype) is a common cause of male hypogonadism.

II. Hypogonadism can be caused by testicular failure (primary hypogonadism) or a loss of gonadotrophic stimuli to the testes (secondary hypogonadism).

Andropause

I. The andropause is a decrease in testosterone with aging (but usually not a complete cessation of androgen production).

SECTION B REVIEW QUESTIONS

1. Describe the sequence of events leading from spermatogonia to sperm.
2. List the functions of the Sertoli cells.
3. Describe the path sperm take from the seminiferous tubules to the urethra.
4. Describe the roles of the prostate gland, seminal vesicles, and bulbourethral glands in the formation of semen.
5. Describe the neural control of erection and ejaculation.
6. Diagram the hormonal chain controlling the testes. Contrast the effects of FSH and LH.

7. What are the feedback controls from the testes to the hypothalamus and pituitary gland?
8. Define *puberty* in the male. When does it usually occur?
9. List the effects of androgens on accessory reproductive organs, secondary sex characteristics, growth, protein metabolism, and behavior.
10. Describe the conversion of testosterone to DHT and estrogen.
11. How does hyperprolactinemia cause hypogonadism?

SECTION B KEY TERMS

SECTION B CLINICAL TERMS

SECTION C
Female Reproductive Physiology

Unlike the continuous sperm production of the male, the maturation of the female gamete (the ovum) followed by its release from the ovary—**ovulation**—is cyclical. The female germ cells, like those of the male, have different names at different stages of development. However, the term **egg** is often used to refer to the female germ cells at any stage, and we will follow that convention unless otherwise noted. The structure and function of certain components of the female reproductive system (e.g., the uterus) are synchronized with these ovarian cycles. In human beings, these cycles are called **menstrual cycles.** The length of a menstrual cycle varies considerably from woman to woman, and even in any particular woman, but averages about 28 days. The first day of menstrual flow (**menstruation**) is designated as day 1.

Menstruation is the result of events occurring in the uterus. However, the uterine events of the menstrual cycle are due to cyclical changes in hormone secretion by the ovaries. The ovaries are also the sites for the maturation of gametes. One oocyte usually becomes fully mature and is ovulated around the middle of each menstrual cycle.

The interactions among the ovaries, hypothalamus, and anterior pituitary gland produce the cyclical changes in the ovaries that result in (1) maturation of a gamete each cycle and (2) hormone secretions that cause cyclical changes in all of the female reproductive organs (particularly the uterus). The interaction of these different structures in the adult female reproductive cycle is an excellent example of the general principle of physiology that the functions of organ systems are coordinated with each other. These changes prepare the uterus to receive and nourish the developing embryo; only when there is no pregnancy does menstruation occur.

17.12 Anatomy

The female reproductive system includes the two ovaries and the female reproductive tract—two **fallopian tubes** (or oviducts), the uterus, the cervix, and the vagina. These structures are termed the **female internal genitalia** (**Figure 17.17**). Unlike in the male, the urinary and reproductive duct systems of the female are entirely separate from each other. Before proceeding with this section, the reader should review Figures 17.2 and 17.3 concerning the development of the internal and external female genitalia.

The ovaries are almond-sized organs in the upper pelvic cavity, one on each side of the uterus. The ends of the fallopian tubes are not directly attached to the ovaries but open into the abdominal cavity close to them. The opening of each fallopian tube is funnel-shaped and surrounded by long, fingerlike projections (the **fimbriae**) lined with ciliated epithelium. The other ends of the fallopian tubes are attached to the uterus and empty directly into its cavity. The **uterus** is a hollow, thick-walled, muscular organ lying between the urinary bladder and rectum. The uterus is the source of menstrual flow and is where the fetus develops during pregnancy. The lower portion of the uterus is the **cervix.** A small opening in the cervix leads to the **vagina,** the canal leading from the uterus to the outside.

The **female external genitalia** (**Figure 17.18**) include the mons pubis, labia majora, labia minora, clitoris, vestibule of the vagina, and vestibular glands. The term **vulva** is another name for all these structures. The mons pubis is the rounded fatty prominence over the junction of the pubic bones. The labia majora, the female homologue of the scrotum, are two prominent skin folds that form the outer lips of the vulva. (The terms *homologous* and *analogous* mean that the two structures are derived embryologically from the same source [see Figures 17.2 and 17.3] and/or have similar functions.) The labia minora are

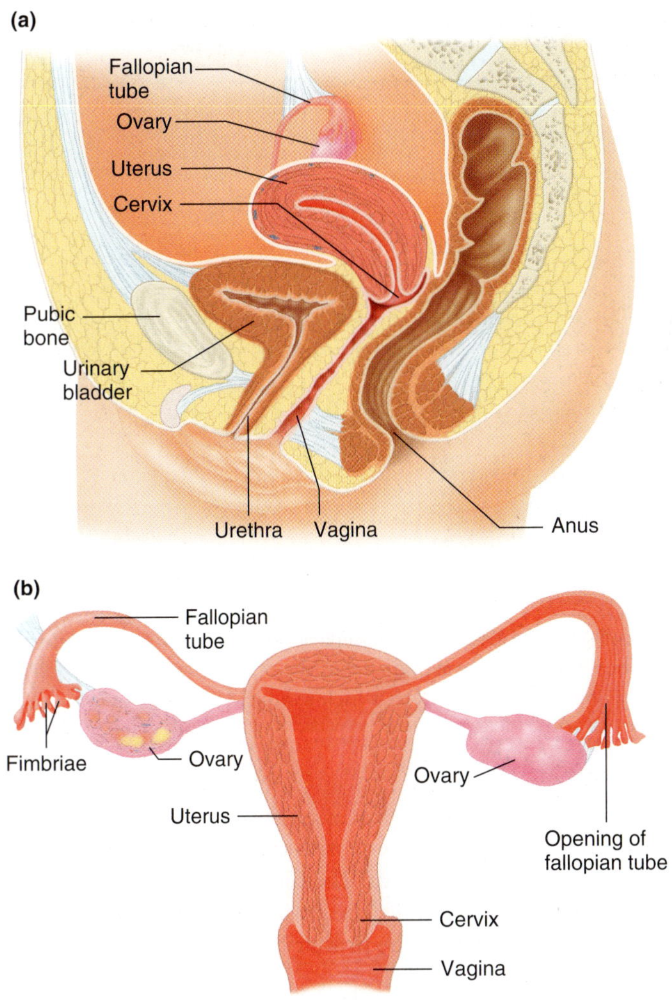

Figure 17.17 AP|R Female reproductive system. (a) Side view of a section through a female pelvis. (b) Frontal view cut away on the right (left side of the body) to show the continuity between the organs of the reproductive duct system—fallopian tubes, uterus, and vagina.

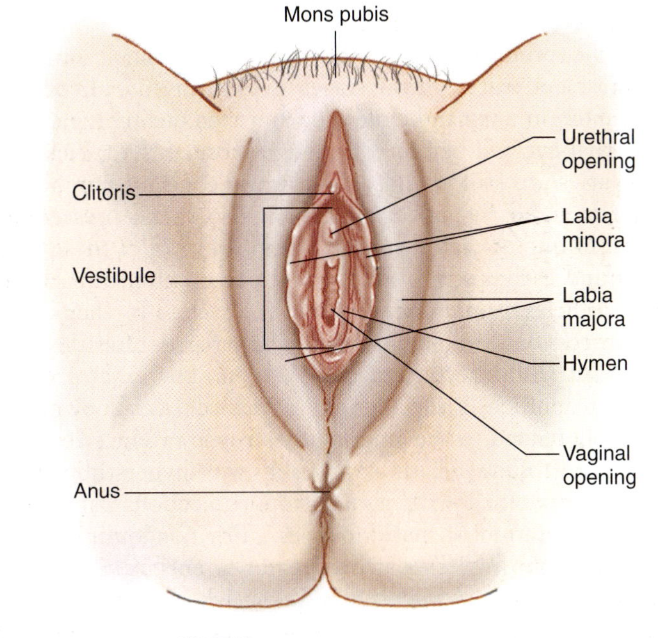

Figure 17.18 AP|R Female external genitalia.

small skin folds lying between the labia majora. They surround the urethral and vaginal openings, and the area thus enclosed is the vestibule, into which secretory glands empty. The vaginal opening lies behind the opening of the urethra. Partially overlying the vaginal opening is a thin fold of mucous membrane, the **hymen.** The **clitoris,** the female homologue of the penis, is an erectile structure located at the top of the vulva.

17.13 Ovarian Functions

As noted at the beginning of this chapter, the ovary, like the testis, serves several functions: (1) **oogenesis,** the production of gametes during the fetal period; (2) maturation of the oocyte; (3) expulsion of the mature oocyte (ovulation); and (4) secretion of the female sex steroid hormones (estrogen and progesterone), as well as the peptide hormone inhibin. Before ovulation, the maturation of the oocyte and endocrine functions of the ovaries take place in a single structure, the follicle. After ovulation, the follicle, now without an egg, differentiates into a corpus luteum, which only has an endocrine function. For comparison, recall that in the testes, the production of gametes and the secretion of sex steroids take place in different compartments—in the seminiferous tubules and in the Leydig cells, respectively.

Oogenesis

At birth, the ovaries contain an estimated total of 2 to 4 million eggs, and no new ones appear after birth. Thus, in marked contrast to the male, the newborn female already has all the germ cells she will ever have. Only a few, perhaps 400, will be ovulated during a woman's lifetime. All the others degenerate at some point in their development so that few, if any, remain by the time a woman reaches approximately 50 years of age. One result of this developmental pattern is that the eggs ovulated near age 50 are 35 to 40 years older than those ovulated just after puberty. It is possible that certain chromosomal defects more common among children born to older women are the result of aging changes in the egg.

During early fetal development, the primitive germ cells, or **oogonia** (singular, **oogonium**) undergo numerous mitotic divisions (**Figure 17.19**). Oogonia are analogous to spermatogonia in the male (see Figure 17.1). Around the seventh month of gestation, the fetal oogonia cease dividing. Current thinking is that from this point on, no new germ cells are generated.

During fetal life, all the oogonia develop into primary oocytes (analogous to primary spermatocytes), which then begin a first meiotic division by replicating their DNA. They do not, however, complete the division in the fetus. Accordingly, all the eggs present at birth are primary oocytes containing 46 chromosomes, each with two sister chromatids. The cells are said to be in a state of **meiotic arrest.**

This state continues until puberty and the onset of renewed activity in the ovaries. Indeed, only those primary oocytes destined for ovulation will ever complete the first meiotic division, for it occurs just before the egg is ovulated. This division is analogous to the division of the primary spermatocyte, and each daughter cell receives 23 chromosomes, each with two chromatids. In this division, however, one of the two daughter cells, the secondary oocyte, retains virtually all the

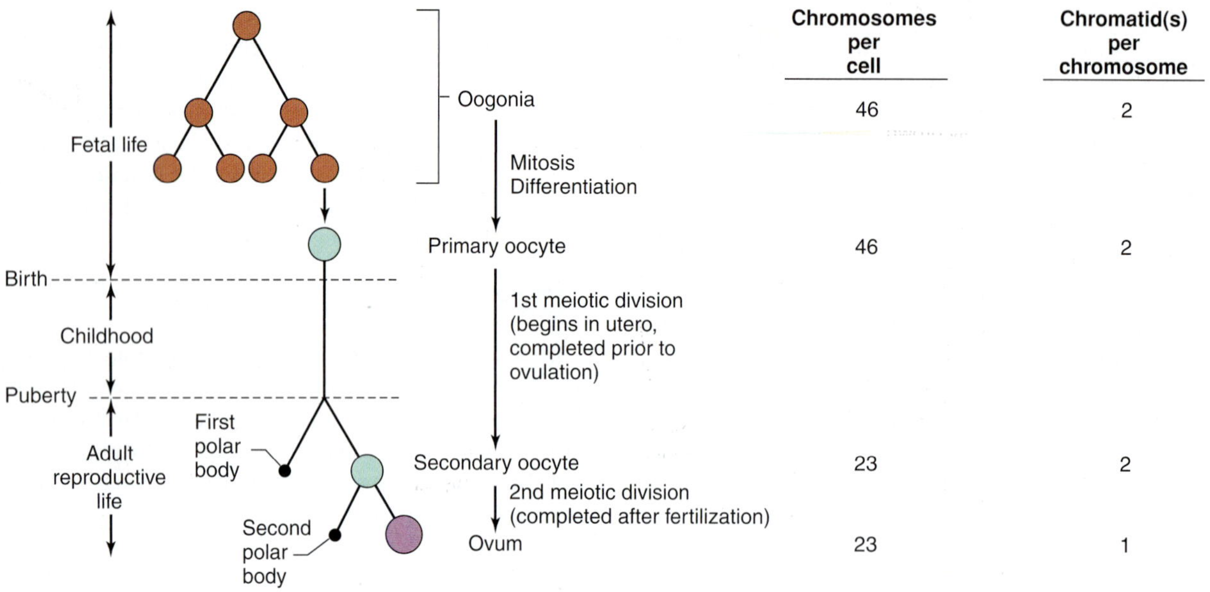

Figure 17.19 APR Summary of oogenesis. Compare with the male pattern in Figure 17.11. The secondary oocyte is ovulated and does not complete its meiotic division unless it is penetrated (fertilized) by a sperm. Thus, it is a semantic oddity that the oocyte is not termed an *egg* or *ovum* until after fertilization occurs. Note that each primary oocyte yields only one secondary oocyte, which can yield only one ovum.

cytoplasm. The other, the first polar body, is very small and nonfunctional. Thus, the primary oocyte, which is already as large as the egg will be, passes on to the secondary oocyte just half of its chromosomes but almost all of its nutrient-rich cytoplasm.

The second meiotic division occurs in a fallopian tube *after ovulation*, but only if the secondary oocyte is fertilized—that is, penetrated by a sperm (see Figure 17.1). As a result of this second meiotic division, the daughter cells each receive 23 chromosomes, each with a single chromatid. Once again, one daughter cell, now called an ovum, retains nearly all the cytoplasm. The other daughter cell, the second polar body, is very small and nonfunctional. The net result of oogenesis is that each primary oocyte can produce only one ovum (see Figure 17.19). In contrast, each primary spermatocyte produces four viable spermatozoa.

Follicle Growth

Throughout their life in the ovaries, the eggs exist in structures known as **follicles.** Follicles begin as **primordial follicles,** which consist of one primary oocyte surrounded by a single layer of cells called **granulosa cells.** The granulosa cells secrete estrogen, small amounts of progesterone just before ovulation, and the peptide hormone inhibin. Further development from the primordial follicle stage (**Figure 17.20**) is characterized by an increase in the size of the oocyte; a proliferation of the granulosa cells into multiple layers; and the separation of the oocyte from the inner granulosa cells by a thick layer of material, the **zona pellucida,** secreted by the surrounding follicular cells. The zona pellucida contains glycoproteins that play a role in the binding of a sperm cell to the surface of an egg after ovulation.

Despite the presence of a zona pellucida, the inner layer of granulosa cells remains closely associated with the oocyte by means of cytoplasmic processes that traverse the zona pellucida and form gap junctions with the oocyte. Through these gap junctions, nutrients and chemical messengers are passed to the oocyte. For example, the granulosa cells produce one or more factors that act on the primary oocytes to maintain them in meiotic arrest.

As the follicle grows by mitosis of granulosa cells, connective-tissue cells surrounding the granulosa cells differentiate and form layers of cells known as the **theca,** which function together with the granulosa cells in the synthesis of estrogen. Shortly after this, the primary oocyte reaches full size (~115μm in diameter), and a fluid-filled space, the **antrum,** begins to form in the midst of the granulosa cells as a result of fluid they secrete.

The progression of some primordial follicles to the preantral and early antral stages (see Figure 17.20) occurs throughout infancy and childhood and then during the entire menstrual cycle. Therefore, although most of the follicles in the ovaries are still primordial, a nearly constant number of preantral and early antral follicles are also always present. At the beginning of each menstrual cycle, 10 to 25 of these preantral and early antral follicles begin to develop into larger antral follicles. About one week into the cycle, a further selection process occurs: only one of the larger antral follicles, the **dominant follicle,** continues to develop. The exact process by which a follicle is selected for dominance is not known, but it is likely related to the amount of estrogen produced locally within the follicle. (This is probably why hyperstimulation of infertile women with gonadotropin injections can result in the maturation of many follicles.) The nondominant follicles (in both ovaries) that had begun to enlarge undergo a degenerative process called **atresia,** which is an example of programmed cell death, or apoptosis. The eggs in the degenerating follicles also die.

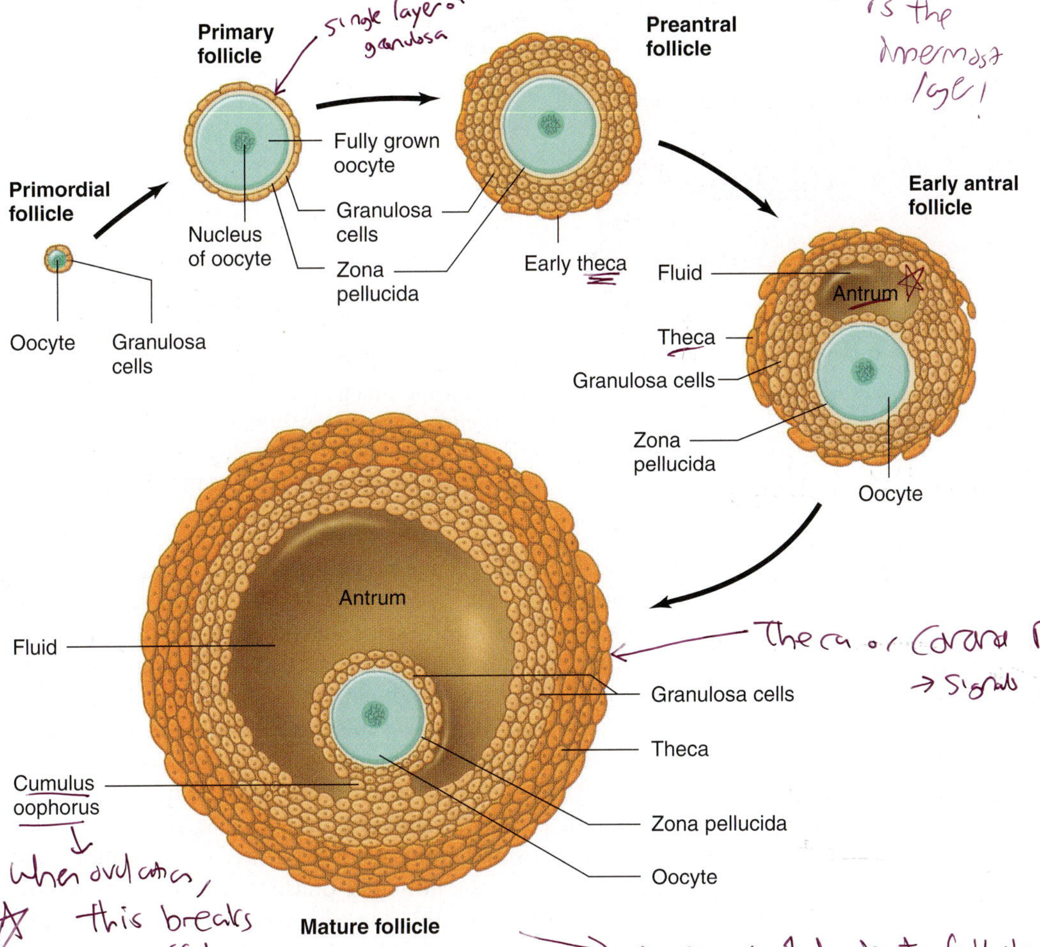

Figure 17.20 AP|R Development of a human oocyte and ovarian follicle. The fully mature follicle is 1.5 cm in diameter. Blood vessels are not shown. Adapted from Erickson et al.

Atresia is not limited to just antral follicles, however, for follicles can undergo atresia at any stage of development. Indeed, this process is already occurring in the female fetus, so that the 2 to 4 million follicles and eggs present at birth represent only a small fraction of those present earlier in gestation. Atresia then continues all through prepubertal life so that only 200,000 to 400,000 follicles remain when active reproductive life begins. Of these, all but about 400 will undergo atresia during a woman's reproductive life. Therefore, 99.99% of the ovarian follicles present at birth will undergo atresia.

The dominant follicle enlarges as a result of an increase in fluid, causing the antrum to expand. As this occurs, the granulosa cell layers surrounding the egg form a mound that projects into the antrum and is called the **cumulus oophorus** (see Figure 17.20). As the time of ovulation approaches, the egg (a primary oocyte) emerges from meiotic arrest and completes its first meiotic division to become a secondary oocyte. The cumulus separates from the follicle wall so that it and the oocyte float free in the antral fluid. The mature follicle (also called a **graafian follicle**) becomes so large (diameter about 1.5 cm) that it balloons out on the surface of the ovary.

Ovulation occurs when the thin walls of the follicle and ovary rupture at the site where they are joined because of enzymatic digestion. The secondary oocyte, surrounded by its tightly adhering zona pellucida and granulosa cells, as well as the cumulus, is carried out of the ovary and onto the ovarian surface by the antral fluid. All this happens on approximately day 14 of the menstrual cycle.

Occasionally, two or more follicles reach maturity, and more than one egg may be ovulated. This is the most common cause of multiple births. In such cases, the siblings are **fraternal (dizygotic) twins,** not identical, because the eggs carry different sets of genes and are fertilized by different sperm. We will describe later how identical twins form.

Formation of the Corpus Luteum

After the mature follicle discharges its antral fluid and egg, it collapses around the antrum and undergoes a rapid transformation. The granulosa cells enlarge greatly, and the entire glandlike structure formed is called the **corpus luteum,** which secretes estrogen, progesterone, and inhibin. If the discharged egg, now in a fallopian tube, is not fertilized by fusing with a sperm cell, the corpus luteum reaches its maximum development within approximately 10 days. It then rapidly degenerates by apoptosis. As we will see, it is the loss of corpus luteum function that leads to menstruation and the beginning of a new menstrual cycle.

In terms of ovarian function, therefore, the menstrual cycle may be divided into two phases approximately equal in length and separated by ovulation (**Figure 17.21**): (1) the **follicular phase,** during which a mature follicle and secondary oocyte develop; and (2) the **luteal phase,** beginning after ovulation and lasting until the death of the corpus luteum. As you will see, these ovarian phases correlate with and control the changes in the appearance of the uterine lining (to be described subsequently).

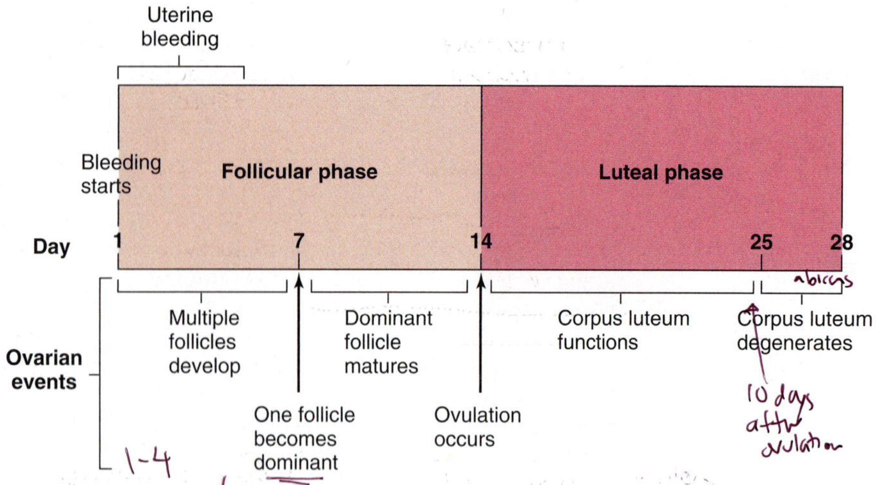

Figure 17.21 AP|R Summary of ovarian events during a menstrual cycle (if fertilization does not occur). The first day of the cycle is named for a uterine event—the onset of bleeding—even though ovarian events are used to denote the cycle phases.

Sites of Synthesis of Ovarian Hormones

The synthesis of gonadal steroids was introduced in Figure 17.6 and can be summarized as follows. Estrogen is synthesized and released into the blood during the follicular phase mainly by the granulosa cells. After ovulation, estrogen is synthesized and released by the corpus luteum. Progesterone, the other major ovarian steroid hormone, is synthesized and released in very small amounts by the granulosa and theca cells just before ovulation, but its major source is the corpus luteum. Inhibin, a peptide hormone, is secreted by both the granulosa cells and the corpus luteum.

17.14 Control of Ovarian Function

The major factors controlling ovarian function are analogous to the controls described for testicular function. They constitute a hormonal system made up of GnRH, the anterior pituitary gland gonadotropins FSH and LH, and gonadal sex hormones—estrogen and progesterone.

As in the male, the entire sequence of controls depends upon the pulsatile secretion of GnRH from hypothalamic neuroendocrine cells. In the female, however, the frequency and amplitude of these pulses during a 24-hour period change over the course of the menstrual cycle. Also, the responsiveness both of the anterior pituitary gland to GnRH and of the ovaries to FSH and LH changes during the cycle.

Let us look first at the patterns of hormone concentrations in systemic plasma during a normal menstrual cycle (**Figure 17.22**). (Plasma GnRH is not shown because it does not reflect GnRH secretion from the hypothalamus into the hypothalamo–hypophyseal portal blood vessels.) In Figure 17.22, the lines are plots of average daily concentrations; that is, the increases and decreases during a single day stemming from episodic secretion have been averaged. For now, ignore both the legend and circled numbers in this figure because we are concerned here only with hormonal patterns and not the explanations of these patterns.

FSH increases in the early part of the follicular phase and then steadily decreases throughout the remainder of the cycle except for a small midcycle peak. LH is constant during most of the follicular phase but then shows a very large midcycle increase—the **LH surge**—peaking approximately 18 h *before* ovulation. This is followed by a rapid decrease and then a further slow decline during the luteal phase.

After remaining fairly low and stable for the first week, estrogen increases rapidly during the second week as the dominant ovarian follicle grows and secretes more estrogen. Estrogen then starts decreasing shortly before LH has peaked. This is followed by a second increase due to secretion by the corpus luteum and, finally, a rapid decrease during the last days of the cycle. Very small amounts of progesterone are released by the ovaries during the follicular phase until just before ovulation. Very soon after ovulation, the developing corpus luteum begins to release large amounts of progesterone; from this point, the progesterone pattern is similar to that for estrogen.

Not shown in Figure 17.22 is the plasma concentration of inhibin. Its pattern is similar to that of estrogen: It increases during the late follicular phase, remains high during the luteal phase, and then decreases as the corpus luteum degenerates.

The following discussion will explain how these hormonal changes are interrelated to produce a self-cycling pattern. The numbers in Figure 17.22 are keyed to the text. The feedback effects of the ovarian hormones to be described in the text are summarized for reference in **Table 17.4**.

Follicle Development and Estrogen Synthesis During the Early and Middle Follicular Phases

Before reading this section, the reader should review Figure 17.20 to appreciate the structure of the developing follicles. There are always a number of preantral and early antral follicles in the ovary between puberty and menopause. Further development of the follicle beyond these stages requires stimulation by FSH. Prior to puberty, the plasma concentration of FSH is too low to induce such development. This changes during puberty, and menstrual cycles commence. The increase in FSH secretion that occurs as one cycle ends and the next begins (numbers 16 to 1 in Figure 17.22) provides this stimulation, and a group of preantral and early antral follicles enlarge 2. The increase in FSH at the end of the cycle (16 to 1) is due to decreased progesterone, estrogen, and inhibin (removal of negative feedback).

During the next week or so, there is a division of labor between the actions of FSH and LH on the follicles: FSH acts

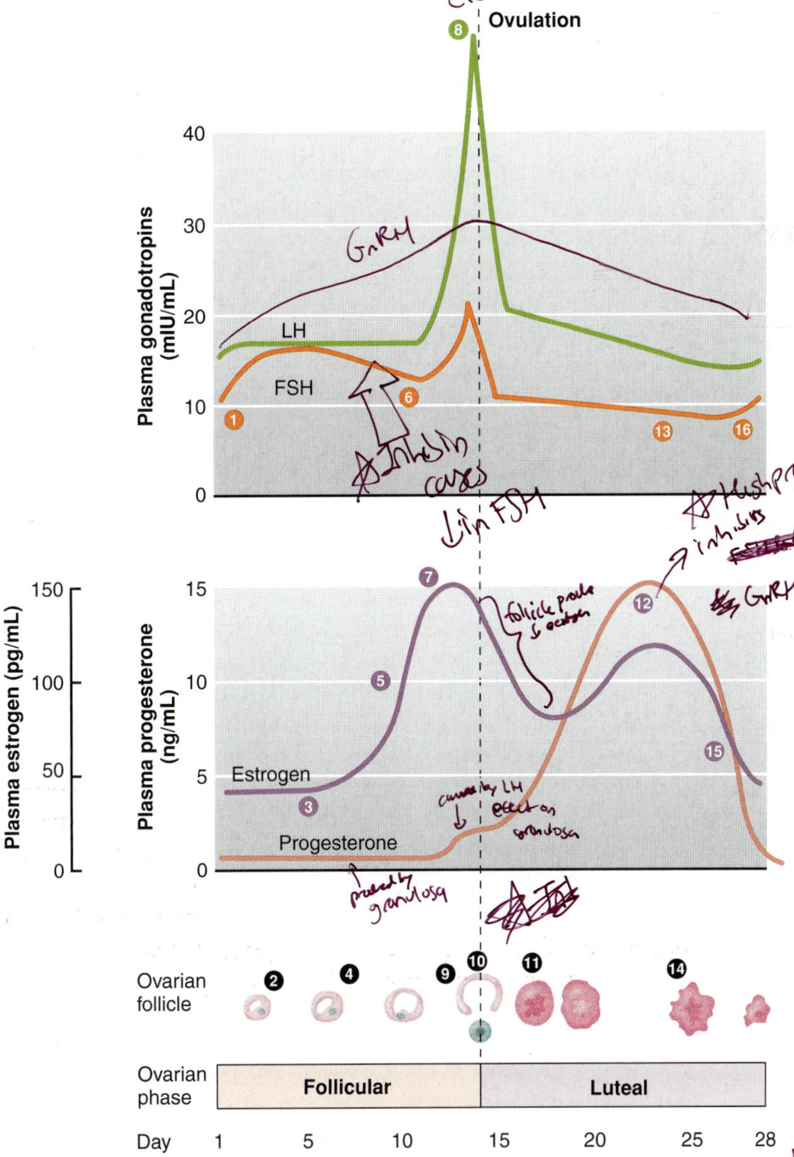

Figure 17.22 AP|R Summary of systemic plasma hormone concentrations and ovarian events during the menstrual cycle. The events marked by the circled numbers are described later in the text and are listed here to provide a summary. The arrows in this legend denote causality. (1) FSH and LH secretion increase (because plasma estrogen concentration is low and exerting little negative feedback). → (2) Multiple antral follicles begin to enlarge and secrete estrogen. → (3) Plasma estrogen concentration begins to rise. (4) One follicle becomes dominant and secretes very large amounts of estrogen. → (5) Plasma estrogen concentration increases markedly. → (6) FSH secretion and plasma FSH concentration decrease, causing atresia of nondominant follicles, but then (7) increasing plasma estrogen exerts a "positive" feedback on gonadotropin secretion. → (8) An LH surge is triggered. → (9) The egg completes its first meiotic division and cytoplasmic maturation while the follicle secretes less estrogen accompanied by some progesterone, (10) ovulation occurs, and (11) the corpus luteum forms and begins to secrete large amounts of both estrogen and progesterone. → (12) Plasma estrogen and progesterone increase. → (13) FSH and LH secretion are inhibited and their plasma concentrations decrease. (14) The corpus luteum begins to degenerate (cause unknown) and decrease its hormone secretion. → (15) Plasma estrogen and progesterone concentrations decrease. → (16) FSH and LH secretions begin to increase, and a new cycle begins (back to (1)).

PHYSIOLOGICAL INQUIRY

- (1) Why do blood FSH concentrations increase at the end of the luteal phase? (2) What naturally occurring event could rescue the corpus luteum and prevent its degeneration starting in the middle of the luteal phase?

Answers can be found at end of chapter.

TABLE 17.4	**Summary of Major Feedback Effects of Estrogen, Progesterone, and Inhibin**
Estrogen, in low plasma concentrations, causes the anterior pituitary gland to secrete less FSH and LH in response to GnRH and also may inhibit the hypothalamic neurons that secrete GnRH. *Result:* Negative feedback inhibition of FSH and LH secretion during the early and middle follicular phase.	
Inhibin acts on the pituitary gland to inhibit the secretion of FSH. *Result:* Negative feedback inhibition of FSH secretion.	
Estrogen, when increasing dramatically, causes anterior pituitary gland cells to secrete more LH and FSH in response to GnRH. Estrogen can also stimulate the hypothalamic neurons that secrete GnRH. *Result:* Positive feedback stimulation of the LH surge, which triggers ovulation.	
High plasma concentrations of progesterone, in the presence of estrogen, inhibit the hypothalamic neurons that secrete GnRH. *Result:* Negative feedback inhibition of FSH and LH secretion and prevention of LH surges during the luteal phase and pregnancy.	

on the granulosa cells, and LH acts on the theca cells. The reasons are that, at this point in the cycle, granulosa cells have FSH receptors but no LH receptors and theca cells have just the reverse. FSH stimulates the granulosa cells to multiply and produce estrogen, and it also stimulates enlargement of the antrum. Some of the estrogen produced diffuses into the blood and maintains a relatively stable plasma concentration (3). Estrogen also functions as a paracrine or autocrine agent within the follicle, where, along with FSH and growth factors, it stimulates the proliferation of granulosa cells, which further increases estrogen production.

The granulosa cells, however, require help to produce estrogen because they are deficient in the enzymes required to produce the androgen precursors of estrogen (see Chapter 11). The granulosa cells are aided by the theca cells. As shown in **Figure 17.23**, LH acts upon the theca cells, stimulating them not only to proliferate but also to synthesize androgens. The androgens diffuse into the granulosa cells and are converted to estrogen by aromatase. Thus, the secretion of estrogen by the granulosa cells requires the interplay of both types of follicle cells and both pituitary gland gonadotropins.

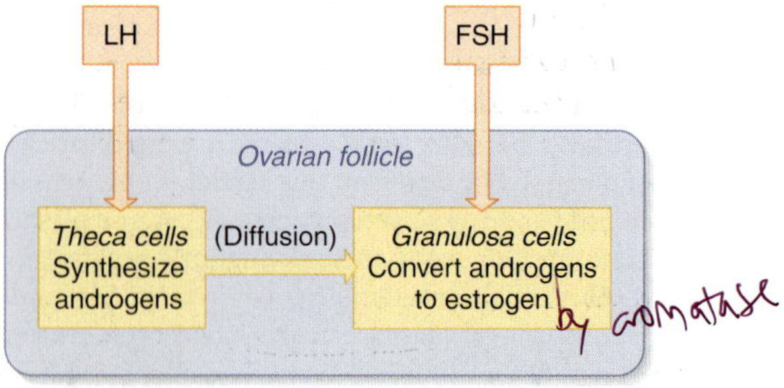

Figure 17.23 APIR Control of estrogen synthesis during the early and middle follicular phases. (The major androgen secreted by the theca cells is androstenedione.) Androgen diffusing from theca to granulosa cell passes through the basement membrane (not shown).

At this point, it is worthwhile to emphasize the similarities that the two types of follicle cells bear to cells of the testes during this period of the cycle. The granulosa cell is similar to the Sertoli cell in that it controls the microenvironment in which the germ cell develops and matures, and it is stimulated by both FSH and the major gonadal sex hormone. The theca cell is similar to the Leydig cell in that it produces mainly androgens and is stimulated to do so by LH. This makes sense when one considers that the testes and ovaries arise from the same embryonic structure (see Figure 17.2).

By the beginning of the second week, one follicle has become dominant (number ❹ in Figure 17.22) and the other developing follicles degenerate. The reason for this is that, as shown in Figure 17.22, the plasma concentration of FSH, a crucial factor necessary for the survival of the follicle cells, begins to decrease and there is no longer enough FSH to prevent atresia. Although it is not known precisely how a specific follicle is selected to become dominant, there are several reasons why this follicle, having gained a head start, is able to continue maturation. First, its granulosa cells have achieved a greater sensitivity to FSH because of increased numbers of FSH receptors. Second, its granulosa cells now begin to be stimulated not only by FSH but by LH as well. We emphasized in the previous section that, during the first week or so of the follicular phase, LH acts only on the theca cells. As the dominant follicle matures, this situation changes, and LH receptors, induced by FSH, also begin to appear in large numbers on the granulosa cells. The increase in local estrogen within the follicle results from these factors.

The dominant follicle now starts to secrete enough estrogen that the plasma concentration of this steroid begins to increase ❺. We can now also explain why plasma FSH starts to decrease at this time. Estrogen, at these still relatively low concentrations, is exerting a *negative feedback* inhibition on the secretion of gonadotropins (Table 17.4 and **Figure 17.24**). A major site of estrogen action is the anterior pituitary gland, where it reduces the amount of FSH and LH secreted in response to any given amount of GnRH. Estrogen probably also acts on the hypothalamus to decrease the amplitude of GnRH pulses and, therefore, the total amount of GnRH secreted over any time period.

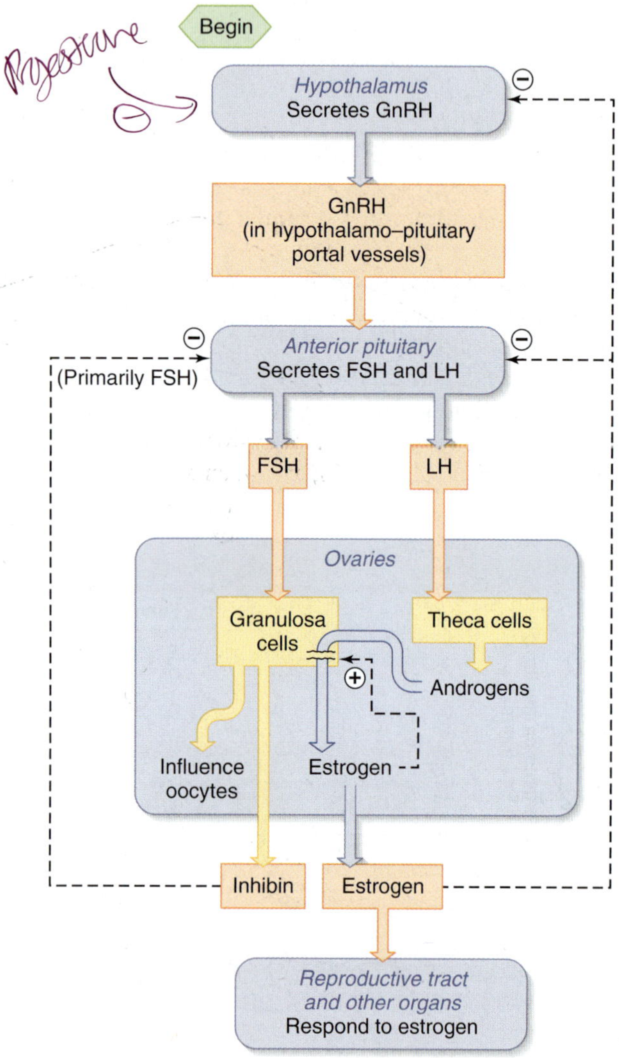

Figure 17.24 APIR Summary of hormonal control of ovarian function during the early and middle follicular phases. Compare with the analogous pattern of the male (see Figure 17.15). Inhibin is a protein hormone that inhibits FSH secretion. The wavy broken lines in the granulosa cells denote the conversion of androgens to estrogen in these cells, as shown in Figure 17.23. The dashed line with an arrow within the ovaries indicates that estrogen increases granulosa cell function (local positive feedback).

PHYSIOLOGICAL INQUIRY

- A 30-year-old woman has failed to have menstrual cycles for the past few months; her pregnancy test is negative. Her plasma FSH and LH concentrations are increased, whereas her plasma estrogen concentrations are low. What is the likely cause of her failure to menstruate?

Answer can be found at end of chapter.

Therefore, as expected from this negative feedback, the plasma concentration of FSH (and LH, to a lesser extent) begins to decrease as a result of the increasing concentration of estrogen as the follicular phase continues (❻ in Figure 17.22). One reason that FSH decreases more than LH is that the granulosa cells also secrete inhibin, which, as in the male, inhibits mainly the secretion of FSH (see Figure 17.24).

LH Surge and Ovulation

The inhibitory effect of estrogen on gonadotropin secretion occurs when plasma estrogen concentration is relatively low, as during the early and middle follicular phases. In contrast, increasing plasma concentrations of estrogen for 1 to 2 days, as occurs during the estrogen peak of the late follicular phase (7 in Figure 17.22), act upon the anterior pituitary gland to enhance the sensitivity of LH-releasing cells to GnRH (Table 17.4 and **Figure 17.25**) and may also stimulate GnRH release from the hypothalamus. The estrogen-induced increase in GnRH release may be mediated by activation of kisspeptin neurons in the hypothalamus described earlier in this chapter. The stimulation of gonadotropin release by estrogen is a particularly important example of *positive feedback* in physiological control systems, and normal menstrual cycles and ovulation would not occur without it.

The net result is that rapidly increasing estrogen leads to the LH surge (8 in Figure 17.22). As shown in Figure 17.22 9, an increase in FSH and progesterone also occurs at the time of the LH surge.

The midcycle surge of LH is the primary event that induces ovulation. The high plasma concentration of LH acts upon the granulosa cells to cause the events, presented in **Table 17.5**, that culminate in ovulation 10, as indicated by the dashed vertical line in Figure 17.22.

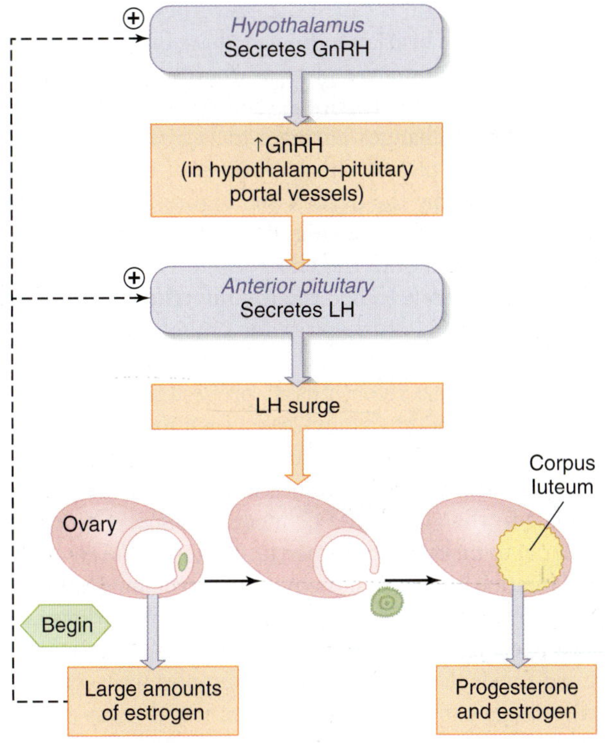

Figure 17.25 APIR In the late follicular phase, the dominant follicle secretes large amounts of estrogen, which act on the anterior pituitary gland and, possibly, the hypothalamus to cause an LH surge. The increased plasma LH then triggers both ovulation and formation of the corpus luteum. These actions of LH are mediated via the granulosa cells.

The function of the granulosa cells in mediating the effects of the LH surge is the last in the series of these cells' functions described in this chapter. They are all summarized in **Table 17.6**. The LH surge peaks and starts to decline just as ovulation occurs. Although the precise signal to terminate the LH surge is not known, it may be due to negative feedback from the small increase in progesterone described earlier (see Figure 17.22) as well as down-regulation of LH receptors in the ovary reducing estrogen-induced positive feedback.

The Luteal Phase

The LH surge not only induces ovulation by the mature follicle but also stimulates the reactions that transform the remaining granulosa and theca cells of that follicle into a

TABLE 17.5 Effects of the LH Surge on Ovarian Function
The primary oocyte completes its first meiotic division and undergoes cytoplasmic changes that prepare the ovum for implantation should fertilization occur. These LH effects on the oocyte are mediated by messengers released from the granulosa cells in response to LH.
Antrum size (fluid volume) and blood flow to the follicle increase markedly.
The granulosa cells begin releasing progesterone and decreasing the release of estrogen, which accounts for the midcycle decrease in plasma estrogen concentration and the small rise in plasma progesterone concentration just before ovulation.
Enzymes and prostaglandins, synthesized by the granulosa cells, break down the follicular–ovarian membranes. These weakened membranes rupture, allowing the oocyte and its surrounding granulosa cells to be carried out onto the surface of the ovary.
The remaining granulosa cells of the ruptured follicle (along with the theca cells of that follicle) are transformed into the corpus luteum, which begins to release progesterone and estrogen.

TABLE 17.6 Functions of Granulosa Cells
Nourish oocyte
Secrete chemical messengers that influence the oocyte and the theca cells
Secrete antral fluid
The site of action for estrogen and FSH in the control of follicle development during early and middle follicular phases
Express aromatase, which converts androgen (from theca cells) to estrogen
Secrete inhibin, which inhibits FSH secretion via an action on the pituitary gland
The site of action for LH induction of changes in the oocyte and follicle culminating in ovulation and formation of the corpus luteum

corpus luteum (⓫ in Figure 17.22). A low but adequate LH concentration maintains the function of the corpus luteum for about 14 days.

During its short life in the nonpregnant woman, the corpus luteum secretes large quantities of progesterone and estrogen ⓬, as well as inhibin. In the presence of estrogen, the high plasma concentration of progesterone causes a decrease in the secretion of the gonadotropins by the pituitary gland. It probably does this by acting on the hypothalamus to *suppress* the pulsatile secretion of GnRH. (The progesterone also prevents any LH surges during the first half of the luteal phase despite the high concentrations of estrogen at this time.) The increase in plasma inhibin concentration in the luteal phase also contributes to the suppression of FSH secretion. Consequently, during the luteal phase of the cycle, plasma concentrations of the gonadotropins are very low ⓭. The feedback suppression of gonadotropins in the luteal phase is summarized in **Figure 17.26**.

The corpus luteum has a finite life in the absence of an increase in gonadotropin secretion. If pregnancy does not occur, the corpus luteum degrades within 2 weeks ⓮.

With degeneration of the corpus luteum, plasma progesterone and estrogen concentrations decrease ⓯. The secretion of FSH and LH (and probably GnRH, as well) increases (⓰ and ❶) as a result of being freed from the inhibiting effects of high concentrations of ovarian hormones. The cycle then begins anew.

This completes the description of the control of ovarian function during a typical menstrual cycle. It should be emphasized that, although the hypothalamus and anterior pituitary gland are essential controllers, events within the *ovary* are the real sources of timing for the cycle. When the ovary secretes enough estrogen, the LH surge is induced, which in turn causes ovulation. When the corpus luteum degenerates, the decrease in hormone secretion allows the gonadotropin concentrations to increase enough to promote the growth of another group of follicles. Thus, ovarian events, via hormonal feedback, control the hypothalamus and anterior pituitary gland.

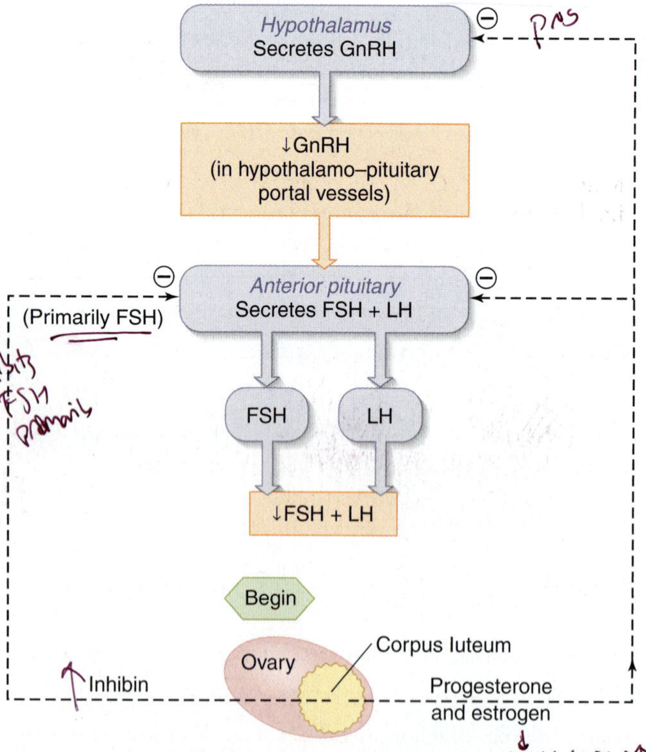

Figure 17.26 APIR Suppression of FSH and LH during luteal phase. If implantation of a developing conceptus does not occur and hCG does not appear in the blood, the corpus luteum dies, progesterone and estrogen decrease, menstruation occurs, and the next menstrual cycle begins.

17.15 Uterine Changes in the Menstrual Cycle

The phases of the menstrual cycle can also be described in terms of uterine events (**Figure 17.27**). Day 1 is, as noted earlier, the first day of menstrual flow, and the entire duration of menstruation is known as the **menstrual phase** (generally about 3 to 5 days in a typical 28-day cycle). During this time, the epithelial lining of the uterus—the **endometrium**—degenerates, resulting in the menstrual flow. The menstrual flow then ceases, and the endometrium begins to thicken as it regenerates under the influence of estrogen. This period of growth, the **proliferative phase,** lasts for the 10 days or so between cessation of menstruation and the occurrence of ovulation. Soon after ovulation, under the influence of progesterone and estrogen, the endometrium begins to secrete glycogen in the glandular epithelium, followed by glycoproteins and mucopolysaccharides. Thus, the part of the menstrual cycle between ovulation and the onset of the next menstruation is called the **secretory phase.** As shown in Figure 17.27, the ovarian follicular phase includes the uterine menstrual and proliferative phases, whereas the ovarian luteal phase is the same as the uterine secretory phase.

The uterine changes during a menstrual cycle are caused by changes in the plasma concentrations of estrogen and progesterone secreted by the ovaries (see Figure 17.22). During the proliferative phase, an increasing plasma estrogen concentration stimulates growth of both the endometrium and the underlying uterine smooth muscle (called the **myometrium**). In addition, it induces the synthesis of receptors for progesterone in endometrial cells. Then, following ovulation and formation of the corpus luteum (during the secretory phase), progesterone acts upon this estrogen-primed endometrium to convert it to an actively secreting tissue. The endometrial glands become coiled and filled with glycogen, the blood vessels become more numerous, and enzymes accumulate in the glands and connective tissue. These changes are essential to make the endometrium a hospitable environment for implantation and nourishment of the developing embryo.

Progesterone also inhibits myometrial contractions, in large part by opposing the stimulatory actions of estrogen and locally generated prostaglandins. This is very important to ensure that a fertilized egg can safely implant once it arrives in the uterus. Uterine quiescence is maintained by progesterone throughout pregnancy and is essential to prevent premature delivery.

Estrogen and progesterone also have important effects on the secretion of mucus by the cervix. Under the influence of estrogen alone, this mucus is abundant, clear, and watery. All of these characteristics are most pronounced at the time of ovulation and allow sperm deposited in the vagina to move easily

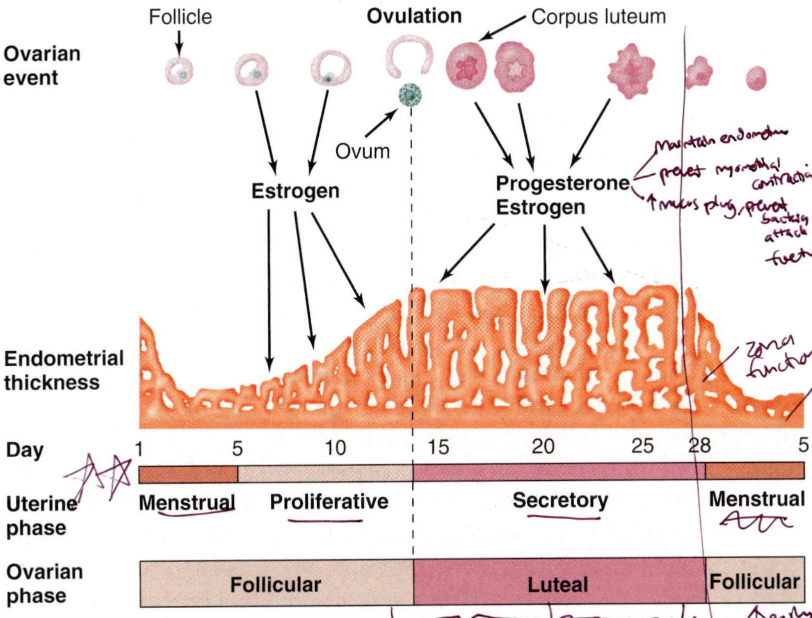

Figure 17.27 APIR Relationships between ovarian and uterine changes during the menstrual cycle. Refer to Figure 17.22 for specific hormonal changes.

through the mucus on their way to the uterus and fallopian tubes. In contrast, progesterone, present in significant concentrations only after ovulation, causes the mucus to become thick and sticky—in essence, a "plug" that prevents bacteria from entering the uterus from the vagina. The antibacterial blockage protects the uterus and the embryo if fertilization has occurred.

The decrease in plasma progesterone and estrogen concentrations that results from degeneration of the corpus luteum deprives the highly developed endometrium of its hormonal support and causes menstruation. The first event is profound constriction of the uterine blood vessels, which leads to a diminished supply of oxygen and nutrients to the endometrial cells. Disintegration starts in the entire lining, except for a thin, underlying layer that will regenerate the endometrium in the next cycle. Also, the uterine smooth muscle begins to undergo rhythmic contractions.

Both the vasoconstriction and uterine contractions are mediated by prostaglandins produced by the endometrium in response to the decrease in plasma estrogen and progesterone concentrations. The major cause of menstrual cramps, ***dysmenorrhea***, is overproduction of these prostaglandins, leading to excessive uterine contractions. The prostaglandins also affect smooth muscle elsewhere in the body, which accounts for some of the systemic symptoms that sometimes accompany the cramps, such as nausea, vomiting, and headache.

After the initial period of vascular constriction, the endometrial arterioles dilate, resulting in hemorrhage through the weakened capillary walls. The menstrual flow consists of this blood mixed with endometrial debris. Typical blood loss per menstrual period is about 50 to 150 mL.

The major events of the menstrual cycle are summarized in **Table 17.7**. This table, in essence, combines the information in Figures 17.22 and 17.27.

TABLE 17.7 Summary of the Menstrual Cycle

Day(s)	Major Events
1–5	Estrogen and progesterone are low because the previous corpus luteum is regressing. *Therefore:* a. Endometrial lining sloughs. b. Secretion of FSH and LH is released from inhibition, and their plasma concentrations increase. *Therefore:* Several growing follicles are stimulated to mature.
7	A single follicle (usually) becomes dominant.
7–12	Plasma estrogen increases because of secretion by the dominant follicle. *Therefore:* Endometrium is stimulated to proliferate.
7–12	LH and FSH decrease due to estrogen and inhibin negative feedback. *Therefore:* Degeneration (atresia) of nondominant follicles occurs.
12–13	LH surge is induced by increasing plasma estrogen. *Therefore:* a. Oocyte is induced to complete its first meiotic division and undergo cytoplasmic maturation. b. Follicle is stimulated to secrete digestive enzymes and prostaglandins.
14	Ovulation is mediated by follicular enzymes and prostaglandins.
15–25	Corpus luteum forms and, under the influence of low but adequate levels of LH, secretes estrogen and progesterone, increasing plasma concentrations of these hormones. *Therefore:* a. Secretory endometrium develops. b. Secretion of FSH and LH from the anterior pituitary gland is inhibited, lowering their plasma concentrations. *Therefore:* No new follicles develop.
25–28	Corpus luteum degenerates (if implantation of the conceptus does not occur). *Therefore:* Plasma estrogen and progesterone concentrations decrease. *Therefore:* Endometrium begins to slough at conclusion of day 28, and a new cycle begins.

17.16 Additional Effects of Gonadal Steroids

Estrogen has other effects in addition to its paracrine function within the ovaries, its effects on the anterior pituitary gland and the hypothalamus, and its uterine actions. They are summarized in **Table 17.8**.

Progesterone also exerts a variety of effects (also shown Table 17.8). Because plasma progesterone concentration is markedly increased only after ovulation has occurred, several of these effects can be used to indicate whether ovulation has taken place. First, progesterone inhibits proliferation of the cells lining the vagina. Second, there is a small increase (approximately 0.5°C) in body temperature that usually occurs after ovulation and persists throughout the luteal phase; this change is probably due to an action of progesterone on temperature regulatory centers in the brain. This is an example of the general principle of physiology that the functions of organ systems are coordinated with each other.

Note that in its myometrial and vaginal effects, as well as several others listed in Table 17.8, progesterone exerts an "antiestrogen effect," probably by decreasing the number of estrogen receptors. In contrast, the synthesis of progesterone receptors is stimulated by estrogen in many tissues (for example, the endometrium), and so responsiveness to progesterone usually requires the presence of estrogen (**estrogen priming**).

Like all steroid hormones, both estrogen and progesterone act in the cell nucleus, and their biochemical mechanism of action is at the level of gene transcription.

Brief mention should be made of the transient physical and emotional symptoms that appear in many women prior to the onset of menstrual flow and disappear within a few days after the start of menstruation. The symptoms—which may include painful or swollen breasts; headache; backache; depression; anxiety; irritability; and other physical, emotional, and behavioral changes—are often attributed to estrogen or progesterone excess. The plasma concentrations of these hormones, however, are usually normal in women having these symptoms, and the cause of the symptoms is not actually known. In order of increasing severity of symptoms, the overall problem is categorized as ***premenstrual tension***, ***premenstrual syndrome*** (***PMS***), or ***premenstrual dysphoric disorder*** (***PMDD***), the last-named being so severe as to be temporarily disabling. These symptoms appear to result from a complex interplay between the sex steroids and brain neurotransmitters.

Androgens are present in the blood of women as a result of production by the adrenal glands and ovaries (see Figure 17.6). These androgens play several important roles in the female, including stimulation of the growth of pubic hair, axillary hair, and, possibly, skeletal muscle, and maintenance of sex drive. Excess androgens may cause ***virilization:*** The female fat distribution lessens, a beard appears along with the male body hair distribution, the voice lowers in pitch, the skeletal muscle mass increases, the clitoris enlarges, and the breasts diminish in size.

TABLE 17.8 Some Effects of Female Sex Steroids

I. Estrogen
- A. Stimulates growth of ovary and follicles (local effects).
- B. Stimulates growth of smooth muscle and proliferation of epithelial linings of reproductive tract. In addition:
  1. Fallopian tubes: Increases contractions and ciliary activity.
  2. Uterus: Increases myometrial contractions and responsiveness to oxytocin. Stimulates secretion of abundant, watery cervical mucus. Prepares endometrium for progesterone's actions by inducing progesterone receptors.
  3. Vagina: Increases layering of epithelial cells.
- C. Stimulates external genitalia growth, particularly during puberty.
- D. Stimulates breast growth, particularly ducts and fat deposition during puberty.
- E. Stimulates female body configuration development during puberty: narrow shoulders, broad hips, female fat distribution (deposition on hips and breasts).
- F. Stimulates fluid secretion from lipid (sebum)-producing skin glands (sebaceous glands). (This "anti-acne" effect opposes the acne-producing effects of androgen.)
- G. Stimulates bone growth and ultimate cessation of bone growth (closure of epiphyseal plates); protects against osteoporosis; does not have an anabolic effect on skeletal muscle.
- H. Vascular effects (deficiency produces "hot flashes").
- I. Has feedback effects on hypothalamus and anterior pituitary gland (see Table 17.4).
- J. Stimulates prolactin secretion but inhibits prolactin's milk-inducing action on the breasts.
- K. Protects against atherosclerosis by effects on plasma cholesterol (Chapter 16), blood vessels, and blood clotting (Chapter 12).

II. Progesterone
- A. Converts the estrogen-primed endometrium to an actively secreting tissue suitable for implantation of an embryo.
- B. Induces thick, sticky cervical mucus.
- C. Decreases contractions of fallopian tubes and myometrium.
- D. Decreases proliferation of vaginal epithelial cells.
- E. Stimulates breast growth, particularly glandular tissue.
- F. Inhibits milk-inducing effects of prolactin.
- G. Has feedback effects on hypothalamus and anterior pituitary gland (see Table 17.4).
- H. Increases body temperature.

17.17 Puberty

Puberty in females is a process similar to that in males (described earlier in this chapter). It usually starts earlier in girls (10 to 12 years old) than in boys. In the female, GnRH, the pituitary gland gonadotropins, and estrogen are all secreted at very low concentrations during childhood. For this reason, there is no follicle maturation beyond the early antral stage and menstrual cycles do not occur. The female accessory sex organs remain small and nonfunctional, and there are minimal secondary sex characteristics. The onset of puberty is caused, in large part, by an alteration in brain function that increases the secretion of GnRH. It is currently thought that activation of kisspeptin neurons in the hypothalamus is involved in the increase in GnRH that occurs early in puberty. GnRH in turn stimulates the secretion of pituitary gland gonadotropins, which stimulate follicle development and estrogen secretion. Estrogen, in addition to its critical role in follicle development, induces the changes in the accessory sex organs and secondary sex characteristics associated with puberty. **Menarche,** the first menstruation, is a late event of puberty (averaging about 12.5 years of age in the United States).

As in males, the mechanism of the brain change that results in increased GnRH secretion in girls at puberty remains unknown. The brain may become less sensitive to the negative feedback effects of gonadal hormones at the time of puberty. Also, the adipose-tissue hormone leptin (see Chapter 16) is known to stimulate the secretion of GnRH and may play a role in puberty. This may explain why the onset of puberty tends to correlate with the attainment of a certain level of energy stores (fat) in the girl's body. The failure to have menstrual flow (menses) is called ***amenorrhea.*** Primary amenorrhea is the failure to initial normal menstrual cycles at puberty (menarche), whereas secondary amenorrhea is defined as the loss of previously normal menstrual cycles. As we will see, the most common causes of secondary amenorrhea are pregnancy and menopause. Excessive exercise and ***anorexia nervosa*** (self-imposed starvation) can cause primary or secondary amenorrhea. There are a variety of theories for why this is so. One unifying theory is that the brain can sense a loss of body fat, possibly via decreased concentrations of the hormone leptin, and that this leads the hypothalamus to cease GnRH pulses. From a teleological view, this makes sense because pregnant women must supply a large caloric input to the developing fetus and a lack of body fat would indicate inadequate energy stores. The prepubertal appearance of female gymnasts who have minimal body fat may indicate hypogonadism and probably amenorrhea, which can persist for many years after menarche would normally take place.

The onset of puberty in both sexes is not abrupt but develops over several years, as evidenced by slowly increasing plasma concentrations of the gonadotropins and testosterone or estrogen. The age of the normal onset of puberty is controversial, although it is generally thought that pubertal onset before the age of 6 to 7 in girls and 8 to 9 in boys warrants clinical investigation. ***Precocious puberty*** is defined as the very premature appearance of secondary sex characteristics and is usually caused by an early increase in gonadal steroid production. This leads to an early onset of the puberty growth spurt, maturation of the skeleton, breast development (in girls), and enlargement of the genitalia (in boys). Therefore, these children are usually taller at an early age. However, because gonadal steroids also stop the pubertal growth spurt by inducing epiphyseal closure, final adult height is usually less than predicted. Although there are a variety of causes for the premature increase in gonadal steroids, *true* (or complete) precocious puberty is caused by the premature activation of GnRH and LH and FSH secretion. This is often caused by tumors or infections in the area of the central nervous system that controls GnRH release. Treatments that decrease LH and FSH release are important to allow normal development.

17.18 Female Sexual Response

The female response to sexual intercourse is characterized by marked increases in blood flow and muscular contraction in many areas of the body. For example, increasing sexual excitement is associated with vascular engorgement of the breasts and erection of the nipples, resulting from contraction of smooth muscle fibers in them. The clitoris, which has a rich supply of sensory nerve endings, increases in diameter and length as a result of increased blood flow. During intercourse, the blood flow to the vagina increases and the vaginal epithelium is lubricated by mucus.

Orgasm in the female, as in the male, is accompanied by pleasurable feelings and many physical events. There is a sudden increase in skeletal muscle activity involving almost all parts of the body; the heart rate and blood pressure increase, and there is a transient rhythmic contraction of the vagina and uterus. Orgasm seems to play a minimal role in ensuring fertilization because fertilization can occur in the absence of an orgasm.

Sexual desire in women is probably more dependent upon androgens, secreted by the adrenal glands and ovaries, than estrogen. Sex drive is also maintained beyond menopause, a time when estrogen concentrations become very low. New studies have suggested that low-dose androgen therapy may be useful for the treatment of decreased libido in women. These effects are mediated by a direct effect of androgen and by conversion of androgens to estrogen by aromatase in the brain.

17.19 Pregnancy

For pregnancy to occur, the introduction of sperm must occur between 5 days before and 1 day after ovulation. This is because the sperm, following their ejaculation into the vagina, remain capable of fertilizing an egg for up to 4 to 6 days, and the ovulated egg remains viable for only 24 to 48 h.

Egg Transport

At ovulation, the egg is extruded onto the surface of the ovary. Recall that the fimbriae at the ends of the fallopian tubes are lined with ciliated epithelium. At ovulation, the smooth muscle of the fimbriae causes them to pass over the ovary while the cilia beat in waves toward the interior of the duct. These ciliary motions sweep the egg into the fallopian tube as it emerges onto the ovarian surface.

Within the fallopian tube, egg movement, driven almost entirely by fallopian-tube cilia, is so slow that the egg takes about 4 days to reach the uterus. Thus, if fertilization is to occur, it must do so in the fallopian tube because of the short viability of the unfertilized egg.

Intercourse, Sperm Transport, and Capacitation

Ejaculation, described earlier in this chapter, results in deposition of semen into the vagina during intercourse. The act of intercourse itself provides some impetus for the transport of sperm out of the vagina to the cervix because of the fluid pressure of the ejaculate. Passage into the cervical mucus by the swimming sperm is dependent on the estrogen-induced changes in consistency of the mucus described earlier. Sperm can enter the uterus within minutes of ejaculation. Furthermore, the sperm can usually survive for up to a day or two within the cervical mucus, from which they can be released to enter the uterus. Transport of the sperm through the length of the uterus and into the fallopian tubes occurs via the sperm's own propulsions and uterine contractions.

The mortality rate of sperm during the trip is huge. One reason for this is that the vaginal environment is acidic, a protection against yeast and bacterial infections. Another is the length and energy requirements of the trip. Of the several hundred million sperm deposited in the vagina in an ejaculation, only about 100 to 200 reach the fallopian tube. This is the major reason there must be so many sperm in the ejaculate for fertilization to occur.

Sperm are not able to fertilize the egg until they have resided in the female tract for several hours and been acted upon by secretions of the tract. This process, called **capacitation**, causes (1) the previously regular wavelike beats of the sperm's tail to be replaced by a more whiplike action that propels the sperm forward in strong surges and (2) the sperm's plasma membrane to become altered so that it will be capable of fusing with the surface membrane of the egg.

Fertilization

Fertilization begins with the fusion of a sperm and egg, usually within a few hours after ovulation. The egg usually must be fertilized within 24 to 48 hours of ovulation. Many sperm, after moving between the granulosa cells of the corona radiata still surrounding the egg, bind to the zona pellucida (**Figure 17.28**). The zona pellucida glycoproteins function

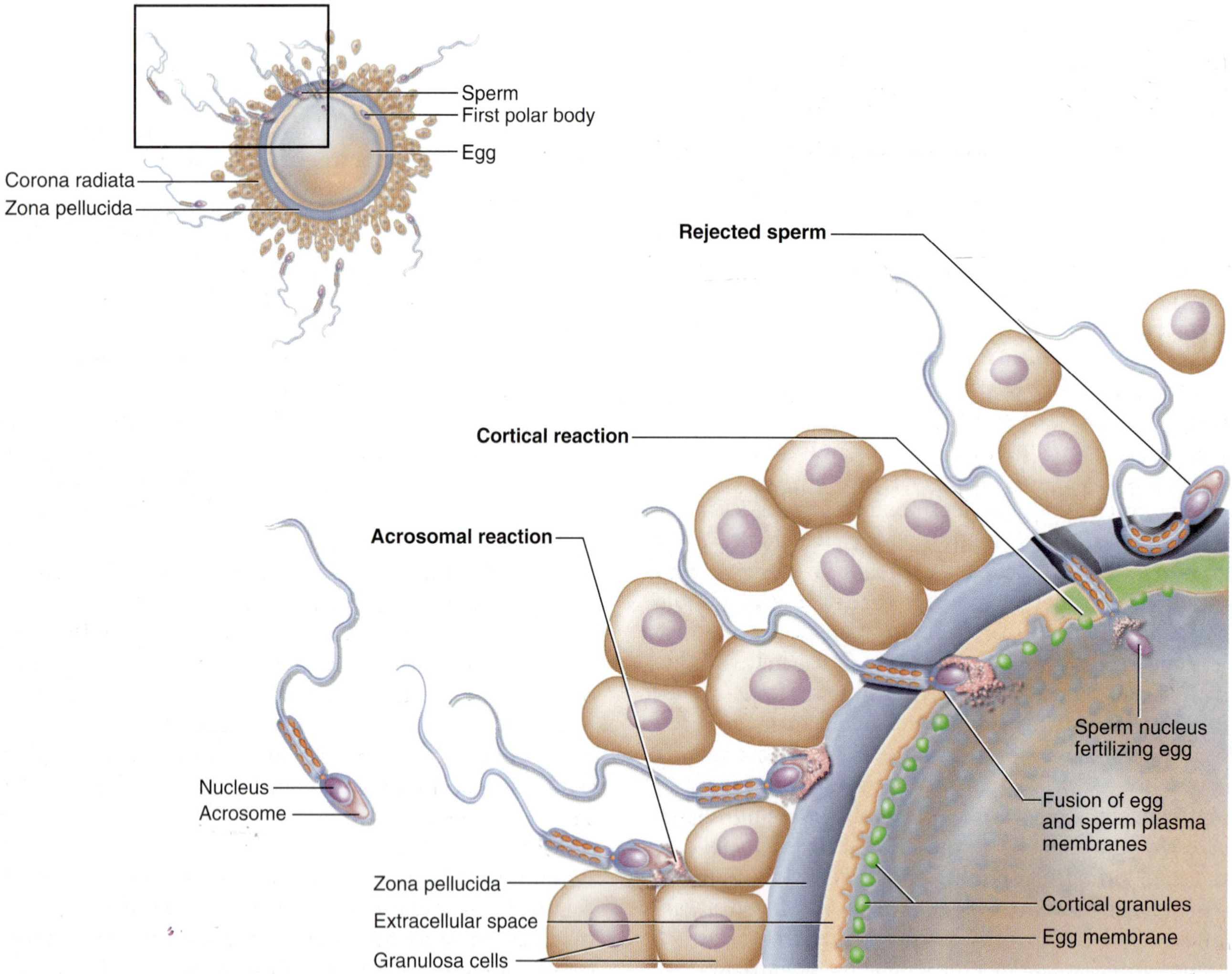

Figure 17.28 AP|R Fertilization and the block to polyspermy. Rectangle on top image indicates area of enlargement below. The size of the sperm is exaggerated for clarity. The photograph on the first page of this chapter shows the actual size relationship between the sperm and the egg.

as receptors for sperm surface proteins. The sperm head has many of these proteins and so becomes bound simultaneously to many sperm receptors on the zona pellucida.

This binding triggers what is termed the **acrosome reaction** in the bound sperm: The plasma membrane of the sperm head is altered so that the underlying membrane-bound acrosomal enzymes are now exposed to the outside—that is, to the zona pellucida. The enzymes digest a path through the zona pellucida as the sperm, using its tail, advances through this coating. The first sperm to penetrate the entire zona pellucida and reach the egg's plasma membrane fuses with this membrane. The head of the sperm then slowly passes into the cytosol of the egg.

Viability of the newly fertilized egg, now called a zygote, depends upon preventing the entry of additional sperm. A specific mechanism mediates this **block to polyspermy.** The initial fusion of the sperm and egg plasma membranes triggers a reaction that changes membrane potential, preventing additional sperm from binding. Subsequently, during the **cortical reaction,** cytosolic secretory vesicles located around the egg's periphery release their contents, by exocytosis, into the narrow space between the egg plasma membrane and the zona pellucida. Some of these molecules are enzymes that enter the zona pellucida and cause both inactivation of its sperm-binding sites and hardening of the entire zona pellucida. This prevents additional sperm from binding to the zona pellucida and those sperm already advancing through it from continuing.

The fertilized egg completes its second meiotic division over the next few hours, and the one daughter cell with practically no cytoplasm—the second polar body—is extruded and disintegrates. The two sets of chromosomes—23 from the egg and 23 from the sperm, which are surrounded by distinct membranes and are known as pronuclei—migrate to the center of the cell. During this period of a few hours, the DNA of the chromosomes in both pronuclei is replicated, the pronuclear membranes break down, the cell is ready to undergo a mitotic division, and fertilization is complete. Fertilization also triggers activation of the egg enzymes required for the ensuing cell divisions and embryogenesis. The major events of fertilization are summarized in **Figure 17.29**. If fertilization had not occurred, the egg would have slowly disintegrated and been phagocytized by cells lining the uterus.

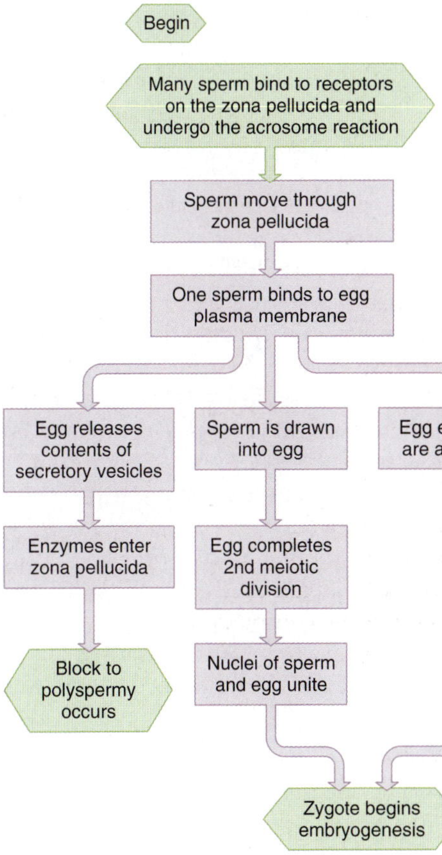

Figure 17.29 Events leading to fertilization, block to polyspermy, and the beginning of embryogenesis.

Rarely, a fertilized egg remains in a fallopian tube and embeds itself in the tube wall. Even more rarely, a fertilized egg may move backward out of the fallopian tube into the abdominal cavity, where implantation can occur. Both kinds of ***ectopic pregnancies*** cannot succeed, and surgery is necessary to end the pregnancy (unless there is a spontaneous abortion) because of the risk of maternal hemorrhage.

Early Development, Implantation, and Placentation

The previously described events from ovulation and fertilization to implantation of the blastocyst are summarized in **Figure 17.30**. The **conceptus**—a collective term for everything ultimately derived from the original zygote (fertilized egg) throughout the pregnancy—remains in the fallopian tube for 3 to 4 days. The major reason is that estrogen maintains the contraction of the smooth muscle near where the fallopian tube enters the wall of the uterus. As plasma progesterone concentrations increase, this smooth muscle relaxes and allows the conceptus to pass. During its stay in the fallopian tube, the conceptus undergoes a number of mitotic cell divisions, a process known as **cleavage.** These divisions, however, are unusual in that no cell growth occurs before each division. Thus, the 16- to 32-cell conceptus that reaches the uterus is essentially the same size as the original fertilized egg.

Each of these cells is **totipotent**—that is, they are **stem cells** that have the capacity to develop into an entire individual. Therefore, identical (monozygotic) twins result when, at some point during cleavage, the dividing cells become completely separated into two independently growing cell masses. In contrast, as described earlier, dizygotic twins result when two eggs are ovulated and fertilized.

After reaching the uterus, the conceptus floats free in the intrauterine fluid, from which it receives nutrients, for approximately 3 days, all the while undergoing further cell divisions to approximately 100 cells. Soon the conceptus reaches the stage known as a **blastocyst,** by which point the cells have lost their totipotentiality and have begun to differentiate. The blastocyst consists of an outer layer of cells called the **trophoblast,** an **inner cell mass,** and a central fluid-filled cavity (**Figure 17.31**). During subsequent development, the inner cell mass will give rise to the developing human—called an **embryo** during the first 2 months and a **fetus** after that—and some of the membranes associated with it. The trophoblast will surround the embryo and fetus throughout development and be involved in its nutrition as well as in the secretion of several important hormones.

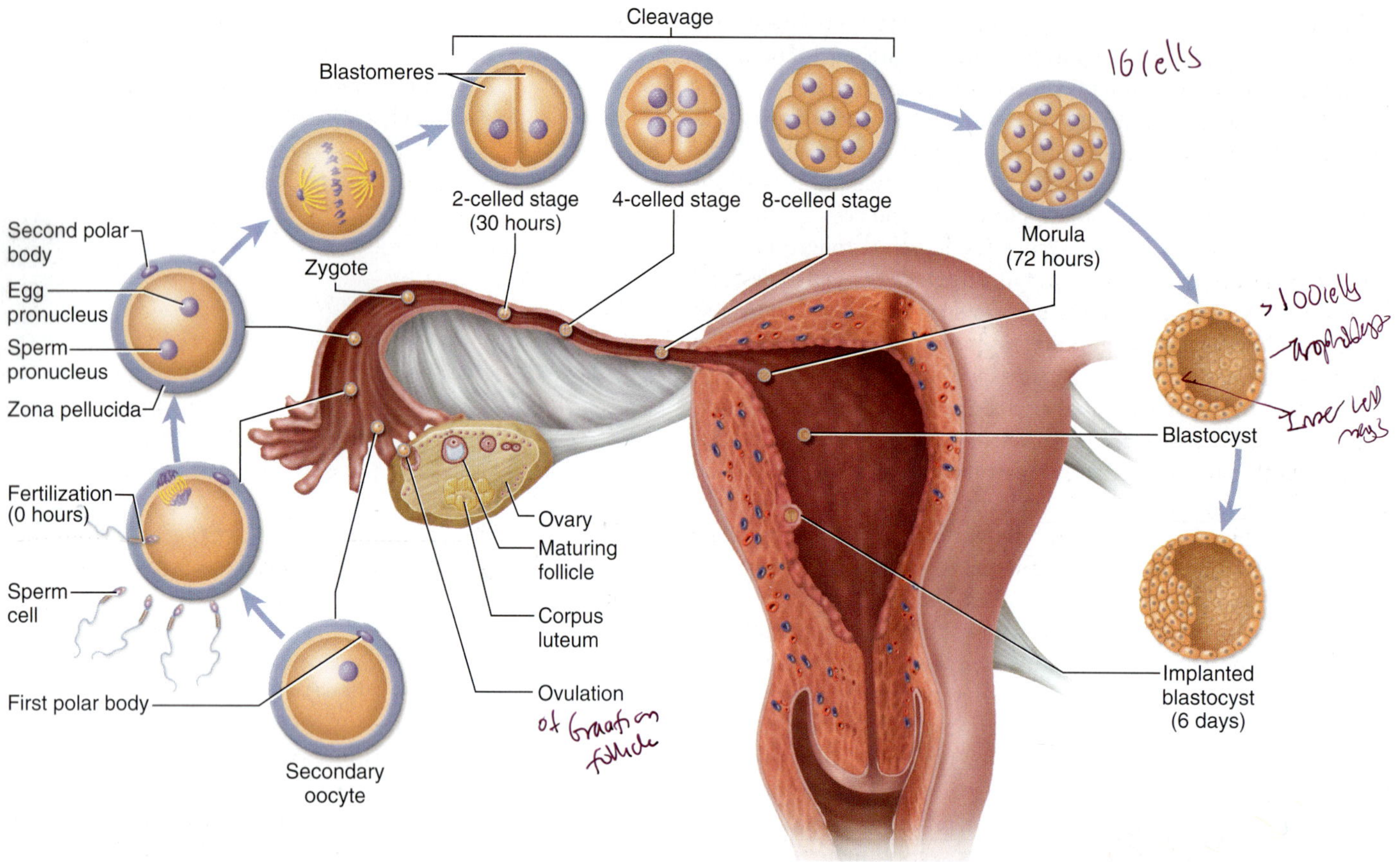

Figure 17.30 AP|R Events from ovulation to implantation. Only one ovary and one fallopian tube are shown (right side of patient).

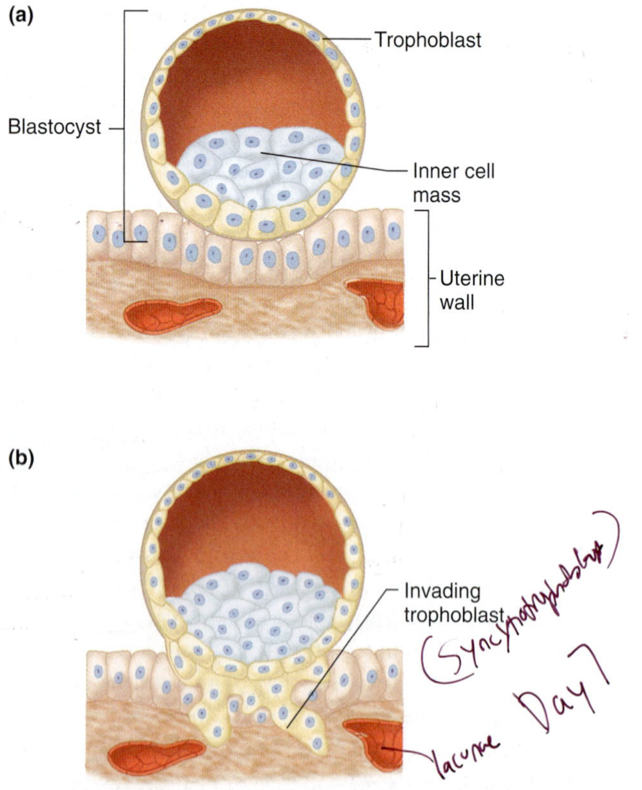

Figure 17.31 AP|R (a) Contact and (b) implantation of the blastocyst into the uterine wall at about 6–7 days after the previous LH peak. The trophoblast cells secrete hCG into the maternal circulation, which rescues the corpus luteum and maintains pregnancy. The trophoblast eventually develops into a component of the placenta.

The period during which the zygote develops into a blastocyst corresponds with days 14 to 21 of the typical menstrual cycle. During this period, the uterine lining is being prepared by progesterone (secreted by the corpus luteum) to receive the blastocyst. By approximately the twenty-first day of the cycle (that is, 7 days after ovulation), **implantation**—the embedding of the blastocyst into the endometrium—begins (see Figure 17.31). The trophoblast cells are quite sticky, particularly in the region overlying the inner cell mass, and it is this portion of the blastocyst that adheres to the endometrium and initiates implantation.

The initial contact between blastocyst and endometrium induces rapid proliferation of the trophoblast, the cells of which penetrate between endometrial cells. Proteolytic enzymes secreted by the trophoblast allow the blastocyst to bury itself in the endometrial layer. The endometrium, too, is undergoing changes at the site of contact. Implantation requires communication—via several paracrine signals—between the blastocyst and the cells of the endometrium. Implantation is soon completed, and the nutrient-rich endometrial cells provide the metabolic fuel and raw materials required for early growth of the embryo.

This simple nutritive system, however, is only adequate to provide for the embryo during the first few weeks, when it is very small. The structure that takes over this function is the **placenta,** a combination of interlocking fetal and maternal tissues, which serves as the organ of exchange between mother and fetus for the remainder of the pregnancy.

The embryonic portion of the placenta is supplied by the outermost layers of trophoblast cells, the **chorion,** and the maternal portion by the endometrium underlying the chorion. Fingerlike projections of the trophoblast cells, called

chorionic villi, extend from the chorion into the endometrium (Figure 17.32). The villi contain a rich network of capillaries that are part of the embryo's circulatory system. The endometrium around the villi is altered by enzymes and other paracrine molecules secreted from the cells of the invading villi so that each villus becomes completely surrounded by a pool, or **sinus,** of maternal blood supplied by maternal arterioles.

The maternal blood enters these placental sinuses via the uterine artery; the blood flows through the sinuses and then exits via the uterine veins. Simultaneously, blood flows from the fetus into the capillaries of the chorionic villi via the **umbilical arteries** and out of the capillaries back to the fetus via the **umbilical vein.** All of these umbilical vessels are contained in the **umbilical cord,** a long, ropelike structure that connects the fetus to the placenta.

Five weeks after implantation, the placenta has become well established; the fetal heart has begun to pump blood; the entire mechanism for nutrition of the embryo and, subsequently, fetus and the excretion of waste products is in operation. A layer of epithelial cells in the villi and of endothelial cells in the fetal capillaries separates the maternal and fetal blood. Waste products move from blood in the fetal capillaries across these layers into the maternal blood; nutrients, hormones, and growth factors move in the opposite direction. Some substances, such as oxygen and carbon dioxide, move by diffusion. Others, such as glucose, use transport proteins in the plasma membranes of the epithelial cells. Still other substances (e.g., several amino acids and hormones) are produced by the trophoblast layers of the placenta itself and added to the fetal and maternal blood. Note that there is an exchange of materials between the two bloodstreams but no actual mixing of the fetal and maternal blood. Umbilical veins carry oxygen and nutrient-rich blood from the placenta to the fetus, whereas umbilical arteries carry blood with waste products and a low oxygen content to the placenta.

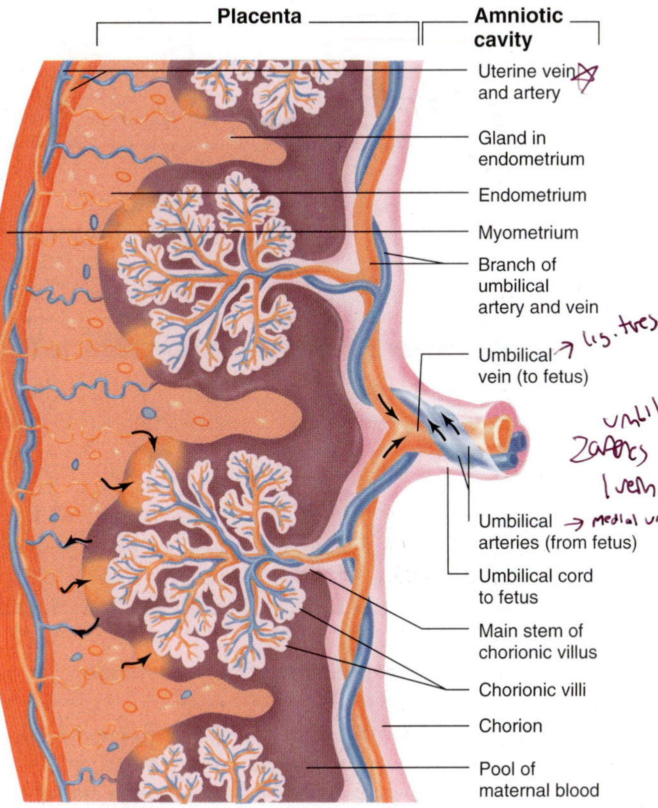

Figure 17.32 Interrelations of fetal and maternal tissues in the formation of the placenta. See Figure 17.33 for the orientation of the placenta. From B. M. Carlson, *Patten's Foundations of Embryology*, 5th ed., McGraw-Hill, New York.

PHYSIOLOGICAL INQUIRY

- How can you determine if a significant amount of fetal blood is leaking into the maternal circulatory system?

Answer can be found at end of chapter.

Meanwhile, a space called the **amniotic cavity** has formed between the inner cell mass and the chorion (Figure 17.33). The epithelial layer lining the cavity is derived from the inner cell mass and is called the **amnion,** or **amniotic sac.** It eventually fuses with the inner surface of the chorion so that only a single combined membrane surrounds the fetus. The fluid in the amniotic cavity, the **amniotic fluid,** resembles the fetal extracellular fluid, and it buffers mechanical disturbances and temperature variations. The fetus, floating in the amniotic cavity and attached by the umbilical cord to the placenta, develops into a viable infant during the next 8 months.

Amniotic fluid can be sampled by ***amniocentesis*** as early as the sixteenth week of pregnancy. This is done by inserting a needle into the amniotic cavity. Some genetic diseases can be diagnosed by the finding of certain chemicals either in the fluid or in sloughed fetal cells suspended in the fluid. The chromosomes of these fetal cells can also be examined for diagnosis of certain disorders as well as to determine the sex of the fetus. Another technique for fetal diagnosis is ***chorionic villus sampling.*** This technique, which can be performed as early as 9 to 12 weeks of pregnancy, involves obtaining tissue from a chorionic villus of the placenta. This technique, however, carries a higher risk of inducing the loss of the fetus (***miscarriage***) than does amniocentesis. A third technique for fetal diagnosis is ultrasound, which provides a "picture" of the fetus without the use of x-rays. A fourth technique for screening for fetal abnormalities involves obtaining only *maternal* blood and analyzing it for several normally occurring substances whose concentrations change in the presence of these abnormalities. For example, particular changes in the concentrations of two hormones produced during pregnancy—human chorionic gonadotropin and estriol—and alpha-fetoprotein (a major fetal plasma protein that crosses the placenta into the maternal blood) can identify many cases of ***Down syndrome,*** a genetic form of intellectual and developmental disability associated with distinct facial and body features.

Maternal nutrition is crucial for the fetus. Malnutrition early in pregnancy can cause specific abnormalities that are **congenital,** that is, existing at birth. Malnutrition retards fetal growth and results in infants with higher-than-normal death rates, reduced growth after birth, and an increased incidence of learning disabilities and other medical problems. Specific nutrients, not just total calories, are also very important. For example, there is an increased incidence of neural defects in the offspring of mothers who are deficient in the

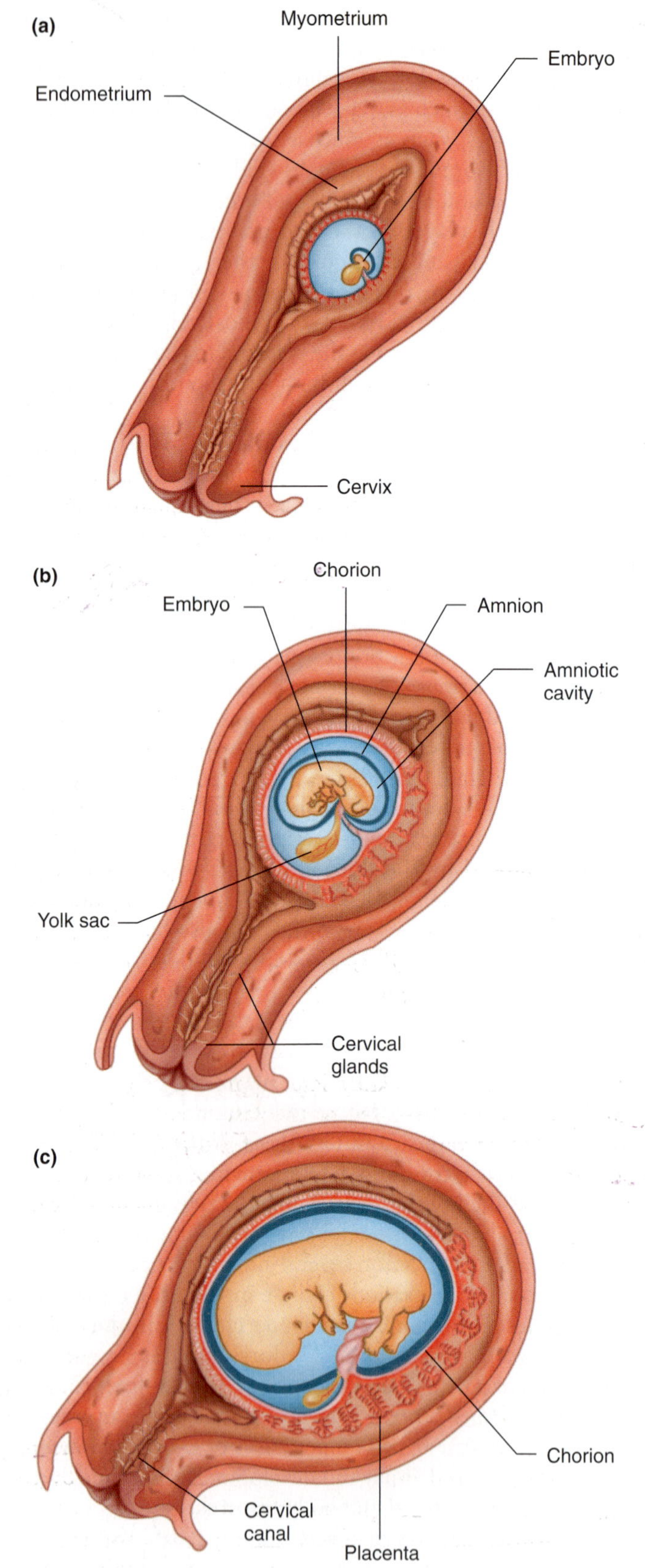

Figure 17.33 The uterus at (a) 3, (b) 5, and (c) 8 weeks after fertilization. Embryos and their membranes are drawn to actual size. Uterus is within actual size range. The yolk sac is formed from the trophoblast. It has no nutritional function in humans but is important in embryonic development. From B. M. Carlson, *Patten's Foundations of Embryology*, 5th ed., McGraw-Hill, New York.

B-vitamin folate (also called folic acid and folacin). Recall from Chapter 11 that normal maternal and fetal thyroid hormone concentrations are necessary for normal fetal development.

The developing embryo and fetus are also subject to considerable influences by a host of nonnutrient factors, such as noise, radiation, chemicals, and viruses, to which the mother may be exposed. For example, drugs taken by the mother can reach the fetus via transport across the placenta and can impair fetal growth and development. In this regard, it must be emphasized that aspirin, alcohol, and the chemicals in cigarette smoke are very potent agents, as are illicit drugs such as cocaine. Any agent that can cause birth defects in the fetus is known as a ***teratogen***.

Because half of the fetal genes—those from the father—differ from those of the mother, the fetus is in essence a foreign transplant in the mother. The integrity of the fetal–maternal blood barrier also protects the fetus from immunologic attack by the mother.

Hormonal and Other Changes During Pregnancy

Throughout pregnancy, plasma concentrations of estrogen and progesterone continually increase (**Figure 17.34**). Estrogen stimulates the growth of the uterine muscle mass,

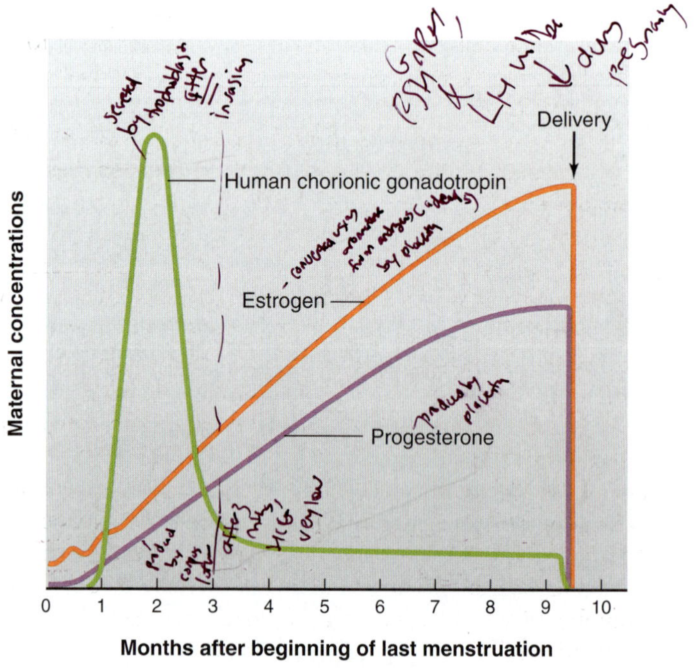

Figure 17.34 Maternal concentrations of estrogen, progesterone, and human chorionic gonadotropin during pregnancy. Curves depicting hormone concentrations are not drawn to scale. Note that the concentrations of estrogen and progesterone achieved in the maternal blood during pregnancy are much higher than during a typical menstrual cycle shown in Figure 17.22.

PHYSIOLOGICAL INQUIRY

- Why do progesterone and estrogen concentrations continue to increase during pregnancy even though human chorionic gonadotropin (hCG) concentration decreases?

Answer can be found at end of chapter.

which will eventually supply the contractile force needed to deliver the fetus. Progesterone inhibits uterine contractility so that the fetus is not expelled prematurely. During approximately the first 2 months of pregnancy, almost all the estrogen and progesterone are supplied by the corpus luteum.

Recall that if pregnancy had not occurred, the corpus luteum would have degenerated within 2 weeks after its formation. The persistence of the corpus luteum during pregnancy is due to a hormone called **human chorionic gonadotropin** (**hCG**), which the trophoblast cells start to secrete around the time they start their endometrial invasion. Human chorionic gonadotropin gains entry to the maternal circulation, and the detection of this hormone in the mother's plasma and/or urine is used as a test for pregnancy. This glycoprotein is very similar to LH, and it not only prevents the corpus luteum from degenerating but strongly stimulates its steroid secretion. Thus, the signal that preserves the corpus luteum comes from the conceptus, not the mother's tissues. The rescue of the corpus luteum by hCG is an example of the general principle of physiology that information flow between organs allows for integration of physiological processes. That is, hCG secreted into maternal blood from the developing trophoblasts of embryonic origin stimulates the maternal ovaries to continue to secrete gonadal steroids. This, via negative feedback on maternal gonadotropin secretion, prevents additional menstrual cycles that would otherwise result in the loss of the implanted embryo.

The secretion of hCG reaches a peak 60 to 80 days after the last menstruation (see Figure 17.34). It then decreases just as rapidly, so that by the end of the third month it has reached a low concentration that changes little for the duration of the pregnancy. Associated with this decrease in hCG secretion, the placenta begins to secrete large quantities of estrogen and progesterone. The very marked increases in plasma concentrations of estrogen and progesterone during the last 6 months of pregnancy are due entirely to their secretion by the trophoblast cells of the placenta, and the corpus luteum regresses after 3 months.

An important aspect of placental steroid secretion is that the placenta has the enzymes required for the synthesis of progesterone but not those required for the formation of androgens, which are the precursors of estrogen. The placenta is supplied with androgens via the maternal ovaries and adrenal glands and by the *fetal* adrenal glands. The placenta converts the androgens into estrogen by expressing the enzyme aromatase.

The secretion of GnRH and, therefore, of LH and FSH is powerfully inhibited by high concentrations of progesterone in the presence of estrogen. Both of these gonadal steroids are secreted in high concentrations by the corpus luteum and then by the placenta throughout pregnancy, so the secretion of the pituitary gland gonadotropins remains extremely low. As a consequence, there are no ovarian or menstrual cycles during pregnancy.

The trophoblast cells of the placenta produce not only hCG and steroids but also inhibin and many other hormones that can influence the mother. One unique hormone that is secreted in very large amounts has effects similar to those of both prolactin and growth hormone. This protein hormone, **human placental lactogen,** mobilizes fats from maternal adipose tissue and stimulates glucose production in the liver (growth-hormone-like) in the mother. It also stimulates breast development (prolactin-like) in preparation for lactation. Some of the many other physiological changes, hormonal and nonhormonal, in the mother during pregnancy are summarized in Table 17.9.

Approximately 5% to 10% of pregnant women retain too much fluid (edema) and have protein in the urine and hypertension. These are the symptoms of ***preeclampsia;*** when convulsions also occur, the condition is termed ***eclampsia.*** These two syndromes are collectively called ***toxemia of pregnancy.*** This can result in decreased growth rate and death of the fetus. The factors responsible for eclampsia are unknown, but the evidence strongly implicates abnormal vasoconstriction of the maternal blood vessels and inadequate invasion of the endometrium by trophoblast cells, resulting in poor blood perfusion of the placenta.

Pregnancy Sickness

Some women suffer from ***pregnancy sickness*** (popularly called morning sickness), which is characterized by nausea and vomiting during the first 3 months (first trimester) of pregnancy. The exact cause is unknown, but high concentrations of estrogen and other substances may be responsible. It may also be linked with increased sensitivity to odors, such as those of certain foods. Whether or not pregnancy sickness has adaptive value is currently being debated. It has been speculated, for example, that pregnancy sickness may prevent ingestion of certain foods that may contain toxic alkaloid compounds or that carry parasites or other infectious organisms that could harm the developing fetus.

Parturition

A normal human pregnancy lasts approximately 40 weeks, counting from the first day of the last menstrual cycle, or approximately 38 weeks from the day of ovulation and conception. Survival of premature infants is now possible from about the twenty-fourth week of pregnancy. Treatment of these infants often requires heroic efforts, often with significant deficits in the infant.

During the last few weeks of pregnancy, a variety of events occur in the uterus and the fetus, culminating in the birth (delivery) of the infant, followed by the placenta. All of these events, including delivery, are collectively called **parturition.** Throughout most of pregnancy, the smooth muscle cells of the myometrium are relatively disconnected from each other and the uterus is sealed at its outlet by the firm, inflexible collagen fibers that constitute the cervix. These features are maintained mainly by progesterone. During the last few weeks of pregnancy, as a result of ever-increasing concentrations of estrogen, the smooth muscle cells synthesize *connexins,* proteins that form gap junctions between the cells, which allow the myometrium to undergo coordinated contractions. Simultaneously, the cervix becomes soft and flexible due to an enzymatically mediated breakdown of its collagen fibers. The synthesis of the enzymes is

TABLE 17.9 Maternal Responses to Pregnancy

Placenta	Secretion of estrogen, progesterone, human chorionic gonadotropin, inhibin, human placental lactogen, and other hormones
Anterior pituitary gland	Increased secretion of prolactin Secretes very little FSH and LH
Adrenal cortex	Increased secretion of aldosterone and cortisol
Posterior pituitary gland	Increased secretion of vasopressin
Parathyroids	Increased secretion of parathyroid hormone
Kidneys	Increased secretion of renin, erythropoietin, and 1,25-dihydroxyvitamin D Retention of salt and water *Cause:* Increased aldosterone, vasopressin, and estrogen
Breasts	Enlarge and develop mature glandular structure *Cause:* Estrogen, progesterone, prolactin, and human placental lactogen
Blood volume	Increased *Cause:* Total erythrocyte number increased by erythropoietin, and plasma volume by salt and water retention; however, plasma volume usually increases more than red cells, thereby leading to small decreases in hematocrit
Bone turnover	Increased *Cause:* Increased parathyroid hormone and 1,25-dihydroxyvitamin D
Body weight	Increased by average of 12.5 kg, 60% of which is water
Circulation	Cardiac output increases, total peripheral resistance decreases (vasodilation in uterus, skin, breasts, GI tract, and kidneys), and mean arterial pressure stays constant
Respiration	Hyperventilation occurs (arterial P_{CO_2} decreases) due to the effects of increased progesterone
Organic metabolism	Metabolic rate increases Plasma glucose, gluconeogenesis, and fatty acid mobilization all increase *Cause:* Hyporesponsiveness to insulin due to insulin antagonism by human placental lactogen and cortisol
Appetite and thirst	Increased (particularly after the first trimester)
Nutritional RDAs*	Increased

*RDA—Recommended daily allowance

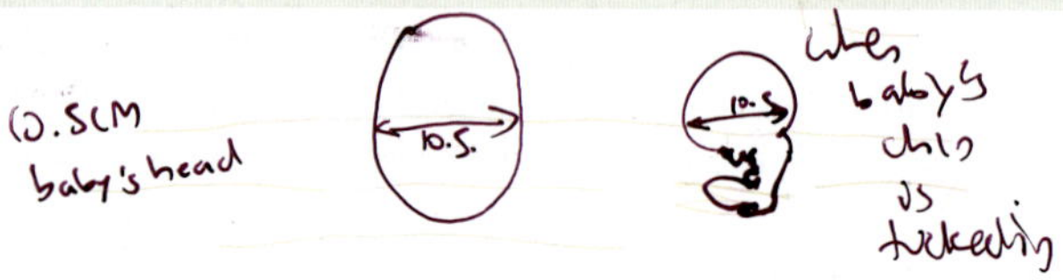

mediated by a variety of messengers, including estrogen and placental prostaglandins, the synthesis of which is stimulated by estrogen. The peptide hormone **relaxin** is secreted by the ovaries, placenta, and uterus and softens cartilaginous joints in the pelvis. Estrogen has yet another important effect on the myometrium during this period: It induces the synthesis of receptors for the posterior pituitary hormone oxytocin, which is a powerful stimulator of uterine smooth muscle contraction.

Delivery is produced by strong rhythmic contractions of the myometrium. Actually, weak and infrequent uterine contractions begin at approximately 30 weeks and gradually increase in both strength and frequency. During the last month, the entire uterine contents shift downward so that the near-term fetus is brought into contact with the cervix. In over 90% of births, the baby's head is downward and acts as the wedge to dilate the cervical canal when labor begins (**Figure 17.35**). Occasionally, a baby is oriented with some other part of the body downward (***breech presentation***). This can require the surgical delivery of the fetus and placenta through an abdominal and uterine incision (***cesarean section***).

At the onset of labor and delivery or before, the amniotic sac ruptures, and the amniotic fluid flows through the vagina. When labor begins in earnest, the uterine contractions become strong and occur at approximately 10 to 15 min intervals. The contractions begin in the upper portion of the uterus and sweep downward.

As the contractions increase in intensity and frequency, the cervix is gradually forced open (dilation) to a maximum

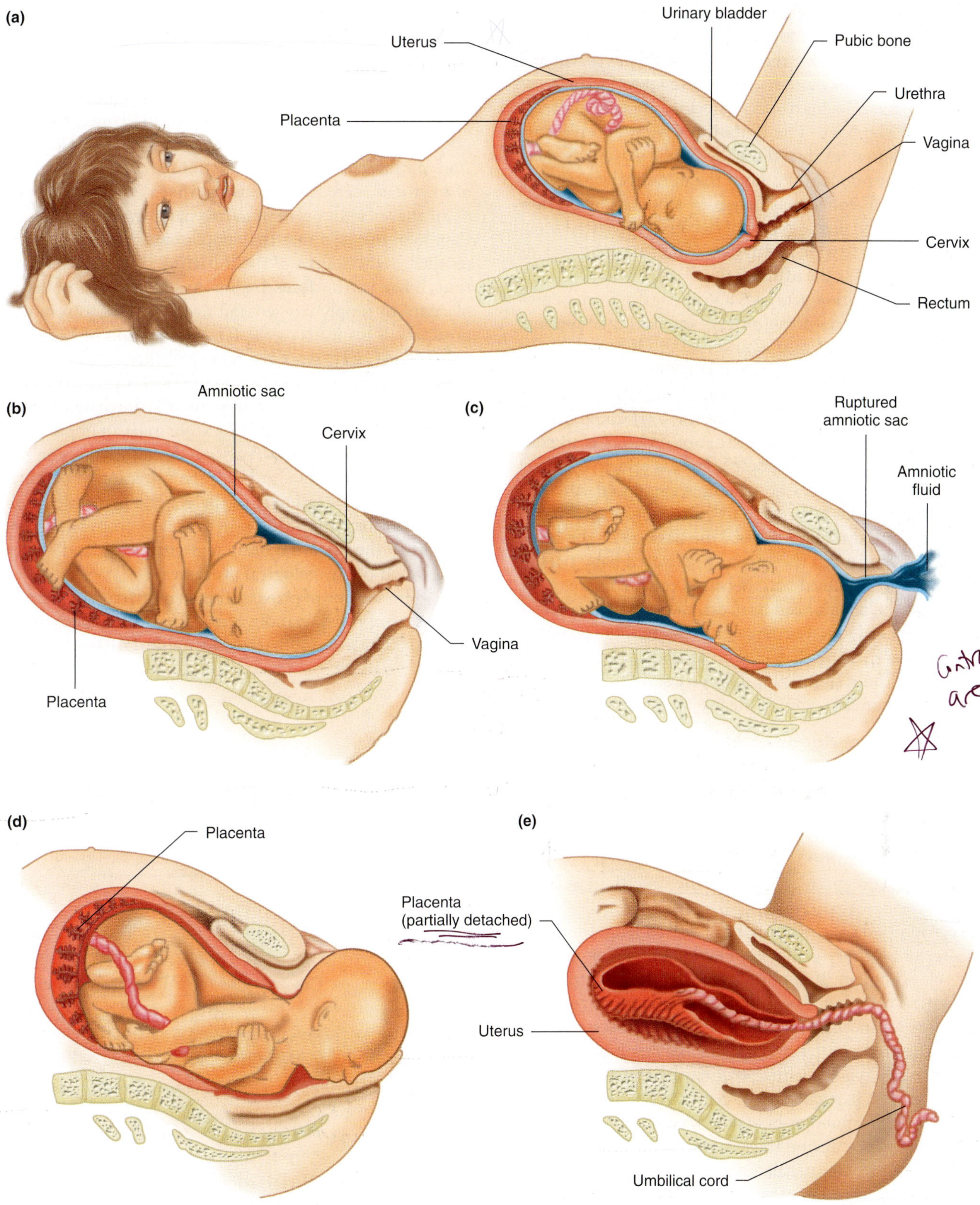

Figure 17.35 Stages of parturition. (a) Parturition has not yet begun. (b) The cervix is dilating. (c) The cervix is completely dilated, and the fetus's head is entering the cervical canal; the amniotic sac has ruptured and the amniotic fluid escapes. (d) The fetus is moving through the vagina. (e) The placenta is coming loose from the uterine wall in preparation for its expulsion.

Contractions are 10–15 mins interval after amniotic sac burst.

diameter of approximately 10 cm (4 in). Until this point, the contractions have not moved the fetus out of the uterus. Now the contractions move the fetus through the cervix and vagina. At this time, the mother—by bearing down to increase abdominal pressure—adds to the effect of uterine contractions to deliver the baby. The umbilical vessels and placenta are still functioning, so that the baby is not yet on its own; but within minutes of delivery, both the umbilical vessels and the placental vessels completely constrict, stopping blood flow to the placenta. The entire placenta becomes separated from the underlying uterine wall, and a wave of uterine contractions delivers the placenta as the **afterbirth.**

Usually, parturition proceeds automatically from beginning to end and requires no significant medical intervention. In a small percentage of cases, however, the position of the baby or some maternal complication can interfere with normal delivery (e.g., breech presentation). The headfirst position of the fetus is important for several reasons. (1) If the baby is not oriented headfirst, another portion of its body is in contact with the cervix and is generally a far less effective wedge. (2) Because of the head's large diameter compared with the rest of the body, if the body were to go through the cervical canal first, the canal might obstruct the passage of the head, leading to problems when the partially delivered baby tries to breathe. (3) If the umbilical cord becomes caught between the canal wall and the baby's head or chest, mechanical compression of the umbilical vessels can result. Despite these potential problems, however, many babies who are not oriented headfirst are born without significant difficulties.

What mechanisms control the events of parturition?

1. The smooth muscle cells of the myometrium have inherent rhythmicity and are capable of autonomous contractions, which are facilitated as the muscle is stretched by the growing fetus.
2. The pregnant uterus near term and during labor secretes several prostaglandins (PGE_2 and $PGF_{2\alpha}$) that are potent stimulators of uterine smooth muscle contraction.
3. **Oxytocin,** one of the hormones released from the posterior pituitary gland, is an extremely potent uterine muscle stimulant. It not only acts directly on uterine smooth muscle but also stimulates it to synthesize the prostaglandins. Oxytocin is reflexively secreted from the posterior pituitary gland as a result of neural input to the hypothalamus, originating from receptors in the uterus, particularly the cervix. Also, as noted previously, the number of oxytocin receptors in the uterus increases during the last few weeks of pregnancy. Therefore, the contractile response to any given plasma concentration of oxytocin is greatly increased at parturition.
4. Throughout pregnancy, progesterone exerts an essential powerful inhibitory effect upon uterine contractions by decreasing the sensitivity of the myometrium to estrogen, oxytocin, and prostaglandins. Unlike the situation in many other species, however, the rate of progesterone secretion does not decrease before or during parturition in women (until after delivery of the placenta, the source of the progesterone); therefore, progesterone withdrawal does not play a role in parturition.

These mechanisms are shown in a unified pattern in **Figure 17.36**. Once started, the uterine contractions exert a positive feedback effect upon themselves via both local facilitation of inherent uterine contractions and reflexive stimulation of oxytocin secretion. Precisely what the relative importance of all these factors is in *initiating* parturition remains unclear. One hypothesis is that the fetoplacental unit, rather than the mother, is the source of the initiating signals to start parturition. That is, the fetus begins to outstrip the ability of the placenta to supply oxygen and nutrients and to remove waste products. This leads to the fetal production of hormonal signals like ACTH. Another theory is that a "placental clock," acting via placental production of CRH, signals the fetal production of ACTH. Either way, ACTH-mediated increases in fetal adrenal steroid production seem to be an important signal to the mother to begin parturition. Whether it is a signal from the fetus, the placenta, or both, the initiation of parturition is another excellent example of the general principle of physiology that information flow—in this case, from the fetoplacental unit to the maternal brain and pituitary gland—allows for integration of physiological processes.

The actions of prostaglandins on parturition are the last in a series of prostaglandin effects on the female reproductive system. They are summarized in **Table 17.10**.

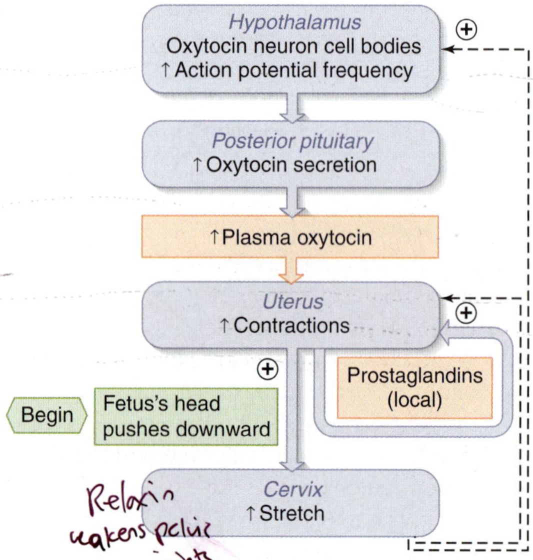

Figure 17.36 Factors stimulating uterine contractions during parturition. Note the positive feedback nature of several of the inputs.

PHYSIOLOGICAL INQUIRY

- If a full-term fetus is oriented feet-first in the uterus, parturition may not proceed in a timely manner. Why?

Answer can be found at end of chapter.

TABLE 17.10	Some Effects of Prostaglandins* on the Female Reproductive System	
Site of Production	**Action of Prostaglandins**	**Result**
Late antral follicle	Stimulate production of digestive enzymes	Rupture of follicle
Corpus luteum	May interfere with hormone secretion and function	Death of corpus luteum
Uterus	Constrict blood vessels in endometrium	Onset of menstruation
	Cause changes in endometrial blood vessels and cells early in pregnancy	Facilitates implantation
	Increase contraction of myometrium	Helps to initiate both menstruation and parturition
	Cause cervical ripening	Facilitates cervical dilation during parturition

*The term *prostaglandins* is used loosely here, as is customary in reproductive physiology, to include all the eicosanoids.

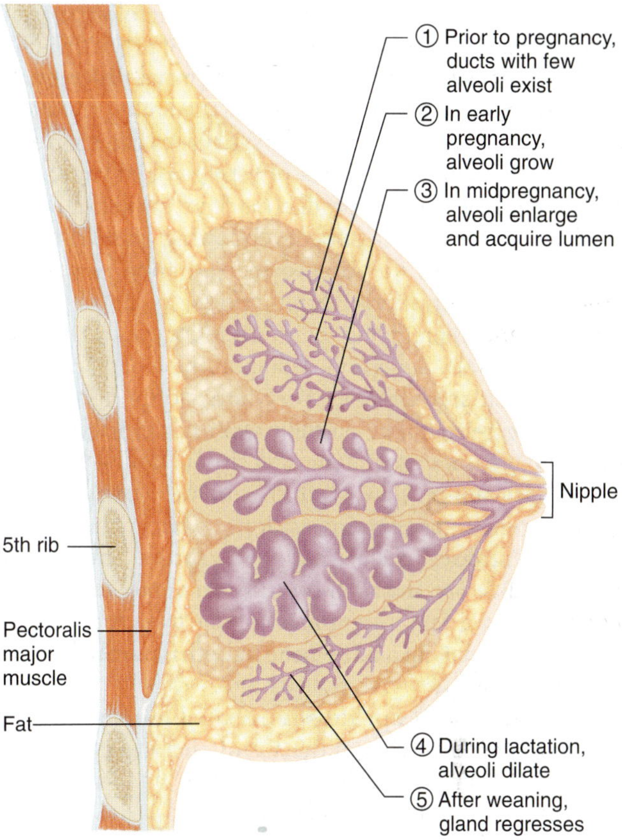

Figure 17.37 APIR Anatomy of the breast. The numbers refer to the sequential changes that occur over time. Adapted from Elias et al.

Lactation

The production and secretion of milk by the **mammary glands,** which are located within the breasts, is called **lactogenesis.** The mammary glands undergo an increase in size and cell number during late pregnancy. After birth of the baby, milk is produced and secreted; this process is also known as **lactation** (or nursing). Each breast contains numerous mammary glands, each with ducts that branch all through the tissue and converge at the nipples (Figure 17.37). These ducts start in saclike structures called **alveoli** (the same term is used to denote the lung air sacs). The breast alveoli, which are the sites of milk secretion, look like bunches of grapes with stems terminating in the ducts. The alveoli and the ducts immediately adjacent to them are surrounded by specialized contractile cells called **myoepithelial cells.**

Before puberty, the breasts are small with little internal glandular structure. With the onset of puberty in females, the increased estrogen concentration stimulates duct growth and branching but relatively little development of the alveoli; much of the breast enlargement at this time is due to fat deposition. Progesterone secretion also commences at puberty during the luteal phase of each cycle, and this hormone contributes to breast growth by stimulating the growth of alveoli.

During each menstrual cycle, the breasts undergo fluctuations in association with the changing blood concentrations of estrogen and progesterone. These changes are small compared with the breast enlargement that occurs during pregnancy as a result of the stimulatory effects of high plasma concentrations of estrogen, progesterone, prolactin, and human placental lactogen. Except for prolactin, which is secreted by the maternal anterior pituitary gland, these hormones are secreted by the placenta. Under the influence of these hormones, both the ductal and the alveolar structures become fully developed.

As described in Chapter 11, other factors influence the anterior pituitary gland cells that secrete prolactin. They are inhibited by **dopamine,** which is secreted by the hypothalamus. They are probably stimulated by at least one **prolactin-releasing factor** (**PRF**), also secreted by the hypothalamus (the chemical identity of PRF in humans is still uncertain). The dopamine and PRF secreted by the hypothalamus are hypophysiotropic hormones that reach the anterior pituitary gland by way of the hypothalamo–hypophyseal portal vessels. This positive and negative hypophysiotropic control of the secretion of prolactin is reminiscent of the dual hypophysiotropic control of growth hormone described in Figure 11.28 and is an example of the general principle of physiology that functions are controlled by multiple regulatory systems, often acting in opposition.

Under the dominant inhibitory influence of dopamine, prolactin secretion is low before puberty. It then increases considerably at puberty in girls but not in boys, stimulated by the increased plasma estrogen concentration that occurs at this time. During pregnancy, there is a further large increase in prolactin secretion due to stimulation by estrogen.

Prolactin is the major hormone stimulating the production of milk. However, despite the fact that prolactin concentrations are increased and the breasts are considerably enlarged and fully developed as pregnancy progresses, there is usually no secretion of milk. This is because estrogen and progesterone, in large concentrations, prevent milk production by inhibiting this action of prolactin on the breasts. Therefore, although estrogen causes an increase in the secretion of prolactin and acts with prolactin in promoting breast growth and differentiation, it—along with progesterone—inhibits the ability of prolactin to induce milk production. Delivery removes the source—the placenta—of the large amounts of estrogen and progesterone and, thereby, releases milk production from inhibition.

The decrease in estrogen following parturition also causes *basal* prolactin secretion to decrease from its peak, late-pregnancy concentrations. After several months, prolactin returns toward prepregnancy concentrations even if the mother continues to nurse. Superimposed upon these basal concentrations, however, are large secretory bursts of prolactin during each nursing period. The episodic pulses of prolactin are signals to the breasts to maintain milk production. These pulses usually cease several days after the mother completely stops nursing her infant but continue as long as nursing continues.

The reflexes mediating the surges of prolactin (**Figure 17.38**) are initiated by afferent input to the hypothalamus from nipple receptors stimulated by suckling. This input's major effect is to inhibit the hypothalamic neurons that release dopamine.

One other reflex process is essential for lactation. Milk is secreted into the lumen of the alveoli, but the infant cannot

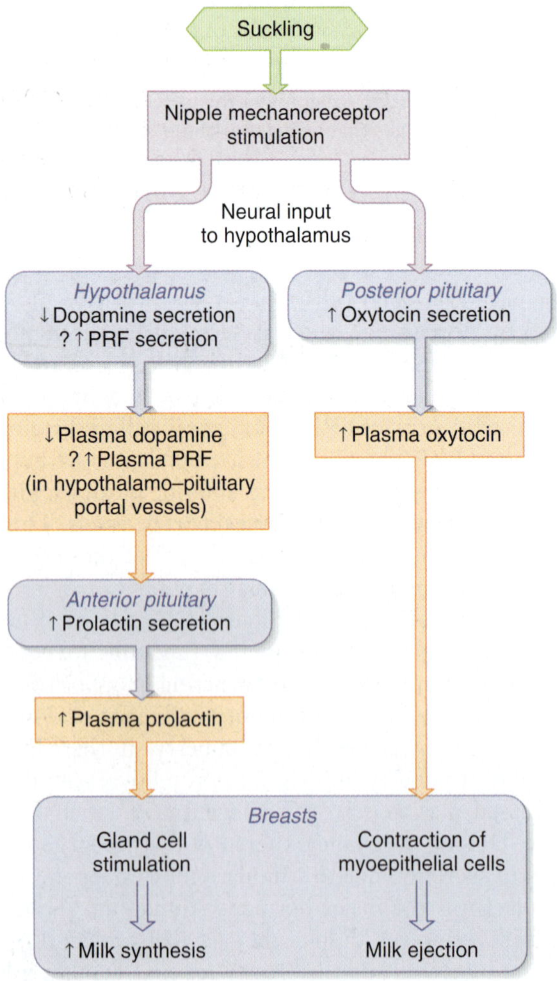

Figure 17.38 Major controls of the secretion of prolactin and oxytocin during nursing. The importance of PRF (prolactin-releasing factors) in humans is not known (indicated by ?).

suck the milk out of the breast. It must first be moved into the ducts, from which it can be suckled. This movement is called the **milk ejection reflex** (also called milk letdown) and is accomplished by contraction of the myoepithelial cells surrounding the alveoli. The contraction is under the control of oxytocin, which is reflexively released from posterior pituitary gland neurons in response to suckling (see Figure 17.38). Higher brain centers can also exert an important influence over oxytocin release; a nursing mother may actually leak milk when she hears her baby cry or even thinks about nursing.

Suckling also inhibits the hypothalamo–hypophyseal–ovarian axis at a variety of steps, with a resultant block of ovulation. This is probably due to increased prolactin, which directly inhibits gonadotropin secretion, and direct effects on the hypothalamic GnRH neurons. If suckling is continued at high frequency, ovulation can be delayed for months to years. This "natural" birth control may help to space out pregnancies. When supplements are added to the baby's diet and the frequency of suckling is decreased, however, most women will resume ovulation even though they continue to nurse. However, ovulation may resume even without a decrease in nursing. Failure to use adequate birth control may result in an unplanned pregnancy in nursing women.

After delivery, the breasts initially secrete a watery, protein-rich fluid called **colostrum.** After about 24 to 48 hours, the secretion of milk itself begins. Milk contains six major nutrients: water, proteins, lipids, the carbohydrate lactose (milk sugar), minerals, and vitamins.

Colostrum and milk also contain antibodies, leukocytes, and other messengers of the immune system, all of which are important for the protection of the newborn, as well as for longer-term activation of the child's own immune system. Milk also contains many growth factors and hormones thought to help in tissue development and maturation, as well as a large number of neuropeptides and endogenous opioids that may subtly shape the infant's brain and behavior. Some of these substances are synthesized by the breasts themselves, not just transported from blood to milk. The reasons the milk proteins can gain entry to the newborn's blood are that (1) the low gastric acidity of the newborn does not denature them, and (2) the newborn's intestinal epithelium is more permeable to proteins than is the adult epithelium.

Unfortunately, infectious agents, including the virus that causes AIDS, can also be transmitted through breast milk, as can some drugs. For example, the concentration of alcohol in breast milk is approximately the same as in maternal plasma.

Breast-feeding for at least the first 6 to 12 months is strongly advocated by health care professionals. In less-developed countries, where alternative formulas are often either contaminated or nutritionally inadequate because of improper dilution or inadequate refrigeration, breast-feeding significantly reduces infant sickness and mortality. In the United States, effects on infant survival are not usually apparent, but breast-feeding reduces the severity of gastrointestinal infections, has positive effects on mother–infant interaction, is economical, and has long-term health benefits. Cow's milk has many but not all of the constituents of mother's milk—and often in very different concentrations, and it is difficult to duplicate mother's milk in a commercial formula.

Contraception

Physiologically, pregnancy is said to begin not at fertilization but after implantation is complete, approximately one week *after* fertilization. Birth control methods that work prior to implantation are called ***contraceptives*** (Table 17.11). Procedures that cause the death of the embryo or fetus after implantation are called ***abortions;*** chemical substances used to induce abortions are called ***abortifacients.***

Some forms of contraception, such as vasectomy, tubal ligation, vaginal diaphragms, vaginal caps, spermicides, and condoms, prevent sperm from reaching the egg. In addition, condoms significantly reduce the risk of ***sexually transmitted diseases*** (***STDs***) such as AIDS, syphilis, gonorrhea, chlamydia, and herpes.

Oral contraceptives are based on the fact that estrogen and progesterone can inhibit pituitary gland gonadotropin release, thereby preventing ovulation. One type of oral contraceptive is a combination of a synthetic estrogen and a progesterone-like substance (a progestogen or progestin). Another type is the so-called minipill, which contains only the progesterone-like substance. In actuality, the oral contraceptives, particularly the minipill, do not always prevent ovulation, but they are still effective because they have other contraceptive effects. For example, progestogens affect the composition of the cervical mucus, reducing the ability of the sperm to pass through the cervix, and they also inhibit the estrogen-induced proliferation of the endometrium, making it inhospitable for implantation. There are now many different other types of oral contraceptive pills that utilize different timing, combinations, and doses of hormones. An extensive discussion of these is beyond the depth of this chapter—more details can be found at www.fda.gov.

Another method of delivering a contraceptive progestogen is via tiny capsules that are implanted beneath the skin and last for 5 years. Yet another method is the intramuscular injection of a different progestogen substance (e.g., ***Depo-Provera*** or ***Lunelle***) every 1 to 3 months. Alternate methods of providing highly efficacious hormonal contraception include skin patches and vaginal rings.

The ***intrauterine device*** (***IUD***) works beyond the point of fertilization but before implantation has begun or is complete. The presence of one of these small objects in the uterus somehow interferes with the endometrial preparation for acceptance of the blastocyst.

In addition to the methods used before intercourse (precoital contraception), there are a variety of drugs used within 72 h *after* intercourse (postcoital or emergency contraception). These most commonly interfere with ovulation, transport of the conceptus to the uterus, or implantation. One approach is a high dose of estrogen, or two large doses (12 h apart) of a combined estrogen–progestin oral contraceptive. Another approach has used the drug ***RU 486*** (***mifepristone***), which has antiprogesterone activity because it binds competitively to progesterone receptors in the uterus but does not activate them. Antagonism of progesterone's effects causes the endometrium to erode and the contractions of the fallopian tubes and myometrium to increase. RU 486 can also be used later in pregnancy as an abortifacient.

The ***rhythm method*** uses abstention from sexual intercourse near the time of ovulation. Unfortunately, it is difficult to time ovulation precisely, even with laboratory techniques. For example, the small increase in body temperature or change in vaginal epithelium, both of which are indicators of ovulation, occur only *after* ovulation. This, combined with the

TABLE 17.11 Some Forms of Contraception

Method	First-Year Failure Rate*	Physiological Mechanism of Effectiveness
Barrier methods Condoms (♂ and ♀) Diaphragm/cervical cap (♀)	12%–23%	Prevent sperm from entering uterus
Spermicides (♀)	20%–50%	Kill sperm in the vagina (after insemination)
Sterilization	<0.5%	
Vasectomy (♂)		Prevents sperm from becoming part of seminal fluid
Tubal ligation (♀)		Prevents sperm from reaching egg
Intrauterine device (IUD) (♀)	<3%	Prevents implantation of blastocyst
Estrogens and/or progestins		Prevent ovulation by suppressing LH surge (negative feedback); thicken cervical mucus (prevents sperm from entering uterus); alter endometrium to prevent implantation of blastocyst
Oral contraceptive pill (♀)	3%	
Emergency oral contraception (♀)	1%	
Injectable or implantable progestins (♀)	<0.5%	
Transdermal (skin patch) (♀)	1%–2%	
Vaginal ring (♀)	1%–2%	

*From Hall, J. E., Infertility and Fertility Control, *Harrison's Principles of Internal Medicine*, McGraw-Hill, 2004; Rosen, M., and Cedars, M. I., Female Reproductive Endocrinology and Infertility, *Basic and Clinical Endocrinology*, 7th ed., McGraw-Hill, 2004; ACOG Practice Bulletin, Emergency Contraception, *Obstet. Gynecol.* 2005, 106:1443–52. See also www.fda.gov. Failure rate assumes proper and consistent use.

Notes:
Spermicides are often used in combination with diaphragm/cervical cap and condoms.
Only condoms are effective in preventing sexually transmitted diseases.
The cervical sponge was made available again in 2009.
Rhythm method (abstinence around time of ovulation) and coitus interruptus (withdrawal) are not listed because they are not reliable.
Only total abstinence is 100% effective in preventing pregnancy.

marked variability of the time of ovulation in many women—from day 5 to day 15 of the cycle, explains why the rhythm method has a high failure rate.

There are still no effective chemical agents for male contraception. One potential approach is to decrease gonadotropin concentrations, which would decrease spermatogenesis. Testosterone would then have to be given to maintain libido.

Infertility

Approximately 12% of men and women of reproductive age in the United States are infertile. The numbers of infertile men and women are approximately equal until about age 30, after which infertility becomes more prevalent in women. In many cases, infertility can be successfully treated with drugs, artificial insemination, or corrective surgery.

When the cause of infertility cannot be treated, it can sometimes be circumvented in women by the technique of ***in vitro fertilization.*** First, the woman is injected with drugs that stimulate multiple egg production. Immediately before ovulation, at least one egg is then removed from the ovary via a needle inserted into the ovary through the top of the vagina or the lower abdominal wall. The egg is placed in a dish for several days with sperm. After the fertilized egg has developed into a cluster of two to eight cells, it is then transferred to the woman's uterus. The success rate of this procedure, when one egg is transferred, is only about 15% to 20%.

17.20 Menopause

When a woman is around the age of 50, on average, menstrual cycles become less regular. Ultimately, they cease entirely in all women; this cessation is known as **menopause,** which is a natural and normal event. The phase of life during which menstrual irregularity begins is termed **perimenopause.** It involves many physical and emotional changes accompanying the cessation of reproductive function.

Menopause and the irregular function leading to it are caused primarily by ovarian failure. The ovaries lose their ability to respond to the gonadotropins, mainly because most, if not all, ovarian follicles and eggs have disappeared by this time through atresia. The hypothalamus and anterior pituitary gland continue to function relatively normally as demonstrated by the fact that the gonadotropins are secreted in greater amounts. The main reason for this is that the decreased plasma estrogen and inhibin do not exert as much negative feedback on gonadotropin secretion.

A small amount of estrogen usually persists in plasma beyond menopause, mainly from the peripheral conversion of adrenal androgens to estrogen by aromatase, but the concentration is inadequate to maintain estrogen-dependent tissues. The breasts and genital organs gradually atrophy to a large degree. Thinning and dryness of the vaginal epithelium can cause sexual intercourse to be painful. Because estrogen is a potent bone-protective hormone, significant decreases in bone mass may occur (***osteoporosis***). This results in an increased risk of bone fractures in postmenopausal women. The ***hot flashes*** so typical of menopause are periodic sudden feelings of warmth, dilation of the skin arterioles, and marked sweating. In addition, the incidence of cardiovascular disease increases after menopause. Women have much less coronary artery disease than men until after menopause, when the incidence becomes similar in both sexes, a pattern that is due to the protective effects of estrogen; estrogen exerts beneficial actions on plasma cholesterol and also exerts multiple direct protective actions on vessel walls. Recent studies, however, have questioned the long-term protective effects of estrogen in the prevention of heart disease.

Many of the symptoms associated with menopause, as well as the development of osteoporosis, can be reduced by the administration of estrogen. Recent studies also indicate that estrogen use may reduce the risk of developing Alzheimer disease and may also be useful in the treatment of this disease.

The desirability of administering estrogen to postmenopausal women is controversial, however, because estrogen administration increases the risk of developing uterine endometrial cancer and breast cancer. The increased risk of endometrial cancer can be reduced by the administration of a progestogen along with estrogen, but the progestogen does not influence the risk of breast cancer. The progestogen only slightly lessens estrogen's protective effect against coronary artery disease.

Relevant to the question of hormone-replacement therapy (as well as to the hormonal treatment of breast and uterine cancer) is the development of drugs, such as ***tamoxifen,*** that exert some proestrogenic and some antiestrogenic effects. These drugs are collectively termed ***selective estrogen receptor modulators*** (***SERMs***) because they activate estrogen receptors in certain tissues but not in others; moreover, in these latter tissues, SERMs act as estrogen antagonists. Obviously, the ideal would be to have a SERM that has the proestrogenic effect of protecting against osteoporosis, heart attacks, and Alzheimer disease but opposes the development of breast and uterine cancers. What makes this type of SERM possible? One important contributor is that there are two distinct forms of estrogen receptors, which are affected differentially by different SERMs.

SECTION C SUMMARY

Anatomy

I. The female internal genitalia are the ovaries, fallopian tubes, uterus, cervix, and vagina.

II. The female external genitalia include the mons pubis, labia, clitoris, and vestibule of the vagina. These are also called the vulva.

Ovarian Functions

I. The female gonads, the ovaries, produce eggs and secrete estrogen, progesterone, and inhibin.

II. The two meiotic divisions of oogenesis result in each ovum having 23 chromosomes, in contrast to the 46 of the original oogonia.

III. The follicle consists of the egg, inner layers of granulosa cells surrounding the egg, and outer layers of theca cells.

IV. At the beginning of each menstrual cycle, a group of preantral and early antral follicles continues to develop, but soon only the dominant follicle continues its development to full maturity and ovulation.

V. Following ovulation, the remaining cells of that follicle differentiate into the corpus luteum, which lasts about 10 to 14 days if pregnancy does not occur.

VI. The menstrual cycle can be divided, according to ovarian events, into a follicular phase and a luteal phase, which each lasts approximately 14 days; they are separated by ovulation.

Control of Ovarian Function

I. The menstrual cycle results from a finely tuned interplay of hormones secreted by the ovaries, the anterior pituitary gland, and the hypothalamus.

II. During the early and middle follicular phases, FSH stimulates the granulosa cells to proliferate and secrete estrogen, and LH stimulates the theca cells to proliferate and produce the androgens that the granulosa cells use to make estrogen.
   a. During this time, estrogen exerts negative feedback on the anterior pituitary gland to inhibit the secretion of the gonadotropins. It probably also inhibits the secretion of GnRH by the hypothalamus.
   b. Inhibin preferentially inhibits FSH secretion.

III. During the late follicular phase, plasma estrogen increases to elicit a surge of LH, which then causes, via the granulosa cells, completion of the egg's first meiotic division and cytoplasmic maturation, ovulation, and formation of the corpus luteum.

IV. During the luteal phase, under the influence of small amounts of LH, the corpus luteum secretes progesterone and estrogen. Regression of the corpus luteum results in a cessation of the secretion of these hormones.

V. Secretion of GnRH and the gonadotropins is inhibited during the luteal phase by the combination of progesterone, estrogen, and inhibin.

Uterine Changes in the Menstrual Cycle

I. The ovarian follicular phase is equivalent to the uterine menstrual and proliferative phases, the first day of menstruation being the first day of the cycle. The ovarian luteal phase is equivalent to the uterine secretory phase.
   a. Menstruation occurs when the plasma estrogen and progesterone concentrations decrease as a result of regression of the corpus luteum.
   b. During the proliferative phase, estrogen stimulates growth of the endometrium and myometrium and causes the cervical mucus to be readily penetrable by sperm.
   c. During the secretory phase, progesterone converts the estrogen-primed endometrium to a secretory tissue and makes the cervical mucus relatively impenetrable to sperm. It also inhibits uterine contractions.

Additional Effects of Gonadal Steroids

I. The many effects of estrogen and progesterone are summarized in Table 17.8.

II. Androgens are produced in women and have several functions including growth of pubic and axillary hair.

III. Excess androgen can cause virilization.

Puberty

I. At puberty, the hypothalamo–pituitary–gonadal axis becomes active as a result of a change in brain function that permits increased secretion of GnRH.

II. The first sign of puberty is the appearance of pubic and axillary hair.

Female Sexual Response

I. Sexual intercourse results in increases in blood flow and muscular contractions throughout the body.

II. Androgens appear to be important in libido in women.

Pregnancy

I. After ovulation, the egg is swept into the fallopian tube, where a sperm, having undergone capacitation and the acrosome reaction, fertilizes it.

II. Following fertilization, the egg undergoes its second meiotic division and the nuclei of the egg and sperm fuse. Reactions in the ovum block penetration by other sperm and trigger cell division and embryogenesis.

III. The conceptus undergoes cleavage, eventually becoming a blastocyst, which implants in the endometrium on approximately day 7 after ovulation.
   a. The trophoblast gives rise to the fetal part of the placenta, whereas the inner cell mass develops into the embryo proper.
   b. Although they do not mix, fetal blood and maternal blood both flow through the placenta, exchanging gases, nutrients, hormones, waste products, and other substances.
   c. The fetus is surrounded by amniotic fluid in the amniotic sac.

IV. The progesterone and estrogen required to maintain the uterus during pregnancy come from the corpus luteum for the first 2 months of pregnancy, their secretion stimulated by human chorionic gonadotropin produced by the trophoblast.

V. During the last 7 months of pregnancy, the corpus luteum regresses and the placenta itself produces large amounts of progesterone and estrogen.

VI. The high concentrations of progesterone, in the presence of estrogen, inhibit the secretion of GnRH and thereby that of the gonadotropins, so that menstrual cycles do not occur.

VII. Delivery occurs by rhythmic contractions of the uterus, which first dilate the cervix and then move the infant, followed by the placenta, through the vagina. The contractions are stimulated in part by oxytocin, released from the posterior pituitary gland in a reflex triggered by uterine mechanoreceptors, and by uterine prostaglandins.

VIII. The breasts develop markedly during pregnancy as a result of the combined influences of estrogen, progesterone, prolactin, and human placental lactogen.
   a. Prolactin secretion is stimulated during pregnancy by estrogen acting on the anterior pituitary gland, but milk is not synthesized because high concentrations of estrogen and progesterone inhibit the milk-producing action of prolactin on the breasts.
   b. As a result of the suckling reflex, large bursts of prolactin and oxytocin are released during nursing. The prolactin stimulates milk production and the oxytocin causes milk ejection.

Menopause

I. When a woman is around the age of 50, her menstrual cycles become less regular and ultimately disappear—menopause.
   a. The cause of menopause is a decrease in the number of ovarian follicles and their hyporesponsiveness to the gonadotropins.
   b. The symptoms of menopause are largely due to the marked decrease in plasma estrogen concentration.

SECTION C REVIEW QUESTIONS

1. Draw the female reproductive tract.
2. Describe the various stages from oogonium to mature ovum.
3. Describe the progression from a primordial follicle to a dominant follicle.
4. Name three hormones produced by the ovaries and name the cells that produce them.
5. Diagram the changes in plasma concentrations of estrogen, progesterone, LH, and FSH during the menstrual cycle.

6. What are the analogies between the granulosa cells and the Sertoli cells and between the theca cells and the Leydig cells?
7. List the effects of FSH and LH on the follicle.
8. Describe the effects of estrogen and inhibin on gonadotropin secretion during the early, middle, and late follicular phases.
9. List the effects of the LH surge on the egg and the follicle.
10. What are the effects of the sex steroids and inhibin on gonadotropin secretion during the luteal phase?
11. Describe the hormonal control of the corpus luteum and the changes that occur in the corpus luteum in a nonpregnant cycle and in a cycle when pregnancy occurs.
12. What happens to the sex steroids and the gonadotropins as the corpus luteum degenerates?
13. Compare the phases of the menstrual cycle according to uterine and ovarian events.
14. Describe the effects of estrogen and progesterone on the endometrium, cervical mucus, and myometrium.
15. Describe the uterine events associated with menstruation.
16. List the effects of estrogen on the accessory sex organs and secondary sex characteristics.
17. List the effects of progesterone on the breasts, cervical mucus, vaginal epithelium, and body temperature.
18. What are the sources and effects of androgens in women?
19. How does the egg get from the ovary to a fallopian tube?
20. Where does fertilization normally occur?
21. Describe the events that occur during fertilization.
22. How many days after ovulation does implantation occur, and in what stage is the conceptus at that time?
23. Describe the structure of the placenta and the pathways for exchange between maternal and fetal blood.
24. State the sources of estrogen and progesterone during different stages of pregnancy. What is the dominant estrogen of pregnancy, and how is it produced?
25. What is the state of gonadotropin secretion during pregnancy, and what is the cause?
26. What anatomical feature permits coordinated contractions of the myometrium?
27. Describe the mechanisms and messengers that contribute to parturition.
28. List the effects of prostaglandins on the female reproductive system.
29. Describe the development of the breasts after puberty and during pregnancy, and list the major hormones responsible.
30. Describe the effects of estrogen on the secretion and actions of prolactin during pregnancy.
31. Diagram the suckling reflex for prolactin release.
32. Diagram the milk ejection reflex.
33. List two main types of amenorrhea and give examples of each.
34. What is the state of estrogen and gonadotropin secretion before puberty and after menopause?
35. List the hormonal and anatomical changes that occur after menopause.

SECTION C KEY TERMS

acrosome reaction 637
afterbirth 644
alveoli 645
amnion 639
amniotic cavity 639
amniotic fluid 639
amniotic sac 639
antrum 626
atresia 626
blastocyst 637
block to polyspermy 637
capacitation 636
cervix 624
chorion 638
chorionic villi 639
cleavage 637
clitoris 625
colostrum 646
conceptus 637
congenital 639
corpus luteum 627
cortical reaction 637
cumulus oophorus 627
dominant follicle 626
dopamine 645
egg 624
embryo 637
endometrium 632
estrogen priming 634
fallopian tube 624
female external genitalia 624
female internal genitalia 624
fertilization 636
fetus 637
fimbria 624
follicle 626
follicular phase 627
fraternal (dizygotic) twins 627
graafian follicle 627
granulosa cell 626
human chorionic gonadotropin (hCG) 641
human placental lactogen 641
hymen 625
implantation 638
inner cell mass 637
lactation 645
lactogenesis 645
LH surge 628
luteal phase 627
mammary gland 645
meiotic arrest 625
menarche 635
menopause 648
menstrual cycle 624
menstrual phase 632
menstruation 624
milk ejection reflex 646
myoepithelial cell 645
myometrium 632
oogenesis 625
oogonium 625
ovulation 624
oxytocin 644
parturition 641
perimenopause 648
placenta 638
primordial follicle 626
prolactin-releasing factor (PRF) 645
proliferative phase 632
relaxin 642
secretory phase 632
sinus 639
stem cells 637
theca 626
totipotent 637
trophoblast 637
umbilical artery 639
umbilical cord 639
umbilical vein 639
uterus 624
vagina 624
vulva 624
zona pellucida 626

SECTION C CLINICAL TERMS

abortifacient 647
abortion 647
amenorrhea 635
amniocentesis 639
anorexia nervosa 635
breech presentation 642
cesarean section 642
chorionic villus sampling 639
contraceptive 647
Depo-Provera 647
Down syndrome 639
dysmenorrhea 633
eclampsia 641
ectopic pregnancy 637
hot flash 648
intrauterine device (IUD) 647
in vitro fertilization 648
Lunelle 647
miscarriage 639
oral contraceptive 647
osteoporosis 648
precocious puberty 635
preeclampsia 641
pregnancy sickness 641
premenstrual dysphoric disorder (PMDD) 634
premenstrual syndrome (PMS) 634
premenstrual tension 634
rhythm method 647
RU 486 (mifepristone) 647
selective estrogen receptor modulators (SERMs) 648
sexually transmitted disease (STD) 647
tamoxifen 648
teratogen 640
toxemia of pregnancy 641
virilization 634

Clinical Case Study: Cessation of Menstrual Cycles in a 21-Year-Old College Student

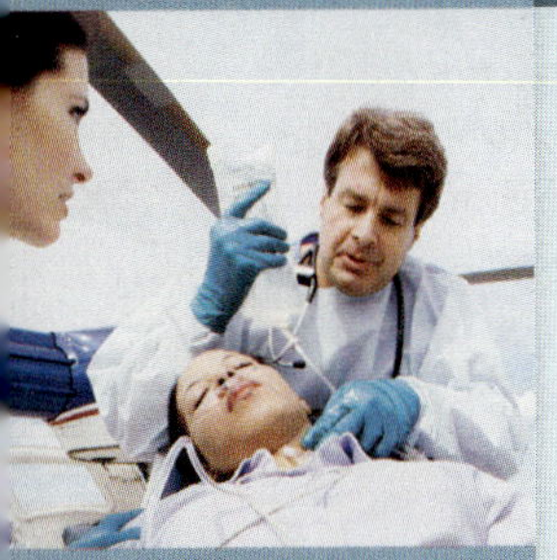

A 21-year-old female college student underwent menarche at 13 years of age. After 5 years of normal menses, her menstrual periods became less frequent and finally stopped (***secondary amenorrhea***). She does not use oral contraception nor is she sexually active, and a urine pregnancy test is negative. She also complains of headaches in the front of her head. During a physical examination by her family practitioner, a milky discharge can be expressed from both nipples. The clinician also finds that the patient has loss of temporal (peripheral) vision in both eyes. A pituitary gland tumor secreting prolactin is suspected. A magnetic resonance image (MRI) reveals the presence of a pituitary gland tumor, and when a blood test for prolactin concentration comes back very high, the diagnosis of *hyperprolactinemia* (excess prolactin in the blood) is confirmed.

Tumors of the lactotrophs of the anterior pituitary gland can hypersecrete prolactin, which in turn suppresses LH and FSH secretion. Thus, menstrual cycles cannot continue because gonadotropin concentrations are low. This is often accompanied by ***galactorrhea***—inappropriate milk production—because prolactin stimulates the mammary gland. Prolactin-secreting tumors (***prolactinomas***) are the most common of the functioning pituitary gland tumors. (Recall from Chapter 11 that pituitary gland tumors arising from different pituitary gland cell types can secrete other pituitary gland hormones—such as growth hormone, causing gigantism and acromegaly, and ACTH, causing Cushing's disease.) If the tumor becomes large enough, it can cause headaches due to stretching of the dura mater near the pituitary gland. The mechanism of the loss of vision in our patient is shown in **Figure 17.39.** The pituitary gland is located just below the optic chiasm. As the tumor grows, it can press on the optic chiasm, interrupting afferent nerve transmission. Because the nerves from the medial parts of the retina cross just above the pituitary gland, they are usually most affected by compression from pituitary gland tumors. As illustrated in the figure, the loss of afferent input from the medial parts of the retina leads to a loss of lateral vision in both eyes. Hyperprolactinemia is usually treated with dopamine agonists such as bromocriptine or

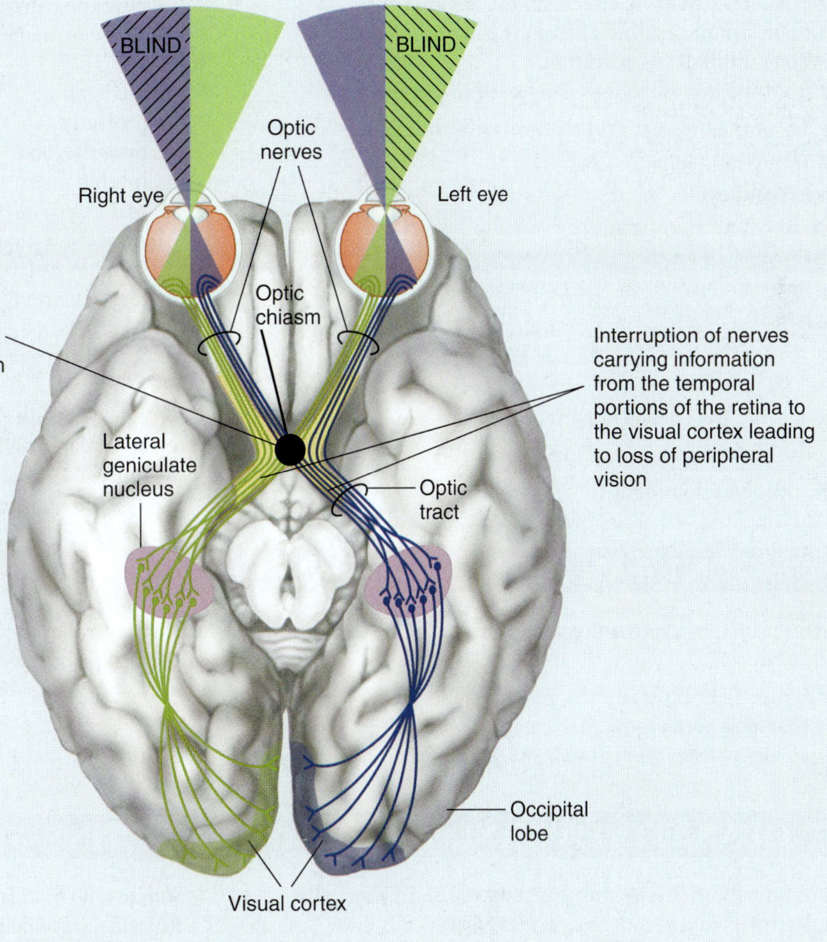

Figure 17.39 Mechanism of loss of lateral visual fields due to a large pituitary gland tumor pressing up from below on the optic chiasm. Refer back to Figure 7.31 for details about the optic tracts and chiasm. This view is from below the brain.

(continued)

(continued)

cabergoline, because prolactin is primarily under the inhibitory control of hypothalamic dopamine. Not only do dopamine agonists decrease the concentrations of prolactin in the blood, but they often lead to a shrinking of the pituitary gland tumor, thus relieving the compression of the optic chiasm with the accompanying restoration of vision. If the pituitary gland tumor is very large or if it does not shrink adequately with medical therapy, pituitary gland surgery may be necessary to remove as much of the tumor as possible. Our patient was treated with cabergoline; fortunately, the tumor gradually got smaller over several months, her visual fields improved, her blood prolactin concentrations normalized, and her menstrual periods returned to normal. Her physician measures her plasma prolactin concentrations every 6 months to monitor for a recurrence of tumor growth.

Clinical terms: galactorrhea, prolactinoma, secondary amenorrhea

See Chapter 19 for complete, integrative case studies.

CHAPTER 17 TEST QUESTIONS

Answers found in Appendix A.

1. Development of normal female internal and external genitalia requires
   a. Müllerian-inhibiting substance.
   b. expression of the *SRY* gene.
   c. insensitivity to circulating testosterone.
   d. complete absence of testosterone.
   e. absence of a Y chromosome.
2. Which is *not* characteristic of a normal postpubertal male?
   a. Inhibin from the Sertoli cells decreases FSH secretion.
   b. Testosterone has paracrine effects on the Sertoli cells.
   c. Testosterone stimulates GnRH from the hypothalamus.
   d. Testosterone inhibits LH secretion.
   e. GnRH from the hypothalamus is released in pulses.

3–7. Match the day of the menstrual cycle (a–e) with the event (3–7; use each answer once).

Day of menstrual cycle:

a. day 1
b. day 7
c. day 13
d. day 23
e. day 26

Event:

3. Progesterone from the corpus luteum peaks.
4. Estrogen positive feedback is peaking.
5. One follicle becomes dominant.
6. Estrogen and progesterone are both decreasing.
7. Increase in FSH stimulates antral follicles to begin to secrete estrogen.
8. The Leydig cell is primarily characterized by
   a. aromatization of testosterone.
   b. secretion of inhibin.
   c. secretion of testosterone.
   d. expression of receptors only to FSH.
   e. transformation into the corpus luteum.
9. During the third trimester of pregnancy, the placenta is *not* the primary source of which hormone in maternal blood?
   a. estrogen
   b. prolactin
   c. progesterone
   d. inhibin
   e. hCG
10. Menopause is characterized primarily by
    a. primary ovarian failure.
    b. loss of estrogen secretion from the ovary due to a decrease in LH.
    c. loss of estrogen secretion from the ovary due to a decrease in FSH.
    d. a decrease in FSH and LH due to increased inhibin.
    e. a decrease in FSH and LH due to a decrease in GnRH pulses.

CHAPTER 17 GENERAL PRINCIPLES ASSESSMENT

Answers found in Appendix A.

1. What general principle of physiology is illustrated in Figures 17.2 and 17.3?
2. How does Figure 17.15 illustrate the general principle of physiology that *most physiological functions are controlled by multiple regulatory systems, often working in opposition?*
3. List several examples from Table 17.9 that demonstrate the general principle of physiology that *the functions of organ systems are coordinated with each other.*

CHAPTER 17 QUANTITATIVE AND THOUGHT QUESTIONS

Answers found at www.mhhe.com/widmaier13.

1. What symptom will be common to a person whose Leydig cells have been destroyed and to a person whose Sertoli cells have been destroyed? What symptom will not be common?
2. A male athlete taking large amounts of an androgenic steroid becomes sterile (unable to produce sperm capable of causing fertilization). Explain.
3. A man who is sterile (infertile) is found to have the following: no evidence of demasculinization, an increased blood concentration of FSH, and a normal plasma concentration of LH. What is the most likely basis of his infertility?
4. If you were a scientist trying to develop a male contraceptive acting on the anterior pituitary gland, would you try to

block the secretion of FSH or LH? Explain the reason for your choice.

5. A 30-year-old man has very small muscles, a sparse beard, and a high-pitched voice. His plasma concentration of LH is elevated. Explain the likely cause of all these findings.
6. There are disorders of the adrenal cortex in which excessive amounts of androgens are produced. If any of these occur in a woman, what will happen to her menstrual cycles?
7. Women with inadequate secretion of GnRH are often treated for their infertility with drugs that mimic the action of this hormone. Can you suggest a possible reason that such treatment is often associated with multiple births?
8. Which of the following would be a signal that ovulation is soon to occur: the cervical mucus becoming thick and sticky, an increase in body temperature, or a marked rise in plasma LH?
9. The absence of what phenomenon would interfere with the ability of sperm obtained by masturbation to fertilize an egg in a test tube?
10. If a woman 7 months pregnant is found to have a marked decrease in plasma estrogen but a normal plasma progesterone for that time of pregnancy, what would you conclude?
11. What types of drugs might you work on if you were trying to develop one to stop premature labor?
12. If a genetic male failed to produce MIS during fetal life, what would the result be?
13. Could the symptoms of menopause be treated by injections of FSH and LH?

CHAPTER 17 ANSWERS TO PHYSIOLOGICAL INQUIRIES

Figure 17.4 These drugs would be absorbed by the pregnant woman and cross the placenta to enter the fetal circulation. These drugs would block production of dihydrotestosterone in target tissues with 5-α-reductase activity, thereby interfering with the development of normal sexual differentiation of the penis, scrotum, and prostate in the male fetus.

Figure 17.7 In the short term, there would be a decrease in sex hormone secretion that, because of a reduction in negative feedback, would result in an increase in GnRH secretion from the hypothalamus and LH and FSH from the anterior pituitary gland. Because of the trophic effects of LH and FSH, in the long term, this would eventually increase the size and function of the remaining gonad. This results in a restoration of sex hormone concentrations in the blood to normal. (See Chapter 11 for a general description of the effects of tropic/trophic anterior pituitary gland hormones.)

Figure 17.15 Testosterone alone usually does not restore spermatogenesis to normal. FSH is necessary to stimulate spermatogenesis from the Sertoli cell independently of local testosterone production. Furthermore, giving testosterone as a drug is usually not sufficient to replace the local production of testosterone in the testes necessary to maintain spermatogenesis. Therefore, gonadotropins with a mixture of activity for receptors to LH (to stimulate local testosterone production) and FSH (to stimulate the Sertoli cells) usually must be given to restore spermatogenesis.

Figure 17.22 (1) FSH increases because the corpus luteum is degenerating. The loss of the negative feedback by progesterone and estrogen from the corpus luteum relieves the pituitary gland of this inhibitory effect and allows FSH to increase, thus stimulating a group of follicles for the next menstrual cycle. (2) If conception occurs and the developing blastocyst implants (pregnancy), the trophoblast cells of the implanted blastocyst release a gonadotropin—human chorionic gonadotropin (hCG)—into the maternal blood, thus rescuing the corpus luteum in very early pregnancy. Production of progesterone from the corpus luteum of pregnancy prevents menses and the loss of the implanted embryo. The measurement of hCG in maternal blood or urine is the basis of the pregnancy test.

Figure 17.24 The increased pituitary gland gonadotropins suggest a lack of estrogen and inhibin negative feedback, pointing to premature ovarian failure as a diagnosis. One cause of premature ovarian failure is autoimmune ovarian destruction. Like Graves' disease and Addison's disease (see Chapters 11 and 19), premature ovarian failure is a form of endocrine autoimmunity.

Figure 17.32 Measurement of a protein specific to fetal blood in a maternal blood sample, such as fetal hemoglobin, would be evidence that fetal blood is leaking into the maternal circulation.

Figure 17.34 hCG stimulates progesterone and estrogen from the corpus luteum early in pregnancy. The placenta takes over this function during the second trimester of pregnancy such that most of the maternal estrogen and progesterone later in pregnancy is from the placenta. Placental production of these steroids does not require gonadotropin stimulation.

Figure 17.36 The feet may not provide sufficient cervical stretch to maintain the positive feedback stimulation of oxytocin and uterine contraction.

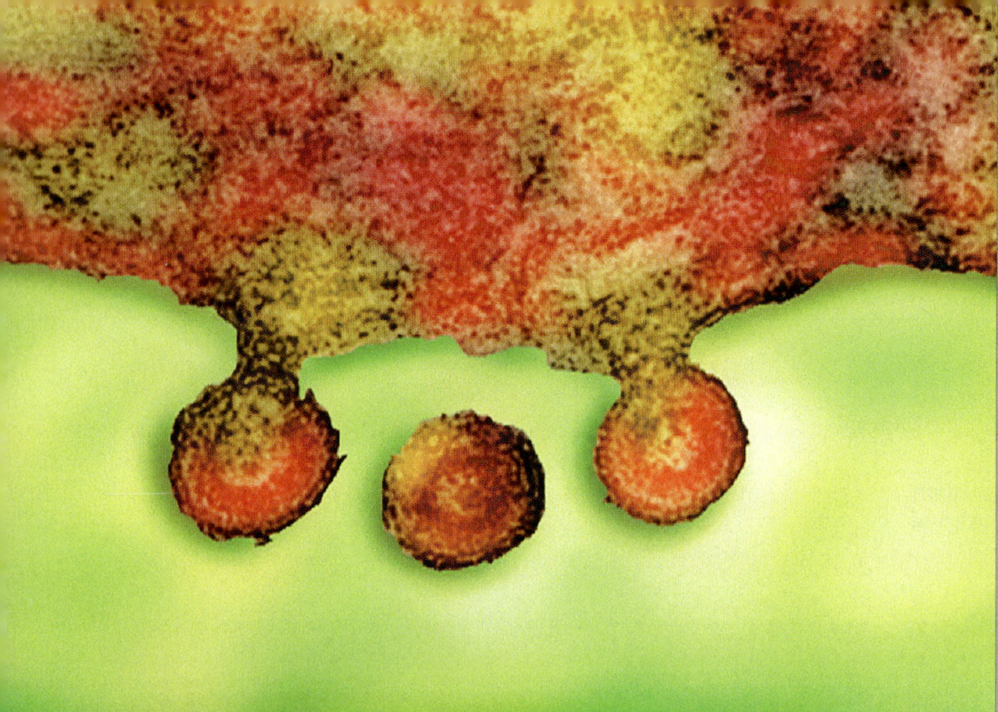

Human immunodeficiency viruses budding from a T cell.

18 The Immune System

You have learned about numerous organ systems in previous chapters, some of which, such as the digestive system, consist of anatomically connected organs. By contrast, the **immune system** consists of a diverse collection of disease-fighting cells found in the blood and lymph and in tissues and organs throughout the body. **Immunology** is the study of the physiological defenses by which the body (the host) recognizes itself from nonself (foreign matter). In the process, foreign matter, both living and nonliving, is destroyed or rendered harmless. In distinguishing self from nonself, immune defenses (1) protect against infection by **pathogens**—viruses, and **microbes** including bacteria, fungi, and eukaryotic parasites; (2) isolate or remove foreign substances; and (3) destroy cancer cells that arise in the body, a function known as **immune surveillance.**

Immune defenses, or immunity, can be classified into two categories, innate and adaptive, which interact with each other. **Innate immune responses** defend against foreign substances or cells without having to recognize their specific identities. The mechanisms of protection used by these defenses are not unique to the particular foreign substance or cell. For this reason, innate immune responses are also known as nonspecific immune responses. **Adaptive immune responses** depend upon specific recognition by lymphocytes of the substance or cell to be attacked. For this reason, adaptive immune responses are also called specific immune responses. Innate and adaptive immune responses function together. For example, components of innate immunity provide instructions that activate the cells that carry out adaptive responses.

The pathogens with which we will be most concerned in this chapter are bacteria and viruses. These are the dominant infectious agents in the United States and other industrialized nations. On a global basis, however, infections with parasitic eukaryotic organisms are responsible for a huge amount of illness and death. For example, several hundred million people now have malaria, a disease caused by infection with protists of the *Plasmodium* genus.

Bacteria are unicellular organisms that have an outer coating (the cell wall) in addition to a plasma membrane but no intracellular membrane-bound organelles. Bacteria can damage tissues at the sites of bacterial replication, or they can release toxins that enter the blood and disrupt physiological functions in other parts of the body.

Viruses are essentially nucleic acids surrounded by a protein coat. Unlike bacteria, viruses lack the enzyme machinery for metabolism and the ribosomes essential for protein synthesis. Consequently, they cannot multiply by themselves but must exist inside other cells and use the molecular apparatuses of those cells. The viral nucleic acid directs the host cell to synthesize the proteins required for viral replication, with the required nucleotides and energy sources also supplied by the host cell. The effect of viral habitation and replication within a cell depends on the type of virus. After entering a cell, some viruses (the common cold virus, for example) multiply rapidly, kill the cell, and then move on to other cells. Other viruses, such as the one that causes genital herpes, can lie dormant in infected cells before suddenly undergoing the rapid replication that causes cell damage. Finally, certain viruses can transform their host cells into cancer cells.

Of the general principles of physiology described in Chapter 1, one that is fundamental to the immune system is the principle that homeostasis is essential for health and survival. Indeed, illness can often be thought of as a disruption in one or more homeostatic processes. A key way in which the immune system regulates homeostasis is via cell-to-cell signaling. As you read this chapter, therefore, consider also how this general principle of physiology applies: Information flow between cells, tissues, and organs is an essential feature of homeostasis and allows for integration of physiological processes.

18.1 Cells and Secretions Mediating Immune Defenses

We begin our survey of the human immune system with an overview of some of the key cells and cellular secretions that make up the innate and adaptive immune responses. The appearance, production, and blood concentrations of immune cells were introduced in Section F of Chapter 12 and should be reviewed at this time.

Immune Cells

The cells of the immune system are the various types of white blood cells collectively known as **leukocytes;** representative histological appearances of some of these can be seen in the human blood smear in **Figure 18.1** (also refer back to Figure 12.67). Unlike erythrocytes, leukocytes can leave the circulatory system to enter the tissues where they function. Leukocytes can be classified into two groups: myeloid cells and lymphoid cells. The myeloid cells include the **neutrophils, basophils, eosinophils,** and **monocytes,** all of whose functions will be described later. Lymphoid cells include several types of **lymphocytes,** including **B lymphocytes (B cells), T lymphocytes (T cells), natural killer (NK) cells,** and **plasma cells.** Plasma cells are not really a distinct cell type but differentiate from B lymphocytes during immune responses. The major functions of plasma cells are to synthesize and secrete antibodies. The functions of the other lymphocytes will be described shortly.

Other immune cells include **macrophages;** these are found in virtually all organs and tissues, their structures varying somewhat from location to location. They are derived from monocytes that pass through the walls of blood vessels to enter the tissues and transform into macrophages. In keeping with one of their major functions, the engulfing of particles and pathogens by **phagocytosis** (the form of endocytosis whereby a cell engulfs and usually destroys particulate matter), macrophages are strategically placed where they will encounter their targets. For example, they are found in large numbers in the various epithelia in contact with the external environment, such as the skin and internal surfaces of respiratory and digestive system tubes. In several organs, they line the vessels through which blood or lymph flows.

There are also cell populations that are not macrophages but exert certain macrophage-like functions such as phagocytosis. These are termed **dendritic cells** because of the characteristic extensions from their plasma membranes at certain stages of their life cycle (not to be confused with the dendrites found on neurons). They are highly motile and are found

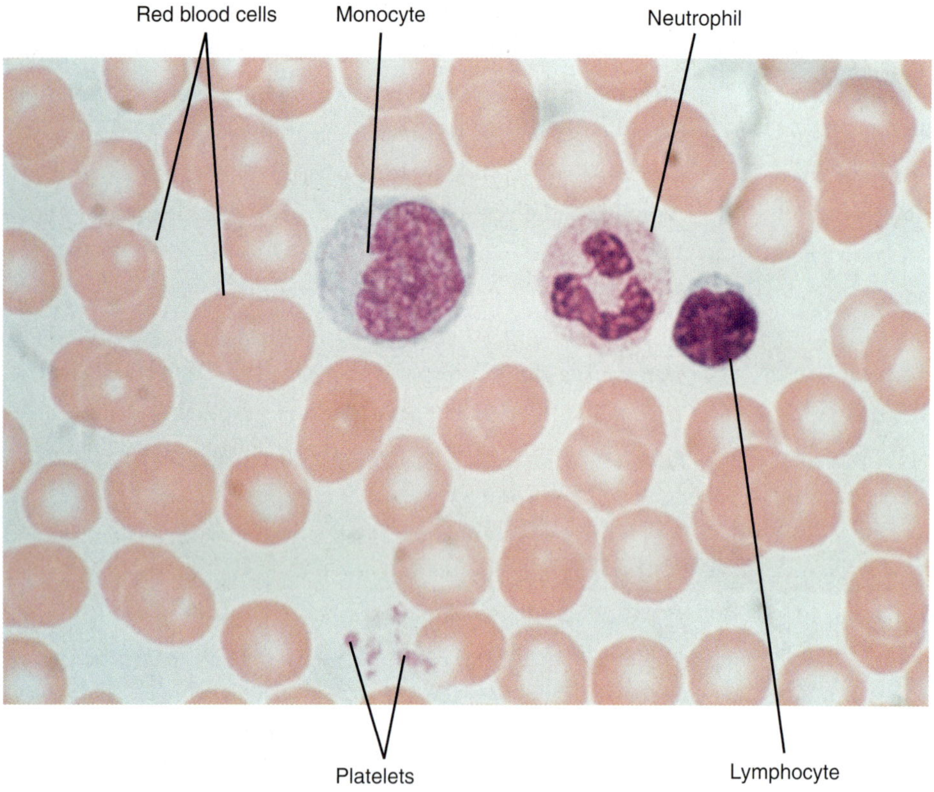

Figure 18.1 AP|R A light micrograph of a human blood smear showing the histological appearance of a few types of leukocytes along with numerous red blood cells and platelets.

scattered in almost all tissues, but particularly at sites where the internal and external environments meet, such as the digestive tract. Upon activation, dendritic cells process phagocytosed pathogens and migrate through the lymphatic vessels to secondary lymphoid organs where they activate T cells.

Mast cells are found throughout connective tissues, particularly beneath the epithelial surfaces of the body. They are derived from the differentiation of a unique set of bone marrow cells that have entered the blood and then left the blood vessels to enter connective tissue, where they differentiate and undergo cell division. Consequently, mature mast cells—unlike basophils, with which they share many characteristics—are not normally found in the blood. The most striking anatomical feature of mast cells is their very large number of cytosolic vesicles, which secrete locally acting chemical messengers such as histamine.

The sites of production and functions of all these cells are briefly listed in **Table 18.1** for reference and will be described in subsequent sections. For now, we emphasize two points. First, lymphocytes serve as recognition cells in adaptive immune responses and are essential for all aspects of these responses. Second, neutrophils, monocytes, macrophages, and dendritic cells have a variety of activities, but particularly important is their ability to secrete inflammatory mediators and to function as **phagocytes.** A phagocyte denotes any cell capable of phagocytosis.

Cytokines

The cells of the immune system secrete a multitude of protein messengers that regulate host cell division (mitosis) and function in both innate and adaptive immune responses. "**Cytokines**" is the collective term for these messengers, each of which has its own unique name. Cytokines are produced not by distinct specialized glands but rather by a variety of individual cells. The great majority of their actions occur at the site at which they are secreted, the cytokine acting as an autocrine or paracrine substance. In some cases, however, the cytokine circulates in the blood to exert hormonal effects on distant organs and tissues involved in host defenses.

Cytokines link the components of the immune system together. They are the chemical communication network that allows different immune system cells to "talk" to one another. This is called *cross talk*, and it is essential for the precise timing of the functions of the immune system. Most cytokines are secreted by more than one type of immune system cell and by nonimmune cells as well (for example, by endothelial cells and fibroblasts). This often produces cascades of cytokine secretion, in which one cytokine stimulates the release of another, and so on. Any given cytokine may exert actions on an extremely broad range of target cells. For example, the cytokine interleukin 2 influences the function of most cells of the immune system. There is great redundancy in cytokine action; that is, different cytokines can have very similar effects. Cytokines are also involved in many nonimmunologic processes, such as bone formation and uterine function.

This chapter will be limited to a discussion of a few of the important cytokines and their most important functions, which are summarized in **Table 18.2**.

18.2 Innate Immune Responses

Innate immune responses defend against foreign cells or matter without having to recognize specific identities. These defenses recognize some *general* molecular property marking the invader as foreign. The most common such identity tags are often found in particular classes of carbohydrates or lipids that are in microbial cell walls. Plasma membrane receptors on certain immune cells, as well as a variety of circulating proteins (particularly a family of proteins called complement), can bind to these carbohydrates and lipids at crucial steps in innate responses. This use of a system based on carbohydrate and lipid for detecting the presence of foreign cells is a key feature that distinguishes innate responses from adaptive ones, which recognize foreign cells mainly by specific proteins the foreign cells produce.

The innate immune responses include defenses at the body surfaces, the response to injury or infection known as *inflammation*, and a family of antiviral proteins called interferons.

TABLE 18.1 Cells Mediating Immune Responses

Name	Site Produced	Functions
Leukocytes (white blood cells)		
Neutrophils	Bone marrow	1. Phagocytosis 2. Release chemicals involved in inflammation (vasodilators, chemotaxins, etc.)
Basophils	Bone marrow	Carry out functions in blood similar to those of mast cells in tissues (see below)
Eosinophils	Bone marrow	1. Destroy multicellular parasites 2. Participate in immediate hypersensitivity reactions
Monocytes	Bone marrow	1. Carry out functions in blood similar to those of macrophages in tissues (see below) 2. Enter tissues and transform into macrophages
Lymphocytes	Mature in bone marrow (B cells and NK cells) and thymus (T cells); activated in peripheral lymphoid organs	Serve as recognition cells in specific immune responses and are essential for all aspects of these responses
B cells		1. Initiate antibody-mediated immune responses by binding specific antigens to the B cell's plasma membrane receptors, which are immunoglobulins 2. Upon activation, are transformed into plasma cells, which secrete antibodies 3. Present antigen to helper T cells
Cytotoxic T cells (CD8 cells)		Bind to antigens on plasma membrane of target cells (virus-infected cells, cancer cells, and tissue transplants) and directly destroy the cells
Helper T cells (CD4 cells)		Secrete cytokines that help to activate B cells, cytotoxic T cells, NK cells, and macrophages
NK cells		1. Bind directly and nonspecifically to virus-infected cells and cancer cells and kill them 2. Function as killer cells in antibody-dependent cellular cytotoxicity (ADCC)
Plasma cells	Peripheral lymphoid organs; differentiate from B cells during immune responses	Secrete antibodies
Macrophages	Bone marrow; reside in almost all tissues and organs; differentiate from monocytes	1. Phagocytosis 2. Extracellular killing via secretion of toxic chemicals 3. Process and present antigens to helper T cells 4. Secrete cytokines involved in inflammation, activation and differentiation of helper T cells, and systemic responses to infection or injury (the acute phase response)
Dendritic cells	Almost all tissues and organs; microglia in the central nervous system	Phagocytosis, antigen presentation
Mast cells	Bone marrow; reside in almost all tissues and organs; differentiate from bone marrow cells	Release histamine and other chemicals involved in inflammation

TABLE 18.2 Features of Selected* Cytokines			
Cytokine	**Source**	**Target Cells**	**Major Functions**
Interleukin 1, tumor necrosis factor-alpha, and interleukin 6	Antigen-presenting cells such as macrophages	Helper T cells; certain brain cells; numerous systemic cells	Stimulate IL-2 receptor expression; induce fever; stimulate systemic responses to inflammation, infection, and injury
Interleukin 2	Most immune cells	Helper T cells; cytotoxic T cells; NK cells; B cells	Stimulate proliferation Promote conversion to plasma cells
Interferons (type I)	Most cell types	Most cell types	Stimulate cells to produce antiviral proteins (innate response)
Interferons (type II)	NK cells and activated helper T cells	NK cells and macrophages	Stimulate proliferation and secretion of cytotoxic compounds
Chemokines	Damaged cells, including endothelial cells	Neutrophils and other leukocytes	Facilitate accumulation of leukocytes at sites of injury and inflammation
Colony-stimulating factors	Macrophages	Bone marrow	Stimulate proliferation of neutrophils and monocytes

**Note:* This list is not meant to be exhaustive. There are >100 known cytokines.

Defenses at Body Surfaces

Though not immune *responses*, the first lines of defense against pathogens are the barriers offered by surfaces exposed to the external environment, because very few pathogens can penetrate the intact skin. Other specialized surface defenses are the hairs at the entrance to the nose and the cough and sneeze reflexes. The various skin glands, salivary glands, and lacrimal (tear) glands play a more active role in immunity by secreting antimicrobial chemicals. These may include antibodies; enzymes such as lysozyme, which destroys bacterial cell walls; and an iron-binding protein called lactoferrin, which prevents bacteria from obtaining the iron they require to function properly.

The mucus secreted by the epithelial linings of the respiratory and upper gastrointestinal tracts also contains antimicrobial chemicals; more importantly, however, mucus is sticky. Particles that adhere to it are prevented from entering the blood. They are either swept by ciliary action up into the pharynx and then swallowed, as occurs in the upper respiratory tract, or are phagocytosed by macrophages in the various linings. Finally, the acid secretion of the stomach can also kill pathogens, although some bacteria can survive to colonize the large intestine where they provide beneficial gastrointestinal functions.

Inflammation

Inflammation is the local response to infection or injury. The functions of inflammation are to destroy or inactivate foreign invaders and to set the stage for tissue repair. The key mediators are the cells that function as phagocytes. As noted earlier, the most important phagocytes are neutrophils, macrophages, and dendritic cells.

In this section, inflammation is described as it occurs in the innate responses induced by the invasion of pathogens. Most of the same responses can be elicited by a variety of other injuries—cold, heat, and trauma, for example. Moreover, we will see later that inflammation accompanies many *adaptive* immune responses in which the inflammation becomes amplified.

The sequence of local events in a typical innate inflammatory response to a bacterial infection—one caused, for example, by a cut with a bacteria-covered splinter—is summarized in **Figure 18.2**. The familiar signs of tissue injury and inflammation are local redness, swelling, heat, and pain.

The events of inflammation that underlie these signs are induced and regulated by a large number of chemical mediators, some of which are summarized for reference in **Table 18.3** (not all of these will be described in this chapter). Note in this table that some of these mediators are cytokines. Any given event of inflammation, such as vasodilation, may be induced by multiple mediators. Moreover, any given mediator may induce more than one event. Based on their origins, the mediators fall into two general categories: (1) peptides (kinins, for example) generated in the infected area by enzymatic actions on proteins that circulate in the plasma and (2) substances secreted into the extracellular fluid from cells that either already exist in the infected area (injured cells or mast cells, for example) or enter it during inflammation (neutrophils, for example).

Let us now go step by step through the process summarized in Figure 18.2, assuming that the bacterial infection in our example is localized to the tissue just beneath the skin. If the invading bacteria enter the blood or lymph, then similar inflammatory responses would take place in any other tissue or organ the blood-borne or lymph-borne microorganisms reach.

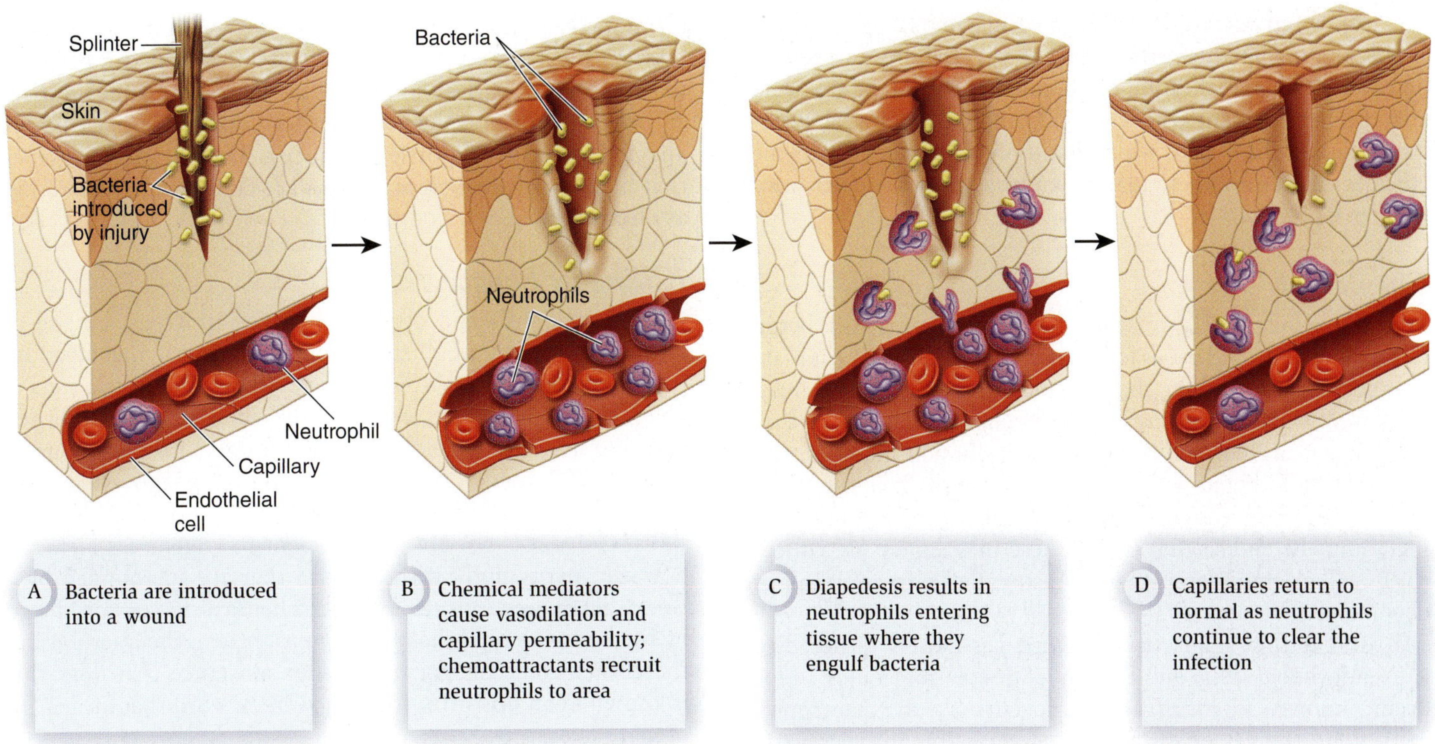

Figure 18.2 APIR The local inflammatory events occurring in response to a wound.

TABLE 18.3 Some Important Local Inflammatory Mediators

Mediator	Source
Kinins	Generated from enzymatic action on plasma proteins
Complement	Generated from enzymatic action on plasma proteins
Products of blood clotting	Generated from enzymatic action on plasma proteins
Histamine	Secreted by mast cells and injured cells
Eicosanoids	Secreted by many cell types including myeloid cells
Platelet-activating factor	Secreted by many cell types including myeloid cells, endothelial cells, platelets, damaged tissue cells
Cytokines, including chemokines	Secreted by activated immune cells, monocytes, macrophages, neutrophils, lymphocytes, and several nonimmune cell types, including endothelial cells and fibroblasts
Lysosomal enzymes, nitric oxide, and other oxygen-derived substances	Secreted by injured cells, neutrophils, and macrophages

Vasodilation and Increased Permeability to Protein

A variety of chemical mediators dilate most of the microcirculation vessels in an infected and/or damaged area. The mediators also cause the local capillaries and venules to become permeable to proteins by inducing their endothelial cells to contract, opening spaces between them through which the proteins can move.

The adaptive value of these vascular changes is twofold: (1) The increased blood flow to the inflamed area (which accounts for the redness and warmth) increases the delivery of proteins and leukocytes; and (2) the increased permeability to protein ensures that the plasma proteins that participate in inflammation—many of which are normally restrained by the intact endothelium—can gain entry to the interstitial fluid.

By mechanisms described in Chapter 12 (see Figure 12.42), the vasodilation and increased permeability to protein, however, cause net filtration of plasma into the interstitial fluid and the development of edema. This accounts for the swelling in an inflamed area, which is simply a consequence of the changes in the microcirculation and has no known adaptive value of its own.

Chemotaxis

With the onset of inflammation, circulating neutrophils begin to move out of the blood across the endothelium of capillaries and venules to enter the inflamed area (see Figure 18.2). This multistage process is known as **chemotaxis.** It involves a variety of protein and carbohydrate adhesion molecules on both the endothelial cell and the neutrophil. It is regulated by messenger molecules released by cells in the injured area, including the endothelial cells. These messengers are collectively called **chemoattractants** (also called **chemotaxins** or chemotactic factors).

In the first stage, the neutrophil is loosely tethered to the endothelial cells by certain adhesion molecules. This event, known as **margination,** occurs as the neutrophil rolls along the vessel surface. In essence, this initial reversible event exposes the neutrophil to chemoattractants being released in the injured area. These chemoattractants act on the neutrophil to induce the rapid appearance of another class of adhesion molecules in its plasma membrane—molecules that bind tightly to their matching molecules on the surface of endothelial cells. As a result, the neutrophils collect along the site of injury rather than being washed away with the flowing blood.

In the next stage, known as **diapedesis,** a narrow projection of the neutrophil is inserted into the space between two endothelial cells, and the entire neutrophil squeezes through the endothelial wall and into the interstitial fluid. In this way, huge numbers of neutrophils migrate into the inflamed area. Once in the interstitial fluid, neutrophils follow a chemotactic gradient and migrate toward the site of tissue damage (chemotaxis). This occurs because pathogen-stimulated innate immune cells release chemoattractants. As a result, neutrophils tend to move toward the pathogens that entered into an injured area.

Movement of leukocytes from the blood into the damaged area is not limited to neutrophils. Monocytes follow later; once in the tissue, they undergo anatomical and functional changes that transform them to macrophages. As we will see later, lymphocytes undergo chemotaxis in adaptive immune responses, as do basophils and eosinophils under certain conditions.

An important aspect of the multistep chemotaxis process is that it provides selectivity and flexibility for the migration of the various leukocyte types. Multiple adhesion molecules that are relatively distinct for the different leukocytes are controlled by different sets of chemoattractants. Particularly important in this regard are those cytokines that function as chemoattractants for distinct subsets of leukocytes. For example, one type of cytokine stimulates the chemotaxis of neutrophils, whereas another stimulates that of eosinophils. Consequently, subsets of leukocytes can be stimulated to enter particular tissues at designated times during an inflammatory response, depending on the type of invader and the cytokine response it induces. The various cytokines that have chemoattractant actions are collectively referred to as **chemokines.**

Killing by Phagocytes

Once neutrophils and other leukocytes arrive at the site of an infection, they begin the process of destroying invading pathogens by phagocytosis (**Figure 18.3**). The initial step in phagocytosis is contact between the surfaces of the phagocyte and microbe. One of the major triggers for phagocytosis during this contact is the interaction of phagocyte receptors with certain carbohydrates or lipids in the microbial cell walls. Contact is not always sufficient to trigger engulfment, however, particularly with bacteria that are surrounded by a thick, gelatinous capsule. Instead, chemical factors produced by the body can bind the phagocyte tightly to the microbe and thereby enhance phagocytosis. Any substance that does this is known as an **opsonin,** from the Greek word that means "to prepare for eating."

As the phagocyte engulfs the microbe (**Figure 18.4**), the internal, microbe-containing sac formed in this step is called a **phagosome.** A layer of plasma membrane separates the microbe from the cytosol of the phagocyte. The phagosome membrane then makes contact with one of the phagocyte's lysosomes, which is filled with a variety of hydrolytic enzymes. The membranes of the phagosome and lysosome fuse, and the combined vesicles are now called a **phagolysosome.** Inside the phagolysosome, the lysosomal enzymes break down the microbe's macromolecules. In addition, other enzymes in the phagolysosome membrane produce **nitric oxide** as well as **hydrogen peroxide** and other oxygen derivatives, all of which are extremely destructive to the microbe's macromolecules.

Such intracellular destruction is not the only way phagocytes can kill pathogens. The phagocytes also release antimicrobial substances into the extracellular fluid, where these chemicals can destroy the pathogens without prior phagocytosis. Some of these substances (for example, nitric oxide) secreted into the extracellular fluid (**Figure 18.5**) also function as inflammatory mediators. Thus, when phagocytes enter the area and encounter pathogens, positive feedback mechanisms cause inflammatory mediators, including chemokines, to be released that bring in more phagocytes.

Complement

The family of plasma proteins known as **complement** provides another means for extracellular killing of pathogens without prior phagocytosis. Certain complement proteins are always circulating in the blood in an inactive state. Upon activation of a complement protein in response to infection or damage, a cascade occurs so that this active protein activates a second complement protein, which activates a third, and so on. In this

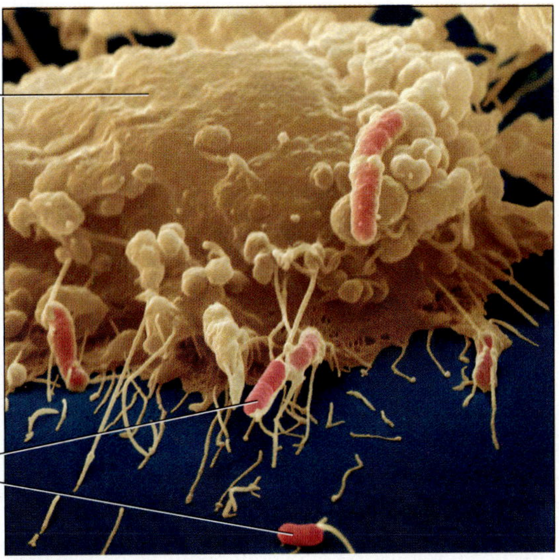

Figure 18.3 APIR Macrophage contacting bacteria and preparing to engulf them.

way, multiple active complement proteins are generated in the extracellular fluid of the infected area from inactive complement molecules that have entered from the blood. Because this system consists of at least 30 distinct proteins, it is extremely complex, and we will identify the roles of only a few of the individual complement proteins.

The central protein in the complement cascade is C3. Activation of C3 initiates a series of events. The first is the deposition of **C3b,** a component of C3, on the microbial surface. C3b acts as an opsonin that is recognized by phagocytes targeting the pathogen for destruction, as shown for a bacterium in **Figure 18.6**. C3b is also part of a proteolytic enzyme that amplifies the complement cascade and leads to the downstream development of a multiunit protein called the **membrane attack complex** (**MAC**). The MAC embeds itself in the bacterial plasma membrane and forms porelike channels in the membrane, making it leaky. Water, ions, and small molecules enter the microbe, which disrupts the intracellular environment and kills the microbe.

In addition to supplying a means for direct killing of pathogens, the complement system serves other important functions in inflammation (**Figure 18.7**). Some of the activated complement molecules along the cascade cause, either directly or indirectly (by stimulating the release of other inflammatory mediators), vasodilation, increased microvessel permeability to protein, and chemotaxis.

As we will see later, antibodies, a class of proteins secreted by certain lymphocytes, are required to activate the very first complement protein (C1) in the full sequence known as the **classical complement pathway.** However, lymphocytes are not involved in *nonspecific* inflammation, our present topic. How, then, is the complement sequence initiated during nonspecific inflammation? The answer is that there is an **alternative complement pathway,** one that is not antibody dependent and that bypasses C1. The alternative pathway is initiated as the result of interactions between carbohydrates on the surface of the microbes and inactive complement molecules beyond C1. These

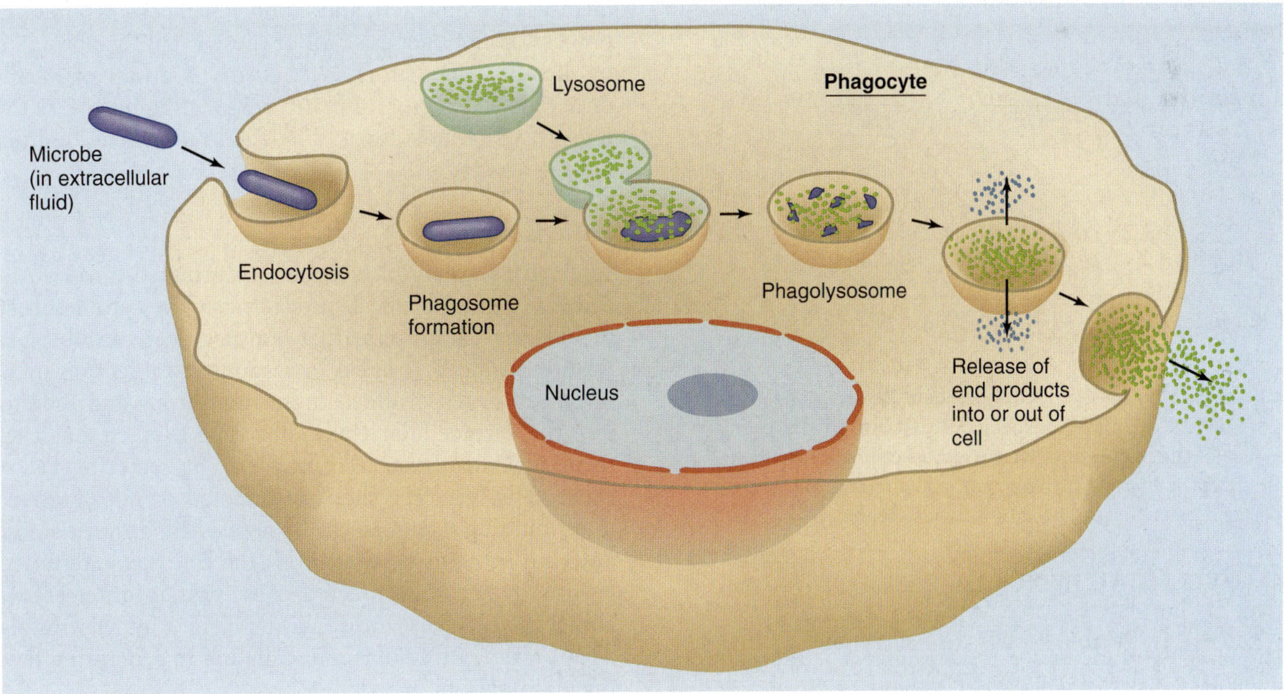

Figure 18.4 APIR Phagocytosis and intracellular destruction of a microbe. After destruction has taken place in the phagolysosome, the end products are released to the outside of the cell by exocytosis or used by the cell for its own metabolism.

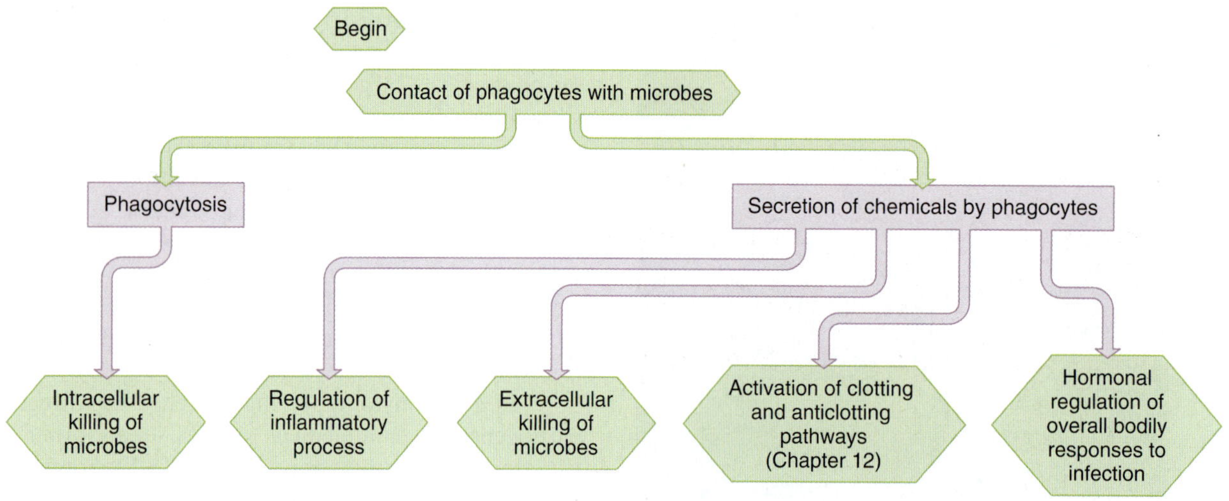

Figure 18.5 APR Role of phagocytes in innate immune responses. Hormonal regulation of overall bodily responses to infection, partly addressed in Chapter 11, will also be discussed later in this chapter.

interactions lead to the formation of active C3b, the opsonin described in the previous paragraph, and the activation of the subsequent complement molecules in the pathway. However, not all microbes have a surface conducive to initiating the alternative pathway.

Other Opsonins in Innate Responses

In addition to complement C3b, other plasma proteins can bind nonspecifically to carbohydrates or lipids in the cell wall of microbes and facilitate opsonization. Many of these—for example, **C-reactive protein**—are produced by the liver and are always found at some concentration in the plasma. Their production and plasma concentrations, however, are greatly increased during inflammation.

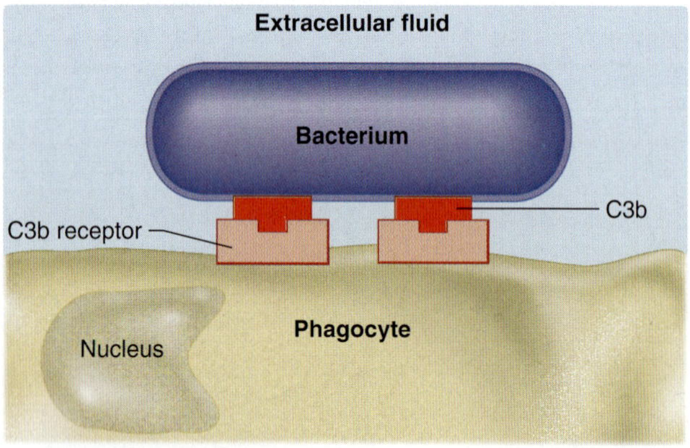

Figure 18.6 Function of complement C3b as an opsonin. One portion of C3b binds nonspecifically to carbohydrates on the surface of the bacterium, whereas another portion binds to specific receptor sites for C3b on the plasma membrane of the phagocyte. The structures are not drawn to scale.

PHYSIOLOGICAL INQUIRY

- In earlier chapters, you learned some of the characteristics of ligand-receptor interactions (e.g., see Figures 3.26 through 3.31). What general features of the C3b receptor may make it suitable for binding C3b and not other ligands?

Answer can be found at end of chapter.

Tissue Repair

The final stage of inflammation is tissue repair. Depending upon the tissue involved, multiplication of organ-specific cells by cell division may or may not occur during this stage. For example, liver cells multiply but skeletal muscle cells do not. In any case, fibroblasts (a type of connective-tissue cell) that reside in the area divide rapidly and begin to secrete large quantities of collagen, and blood vessel cells proliferate in the process of angiogenesis. All of these events are brought about by chemical mediators, particularly a group of locally produced growth factors. Finally, remodeling occurs as the healing process winds down. The final repair may be imperfect, leaving a scar.

Interferons

Interferons are cytokines and are grouped into two families called type I and type II interferons. The **type I interferons** include several proteins that nonspecifically inhibit viral replication inside host cells. In response to infection by a virus, most cell types produce these interferons and secrete them into the extracellular fluid. The type I interferons then bind to plasma membrane receptors on the secreting cell and on other cells, whether they are infected or not (**Figure 18.8**). This binding triggers the synthesis of dozens of different antiviral proteins by the cell. If the cell is already infected or eventually becomes infected, these proteins interfere with the ability of the viruses to replicate. Type I interferons also play a role in the killing of tumor cells and in generating fever during an infection.

The actions of type I interferons just described are not specific. Many kinds of viruses induce interferon synthesis, and interferons in turn can inhibit the multiplication of

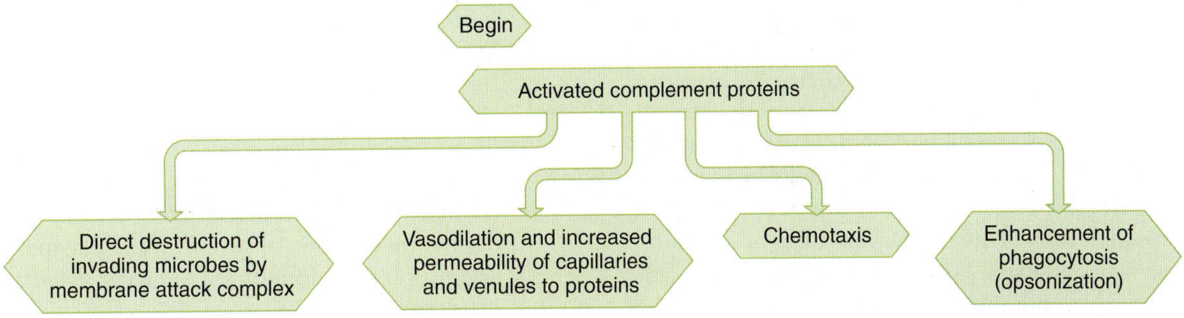

Figure 18.7 Functions of complement proteins. The effects on blood vessels and chemotaxis are exerted both directly by complement molecules and indirectly via other inflammatory mediators (for example, histamine) that are released by the complement molecules.

many kinds of viruses. Recent research, however, has revealed that type I interferons also influence the nature of certain aspects of the adaptive immune response.

The one member of the **type II interferons**—called **interferon-gamma**—is produced by immune cells. This interferon potentiates some of the actions of type I interferons, enhances the bacteria-killing activity of macrophages, and acts as a chemokine in the inflammatory process.

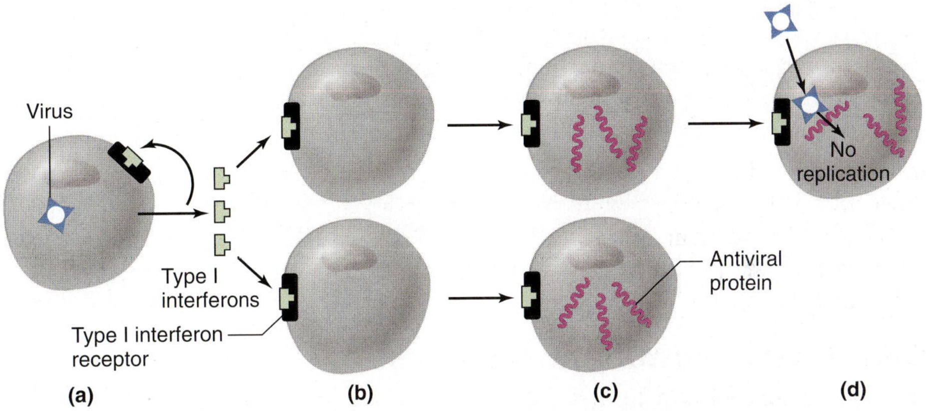

Figure 18.8 Role of type I interferon in preventing viral replication. (a) Most cell types, when infected with viruses, secrete type I interferons, which enter the interstitial fluid and (b) bind to type I interferon receptors on the secreting cells themselves (autocrine function) and adjacent cells (paracrine function). In addition, some type I interferons enter the blood and bind to type I interferon receptors on far-removed cells (endocrine function). (c) The binding of type I interferons to their receptors induces the synthesis of proteins that (d) inhibit viral replication should viruses enter the cell.

PHYSIOLOGICAL INQUIRY

- Are there other examples besides immune secretions in which a single substance may act as both an endocrine and paracrine substance? (*Hint:* Refer back to Chapters 11, 15, and 17 for help if necessary.)

Answer can be found at end of chapter.

Toll-Like Receptors

At the beginning of this section, we mentioned that innate immunity often depends upon an immune cell recognizing some general molecular feature common to many types of pathogens. These features are called **pathogen-associated molecular patterns (PAMPs)**. We now ask, How is that recognition accomplished? In 1985, researchers interested in how embryonic animals differentiate into mature organisms discovered a protein they named Toll (now called Toll-1) that was required for the proper dorsoventral orientation of fruit flies. In 1996, however, it was discovered that Toll-1 also conferred upon *adult* fruit flies the ability to fight off fungal infections, a discovery that was recognized in 2011 with the awarding of the Nobel Prize in Physiology or Medicine. Since that time, a family of Toll proteins has been discovered in animals from nematodes to mammals, including humans, expressed in the plasma and endosomal membranes of macrophages and dendritic cells, among others. One function of these proteins is to recognize and bind to highly conserved molecular features associated with pathogens (that is, PAMPs); these include lipopolysaccharide and other lipids and carbohydrates, viral and bacteria nucleic acids, and a protein found in the flagellum of many bacteria. When binding of one of these ligands occurs on the plasma membrane, second messengers are generated within the immune cell, which leads to secretion of inflammatory mediators such as IL-1, IL-12, and TNF-α. These in turn stimulate the activity of immune cells involved in the innate immune response. Some of these signals also activate cells involved in the adaptive immune response. Because many of the Toll proteins are plasma-membrane-bound, bind to extracellular ligands, and induce second-messenger formation, they are referred to as *receptors;* the family of proteins is known as **Toll-like receptors (TLRs)**. Despite this, not all TLRs generate intracellular signals when bound to a ligand; some TLRs induce attachment of a microbe to a macrophage, for example, and thereby its phagocytosis and subsequent destruction.

TLRs belong to a family of proteins called **pattern-recognition receptors** (**PRRs**), all of which recognize and bind to a variety of pathogen ligands. These ligands have conserved molecular features that are generally considered to be vital to the survival or function of that pathogen. It is estimated that as many as a thousand such molecular features are recognized by PRRs.

The importance of TLRs in mammals has been demonstrated in mice with a mutated form of one member of the family called Toll-4. These mice are hypersensitive to the effects of injections with lipopolysaccharide (to mimic a bacterial infection) and are less able to ward off bacterial infection. In humans, recent studies suggest that certain naturally occurring variants in a specific TLR are associated with increased risk of certain diseases.

TLRs are currently an active area of investigation among biologists because of their importance as developmental factors in invertebrates and their immune significance in some adult invertebrates and possibly all vertebrates. Certain domains of these receptors have even been identified in plants, where they seem also to be involved in disease resistance. Therefore, TLRs may be among the first mechanisms to ever evolve in living organisms to protect against pathogen infection.

18.3 Adaptive Immune Responses

Because of the complexity of adaptive immune responses, the following is presented as a brief orientation before more detail is given regarding the various components of the response.

Overview

Lymphocytes are the essential cells in adaptive immune responses. Unlike innate response mechanisms, lymphocytes must recognize the specific foreign material to be attacked. Any molecule that can trigger an adaptive immune response against itself or the cell bearing it is called an **antigen.** (Immunologists prefer the more technically correct term *immunogen.*) Most antigens are either proteins or very large polysaccharides. The term *antigen* is a functional term; that is, any molecule, regardless of its location or function, that can induce a specific immune response against itself is by definition an antigen. Therefore, an antigen is any molecule that the host does not recognize as self. Antigens include the protein coats of viruses, specific proteins on foreign cells, some cancer cells, transplanted cells, and toxins. The ability of lymphocytes to distinguish one antigen from another confers specificity upon the immune responses in which they participate.

A typical adaptive immune response can be divided into three stages:

1. *The encounter and recognition of an antigen by lymphocytes.* During its development, each lymphocyte synthesizes and inserts into its plasma membrane multiple copies of a single type of receptor that can bind to a specific antigen. If, at a later time, the lymphocyte ever encounters that antigen, the antigen becomes bound to the receptors. This binding is the physicochemical meaning of the word *recognize* in immunology. As a result, the ability of lymphocytes to distinguish one antigen from another is determined by the nature of their plasma membrane receptors. *Each lymphocyte is specific for just one type of antigen.*
2. *Lymphocyte activation.* The binding of an antigen to a receptor must occur for **lymphocyte activation.** Upon binding to an antigen, the lymphocyte becomes activated and undergoes multiple rounds of cell division. As a result, many daughter lymphocytes develop from a single progenitor that are identical in their ability to recognize a specific antigen; this is called **clonal expansion.** It is estimated that in a typical person the lymphocyte population expresses more than 100 million distinct antigen receptors. After activation, some lymphocytes will function as effector lymphocytes to carry out the attack response. Others will be set aside as **memory cells,** poised to recognize the antigen if it returns in the future.
3. *The attack launched by the activated lymphocytes and their secretions.* The activated effector lymphocytes launch an attack against the antigens that are recognized by the antigen-specific receptor. Activated B cells, which comprise one group of lymphocytes, differentiate into plasma cells that secrete antibodies into the blood. These antibodies opsonize pathogens or foreign substances and target them for attack by innate immune cells. Activated cytotoxic T cells, another type of lymphocyte, directly attack and kill the cells bearing the antigens. Once the attack is successfully completed, the great majority of the B cells, plasma cells, and T cells that participated in it die by apoptosis. The timely death of these effector cells is a homeostatic response that prevents the immune response from becoming excessive and possibly destroying its own tissues. However, memory cells persist even after the immune response has been successfully completed.

Lymphoid Organs and Lymphocyte Origins

Our first task is to describe the organs and tissues in which lymphocytes originate and come to reside. Then the various types of lymphocytes alluded to in the overview and summarized in Table 18.1 will be described.

Lymphoid Organs

Like all leukocytes, lymphocytes circulate in the blood. At any moment, the great majority of lymphocytes are not actually in the blood, however, but in a group of organs and tissues collectively called the **lymphoid organs.** These are subdivided into primary and secondary lymphoid organs.

The **primary lymphoid organs** are the bone marrow and thymus. These organs are the initial sites of lymphocyte development. They supply the body with mature but naive lymphocytes—that is, lymphocytes that have not yet been activated by specific antigen. The bone marrow and thymus are not normally sites in which naive lymphocytes undergo activation during an immune response.

The **secondary lymphoid organs** include the lymph nodes, spleen, tonsils, and lymphocyte accumulations in the linings of the intestinal, respiratory, genital, and urinary tracts. It is in the secondary lymphoid organs that naive lymphocytes are activated to participate in adaptive immune responses.

We have stated that the bone marrow and thymus supply mature lymphocytes to the secondary lymphoid organs. Most of the lymphocytes in the secondary organs are not, however, the same cells that originated in the primary lymphoid organs. The explanation of this seeming paradox is that, once in the secondary organ, a mature lymphocyte coming from the bone marrow or thymus can undergo cell division to produce additional identical lymphocytes, which in turn undergo cell division, and so on. In other words, all lymphocytes are *descended* from ancestors that matured in the bone marrow or thymus but may not themselves have arisen in those organs. All the progeny cells derived by cell division from a single lymphocyte constitute a lymphocyte **clone.**

There are no anatomical links, other than via the cardiovascular system, between the various lymphoid organs. Let us look briefly at these organs—with the exception of the bone marrow, which was described in Section F of Chapter 12.

The **thymus** lies in the upper part of the chest. Its size varies with age, being relatively large at birth and continuing to grow until puberty, when it gradually atrophies and is replaced by fatty tissue. Before its atrophy, the thymus consists mainly of immature lymphocytes that will develop into mature T cells that will eventually migrate via the blood to the secondary lymphoid organs.

Recall from Chapter 12 that the fluid flowing in the lymphatic vessels is called *lymph*, which is interstitial fluid that has entered the lymphatic capillaries and is routed to the large lymphatic vessels that drain into systemic veins. During this trip, the lymph flows through **lymph nodes** scattered along the vessels. Lymph, therefore, is the route by which lymphocytes in the lymph nodes encounter the antigens that activate them. Each node is a honeycomb of lymph-filled sinuses (**Figure 18.9**) with large clusters of lymphocytes (the lymphatic nodules) between the sinuses. The lymph nodes also contain many macrophages and dendritic cells.

The **spleen** is the largest of the secondary lymphoid organs and lies in the left part of the abdominal cavity between the stomach and the diaphragm. The spleen is to the circulating blood what the lymph nodes are to the lymph. Blood percolates through the vascular meshwork of the spleen's interior, where large collections of lymphocytes, macrophages, and dendritic cells are found. The macrophages of the spleen, in addition to interacting with lymphocytes, also phagocytose aging or dead erythrocytes.

The **tonsils** and **adenoids** are a group of small, rounded lymphoid organs in the pharynx. They are filled with lymphocytes, macrophages, and dendritic cells, and they have openings called crypts to the surface of the pharynx. Their lymphocytes respond to microbes that arrive by way of ingested food as well as through inspired air.

At any moment in time, some lymphocytes are on their way from the bone marrow or thymus to the secondary lymphoid organs. The vast majority, though, are cells that are participating in lymphocyte traffic *between* the secondary lymphoid organs, blood, lymph, and all the tissues of the body. Lymphocytes from all the secondary lymphoid organs constantly enter the lymphatic vessels that drain them (all lymphoid organs, not just lymph nodes, are drained by lymphatic vessels) and are carried to the blood. Simultaneously, some blood lymphocytes are pushing through the endothelium of venules all over the body to enter the interstitial fluid. From there, they move into lymphatic capillaries and along the lymphatic vessels to lymph nodes. They may then leave the lymphatic vessels to take up residence in the node.

This recirculation is going on all the time, not just during an infection, although the migration of lymphocytes into an inflamed area is greatly increased by the chemotaxis process (see Figure 18.2). Lymphocyte trafficking greatly increases the likelihood that any given lymphocyte will encounter the antigen it is specifically programmed to recognize. (In contrast to the lymphocytes, polymorphonuclear granulocytes and monocytes do not recirculate; once they leave the bloodstream and enter a tissue, they remain there or die.)

Lymphocyte Origins

The multiple populations and subpopulations of lymphocytes are summarized in Table 18.1. *B lymphocytes* (*B cells*) mature in the bone marrow and then are carried by the blood to the secondary lymphoid organs (**Figure 18.10**). This process of maturation and migration continues throughout a person's life. All generations of lymphocytes that subsequently arise from these cells by cell division in the secondary lymphoid organs will be identical to the parent cells; that is, they will be B-cell clones.

In contrast to the B cells, other lymphocytes leave the bone marrow in an immature state during fetal and early neonatal life. They are carried to the thymus and mature there before moving to the secondary lymphoid organs. These cells are called *T lymphocytes* (or *T cells*). Like B cells, T cells also undergo cell division in secondary lymphoid organs, the progeny being identical to the original T cells and thereby part of that T-cell clone.

In addition to the B and T cells, there is another distinct population of lymphocytes called *natural killer* (*NK*) *cells*. These cells arise in the bone marrow, but their precursors and life history are still unclear. As we will see, NK cells, unlike B and T cells, are not specific to a given antigen.

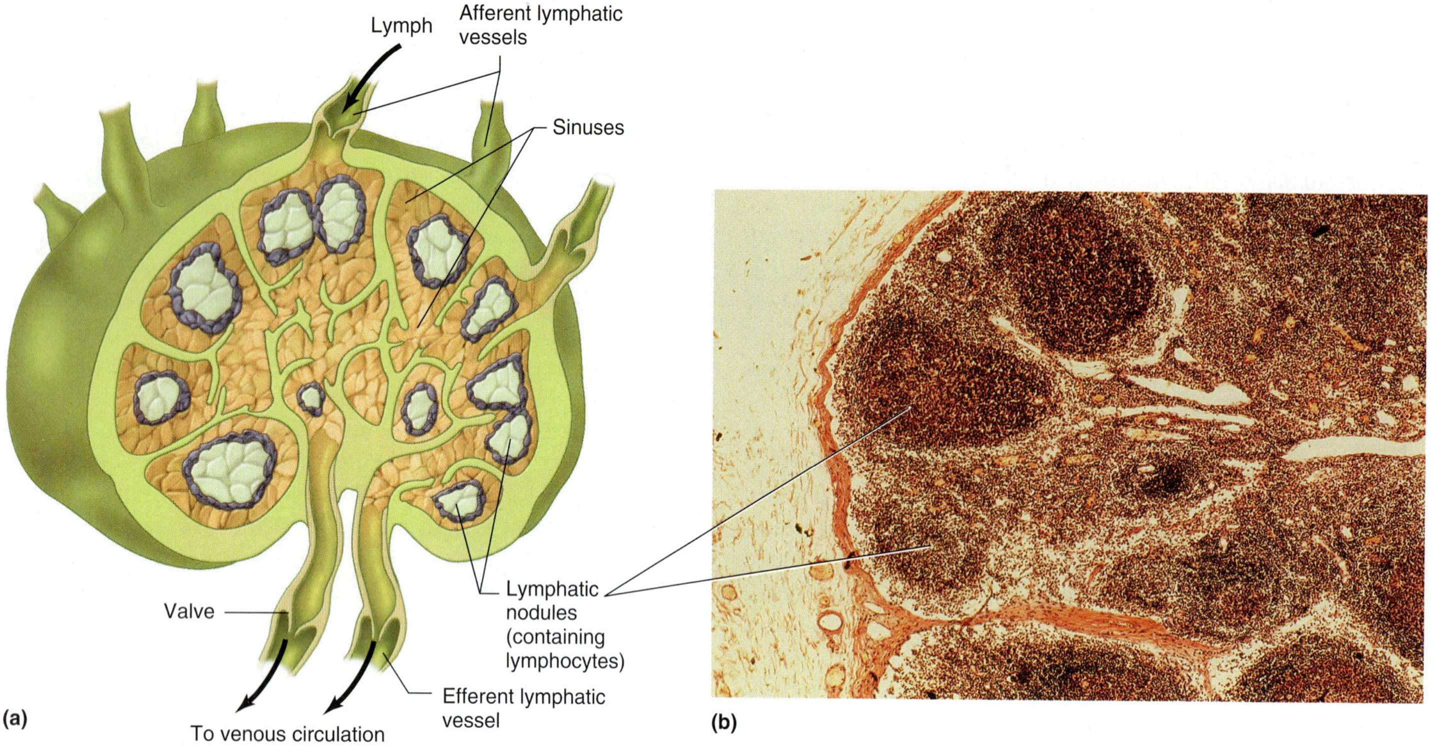

Figure 18.9 APIR Anatomy of a lymph node as seen in (a) a sketch and in (b) a section viewed by light microscopy.

PHYSIOLOGICAL INQUIRY

- The innate immune response includes vasodilation of the microcirculation and an increase in protein permeability of the capillaries (see Figure 18.2). How might these changes enhance the adaptive immune response during an infection? (*Hint:* What effect would these circulatory changes have on the volume of fluid in the interstitial space and, therefore, lymph flow?)

Answer can be found at end of chapter.

Functions of B Cells and T Cells

Upon activation, B cells differentiate into plasma cells, which secrete **antibodies**, proteins that travel all over the body to reach antigens identical to those that stimulated their production. In the body fluids outside of cells, the antibodies combine with these antigens and guide an attack that eliminates the antigens or the cells bearing them.

Antibody-mediated responses are also called *humoral* responses, the adjective *humoral* denoting communication "by way of soluble chemical messengers" (in this case, antibodies in the blood). Antibody-mediated responses have an extremely wide diversity of targets and are the major defense against bacteria, viruses, and other pathogens in the extracellular fluid and against toxic molecules (toxins).

In contrast to humoral responses, T-cell responses are *cell-mediated* responses. T cells constitute a family that has at least two major functional subsets, **cytotoxic T cells** and **helper T cells.** Recently, it has become clear that a third subset—called suppressor or **regulatory T cells**—inhibits the function of both B cells and cytotoxic T cells.

Another way to categorize T cells is not by function but rather by the presence of certain proteins, called CD4 and CD8, in their plasma membranes. Cytotoxic T cells have CD8 and so are also commonly called CD8+ cells; helper T cells and regulatory T cells express CD4 and so are also commonly called CD4+ cells.

Cytotoxic T cells are "attack" cells. Following activation, they travel to the location of their target, bind to them via antigen on these targets, and directly kill their targets via secreted chemicals. Responses mediated by cytotoxic T cells are directed against the body's own cells that have become cancerous or infected with viruses (or certain bacteria and parasites that, like viruses, take up residence inside host cells).

It is worth emphasizing the important geographic difference in antibody-mediated responses and responses mediated by cytotoxic T cells. The B cells (and plasma cells derived from them) remain in whatever location the recognition and activation steps occurred. The plasma cells send their antibodies forth via the blood to seek out antigens identical to those that triggered the response. Cytotoxic T cells must enter the blood and seek out the targets.

We have now assigned general roles to the B cells and cytotoxic T cells. What role is performed by the helper T cells? As their name implies, these cells do not themselves

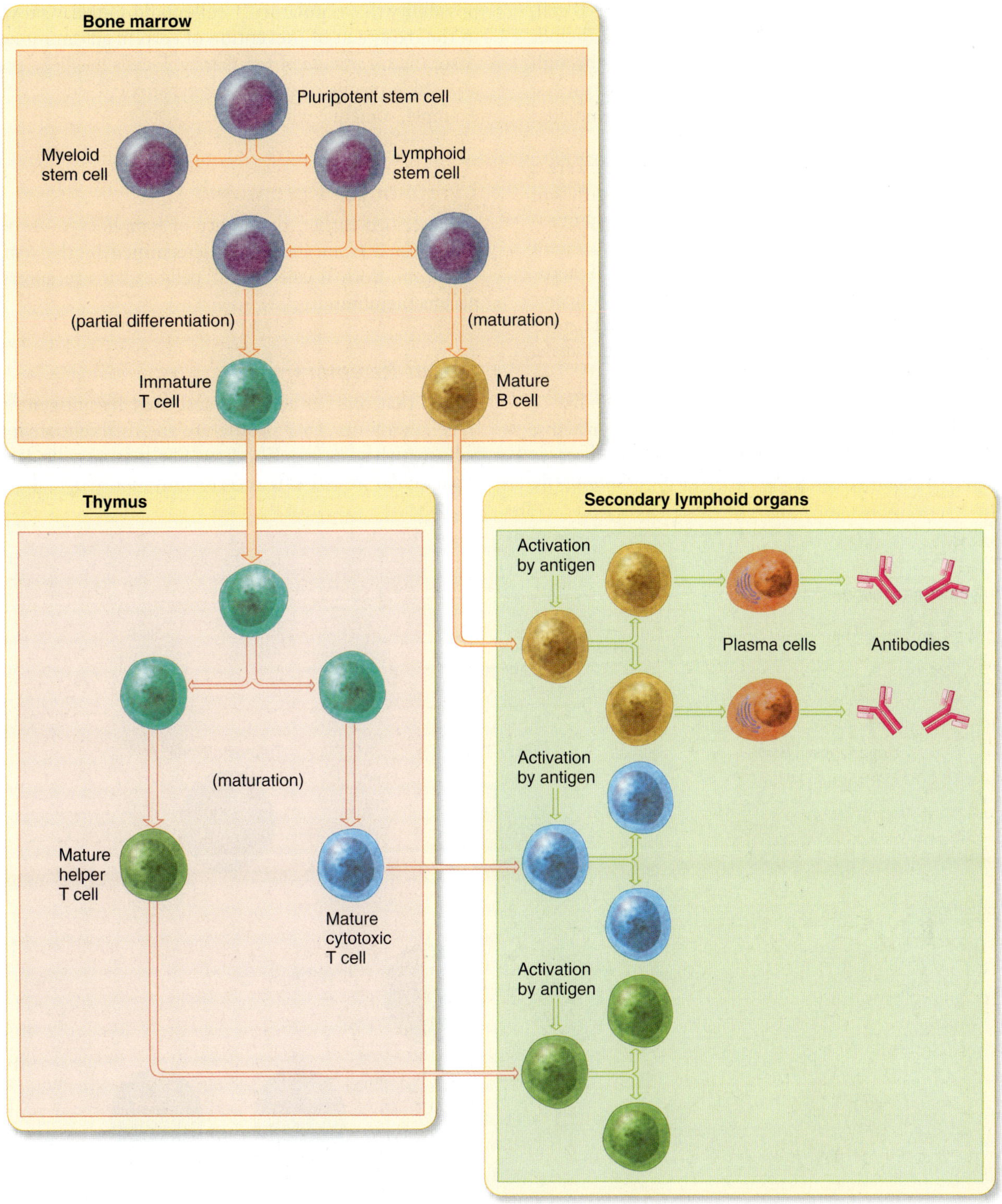

Figure 18.10 APIR Derivation of B cells and T cells. NK cells are not shown because their transformations, if any, after leaving the bone marrow are still not clear.

function as attack cells but, rather, assist in the activation and function of B cells, macrophages, and cytotoxic T cells. Helper T cells go through the usual first two stages of the immune response. First, they combine with antigen and then undergo activation. Once activated, they migrate to the site of B-cell activation. B cells that have bound antigen present it to activated helper cells. Antigen-specific helper T cells make direct contact with the B cell, and the communication given by surface receptors—along with the secretion of cytokines—induces B-cell activation. The role of helper T cells in cytotoxic T-cell activation is more complex. To activate cytotoxic T cells, activated helper T cells help other cells, most likely dendritic cells, to activate cytotoxic T cells. Unlike the B cell, which directly interacts with the helper T cell, the helper T cell assists cytotoxic T-cell activation indirectly through other cells. With only a few exceptions, B cells and cytotoxic T cells cannot function adequately unless they are stimulated by cytokines from helper T cells.

Helper T cells will be considered as though they were a homogeneous cell population, but in fact, there are different subtypes of helper T cells, distinguished by the different cytokines they secrete when activated. By means of these different cytokines, they help different sets of lymphocytes, macrophages, and NK cells. Some of the cytokines secreted by helper T cells also act as inflammatory mediators. **Figure 18.11** summarizes the basic interactions among B cells, cytotoxic T cells, and helper T cells.

Regulatory T cells are believed to suppress the ability of certain B and cytotoxic T cells to attack a person's own proteins, which can occur in diseases known as autoimmune diseases (described later). As such, investigators are actively pursuing the possibility that regulatory T cells could someday prove effective in the treatment or prevention of certain autoimmune diseases. Also, the *suppression* of regulatory T cells has been proposed as a possible means of increasing cytotoxic T-cell activity in, for example, someone with cancer.

Lymphocyte Receptors

As described earlier, the ability of lymphocytes to distinguish one antigen from another is determined by the lymphocytes' receptors. Both B cells and T cells express receptors on their plasma membrane.

B-Cell Receptors

Recall that once B cells are activated by antigen and helper T-cell cytokines, they proliferate and differentiate into plasma cells, which secrete antibodies. The plasma cells derived from a particular B cell can secrete only one particular antibody.

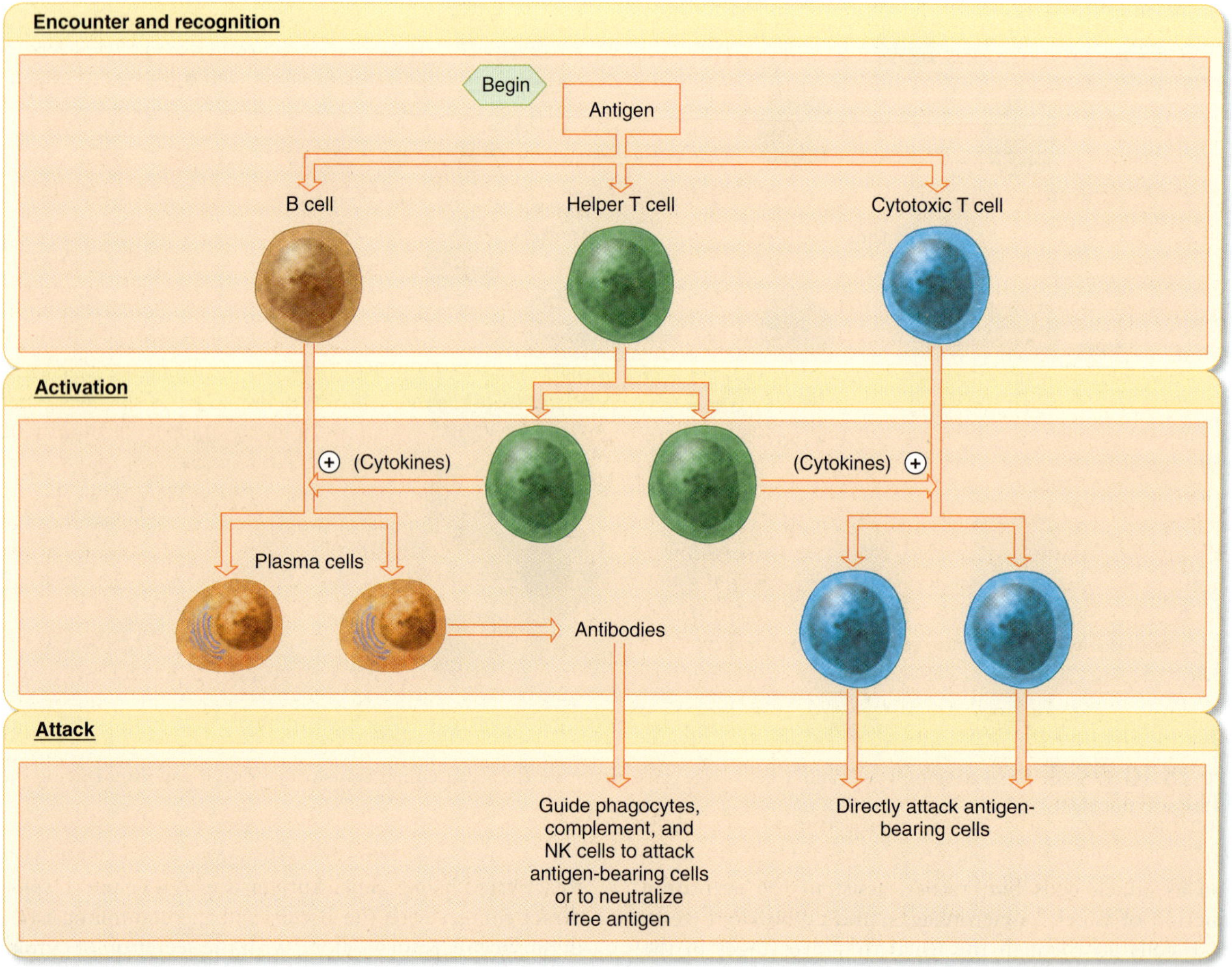

Figure 18.11 AP|R Summary of the roles of B, cytotoxic T, and helper T cells in immune responses. Events of the attack phase are described in later sections. The ⊕ symbol denotes a stimulatory effect (activation) of cytokines.

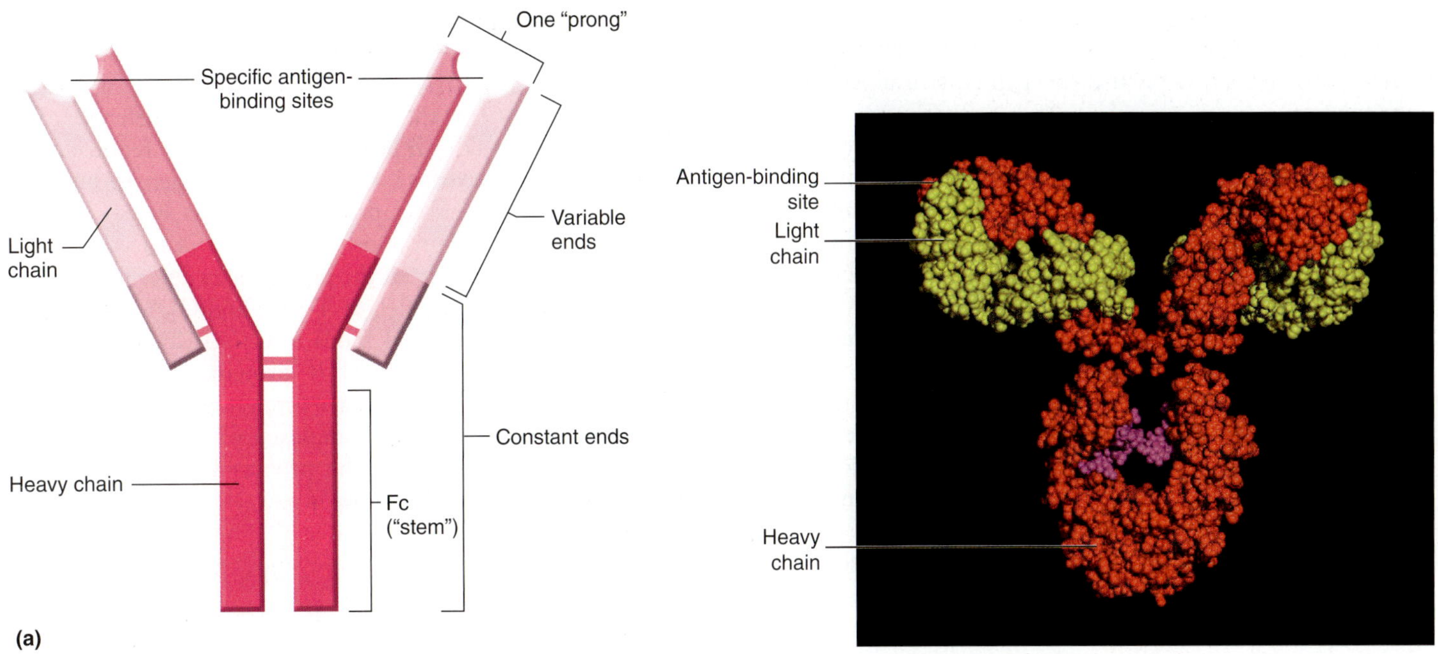

Figure 18.12 AP|R Immunoglobulin structure. (a) The Fc portions and an extended region of the heavy chains are the same for all immunoglobulins of a particular class. A small portion of the light chains are also the same for a given immunoglobulin class. Collectively, these portions of the heavy and light chains are called "constant ends." Each "prong" contains a variable amino acid sequence, which represents the single antigen-binding site. The links between chains represent disulfide bonds. (b) Three-dimensional simulation of an immunoglobulin showing antigen-binding sites and the light and heavy chains. The purple region represents associated carbohydrate, the function of which is uncertain but may be related to binding of immunoglobulins to substrates.

Each B cell always displays on its plasma membrane copies of the particular antibody its plasma cell progeny can produce. This surface protein (glycoprotein, to be more accurate) acts as the receptor for the antigen specific to it.

B-cell receptors and plasma cell antibodies constitute the family of proteins known as **immunoglobulins.** The receptors themselves, even though they are identical to the antibodies to be secreted by the plasma cell derived from the activated B cell, are technically not antibodies because only *secreted* immunoglobulins are called antibodies. Each immunoglobulin molecule is composed of four interlinked polypeptide chains (**Figure 18.12**). The two long chains are called heavy chains, and the two short ones, light chains. There are five major classes of immunoglobulins, determined by the amino acid sequences in the heavy chains and a portion of the light chains. The classes are designated by the letters A, D, E, G, and M following the symbol Ig for immunoglobulin; thus, we have IgA, IgD, and so on.

As illustrated in Figure 18.12, immunoglobulins have a "stem" called the **Fc** portion and comprising the lower half of the two heavy chains. The upper part of each heavy chain and its associated light chain form an **antigen-binding site**—the amino acid sequences that bind antigen. The amino acid sequences of the Fc portion plus an additional portion of the heavy chains and part of the light chains are identical for all immunoglobulins of a single class (IgA, IgD, and so on). In contrast to the identical (or "constant") regions of the heavy and light chains, the amino acid sequences of the antigen-binding sites vary from immunoglobulin to immunoglobulin in a given class and are therefore known as variable ends. Each of the five classes of antibodies, therefore, could contain up to millions of unique immunoglobulins, each capable of combining with only one specific antigen (or, in some cases, several antigens whose structures are very similar). The interaction between an antigen-binding site of an immunoglobulin and an antigen is analogous to the lock-and-key interactions that apply generally to the binding of ligands by proteins.

One more point should be mentioned: B-cell receptors can bind antigen whether the antigen is a molecule dissolved in the extracellular fluid or is present on the surface of a foreign cell, such as a microbe, floating free in the fluids. In the latter case, the B cell becomes linked to the foreign cell via the bonds between the B-cell receptor and the surface antigen.

To summarize so far, any given B cell or clone of identical B cells possesses unique immunoglobulin receptors—that is, receptors with unique antigen-binding sites. Consequently, the body arms itself with millions of clones of different B cells to ensure that specific receptors exist for the vast number of different antigens the organism *might* encounter during its lifetime. The particular immunoglobulin that any given B cell displays as a receptor on its plasma membrane (and that its plasma cell progeny will secrete as antibodies) is determined during the cell's maturation in the bone marrow.

This raises a very interesting question. In the human genome, there are only about 200 genes that code for immunoglobulins. How, then, can the body produce immunoglobulins having millions of different antigen-binding sites, given that each immunoglobulin requires coding by a distinct gene? This diversity arises as the result of a genetic process unique to developing lymphocytes because only these cells express the enzymes required to catalyze the process. The DNA in each of the genes that code for immunoglobulin antigen-binding sites is cut into small segments, randomly rearranged along the gene, and then rejoined to form new DNA molecules. This cutting and rejoining varies from B cell to B cell, thereby resulting in great diversity of the genes coding for the immunoglobulins of all the B cells taken together.

T-Cell Receptors

T-cell receptors for antigens are two-chained proteins that, like immunoglobulins, have specific regions that differ from one T-cell clone to another. However, T-cell receptors remain embedded in the T-cell membrane and are not secreted like antibodies. As in B-cell development, multiple DNA rearrangements occur during T-cell maturation, leading to millions of distinct T-cell clones—distinct in that the cells of any given clone possess receptors of a single specificity. For T cells, this maturation occurs during their residence in the thymus.

In addition to their general structural differences, the B-cell and T-cell receptors differ in a much more important way: *The T-cell receptor cannot combine with antigen unless the antigen is first complexed with certain of the body's own plasma membrane proteins.* The T-cell receptor then combines with the entire complex of antigen and body (self) protein.

The self plasma membrane proteins that must be complexed with the antigen in order for T-cell recognition to occur constitute a group of proteins coded for by genes found on a single chromosome (chromosome 6) and known collectively as the **major histocompatibility complex** (**MHC**). The proteins are therefore called **MHC proteins** (in humans, also known as the human leukocyte antigens, or HLAs). Because no two persons other than identical twins have the same sets of MHC genes, no two individuals have the same MHC proteins on the plasma membranes of their cells. MHC proteins are, in essence, cellular "identity tags"—that is, genetic markers of biological self.

The MHC proteins are often called "restriction elements" because the ability of a T cell's receptor to recognize an antigen is restricted to situations in which the antigen is first complexed with an MHC protein. There are two classes of MHC proteins: I and II. **Class I MHC proteins** are found on the surface of virtually all cells of the body except erythrocytes. **Class II MHC proteins** are found mainly on the surface of macrophages, B cells, and dendritic cells. Under certain conditions, other cell types are induced to express class II MHC.

Another important point is that the different subsets of T cells do not all have the same MHC requirements (**Table 18.4**). Cytotoxic T cells require antigen to be associated with class I MHC proteins, whereas helper T cells require class II MHC proteins. One reason for this difference in requirements stems from the presence, as described earlier, of CD4 proteins on the helper T cells and CD8 proteins on the cytotoxic T cells; CD4 binds to class II MHC proteins, whereas CD8 binds to class I MHC proteins.

How do antigens, which are foreign, end up on the surface of the body's own cells complexed with MHC proteins? The answer is provided by the process known as **antigen presentation,** to which we now turn.

Antigen Presentation to T Cells

T cells can bind antigen only when the antigen appears on the plasma membrane of a host cell complexed with the cell's MHC proteins. Cells bearing these complexes, therefore, function as **antigen-presenting cells** (**APCs**).

Presentation to Helper T Cells

Helper T cells require class II MHC proteins to function. Only macrophages, B cells, and dendritic cells express class II MHC proteins and therefore can function as APCs for helper T cells.

The function of the macrophage or dendritic cell as an APC for helper T cells is depicted in **Figure 18.13**, which shows that the cells form a link between innate and adaptive immune responses. After a microbe or noncellular antigen has been phagocytosed by a macrophage or dendritic cell in a *nonspecific* response, it is partially broken down into smaller peptide fragments by the cell's proteolytic enzymes. The resulting digested fragments then bind (within endosomes) to class II MHC proteins synthesized by the cell. This entire complex is then transported to the cell surface, where it is displayed in the plasma membrane. It is to this complex on the cell surface of the macrophage or dendritic cell that a specific helper T cell binds.

TABLE 18.4 MHC Restriction of the Lymphocyte Receptors

Cell Type	MHC Restriction
B	Do not interact with MHC proteins
Helper T	Class II, found only on macrophages, dendritic cells, and B cells
Cytotoxic T	Class I, found on all nucleated cells of the body
NK	Interaction with MHC proteins not required for activation

Note that it is not the intact antigen but rather the peptide fragments, called antigenic determinants or **epitopes,** of the antigen that are complexed to the MHC proteins and presented to the T cell. Despite this, it is customary to refer to "antigen" presentation rather than "epitope" presentation.

How B cells process antigen and present it to helper T cells is essentially the same as just described for dendritic cells and macrophages (**Figure 18.13b**). The ability of B cells to present antigen to helper T cells is a *second* function of B cells in response to antigenic stimulation, the other being the differentiation of the B cells into antibody-secreting plasma cells.

The binding between a helper T-cell receptor and an antigen bound to class II MHC proteins on an APC is the essential *antigen-specific* event in helper T-cell activation. However, this binding by itself will not result in T-cell activation. In addition, interactions occur between other (nonantigenic) pairs of proteins on the surfaces of the attached helper T cell and APC, and these provide a necessary **costimulus** for T-cell activation (**Figure 18.14**).

Finally, the antigenic binding of the APC to the T cell—along with the costimulus—causes the APC to secrete large amounts of the cytokines **interleukin 1 (IL-1)** and **tumor necrosis factor-alpha (TNF-α)**, which act as paracrine substances on the attached helper T cell to provide yet another important stimulus for activation.

Thus, the APC participates in the activation of a helper T cell in three ways: (1) antigen presentation; (2) provision of a costimulus in the form of a matching nonantigenic plasma membrane protein; and (3) secretion of IL-1, TNF-α, and other cytokines (see Figure 18.14).

The activated helper T cell itself now secretes various cytokines that have both autocrine effects on the helper T cell and paracrine effects on adjacent B cells and any nearby

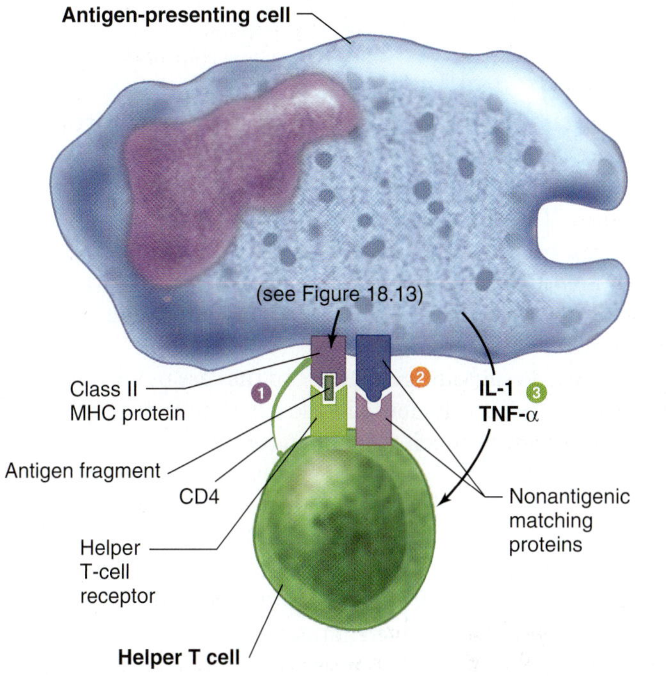

Figure 18.14 APR Three events are required for the activation of helper T cells: (1) presentation of the antigen bound to a class II MHC protein on an antigen-presenting cell (APC); (2) the binding of matching nonantigenic proteins in the plasma membranes of the APC and the helper T cell (costimulus); and (3) secretion by the APC of the cytokines interleukin 1 (IL-1), tumor necrosis factor-alpha (TNF-α), and other cytokines, which act on the helper T cell.

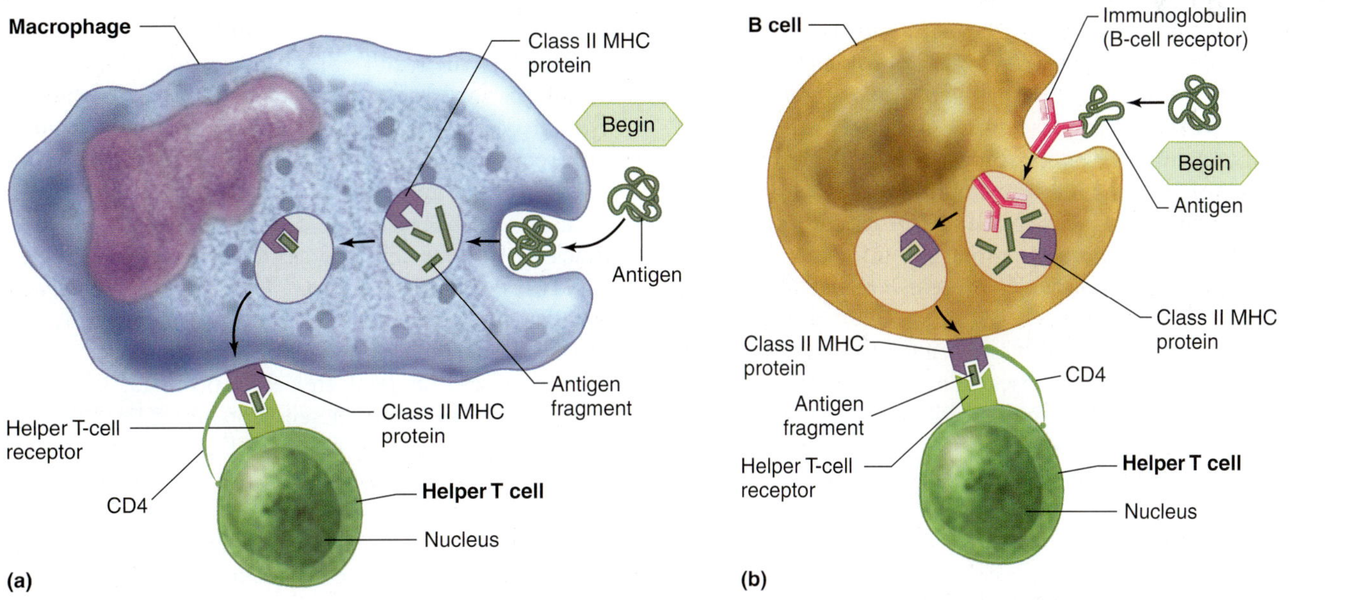

Figure 18.13 APR Sequence of events by which antigen is processed and presented to a helper T cell by (a) a macrophage or (b) a B cell. In both cases, begin the figure with the antigen in the extracellular fluid.

cytotoxic T cells, NK cells, and still other cell types. Recent evidence suggests that helper T cells may program dendritic cells to activate CD8+ T cells. These processes will be described in later sections.

Presentation to Cytotoxic T Cells

Because class I MHC proteins are synthesized by virtually all nucleated cells, any such cell can act as an APC for a cytotoxic T cell. This distinction helps explain the major function of cytotoxic T cells—destruction of *any* of the body's own cells that have become cancerous or infected with viruses. The key point is that the antigens that complex with class I MHC proteins arise *within* body cells. They are endogenous antigens, synthesized by a body cell.

How do such antigens arise? In the case of viruses, once a virus has taken up residence inside a host cell, the viral nucleic acid causes the host cell to manufacture viral proteins that are foreign to the cell. A cancerous cell has had one or more of its genes altered by chemicals, radiation, or other factors. The altered genes, called ***oncogenes***, code for proteins that are not normally found in the body. Such proteins act as antigens.

In both virus-infected cells and cancerous cells, some of the endogenously produced antigenic proteins are hydrolyzed by cytosolic enzymes (in proteasomes) into peptide fragments, which are transported into the endoplasmic reticulum. There, they are complexed with the host cell's class I MHC proteins and then shuttled by exocytosis to the plasma membrane surface, where a cytotoxic T cell specific for the complex can bind to it (**Figure 18.15**).

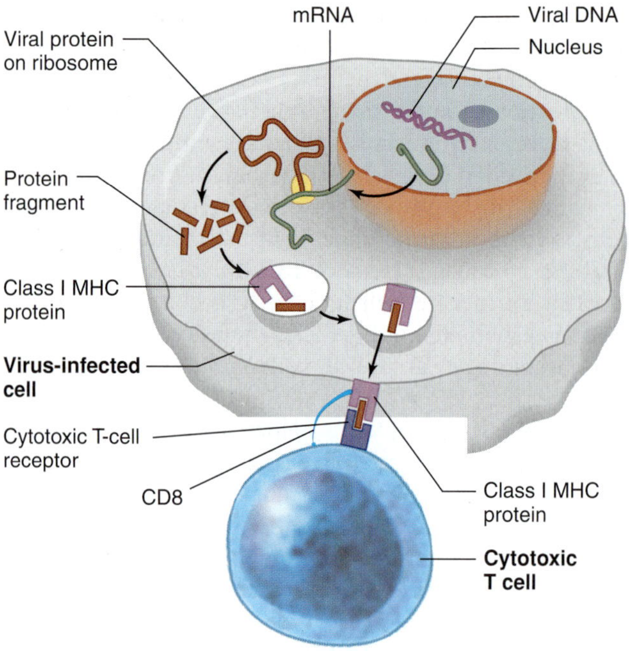

Figure 18.15 AP|R Processing and presentation of viral antigen to a cytotoxic T cell by an infected cell. Begin this figure with the viral DNA in the cell's nucleus. The viral DNA induces the infected cell to produce viral protein, which is then hydrolyzed (by proteasomes). The fragments are complexed to the cell's class I MHC proteins in the endoplasmic reticulum, and these complexes are then shuttled to the plasma membrane.

NK Cells

As noted earlier, NK (natural killer) cells constitute a distinct class of lymphocytes. They have several functional similarities to those of cytotoxic T cells. For example, their major targets are virus-infected cells and cancer cells, and they attack and kill these target cells directly after binding to them. However, unlike cytotoxic T cells, NK cells are not antigen-specific; that is, each NK cell can attack virus-infected cells or cancer cells without recognizing a specific antigen. They have neither T-cell receptors nor the immunoglobulin receptors of B cells, and the exact nature of the NK-cell surface receptors that permits the cells to identify their targets is unknown (except in one case presented later). MHC proteins are not involved in the activation of NK cells.

Why, then, do we deal with them in the context of *specific* (adaptive) immune responses? The reason is that, as will be described subsequently, their participation in an immune response is greatly enhanced either by certain antibodies or by cytokines secreted by helper T cells activated during adaptive immune responses.

Development of Immune Tolerance

Our basic framework for understanding adaptive immune responses requires consideration of one more crucial question. How does the body develop what is called **immune tolerance**—lack of immune responsiveness to self? This may seem a strange question given the definition of an antigen as a foreign molecule that can generate an immune response. How is it, though, that the body "knows" that its own molecules, particularly proteins, are not foreign but are self molecules?

Recall that the huge diversity of lymphocyte receptors is ultimately the result of multiple, random DNA cutting and recombination processes. It is virtually certain, therefore, that in each person, clones of lymphocytes would have emerged with receptors that could bind to that person's own proteins. The existence and functioning of such lymphocytes would be disastrous because such binding would launch an immune attack against the cells expressing these proteins. There are at least two mechanisms—*clonal deletion* and *clonal inactivation*—that explain why normally there are no active lymphocytes that respond to self components.

First, during fetal and early postnatal life, T cells are exposed to a wide mix of self proteins in the thymus. Those T cells with receptors capable of binding self proteins are destroyed by apoptosis (programmed cell death). This process is called **clonal deletion.** The second process, **clonal inactivation**, occurs not in the thymus but in the periphery and causes potentially self-reacting T cells to become nonresponsive.

What are the mechanisms of clonal deletion and inactivation during fetal and early postnatal life? Recall that full activation of a helper T cell requires not only an antigen-specific stimulus but a nonspecific costimulus (interaction between complementary nonantigenic proteins on the APC and the T cell). If this costimulus is *not* provided, the helper T cell not only fails to become activated by antigen but dies or becomes inactivated forever. This is the case during early life. The induction of costimulatory molecules requires activated, antigen-presenting cells. Signaling through TLRs and secretion of inflammatory cytokines are two mechanisms of activating antigen-presenting cells to express costimulatory molecules that provide costimulus for T-cell activation.

This completes the framework for understanding adaptive immune responses. The next two sections utilize this framework in presenting typical responses from beginning to end, highlighting the interactions between lymphocytes and describing the attack mechanisms used by the various pathways.

Antibody-Mediated Immune Responses: Defenses Against Bacteria, Extracellular Viruses, and Toxins

A classical antibody-mediated response is one that results in the destruction of bacteria. The sequence of events, which is quite similar to the response to a virus in the extracellular fluid, is summarized in **Table 18.5** and **Figure 18.16**.

Antigen Recognition and B-Cell Activation

This process starts the same way as for nonspecific responses, with the bacteria penetrating one of the body's linings and entering the interstitial fluid. The bacteria then enter the lymphatic system and/or the bloodstream and are taken up by the lymph nodes and/or the spleen, respectively. There, a B cell, using its immunoglobulin receptor, recognizes the bacterial surface antigen and binds the bacterium.

In a few cases (notably, bacteria with cell-wall polysaccharide capsules), this binding is all that is needed to trigger B-cell activation. For the great majority of antigens, however, antigen binding is not enough, and signals in the form of cytokines released into the interstitial fluid by helper T cells near the antigen-bound B cells are also required.

For helper T cells to react against bacteria by secreting cytokines, they must bind to a complex of antigen and class II MHC protein on an APC. Let us assume that in this case the APC is a macrophage that has phagocytosed one of the bacteria, hydrolyzed its proteins into peptide fragments, complexed them with class II MHC proteins, and displayed the complexes on its surface. A helper T cell specific for the complex then binds to it, beginning the activation of the helper T cell. Moreover, the macrophage helps this activation process in two other ways: (1) It provides a costimulus via nonantigenic plasma membrane proteins, and (2) it secretes IL-1 and TNF-α.

The costimulus activates the helper T cell to secrete another cytokine named **interleukin-2** (**IL-2**). Among other functions, IL-1 and TNF-α stimulate the helper T cell to express more receptors for IL-2. IL-2, acting in an autocrine manner, then provides a proliferative stimulus to the activated helper T cell (see Figure 18.16). The cell divides, beginning the mitotic cycles that lead to the formation of a clone of activated helper T cells; these cells then release not only IL-2 but other cytokines as well.

Once activated, helper T cells migrate to lymph nodes where they interact with antigen-presenting B cells. The helper T cell stimulates B-cell activation by direct contact and cytokine release. Other cytokines—notably, IL-4 possibly produced by basophils—are also important in this step. Once activated, the B cell differentiates into a plasma cell that secretes antibodies that recognize the specific antigen. Thus, as shown in Figure 18.16, a series of protein messengers interconnects the various cell types, the helper T cells serving as the central coordinators.

As stated earlier, however, some of the B-cell progeny differentiate not into plasma cells but instead into memory cells, whose characteristics permit them to respond more

TABLE 18.5 Summary of Events in Antibody-Mediated Immunity Against Bacteria

I. In secondary lymphoid organs, bacterial antigen binds to specific receptors on the plasma membranes of B cells.

II. Antigen-presenting cells (APCs)—most likely the dendritic cells but macrophages and B cells—
   A. Present to helper T cells' processed antigen complexed to class II MHC proteins on the APCs;
   B. Provide a costimulus in the form of another membrane protein; and
   C. Secrete IL-1, TNF-α, and other cytokines, which act on the helper T cells.

III. In response, the helper T cells secrete IL-2, which stimulates the helper T cells themselves to proliferate and secrete IL-2 and other cytokines. These activate antigen-bound B cells to proliferate and differentiate into plasma cells. Some of the B cells differentiate into memory cells rather than plasma cells.

IV. The plasma cells secrete antibodies specific for the antigen that initiated the response, and the antibodies circulate all over the body via the blood.

V. These antibodies combine with antigen on the surface of the bacteria anywhere in the body.

VI. Presence of antibody bound to antigen facilitates phagocytosis of the bacteria by neutrophils and macrophages. It also activates the complement system, which further enhances phagocytosis and can directly kill the bacteria by the membrane attack complex. It may also induce antibody-dependent cellular cytotoxicity mediated by NK cells that bind to the antibody's Fc portion.

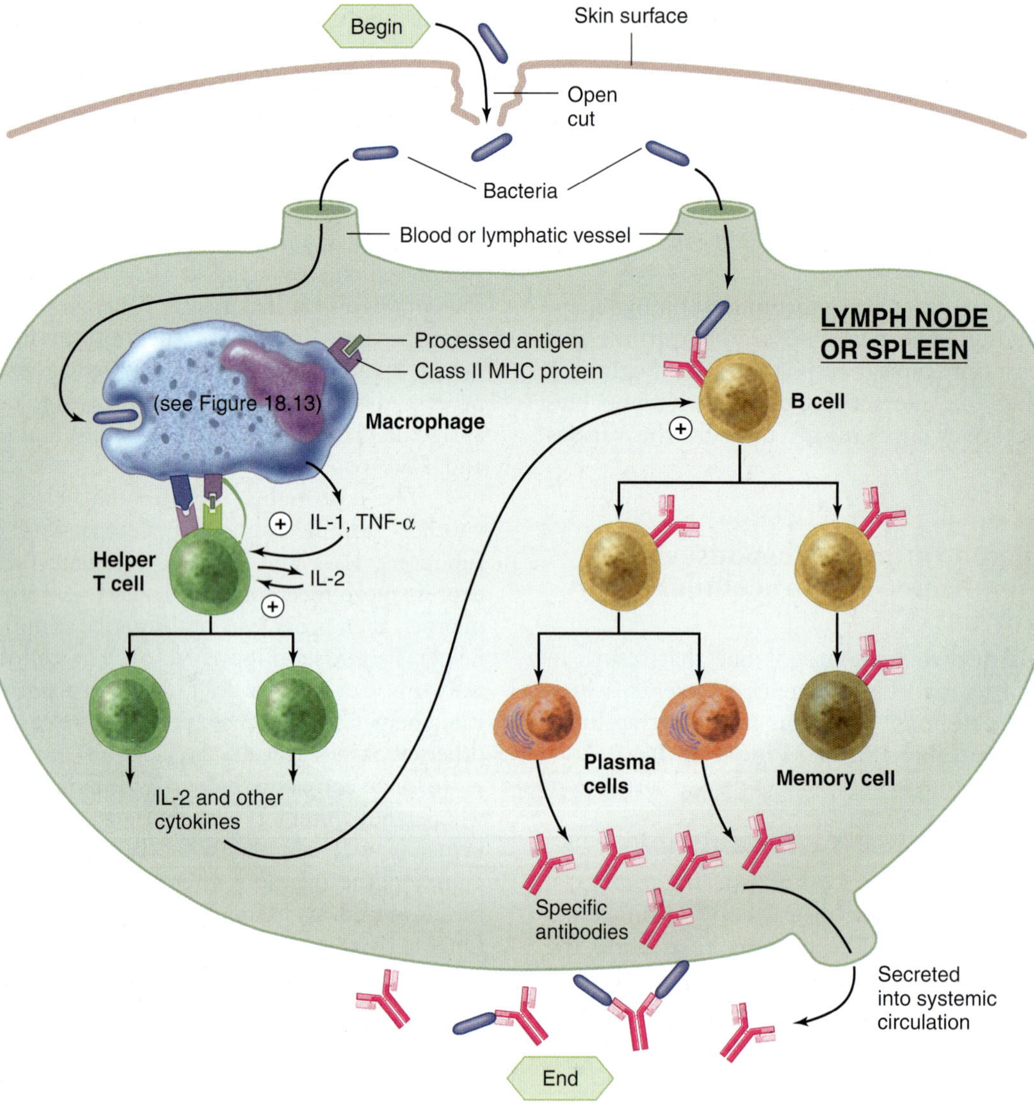

Figure 18.16 APR Summary of events by which a bacterial infection leads to antibody synthesis in secondary lymphoid organs. Refer back to Figure 18.13 for additional details about intracellular processing of antigen. The secreted antibodies travel by the blood to the site of infection, where they bind to bacteria of the type that induced the response. The attack triggered by antibodies' binding to bacteria is described in the text.

rapidly and vigorously should the antigen reappear at a future time (see Figure 18.16).

The example we have been using employed a macrophage as the APC to helper T cells, but B cells can also serve in this role (see Figure 18.13). The binding of the helper T cell to the antigen-bound B cell ensures maximal stimulation of the B cell by the cytokines secreted by that helper T cell and any of its progeny that remain nearby.

Antibody Secretion

After their differentiation from B cells, plasma cells produce thousands of antibody molecules per second before they die in a day or so. We mentioned earlier that there are five major classes of antibodies. The most abundant are the **IgG** antibodies, commonly called **gamma globulin,** and **IgM** antibodies. These two groups together provide the bulk of specific immunity against bacteria and viruses in the extracellular fluid. **IgE** antibodies participate in defenses against multicellular parasites and also mediate allergic responses. **IgA** antibodies are secreted by plasma cells in the linings of the gastrointestinal, respiratory, and genitourinary tracts; these antibodies generally act locally in the linings or on their surfaces. They are also secreted by the mammary glands and, therefore, are the major antibodies in milk. The functions of **IgD** are still unclear.

In the kind of infection described in this chapter, the B cells and plasma cells, sitting on the nodes near the infected tissues, recognize antigen and are activated to make antibodies. The antibodies (mostly IgG and IgM) circulate through the lymph and blood to return to the infected site. At sites of infection, the antibodies leave the blood (recall that nonspecific inflammation has already made capillaries and venules leaky at these sites) and combine with the type of bacterial surface antigen that initiated the immune response (see Figure 18.16). These antibodies then direct the attack (see following discussion) against the bacteria to which they are now bound.

Consequently, immunoglobulins play two distinct roles in immune responses during the initial recognition step: (1) Those on the surface of B cells bind to antigen brought to them; and (2) those secreted by the plasma cells (antibodies) bind to bacteria bearing the same antigens, "marking" them as the targets to be attacked.

The Attack: Effects of Antibodies

The antibodies bound to antigen on the microbial surface do not directly kill the microbe but instead link up the microbe physically to the actual killing mechanisms—phagocytes (neutrophils and macrophages), complement, or NK cells. This linkage not only triggers the attack mechanism but ensures that the killing effects are restricted to the microbe. Linkage to specific antibodies helps protect adjacent normal structures from the toxic effects of the chemicals employed by the killing mechanisms.

Direct Enhancement of Phagocytosis Antibodies can act directly as opsonins. The mechanism is analogous to that for complement C3b (see Figure 18.6) in that the antibody links the phagocyte to the antigen. As shown in **Figure 18.17**, the phagocyte has membrane receptors that bind to the Fc portion of an antibody. This linkage promotes attachment of the antigen to the phagocyte and the triggering of phagocytosis of the bacterium.

Activation of the Complement System As described earlier in this chapter, the plasma complement system is activated in *nonspecific* (innate) inflammatory responses via the alternative complement pathway. In contrast, in *adaptive* immune responses, the presence of antibody of the IgG or IgM class bound to antigen activates the *classical complement pathway*. The first molecule in this pathway, C1, binds to the Fc portion of an antibody that has combined with antigen (**Figure 18.18**). This results in activation of the enzymatic portions of C1, thereby initiating the entire classical pathway. The end product of this cascade, the membrane attack complex (MAC), can kill the cells the antibody is bound to by making their membranes leaky. In addition, as we saw in Figure 18.6, another activated complement molecule (C3b) functions as an opsonin to enhance phagocytosis of the microbe by neutrophils and macrophages (see Figure 18.18). As a result, antibodies enhance phagocytosis both directly (see Figure 18.17) and via activation of complement C3b.

It is important to note that C1 binds not to the unique antigen-binding sites in the antibody's prongs but rather to complement-binding sites in the Fc portion. Because the latter are the same in virtually all antibodies of the IgG and IgM classes, the complement molecule will bind to *any* antigen-bound antibodies belonging to these classes. In other words, there is only one set of complement molecules and, once activated, they do essentially the same thing regardless of the specific identity of the invader.

Antibody-Dependent Cellular Cytotoxicity We have seen that both a particular complement molecule (C1) and a phagocyte can bind nonspecifically to the Fc portion of an antibody bound to antigen. NK cells can also do this (just substitute an NK cell for the phagocyte in Figure 18.17). Thus, antibodies can link target cells to NK cells, which then kill the targets directly by secreting toxic chemicals. This is called **antibody-dependent cellular cytotoxicity (ADCC)**, because killing (cytotoxicity) is carried out by cells (NK cells) but the process depends upon the presence of antibody. Note that the antibodies confer specificity upon ADCC, just as they do on antibody-dependent phagocytosis and complement activation. This mechanism for bringing NK cells into play is the one exception, mentioned earlier, to the generalization that the mechanism by which NK cells identify their targets is unclear.

Direct Neutralization of Bacterial Toxins and Viruses Toxins secreted by bacteria into the extracellular fluid can act as antigens to induce antibody production. The antibodies then combine with the free toxins, thereby preventing interaction of the toxins with susceptible cells. Because each antibody has two binding sites for antigen, clumplike chains of antibody–antigen complexes form, and these clumps are then phagocytosed.

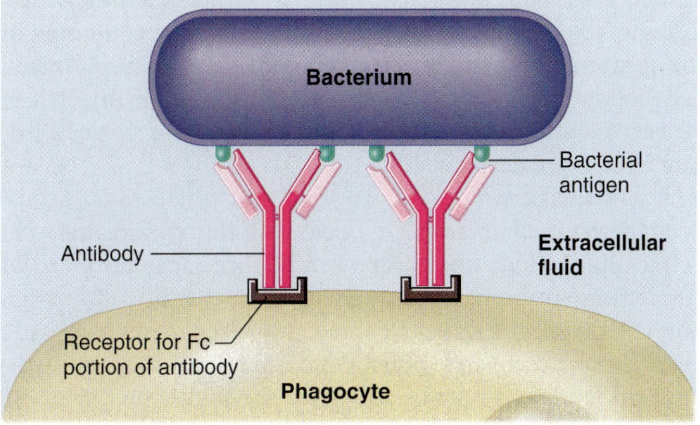

Figure 18.17 APIR Direct enhancement of phagocytosis by antibody. The antibody links the phagocyte to the bacterium. Compare this mechanism of opsonization to that mediated by complement C3b (see Figure 18.6).

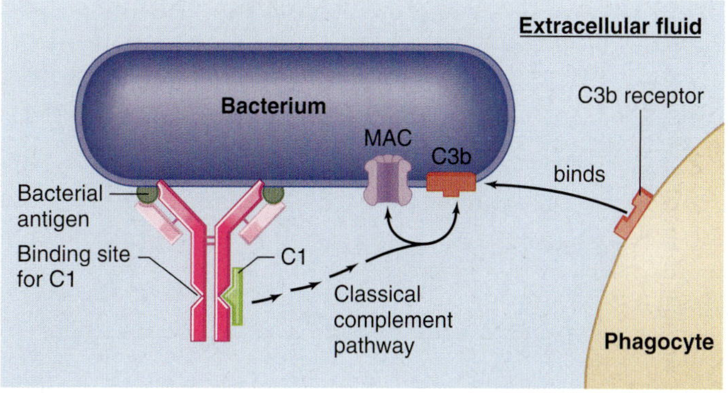

Figure 18.18 Activation of classical complement pathway by binding of antibody to bacterial antigen. C1 is activated by its binding to the Fc portion of the antibody. The membrane attack complex (MAC) is then generated, along with C3b, which acts as an opsonin by binding the bacteria to a phagocyte. C3b also plays a role in initiating the MAC (not shown here).

A similar binding process occurs as part of the major antibody-mediated mechanism for eliminating viruses in the extracellular fluid. Certain of the viral surface proteins serve as antigens, and the antibodies produced against them combine with them, preventing attachment of the virus to plasma membranes of potential host cells. This prevents the virus from entering a cell. As with bacterial toxins, chains of antibody–virus complexes are formed and can be phagocytosed.

Active and Passive Humoral Immunity

The response of the antibody-producing machinery to invasion by a foreign antigen varies enormously, depending upon whether the machinery has previously been exposed to that antigen. Antibody production occurs slowly over several weeks following the first contact with an antigen, but any subsequent infection by the same invader elicits an immediate and considerable outpouring of additional specific antibodies (**Figure 18.19**). This response, which is mediated by the memory B cells described earlier, is one of the key features that distinguishes innate and adaptive immunity. It confers a greatly enhanced resistance toward subsequent infection with that particular microorganism. Resistance built up as a result of the body's contact with microorganisms and their toxins or other antigenic components is known as **active immunity.**

Until the twentieth century, the only way to develop active immunity was to suffer an infection, but now the injection of microbial derivatives in vaccines is used. A ***vaccine*** may consist of small quantities of living or dead pathogens, small quantities of toxins, or harmless antigenic molecules derived from the microorganism or its toxin. The general principle is always the same: Exposure of the body to the antigenic substance results in an active immune response along with the induction of the memory cells required for rapid, effective response to possible future infection by that particular organism.

A second kind of immunity, known as **passive immunity**, is simply the direct transfer of antibodies from one person to another, the recipient thereby receiving preformed antibodies. Such transfers occur between mother and fetus because IgG can move across the placenta. Also, a breast-fed child receives IgA antibodies in the mother's milk; the intestinal mucosa is permeable to IgA antibodies during early life. These are important sources of protection for the infant during the first months of life, when the antibody-synthesizing capacity is relatively poor.

The same principle is used clinically when specific antibodies (produced by genetic engineering) or pooled gamma globulin injections are given to patients exposed to or suffering from certain infections such as hepatitis. Because antibodies are proteins with a limited life span, the protection afforded by this transfer of antibodies is relatively short-lived, usually lasting only a few weeks or months.

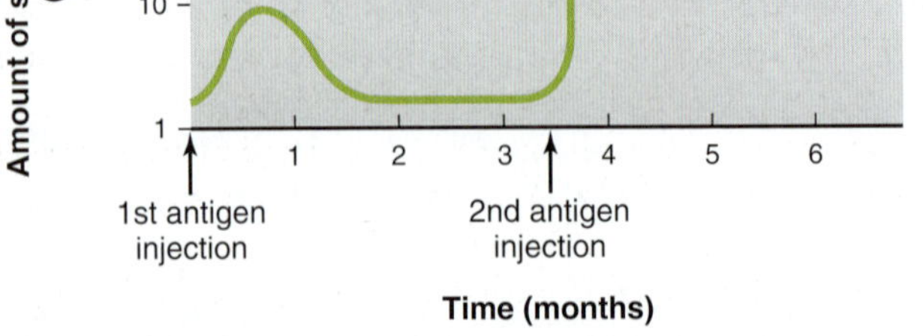

Figure 18.19 Rate of antibody production following initial exposure to an antigen and subsequent exposure to the same antigen. Note that the *y*-axis is a log scale.

Summary

It is now possible to summarize the interplay between innate and adaptive immune responses in resisting a bacterial infection. When a particular bacterium is encountered for the first time, *innate* defense mechanisms resist its entry and, if entry is gained, attempt to eliminate it by phagocytosis and nonphagocytic killing in the inflammatory process. Simultaneously, bacterial antigens induce the relevant specific B-cell clones to differentiate into plasma cells capable of antibody production. If the innate defenses are rapidly successful, these slowly developing *specific* immune responses may never play an important role. If the innate responses are only partly successful, the infection may persist long enough for significant amounts of antibody to be produced. The presence of antibody leads to both enhanced phagocytosis and direct destruction of the foreign cells, as well as to neutralization of any toxins the bacteria secrete. All subsequent encounters with that type of bacterium will activate the specific responses much sooner and with greater intensity. That is, the person may have active immunity against those bacteria.

The defenses against viruses in the extracellular fluid are similar, resulting in destruction or neutralization of the virus.

Defenses Against Virus-Infected Cells and Cancer Cells

The previous section described how antibody-mediated immune responses constitute the major long-term defense against exogenous antigens—bacteria, viruses, and individual foreign molecules that enter the body and are encountered by the immune system in the extracellular fluid. This section now details how the body's own cells that have become infected by viruses (or other intracellular pathogens) or transformed into cancer cells are destroyed.

What is the value of destroying virus-infected host cells? Such destruction results in release of the viruses into the extracellular fluid, where they can be directly neutralized by circulating antibody, as just described. Generally, only a few host cells are sacrificed in this way, but once viruses have had a chance to replicate and spread from cell to cell, so many virus-infected host cells may be killed by the body's own defenses that organ malfunction may occur.

Role of Cytotoxic T Cells

Figure 18.20 summarizes a typical cytotoxic T-cell response triggered by viral infection of body cells. The response

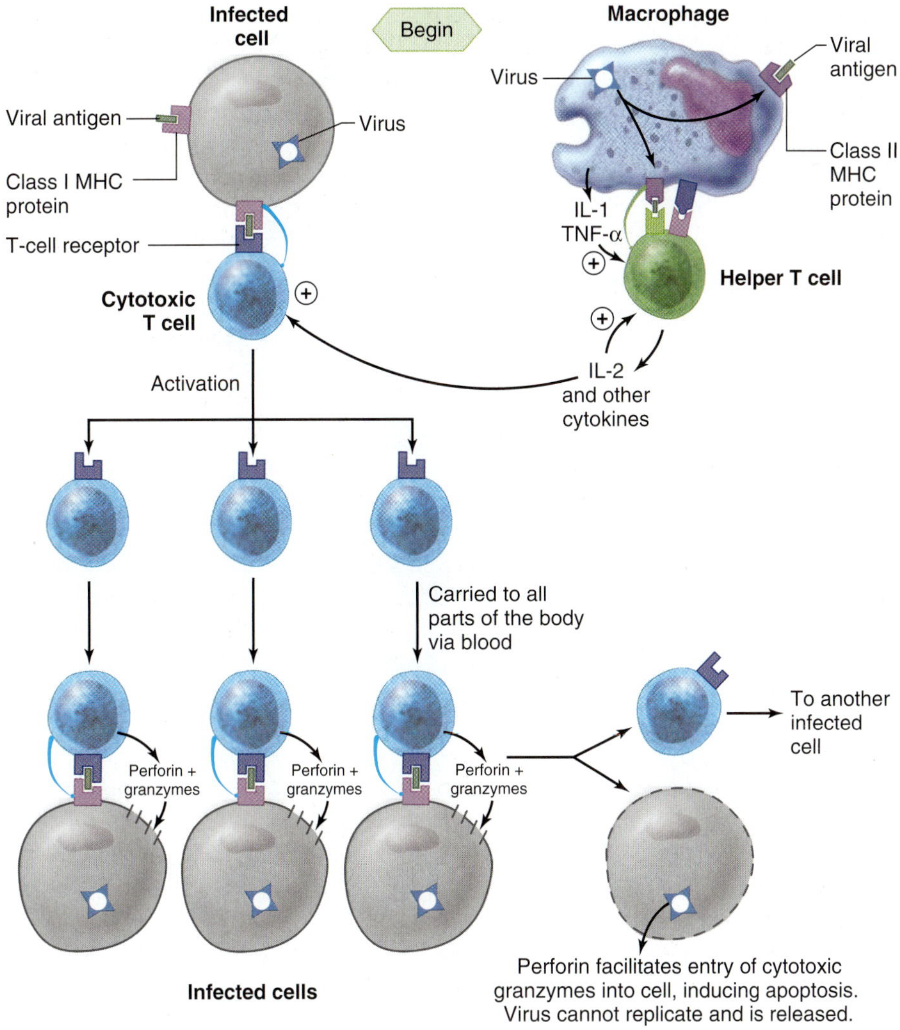

Figure 18.20 APIR Summary of events in the killing of virus-infected cells by cytotoxic T cells. The released viruses can then be phagocytosed. The precise mechanism of action of perforin is uncertain. The sequence would be similar if the inducing cell were a cancer cell rather than a virus-infected cell.

triggered by a cancer cell would be similar. As described earlier, a virus-infected or cancer cell produces foreign proteins, "endogenous antigens," which are processed and presented on the plasma membrane of the cell complexed with class I MHC proteins. Cytotoxic T cells specific for the particular antigen can bind to the complex; just as with B cells, however, binding to antigen alone does not cause activation of the cytotoxic T cell. Cytokines from adjacent activated helper T cells are also required.

What role do the helper T cells play in these cases? Figure 18.20 illustrates the most likely mechanism. Macrophages phagocytose free extracellular viruses (or, in the case of cancer, antigens released from the surface of the cancerous cells) and then process and present antigen, in association with class II MHC proteins, to the helper T cells. In addition, the macrophages provide a costimulus and also secrete IL-1 and TNF-α. The activated helper T cell releases IL-2 and other cytokines. IL-2 then acts as an autocrine substance to stimulate proliferation of the helper T cell.

The IL-2 also acts as a paracrine substance on the cytotoxic T cell bound to the surface of the virus-infected or cancer cell, stimulating this attack cell to proliferate. Other cytokines secreted by the activated helper T cell perform the same functions. Why is proliferation important if a cytotoxic T cell has already found and bound to its target? The answer is that there is rarely just one virus-infected cell or one cancer cell. By expanding the clone of cytotoxic T cells capable of recognizing the particular antigen, proliferating attack cells increase the likelihood that other virus-infected or cancer cells will be encountered by the specific type of cytotoxic T cell.

There are several mechanisms of target-cell killing by activated cytotoxic T cells, but one of the most important is as follows (see Figure 18.20). The cytotoxic T cell releases, by exocytosis, the contents of its secretory vesicles into the extracellular space between itself and the target cell to which it is bound. These vesicles contain a protein, **perforin,** which is similar in structure to the proteins of the complement system's membrane attack complex. Exactly how perforin acts is currently uncertain. However, it is believed that at least one mechanism by which perforin acts is to facilitate the transport of cytotoxic enzymes called granzymes, released by the cytotoxic T cells, into the infected cell. These enzymes then activate intracellular enzymes that induce apoptosis, killing the cell. The fact that perforin is released directly into the space between the tightly attached cytotoxic T cell and the target ensures that uninfected host bystander cells will not be killed, because perforin is not at all specific.

Some cytotoxic T cells generated during proliferation following an initial antigenic stimulation do not complete their full activation at this time but remain as memory cells. Thus, active immunity exists for cytotoxic T cells just as for B cells.

Role of NK Cells and Activated Macrophages

Although cytotoxic T cells are very important attack cells against virus-infected and cancer cells, they are not the only ones. NK cells and activated macrophages also destroy such cells by secreting toxic chemicals.

In the section on antibody-dependent cellular cytotoxicity (ADCC), we pointed out that NK cells can be linked to target cells by antibodies; this constitutes one potential method of bringing them into play against virus-infected or cancer cells. In most cases, however, strong antibody responses are not triggered by virus-infected or cancer cells, and the NK cell must bind *directly* to its target, without the help of antibodies. As noted earlier, NK cells do not have antigen specificity; rather, they nonspecifically bind to any virus-infected or cancer cell.

The major signals for NK cells to proliferate and secrete their toxic chemicals are IL-2 and interferon-gamma, secreted by the helper T cells that have been activated specifically by the targets (**Figure 18.21**). (Whereas essentially all body cells can produce the type I interferons, as described earlier, only activated helper T cells and NK cells can produce interferon-gamma.)

Thus, the attack by the NK cells is nonspecific, but a specific immune response on the part of the helper T cells is required to bring the NK cells into play. Moreover, there is a positive feedback mechanism at work here because activated NK cells can themselves secrete interferon-gamma (see Figure 18.21).

IL-2 and interferon-gamma act not only on NK cells but on macrophages in the vicinity to enhance their ability to kill cancer cells and cells infected with viruses and other pathogens. Macrophages stimulated by IL-2 and interferon-gamma are called **activated macrophages** (see Figure 18.21). In addition to phagocytosis, they secrete large amounts of many chemicals that are capable of killing cells by a variety of mechanisms. As long as there is a pathogen at the site of infection, activated macrophages will continue to present antigens to T cells that will maintain the ensuing immune response. Once cleared of infection, tissue repair will continue and the immune response will wane as T cells are no longer being activated against the pathogen.

Table 18.6 summarizes the multiple defenses against viruses described in this chapter.

18.4 Systemic Manifestations of Infection

There are many *systemic* responses to infection, that is, responses of organs and tissues distant from the site of infection or immune response. These systemic responses are collectively known as the **acute phase response** (**Figure 18.22**). It is natural to think of these responses as part of the disease, but the fact is that most of them actually represent the body's own adaptive responses to the infection.

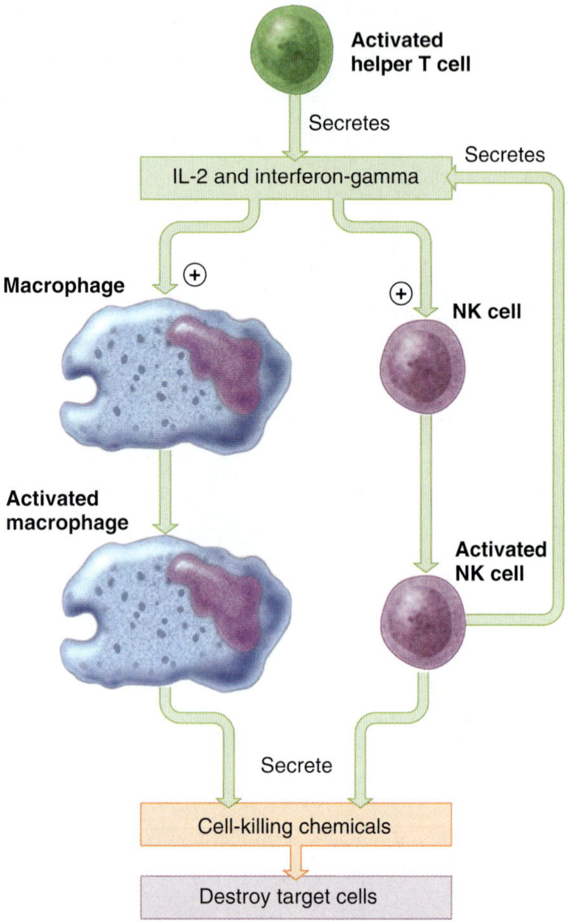

Figure 18.21 AP|R Role of IL-2 and interferon-gamma, secreted by activated helper T cells, in stimulating the killing ability of NK cells and macrophages.

The single most common and striking systemic sign of infection is fever, the mechanism of which is described in Chapter 16. Present evidence suggests that moderate fever can be beneficial because an increase in body temperature enhances many of the protective responses described in this chapter.

Decreases in the plasma concentrations of iron and zinc occur in response to infection and are due to changes in the uptake and/or release of these elements by liver, spleen, and other tissues. The decrease in plasma iron concentration has adaptive value because bacteria require a high concentration of iron to multiply. The role of the decrease in zinc is not known.

Another adaptive response to infection is the secretion by the liver of a group of proteins known collectively as **acute phase proteins.** These proteins exert many effects on the inflammatory process that serve to minimize the extent of local tissue damage. In addition, they are important for tissue repair and for clearance of cell debris and the toxins released from microbes. An example of an acute phase protein is C-reactive protein, which functions as a nonspecific opsonin to enhance phagocytosis.

Another response to infection, increased production and release of neutrophils and monocytes by the bone marrow, is of obvious value. Also occurring is a release of amino acids from muscle; the amino acids provide the building blocks for the

TABLE 18.6 Summary of Host Responses to Viruses

	Main Cells Involved	Comment on Action
Innate responses		
Anatomical barriers	Body surface linings	Provide physical barrier; antiviral chemicals
Inflammation	Tissue macrophages	Provide phagocytosis of extracellular virus
Interferon (type I)	Most cell types after viruses enter them	Type I interferon nonspecifically prevents viral replication inside host cells
Adaptive responses		
Antibody-mediated	Plasma cells (derived from B cells) that secrete antibodies	Antibodies neutralize virus and thus prevent viral entry into cell Antibodies activate complement, which leads to enhanced phagocytosis of extracellular virus Antibodies recruit NK cells via antibody-mediated cellular cytotoxicity
Helper	Helper T cells	Secrete interleukins; keep NK cells, macrophages, cytotoxic T cells, and helper T cells active; also help convert B cells to plasma cells
Direct cell killing	Cytotoxic T cells, NK cells, and activated macrophages	Destroy host cell via secreted chemicals and thus induce release of virus into extracellular fluid where it can be phagocytosed Activity stimulated by IL-2 and interferon-gamma

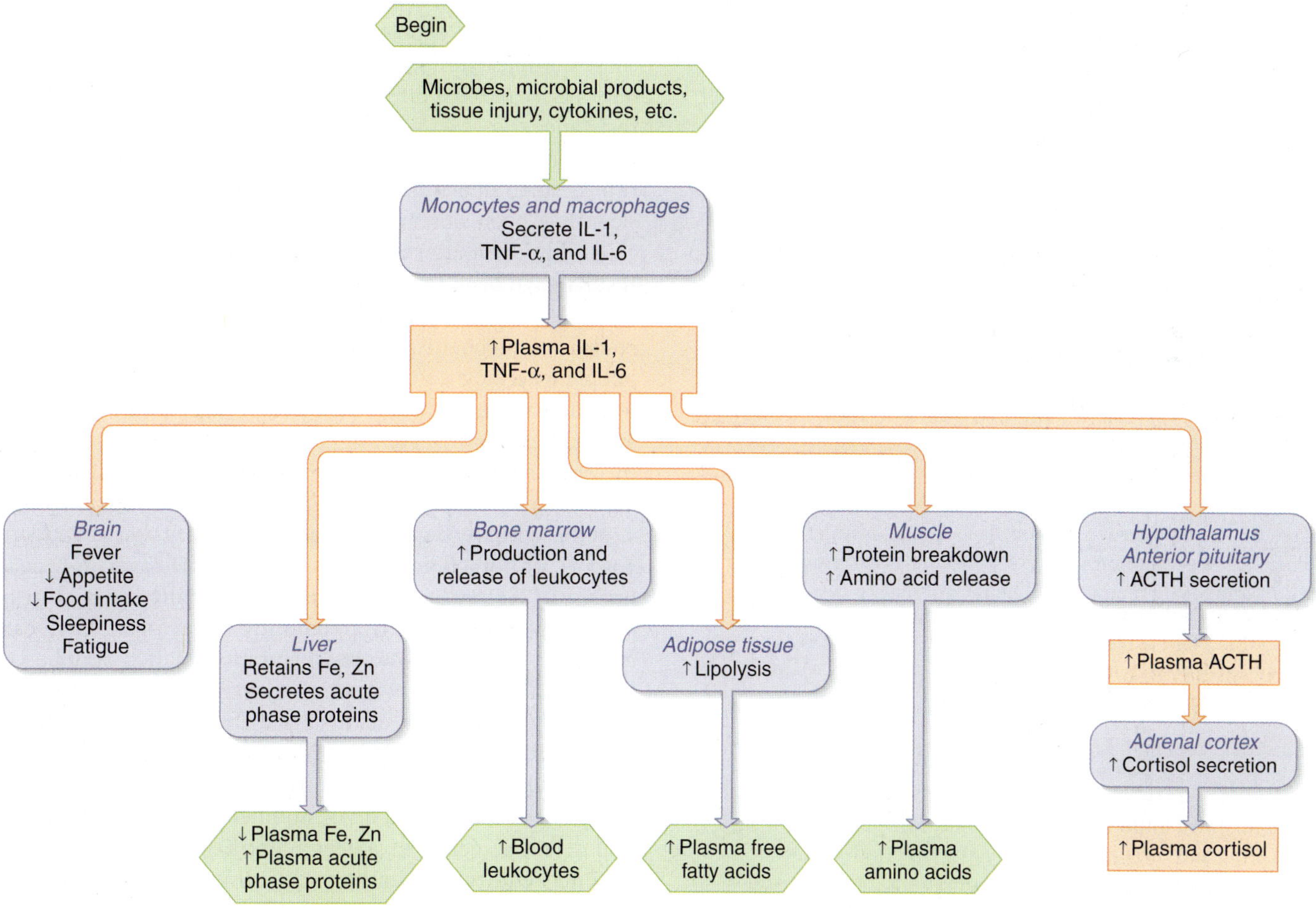

Figure 18.22 Systemic responses to infection or injury (the acute phase response). Other cytokines probably also participate. This figure does not include all the components of the acute phase response; for example, IL-1 and several other cytokines also stimulate the secretion of insulin and glucagon. The effect of cortisol on the immune response is inhibitory; cortisol provides a negative feedback action to prevent excessive immune activity (see Chapter 11 for the control mechanisms and basic functions of cortisol).

synthesis of proteins required to fight the infection and for tissue repair. Increased release of fatty acids from adipose tissue also occurs, providing a source of energy. The secretion of many hormones—notably, cortisol—is increased in the acute phase response, exerting negative feedback actions on immune function.

All of these systemic responses to infection and many others are elicited by one or more of the cytokines released from activated macrophages and other cells (see Figure 18.22). In particular, IL-1, TNF-α, and another cytokine—**interleukin 6 (IL-6)**, all of which serve local roles in immune responses, also serve as hormones to elicit distant responses such as fever.

Several other cytokines are also known to participate in the acute phase response. For example, colony-stimulating factors, which are secreted by macrophages, lymphocytes, endothelial cells, and fibroblasts, provide a major stimulus to the bone marrow to produce more neutrophils and monocytes.

The participation of macrophages in the acute phase response completes our discussion of these cells, the various functions of which are summarized in **Table 18.7**.

18.5 Factors That Alter the Resistance to Infection

Many factors determine the capacity to resist infection; a few important examples are presented here. Protein–calorie malnutrition is, worldwide, the single greatest contributor to decreased resistance to infection. Because inadequate amino acids are available to synthesize essential proteins, immune function is impaired. Deficits of specific nutrients other than protein can also lower resistance to infection.

A preexisting disease, infectious or noninfectious, can also predispose the body to infection. People with diabetes mellitus, for example, are more likely to develop infections, at least partially explainable on the basis of defective leukocyte function. Moreover, any injury to a tissue lowers its resistance, perhaps by altering the chemical environment or interfering with the blood supply.

TABLE 18.7 Role of Macrophages in Immune Responses
In innate inflammation, macrophages phagocytose particulate matter, including microbes. They also secrete antimicrobial chemicals and protein messengers (cytokines) that function as local inflammatory mediators. The inflammatory cytokines include IL-1 and TNF-α.
Macrophages process and present antigen to cytotoxic T cells and helper T cells.
The secreted IL-1 and TNF-α stimulate helper T cells to secrete IL-2 and to express the receptor for IL-2.
During adaptive immune responses, macrophages perform the same killing and inflammation-inducing functions as above but are more efficient because antibodies act as opsonins and because the cells are transformed into activated macrophages by IL-2 and interferon-gamma, both secreted by helper T cells.
The secreted IL-1, TNF-α, and IL-6 mediate many of the systemic responses to infection or injury.

Both stress and a person's state of mind can either enhance or reduce resistance to infection (and cancer). There are multiple mechanisms that constitute the links in these "mind–body" interactions. For example, lymphoid tissue is innervated, and the cells that mediate immune defenses have receptors for many neurotransmitters and hormones. Conversely, as we have seen, some of the cytokines the immune cells release have important effects on the brain and endocrine system. Moreover, lymphocytes secrete several of the same hormones produced by endocrine glands. Thus, the immune system can alter neural and endocrine function; in turn, neural and endocrine activity can modify immune function. For example, it has been shown in mice and rats that the production of antibodies can be altered by psychological conditioning. If this proves to be the case in humans, it could someday partially replace the requirement for medications to control the immune activity of persons with autoimmune disease.

The influence of physical exercise on the body's resistance to infection and cancer has been debated for decades. Present evidence indicates that the intensity, duration, chronicity, and psychological stress of the exercise all have important influences, both negative and positive, on a host of immune functions (for example, the number of circulating NK cells). Most experts in the field believe that, despite all these complexities, modest exercise and physical conditioning have net beneficial effects on the immune system and on host resistance.

Another factor associated with decreased immune function is sleep deprivation. For example, loss of a single night's sleep has been observed to reduce the activity of blood NK cells. The mechanism of this response is uncertain, but the results have been replicated by numerous investigators.

Resistance to infection will be impaired if one of the basic resistance mechanisms itself is deficient, as, for example, in people who have a genetic deficiency that impairs their ability to produce antibodies. These people experience frequent and sometimes life-threatening infections that can be prevented by regular replacement injections of gamma globulin. Another genetic defect is ***severe combined immunodeficiency (SCID)***, which is actually a group of related diseases that arise from an absence of both B and T cells and, in some cases, NK cells. If untreated, infants with this disorder usually die within their first year of life from overwhelming infections. SCID can be cured by bone marrow transplantation, which supplies both B cells and cells that will migrate to the thymus and become T cells, but these transplants are difficult and not always successful. Recently, gene therapy to restore the defective gene using a viral vector targeted to hematopoietic stem cells has proven successful in a small number of SCID patients. Several defective genes have been identified, including one for an enzyme required for immunoglobulin production and one for an enzyme that protects immature lymphocytes against toxic by-products of purine metabolism.

An environmentally induced decrease in the production of leukocytes is also an important cause of lowered resistance. This can occur, for example, in patients given drugs to inhibit the rejection of tissue or organ transplants (see the section on graft rejection that follows).

In terms of the numbers of people involved, the most important example of the lack of a basic resistance mechanism is the disease called *acquired immune deficiency syndrome* (*AIDS*).

Acquired Immune Deficiency Syndrome (AIDS)

Acquired immune deficiency syndrome (***AIDS***) is caused by the ***human immunodeficiency virus*** (***HIV***), which incapacitates the immune system. HIV belongs to the retrovirus family, whose nucleic acid core is RNA rather than DNA. Retroviruses possess an enzyme called reverse transcriptase, which, once the virus is inside a host cell, transcribes the virus's RNA into DNA, which is then integrated into the host cell's chromosomes. Replication of the virus inside the cell causes the death of the cell.

The cells that HIV preferentially (but not exclusively) enters are helper T cells. HIV infects these cells because the CD4 protein on the plasma membrane of helper T cells acts as a receptor for one of the HIV's surface proteins called gp120. As a result, the helper T cell binds the virus, making it possible for the virus to enter the cell. Very importantly, this binding of the HIV gp120 protein to CD4 is not sufficient to grant the HIV entry into the helper T cell. In addition, another surface protein on the helper T cell, one that serves normally as a receptor for certain chemokines, must serve as a coreceptor for the gp120. It has been found that persons who have a mutation in this chemokine receptor are highly resistant to infection with HIV. Much research is now focused on the possible therapeutic use of chemicals that can interact with and block this coreceptor.

Once in the helper T cell, the replicating HIV can directly kill the helper T cell but also indirectly causes its death via the body's usual immune attack. The attack is mediated in this case mainly by cytotoxic T cells attacking the virus-infected cells. In addition, by still poorly understood mechanisms, HIV causes the death of many *uninfected* helper T cells by apoptosis. Without adequate numbers of helper T cells, neither B cells nor cytotoxic T cells can function normally. As a result, the AIDS patient dies from infections and cancers that the immune system would ordinarily readily handle.

AIDS was first described in 1981, and it has since reached epidemic proportions worldwide. The great majority of persons now infected with HIV have no symptoms of AIDS. It is important to distinguish between the presence of the symptomatic disease—AIDS—and asymptomatic infection with HIV. The latter is diagnosed by the presence of anti-HIV antibodies or HIV RNA in the blood. It is thought, however, that most infected persons will eventually develop AIDS, although at highly varying rates.

The path from HIV infection to AIDS commonly takes about 10 years in untreated persons. Typically, during the first 5 years, the rapidly replicating viruses continually kill large numbers of helper T cells in lymphoid tissues, but these are replaced by new cells. Therefore, the number of helper T cells stays relatively normal (about 1000 cells/mm^3 of blood) and the person is asymptomatic. During the next 5 years, this balance is lost; the number of helper T cells, as measured in blood, decreases to about half the normal level but many people still remain asymptomatic. As the helper T-cell count continues to decrease, however, the symptoms of AIDS begin—infections with bacteria, viruses, fungi, and parasites. These are accompanied by systemic symptoms of weight loss, lethargy, and fever—all caused by high concentrations of the cytokines that induce the acute phase response. Certain unusual cancers (such as ***Kaposi's sarcoma***) also occur with relatively high frequency. In untreated persons, death usually ensues within 2 years after the onset of AIDS symptoms.

The major routes of transmission of HIV are through (1) transfer of contaminated blood or blood products from one person to another, (2) unprotected sexual intercourse with an infected partner, (3) transmission from an infected mother to her fetus across the placenta during pregnancy and delivery, or (4) transfer via breast milk during nursing.

Two components to the therapeutic management of HIV-infected persons include one directed against the virus itself to delay progression of the disease and one to prevent or treat the opportunistic infections and cancers that ultimately cause death. The present recommended treatment for HIV infection itself is a simultaneous battery of at least four drugs. Two of these inhibit the action of the HIV enzyme (reverse transcriptase) that converts the viral RNA into the host cell's DNA; a third drug inhibits the HIV enzyme (α-protease) that cleaves a large protein into smaller units required for the assembly of new HIV; and a fourth drug blocks fusion of the virus with the T cell. The use of this complex and expensive regimen (called ***HAART***, for *highly active anti-retroviral therapy*) greatly reduces the replication of HIV in the body and ideally should be introduced very early in the course of HIV infection, not just after the appearance of AIDS.

The ultimate hope for prevention of AIDS is the development of a vaccine. For a variety of reasons related to the nature of the virus (it generates large numbers of distinct subspecies) and the fact that it infects helper T cells, which are crucial for immune responses, vaccine development is not an easy task.

Antibiotics

The most important of the drugs employed in helping the body to resist microbes, mainly bacteria, are antibiotics. An ***antibiotic*** is any molecule or substance that kills bacteria. Antibiotics may be produced by one strain of bacteria to defend against other strains. Since the mid-twentieth century, commercial manufacture of antibiotics such as ***penicillin*** has revolutionized our ability to treat disease.

Antibiotics inhibit a wide variety of processes, including bacterial cell-wall synthesis, protein synthesis, and DNA replication. Fortunately, a number of the reactions involved in the synthesis of protein by bacteria and the proteins themselves are sufficiently different from those in human cells that certain antibiotics can inhibit them without interfering with the body's own protein synthesis. For example, the antibiotic ***erythromycin*** blocks the movement of ribosomes along bacterial messenger RNA.

Antibiotics, however, must not be used indiscriminately. They may exert allergic reactions, and they may exert toxic effects on the body's cells. Another reason for judicious use is the escalating and very serious problem of drug resistance. Most large bacterial populations contain a few mutants that are resistant to the drug, and these few may be capable of multiplying into large populations resistant to the effects of that particular antibiotic. Alternatively, the antibiotic can induce the expression of a latent gene that confers resistance. Finally, resistance can be transferred from one resistant microbe directly to another previously nonresistant microbe by means of DNA passed between them. (One example of how drug resistance can spread by these phenomena is that many bacterial strains that were once highly susceptible to penicillin now produce an enzyme that cleaves the penicillin molecule.) Yet another reason for the judicious use of antibiotics is that these substances may actually contribute to a new infection by eliminating certain species of relatively harmless bacteria that ordinarily prevent the growth of more dangerous ones. One site in which this may occur is the large intestine, where the loss of harmless bacteria may account for the symptoms of cramps and diarrhea that occur in some individuals taking certain types of antibiotics.

18.6 Harmful Immune Responses

Until now, we have focused on the mechanisms of immune responses and their protective effects. The following section discusses how immune responses can sometimes actually be harmful or unwanted.

Graft Rejection

The major obstacle to successful transplantation of tissues and organs is that the immune system recognizes the transplants, called grafts, as foreign and launches an attack against them. This is called ***graft rejection.*** Although B cells and macrophages play some role, cytotoxic T cells and helper T cells are mainly responsible for graft rejection.

Except in the case of identical twins, the class I MHC proteins on the cells of a graft differ from the recipient's as do the class II molecules present on the macrophages in the graft (recall that virtually all organs and tissues have macrophages). Consequently, the MHC proteins of both classes are recognized as foreign by the recipient's T cells, and the cells bearing these proteins are destroyed by the recipient's cytotoxic T cells with the aid of helper T cells.

Some of the tools aimed at reducing graft rejection are radiation and drugs that kill actively dividing lymphocytes and thereby decrease the recipient's T-cell population. A very effective drug, however, is ***cyclosporin,*** which does not kill lymphocytes but rather blocks the production of IL-2 and other cytokines by helper T cells. This eliminates a critical signal for proliferation of both the helper T cells themselves and the cytotoxic T cells. Synthetic adrenal corticosteroids are also used to reduce the rejection.

Problems with the use of drugs like cyclosporin and potent synthetic adrenal corticosteroids include the following: (1) Immunosuppression with them is nonspecific, so patients taking them are at increased risk for infections and cancer; (2) they exert other toxic side effects; and (3) they must be used continuously to inhibit rejection. An important new kind of therapy, one that may be able to avoid these problems, is under study. Recall that immune tolerance for self proteins is achieved by clonal deletion and/or inactivation and that the mechanism for this is absence of a nonantigenic costimulus at the time the antigen is first encountered. The hope is that, at the time of graft surgery, treatment with drugs that block the complementary proteins constituting the costimulus may induce a permanent state of immune tolerance toward the graft.

The Fetus as a Graft

During pregnancy, the fetal trophoblast cells of the placenta lie in direct contact with maternal immune cells. Because half of the fetal genes are paternal, all proteins coded for by these genes are foreign to the mother. Why does the mother's immune system refrain from attacking the trophoblast cells, which express such proteins, and thereby fail to reject the placenta? This issue is far from solved, but one critical mechanism (there are certainly others) is as follows. Trophoblast cells, unlike virtually all other nucleated cells, do not express the usual class I MHC proteins. Instead, they express a unique class I MHC protein that maternal immune cells do not recognize as foreign.

Transfusion Reactions

Transfusion reaction, the illness caused when erythrocytes are destroyed during blood transfusion, is a special example of tissue rejection, one that illustrates the fact that antibodies rather than cytotoxic T cells can sometimes be the major factor in rejection. Erythrocytes do not have MHC proteins, but they do have plasma membrane proteins and carbohydrates (the latter linked to the membrane by lipids) that can function as antigens when exposed to another person's blood. There are more than 400 erythrocyte antigens, but the ABO system of carbohydrates is the most important for transfusion reactions.

Some people have the gene that results in synthesis of the A antigen, some have the gene for the B antigen, some have both genes, and some have neither gene. (Genes cannot code for the carbohydrates that function as antigens; rather, they code for the particular enzymes that catalyze the formation of the carbohydrates.) The erythrocytes of those with neither gene are said to have O-type erythrocytes. Consequently, the possible blood types are A, B, AB, and O (**Table 18.8**).

Type A individuals always have anti-B antibodies in their plasma. Similarly, type B individuals have plasma anti-A antibodies. Type AB individuals have neither anti-A nor anti-B antibody, and type O individuals have both. These antierythrocyte antibodies are called natural antibodies. How they arise naturally—that is, without exposure to the appropriate antigen-bearing erythrocytes—is not clear.

With this information as background, we can predict what happens if a type A person is given type B blood. There are two incompatibilities: (1) The recipient's anti-B antibodies cause the transfused cells to be attacked; and (2) the anti-A antibodies in the transfused plasma cause the recipient's cells to be attacked. The latter is generally of little consequence, however, because the transfused antibodies become so diluted in the recipient's plasma that they are ineffective in inducing a response. It is the destruction of the transfused cells by the recipient's antibodies that produces the problem.

TABLE 18.8 Human ABO Blood Groups

Blood Group	Percentage*	Antigen on RBC	Genetic Possibilities Homozygous	Heterozygous	Antibody in Blood
A	42	A	AA	AO	Anti-B
B	10	B	BB	BO	Anti-A
AB	3	A and B	—	AB	Neither anti-A nor anti-B
O	45	Neither A nor B	OO	—	Both anti-A and anti-B

*In the United States.

Similar analyses show that the following situations would result in an attack on the transfused erythrocytes: a type B person given either A or AB blood; a type A person given either B or AB blood; a type O person given A, B, or AB blood. Type O people are, therefore, sometimes called universal donors, whereas type AB people are universal recipients. These terms are misleading, however, because besides antigens of the ABO system, many other erythrocyte antigens and plasma antibodies exist. Therefore, except in a dire emergency, the blood of the donor and recipient must be tested for incompatibilities directly by the procedure called ***cross-matching.*** The recipient's serum is combined on a glass slide with the prospective donor's erythrocytes (a "major" cross-match), and the mixture is observed for rupture (hemolysis) or clumping (agglutination) of the erythrocytes, either of which indicates a mismatch. In addition, the recipient's erythrocytes can be combined with the prospective donor's serum (a "minor" cross-match), looking again for mismatches.

Another group of erythrocyte membrane antigens of medical importance is the Rh system of proteins. There are more than 40 such antigens, but the one most likely to cause a problem is called Rh_o, known commonly as the **Rh factor** because it was first studied in rhesus monkeys. Human erythrocytes either have the antigen (Rh-positive) or lack it (Rh-negative). About 85% of the U.S. population are Rh-positive.

Antibodies in the Rh system, unlike the "natural antibodies" of the ABO system, follow the classical immunity pattern in that no one has anti-Rh antibodies unless exposed to Rh-positive cells from another person. This can occur if an Rh-negative person is subjected to multiple transfusions with Rh-positive blood, but its major occurrence involves the mother–fetus relationship. During pregnancy, some of the fetal erythrocytes may cross the placental barriers into the maternal circulation. If the mother is Rh-negative and the fetus is Rh-positive, this can induce the mother to synthesize anti-Rh antibodies. This occurs mainly during separation of the placenta at delivery. Consequently, a first Rh-positive pregnancy rarely offers any danger to the fetus because delivery occurs before the mother makes the antibodies. In future pregnancies, however, these antibodies will already be present in the mother and can cross the placenta to attack and hemolyze the erythrocytes of an Rh-positive fetus. This condition, which can cause an anemia severe enough to cause the death of the fetus in utero or of the newborn, is called ***hemolytic disease of the newborn.*** The risk increases with each Rh-positive pregnancy as the mother becomes more and more sensitized.

Fortunately, this disease can be prevented by giving an Rh-negative mother human gamma globulin against Rh-positive erythrocytes within 72 h after she has delivered an Rh-positive infant. These antibodies bind to the antigenic sites on any Rh-positive erythrocytes that might have entered the mother's blood during delivery and prevent them from inducing antibody synthesis by the mother. The administered antibodies are eventually metabolized.

You may be wondering whether ABO incompatibilities are also a cause of hemolytic disease of the newborn. For example, a woman with type O blood has antibodies to both the A and B antigens. If her fetus is type A or B, this theoretically should cause a problem. Fortunately, it usually does not, partly because the A and B antigens are not strongly expressed in fetal erythrocytes and partly because the antibodies, unlike the anti-Rh antibodies, are of the IgM type, which do not readily cross the placenta.

Allergy (Hypersensitivity)

Allergy (***hypersensitivity***) refers to diseases in which immune responses to environmental antigens cause inflammation and damage to the body itself. Antigens that cause allergy are called ***allergens;*** common examples include those in ragweed pollen and poison ivy. Most allergens themselves are relatively or completely harmless—the immune responses to them cause the damage. In essence, then, allergy is immunity gone wrong, for the response is inappropriate to the stimulus.

A word about terminology is useful here. There are four major types of hypersensitivity, as categorized by the different immunologic effector pathways involved in the inflammatory response. The term *allergy* is sometimes used popularly to denote only one of these types, that mediated by IgE antibodies. We will follow the common practice, however, of using the term *allergy* in its broader sense as synonymous with *hypersensitivity.*

To develop a particular allergy, a genetically predisposed person must first be exposed to the allergen. This initial exposure causes "sensitization." The subsequent exposures elicit the damaging immune responses that we recognize as the disease. The diversity of allergic responses reflects the different immunologic effector pathways elicited. The classification of allergic diseases is based on these mechanisms (**Table 18.9**).

TABLE 18.9 Major Types of Hypersensitivity
I. Delayed hypersensitivity A. Mediated by helper T cells and macrophages B. Independent of antibodies
II. Immune-complex hypersensitivity A. Mediated by antigen–antibody complexes deposited in tissue
III. Cytotoxic hypersensitivity A. Mediated by antibodies that lead to damage or destruction of cells, as in hemolytic disease of the newborn
IV. Immediate hypersensitivity A. Mediated by IgE antibodies, mast cells, and eosinophils

In one type of allergy, the inflammatory response is independent of antibodies. It is due to pronounced secretion of cytokines by helper T cells activated by antigen in the area. These cytokines themselves act as inflammatory mediators and also activate macrophages to secrete their potent mediators. Because it takes several days to develop, this type of allergy is known as ***delayed hypersensitivity.*** The tuberculin skin test is an example.

In contrast to this are the various types of antibody-mediated allergic responses. One important type is called ***immune-complex hypersensitivity.*** It occurs when so many antibodies (of either the IgG or IgM types) combine with free antigens that large numbers of antigen–antibody complexes precipitate out on the surface of endothelial cells or are trapped in capillary walls, particularly those of the renal corpuscles. These immune complexes activate complement, which then induces an inflammatory response that damages the tissues immediately surrounding the complexes.

A third type of hypersensitivity or ***cytotoxic hypersensitivity*** occurs when antibodies bind to cell-surface-associated antigens that lead to tissue injury or altered receptor function. An example of this type of hypersensitivity, just discussed, is hemolytic disease of the newborn.

Immediate Hypersensitivity

The more common type of antibody-mediated allergic response is called ***immediate hypersensitivity,*** because the response is usually very rapid in onset. It is also called ***IgE-mediated hypersensitivity*** because it involves IgE antibodies. In immediate hypersensitivity, initial exposure to the antigen leads to some antibody synthesis and, more important, to the production of memory B cells that mediate active immunity. Upon reexposure, the antigen elicits a more powerful antibody response. So far, none of this is unusual; the difference is that the particular antigens that elicit immediate hypersensitivity reactions stimulate, in genetically susceptible persons, the production of type IgE antibodies. Production of IgE requires the participation of a particular subset of helper T cells that are activated by the allergens presented by B cells. These activated helper T cells then release cytokines that preferentially stimulate differentiation of the B cells into IgE-producing plasma cells.

Upon their release from plasma cells, IgE antibodies circulate throughout the body and become attached via binding sites on their Fc portions to connective-tissue mast cells (**Figure 18.23**). When the same antigen type subsequently enters the body and combines with the IgE bound to the mast

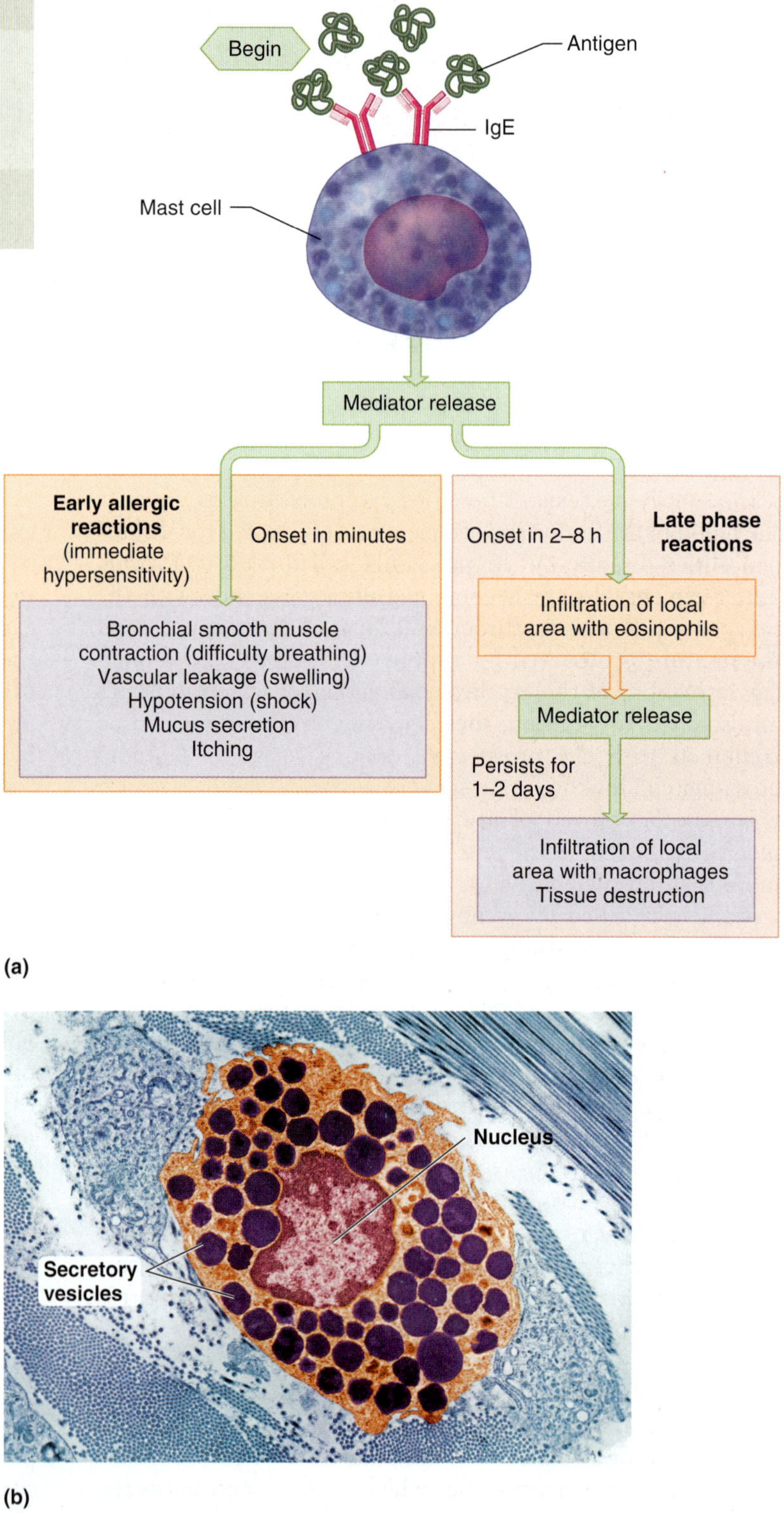

Figure 18.23 APR Immediate hypersensitivity allergic response. (a) Sequence of events. (b) Colorized electron micrograph of a mast cell, showing numerous secretory vesicles.

cell, this triggers the mast cell to secrete many inflammatory mediators, including **histamine,** various eicosanoids, and chemokines. All of these mediators then initiate a local inflammatory response. (The entire sequence of events just described for mast cells can also occur with basophils in the circulation.)

Consequently, the symptoms of IgE-mediated allergy reflect the various effects of these inflammatory mediators and the body site in which the antigen–IgE–mast cell combination occurs. For example, when a previously sensitized person inhales ragweed pollen, the antigen combines with IgE on mast cells in the respiratory passages. The mediators released cause increased secretion of mucus, increased blood flow, swelling of the epithelial lining, and contraction of the smooth muscle surrounding the airways. As a result, the symptoms that characterize hay fever follow—congestion, runny nose, sneezing, and difficulty breathing. Immediate hypersensitivities to penicillin and insect venoms sometimes occur, and these are usually correlated with IgE production.

Allergic symptoms are usually localized to the site of antigen entry. If very large amounts of the chemicals released by the mast cells (or blood basophils) enter the circulation, however, systemic symptoms may result and cause severe hypotension and bronchiolar constriction. This sequence of events, called ***anaphylaxis,*** can cause death due to circulatory and respiratory failure; it can be elicited in some sensitized people by the antigen in a single bee sting.

The very rapid components of immediate hypersensitivity often proceed to a ***late phase reaction*** lasting many hours or days, during which large numbers of leukocytes, particularly eosinophils, migrate into the inflamed area. The chemoattractants involved are cytokines released by mast cells and helper T cells activated by the allergen. The eosinophils, once in the area, secrete mediators that prolong the inflammation and sensitize the tissues so that less allergen is required the next time to evoke a response.

Given the inappropriateness of most immediate hypersensitivity responses, how did such a system evolve? The normal physiological function of the IgE–mast cell–eosinophil pathways is to repel invasion by multicellular parasites that cannot be phagocytosed. The mediators released by the mast cells stimulate the inflammatory response against the parasites, and the eosinophils serve as the major killer cells against them by secreting several toxins. How this system also came to be inducible by harmless substances is not clear.

Autoimmune Disease

Whereas allergy is due to an inappropriate response to an environmental antigen, ***autoimmune disease*** is due to an inappropriate immune attack triggered by the body's own proteins acting as antigens. The immune attack, mediated by autoantibodies and self-reactive T cells, is directed specifically against the body's own cells that contain these proteins.

We explained earlier how the body is normally in a state of immune tolerance toward its own cells. Unfortunately, there are situations in which this tolerance breaks down and the body does in fact launch antibody-mediated or killer cell–mediated attacks against its own cells and tissues. A growing number of human diseases are being recognized as autoimmune in origin, some of which have been described elsewhere in this textbook. Examples are ***multiple sclerosis,*** in which myelin is attacked (see Chapter 6); ***myasthenia gravis,*** in which the nicotinic receptors for acetylcholine on skeletal muscle cells are the target (see Chapter 9); ***rheumatoid arthritis,*** in which connective tissues in joints are damaged; and ***type 1 diabetes mellitus,*** in which the insulin-producing cells of the pancreas are destroyed (see Chapter 16). Some possible causes for the body's failure to recognize its own cells are summarized in **Table 18.10**.

Excessive Inflammatory Responses

Recall that complement, other inflammatory mediators, and the toxic chemicals secreted by neutrophils and macrophages are not specific with regard to their targets. Consequently, during an inflammatory response directed against pathogens, there can be so much generation or release of these substances that adjacent normal tissues may be damaged. These substances can also cause potentially lethal systemic responses. For example, macrophages release very large amounts of IL-1 and TNF-α, both of which are powerful inflammatory mediators (in addition to their other effects) in response to an infection with certain types of bacteria. These cytokines can cause profound vasodilation throughout the body, precipitating a type of hypotension called ***septic shock.*** This is often accompanied by dangerously high fevers. In other words, the cytokines released in response to the bacteria, not the bacteria themselves, cause septic shock.

Another important example of damage produced by excessive inflammation in response to pathogens is the dementia that occurs in AIDS. HIV does not itself attack neurons, but it does infect microglia. Such invasion causes the microglia, which function as macrophage-like cells, to produce very high concentrations of inflammatory cytokines and other

TABLE 18.10 Some Possible Causes of Autoimmune Attack
There may be failure of clonal deletion in the thymus or of clonal inactivation in the periphery. This is particularly true for "sequestered antigens," such as certain proteins that are unavailable to the immune system during critical early-life periods.
Normal body proteins may be altered by combination with drugs or environmental chemicals. This leads to an attack on the cells bearing the now "foreign" protein.
In immune attacks on virus-infected bodily cells, so many cells may be destroyed that disease results.
Genetic mutations in the body's cells may yield new proteins that serve as antigens.
The body may encounter pathogens whose antigens are so close in structure to certain of the body's own proteins that the antibodies or cytotoxic T cells produced against these microbial antigens also attack cells bearing the self proteins.
Proteins normally never encountered by lymphocytes may become exposed as a result of some other disease.

molecules that are toxic to neurons. (Microglia are also implicated in noninfectious brain disorders, like ***Alzheimer disease,*** that are characterized by inflammation.)

Excessive chronic inflammation can also occur in the absence of pathogen infection. Thus, various major diseases, including ***asthma,*** rheumatoid arthritis, and ***inflammatory bowel disease,*** are categorized as ***chronic inflammatory diseases.*** The causes of these diseases and the interplay between genetic and environmental factors are still poorly understood (see Chapters 13 and 15 for additional details on the nature of asthma and inflammatory bowel disease, respectively). Some, like rheumatoid arthritis, are mainly autoimmune in nature, but all appear to be associated with positive feedback increases in the production of cytokines and other inflammatory mediators.

Yet another example of excessive inflammation in a noninfectious state is the development of atherosclerotic plaques in blood vessels (see Figure 12.66). It is likely that, in response to endothelial cell dysfunction, the vessel wall releases inflammatory cytokines (IL-1, for example) that promote all stages of atherosclerosis—excessive clotting, chemotaxis of various leukocytes (as well as smooth muscle cells), and so on. The endothelial-cell dysfunction is caused by initially subtle vessel-wall injury by lipoproteins and other factors, including elevated blood pressure and homocysteine (see Chapter 12).

In summary, the various mediators of inflammation and immunity are a double-edged sword. In usual amounts, they are essential for normal resistance; in excessive amounts, however, they can cause illness.

This completes the section on immunology. **Table 18.11** presents a summary of immune mechanisms in the form of a mini-glossary of cells and chemical mediators involved in immune responses. All of the material in this table has been covered in this chapter.

TABLE 18.11 A Mini-Glossary of Chemical Mediators and Cells Involved in Immune Functions

Chemical Mediators

Acute phase proteins Group of proteins secreted by the liver during systemic response to injury or infection; stimuli for their secretion are IL-1, IL-6, and other cytokines.

Antibodies Immunoglobulins secreted by plasma cells; combine with the type of antigen that stimulated their production and direct an attack against the antigen or a cell bearing it.

C1 The first protein in the classical complement pathway.

Chemoattractants A general name given to any chemical mediator that stimulates chemotaxis of neutrophils or other leukocytes.

Chemokines Any cytokine that functions as a chemoattractant.

Chemotaxin A synonym for chemoattractant.

Complement A group of plasma proteins that, upon activation, kill pathogens directly and facilitate the various steps of the inflammatory process, including phagocytosis; the classical complement pathway is triggered by antigen–antibody complexes, whereas the alternative pathway can operate independently of antibody.

C-reactive protein One of several proteins that function as nonspecific opsonins; production by the liver is increased during the acute phase response.

Cytokines General term for protein messengers that regulate immune responses; secreted by macrophages, monocytes, lymphocytes, neutrophils, and several nonimmune cell types; function both locally and as hormones.

Eicosanoids General term for products of arachidonic acid metabolism (prostaglandins, thromboxanes, leukotrienes); function as important inflammatory mediators.

Histamine An inflammatory mediator secreted mainly by mast cells; acts on microcirculation to cause vasodilation and increased permeability to protein.

IgA The class of antibodies secreted by cells lining the GI, respiratory, and genitourinary tracts.

IgD A class of antibodies whose function is unknown.

IgE The class of antibodies that mediates immediate hypersensitivity and resistance to parasites.

IgG The most abundant class of plasma antibodies.

IgM A class of antibodies that is produced first in all immune responses. Along with IgG, it provides the bulk of specific humoral immunity against bacteria and viruses.

Immunoglobulin (Ig) Proteins that function as B-cell receptors and antibodies; the five major classes are IgA, IgD, IgE, IgG, and IgM.

Interferons (type I) Group of cytokines that nonspecifically inhibit viral replication.

TABLE 18.11 A Mini-Glossary of Chemical Mediators and Cells Involved in Immune Functions *(continued)*

Chemical Mediators

Interferon (type II) Also called interferon-gamma, it stimulates the killing ability of NK cells and macrophages.

Interleukin 1 (IL-1) Cytokine secreted by macrophages (and other cells) that activates helper T cells, exerts many inflammatory effects, and mediates many of the systemic acute phase responses, including fever.

Interleukin 2 (IL-2) Cytokine secreted by activated helper T cells that causes helper T cells, cytotoxic T cells, and NK cells to proliferate, and causes activation of macrophages.

Interleukin 6 (IL-6) Cytokine secreted by macrophages (and other cells) that exerts multiple effects on immune system cells, inflammation, fever, and the acute phase response.

Kinins Peptides that split from kininogens in inflamed areas and facilitate the vascular changes associated with inflammation; they also activate neuronal pain receptors.

Membrane attack complex (MAC) Group of complement proteins that forms channels in the surface of a microbe, making it leaky and killing it.

Natural antibodies Antibodies to the erythrocyte antigens (of the A or B type).

Opsonin General name given to any chemical mediator that promotes phagocytosis.

Perforin Protein secreted by cytotoxic T cells and NK cells that forms channels in the plasma membrane of the target cell, making it leaky and killing it; its structure and function are similar to that of the MAC in the complement system.

Tumor necrosis factor-alpha (TNF-α) Cytokine secreted by macrophages (and other cells) that has many of the same actions as IL-1.

Cells

Activated macrophages Macrophages whose killing ability has been enhanced by cytokines, particularly IL-2 and interferon-gamma.

Antigen-presenting cell (APC) Cell that presents antigen, complexed with MHC proteins, on its surface to T cells.

B cells Lymphocytes that, upon activation, proliferate and differentiate into antibody-secreting plasma cells; provide major defense against bacteria, viruses in the extracellular fluid, and toxins; and can function as antigen-presenting cells to helper T cells.

Cytotoxic T cells The class of T lymphocytes that, upon activation by specific antigen, directly attack the cells bearing that type of antigen; are major killers of virus-infected cells and cancer cells; and bind antigen associated with class I MHC proteins.

Dendritic cells Cells that carry out phagocytosis and serve as antigen-presenting cells.

Eosinophils Leukocytes involved in destruction of parasites and in immediate hypersensitivity responses.

Helper T cells The class of T cells that, via secreted cytokines, play a stimulatory role in the activation of B cells and cytotoxic T cells; also can activate NK cells and macrophages; and bind antigen associated with class II MHC proteins.

Lymphocytes The type of leukocyte responsible for adaptive immune responses; categorized mainly as B cells, T cells, and NK cells.

Macrophages Cell type that (1) functions as a phagocyte, (2) processes and presents antigen to helper T cells, and (3) secretes cytokines involved in inflammation, activation of lymphocytes, and the systemic acute phase response to infection or injury.

Mast cells Tissue cells that bind IgE and release inflammatory mediators in response to parasites and immediate hypersensitivity reactions.

Memory cells B cells and cytotoxic T cells that differentiate during an initial immune response and respond rapidly during a subsequent exposure to the same antigen.

Monocytes A type of leukocyte; leaves the bloodstream and is transformed into a macrophage.

Natural killer (NK) cells Class of lymphocytes that bind to cells bearing foreign antigens without specific recognition and kill them directly; major targets are virus-infected cells and cancer cells; participate in antibody-dependent cellular cytotoxicity (ADCC).

Neutrophils Leukocytes that function as phagocytes and also release chemicals involved in inflammation.

Plasma cells Cells that differentiate from activated B lymphocytes and secrete antibodies.

T cells Lymphocytes derived from precursors that differentiated in the thymus; see *Cytotoxic T cells* and *Helper T cells.*

SUMMARY

Cells and Secretions Mediating Immune Defenses

I. Immune defenses may be nonspecific, so that the identity of the target is not recognized, or they may be specific, so that it is recognized.

II. The cells of the immune system are leukocytes (neutrophils, eosinophils, basophils, monocytes, and lymphocytes), plasma cells, macrophages, dendritic cells, and mast cells. The leukocytes use the blood for transportation but function mainly in the tissues.

III. Cells of the immune system (as well as some other cells) secrete protein messengers that regulate immune responses and are collectively called cytokines.

Innate Immune Responses

I. External barriers to infection are the skin; the linings of the respiratory, gastrointestinal, and genitourinary tracts; the cilia of these linings; and antimicrobial chemicals in glandular secretions.

II. Inflammation, the local response to infection, includes vasodilation, increased vascular permeability to protein, phagocyte chemotaxis, destruction of the invader via phagocytosis or extracellular killing, and tissue repair.
   a. The mediators controlling these processes, summarized in Table 18.3, are either released from cells in the area or generated extracellularly from plasma proteins.
   b. The main cells that function as phagocytes are the neutrophils, monocytes, macrophages, and dendritic cells. These cells also secrete many inflammatory mediators.
   c. One group of inflammatory mediators—the complement family of plasma proteins activated during nonspecific inflammation by the alternative complement pathway—not only stimulates many of the steps of inflammation but mediates extracellular killing via the membrane at tack complex.
   d. The final response to infection or tissue damage is tissue repair.

III. Interferons stimulate the production of intracellular proteins that nonspecifically inhibit viral replication.

IV. Toll-like receptors are evolutionarily ancient proteins that recognize pathogen-associated molecular patterns that are highly conserved features of pathogens. TLRs belong to a family of proteins called pattern-recognition receptors and may be among the first molecules to have evolved in eukaryotic organisms to combat microbial diseases.

Adaptive Immune Responses

I. Lymphocytes mediate adaptive immune responses.

II. Adaptive immune responses occur in three stages.
   a. A lymphocyte programmed to recognize a specific antigen encounters it and binds to it via plasma membrane receptors specific for the antigen.
   b. The lymphocyte undergoes activation—a cycle of cell divisions and differentiation.
   c. The multiple active lymphocytes produced in this manner launch an attack all over the body against the specific antigens that stimulated their production.

III. The lymphoid organs are categorized as primary (bone marrow and thymus) or secondary (lymph nodes, spleen, tonsils, and lymphocyte collections in the linings of the body's tracts).
   a. The primary lymphoid organs are the sites of maturation of lymphocytes that will then be carried to the secondary lymphoid organs, which are the major sites of lymphocyte cell division and adaptive immune responses.
   b. Lymphocytes undergo a continuous recirculation among the secondary lymphoid organs, lymph, blood, and all the body's organs and tissues.

IV. The three broad populations of lymphocytes are B, T, and NK cells.
   a. B cells mature in the bone marrow and are carried to the secondary lymphoid organs, where additional B cells arise by cell division.
   b. T-cell precursors leave the bone marrow, migrate to the thymus, and undergo maturation there. These cells then circulate between the blood and secondary lymphoid organs. Stimulation with antigen and costimulatory molecules lead to T cells' expansion by cell division.
   c. NK cells originate in the bone marrow.

V. B cells and T cells have different functions.
   a. B cells, upon activation, differentiate into plasma cells, which secrete antibodies. Antibody-mediated responses constitute the major defense against bacteria, viruses, and toxins in the extracellular fluid.
   b. Cytotoxic T cells directly attack and kill virus-infected cells and cancer cells, without the participation of antibodies.
   c. Helper T cells stimulate B cells and cytotoxic T cells via the cytokines they secrete. With few exceptions, this help is essential for activation of the B cells and cytotoxic T cells.

VI. B-cell plasma membrane receptors are copies of the specific antibody (immunoglobulin) that the cell is capable of producing.
   a. Any given B cell or clone of B cells produces antibodies that have a unique antigen-binding site.
   b. Antibodies are composed of four interlocking polypeptide chains; the variable regions of the antibodies are the sites that bind antigen.

VII. T-cell surface plasma membrane receptors are not immunoglobulins, but they do have specific antigen-binding sites that differ from one T-cell clone to another.
   a. The T-cell receptor binds antigen only when the antigen is complexed to one of the body's own plasma membrane MHC proteins.
   b. Class I MHC proteins are found on all nucleated cells of the body, whereas class II MHC proteins are found only on macrophages, B cells, and dendritic cells. Cytotoxic T cells require antigen to be complexed to class I proteins, whereas helper T cells require class II proteins.

VIII. Antigen presentation is required for T-cell activation.
   a. Only macrophages, B cells, and dendritic cells function as antigen-presenting cells (APCs) for helper T cells. The antigen is internalized by the APC and hydrolyzed to peptide fragments, which are complexed with class II MHC proteins. This complex is then shuttled to the plasma membrane of the APC, which also delivers a nonspecific costimulus to the T cell and secretes interleukin 1 (IL-1) and tumor necrosis factor-alpha (TNF-α).

b. A virus-infected cell or cancer cell can function as an APC for cytotoxic T cells. The viral antigen or cancer-associated antigen is synthesized by the cell itself and hydrolyzed to peptide fragments, which are complexed to class I MHC proteins. The complex is then shuttled to the plasma membrane of the cell.

IX. NK cells have the same targets as cytotoxic T cells, but they are not antigen-specific; most of their mechanisms of target identification are not understood.

X. Immune tolerance is the result of clonal deletion and clonal inactivation.

XI. In antibody-mediated responses, the membrane receptors of a B cell bind antigen, and at the same time a helper T cell also binds antigen in association with a class II MHC protein on a macrophage or other APC.

a. The helper T cell, activated by the antigen, by a nonantigenic protein costimulus, and by IL-1 and TNF-α secreted by the APC, secretes IL-2, which then causes the helper T cell to proliferate into a clone of cells that secrete additional cytokines.

b. These cytokines then stimulate the antigen-bound B cell to proliferate and differentiate into plasma cells, which secrete antibodies. Some of the activated B cells become memory cells, which are responsible for active immunity.

c. There are five major classes of secreted antibodies: IgG, IgM, IgA, IgD, and IgE. The first two are the major antibodies against bacterial and viral infection.

d. The secreted antibodies are carried throughout the body by the blood and combine with antigen. The antigen–antibody complex enhances the inflammatory response, in large part by activating the complement system. Complement proteins mediate many steps of inflammation, act as opsonins, and directly kill antibody-bound cells via the membrane attack complex.

e. Antibodies of the IgG class also act directly as opsonins and link target cells to NK cells, which directly kill the target cells.

f. Antibodies also neutralize toxins and extracellular viruses.

XII. Virus-infected cells and cancer cells are killed by cytotoxic T cells, NK cells, and activated macrophages.

a. A cytotoxic T cell binds via its membrane receptor to cells bearing a viral antigen or cancer-associated antigen in association with a class I MHC protein.

b. Activation of the cytotoxic T cell also requires cytokines secreted by helper T cells, themselves activated by antigen presented by a macrophage. The cytotoxic T cell then releases perforin, which kills the attached target cell by making it leaky.

c. NK cells and macrophages are also stimulated by helper T-cell cytokines, particularly IL-2 and interferon-gamma, to attack and kill virus-infected or cancer cells.

Systemic Manifestations of Infection

I. The acute phase response is summarized in Figure 18.22.

II. The major mediators of this response are IL-1, TNF-α, and IL-6.

Factors That Alter the Resistance to Infection

I. The body's capacity to resist infection is influenced by nutritional status, the presence of other diseases, psychological factors, and the intactness of the immune system.

II. AIDS is caused by a retrovirus that destroys helper T cells and therefore reduces the body's ability to resist infection and cancer.

III. Antibiotics interfere with the synthesis of macromolecules by bacteria.

Harmful Immune Responses

I. Rejection of tissue transplants is initiated by MHC proteins on the transplanted cells and is mediated mainly by cytotoxic T cells.

II. Transfusion reactions are mediated by antibodies.

a. Transfused erythrocytes will be destroyed if the recipient has natural antibodies against the antigens (type A or type B) on the cells.

b. Antibodies against Rh-positive erythrocytes can be produced following the exposure of an Rh-negative person to such cells.

III. Allergies (hypersensitivity reactions) caused by allergens are of several types.

a. In delayed hypersensitivity, the inflammation is due to the interplay of helper T-cell cytokines and macrophages. Immune-complex hypersensitivity is due to complement activation by antigen–antibody complexes.

b. In immediate hypersensitivity, antigen binds to IgE antibodies, which are themselves bound to mast cells. The mast cells then release inflammatory mediators, such as histamine, that produce the symptoms of allergy. The late phase of immediate hypersensitivity is mediated by eosinophils.

IV. Autoimmune attacks are directed against the body's own proteins acting as antigens. Reasons for the failure of immune tolerance are summarized in Table 18.10.

V. Normal tissues can be damaged by excessive inflammatory responses to pathogens.

REVIEW QUESTIONS

1. What are the major cells of the immune system and their general functions?
2. Describe the major anatomical and biochemical barriers to infection.
3. Name the three cell types that function as phagocytes.
4. List the sequence of events in an inflammatory response and describe each step.
5. Name the sources of the major inflammatory mediators.
6. What triggers the alternative pathway for complement activation? What roles does complement play in inflammation and cell killing?
7. Describe the antiviral role of type I interferon.
8. Name the lymphoid organs. Contrast the functions of the bone marrow and thymus with those of the secondary lymphoid organs.
9. Name the various populations and subpopulations of lymphocytes and discuss their roles in adaptive immune responses.
10. Contrast the major targets of antibody-mediated responses and responses mediated by cytotoxic T cells and NK cells.
11. How do the Fc and variable regions of antibodies differ?
12. What are the differences between B-cell receptors and T-cell receptors? Between cytotoxic T-cell receptors and helper T-cell receptors?

13. Compare and contrast antigen presentation to helper T cells and cytotoxic T cells.
14. Compare and contrast cytotoxic T cells and NK cells.
15. What two processes contribute to immune tolerance?
16. Diagram the sequence of events in an antibody-mediated response, including the role of helper T cells, interleukin 1, and interleukin 2.
17. Contrast the general functions of the different antibody classes.
18. How is complement activation triggered in the classical complement pathway, and how does complement "know" what cells to attack?
19. Name two ways in which the presence of antibodies enhances phagocytosis.
20. How do NK cells recognize which cells to attack in ADCC?
21. Diagram the sequence of events by which a virus-infected cell is attacked and destroyed by cytotoxic T cells. Include the roles of cytotoxic T cells, helper T cells, interleukin 1, and interleukin 2.
22. Contrast the extracellular and intracellular phases of immune responses to viruses, discussing the role of interferons.
23. List the systemic responses to infection or injury and the mediators responsible for them.
24. What factors influence the body's resistance to infection?
25. What is the major defect in AIDS, and what causes it?
26. What is the major cell type involved in graft rejection?
27. Diagram the sequences of events in immediate hypersensitivity.

KEY TERMS

activated macrophage 676
active immunity 674
acute phase protein 676
acute phase response 676
adaptive immune response 652
adenoid 663
alternative complement pathway 659
antibody 664
antibody-dependent cellular cytotoxicity (ADCC) 673
antibody-mediated response 664
antigen 662
antigen-binding site 667
antigen presentation 668
antigen-presenting cell (APC) 668
basophil 653
B lymphocyte (B cell) 653
chemoattractant 658
chemokine 658
chemotaxin 658
chemotaxis 658
classical complement pathway 659
class I MHC protein 668
class II MHC protein 668
clonal deletion 670
clonal expansion 662
clonal inactivation 670
clone 663
complement 658
costimulus 669
C3b 659
C-reactive protein 660
cytokine 654
cytotoxic T cell 664
dendritic cell 653
diapedesis 658
eosinophil 653
epitope 669
Fc 667
gamma globulin 672
helper T cell 664
histamine 683
hydrogen peroxide 658
IgA 672
IgD 672
IgE 672
IgG 672
IgM 672
immune surveillance 652
immune system 652
immune tolerance 670
immunoglobulin 667
immunology 652
inflammation 656
innate immune response 652
interleukin 1 (IL-1) 669
interleukin 2 (IL-2) 671
interleukin 6 (IL-6) 678
leukocyte 653
lymph node 663
lymphocyte 653
lymphocyte activation 662
lymphoid organ 662
macrophage 653
major histocompatibility complex (MHC) 668
margination 658
mast cell 654
membrane attack complex (MAC) 659
memory cell 662
MHC proteins 668
microbes 652
monocyte 653
natural killer (NK) cell 653
neutrophil 653
nitric oxide 658
opsonin 658
passive immunity 674
pathogen-associated molecular patterns (PAMPs) 661
pathogens 652
pattern-recognition receptors (PRRs) 662
perforin 675
phagocyte 654
phagocytosis 653
phagolysosome 658
phagosome 658
plasma cell 653
primary lymphoid organ 663
regulatory T cell 664
Rh factor 681
secondary lymphoid organ 663
spleen 663
T lymphocyte (T cell) 653
thymus 663
Toll-like receptors (TLRs) 661
tonsil 663
tumor necrosis factor-alpha (TNF-α) 669
type I interferon 660
type II interferon (interferon-gamma) 661

CLINICAL TERMS

Because of the subject matter of this chapter, it is difficult to distinguish between physiological key terms and "clinical" terms. This list is limited largely to specific diseases, their causes, symptoms and signs, and treatments.

acquired immune deficiency syndrome (AIDS) 679
allergen 681
allergy (hypersensitivity) 681
Alzheimer disease 684
anaphylaxis 683
antibiotic 679
asthma 684
autoimmune disease 683
bacteria 653
chronic inflammatory disease 684
cross-matching 681
cyclosporin 680
cytotoxic hypersensitivity 682
delayed hypersensitivity 682
erythromycin 679
graft rejection 680
HAART 679
hemolytic disease of the newborn 681
human immunodeficiency virus (HIV) 679
IgE-mediated hypersensitivity 682
immediate hypersensitivity 682
immune-complex hypersensitivity 682
inflammatory bowel disease 684
Kaposi's sarcoma 679
late phase reaction 683
multiple sclerosis 683
myasthenia gravis 683
oncogene 670
penicillin 679
rheumatoid arthritis 683
septic shock 683
severe combined immunodeficiency (SCID) 678
transfusion reaction 680
type 1 diabetes mellitus 683
vaccine 674
virus 653

CHAPTER 18

Clinical Case Study: A Teenage Girl with Widespread Pain and Severe Facial Rash

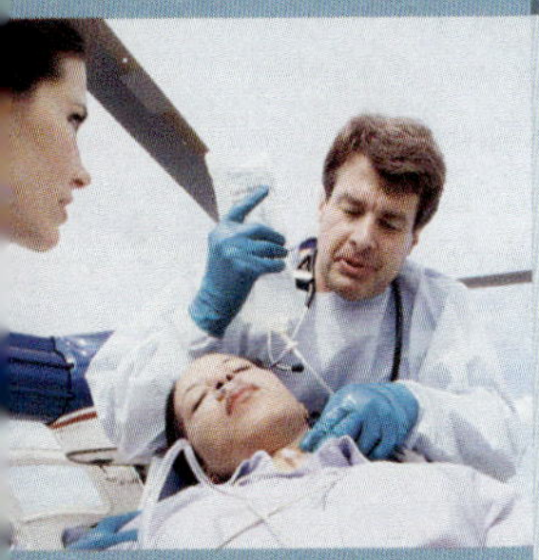

A 17-year-old Caucasian girl returned from a long day at the beach one sunny, late-summer day complaining of a sunburn and fatigue. Over the next few days, the "sunburn" took on the form of a rash across her cheeks and the bridge of her nose, and the girl began to feel sick, tired, and "achy all over." She assumed her symptoms were from severe sunburn. After a few days, the rash subsided a bit, but over the next several weeks she regularly felt pain and stiffness in her knees, wrists, and fingers. She did not alert her parents of this, however, thinking it was of no importance and would eventually subside. During this time, she spent considerable time outdoors in after-school activities and on weekends, being exposed to the sun. One day, while sitting at the computer, her fingers became so stiff that she had to stop typing. She could see that her fingers were swollen. She also felt nauseated, and upon standing, her knees felt stiff and very painful. At this point, she told her parents she was feeling very ill, and a visit was scheduled to see her physician.

The physician noted that the girl had an unremarkable medical history with no chronic illnesses, had until recently been very fit and active, and had no history of major allergies or disease; upon examination, however, she did appear extremely fatigued and weak. The joints in her fingers, wrists, knees, and toes were slightly swollen and had restricted movement. The rash had also reappeared on her face. At the time of her visit, the girl had a slightly elevated body temperature of 37.6°C (99.7°F). Also, the girl indicated that recently it "hurt to breathe" and that she felt "winded" all the time, which the physician took to mean that the girl was experiencing ***dyspnea*** (shortness of breath). The physician listened to her heart and chest sounds through a stethoscope and detected sounds that suggested inflammation. A chest radiograph revealed fluid buildup in the pleural membranes around the lungs and in the pericardium around the heart. Blood tests indicated an increased concentration of liver enzymes, suggesting that some liver cells were damaged and had released their contents into the blood. The concentration of albumin, the major protein in blood, was lower than normal. Because albumin is made in the liver, this was another sign that the liver was not functioning normally. The tests also revealed that the concentration of creatinine in the blood was slightly elevated (see Chapter 14), and a urinalysis revealed trace amounts of protein and blood in the urine. This suggested that the girl's kidneys were not functioning properly. Finally, the girl's hematocrit was 34.1%, which is below normal (see Chapter 12). Taken together, these test results were sufficiently serious that the physician admitted the girl to the hospital so that her condition could be carefully monitored and treated and additional tests could be performed.

The physician concluded that the girl may have an autoimmune disease known as ***systemic lupus erythematosus*** (***SLE***). Although a relatively uncommon disease (about 1.5 million total cases in the United States), all of the signs in this girl were consistent with a diagnosis of SLE. As with most autoimmune diseases, the majority (>90%) of SLE sufferers are female. The disease can occur at any age, but it most commonly appears in women of childbearing age and its onset can be quite sudden.

The two major immune dysfunctions in SLE are hyperactivity of T and B cells, with overexpression of "self" antibodies, and decreased negative regulation of the immune response. In some other autoimmune diseases, one or a small number of antigens appear to be the target of the immune attack, and these are often localized to one or a few organs. In SLE, however, the reaction is much more widespread. The most common antigens are proteins and double-stranded DNA in the nuclei of all nucleated cells. Because all nucleated cells share most of the same DNA and nuclear proteins, few—if any—parts of the body are not susceptible to immune attack in SLE. A subsequent blood test in this patient was positive for the presence of circulating antibodies that recognize cell nuclear material, confirming the diagnosis of SLE.

Exactly what initiates the immune response in SLE is unclear. However, it is known that most people with this disease are photosensitive—that is, their skin cells are readily damaged by ultraviolet light from the sun. When these cells die, their nuclear contents become exposed to phagocytes and other components of the immune system. It is also believed that UV light induces intact skin cells to express certain proteins that are antigenic in SLE. As a result, symptoms of SLE tend to flare up when a person with the disease is exposed to excessive sunlight. This is what happened to our patient after a day at the beach without sunscreen and as she continued to spend considerable time outdoors thereafter.

SLE has a strong genetic component, as evidenced by the fact that approximately 40% to 50% of identical twins share the disease when one is afflicted. Moreover, there is an increased frequency of five specific class II MHC variants in people with SLE, as well as deficient or abnormal complement proteins. Still, environmental triggers almost certainly elicit the disease in genetically susceptible people (because, as stated, in half the cases in which one twin has SLE, the other does not). There is no conclusive evidence that infections due to viral invasion are a trigger for the development of SLE. In addition to sunlight, other triggers associated with the appearance of SLE are certain chemicals and foods, such as alfalfa sprouts.

SLE can be mild or severe, intermittent or chronic. In most cases, though, the effects are widespread. Typically, connective-tissue involvement is extensive, with repeated episodes of inflammation in joints and skin. The outer covering of the heart (pericardium) and the pleural membranes of the lungs may become inflamed. Gastrointestinal function may be affected, resulting in nausea or diarrhea, and retinal damage is sometimes observed. Even the brain is not spared, as cognitive dysfunction and even seizures may arise in severe cases. The skin often develops inflamed patches, notably on the face along the cheeks and bridge of the nose, forming the so-called ***butterfly*** (***malar***) ***rash*** seen in some patients with SLE (**Figure 18.24**). One of the most serious manifestations of SLE occurs when immune complexes and immunoglobulins accumulate in the glomeruli of the nephrons of the kidney (see Chapter 14 for description of nephrons). This often leads to ***nephritis*** (inflammation of the nephrons) and results in damaged, leaky glomeruli. The appearance of protein or blood in the urine, therefore, is a clinical finding often associated with SLE.

(continued)

(continued)

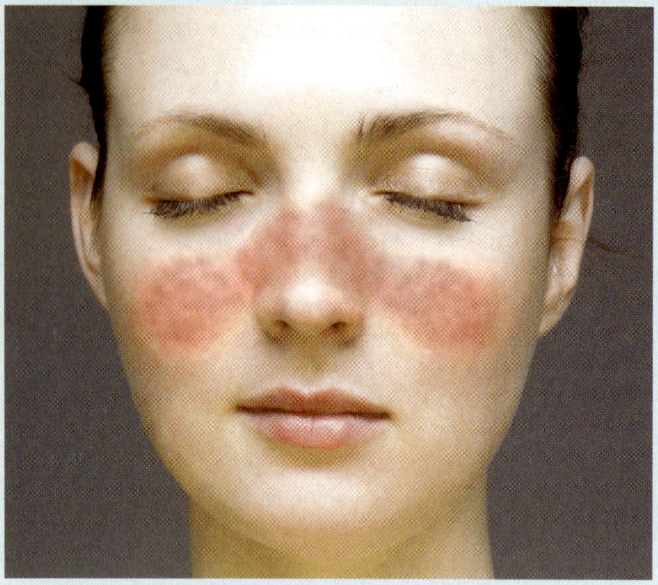

Figure 18.24 Characteristic butterfly or malar rash in a patient with systemic lupus erythematosus.

Finally, certain proteins on the plasma membranes of red blood cells and platelets may also become antigenic in SLE. When the immune system attacks these structures, the results are lysis of red blood cells and destruction and loss of platelets (***thrombocytopenia***). Loss of red blood cells in this manner contributes to the condition known as ***hemolytic anemia,*** a common manifestation of SLE. Our patient demonstrated widespread organ malfunction, evidenced by blood tests assessing liver and kidney function, radiograph results, and urinalysis. She also had mild hemolytic anemia. Considering the extent to which her disease affected her skin and other organs, it is not surprising that she felt ill and "achy all over."

In addition to the production of self antibodies in large numbers, there also appears to be a failure of the immune system to regulate itself in SLE. Consequently, the immune attacks, once begun, do not stop after a few days but instead continue. Some investigators believe this may be related to a deficiency or inactivity of regulatory T cells, but this has not been proven. It is clear, however, that the circulating concentrations of numerous cytokines—notably, IL-10, IL-12, and TNF-α—are abnormal in persons with SLE.

The treatments for SLE depend on its severity and the overall physical condition of the patient. In mild flare-ups, nonsteroidal anti-inflammatory drugs (NSAIDs) may be sufficient to control pain and inflammation, together with changes in lifestyle to avoid potential triggers. In more advanced cases, immunosuppression with high doses of synthetic adrenal corticosteroids (such as prednisone) or other potent immunosuppressant drugs is employed. Our patient was started on prednisone at an initially high dosage to control the widespread inflammation and immune attacks. The dose was tapered off once her blood tests were restored to nearly normal, because chronic high dosages of prednisone can have severe side effects (see Section D of Chapter 11 for a discussion of the effects of high concentrations of glucocorticoids). She was additionally started on ***hydroxychloroquine,*** an antimalarial drug commonly used in treatment of SLE due to its immunomodulatory effects. She was advised to immediately begin taking ibuprofen (an NSAID) whenever her symptoms worsened in the future and to use hydrocortisone skin cream if she developed rashes again. She was counseled on lifestyle changes that she would need to follow for the rest of her life. These included eating a healthy diet and exercising to promote cardiovascular health, to avoid smoking (which is a major risk factor for blood vessel disease and hypertension), and most significantly to avoid exposure to the sun when possible. This meant using sunscreen and a wide-brimmed hat at all times when outdoors, not just when at the beach, and even indoors because fluorescent and halogen lights emit sufficient UV light to trigger symptoms in some SLE patients. As she was of reproductive age, she was counseled about the possible effects of SLE on pregnancy and was advised against the use of estrogen-containing oral contraceptives, as estrogen has been reported to trigger or worsen flare-ups of SLE. After several days, a follow-up urinalysis indicated an absence of protein; therefore, kidney damage was minimal. Additional blood tests were near normal for liver and kidney function, and a chest radiograph was normal. She was released from the hospital but returned 2 weeks later for follow-up tests, which were all nearly or completely normal. One month after beginning treatment, she was able to resume normal activities and most of the stiffness in her joints had disappeared. Her steroid dosage was reduced to a very low dose every other day and then stopped. She was advised to call her physician if and when symptoms flared so that a new course of therapy could be initiated quickly.

Clinical terms: butterfly (malar) rash, dyspnea, hemolytic anemia, hydroxychloroquine, nephritis, systemic lupus erythematosus (SLE), thrombocytopenia,

See Chapter 19 for complete, integrative case studies.

CHAPTER 18 TEST QUESTIONS

Answers found in Appendix A.

1. Which of the following is an opsonin?
   a. IL-2
   b. C1 protein
   c. C3b protein
   d. C-reactive protein
   e. membrane attack complex

2. Which is/are important in innate immune responses?
   a. interferons
   b. clonal inactivation
   c. lymphocyte activation
   d. secretion of antibodies from plasma cells
   e. class 1 MHC proteins

3. A second exposure to a given foreign antigen elicits a rapid and pronounced immune response because
   a. passive immunity occurs after the first exposure.
   b. some B cells differentiate into memory B cells after the first exposure.
   c. a greater number of antigen-presenting cells are available due to the earlier exposure.
   d. the array of class II MHC proteins expressed by antigen-presenting cells is permanently altered by the first exposure.
   e. Both a and b are correct.
4. Which statement is incorrect?
   a. The most abundant immunoglobulins in serum are IgG and IgM antibodies.
   b. IgG antibodies are involved in adaptive immune responses against bacteria and viruses in the extracellular fluid.
   c. IgM antibodies are primarily involved in immune defense mechanisms found in the surface or lining of the gastrointestinal, respiratory, and genitourinary tracts.
   d. All antibodies of a given class have an Fc portion that is identical in amino acid sequence.
   e. Antibodies can exist at the surface of a B cell or be circulating freely in the blood.

True or False

5. Antibiotics are useful for treating illnesses caused by viruses.
6. Chronic inflammatory diseases may occur even in the absence of any infection.
7. All T cells are lymphocytes, but not all lymphocytes are T cells.
8. Edema (swelling), which occurs during inflammation, has important adaptive value in helping defend against infection or injury.
9. Bone marrow and the thymus are examples of secondary lymphoid organs.

CHAPTER 18 GENERAL PRINCIPLES ASSESSMENT

Answer found in Appendix A.

1. *Homeostasis is essential for health and survival.* Using Figure 18.22 as your guide, describe several ways in which infection may result in a disruption of homeostasis.

CHAPTER 18 QUANTITATIVE AND THOUGHT QUESTIONS

Answers found at www.mhhe.com/widmaier13.

1. If an individual failed to develop a thymus because of a genetic defect, what would happen to the immune responses mediated by antibodies and those mediated by cytotoxic T cells?
2. What abnormalities would a person with a neutrophil deficiency display? A person with a monocyte deficiency?
3. An experimental animal is given a drug that blocks phagocytosis. Will this drug prevent the animal's immune system from killing foreign cells via the complement system?
4. If the Fc portion of a patient's antibodies is abnormal, what effects could this have on antibody-mediated responses?
5. Would you predict that patients with AIDS would develop fever in response to an infection? Explain.

CHAPTER 18 ANSWERS TO PHYSIOLOGICAL INQUIRIES

Figure 18.6. The C3b receptor should have a ligand-binding site that is *specific* for C3b and that binds C3b with high *affinity.*

Figure 18.8 Many molecules in the body act this way. For example, somatostatin acts locally in the stomach to control acid production (paracrine) and is secreted into the hypothalamo–pituitary portal veins to control growth hormone secretion (endocrine). Testosterone acts locally within the testes (paracrine) and reaches other targets through the blood (endocrine).

Figure 18.9 Vasodilation and increased protein permeability of the microcirculation both contribute to an increase in the rate of filtration of fluid from the plasma into the interstitial space. Because lymph vessels are the main route by which fluid and protein are returned from the interstitial space to the circulatory system (see Figure 12.47), these changes will lead to increased flow of lymph. As that fluid flows through the lymph nodes, lymphocytes are exposed to antigens from the invading pathogen, thus activating the adaptive immune response.

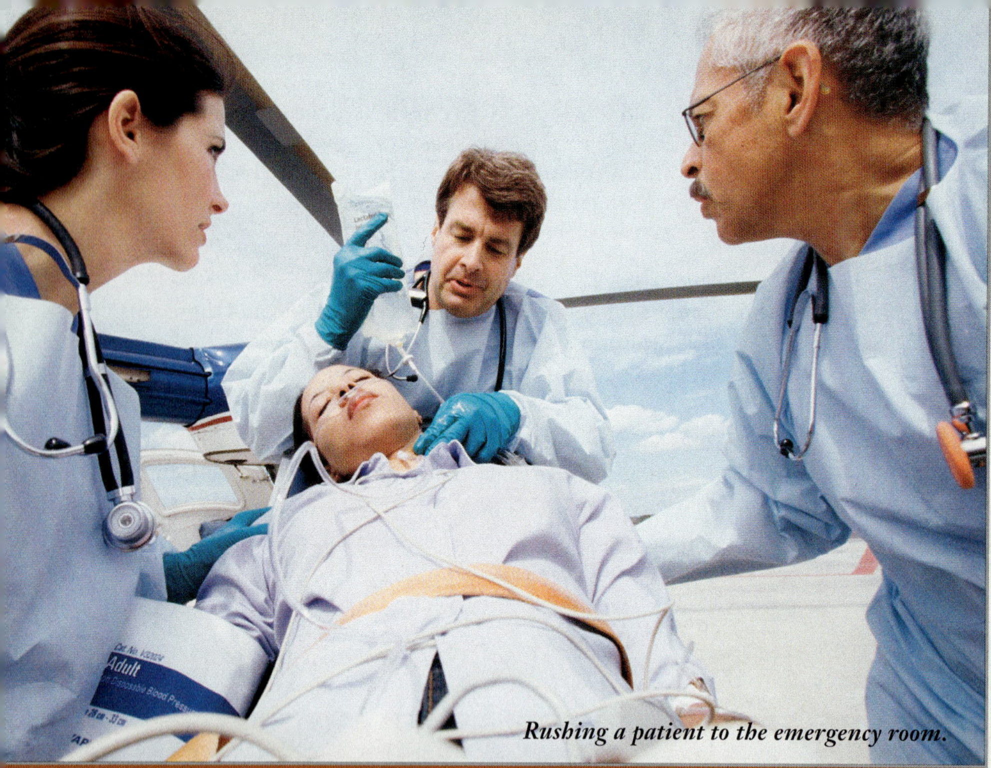

Rushing a patient to the emergency room.

19 Medical Physiology

INTEGRATION USING CLINICAL CASES

Physiology is one of the pillars of the health-related professions, including nursing, occupational health, physical therapy, dentistry, and medicine. In fact, the term *pathophysiology*—the changes in function associated with disease—highlights the intertwining of physiology and medicine. You need a thorough understanding of the general principles of physiology to properly diagnose and treat diseases and disorders. We are aware that many users of this textbook may not be planning a career in the health professions. However, teachers of physiology can attest to the use of clinical examples as an effective approach to highlight and reinforce the understanding of the functions and interactions of the organ systems of the body.

This chapter uses clinical cases to allow you to continue to explore the material you learned from this book and, at the same time, review some of the general principles of physiology that were first introduced in Chapter 1. You have been introduced to the educational power of clinical cases at the end of each chapter of this book. This chapter continues this theme with more extensive cases. More importantly, this chapter illustrates the concept of *integrative physiology*. In real life, complicated clinical cases involve multiple organ systems. The true art of medicine is the ability of clinicians to recall these basic principles and put them together in the evaluation of the patient. Each case in this chapter has a section called "Physiological Integration" to highlight this fact. As you read these sections, you should consider the relationships among disease, integrative physiology, and homeostasis, the last of which has been a theme throughout this textbook.

Some of the conditions and physiological interactions described in this chapter are not explicitly described in the book and may be new to you. Interspersed at key points in the chapter are several places where you will be asked to "Reflect and Review." In some cases, specific answers to these questions are not provided in the case itself. We encourage you to answer these questions as the case unfolds by, if necessary, referring back to the appropriate section of the book. Furthermore, we have annotated each case with figure and table numbers to facilitate review of material covered in previous chapters. In some cases, the figures and tables from previous chapters do not specifically answer the question but provide an opportunity to review the control system in question to allow the student to propose potential answers.

We hope that the cases in this chapter will motivate you to synthesize and integrate information from throughout the book and perhaps even go beyond what you have learned. In fact, you may enjoy consulting other sources to answer some of the more challenging questions or learn more about specific aspects of each case that interests you.

We hope you enjoy this chapter and encourage you as readers of the book to send us comments and suggestions for additional cases.

CASE A

Woman with Palpitations and Heat Intolerance

19.A1 Case Presentation

A 23-year-old woman visits her family physician with complaints of a 12-month history of increasing nervousness, irritability, and ***palpitations*** (a noticeable increase in the force of her heartbeat). Furthermore, she feels very warm in a room when everyone else feels comfortable. Her skin is unusually warm and moist to the touch. She has lost 30 pounds of body weight over this period despite having a voracious appetite and increased food intake.

Reflect and Review #1

- Describe the general principles of the control of body temperature (see Figures 16.16 through 16.18). What may have caused her skin to feel warm and moist?

Two years ago, she was jogging about 20 miles per week. However, she had not done any running for the past year because she "didn't feel up to it" and complained of general muscle weakness. She said she often felt irritable and had mood swings. Her menstrual periods have been less frequent over the past year. Her previous medical history was normal for a person her age. She states that she has double vision when looking to the side but does not have any loss of vision when using only one eye or the other.

Reflect and Review #2

- Which hypothalamic, anterior pituitary gland, and ovarian hormones control the menstrual cycle? (See Figure 17.22 and Table 17.7.)
- What anterior pituitary gland disorder can cause a decrease in menstrual cycle frequency and loss of vision? (See Figure 17.39.)

19.A2 Physical Examination

The patient is a 5' 7" (170 cm), 110-pound (50 kg) woman. Her systolic/diastolic blood pressure is 140/60 mmHg (normal for a young, healthy woman is about 110/70 mmHg). Her resting pulse rate is 100 beats per minute. Before she became ill, her resting heart rate was about 60–70 beats per minute. Her respiratory rate is 17 breaths per minute (normal for her was approximately 12–14 breaths per minute). Her skin is warm and moist. Her eyes are bulging out (***proptosis*** or ***exophthalmos***) (**Figure 19.1a**). Finally, when she is asked to gaze to the far right, her right eye does not move as far as does her left eye and she says she has double vision (***diplopia***).

Reflect and Review #3

- Briefly describe the control of systemic blood pressure, heart rate, and respiratory rate (see Figures 12.23 and 12.51 and Figure 13.32). What might be causing her hypertension, ***tachycardia*** (increased heart rate), and ***tachypnea*** (increased respiratory rate)?
- Describe the muscles that control eye movement (see Figure 7.35).

Upon further examination, the physician notes an enlargement of a structure in the front, lower part of her neck (**Figure 19.1b**). It is smooth (no bumps or nodules felt) and painless. When the patient swallows, this enlarged structure moves up and down. When a stethoscope is placed over this structure, the physician can hear a swishing sound (called a ***bruit*** [BREW-ee]) with each heartbeat.

Reflect and Review #4

- What structure might be responsible for the swelling in the patient's lower neck? (See Figures 11.20a and 15.16.) What are the major functions of this structure?

Her patellar tendon (knee-jerk) reflexes are hyperactive. When she holds her hands out straight, she exhibits fine tremors (shaking).

Reflect and Review #5

- What are the neural pathways involved in the knee-jerk reflex? (See Figure 10.6.) Could the enlarged structure in her neck account for the abnormal reflexes observed?

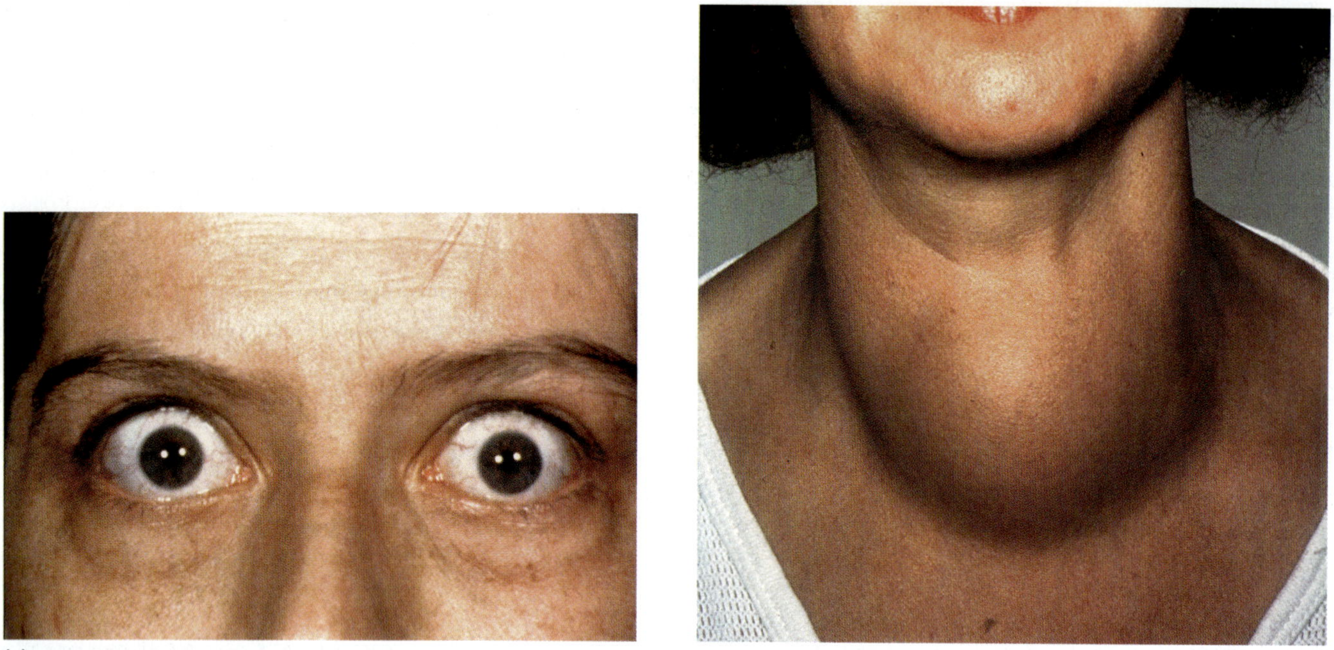

(a) (b)

Figure 19.1 (a) Proptosis and (b) goiter.

19.A3 Laboratory Tests

The family physician considers the history and physical exam and decides to order some blood tests. The results are shown in **Table 19.1**.

Reflect and Review #6

- Describe the feedback control loops of the hormones whose values were abnormal (see Figure 11.22 and Figure 17.24). Which, if any, of these hormones might account for the symptoms in this patient? What might have contributed to the woman's feelings of excessive warmth?
- Why is the serum glucose sample obtained in the fasted state? (See Figure 16.8.) Does the serum glucose concentration rule out diabetes mellitus as a factor in this patient's illness?

19.A4 Diagnosis

The most likely explanation for the findings is an increase in thyroid hormone in the patient's blood. When increased thyroid hormone causes significant symptoms, it is part of a condition called ***hyperthyroidism*** or ***thyrotoxicosis.*** The enlarged organ in the neck is likely the thyroid gland, although large thyroid glands (***goiters***) also occur in hypothyroidism (see Figure 11.23 for an extreme example). In order to interpret the thyroid function tests shown in Table 19.1, first review the control of thyroid hormone synthesis and release (see Figures 11.20 through 11.22).

There are two circulating thyroid hormones—thyroxine (T_4) and triiodothyronine (T_3). Whereas T_4 is the main secretory product of the thyroid gland, T_3 is actually more potent and is actively produced in target tissues by the removal of one

TABLE 19.1 Laboratory Results for Patient

Blood Measurements*	Result	Normal Range
Sodium	136 mmol/L	135–146 mmol/L
Potassium	5.0 mmol/L	3.8–5.0 mmol/L
Chloride	102 mmol/L	97–110 mmol/L
pH	7.39	7.38–7.45
Calcium (total)	9.6 mg/dL	9.0–10.5 mg/dL
Parathyroid hormone	15 pg/mL	10–75 pg/mL
Glucose (fasting)	80 mg/dL	70–110 mg/dL
Prolactin	10.4 ng/mL	1.4–24.2 ng/mL
Estrogen (midcycle)	100 pg/mL	150–750 pg/mL
Total T_4†	20 μg/dL	5–11 μg/dL
Free T_4	2.8 ng/dL	0.8–1.6 ng/dL
Thyroid-stimulating hormone (TSH)	0.01 μU/mL	0.3–4.0 μU/mL

*In actuality, these measurements are performed in blood serum or plasma.

†T_4, thyroxine

iodine molecule from T_4. Nonetheless, for practical reasons, T_4 is the form of thyroid hormone that is routinely measured in clinical situations. The release of T_4 by the thyroid gland is normally controlled by thyroid-stimulating hormone (TSH) secreted by the anterior pituitary gland. Binding of TSH to its G-protein-coupled plasma membrane receptor activates adenylyl cyclase and cAMP formation, which then stimulates cAMP-dependent protein kinase (see Figure 5.6). Like most anterior pituitary gland tropic/trophic hormones, TSH not only stimulates the activity of the thyroid gland but also stimulates its growth. As with most other pituitary gland–target hormone systems, the target-gland hormone (T_4) inhibits the release of the anterior pituitary gland hormone controlling it (in this case, TSH) via negative feedback (see Figure 11.22).

There are several reasons why the thyroid gland in this patient could be producing too much thyroid hormone, leading to thyrotoxicosis. The most common condition to focus on here is called ***Graves' disease.*** In this condition, the thyroid gland is stimulated by antibodies that activate the receptor for TSH on the follicular cell of the thyroid (**Figure 19.2**). Therefore, these TSH receptor-stimulating antibodies mimic the action of TSH but are distinct from authentic TSH from the anterior pituitary gland. These ***thyroid-stimulating immunoglobulins (TSIs)*** are characteristic of an autoimmune disorder in which the patient makes antibodies that bind to one or more proteins expressed in his or her own tissues (see Table 18.10). The exact cause of an increase in TSIs in individual patients is usually not known. TSIs are produced by B lymphocytes that, in addition to residing in lymph nodes, can actually infiltrate the thyroid gland in Graves' disease. In Chapter 9, you learned about a disease called myasthenia gravis, in which autoantibodies bind to and destroy the nicotinic acetylcholine receptor in the neuromuscular junction. This is typical of antibody–antigen reactions, in which antigens are removed from the body (see Chapter 18). In Graves' disease, however, the autoantibodies are highly unusual in that they not only recognize and bind to the TSH receptor on thyroid follicular cells but this binding *stimulates* rather than destroys the receptor. Therefore, TSIs stimulate the thyroid gland to synthesize and secrete excess T_4 independently of TSH. The increase in T_4 would be predicted to suppress the secretion of TSH from the anterior pituitary gland by negative feedback, which is consistent with the low serum TSH concentration measured in the patient's blood. The increased serum T_4 probably also suppressed the synthesis and release of thyrotropin-releasing hormone (TRH) from the hypothalamus via negative feedback. (Serum TRH concentrations are not determined in such situations because TRH is secreted directly into the hypothalamo–pituitary portal circulation. The actual amount of TRH from the hypothalamus that reaches the systemic circulation is too small for its measurement in a blood sample from a peripheral vein to be useful.)

The total and free (not bound to plasma proteins) T_4 concentrations in the blood of this patient are increased, confirming the diagnosis of hyperthyroidism. Measurement of free T_4 is helpful because most of the circulating thyroid hormone in the blood is bound to plasma proteins, so measuring the serum T_4 that is not bound to plasma proteins proves that

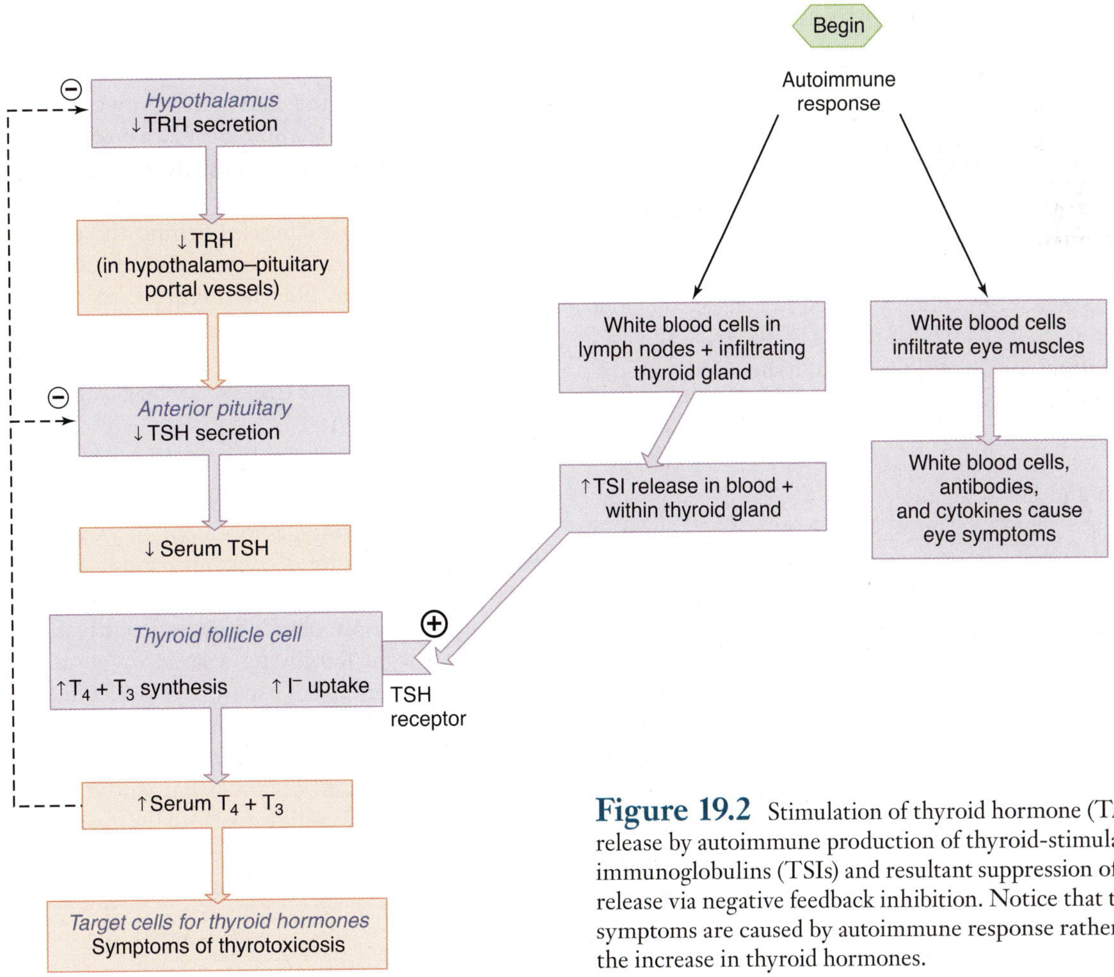

Figure 19.2 Stimulation of thyroid hormone (T_4 and T_3) release by autoimmune production of thyroid-stimulating immunoglobulins (TSIs) and resultant suppression of TSH release via negative feedback inhibition. Notice that the eye symptoms are caused by autoimmune response rather than by the increase in thyroid hormones.

there is an increase in the amount of biologically active T_4. The suppressed TSH confirms that the T_4 is increased independently of stimulation from the anterior pituitary gland. This suppression of serum TSH, as in our patient, is one of the hallmarks of Graves' disease. The measurement of serum TSH concentration is used as a screening test for many disorders of the thyroid gland. Although TSI concentrations can be measured in the serum in some patients, it is often not necessary because the diagnosis of Graves' disease is the most likely, considering that it causes the majority of cases of hyperthyroidism. It was not necessary to measure TSIs in our patient.

Although Graves' disease was by far the most likely diagnosis, the physician ordered some additional tests to rule out other possible causes of the symptoms. Serum electrolytes were measured because they are important in the generation and maintenance of membrane potentials (Chapter 6) and their abnormalities can lead to weakness and palpitations. Serum calcium and parathyroid hormone were measured because weakness is a common finding in primary hyperparathyroidism (Chapter 11). A normal fasting serum glucose and pH indicated that diabetes mellitus was probably not the cause of the patient's weakness and fatigue. A normal prolactin concentration indicated that she does not have hyperprolactinemia, which can cause abnormalities in the menstrual cycle and visual disturbances (see Chapter 17 Clinical Case Study).

19.A5 Physiological Integration

Thyroid diseases are common. Up to 10% of women will develop hyperthyroidism or hypothyroidism by the age of 60 to 65. Thyroid hormone has a wide range of effects throughout the body; therefore, an understanding of all the organ systems is extremely useful in understanding the symptoms of thyroid disease.

One of the main effects of thyroid hormone is calorigenic—it increases the basal metabolic rate (BMR). This increase in metabolic rate is caused by activation of intracellular thyroid hormone receptors (see Figure 5.4) that are expressed in cells throughout the body. This leads to increased expression of Na^+/K^+-ATPases as well as the synthesis of other cellular proteins involved in oxidative phosphorylation, oxygen consumption, and metabolic rate in many tissues (see Figures 3.44 and 3.45). The resultant increase in heat production by our patient explains the warmness and moistness of her skin and her heat intolerance. It also explains why, despite eating more, she is losing weight because she is burning more fuel than she is ingesting.

The nervousness, irritability, and emotional swings are likely due to effects of thyroid hormone on the central nervous system, although the exact cellular mechanism of this is not well understood. The symptoms also appear to be due to an increased sensitivity within the central nervous system to circulating catecholamines. The muscle weakness is probably due to a thyroid hormone–induced increase in muscle protein turnover, local metabolic changes, and loss of muscle mass. Despite this, there appears to be an increase in the speed of muscle contraction and relaxation, contributing to the hyperactive reflexes observed in our patient. The normal fasting blood glucose rules out diabetes mellitus as a cause of her muscle weakness.

Her thyroid gland is enlarged because TSIs are mimicking the actions of TSH to stimulate the thyroid gland to grow. The enlarged thyroid with increased metabolic activity explains why a bruit was heard over the thyroid gland. The thyroid gland has a high blood flow per gram of tissue even in healthy individuals. The increase in thyroid function in Graves' disease leads to a large increase in blood flow to the thyroid—so much so that it is audible with a stethoscope during systole in some patients.

Her increased systolic blood pressure and heart rate can be explained in several ways. First, there are direct effects of thyroid hormones on the heart, such as an increase in transcription of the myosin genes. Second, as described in Chapter 11, Section C, thyroid hormone has permissive effects to potentiate the effects of catecholamines on the cardiovascular system. Finally, the small decrease in diastolic pressure may result from arteriolar vasodilation and reduced total peripheral resistance in response to increased tissue temperature and metabolite concentrations (see Figure 12.51).

Increased thyroid hormone can directly inhibit the release of the pituitary gland gonadotropins FSH and LH, particularly in the middle of the menstrual cycle when the LH and FSH surge that stimulates ovulation occurs. This can lead to a decrease in release of gonadal steroids from the ovaries, an irregular pattern or complete loss of menstrual periods, and a lack of ovulation. This also explains the lower serum estrogen concentrations at the middle of the menstrual cycle in our patient.

The eye findings are among the most striking in many patients with Graves' disease (see Figure 19.1). The proptosis (bulging out of the eye) is likely due to the autoimmune component of the disease, rather than to a direct effect of thyroid hormone. Supporting this idea is that proptosis can occur before the development of hyperthyroidism, and excessive thyroid hormone therapy for hypothyroidism usually does not cause proptosis. Furthermore, proptosis is caused by infiltration of white blood cells into the extraocular muscles behind the eye, rather than being caused by TSIs. These cells release chemicals that result in inflammation (see Figure 19.1 and Figure 7.35), causing the muscles to swell and forcing the eyeball forward. Sometimes, particular muscles of the eye are more affected than others, which explains the double vision of our patient when she gazes to one side.

19.A6 Therapy

The most important component of treatment is to decrease the thyroid hormone concentrations. There are three general approaches to accomplish this. Removal of the thyroid gland is the most obvious but currently the least frequently used approach. Removing a large, hyperactive thyroid gland has surgical risk and is usually not performed unless absolutely necessary. The drugs ***methimazole*** and ***propylthiouracil*** can be used because they block the synthesis of thyroid hormone by reducing organification—that is, the oxidation and subsequent binding of iodide to tyrosine residues in the colloidal thyroglobulin molecule (see Figure 11.21). Although these drugs are effective in some patients, they sometimes lose effectiveness, can have side effects, and do not provide a definitive, permanent cure.

In the United States, a common approach is a more permanent, nonsurgical treatment. This involves the partial destruction of the thyroid gland with a high dose of orally administered ***radioactive iodine.*** Remember that iodide (the active anion of iodine) is a critical component of thyroid hormone (see Figure 11.21) and the thyroid gland has a mechanism to trap iodide by secondary active transport from the blood into the follicular cell. Radioactive iodide is trapped by the thyroid; the local emission of radioactive decay destroys most of the thyroid gland over time. However, the procedure does not work equally well in all people. In fact, sometimes patients have so much of their thyroid gland destroyed that they develop permanent hypothyroidism. Such people must take T_4 pills for the rest of their lives to maintain thyroid hormones in the normal range.

In the short term, while waiting for the treatments to take effect, patients benefit from treatment with beta-adrenergic receptor blockers (see Table 12.9) to reduce the effects of increased sensitivity to circulating catecholamines. This often helps control the palpitations and increased heart rate, as well as some of the other symptoms such as nervousness and tremors. Because proptosis is not caused by the increase in T_4, its treatment can be accomplished, if necessary, with anti-inflammatory drugs, such as glucocorticoids, or surgery or radiation therapy of the eye muscles.

With adequate treatment, patients generally get better over time with most, if not all, of the symptoms resolving. Our patient was treated with radioactive iodide, and her symptoms slowly resolved over several months.

CASE **B**

Man with Chest Pain After a Long Airplane Flight

19.B1 Case Presentation

A 50-year-old, obese man has just returned from vacationing in Hawaii. He took an 8 h flight during which he sat by the window and did not leave his seat. In the taxi on the way home from the airport, he starts to feel chest pain and has shortness of breath, increased respiratory rate, and nausea. Thinking he is having a heart attack (***myocardial infarction***), he asks the taxi driver to take him to the nearest hospital.

19.B2 Physical Examination

An examination of the patient at the hospital emergency room indicates that he has dull, aching chest pain and is clearly upset and anxious, short of breath, and overweight. He is 68 in (173 cm) tall and weighs 300 pounds (136 kg). The emergency room nurse practitioner performs an electrocardiogram (ECG), primarily to rule out a heart attack. The ECG shows an increased heart rate (105 beats per min) but does not show changes consistent with a heart attack or with left heart failure.

Reflect and Review #7

- What are the main factors that control heart rate? (See Figure 12.23.) Might any of them explain the increased heart rate in our patient?
- How might damage to the heart be detected in an ECG? (See Figures 12.15 and 12.16 for a general discussion of ECG.)

A chest x-ray is performed in an attempt to determine the cause of the patient's chest pain and shortness of breath. The results indicate no abnormalities such as pneumonia or collapse of lung lobes (***atelectasis***).

19.B3 Laboratory Tests

Based on the patient's history and symptoms, the physician obtains a sample of the patient's arterial blood in order to measure the levels of oxygen, carbon dioxide, bicarbonate, hydrogen ions (pH), and hemoglobin. The findings are shown in Table 19.2.

TABLE 19.2 Blood Gas, Bicarbonate, and Hemoglobin Results While Patient Breathes Room Air

Blood Measurement	Result	Normal Range
Arterial P_{O_2}	60 mmHg	80–100 mmHg
Arterial P_{CO_2}	30 mmHg	35–45 mmHg
Arterial pH	7.50	7.38–7.45
Bicarbonate	22 mmol/L	23–27 mmol/L
Hemoglobin	15 g/dL	12–16 g/dL

Reflect and Review #8

- What is the cause of the change in arterial pH in our patient? (See Table 14.8.)

The results of these tests reveal that the patient has hypoxic hypoxia (hypoxemia), as indicated by the low arterial P_{O_2}, and is hyperventilating, leading to respiratory alkalosis (see Figure 13.22), as indicated by the low arterial P_{CO_2} and bicarbonate, and high arterial pH. The normal hemoglobin concentration indicates that the patient is not anemic.

Reflect and Review #9

- What are some possible causes of hypoxemia? (See Table 13.10.)
- What are the two main types of alkalosis? (See Table 14.8.)
- How do we know the alkalosis in our patient was acute (of recent, short-term origin)? (See Table 14.8.)

The patient is given 100% oxygen to breathe through a mask over his mouth and nose. This results in an increase in arterial P_{O_2} to 205 mmHg, a small increase in arterial P_{CO_2} to 32 mmHg, and a small decrease in arterial pH to 7.48. The normal response to breathing 100% oxygen in a healthy person is an increase in arterial P_{O_2} to greater than 600 mmHg, with no change in arterial P_{CO_2} or pH.

Reflect and Review #10

- Explain why increasing arterial P_{O_2} with supplemental oxygen caused the observed changes in arterial P_{CO_2} and pH (see Figures 13.35 and 13.40).

19.B4 Diagnosis

Because a heart attack has been ruled out, the physician suspects that the patient has at least one ***pulmonary embolism***. An ***embolism*** (plural, *emboli*) is a blockage of blood flow through a blood vessel produced by an obstruction. It is often caused by a blood clot—or ***thrombus***—in the pulmonary arteries/arterioles. These clots usually arise from larger clots in leg veins.

To confirm his diagnosis, the physician orders a ***ventilation–perfusion scan***, which is actually the combination of two different scans. In the ventilation scan, the patient inhales a small amount of radioactive gas. Special imaging devices are then used to detect the inhaled radioactive molecules and visualize which parts of the lung are adequately ventilated. Poorly ventilated areas of the lung will contain less radioactive gas. In the perfusion scan, a small amount of albumin, a naturally occurring plasma protein, tagged with a radioactive tracer, is injected into a vein. As the radioactive protein enters the pulmonary circulation, its distribution can be monitored using the same imaging device as just described. This procedure allows the physician to determine if parts of the lungs are receiving less than their normal share of blood flow because poorly perfused areas of the lungs will contain less radioactive albumin. The ventilation scan was normal, but the perfusion scan showed abnormalities. **Figure 19.3** shows the results of the perfusion scan, demonstrating dramatic decreases in perfusion in specific regions of the lung. These results supported the physician's diagnosis of several pulmonary emboli.

A variety of materials can occlude pulmonary arterial blood vessels, including air, fat, foreign bodies, parasite eggs, and tumor cells. The most common embolus is a thrombus that can theoretically come from any large vein but usually comes from the deep veins of the muscles in the calves (***deep vein thrombosis***). The fact that our patient sat on an 8 h flight without moving around greatly increased the chances for the formation of a deep vein thrombosis in the leg. This is because without skeletal muscle contractions, blood is not adequately pushed back toward the heart (see Figure 12.45). This allows blood to pool in the leg veins, which increases the chance for the formation of clots. After the abnormal lung perfusion scan, an ultrasound examination of the legs was performed to confirm whether clots were present in the leg veins. The results showed a large clot in the femoral and popliteal veins in the right leg.

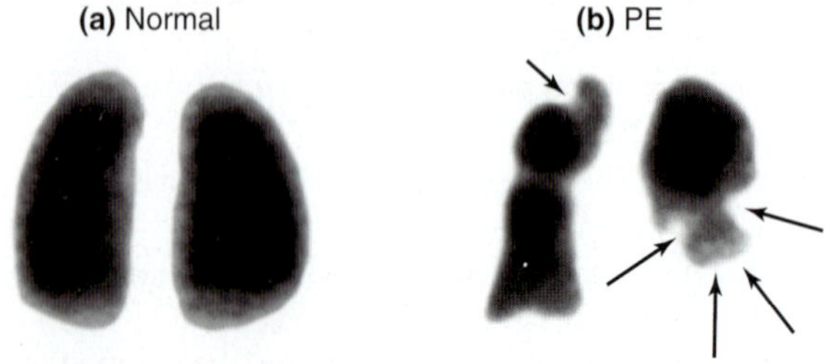

Figure 19.3 Pulmonary embolism (PE) from a deep vein thrombosis shown on a lung perfusion scan (posterior) with radiolabeled albumin. (a) A normal perfusion scan. (b) Multiple perfusion defects are shown (arrows).

Pulmonary embolism is a common and potentially fatal result of deep vein thrombosis. In fact, pulmonary embolism and deep vein thrombosis can be considered part of one syndrome. It may cause as many as 200,000 deaths each year in the United States. Most cases are not diagnosed until after death (on postmortem examination) either because the symptoms are initially mild or because the syndrome is misdiagnosed. Most small clots that form in small veins in the calves of the lower legs remain fixed in place, associated with the lining of the vein, and do not cause symptoms. However, if a clot enlarges and migrates into larger veins such as the femoral and popliteal veins, as in our patient, it can break off and migrate up the vena cava, through the right atrium and right ventricle, and into the pulmonary arterial circulation, where it can become lodged (see Figure 12.2 for an overview of the circulatory system). When this happens, blood flow is reduced or cut off to one or more large segments of the lung.

Reflect and Review #11

- Why will regional decreases in pulmonary blood flow lead to hypoxemia? (See Figure 13.24 and Table 13.10.)

Fortunately, these clots are too large to pass through the pulmonary circulation into the systemic circulation. When clots do form in the systemic circulation, they can occlude arteries and arterioles, thereby depriving vital organs of oxygen and nutrients and preventing the removal of toxic waste products. If this occurs in the cerebral arterial circulation, it can lead to a stroke. If this occurs in the coronary arteries, it can lead to a heart attack (see Chapter 12, Section E).

19.B5 Physiological Integration

The presence of hypoxemia and hyperventilation (the cause of the acute respiratory alkalosis), the history, and symptoms suggest that the patient is suffering from an acute decrease in pulmonary blood flow to some parts of the lung. Remember that hyperventilation is defined as a decrease in the ratio of CO_2 production to alveolar ventilation (see Figure 13.22). That is, if whole-body CO_2 production stays the same and alveolar ventilation increases as in our patient, arterial P_{CO_2} will decrease resulting in an increase in arterial pH. The acute decrease in pulmonary blood flow in some regions of the lung results in a clinically significant ventilation–perfusion inequality (see Table 13.10). The hyperventilation is only partly due to the mild hypoxemia, because the arterial P_{O_2} of 60 mmHg in our patient, although low, is just at the threshold oxygen level that stimulates the peripheral chemoreceptors (see Figures 13.33 and 13.34). Other causes of hyperventilation may be anxiety and pain, which may also explain the increased heart rate observed in the patient at the emergency room.

The ventilation–perfusion inequality means that the patient is ventilating areas of the lung to which blood is not flowing, leading to increased alveolar dead space (see Figure 13.19). The extra blood flows to other nearby lung regions leading to a local decrease in the ratio of ventilation to perfusion (physiological shunt). This results in some blood leaving the lung without adequate oxygenation. Remember that disruption of the delicate balance between regional ventilation and perfusion throughout the lung results in a failure to fully oxygenate the blood leaving the lung. In addition, hypoxia within the pulmonary circulation leads to vasoconstriction of the arterioles in the lungs and an increase in pulmonary artery pressure (see Figure 13.24).

We know that the hyperventilation was acute and not a long-standing problem because the arterial pH was still alkaline from the decrease in P_{CO_2}. This indicates that the kidneys did not have time to respond to the change in pH by increasing bicarbonate excretion in the urine (see Table 14.7). When the kidney has time to compensate, the condition is called respiratory alkalosis with metabolic compensation.

Why did the pulmonary embolism cause a decrease in arterial P_{O_2} but did not increase and, in fact, decreased arterial P_{CO_2}? Remember from Chapter 13 that the relationship between partial pressure and content is sigmoidal for oxygen but relatively linear for CO_2. Because of the plateau of O_2 content as P_{O_2} increases above 60 mmHg (see Figure 13.26), increasing alveolar O_2 in over-ventilated regions of the lung does not significantly increase O_2 content of the blood leaving that region. Therefore, although hyperventilation does increase O_2 in some alveoli, it does not compensate for the significant decrease in O_2 content in some pulmonary capillaries due to ventilation–perfusion inequalities. Increasing ventilation can decrease the CO_2 content of blood due to the linearity of the relationship between P_{CO_2} and CO_2 content of the blood. The overall net effect is acute respiratory alkalosis due to decreased arterial P_{CO_2}. Interestingly, the hypoxemia can be partially overcome if the patient breathes gas that is enriched in oxygen because, although ventilation and perfusion are not well matched, there is not complete shunting of blood in the lungs. Thus, increasing alveolar P_{O_2} can still increase oxygenation of some areas of the lung with ventilation–perfusion mismatching, at least somewhat. The arterial P_{CO_2} may have increased a little and pH decreased a little on supplemental O_2 because the improved arterial P_{O_2} decreased peripheral chemoreceptor stimulation and the degree of hyperventilation lessened (see Figure 13.34).

Our patient's initial complaint was chest pain, which made him think he was having a heart attack. He was actually fortunate to have chest pain because it caused him to go to the emergency room, which may have saved his life. Although the exact reasons for chest pain in pulmonary embolism are uncertain, one possibility is that the clots result in an acute increase in pulmonary artery pressure, which can result in pain.

Why did this man have a pulmonary embolism? Several risk factors for the development of deep vein thrombosis can result in pulmonary embolism. Prolonged sitting often causes a stagnant pooling of blood in the lower legs (see Figures 12.45 and 12.60). That is why it is highly recommended to avoid sitting for extended periods of time. Even sitting at a computer for just a few hours is discouraged. Contraction of the leg skeletal muscles compresses the leg veins. This results in intermittent emptying of the veins, decreasing the chances for clot formation. Obesity also increased the risk of deep vein thrombosis in our patient by further increasing the pooling of blood in the leg veins (due to obstruction of venous outflow and weakening of venous valves), increasing the amount of certain clotting factors in the blood, and changing platelet function.

A number of gene defects can also lead to an increased tendency to form clots, a condition called inherited ***hypercoagulability***. The most common is resistance to activated protein C (see Figure 12.78), which can occur in up to 3% of healthy adults in the United States. In fact, our patient was tested and found to have resistance to activated protein C. Therefore, the combination of obesity, sitting for a prolonged period of time, and hypercoagulability is the likely cause of deep vein thrombosis and pulmonary embolism in our patient.

19.B6 Therapy

As soon as the diagnosis of pulmonary embolism was made, our patient was immediately started on intravenous heparin and ***recombinant tissue plasminogen activator*** (***rec-tPA***). Heparin is an anticlotting factor that counteracts the hypercoagulability. Rec-tPA is a synthetic form of a naturally occurring molecule that helps dissolve clots. The ventilation–perfusion scan was repeated a few days later and lung blood flow was almost normal. Supplemental oxygen was reduced over this time and then stopped when blood gases normalized.

Considering that this patient has an inherited cause of hypercoagulability, he has an increased probability to have another deep vein thrombosis and even pulmonary embolism in the near future. It is also possible that some of his family members have the same defect, for which they should be tested and adequately counseled. Our patient was sent home and continued to receive oral anticoagulants for 6 months (see description of anticlotting drugs in Chapter 12, Section F) and was actively followed by his primary care physician. He was encouraged to lose weight because obesity increases the risk of a deep vein thrombosis occurring again. Some physicians even advocate lifelong anticoagulation therapy for a patient such as ours.

CASE C

Man with Abdominal Pain, Fever, and Circulatory Failure

19.C1 Case Presentation

A 21-year-old healthy college student and his friends were canoeing deep in the Alaskan wilderness when he felt the first twinge of abdominal pain. Thinking that he either ate some undercooked fish or strained a muscle while paddling, he stopped to rest for a day, but the pain steadily intensified. He began to shiver and felt extremely cold even though it was a warm day. These symptoms worsened during the 36 hours it took to paddle to the outpost camp and be airlifted to the nearest medical center.

Reflect and Review #12

- Based on your knowledge of the homeostatic control of body temperature, why might this young man feel cold despite the signs that his body temperature is increased? (See Figures 16.17 through 16.19.)
- What might be the cause of the abdominal pain?

19.C2 Physical Examination

On arrival at the hospital emergency room, the young man is confused and lapsing into and out of consciousness. His temperature is 39.2°C (normal range ~36.5°C–37.5°C), heart rate is 140 beats per min (normal range 65–85), respiration rate is 34 breaths per min (normal ~12), and blood pressure is 84/44 mmHg (normal for a young man ~120/80). He is taking deep breaths, but his lungs are clear when listened to with a stethoscope. His abdomen is rigid and extremely tender when gently pressed on, especially in the lower-right quadrant. Upon questioning, his friends state that he has not urinated in over 24 hours. Therefore, a hollow tube called a ***catheter*** is inserted through the urethra into the urinary bladder to collect his urine. However, an abnormally small amount of urine (10 mL) is collected (see Figures 14.22 through 14.28 for a review of the control of urine output).

Reflect and Review #13

- What mechanisms link low systemic blood pressure in this patient to the low urine output? (See Figure 14.22.)
- What organs are located in the lower-right quadrant of the abdominal cavity? (See Figures 15.1 and 15.35.)

19.C3 Laboratory Tests

Additional measurements are then performed, and the results are shown in **Table 19.3**.

TABLE 19.3 Initial Laboratory Results with the Patient Breathing Room Air

Blood Measurement*	Result	Normal Range
White blood cells	$25.0 \times 10^3/\text{mm}^3$	$4.3\text{–}10.8 \times 10^3/\text{mm}^3$
Arterial P_{O_2}	90 mmHg	80–100 mmHg
Arterial P_{CO_2}	28 mmHg	35–45 mmHg
Arterial pH	7.25	7.38–7.45
Arterial bicarbonate	13 mmol/L	23–27 mmol/L
Lactate	8 mmol/L	0.5–2.2 mmol/L
Glucose	90 mg/dL	70–110 mg/dL
Creatinine	2.2 mg/dL	0.8–1.4 mg/dL

*In actuality, these measurements are done in whole blood or blood serum.

Reflect and Review #14

- Explain the relationship between arterial P_{CO_2} and pH values. Why is his arterial bicarbonate so low? (See Table 14.8.)
- What functions do white blood cells serve? What might be the cause of their abnormal values in this patient? (See Figure 12.67 and Table 18.1.)
- What metabolic processes produce lactate (lactic acid)? Under what circumstances would lactate production be increased above normal? (See Figures 3.41 and 3.42.)
- What effect does an increase in lactate have on alveolar ventilation? (See Figure 13.38.)
- Why did creatinine concentration in the blood increase? (See the discussion of Figure 14.12.)

19.C4 Diagnosis

A catheter is placed into an arm vein so that an intravenous infusion of isotonic saline (NaCl) can be started. Antibiotics are added to the saline to fight the apparent infection. A ***computed tomography*** (***CT***) scan of the abdomen is performed, which reveals an inflamed appendix (**Figure 19.4**). The patient is admitted to the intensive care unit (ICU) for continued intravenous fluid replacement, physiological monitoring, and the insertion of additional catheters that can be used for the measurement of arterial and right atrial blood pressures.

The patient is then taken to the operating room for abdominal exploration. Surgeons remove an inflamed appendix that is found to have a small hole (***perforation***) and shows signs of ***necrosis*** (dying or dead tissue).

Reflect and Review #15

- Where is the appendix located? (See Figure 15.35.)

A bacterial infection of the membranes surrounding the abdominal organs is found. This type of infection, called ***peritonitis***, results in ***pus*** (yellow liquid made up of white blood cells, bacteria, and cellular debris) being produced. The pus is removed, the abdominal organs are thoroughly washed with saline and antibiotics, and the patient is returned to the ICU where arterial and central venous blood pressures and urine output are monitored.

Reflect and Review #16

- What is the purpose of monitoring right atrial blood pressure? (See Figure 12.46.) Suggest other variables to monitor in this patient.

In the hours after surgery, the patient is maintained on mechanical ventilation. Gurgling breath sounds and decreasing arterial oxygen partial pressure indicate the presence of fluid in his lungs. Supplemental oxygen is provided to minimize the decrease in arterial oxygen by having the patient breathe a mixture of air enriched in oxygen. Widespread swelling of body tissues indicates that interstitial fluid volume is increasing, and his blood pressure and urine output remain dangerously below normal. In addition to providing continued intravenous fluids and antibiotic therapy, the ICU staff infuses norepinephrine and vasopressin (vasoconstrictors), and methylprednisolone (a synthetic glucocorticoid given at pharmacological doses).

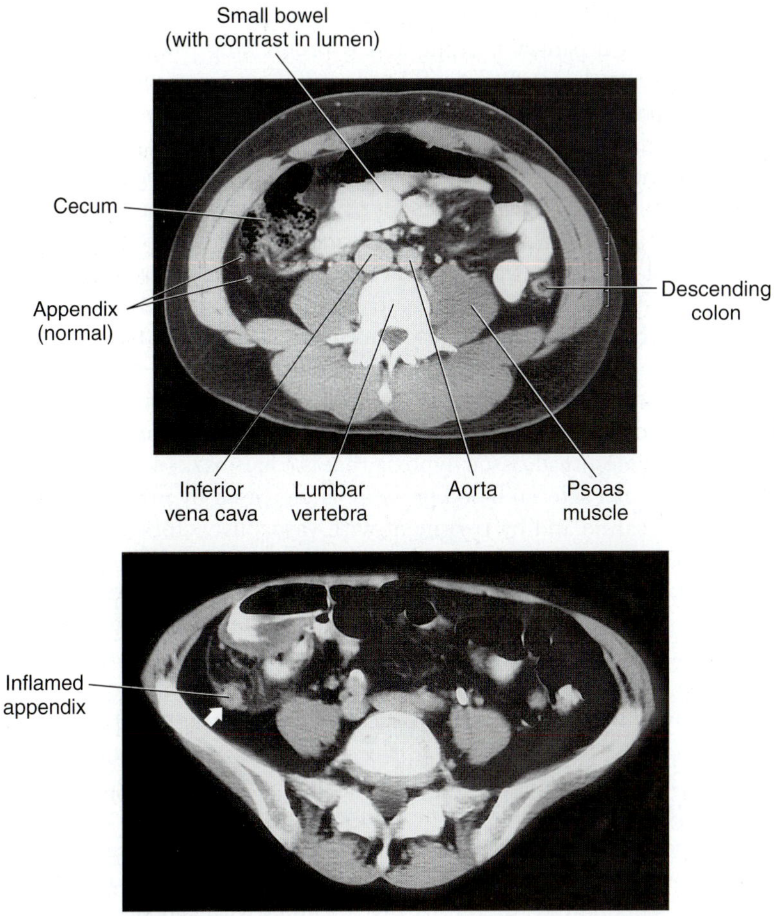

Figure 19.4 Normal abdominal CT scan (top) identifying major structures. CT scan on the bottom shows an inflamed appendix (arrow).

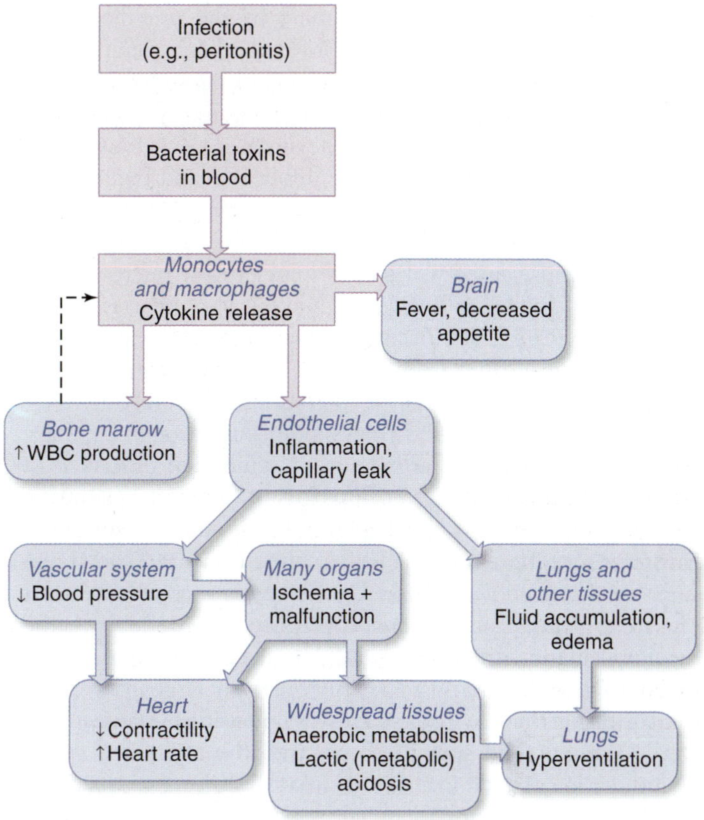

Figure 19.5 Cascade of some of the events from a serious infection to widespread organ failure in septic shock.

For the next several days, the patient is critically ill while his condition is continuously monitored. Appropriate treatment adjustments are implemented as needed to attempt to normalize his blood volume, blood pressure, serum lactate, blood pH, and gas partial pressures in his blood.

This patient's condition began as acute ***appendicitis,*** but the delay in treatment allowed it to progress to the potentially lethal condition known as ***septic shock.*** Although *Escherichia coli* and other bacterial species are normally present in the large intestine and its associated appendix, blockage of the lumen of the appendix or the blood supply to the appendix can allow those normally harmless bacteria to multiply out of control. When this happens, the appendix becomes distended and the pressure inside the appendix increases significantly due to inflammation. Eventually, these factors can lead to ulceration of the mucosa of the appendix, followed by perforation and ultimately rupture of the organ. This releases bacteria into the peritoneal cavity. The bacteria then release toxins that diffuse into the blood vessels in the abdomen, leading to a dramatic cascade of events (**Figure 19.5**). When a bacterial infection is accompanied by a ***systemic inflammatory response*** (defined by symptoms such as increases in body temperature, pulse rate, respiratory rate, and white blood cell count), the condition is referred to as ***sepsis.*** The most common sites of bacterial infections leading to sepsis are the lungs, abdomen (as in our patient), urinary tract, and sites where catheters penetrate the skin or blood vessels. If sepsis progresses to septic shock, patients also develop a significant decrease in blood pressure (a decrease in systolic pressure of greater than 40 mmHg or a mean arterial pressure less than 65 mmHg) that is not reversible by intravenous infusion of large volumes of isotonic saline solution. This type of circulatory failure is an example of ***low-resistance shock,*** defined as a decrease in total peripheral resistance and blood pressure due to an excessive release of vasodilatory substances (see Chapter 12, Section E).

19.C5 Physiological Integration

Bacterial infections stimulate the body to mount a rapid and widespread defense reaction (see Figures 18.16 through 18.19 and 18.22). Monocytes and macrophages (two types of white blood cells) secrete a variety of signaling molecules known generally as cytokines (see Table 18.2), which include substances such as interleukins and tumor necrosis factor. Target tissues for cytokines include (1) the brain, where they mediate the onset of fever, a decrease in appetite, fatigue, and an increase in ACTH secretion; (2) the bone marrow, where they stimulate an increase in the rate of white blood cell production; and (3) endothelial cells throughout the vasculature, where they stimulate processes leading to inflammation and increased capillary leakiness. Many species of bacteria release toxins, which greatly accelerate and exaggerate cytokine release and effects, often resulting in a maladaptive or life-threatening overreaction. The systemic inflammatory response has far-reaching effects on all body systems.

Such was the case of our patient by the time he finally reached the hospital. The set point for his body temperature was reset upward by circulating cytokines, resulting in ***fever***, and he shivered and felt chilled as his body attempted to warm itself toward the new, higher set point. The onslaught of cytokines and other inflammatory mediators (see Table 18.3 and Figure 18.2) accelerated as his white blood cell count increased and bacterial toxins were released into his circulation. Excessive amounts of those chemicals caused widespread injury to the microvascular endothelium and led to leakage of fluid out of capillaries.

When capillaries become excessively leaky, bulk flow favors the exit of fluid from the circulation (see Figure 12.41). Plasma proteins escape into the interstitial fluid, creating a significant osmotic force that draws fluid out through capillary pores. This is due to Starling forces, which are described in Chapter 12 (see Figure 12.42). This loss of fluid causes a drastic reduction in circulating blood volume, to the point at which even baroreceptor reflexes are unable to maintain arterial blood pressure (see Chapter 12, Section D). Dramatic increases in heart rate are evidence of activation of the baroreceptor reflexes via the cardiovascular control centers in the brain attempting to restore blood pressure toward normal. Even relatively large intravenous fluid infusions fail to reverse this hypotension because much of the infused fluid simply escapes into the interstitial space. Accumulation of fluid in the interstitial space leads to the tissue edema observed in our patient, and leakiness of pulmonary capillaries eventually led to fluid in his lungs (***pulmonary edema***).

Decreased systemic arterial blood pressure makes it difficult to produce adequate blood flow through the tissues. When blood flow is inadequate to meet demands for oxygen and nutrients (***ischemia***), tissues, organs, and organ systems malfunction. For example, our patient's inability to form urine resulted from low blood flow through his kidneys (see Figure 14.22). The increase in serum creatinine concentration was evidence that glomerular filtration rate was decreased (see discussion of Figure 14.12).

A more general consequence of reduced oxygen availability is that cells must resort to anaerobic pathways to manufacture ATP, and lactic acid (lactate) is produced as a by-product (see Figure 3.41 and Figure 9.22). This led to the marked metabolic acidosis seen in our patient. His hyperventilation was driven by the peripheral chemoreceptors (primarily the carotid bodies), in an attempt to compensate by removing CO_2-derived acid from the plasma (see Figure 13.37). Another mechanism designed to combat acidosis is the addition of new bicarbonate to the plasma and the excretion of H^+ via the kidney (Chapter 14, Section C), but the decrease in renal blood flow and glomerular filtration rate rendered this mechanism ineffective. His oxygen delivery to tissues was further compromised by the fluid buildup in his lungs. The added barrier to oxygen diffusion from lung alveoli into pulmonary capillaries (see Figure 13.28) reduced the oxygen partial pressure of his systemic arterial blood.

19.C6 Therapy

Septic shock is an extremely challenging condition to treat, with mortality rates of 40% to 60%. One of the most important factors in determining patient survival is early recognition of the condition and onset of treatment. As soon as it has been determined that a patient is septic and is progressing toward septic shock, survival depends on rapid and continuous assessment of his or her physiological condition and timely therapeutic responses to changing conditions. Among the variables monitored, in addition to those listed in Table 19.3, are body temperature, heart rate, blood pressure, arterial and venous oxygen saturation, mean arterial and right atrial blood pressures, urine output, and specific biochemical plasma indicators of the function of other organs, such as the liver. Using this information, clinicians can take steps to improve cardiovascular and respiratory function while at the same time battling the infection that is the root cause of the condition.

Immediate interventions in the treatment of septic shock are aimed at restoring systemic oxygen delivery and thus relieving the widespread tissue hypoxia that is a hallmark of the condition. Mean arterial blood pressure is increased by infusion of isotonic saline and by treatment with vasoconstrictors such as norepinephrine and vasopressin (see Figure 12.51). The extra circulating fluid volume increases cardiac output by increasing venous pressure and cardiac filling (see Figure 12.46), whereas norepinephrine (the neurotransmitter normally released from postsynaptic sympathetic nerve endings) increases cardiac contractility and arteriolar vasoconstriction (see Figure 12.51). Maintaining mean arterial pressure between 65 and 90 mmHg is necessary to ensure adequate flow of blood through the tissues. Right atrial pressure is monitored because it is a good index of venous return and the volume of fluid within the cardiovascular system (see Figure 12.57). The oxygen content of the blood is maintained by ventilating the lungs with supplemental oxygen to make sure that hemoglobin is saturated with oxygen (see Figure 13.26). It is also helpful to reduce the patient's demand for oxygen by paralyzing the respiratory muscles with drugs and providing mechanical ventilation, usually through a tube placed in the trachea attached to a positive-pressure pump. Otherwise, the increase in rate and depth of breathing that is typical of a patient in septic shock causes a marked increase in oxygen use by the respiratory muscles and directs blood flow away from other organs already suffering from lack of oxygen.

The infection must be treated while also restoring cardiovascular function. Antibiotics that act on a wide variety of types of bacteria are administered as soon as possible after sepsis is diagnosed. The source of the infection is then located, accumulated pus and dead tissue are removed, and the surrounding tissue is thoroughly cleaned. Ideally, samples of blood and/or pus from the site of infection can be grown in culture, and within 48 hours the specific bacterial species involved in the infection can be identified. The intravenous antibiotic therapy can then be altered to use drugs known to specifically target the invading species.

Recent clinical studies have suggested other therapeutic measures that can increase the survival rate of patients with septic shock. Pharmacological doses of glucocorticoid injections have also shown promise in some patients with septic shock. These hormones activate mechanisms throughout many tissues of the body that help the body cope with stress (see Table 11.3). Important among those effects are the inhibition of the inflammatory response and the enhancement of the sensitivity of vascular smooth muscle to adrenergic agents like norepinephrine.

Over a 6-day period, the condition of our patient gradually improved. His blood pressure increased and stabilized, and the intravenous fluid and norepinephrine infusions were gradually reduced and then stopped. The edema in his lungs and tissues slowly subsided, he regained consciousness, and he was eventually able to maintain oxygen saturation in his arterial blood without mechanical ventilation. During his 2-week hospital stay, the brain, liver, and kidney function returned to normal, and he had no apparent long-term organ damage from his ordeal. He has been extremely fortunate; approximately 500,000 cases of severe septic shock occur in the United States each year, and less than half of those patients survive. His youth and relatively good initial physical condition were most likely instrumental in helping him beat the odds.

CASE D

College Student with Nausea, Flushing, and Sweating

19.D1 Case Presentation

A 21-year-old female Caucasian college student visits the student health clinic because of several episodes of nausea (without vomiting), flushing (redness and warmth in the face), and sweating. Although she admits to some binge drinking in the past, her recent episodes of nausea do not correlate with those events and occur without any identifiable trigger. Following the onset of her symptoms, she also notices mild tingling ("pins and needles") and rhythmic jerking beginning in the left side of her face and progressively marching down her body to include the left arm and left leg. These symptoms persist for about 3–4 minutes and then completely go away. The student health service physician assistant asks the patient if she has had any recent head injuries that could account for her symptoms. The patient reports that no such injuries have occurred. During the physical exam, the patient becomes nauseated, visibly flushed in the face, and sweaty. After a few seconds, twitching of the left side of her face occurs, with progressive involvement of the left arm, followed by the left leg. After a minute or so, the student loses consciousness and starts to have rhythmic ***convulsions*** (violent spasms) of both arms and legs that look like an ***epileptic seizure*** (see Figure 8.2). A seizure is a storm of uncontrolled electrical activity in the brain that in some cases can become rhythmic. In addition, her back becomes arched and stiff, and her eyes roll back into their sockets. The physician assistant applies a ***transcutaneous*** (through the skin) ***oxygen monitor***, which is placed on the patient's finger. The patient's oxygen saturation is found to be low at 83% (normal is 95%). The convulsions stop after about 2–3 min, but the patient does not regain consciousness and soaks her pants with urine. The physician assistant immediately calls an ambulance, and the student is rushed to a nearby hospital emergency room.

Reflect and Review #17

- What can cause a sudden decrease in oxygen saturation? (See Figure 13.26 and Table 13.10.)
- What could be causing the flushing and sweating? (See Table 6.11 and Figures 16.17 and 16.18.)
- What controls micturition (urination)? (See Figure 14.13.)

19.D2 Physical Examination

The emergency room physician assesses the vital signs of the patient. Her blood pressure is increased at 159/83 mmHg, her heart rate is increased at 114 beats per minute, and her body temperature is normal at 98.8°F (37.1°C). A thin tube called a catheter is placed in the antecubital vein in one of her arms; a blood sample is drawn for the measurement of hematocrit, white blood cell count, electrolytes, glucose, and creatinine (**Table 19.4**). A slow infusion of 0.9% normal saline containing 150 mmol/L of sodium and 150 mmol/L of chloride (300 mOsm/L) is then started. A cursory neurological exam shows that the patient can be aroused but does not follow commands consistently and seems somewhat dazed. The pupils are similar in size and constrict symmetrically when a light is shone in either eye, which is normal. The patient does not seem to be moving the left arm and leg as much as the extremities on the right side. When the physician taps on the elbows and knees with a reflex hammer, the reflexes at the joints on the left side are more active, or brisker, than those of the right side. Based on this neurological exam, the physician orders an MRI scan of the head.

Reflect and Review #18

- What could cause her increase in heart rate? (See Figures 12.23, 12.27, and 12.51.)
- What does hematocrit measure? (See Figure 12.1.)

TABLE 19.4 Laboratory Tests in the Emergency Room

Blood Measurement*	Result	Normal Range
Hematocrit	47%	37%–48%
White blood cell count	$5.8 \times 10^3/mm^3$	$4.3–10.8 \times 10^3/mm^3$
Sodium	140 mmol/L	135–146 mmol/L
Potassium	4.0 mmol/L	3.5–5.0 mmol/L
Chloride	101 mmol/L	97–110 mmol/L
Calcium (total)	9.5 mg/dL	9.0–10.5 mg/dL
Glucose	130 mg/dL	70–110 mg/dL
Creatinine	0.9 mg/dL	0.8–1.4 mg/dL

*In actuality, sodium, potassium, chloride, calcium, glucose, and creatinine are measured in blood serum or plasma.

- Why was blood glucose measured? (See Figure 16.11 and the description of hypoglycemia in Chapter 16.)
- Why was blood creatinine concentration measured? (See section on renal clearance in Chapter 14.)
- Why was 0.9% normal saline infused? (See Table 4.1.)
- What is the significance of the increased reflexes in the left arm and leg? (See Figures 10.3 and 10.6.)

19.D3 Laboratory Tests

Magnetic resonance imaging (***MRI***) uses a powerful magnet to create a strong magnetic field around a patient's body (**Figure 19.6**). This field acts on the spin—or resonance—of the nuclei (protons) of hydrogen atoms in the body, aligning them in the same direction. The part of the body being examined—in this case, the brain—is then subjected to a pulse of radio waves. The atoms of the brain absorb the energy of the waves and the resonance of their nuclei changes, thus altering their alignment with the magnetic field. The realignment of the hydrogen nuclei within the magnetic field is dependent on the type of tissue and is detected as a change in the characteristics of an electrical current passing through the radio frequency coils. Protons in different tissues like brain, adipose, and muscle behave differently, because their behavior is dependent upon the local environment such as the content of fat and water. Therefore, the different behavior of protons in different tissues can be analyzed by a computer to generate an image of the internal structures of the brain and many abnormalities and disease states.

19.D4 Diagnosis

The MRI shows a lesion in the right temporal lobe of the brain. (See Figure 6.38 and **Figure 19.7** for the location of the temporal lobe.) There are at least two possible explanations for this lesion. First, an infection may have led to the formation of an ***abscess***, which is an inflammation characterized by a collection of neutrophils, bacteria, and fluid. Second, the lesion may be a ***neoplasm***, which means "new growth," or tumor. Some neoplasms are malignant, that is, they are cancerous and may spread to other parts of the brain. Many CNS tumors are benign or noncancerous. Benign tumors are generally less dangerous because they usually do not grow as rapidly or spread to other organs, but they can still cause problems due to local growth. The only way to determine the tissue diagnosis is by surgical removal of the abnormal tissue via a ***craniotomy***, in which a part of the skull is removed to give access to underlying brain tissue. This is performed on the patient and a histological diagnosis of a tumor of astrocytes (***astrocytoma***) is made (see Figure 6.6). Specifically, the pathologist examining the stained histological sections of this tumor under a microscope determines that the patient has a ***glioblastoma multiforme***. These tumors get their name because they arise from glia cells (in this case, astrocytes) that are not fully differentiated; such cells are known as blast cells. The tumors are "multiforme" because they can attain varied appearances depending on their age, location, and the extent of surrounding damage to the brain. Unfortunately, glioblastoma multiforme is a cancerous form of tumor.

Reflect and Review #19

- What is the significance of the anatomical location of this lesion? (See Figure 7.13.)
- What might possibly explain the appearance of the lesion found in the MRI?

19.D5 Physiological Integration

Glioblastoma multiforme is a fast-growing and potentially lethal form of brain cancer. Of the approximately 13,000 new cases of brain tumors in the United States each year, about

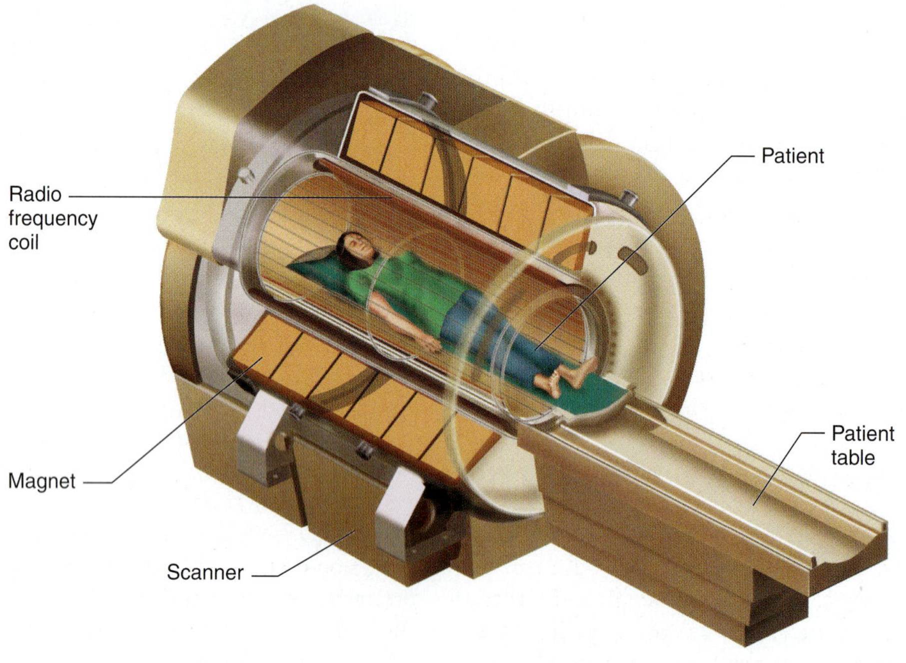

Figure 19.6 Cutaway diagram of an MRI scanner. Figure 19.6 was modified from an image on the following website: www.magnet.fsu.edu.

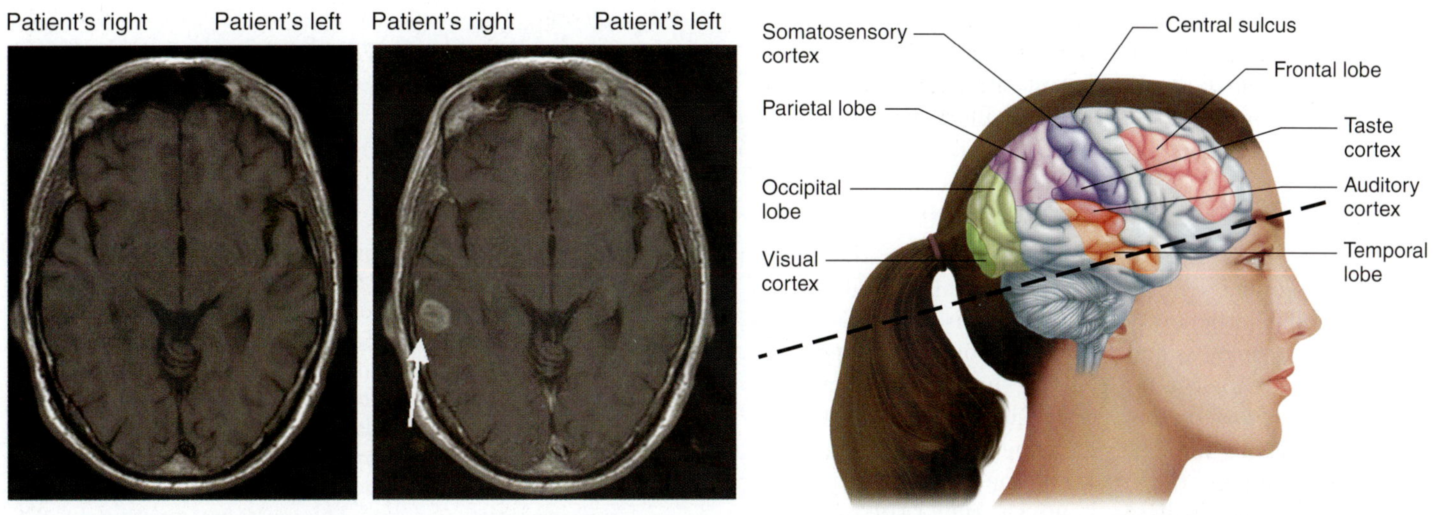

Figure 19.7 In these images, the settings on the MRI scanner are first set so that the brain tissue looks homogeneously gray, the fat surrounding the brain is lighter, and the water within the cerebral ventricles is dark (left scan). By convention, the MRI images are reversed so that the right side of the brain appears on the left side of the image. A contrast agent containing the element gadolinium is then infused intravenously into the patient and a repeat scan is taken (right scan). Gadolinium has paramagnetic properties, which are magnetic properties that only arise in the presence of an externally applied magnetic field. When infused intravenously, the contrast agent can enter the brain in regions where the blood–brain barrier (see Figure 6.6) is absent or damaged, as is sometimes the case in sites of brain injury or disease. Once inside the brain, the association of gadolinium with water and fat changes the local environment and causes an area of higher intensity. This MRI scan demonstrates an area of signal abnormality in the right temporal lobe of the brain that measures about 2 cm in diameter (white arrow). The dashed line on the right image shows the plane of the MRI image. MRI images courtesy of Douglas Woo, M.D., Medical College of Wisconsin.

65% are of glial origin and are known collectively as gliomas. These tumors arise from astrocytes and invade normal brain tissue. As they grow, these tumors can infiltrate, compress, and destroy the healthy brain tissue surrounding the tumor. In addition, these invading tumor cells can irritate the brain, causing seizures. In fact, like our patient, approximately 20–30% of patients with brain neoplasms experience epileptic-like seizures (see Figure 8.2). During seizures, there is often a large increase in sympathetic nerve activity that was, at least in part, the cause of the nausea, facial flushing, sweatiness, and increase in blood pressure and heart rate that occurred in our patient. The decrease in oxygen saturation was due to a rigid and prolonged contraction of the respiratory muscles during the seizure leading to hypoventilation (see Table 13.10). The patient urinated after the seizure because, when the increased sympathetic activity from the seizure subsided, the remaining parasympathetic tone resulted in micturition (see Figure 14.13).

Until the brain MRI was done, the physicians did not know the cause of the seizures. A variety of metabolic disturbances can cause seizures. Abnormalities in blood electrolytes such as Na^+, K^+, and Ca^{2+} can interfere with normal neuronal resting membrane and action potentials (see Section B of Chapter 6). This could not explain the patient's seizures, however, as blood electrolytes were normal (see Table 19.4). The patient was given an infusion of 0.9% normal saline because its osmolarity is very similar to that of plasma. This fluid infusion helps to maintain blood volume and also ensures that the intravenous line stays open in case drugs need to be infused. Renal failure can also cause metabolic and fluid-balance abnormalities leading to abnormal brain activity. Because the concentration of creatinine in the blood is a good estimate for glomerular filtration rate in the kidney, we know that this patient had normal renal function (see Table 19.4). Severe hypoglycemia can decrease the amount of glucose available for brain metabolism, which can cause seizures. This did not occur in our patient (see Table 19.4). In fact, she had a small increase in blood glucose concentration that was probably due to an increase in the blood concentrations of stress hormones such as cortisol and epinephrine (see Section D of Chapter 11, Figure 16.11, and Table 16.3).

Another problem with intracranial lesions is that they may interfere with the drainage of cerebrospinal fluid from the lateral and third ventricles. If this were to happen, it could result in an increase in pressure within the cerebral ventricles. This leads to an enlargement of the ventricles that results in compression of the brain within the cranium. This is called ***hydrocephalus*** (from the Greek words for "water" and "head"; see Figure 6.47). It can cause many functional abnormalities including the convulsions that occurred in our patient. The MRI scan of our patient, however, did not show signs of hydrocephalus such as increases in the size of the cerebral ventricles.

A revealing aspect of this patient's condition was that most of the neurological symptoms were localized to one side of her body—in this case, the left. This included tingling, rhythmic jerking, and loss of motion. Just as sensory afferent information crosses from one side of the body to the other side of the brain (see Figure 7.19), motor control by descending pathways from the cerebral cortex to skeletal muscles also crosses from one side of the body to the other (see Figure 10.12). Therefore, the lesion on the right side of the temporal lobe caused seizures primarily on the right side of the brain leading to increased rhythmic motor activity on the left side of the body. Furthermore, the increase in reflexes on the left side was due to a loss of descending inhibition of spinal reflexes from the right side of the cortex to the motor neurons on the left side of the spinal cord (see Figures 10.3 and 10.6). Without the restraint provided by these descending pathways, the spinal reflexes were free from inhibition and were brisker than normal.

19.D6 Therapy

This patient underwent brain surgery to have the tumor removed, followed by radiation therapy and a number of courses of chemotherapy. Chemotherapy is usually administered by an oncologist and typically involves administration of drugs that are toxic to fast-growing tumors. However, these drugs also have toxicity to normal tissue in which growth continues throughout life, such as blood cell–producing tissue and the epithelium of the small intestine. In radiation therapy, a beam of radiation is directed onto the tumor site to kill the tumor cells. In addition to these treatments, the patient was given an antiepileptic drug to prevent more seizures. One such drug is ***phenytoin* (*Dilantin*)**, which acts by blocking voltage-gated Na^+ channels (see Figure 6.18), particularly in neurons that are very active and firing with a high frequency. The patient was also treated with high doses of potent synthetic glucocorticoids because of their anti-inflammatory and anti-edema properties; these hormones, therefore, were given to reduce the swelling in the region of the patient's brain that was affected by the tumor.

After removal of the tumor and a small part of the surrounding right temporal lobe, our patient's right auditory cortex was damaged (see Figure 7.13) and she had trouble recognizing familiar musical melodies. Discrimination of melody (as opposed to rhythm) is a function that has been localized by researchers to the right temporal lobe of the human brain. Our patient remained stable for 16 months after her diagnosis but subsequently had a recurrence of the tumor that could not be surgically removed because of its position and size. She underwent further rounds of chemotherapy and radiation therapy. Sadly, however, only about 25% of patients survive more than 2 years from the time of diagnosis of glioblastoma multiforme.

SUMMARY

Case A: Woman with Palpitations and Heat Intolerance

I. Case Presentation
   a. Her symptoms are nervousness, palpitations, feelings of warmth in a cool room, and significant weight loss despite eating a lot.

II. Physical Examination
   a. Her systolic blood pressure is increased, and her diastolic pressure is decreased. Her resting heart rate is 100 beats per minute.
   b. She has an enlarged thyroid gland (goiter) and her eyes bulge out (proptosis).
   c. She has hyperactive knee-jerk reflexes and her hands are shaking.

III. Laboratory Tests
   a. She has increased thyroid hormone and decreased thyroid-stimulating hormone in the blood.

IV. Diagnosis
   a. She is diagnosed with hyperthyroidism (excess thyroid hormone activity).
   b. Hyperthyroidism is usually caused by Graves' disease—an autoimmune disease.

V. Physiological Integration
   a. Autoimmune production of thyroid-stimulating immunoglobulins (TSIs) stimulates the thyroid gland to produce too much thyroid hormone and to enlarge. The excess thyroid hormone suppresses the release of thyroid-stimulating hormone from the anterior pituitary gland.
   b. Infiltration of the muscles controlling eye movement by white blood cells leads to inflammation and proptosis.
   c. Increased thyroid hormone in the blood leads to an increase in sensitivity to catecholamines, resulting in an increase in systolic blood pressure and heart rate.
   d. Increased thyroid hormone leads to increased metabolic rate in a variety of tissues. This causes heat intolerance, hyperactive reflexes, and a small decrease in diastolic pressure.

VI. Therapy
   a. Three possible therapies include radioactive iodide administration to destroy much of the thyroid gland, drugs that block the synthesis of thyroid hormone, or surgical removal of the thyroid gland.

Case B: Man with Chest Pain After a Long Airplane Flight

I. Case Presentation
   a. A man has chest pain and shortness of breath after an 8 h flight.

II. Physical Examination
   a. He has an increased heart rate, but his ECG does not show evidence of a heart attack.
   b. His chest x-ray is essentially normal.

III. Laboratory Tests
   a. He is hypoxemic and has an acute respiratory alkalosis.

IV. Diagnosis
   a. His ventilation–perfusion scan shows evidence of a pulmonary embolism (blockage of pulmonary blood flow).
   b. An ultrasound of his legs shows a deep vein thrombosis.
   c. A clot formed in his leg veins because he sat for a long period of time. In addition, there is evidence that he has a genetic disorder of coagulation. The clot migrated to the lung, causing a pulmonary embolus.

V. Physiological Integration
   a. Hypoxemia is caused by a dramatic disruption of the regional balance between ventilation and perfusion throughout the lung.
   b. Hyperventilation due to anxiety and pain, as well as hypoxemia, caused an acute respiratory alkalosis.

VI. Therapy
   a. Treatment focuses on anticoagulation with heparin (to prevent clotting) and recombinant tissue plasminogen activator (to dissolve the clots).
   b. Long-term anticoagulation therapy is recommended.

Case C: Man with Abdominal Pain, Fever, and Circulatory Failure

I. Case Presentation
   a. A young man has increasing abdominal pain over 3 days.

II. Physical Examination
   a. He has a fever, increased heart and respiratory rates, and low blood pressure.

b. He has pain and rigidity localized to the lower-right quadrant of his abdomen.
c. His urine output is low.

III. Laboratory Tests
a. His white blood cell count is increased, suggesting an infection.
b. He has a metabolic (lactic) acidosis with a respiratory compensation (low arterial P_{CO_2}).
c. His blood creatinine concentration is increased, which indicates a decrease in glomerular filtration rate.

IV. Diagnosis
a. A computed tomography (CT) scan shows an inflamed appendix, suggesting a diagnosis of appendicitis. The low blood pressure suggests septic shock due to peritonitis (caused by a ruptured appendix).
b. The diagnosis is confirmed in an abdominal exploration during which a perforated appendix is removed. The membranes near it are infected, proving peritonitis.

V. Physiological Integration
a. Toxins from the bacteria have caused the low blood pressure because of vasodilation.
b. The decreased glomerular filtration rate is due to low blood pressure and decreased renal perfusion.

VI. Therapy
a. Therapy consists of intravenous fluids before and after surgery to support cardiac output and blood pressure and vasoconstrictor drugs to maintain blood pressure.
b. Antibiotic therapy is given to fight the peritoneal infection.

Case D: College Student with Nausea, Flushing, and Sweating

I. Case Presentation
a. A 21-year-old woman has several episodes of nausea, flushing, and sweating.
b. She also has tingling and jerking on the left side of her face, which progresses to the left arm and leg. This is followed by a loss of consciousness and convulsions.

II. Physical Examination
a. She has a decrease in motion on her left side.
b. She has an increase in her reflexes in the left arm and leg.

III. Laboratory Tests
a. Her blood tests are essentially normal except for a small increase in blood glucose.
b. An MRI of the brain is administered with gadolinium contrast injected intravenously.

IV. Diagnosis
a. The MRI of the brain reveals a bright 2-cm-diameter lesion in the right temporal lobe.
b. A craniotomy is performed to obtain a tissue sample of the lesion, which the pathologist identifies as a glioblastoma multiforme, a malignant brain tumor arising from astrocytes.

V. Physiological Integration
a. The tumor in the right temporal lobe causes seizures on the left side of the body because descending motor pathways cross from one side of the brain to the other side of the body.
b. Increased reflexes on the left side are due to a loss of descending inhibition from the right side of the brain to the spinal motor nerves on the left.

VI. Therapy
a. After as much of the tumor as possible is removed, the patient is treated with radiation and chemotherapy.
b. In addition, antiepileptic medicine and glucocorticoid therapy to decrease swelling and edema are administered.

CLINICAL TERMS

Appendix A ANSWERS TO TEST QUESTIONS AND GENERAL PRINCIPLES ASSESSMENTS

CHAPTER 1

Test Questions

1.1 b The four basic cell types are epithelial, muscle, nervous, and connective.

1.2 a Steady state requires energy input, but equilibrium does not.

1.3 c Muscles carry out the response (removing the hand from the stove).

1.4 c Circadian rhythms are typically entrained by the light–dark cycle, but in the absence of such cues, the rhythms "free-run" with their own endogenous cycle length.

1.5 b Intracellular fluid volume is greater than the sum of plasma and interstitial fluid.

Quantitative and Thought Questions

1.1 No. There may in fact be a genetic difference, but there is another possibility: The altered skin blood flow in the cold could represent an *acclimatization* undergone by each Inuit during his or her lifetime as a result of performing such work repeatedly.

1.2 This could occur in many ways. For example, suppose that an individual were to become dehydrated. What would happen to his or her plasma Na^+ *concentration?* Initially, the loss of fluid would result in an increased Na^+ concentration, even though the absolute amount of sodium may not have changed much. The increase in Na^+ concentration would trigger endocrine and renal responses that return the Na^+ concentration to normal. Another example occurs during mountain climbing. At high altitude, a person who is not acclimatized to low oxygen pressures will greatly increase the rate and depth of breathing to get more oxygen into his or her blood. One consequence of this, though, is that more of the carbon dioxide in the body is exhaled. Carbon dioxide tends to produce hydrogen ions in the blood (Chapters 13 and 14). Thus, ascent to high altitude leads to alkaline blood, which must then be compensated for by renal, endocrine, and other responses.

CHAPTER 2

Test Questions

2.1 e The continued creation of new free radicals is a chain reaction and contributes to the potentially damaging effects of a given free radical.

2.2 d

2.3 b This is a dehydration reaction. The reverse reaction would be hydrolysis.

2.4 b Uracil is found in RNA; thymine is found in DNA.

2.5 b

2.6 Sucrose (b); Glucose (a); Glycogen (c); Fructose (a); Starch (c)

2.7 c The other reactions in which larger molecules are formed occur via dehydration reactions.

Quantitative and Thought Questions

2.1 0.79 mol/L. The molecular weight of fructose can be calculated by adding up the weights of the individual atoms. However, since it is an isomer of glucose, you know that it must have the same molecular weight—180 daltons—as glucose. Thus, $[100g/0.7L] \times [1mole/180g] = 0.79$ mol/L.

2.2 Using a calculator, simply enter –1.5 and select the inverse log function. The answer is approximately 0.03 mol/L or 3×10^{-2} M.

2.3 Recall that atomic mass is the sum of the protons and neutrons in a nucleus. Regardless of its ionization state, potassium has (39 – 19) or 20 neutrons. The number of electrons is equal to the number of protons in a nonionized atom; therefore, K has 19 electrons. When ionized, K^+ has a single positive charge; it still has 19 protons and 20 neutrons, but it now has only 18 electrons.

General Principles Assessment

2.1 The chemical and physical properties of atoms, such as the number of electrons in their outer shells or their solubility in water, determine their reactivity with other atoms and molecules. For example, proteins are made by the linkage of amino acids through peptide bonds, which depend on the reactivity between amino and carboxyl groups. Further chemical and physical interactions, such as electrostatic attraction or repulsion, and hydrophobicity of amino acid side groups, bend and twist the protein into its final three-dimensional shape. Some of these same forces may in certain cases create a larger protein from several subunits. Without the correct chemical and physical properties, proteins would not assume a proper shape; this is extremely important in physiology because the shape of a protein is critically linked with its function.

CHAPTER 3

Test Questions

3.1 a

3.2 b Transcription refers to the conversion of a gene's DNA into RNA; translation is the conversion of mRNA into protein.

3.3 a Allosteric modulation occurs at a site separate from the ligand-binding site. The resulting change in three-dimensional structure of the protein may enhance or reduce the ability of the protein to bind its ligand.

3.4 b

3.5 c

3.6 d Catabolism refers to the breakdown of fatty acids into usable forms for the production of ATP.

Quantitative and Thought Questions

3.1 Nucleotide bases in DNA pair A to T and G to C. Given the base sequence of one DNA strand as

A—G—T—G—C—A—A—G—T—C—T

a. The complementary strand of DNA would be

T—C—A—C—G—T—T—C—A—G—A

b. The sequence in RNA transcribed from the first strand would be

U—C—A—C—G—U—U—C—A—G—A

Recall that uracil (U) replaces thymine (T) in RNA.

3.2 The triplet code G—T—A in DNA will be transcribed into mRNA as C—A—U, and the anticodon in tRNA corresponding to C—A—U is G—U—A.

3.3 If the gene were only composed of the triplet exon code words, the gene would be 300 nucleotides in length because a triplet of three nucleotides codes for one amino acid. However, because of the presence of intron segments in most genes, which account for 75% to 90% of the nucleotides in a gene, the gene would be between 1200 and 3000 nucleotides long; moreover, it would also contain termination codons. Thus, the exact size of a gene cannot be determined by knowing the number of amino acids in the protein for which the gene codes.

3.4 A drug could decrease acid secretion by (a) binding to the membrane sites that normally inhibit acid secretion, which would produce the same effect as the body's natural messengers that inhibit acid secretion; (b) binding to a membrane protein that normally stimulates acid secretion but not itself triggering acid secretion, thereby preventing the body's natural messengers from binding (competition); or (c) having an allosteric effect on the binding sites, which would increase the affinity of the sites that normally bind inhibitor messengers or decrease the affinity of those sites that normally bind stimulatory messengers.

3.5 The reason for a lack of insulin effect could be either a decrease in the number of available binding sites insulin can bind to or a decrease in the affinity of the binding sites for insulin so that less insulin is bound. A third possibility, which does not involve insulin binding, would be a defect in the way the binding site triggers a cell response once it has bound insulin.

3.6 (a) Acid secretion could be increased to 40 mmol/h by (1) increasing the concentration of compound X from 2 pM to 8 pM, thereby increasing the number of binding sites occupied; or (2) increasing the affinity of the binding sites for compound X, thereby increasing the amount bound without changing the concentration of compound X. (b) Increasing the concentration of compound X from 20 pM to 28 pM will not increase acid secretion because, at 20 pM, all the binding sites are occupied (the system is saturated) and there are no further binding sites available.

3.7 The maximum rate at which the end product E can be formed is 5 molecules per second, the rate of the slowest (rate-limiting) reaction in the pathway.

3.8 Under normal conditions, the concentration of oxygen at the level of the mitochondria in cells, including muscle at rest, is sufficient to saturate the enzyme that combines oxygen with hydrogen to form water. The rate-limiting reactions in the electron-transport chain depend on the available concentrations of ADP and P_i, which are combined to form ATP.

Thus, increasing the oxygen concentration above normal will not increase ATP production. If a muscle is contracting, it will break down ATP into ADP and P_i, which become the major rate-limiting substrates for increasing ATP production. With intense muscle activity, the level of oxygen may fall below saturating levels, limiting the rate of ATP production, and intensely active muscles must then use anaerobic glycolysis to provide additional ATP. Under these circumstances, increasing the oxygen concentration in the blood will increase the rate of ATP production. As discussed in Chapter 12, it is not the concentration of oxygen in the blood that is increased during exercise but the rate of blood flow to a muscle, resulting in greater quantities of oxygen delivery to the tissue.

3.9 During starvation, in the absence of ingested glucose, the body's stores of glycogen are rapidly depleted. Glucose, which is the major fuel used by the brain, must now be synthesized from other types of molecules. Most of this newly formed glucose comes from the breakdown of proteins to amino acids and their conversion to glucose. To a lesser extent, the glycerol portion of fat is converted to glucose. The fatty acid portion of fat cannot be converted to glucose.

3.10 Ammonia is formed in most cells during the oxidative deamination of amino acids and then travels to the liver via the blood. The liver detoxifies the ammonia by converting it to the nontoxic compound urea. Because the liver is the site in which ammonia is converted to urea, diseases that damage the liver can lead to an accumulation of ammonia in the blood, which is especially toxic to neurons. Note that it is not the liver that produces the ammonia.

General Principles Assessments

3.1 The extensive folding of the inner mitochondrial membrane increases the total surface area of the membrane. As shown in Figure 3.45, this is where the enzymes are located that are required for the generation of ATP. Thus, the structure of this membrane increases the ability of mitochondria to carry out their major function. The general principle that *structure is a determinant of—and has coevolved with—function* is also evident at the molecular (protein) level. In Figure 3.28, for example, it is clear that a protein's structure determines its function—in this case, its ability to bind particular ligands. Figure 3.32b shows how a protein's function is altered due to allosteric changes in its structure.

3.2 Proteins and ligands interact due to a variety of forces and molecular features, including complementary shapes. In addition, however, chemical or physical properties of molecules often strongly influence their ability to interact or bind with each other. In Figure 3.27, you can see how the structure of the protein results in an arrangement of certain charged amino acids. The fundamental property of physics that opposite charges attract one another means that a ligand with the correct electrical charges will be more likely to bind to this protein than another ligand without those charges.

3.3 Figure 3.53 summarizes how nutrients such as amino acids, glucose, and small lipids can be metabolized by a variety of mechanisms leading to the production of smaller molecules, which in turn can be used to eventually generate ATP. It is ATP that provides the energy required for the events that mediate all homeostatic processes, such as muscle contraction, neuron signaling, and so on. Recall from Chapter 1 (see Figure 1.6) that the generation of ATP is under negative feedback control, such that cells generate more ATP when required, and less when not required. Negative feedback is an essential component of homeostasis.

CHAPTER 4

Test Questions

4.1 c Channels are proteins that span the membrane and are opened by ligands, voltage, or mechanical stimuli.

4.2 d Facilitated diffusion does not require ATP. Recall that secondary active transport *indirectly* requires ATP because ion pumps were required to establish the electrochemical gradient for a particular ion (such as Na^+).

4.3 b After the initial movement of water out of the cells due to osmosis, the urea concentration quickly equilibrates across each cell's plasma membrane, removing any osmotic stimulus.

4.4 e Segregation of function on different surfaces of the cell, and the ability to secrete chemicals (e.g., from the pancreas), are two of the most important features of epithelial cells.

4.5 a Diffusion is slowed by the resistance of a membrane.

4.6 e Because ions are charged, both the chemical and the electrical gradients determine their rate and direction of diffusion.

Quantitative and Thought Questions

4.1 (a) During diffusion, the net flux always occurs from high to low concentration. Therefore, it will be from 2 to 1 in A and from 1 to 2 in B. (b) At equilibrium, the concentrations of solute in the two compartments will be equal: 4 mM in case A and 31 mM in case B. (c) Both will reach diffusion equilibrium at the same rate because the absolute difference in concentration across the membrane is the same in each case, 2 mM [$(3 - 5) = -2$, and $(32 - 30) = 2$]. The two one-way fluxes will be much larger in B than in A, but the net flux has the same magnitude in both cases, although it is oriented in opposite directions.

4.2 The ability of one amino acid to decrease the flux of a second amino acid across a cell membrane is an example of the competition of two molecules for the same binding site, as explained in Chapter 3. The binding site for alanine on the transport protein can also bind leucine. The higher the concentration of alanine, the greater the number of binding sites that it occupies and the fewer available for binding leucine. Consequently, less leucine will move into the cell.

4.3 The net transport will be out of the cell in the direction from the higher-affinity site on the intracellular surface to the lower-affinity site on the extracellular surface. More molecules will be bound to the transporter on the higher-affinity side of the membrane, and therefore more will move out of the cell than into it, until the concentration in the extracellular fluid becomes great enough that the number of molecules bound to transporters at the extracellular surface is equal to the number bound at the intracellular surface.

4.4 Although ATP is not used directly in secondary active transport, it is necessary for the primary active transport of Na^+ out of cells. Because it is the Na^+ concentration gradient across the plasma membrane that provides the energy for most secondary active transport systems, a decrease in ATP production will decrease primary active Na^+ transport, leading to a decrease in the sodium ion concentration gradient and therefore to a decrease in secondary active transport.

4.5 The solution with the greatest osmolarity will have the lowest water concentration. Recall that NaCl forms two ions in solution and $CaCl_2$ forms three. Thus, the osmolarities are

A. $20 + 30 + (2 \times 150) + (3 \times 10) = 380$ mOsm
B. $10 + 100 + (2 \times 20) + (3 \times 50) = 300$ mOsm
C. $100 + 200 + (2 \times 10) + (3 \times 20) = 380$ mOsm
D. $30 + 10 + (2 \times 60) + (3 \times 100) = 460$ mOsm

Solution D has the lowest water concentration. Solution B is isoosmotic because it has the same osmolarity as intracellular fluid. Solutions A and C have the same osmolarity.

4.6 Initially, the osmolarity of compartment 1 is $(2 \times 200) + 100 = 500$ mOsm and that of 2 is $(2 \times 100) + 300 = 500$ mOsm. The two solutions therefore have the same osmolarity, and there is no difference in water concentration across the membrane. Because the membrane is permeable to urea, this substance will undergo net diffusion until it reaches the same concentration (200 mM) on the two sides of the membrane. In other words, in the steady state, it will not affect the volumes of the compartments. In contrast, the higher initial NaCl concentration in compartment 1 than in compartment 2 will cause, by osmosis, the movement of water from compartment 2 to compartment 1 until the concentration of NaCl in both is 150 mM. Note that the same volume change would have occurred if there were no urea present in either compartment. It is only the concentration of nonpenetrating solutes (NaCl in this case) that determines the volume change, regardless of the concentration of any penetrating solutes that are present.

4.7 The osmolarities and nonpenetrating solute concentrations are

Solution	Osmolarity (mOsm)	Nonpenetrating Solute Concentration (mOsm)
A	$(2 \times 150) + 100 = 400$	$2 \times 150 = 300$
B	$(2 \times 100) + 150 = 350$	$2 \times 100 = 200$
C	$(2 \times 200) + 100 = 500$	$2 \times 200 = 400$
D	$(2 \times 100) + 50 = 250$	$2 \times 100 = 200$

Only the concentration of nonpenetrating solutes (NaCl in this case) will determine the change in cell volume. The intracellular concentration of nonpenetrating solute is typically about 300 mOsm, so solution A will produce no change in cell volume. Solutions B and D will cause cells to swell because they have a lower concentration of nonpenetrating solute (higher water concentration) than the intracellular fluid. Solution C will cause cells to shrink because it has a higher concentration of nonpenetrating solute than the intracellular fluid.

4.8 Solution A is isotonic because it has the same concentration of nonpenetrating solutes as intracellular fluid (300 mOsm). Solution A is also hyperosmotic because its total osmolarity is greater than 300 mOsm, as is also true for solutions B and C. Solution B is hypotonic because its concentration of nonpenetrating solutes is less than 300 mOsm. Solution C is hypertonic because its concentration of nonpenetrating solutes is greater than 300 mOsm. Solution D is hypotonic (less than 300 mOsm of nonpenetrating solutes) and also hypoosmotic (having a total osmolarity of less than 300 mOsm).

4.9 Exocytosis is triggered by an increase in cytosolic Ca^{2+} concentration. Calcium ions are actively transported out of cells, in part by secondary countertransport coupled to the downhill entry of sodium ions on the same transporter (see Figure 4.15). If the intracellular concentration of sodium ions were increased, the sodium ion concentration gradient across the membrane would be decreased, and this would decrease the secondary active transport of Ca^{2+} out of the cell. This would lead to an increase in cytosolic Ca^{2+} concentration, which would trigger increased exocytosis.

General Principles Assessments

4.1 One example of the general principle that *homeostasis is essential for health and survival* illustrated in Figures 4.8–4.10 is mediated transport across plasma membranes. For example, the controlled movement of glucose transporters (GLUTs) to plasma membranes in response to the hormone insulin helps maintain homeostatic concentrations of glucose in the extra- and intracellular fluids. This is important because glucose is the major source of energy for cells. Also, the regulated changes in aquaporin numbers in the epithelial cells of the kidneys help maintain water homeostasis by controlling the rate at which water is lost in the urine; this is particularly important in situations such as dehydration. A third example is osmosis, which regulates water flux across membranes (see Figure 4.17); this, in turn, helps maintain proper cell shape and size and the ability of cells to perform signaling functions.

4.2 The general principle that *controlled exchange of materials occurs between compartments and across cellular membranes* is apparent from the many diverse types of mechanisms by which solutes may cross plasma membranes. The control arises from such mechanisms as gates in ion channels that may open or close depending on cell requirements, and the just-mentioned glucose transporters and aquaporins, the concentrations of which can increase or decrease in plasma membranes under different conditions.

4.3 The general principle that *physiological processes are dictated by the laws of chemistry and physics* is evident from the relationship between the chemical nature (e.g., degree of hydrophobicity) of solutes and the ease with which they can diffuse through a lipid bilayer. The greater a molecule's hydrophobicity, the more likely it is to dissolve in the lipid bilayer of membranes and thus diffuse across cells. Electrochemical gradients aid in the diffusion of charged molecules (ions) through membrane channels because of the basic physical principle that like charges repel and opposite charges attract each other. Finally, molecular movement (and therefore potential interactions between molecules) is directly related to heat energy; solutes move through solution at faster rates at higher temperatures.

CHAPTER 5

Test Questions

5.1 b
5.2 a
5.3 e

5.4 a Calmodulin is a calcium-binding protein that is inactive in the absence of Ca^{2+}.

5.5 d Lipid-soluble messengers cross the plasma membrane and act primarily on cytosolic and nuclear receptors.

5.6 b

5.7 d

5.8 a

5.9 e Neurotransmitters and hormones are just two of many types of ligands that act as signaling molecules and first messengers, via their binding to a receptor.

5.10 b

Quantitative and Thought Questions

5.1 Patient A's drug very likely acts to block phospholipase A_2, whereas patient B's drug blocks lipoxygenase (see Figure 5.12).

5.2 The chronic loss of exposure of the heart's receptors to norepinephrine causes an up-regulation of this receptor type (i.e., more receptors in the heart for norepinephrine). The drug, being an agonist of norepinephrine (i.e., able to bind to norepinephrine's receptors and activate them) is now more effective because there are more receptors for it to combine with.

5.3 None. You are told that all six responses are mediated by the cAMP system; consequently, blockage of any of the steps listed in the question would eliminate all six of the responses. This is because the cascade for all six responses is identical from the receptor through the formation of cAMP and activation of cAMP-dependent protein kinase. Therefore, the drug must be acting at a point beyond this kinase (e.g., at the level of the phosphorylated protein mediating this response).

5.4 Not in most cells, because there are other physiological mechanisms by which signals impinging on the cell can increase cytosolic Ca^{2+} concentration. These include (a) second-messenger-induced release of Ca^{2+} from the endoplasmic reticulum and (b) voltage-sensitive Ca^{2+} channels.

5.5 Intracellular second messengers do not disappear immediately upon removal of a first messenger. Instead, some second messengers (such as cAMP) may linger inside the cell for seconds, minutes, or even longer after the first messenger is gone.

General Principles Assessments

5.1 Figures 5.5a and 5.9 illustrate ways in which movement of ions, for example, is controlled by first and second messengers. These messengers may open ion channels or activate or induce production of ion transporters in plasma membranes. In this way, ions may move between fluid compartments in the body—for example, from interstitial fluid to intracellular fluid.

5.2 Certain forms of cell signaling require a supply of ATP to form cAMP, a major second messenger, and to phosphorylate proteins. Without a homeostatic balance of cellular energy stored in the terminal bond of ATP molecules, most cell signaling pathways would be deficient or impossible.

CHAPTER 6

Test Questions

6.1 b Afferent neurons have peripheral axon terminals associated with sensory receptors, cell bodies in the dorsal root ganglion of the spinal cord, and central axon terminals that project into the spinal cord.

6.2 c Oligodendrocytes form myelin sheaths in the central nervous system.

6.3 d Insert the given chloride ion concentrations into the Nernst equation; remember to use -1 as the valence (Z).

6.4 d A, B, and C all are correct. Using the Nernst equation to calculate the Na^+ equilibrium potential gives values of +31, +36, and +40 mV for A, B, and C. If the membrane potential was +42 mV, the outward electrical force on Na^+ would be greater than the inward concentration gradient, so Na^+ would move out of the cell in each of these cases.

6.5 e Neither Na^+ nor K^+ is in equilibrium at the resting membrane potential, but the action of the Na^+/K^+-ATPase pump prevents the small but steady leak of both ions from dissipating the concentration gradients.

6.6 a Because Na^+ is farther away from its electrochemical equilibrium than is K^+, there would be more Na^+ entry than K^+ exit, causing local depolarization and local current flow that would decrease with distance from the site of the stimulus.

6.7 c Due to the persistent open state of the voltage-gated K^+ channels, for a brief time at the end of an action potential the membrane is hyperpolarized. When the voltage-gated K^+ channels eventually close, the K^+ leak channels once again determine the resting membrane potential.

6.8 d The IPSP caused by neuron B would summate with (subtract from) the amplitude of the EPSP caused by neuron A's firing.

6.9 a Dopamine, like norepinephrine and epinephrine, is a catecholamine neurotransmitter manufactured by enzymatic modification of the amino acid tyrosine.

6.10 b Norepinephrine is the neurotransmitter released by postganglionic neurons onto smooth muscle cells.

Quantitative and Thought Questions

6.1 Little change in the resting membrane potential would occur when the pump first stops because the pump's *direct* contribution to charge separation is very small. With time, however, the membrane potential would depolarize progressively toward zero because the Na^+ and K^+ concentration gradients, which depend on the Na^+/K^+-ATPase pumps and which give rise to the membrane potential, run down.

6.2 The resting potential would decrease (i.e., become less negative) because the concentration gradient causing net diffusion of this positively charged ion out of the cell would be smaller. The action potential would fire more easily (i.e., with smaller stimuli) because the resting potential would be closer to threshold. It would repolarize more slowly because repolarization depends on net K^+ diffusion from the cell, and the concentration gradient driving this diffusion is lower. Also, the after hyperpolarization would be smaller.

6.3 The hypothalamus was probably damaged. It plays a critical role in appetite, thirst, and sexual capacity.

6.4 The drug probably blocks cholinergic muscarinic receptors. These receptors on effector cells mediate the actions of parasympathetic nerves. Therefore, the drug would remove the slowing effect of these nerves on the heart, allowing the heart to speed up. Blocking their effect on the salivary glands would cause the dry mouth. We know that the drug is not blocking cholinergic nicotinic receptors because the skeletal muscles are not affected.

6.5 Because the membrane potential of the cells in question depolarizes (i.e., becomes less negative) when Cl^- channels are blocked, we can assume there was net Cl^- diffusion into the cells through these channels prior to treatment with the drug. Therefore, we can also predict that this passive inward movement was being exactly balanced by active transport of Cl^- out of the cells.

6.6 Without acetylcholinesterase, more acetylcholine would remain bound to the receptors, and all the actions normally caused by acetylcholine would be accentuated. Consequently, there would be significant narrowing of the pupils, airway constriction, stomach cramping and diarrhea, sweating, salivation, slowing of the heart, and decrease in blood pressure. On the other hand, in skeletal muscles, which must repolarize after excitation in order to be excited again, there would be weakness, fatigue, and finally inability to contract. In fact, lethal poisoning by high doses of cholinesterase inhibitors occurs because of paralysis of the muscles involved in respiration. Low doses of these compounds are used therapeutically.

6.7 These K^+ channels, which open after a short delay following the initiation of an action potential, increase K^+ diffusion out of the cell, hastening repolarization. They also account for the increased K^+ permeability that causes the after hyperpolarization. Therefore, the action potential would be broader (that is, longer in duration) and would return to resting level more slowly, and the after hyperpolarization would be absent.

General Principles Assessments

6.1 The autonomic nervous system controls many physiological functions through its sympathetic and parasympathetic subdivisions. The most common structural pattern is dual innervation—organs receive signals along neurons from both the sympathetic and parasympathetic division—and typically the effects of those signals are opposite. For example, action potentials along parasympathetic neurons increase secretions and contractions of the gastrointestinal tract, while action potentials along sympathetic pathways tend to decrease them. By having such dual regulatory control, more precise regulation of organ function is made possible. Other examples of dual sympathetic/parasympathetic regulatory control can be found in Figure 6.44.

6.2 The establishment of neuronal resting membrane potential clearly demonstrates at least two general principles of physiology: *Controlled exchange of materials occurs between compartments and across cellular membranes,* and *Physiological processes are dictated by the laws of chemistry and physics.* The concentration and movement of Na^+ and K^+ ions across the plasma membrane are carefully controlled as a result of the hydrophobic properties of the phospholipid bilayer, the action of Na^+/K^+ ATPase pumps, and the gating of ion-specific channels. Given the establishment of concentration gradients for these ions (and associated anions) across the membrane, Fick's diffusion equation (Chapter 4) and the electrical repulsion and attraction between charged ions then enable the storage of energy (electrical potential) across the membrane. The potential energy stored in this gradient is the basis of a substantial amount of cellular activity in nerve, skeletal muscle, cardiac muscle, and many other tissues.

6.3 As discussed in Section A, 6.1, some neurons have a large number of dendrites—as many as 400,000—that vastly increase the surface area over which the cell can receive inputs from other neurons. Additionally, the human cerebral cortex is elaborately folded into sulci and gyri, which vastly increases the surface area. As Figure 6.39 shows, the majority of the cells of the cerebral hemispheres lie within a few millimeters of the surface. The tortuous folding of the cortex allows far more cells to fit within the confines of the cranium, and along with a greater number of cells comes a greater potential for neural processing power. This accounts in part for the advanced cognitive capabilities and complex behaviors of humans as compared to animals with less complex folding of the cerebral cortex.

CHAPTER 7

Test Questions

7.1 a For example, photons of light are the adequate stimulus for photoreceptors of the eye, and sound is the adequate stimulus for hair cells of the ear.

7.2 b Receptor potentials generate only local currents in the receptor membrane that transduces the stimulus, but when they reach the first node of Ranvier, they depolarize the membrane to threshold, and there the voltage-gated Na^+ channels first initiate action potentials. Beyond that point, the receptor potential decreases with distance, whereas action potentials propagate all the way to the central axon terminals.

7.3 d Lateral inhibition increases the contrast between the region at the center of a stimulus and regions at the edges of the stimulus, which increases the acuity of stimulus localization.

7.4 a The occipital lobe of the cortex is the initial site of visual processing. (Review Figure 7.13.)

7.5 e Somatic sensations include those from the skin, muscles, bones, tendons, and joints, but not encoding of sound by cochlear hair cells.

7.6 b A myopic (nearsighted) person has an eyeball that is too long. When the ciliary muscles are relaxed and the lens is as flat as possible, parallel light rays from distant objects focus in front of the retina, whereas diverging rays from near objects are able to focus on the retina. (Recall that with normal vision, it takes ciliary muscle contraction and a rounded lens to focus on near objects.)

7.7 d When the right optic tract is destroyed, perception of images formed on the right half of the retina in both eyes is lost, so nothing is visible at the left side of a person's field of view. (Review Figure 7.31.)

7.8 a Pressure waves traveling down the cochlea make the cochlear duct vibrate, moving the basilar membrane against the stationary tectorial membrane and bending the hair cells that bridge the gap between the two.

7.9 c With the sudden head rotation from left to right, inertia of the endolymph causes it to rotate from right to left with respect to the semicircular canal that lies in the horizontal plane. This fluid flow bends the cupula and embedded hair cells within the ampulla, which influences the firing of action potentials along the vestibular nerve.

7.10 d "Umami" is derived from the Japanese word meaning "delicious" or "savory"; the stimulation of these taste receptors by glutamate produces the perception of a rich, meaty flavor.

Quantitative and Thought Questions

7.1 (a) Use drugs to block transmission in the pathways that convey information about pain to the brain. For example, if substance P is the neurotransmitter at the central endings of the nociceptor afferent fibers, give a drug that blocks the substance P receptors. (b) Cut the dorsal root at the level of entry of the nociceptor fibers to prevent transmission of their action potentials into the central nervous system. (c) Give a drug that activates receptors in the descending pathways that block transmission of the incoming or ascending pain information. (d) Stimulate the neurons in these same descending pathways to increase their blocking activity (stimulation-produced analgesia or, possibly, acupuncture). (e) Cut the ascending pathways that transmit information from the nociceptor afferents. (f) Deal with emotions, attitudes, memories, and so on to decrease sensitivity to the pain. (g) Stimulate nonpain, low-threshold afferent fibers to block transmission through the pain pathways (TENS). (h) Block transmission in the afferent nerve with a local anesthetic such as Novocaine or Lidocaine.

7.2 Information regarding temperature is carried via the anterolateral system to the brain. Fibers of this system cross to the opposite side of the body in the spinal cord at the level of entry of the afferent fibers (see Figure 7.19a). Damage to the left side of the spinal cord or any part of the left side of the brain that contains fibers of the pathways for temperature would interfere with awareness of a heat stimulus on the right. Thus, damage to the somatosensory cortex of the left cerebral hemisphere (i.e., opposite the stimulus) would interfere with awareness of the stimulus. Injury to the spinal cord at the point at which fibers of the anterolateral system from the two halves of the spinal cord cross to the opposite side would interfere with the awareness of heat applied to either side of the body, as would the unlikely event that damage occurred to relevant areas of both sides of the brain.

7.3 Vision would be restricted to the rods; therefore, it would be normal at very low levels of illumination (when the cones would not be stimulated anyway). At higher levels of illumination, however, clear vision of fine details would be lost, and everything would appear in shades of gray, with no color vision. In very bright light, there would be no vision because of bleaching of the rods' rhodopsin.

7.4 (a) The individual lacks a functioning primary visual cortex. (b) The individual lacks a functioning visual association cortex.

7.5 Because it is common for somatic receptors in visceral organs to converge onto ascending pathways for receptors in the skin, muscles, and joints (see Figure 7.17), physicians must be aware that complaints about pain in superficial structures may indicate a deeper problem. For example, a person having a heart attack may complain of pain in the left arm, a patient with stomach cancer may experience pain in the middle of the back, and a patient with kidney stones may complain of an ache in the upper thigh or hip. Review Figure 7.18 for a map of surface regions of the body where referred pain from deeper organs can be perceived.

General Principles Assessments

7.1 Nociceptors detect stimuli indicating potential or actual damage to tissues, which could threaten homeostasis. By allowing us to perceive those stimuli, nociceptors not only help us to learn to avoid them but also let us respond quickly to minimize damage when they occur (like quickly removing your hand from a hot stove burner). In these ways, we can avoid injuries like burns or cuts that may threaten homeostasis by causing fluid loss from the body. As another example, pain stops us temporarily from overusing injured limbs, giving them time to heal so that our ability to move and obtain food or avoid life-threatening situations is not permanently impaired.

7.2 A good example of the importance of controlled exchange between extracellular compartments in the vestibular and auditory systems is the endolymph found within the cochlear duct and vestibular apparatus. The unusually high K^+ concentration allows current to flow into the cells when tip links are stretched, generating a receptor potential that leads to neurotransmitter release from the hair cells. This, in turn, generates action potentials in the afferent neuron (review Figure 7.41). In addition, like in all neurons and excitable cells, the maintenance of Na^+ and K^+ concentration gradients between the intracellular and extracellular fluid compartments by Na^+/K^+-ATPase pumps is essential for the transmission of action potentials in the auditory and vestibular afferent neurons (review Chapter 6, Section B).

7.3 An excellent example of a body structure that has maximized surface area to maximize function is a photoreceptor cell. Repeated foldings of the membranous discs in rods and cones greatly increases the surface area available for the retinal-containing photopigments, making the eye exquisitely sensitive to light.

CHAPTER 8

Test Questions

8.1 d

8.2 c

8.3 a

8.4 b

8.5 e See Figures 8.6 and 8.7.

8.6 b If by experience you discover that a persistent stimulus like the noise from a fan does not have relevance, there is a reduction in conscious attention directed toward that stimulus. This is an example of "habituation."

8.7 c The mesolimbic dopamine pathway mediates the perception of reward that is associated with adaptive behaviors, including goal-directed behaviors related to preserving homeostasis, like eating and drinking.

8.8 d Serotonin-specific reuptake inhibitors (SSRIs), also called selective serotonin reuptake inhibitors, are the most widely used antidepressant drugs, although other types of antidepressants additionally enhance signaling by norepinephrine.

8.9 a Short-term, or "working" memories are transferred into new long-term memories in the process of consolidation, which requires a functional hippocampus. When the hippocampus is destroyed, previously formed long-term memories remain intact, but the ability to form new memories is lost.

8.10 c Broca's area is located near the region of the left frontal lobe motor cortex that controls the face; when it is damaged, individuals have "expressive aphasia." This means that they comprehend language but are unable to articulate their own thoughts into words.

Quantitative and Thought Questions

8.1 Dopamine is depleted in the basal ganglia of people with Parkinson disease, and they are therapeutically given dopamine agonists, usually L-dopa. This treatment raises dopamine concentrations in other parts of the brain, however, where the dopamine concentrations were previously normal. Schizophrenia is associated with increased brain dopamine concentrations, and symptoms of this disease appear when dopamine concentrations are high. The converse therapeutic problem can occur during the treatment of schizophrenics with dopamine-lowering drugs, which sometimes cause the symptoms of Parkinson disease to appear.

8.2 Experiments on anesthetized animals often involve either stimulating a brain part to observe the effects of increased neuronal activity, or damaging ("lesioning") an area to observe resulting deficits. Such experiments on animals, which lack the complex language mechanisms humans have, cannot help with language studies. Diseases sometimes mimic these two experimental situations, and behavioral studies of the resulting language deficits in people with aphasia, coupled with study of their brains after death, have provided a wealth of information.

General Principles Assessments

8.1 A general principle of physiology demonstrated very well by Figure 8.7 states that *most physiological functions are controlled by multiple regulatory systems, often working in opposition.* The orexin and monoaminergic RAS neurons compete with the sleep center in regulating the state of consciousness. When the orexin/RAS neurons are active, not only do they arouse the cortex and cause wakefulness, but they also inhibit the sleep center. When the sleep center neurons become active, the exact opposite occurs.

8.2 There seems to be a homeostatic set point for the amount of sleep we need. In addition to a daily increase in activity of the SCN that wakes us up, inputs related to energy homeostasis also prevent sleep from being prolonged (see Figure 8.7). On the other hand, sleep deprivation impairs the immune system, causes cognitive and memory defects, can result in decreased growth hormone secretion and growth velocity in children, and if prolonged can lead to psychosis and even death. When sleep is disrupted or postponed for even one day, we respond with bouts of "make-up" sleep, as though some chemical or factor has gone too far from its homeostatic set point and needs to be restored toward normal. Adenosine has been proposed to be a homeostatic sleep regulator.

CHAPTER 9

Test Questions

9.1 a A single skeletal muscle fiber, or cell, is composed of many myofibrils.

9.2 e The dark stripe in a striated muscle that constitutes the A band results from the aligned thick filaments within myofibrils, so thick filament length is equal to A-band width.

9.3 b As filaments slide during a shortening contraction, the I band becomes narrower, so the distance between the Z line and the thick filaments (at the end of the A band) must decrease.

9.4 d DHP receptors act as voltage sensors in the T-tubule membrane and are physically linked to ryanodine receptors in the sarcoplasmic reticulum membrane. When an action potential depolarizes the T-tubule membrane, DHP receptors change conformation and trigger the opening of the ryanodine receptors. This allows Ca^{2+} to diffuse from the interior of the sarcoplasmic reticulum into the cytosol.

9.5 c In an isometric twitch, tension begins to rise as soon as excitation–contraction is complete and the first cross-bridges begin to attach. In an isotonic twitch, excitation–contraction coupling takes the same amount of time, but the fiber is delayed from shortening until after enough cross-bridges have attached to move the load.

9.6 b In the first few seconds of exercise, mass action favors transfer of the high-energy phosphate from creatine phosphate to ADP by the enzyme creatine kinase.

9.7 d Fast-oxidative-glycolytic fibers are an intermediate type that are designed to contract rapidly but to resist fatigue. They utilize both aerobic and anaerobic energy systems; thus, they are red fibers with high myoglobin (which facilitates production of ATP by oxidative phosphorylation), but they also have a moderate ability to generate ATP through glycolytic pathways. (Refer to Table 9.3.)

9.8 c In smooth muscle cells, dense bodies serve the same functional role as Z lines do in striated muscle cells—they serve as the anchoring point for the *thin* filaments.

9.9 b When myosin-light-chain kinase transfers a phosphate group from ATP to the myosin light chains of the cross-bridges, binding and cycling of cross-bridges are activated.

9.10 d Stretching a sheet of single-unit smooth muscle cells opens mechanically gated ion channels, which causes a depolarization that propagates through gap junctions, followed by Ca^{2+} entry and contraction. This does not occur in multiunit smooth muscle.

9.11 e The amount of Ca^{2+} released during a typical resting heart beat exposes less than half of the thin filament cross-bridge binding sites. Autonomic neurotransmitters and hormones can increase or decrease the amount of Ca^{2+} released to the cytosol during EC coupling.

Quantitative and Thought Questions

9.1 Under resting conditions, the myosin has already bound and hydrolyzed a molecule of ATP, resulting in an energized molecule of myosin ($M \cdot ADP \cdot P_i$). Because ATP is necessary to detach the myosin cross-bridge from actin at the end of cross-bridge movement, the absence of ATP will result in rigor mortis, in which case the cross-bridges become bound to actin but do not detach, leaving myosin bound to actin ($A \cdot M$).

9.2 The distance from the elbow joint to the hand (30 cm) is 10 times greater than the distance from the elbow joint to the biceps insertion (3 cm), so her hand will move 20 m/sec when her biceps contracts at 2 m/sec (see Figure 9.30).

9.3 The length–tension relationship states that the maximum tension developed by a muscle decreases at lengths below L_0. During normal shortening, as the sarcomere length becomes shorter than the optimal length, the maximum tension that can be generated decreases. With a light load, the muscle will continue to shorten until its maximal tension just equals the load. No further shortening is possible because at shorter sarcomere lengths the tension would be less than the load. The heavier the load, the less the distance shortened before reaching the isometric state.

9.4 Maximum tension is produced when the fiber is (a) stimulated by an action potential frequency that is high enough to produce a maximal tetanic tension and (b) at its optimum length L_0, where the thick and thin filaments have overlap sufficient to provide the greatest number of cross-bridges for tension production.

9.5 Moderate tension—for example, 50% of maximal tension—is accomplished by recruiting sufficient numbers of motor units to produce this degree of tension. If activity is maintained at this level for prolonged periods, some of the active fibers will begin to fatigue and their contribution to the total tension will decrease. The same level of total tension can be maintained, however, by recruiting new motor units as some of the original ones fatigue. At this point, for example, one may have 50% of the fibers active, 25% fatigued, and 25% still unrecruited. Eventually, when all the fibers have fatigued and there are no additional motor units to recruit, the whole muscle will fatigue.

9.6 The oxidative motor units, both fast and slow, will be affected first by a decrease in blood flow because they depend on blood flow to provide both the fuel—glucose and fatty acids—and the oxygen required to metabolize the fuel. The fast-glycolytic motor units will be affected more slowly because they rely predominantly on internal stores of glycogen, which is anaerobically metabolized by glycolysis.

9.7 Two factors lead to the recovery of muscle force. (a) Some new fibers can be formed by the fusion and development of undifferentiated satellite cells. This will replace some, but not all, of the fibers that were damaged. (b) Some of the restored force results from hypertrophy of the surviving fibers. Because of the loss of fibers in the accident, the remaining fibers must produce more force to move a given load. The remaining fibers undergo increased synthesis of actin and myosin, resulting in increases in fiber diameter and, consequently, their force of contraction.

9.8 In the absence of extracellular Ca^{2+}, skeletal muscle contracts normally in response to an action potential generated in its plasma membrane because the Ca^{2+} required to trigger contraction comes entirely from the sarcoplasmic reticulum within the muscle fibers. If the motor neuron to the muscle is stimulated in a Ca^{2+}-free medium, however, the muscle will not contract because the influx of Ca^{2+} from the extracellular fluid into the motor nerve terminal is necessary to trigger the release of acetylcholine that in turn triggers an action potential in the muscle.

In a Ca^{2+}-free solution, smooth muscles would not respond either to stimulation of the nerve or to the plasma membrane. Stimulating the nerve would have no effect because Ca^{2+} entry into presynaptic terminals is necessary for neurotransmitter release. Stimulating the smooth muscle cell membrane would also not cause a response in the absence of Ca^{2+} because in all of the various types of smooth muscle, Ca^{2+} must enter from outside the cell to trigger contraction. In some cases, the external Ca^{2+} directly initiates contraction, and in others it triggers the release of Ca^{2+} from the sarcoplasmic reticulum (Ca^{2+}-induced Ca^{2+} release).

9.9 The simplest model to explain the experimental observations is as follows. Upon parasympathetic nerve stimulation, a neurotransmitter is released that binds to receptors on the membranes of smooth muscle cells and triggers contraction. The substance released, however, is not acetylcholine (ACh) for the following reason.

Action potentials in the parasympathetic nerves are essential for initiating nerve-induced contraction. When the nerves were prevented from generating action potentials by blockage of their voltage-gated Na^+ channels, there was no response to nerve stimulation. ACh is the neurotransmitter released from most, but not all, parasympathetic endings. When the muscarinic receptors for ACh were blocked, however, stimulation of the parasympathetic nerves still produced a contraction, providing evidence that some substance other than ACh is being released by the neurons and producing contraction.

9.10 Elevation of extracellular fluid Ca^{2+} concentration would increase the amount of Ca^{2+} entering the cytosol through L-type Ca^{2+} channels. This would result in a greater depolarization of cardiac muscle cell membranes during action potentials. The strength of cardiac muscle contractions would also be increased because this larger Ca^{2+} entry would trigger more Ca^{2+} release through ryanodine receptor channels, and consequently there would be a greater activation of cross-bridge cycling.

9.11 In order for unfused tetanus to occur, action potentials must occur more closely in time than the duration of a twitch cycle. Frequency is the inverse of cycle duration, so to produce unfused tetanus, action potentials must occur at a frequency greater than 1/0.04 seconds, or 25 action potentials per second.

General Principles Assessments

9.1 The control of cardiac muscle pacemaker cell activity by sympathetic and parasympathetic neurotransmitters is an excellent example of the general principle that *most physiological functions are controlled by multiple regulatory systems, often working in opposition.*

9.2 The forward motion of cross-bridges during the cross-bridge cycle (power stroke) is associated with a chemical reaction in which ADP and P_i are released as products (see step 2 in Figure 9.15). During high-frequency stimulation of muscles when cross-bridges cycle repeatedly, the concentrations of ADP and P_i build up in the muscle cytosol. Due to the law of mass action, the buildup of these products inhibits the rate of the chemical reaction and, thus, the power stroke of the cross-bridge cycle. This contributes to the reduction of contraction speed and force that occurs when muscles are fatigued.

9.3 The general principle that *controlled exchange of materials occurs between compartments and across cellular membranes* is demonstrated by the movements of Ca^{2+} and other ions involved in the skeletal muscle excitation–contraction coupling mechanism (see Figure 9.40). Controlled movement of Na^+, K^+ and Ca^{2+} across muscle cell plasma membranes maintains the resting membrane potential and allows the generation and propagation of action potentials. Sequestering Ca^{2+} in the sarcoplasmic reticulum allows the resting state of muscle to be maintained until controlled release of Ca^{2+} into the cytosol activates cross-bridge cycling and muscle contraction. The termination of muscle contraction requires the return of Ca^{2+} into the sarcoplasmic reticulum and extracellular fluid.

CHAPTER 10

Test Questions

10.1 b The basal nuclei, sensorimotor cortex, thalamus, brainstem, and cerebellum are all middle-level structures that create a motor program based on the intention to carry out a voluntary movement.

10.2 c When a given muscle is stretched, muscle-spindle stretch receptors send action potentials along afferent fibers that synapse directly on alpha motor neurons to extrafusal fibers to that muscle, causing it to contract back toward the prestretched length.

10.3 a Afferent action potentials from pain receptors in the injured left foot would stimulate the withdrawal reflex of the left leg (activation of flexor muscles and inhibition of extensors) and the opposite pattern in the right leg (the crossed-extensor reflex).

10.4 d Activating the gamma motor neurons would cause contraction of the ends of intrafusal muscle fibers, stretching the muscle-spindle receptors, and the resulting action potentials would monosynaptically excite the alpha motor neurons innervating the extrafusal fibers of the stretch receptors.

10.5 c See Figure 10.10.

10.6 T Most descending corticospinal pathways cross the midline of the body in the medulla oblongata.

10.7 F Upper motor neuron disorders are typically characterized by hypertonia and spasticity.

10.8 F The reverse is actually true.

10.9 F In Parkinson disease, a deficit of dopamine from neurons of the substantia nigra results in "resting tremors."

10.10 T *Clostridium tetani* toxin specifically blocks the release of neurotransmitter from neurons that normally inhibit motor neurons. The resulting imbalance of excitatory and inhibitory inputs causes spastic contractions of muscles.

Quantitative and Thought Questions

10.1 None. The gamma motor neurons are important in preventing the muscle-spindle stretch receptors from going slack, but when this reflex is tested, the intrafusal fibers are not flaccid. The test is performed with a bent knee, which stretches the extensor muscles in the thigh (and the intrafusal fibers within the stretch receptors). The stretch receptors are therefore responsive.

10.2 The efferent pathway of the reflex arc (the alpha motor neurons) would not be activated, the effector cells (the extrafusal muscle fibers) would not be activated, and there would be no reflexive response.

10.3 The drawing must have excitatory synapses on the motor neurons of both ipsilateral extensor and ipsilateral flexor muscles.

10.4 A toxin that interferes with the inhibitory synapses on motor neurons would leave unbalanced the normal excitatory input to these neurons. Thus, the otherwise normal motor neurons would fire excessively, which would result in increased muscle contraction. This is exactly what happens in lockjaw as a result of the toxin produced by the tetanus bacillus.

10.5 In mild cases of tetanus, agonists (stimulators) of the inhibitory interneuron neurotransmitter gamma-aminobutyric acid (GABA) can shift the balance back toward the inhibition of alpha motor neurons. In more severe cases, paralysis can be induced by administering long-lasting drugs that block the nicotinic acetylcholine receptors at the neuromuscular junction.

10.6 Having a person pull the arms apart during the performance of the knee-jerk test is called the Jendrassik maneuver (named for a Hungarian physician who first described it). The exact mechanism by which the reflex increases is unknown. It is most commonly thought that performing a task with the arms simply distracts the person so that there is less descending inhibition of the motor neurons to the leg muscles. In other words, a person may be more able to truly relax the leg muscles (thus allowing the reflex to more fully occur) when her attention is not focused on the legs or anticipating the strike of the reflex hammer. Another possible explanation is that voluntarily flexing arm muscles produces a general activation and increase in excitability of interneurons in the spinal cord that integrate synchronized arm and leg movements; those inputs add to those from the stretch receptors to enhance activation of the motor neurons to leg extensors.

General Principles Assessments

10.1 Unlike smooth and cardiac muscle cells, which are regulated directly by both excitatory and inhibitory inputs, skeletal muscle fibers only have excitatory inputs, so must be inhibited indirectly. They are inhibited from contracting when there are no action potentials arriving along their associated alpha motor neurons, so inhibition must occur at the level of the alpha motor neurons. The dendrites and cell bodies of alpha motor neurons found in the brainstem and spinal cord receive both excitatory and inhibitory inputs from interneurons, sensory neurons, and neurons in descending pathways. When the inhibitory inputs predominate, the alpha motor neuron does not generate action potentials and the muscle fibers it innervates remain relaxed.

10.2 One way that the withdrawal reflex contributes to homeostasis is by minimizing the extent of tissue injury that could potentially result from prolongation of a painful stimulus. Rapidly withdrawing a limb from a position where it is being cut, burned, or crushed helps to minimize the loss of blood, tissue fluid, and tissue function that could compromise homeostasis.

CHAPTER 11

Test Questions

11.1 c

11.2 a

11.3 e

11.4 b

11.5 d

11.6 a At any given concentration of hormone, more A is bound to receptor than B.

11.7 d Goiter results from dysfunction of the thyroid gland.

11.8 e Recall that thyroid hormone potentiates the effects of epinephrine and the sympathetic nervous system.

11.9 b

11.10 e Recall that there exists a large store of iodinated thyroglobulin in thyroid follicles.

11.11 c Low plasma Ca^{2+} decreases the filtered load of Ca^{2+}. It also stimulates parathyroid hormone, which increases Ca^{2+} reabsorption from the distal tubule. This helps to prevent the further loss of Ca^{2+} in the urine.

11.12 d Parathyroid hormone is a potent stimulator of Ca^{2+} resorption from bone.

11.13 T T_4 is the chief circulating form, but T_3 is more active.

11.14 F Acromegaly is associated with hyperglycemia and hypertension.

11.15 T

Quantitative and Thought Questions

11.1 Epinephrine decreases to very low concentrations during rest and fails to increase during stress. The sympathetic preganglionics provide the only major control of the adrenal medulla.

11.2 The increased concentration of binding protein causes more T_3 and T_4 to be bound, thereby lowering the plasma concentration of *free* T_3 and T_4. This causes less negative feedback inhibition of TSH secretion by the anterior pituitary gland, and the increased TSH causes the thyroid to secrete more T_3 and T_4 until the free concentration has returned to normal. The end result is an increased *total* plasma T_3 and T_4—most bound to the protein—but a normal free T_3 and T_4. There is no hyperthyroidism because it is only the free concentration that exerts effects on T_3 and T_4 target cells.

11.3 Destruction of the anterior pituitary gland or hypothalamus. These symptoms reflect the absence of, in order, growth hormone, the gonadotropins, and ACTH (the symptom is due to the resulting decrease in cortisol secretion). The problem is either primary hyposecretion of anterior pituitary gland hormones or secondary hyposecretion because the hypothalamus is not secreting hypophysiotropic hormones normally.

11.4 Vasopressin and oxytocin (the posterior pituitary gland hormones) secretion would decrease. The anterior pituitary gland hormones would not be affected because the influence of the hypothalamus on these hormones is exerted not by connecting nerves but via the hypophysiotropic hormones in the portal vascular system.

11.5 The secretion of GH increases. Somatostatin, coming from the hypothalamus, normally exerts an inhibitory effect on the secretion of this hormone.

11.6 Norepinephrine and many other neurotransmitters are released by neurons that terminate on the hypothalamic neurons that secrete the hypophysiotropic hormones. Therefore, manipulation of these neurotransmitters will alter secretion of the hypophysiotropic hormones and thereby the anterior pituitary gland hormones.

11.7 The high dose of the cortisol-like substance inhibits the secretion of ACTH by feedback inhibition of (1) hypothalamic corticotropin releasing hormone and (2) the response of the anterior pituitary gland to this hypophysiotropic hormone. The lack of ACTH causes the adrenal to atrophy and decrease its secretion of cortisol.

11.8 The hypothalamus. The low basal TSH indicates either that the pituitary gland is defective or that it is receiving inadequate stimulation (TRH) from the hypothalamus. If the thyroid itself were defective, basal TSH would be elevated because of less negative feedback inhibition by T_3 and T_4. The TSH increase in response to TRH shows that the pituitary gland is capable of responding to a stimulus and so is unlikely to be defective. Therefore, the problem is that the hypothalamus is secreting too little TRH (in reality, this is very rare).

11.9 In utero malnutrition. Neither growth hormone nor the thyroid hormones influence in utero growth.

11.10 Androgens stimulate growth but also cause the ultimate cessation of growth by closing the epiphyseal plates. Therefore, there might be a rapid growth spurt in response to the androgens but a subsequent premature cessation of growth. Estrogens exert similar effects.

General Principles Assessments

11.1 Despite having many different actions, epinephrine, cortisol, and growth hormone all act on adipocytes and the liver to regulate energy balance. They do this by stimulating the production and/or release of glucose from liver cells, and the breakdown in adipocytes of triglycerides into usable substrates for energy that can enter the bloodstream. It should not be surprising that a function as critical as energy homeostasis would be regulated by multiple factors; indeed, these three hormones are only one part of a larger control mechanism that regulates energy balance (see Chapter 16).

11.2 The structure of the thyroid gland differs from most other endocrine glands in that it consists of colloid-filled follicles that contain hormone precursors. These precursors can be metabolized to produce thyroid hormones as required. This structure most likely evolved as an adaptation to the relative rarity of iodine in animal diets, including our own. Because iodine is required for the synthesis of thyroid hormones, having a large store of iodinated precursors available in the thyroid gland ensures that even with prolonged absences of dietary intake of the element, thyroid hormones can still be produced.

11.3 Parathyroid hormone is a key part of the mechanism that regulates calcium ion homeostasis. The absence of PTH would have devastating health consequences, because it would result in decreased Ca^{2+} concentrations in the blood; Ca^{2+} is vitally important for proper functioning of all types of muscle tissue, including the heart, and also regulates neuronal function, among other actions. Antidiuretic hormone (vasopressin) contributes to the control of blood pressure and to water balance, because of its actions on kidney tubules. In its absence, blood pressure would be difficult to maintain, and the body would lose considerable volumes of water in the urine. That, in turn, would further compromise blood pressure and would also alter solute concentrations in the extracellular fluid. T_3 (thyroid hormone), through its calorigenic actions, is a major part of the mechanism by which body temperature homeostasis is maintained. In the absence of T_3, most people generally develop cold intolerance.

CHAPTER 12

Test Questions

12.1 c Blood in the right ventricle is relatively deoxygenated after returning from the tissues.

12.2 e Resistance decreases as the fourth power of an increase in radius, and in direct proportion to a decrease in vessel length.

12.3 d See Figure 12.19.

12.4 d The large total cross-sectional area of capillaries results in very slow blood velocity.

12.5 a Increasing colloid osmotic pressure would decrease filtration of fluid from capillaries into the tissues.

12.6 d Pressures are higher in the systemic circuit, but because the cardiovascular system is a closed loop, the flow must be the same in both.

12.7 b The AV node is the only conduction point between atria and ventricles, and the slow propagation through it delays the beginning of ventricular contraction.

12.8 c The diastolic pressure in this example is 85; adding 1/3 of the pulse pressure gives a *MAP* of 101.7 mmHg.

12.9 d Reduced firing to arterioles would reduce total peripheral resistance and thereby reduce mean arterial pressure toward normal.

12.10 e Ventricular muscle cells do not have a pacemaker potential, and the L-type Ca^{2+} channel is not open during this phase of the action potential even in autorhythmic cells.

12.11 c

12.12 a Increased sympathetic nerve firing and norepinephrine release during exercise constrict vascular beds in the kidneys, GI tract, and other tissues to compensate for the large dilation of muscle vascular beds.

12.13 b Reduced oxygen delivery to the kidneys increases the secretion of erythropoietin, which stimulates bone marrow to increase production of erythrocytes.

12.14 c

12.15 e t-PA is part of the fibrinolytic system that dissolves clots.

Quantitative and Thought Questions

12.1 No. Decreased erythrocyte volume is certainly one possible explanation, but there is a second: The person may have a normal erythrocyte volume but an abnormally increased plasma volume. Convince yourself of this by writing the hematocrit equation as

Erythrocyte volume/(Erythrocyte volume + Plasma volume)

12.2 A halving of tube radius. Resistance is directly proportional to blood viscosity but inversely proportional to the *fourth power* of tube radius.

12.3 The plateau of the action potential and the contraction would be absent. You may think that contraction would persist because most Ca^{2+} in excitation–contraction coupling in the heart comes from the sarcoplasmic reticulum. However, the signal for the release of this Ca^{2+} is the Ca^{2+} entering across the plasma membrane.

12.4 The SA node is not functioning, and the ventricles are being driven by a pacemaker in the AV node or the bundle of His.

12.5 The person has a narrowed aortic valve. Normally, the resistance across the aortic valve is so small that there is only a tiny pressure difference between the left ventricle and the aorta during ventricular ejection. In the example given here, the large pressure difference indicates that resistance across the valve must be very high.

12.6 This question is analogous to question 12.5 in that the large pressure difference across a valve while the valve is open indicates an abnormally narrowed valve—in this case, the left AV valve.

12.7 Decreased heart rate and contractility. These are effects mediated by the sympathetic nerves on beta-adrenergic receptors in the heart.

12.8 120 mmHg. $MAP = DP + 1/3\ (SP - DP)$.

12.9 The drug must have caused the arterioles in the kidneys to dilate enough to reduce their resistance by 50%. Blood flow to an organ is determined by mean arterial pressure and the organ's resistance to flow. Another important point can be deduced here: If mean arterial pressure has not changed even though renal resistance has dropped 50%, then either the resistance of some other organ or actual cardiac output has gone up.

12.10 The experiment suggests that acetylcholine causes vasodilation by releasing nitric oxide or some other vasodilator from endothelial cells.

12.11 A low plasma protein concentration. Capillary pressure is, if anything, lower than normal and so cannot be causing the edema. Another possibility is that capillary permeability to plasma proteins has increased, as occurs in burns.

12.12 20 mmHg/L per minute. $TPR = MAP/CO$.

12.13 Nothing. Cardiac output and *TPR* have remained unchanged, so their product, *MAP*, also remains unchanged. This question emphasizes that *MAP* depends on cardiac output but not on the combination of heart rate and stroke volume that produces the cardiac output.

12.14 It increases. There are a certain number of impulses traveling up the nerves from the arterial baroreceptors. When these nerves are cut, the number of impulses reaching the medullary cardiovascular center goes to zero, just as it would physiologically if the mean arterial pressure were to decrease markedly. Accordingly, the medullary cardiovascular center responds to the absent impulses by reflexively increasing arterial pressure.

12.15 It decreases. The hemorrhage causes no immediate change in hematocrit because erythrocytes and plasma are lost in the same proportion. As interstitial fluid starts entering the capillaries, however, it expands the plasma volume and decreases hematocrit. (This is too soon for any new erythrocytes to be synthesized.)

12.16 Using the following equation, $MAP = DP + 1/3(SP - DP)$, inserting 85 for *MAP* and 105 for *SP*, solving for *DP* gives a value of 75 mmHg. Pulse pressure $= SP - DP$, or in this case, $105 - 75 = 30$ mmHg.

12.17 Transplant recipients can increase cardiac output during exercise in two ways. When exercise begins, epinephrine is released from the adrenal medulla and stimulates β-adrenergic receptors on the heart. This increases heart rate and contractility just like would happen in response to norepinephrine released directly from sympathetic neurons; only the response will be delayed in onset. Also, when the individual starts to exercise and venous return to the heart is increased, end-diastolic volume is increased. This initiates the Frank–Starling mechanism, increasing stroke volume and contributing to an increased cardiac output.

12.18 In lead aVR, the electrical poles of the leads are oriented nearly the opposite of lead 1: Lead 1 is a vector oriented from the right side of the body toward a positive pole on the left arm, while lead aVR is a vector oriented from the left side of the body toward a positive pole on the right arm. Thus, if the sweep of depolarization toward the positive pole in lead 1 generates an upright P wave, you can expect that same sweep of depolarization away from the positive pole in lead aVR to produce a downward P wave.

12.19 The stroke volume can be determined by inserting cardiac output and heart rate into the equation $CO = HR \times SV$: 5400 mL/min $= 75$ beats/min $\times SV$; so $SV = 72$ mL. Next, the end-diastolic volume (*EDV*) can be determined using the equation $SV = EDV - ESV$: 72 mL $= EDV - 60$; so $EDV = 132$ mL. Finally, the ejection fraction (*EF*) is $EF = SV/EDV$, so $EF = 72$ mL/132 mL $= 54.5\%$.

12.20 A small blood clot (thrombus) that results in a blockage of blood flow (embolism) is more dangerous if it forms in the pulmonary veins, because after returning to the heart and being pumped into the systemic arteries, it could lodge in a coronary artery, leading to a heart attack, or in a brain artery, causing a stroke; it could also cause ischemic damage to other organs. A small clot that formed in the systemic circuit will be trapped in the lungs, where the blockage of a small pulmonary artery will do little harm, because blood can flow through alternate branches to pick up fresh O_2 and eliminate CO_2. Small clots trapped in the lungs are eventually dissolved by the fibrinolytic mechanisms without causing much harm. See Chapter 19 for a case study discussion of the dangers of large clots forming in systemic veins.

General Principles Assessments

12.1 Hormones of the endocrine system represent vital information that integrates the function of cells and organs that are widely distributed in the body. The circulatory system delivers blood and any hormones it may contain rapidly and efficiently to all cells throughout the body. Without this information-delivery system, the endocrine system could not function in the regulation of homeostasis.

12.2 Although it is possible that the difference in valve leaflet number is simply a random quirk of how the heart develops, a clear difference in the functional demands on the two AV valves is the amount of pressure they must withstand. At the peak of systole, the typical pressure gradient across the right AV valve is approximately 25 mmHg (pulmonary systolic pressure), while across the left AV valve it is approximately 120 mmHg (systemic systolic pressure). Having one less valve leaflet, the left AV valve has a smaller area where the edges of valve leaflets must seal. It seems likely that this structure makes it less susceptible to failure despite the greater pressure it encounters.

12.3 The liver produces plasma proteins at a rate that keeps their concentration in the plasma within a narrow range. Plasma proteins do not freely exchange across capillary walls, and their concentration determines the value of π_C, the main force that opposes bulk flow of fluid from the plasma to the interstitial fluid (see Figure 12.42). Maintaining balance in the bulk flow forces is essential for controlling the movement of fluid between the interstitial and plasma compartments. The failure of the liver to maintain plasma protein concentration in individuals who are protein starved (kwashiorkor) results in excessive filtration of fluid from the plasma and tissue edema.

CHAPTER 13

Test Questions

13.1 e If alveolar pressure (P_{alv}) is negative with respect to atmospheric pressure (P_{atm}), the driving force for airflow is inward (from the atmosphere into the lung).

13.2 a For the same change in transpulmonary pressure, a less compliant (i.e., stiffer) lung will have a smaller change in lung volume.

13.3 a Total minute ventilation is comprised of dead space plus alveolar ventilation. Minute ventilation is respiratory frequency (12 breaths per minute) multiplied by tidal volume (500 mL/breath) = 6000 mL/min. Subtract from that alveolar ventilation (4200 mL/min) and one gets 1800 mL/min.

13.4 d An increase in alveolar P_{O_2} results from an increase in alveolar ventilation (supply of oxygen) relative to metabolic rate (consumption of oxygen).

13.5 c The relationship between arterial P_{O_2} and arterial oxygen saturation is described by the oxygen–hemoglobin dissociation curve. The greatest increase in oxygen saturation for the same change in P_{O_2} occurs at the steepest part of the curve—a P_{O_2} of between 40 and 60 mmHg.

13.6 b Increases in blood temperature, decreases in blood pH, and increases in DPG shift the oxygen–hemoglobin curve downward, leading to a lower oxygen saturation at the same P_{O_2}.

13.7 b There are forms of asthma that are not primarily due to the presence of allergens. Examples are exercise-induced or cold-air-induced asthma.

13.8 e Respiratory acidosis (increase in blood P_{CO_2} and decrease in pH) is a major stimulus to ventilation—this is mediated both by afferents from the peripheral chemoreceptors and by an increase in central chemoreceptor activity.

13.9 c Because of the shape of the oxygen–hemoglobin dissociation curve, small increases in P_{O_2} due to increases in ventilation cannot fully saturate hemoglobin. When the desaturated blood mixes with saturated blood, the average is still hypoxemic.

13.10 c Remember that a lung capacity is the sum of at least two volumes. Inspiratory capacity is the sum of tidal volume and inspiratory reserve volume.

Quantitative and Thought Questions

13.1 200 mL/mmHg.

$$\text{Lung compliance} = \Delta\ \text{lung volume}/\Delta\ (P_{alv} - P_{ip})$$
$$= 800\ \text{mL}/[0 - (-8)]\ \text{mmHg} - [0 - (-4)]\ \text{mmHg}$$
$$= 800\ \text{mL}/4\ \text{mmHg} = 200\ \text{mL/mmHg}$$

13.2 More subatmospheric than normal. A decreased surfactant level causes the lungs to be less compliant (i.e., more difficult to expand). Therefore, a greater transpulmonary pressure ($P_{alv} - P_{ip}$) is required to expand them a given amount.

13.3 No.

$$\text{Alveolar ventilation} = (\text{Tidal volume} - \text{Dead space}) \times \text{Breathing rate}$$
$$= (250\ \text{mL} - 150\ \text{mL})/\text{breath} \times 20\ \text{breaths/min}$$
$$= 2000\ \text{mL/min}$$

Normal alveolar ventilation is approximately 4000 mL/min in a 70 kg adult.

13.4 The volume of the snorkel constitutes an additional dead space, so total pulmonary ventilation must be increased if alveolar ventilation is to remain constant.

13.5 The alveolar P_{O_2} will be higher than normal, and the alveolar P_{CO_2} will be lower. To better understand why, review the factors that determine the alveolar gas pressures (see Table 13.5).

13.6 No. Hypoventilation reduces arterial P_{O_2} but only because it reduces alveolar P_{O_2}. That is, in hypoventilation, *both* alveolar and arterial P_{O_2} are decreased to essentially the same degree. In this problem, alveolar P_{O_2} is normal, and so the person is not hypoventilating. The low arterial P_{O_2} must therefore represent a defect that causes a discrepancy between alveolar P_{O_2} and arterial P_{O_2}. Possibilities include impaired diffusion, a shunting of blood from the right side of the heart to the left through a hole in the heart wall, and a mismatch between airflow and blood flow in the alveoli.

13.7 Not at rest, if the defect is not too severe. Recall that equilibration of alveolar air and pulmonary capillary blood is normally so rapid that it occurs well before the end of the capillaries. Therefore, even though diffusion may be slowed as in this problem, there may still be enough time for equilibration to be reached. In contrast, the time for equilibration is decreased during exercise, and failure to equilibrate is much more likely to occur, resulting in a lowered arterial P_{O_2}.

13.8 Only a few percent (specifically, from approximately 200 mL O_2/L blood to approximately 215 mL O_2/L blood). The reason the increase is so small is that almost all the oxygen in blood is carried bound to hemoglobin, and hemoglobin is almost 100% saturated at the arterial P_{O_2} achieved by breathing room air. The high arterial P_{O_2} achieved by breathing 100% oxygen does cause a directly proportional increase in the amount of oxygen *dissolved* in the blood (the additional 15 mL), but this still remains a small fraction of the total oxygen in the blood. Review the numbers given in the chapter.

13.9 All. Venous blood contains products of metabolism released by cells, such as carbon dioxide.

13.10 It would cease. Respiration depends on descending input from the medulla to the nerves supplying the diaphragm and the inspiratory intercostal muscles.

13.11 (a) The combination of hypercapnia (increased P_{CO_2} due to increased inspired CO_2) and hypoxia (due to decreased inspired O_2) greatly augments ventilation by stimulating central and peripheral chemoreceptors. Although CO decreases O_2 content, chemoreceptors are not stimulated and ventilation does not increase.

13.12 These patients have profound hyperventilation, with large increases in both the depth and rate of ventilation. The stimulus, mainly via the peripheral chemoreceptors, is the large increase in their arterial hydrogen ion concentration due to the acids produced. The hyperventilation causes an increase in their arterial P_{O_2} and a decrease in their arterial P_{CO_2}.

13.13 In pure anatomical shunt, blood passes through the lung without exposure to any alveolar air. Therefore, increases in alveolar P_{O_2} caused by increased inspired O_2 will not affect the P_{O_2} of the shunt blood. By contrast, there is still some blood flowing through a region of the lung with a ventilation–perfusion mismatch. Therefore, an increase in P_{O_2} in the alveoli can increase the P_{O_2} in this blood, which, when mixing with blood leaving other areas of the lung, can increase the blood in the pulmonary vein and hence the arterial circulation.

General Principles Assessments

13.1 Boyle's law (see Figure 13.8) explains that the pressure exerted by a constant number of gas molecules (at constant temperature) is inversely proportional to the volume of a container. Therefore, when the volume of the lung increases during negative pressure breathing, the resultant decrease in pressure draws air into the lungs (inspiration). Conversely, when the lung deflates, the pressure in it increases pushing air out of the lung (expiration). The Law of Laplace (Figure 13.17) demonstrates that the larger the radius of a sphere (e.g., an alveolus), the lower the surface tension. This explains the need for pulmonary surfactant, which lowers the surface tension of smaller alveoli, thereby preventing smaller alveoli from collapsing. Dalton's law states that, in a mixture of gases, the pressure each gas exerts is independent of the pressure the others exert and is proportional to the percentage of that gas in the mixture. This explains, therefore, why the partial pressure of oxygen in air at sea level is equal to 0.21×760 mmHg, or 160 mmHg. Henry's law states that the amount of gas dissolved in a liquid will be directly proportional to the partial pressure of the gas with which the liquid is in equilibrium. This is extremely important in understanding the transfer of oxygen from the alveolar gas to the blood. Finally, the unique allosteric properties of hemoglobin shown in Figures 13.26 and 13.29 allow the appropriate delivery of oxygen from the lungs to the tissues. As the CO_2 diffuses out of the pulmonary capillaries, the decrease in CO_2 in the blood shifts the oxygen dissociation curve to the left allowing more oxygen uptake. Conversely, as the blood enters the tissue, CO_2 diffuses into the blood and shifts the oxygen dissociation curve to the right allowing a greater unloading of oxygen to the tissues.

13.2 The thinness of the alveolar wall minimizes the barrier for oxygen and carbon dioxide diffusion allowing an efficient transfer of gases to and from the blood (Figure 13.4). The multiple branching of the airways into respiratory bronchioles and alveoli and the branching of the pulmonary artery into the pulmonary arterioles and capillaries greatly increase the surface area for gas exchange (Figure 13.3).

13.3 Some of the factors that influence alveolar ventilation are summarized in Figure 13.40. The three major stimulatory factors in the blood are a decrease in P_{O_2}, an increase in nonvolatile acids, and an increase in P_{CO_2}. Conversely, a decrease in acids and P_{CO_2} in the blood inhibit ventilation. These factors often work in opposition during the adaptation to hypoxia due, for example, to high altitude. In this case, P_{O_2} decreases due to a decrease in barometric pressure. The resulting increase in alveolar ventilation (Figure 13.35) leads to a decrease in P_{CO_2} (hyperventilation). This respiratory alkalosis attenuates the increase in alveolar ventilation that would have otherwise occurred with arterial hypoxia.

CHAPTER 14

Test Questions

14.1 c The main driving force favoring fluid filtration from the glomerular capillary to Bowman's space is glomerular capillary blood pressure (P_{GC}).

14.2 c In order for a substance to appear in the urine at a faster rate than its filtration rate, it must also be actively secreted into the tubular fluid.

14.3 a Excessive sweating will decrease blood volume. This will lead to compensatory mechanisms to preserve total-body water, including a decrease in urine production (antidiuresis).

14.4 e Urea is trapped in the medullary interstitium and is an osmotically active solute. The resultant increase in tonicity helps to maintain the gradient for medullary passive water reabsorption.

14.5 a A decrease in sodium intake stimulates renin because of the decrease in Na^+ delivery to the macula densa. This is detected and results in an increase in renin release from the juxtaglomerular cells.

14.6 c Parathyroid hormone stimulates Ca^{2+} reabsorption in the distal tubules of the nephron, thereby decreasing Ca^{2+} excretion. Because parathyroid hormone is increased in hypocalcemic states, the resulting decrease in Ca^{2+} excretion helps to restore blood Ca^{2+} to normal.

14.7 c Secretion of ammonium into the renal tubule is one way to rid the body of excess hydrogen ion (metabolic acidosis).

14.8 b Increases in ventilation greater than metabolic rate "blow off" CO_2 and result in a decrease in arterial P_{CO_2}. Because of the buffering of bicarbonate ions, this increases arterial pH (respiratory alkalosis).

14.9 e Cortical nephrons either have short or absent loops of Henle. Only juxtamedullary nephrons have long loops of Henle, which plunge into the renal medulla and create a hyperosmotic interstitium via countercurrent multiplication.

14.10 a When the renal corpuscles become diseased, they greatly increase their permeability to protein. Furthermore, diseased proximal tubules cannot remove the filtered protein from the tubular lumen. This results in increased protein in the urine (proteinuria).

Quantitative and Thought Questions

14.1 No. This is a possible answer, but there is another. Substance T may be secreted by the tubules.

14.2 No. It is a possibility, but there is another. Substance V may be filtered and/or secreted, but the substance V entering the lumen via these routes may be completely reabsorbed.

14.3 125 mg/min. The amount of any substance filtered per unit time is given by the product of the *GFR* and the filterable plasma concentration of the substance—in this case, 125 mL/min $\times$ 100 mg/100 mL = 125 mg/min.

14.4 The plasma concentration may be so high that the T_m for the amino acid is exceeded, so all the filtered amino acid is not reabsorbed. A second possibility is that there is a specific defect in the tubular transport for this amino acid. A third possibility is that some other amino acid is present in the plasma in high concentration and is competing for reabsorption.

14.5 No. Urea is filtered and then partially reabsorbed. The reason its concentration in the tubule is higher than in the plasma is that relatively more water is reabsorbed than urea. Therefore, the urea in the tubule becomes concentrated. Despite the fact that urea *concentration* in the urine is greater than in the plasma, the *amount excreted* is less than the filtered load (that is, net reabsorption has occurred).

14.6 They would all be decreased. The transport of all these substances is coupled, in one way or another, to that of Na^+.

14.7 *GFR* would not decrease as much, and renin secretion would not increase as much as in a person not receiving the drug. The sympathetic nerves are a major pathway for both responses during hemorrhage.

14.8 There would be little if any increase in aldosterone secretion. The major stimulus for increased aldosterone secretion is angiotensin II, but this substance is formed from angiotensin I by the action of angiotensin-converting enzyme, and so blockade of this enzyme would block the pathway.

14.9 (b) Urinary excretion in the steady state must be less than ingested sodium chloride by an amount equal to that lost in the sweat and feces. This is normally quite small, less than 1 g/day, so that urine excretion in this case equals approximately 11 g/day.

14.10 If the hypothalamus had been damaged, there may be inadequate secretion of ADH. This would cause loss of a large volume of urine, which would tend to dehydrate the person and make her thirsty. Of course, the area of the brain involved in thirst might have suffered damage.

14.11 This is primary hyperaldosteronism or Conn's syndrome. Because aldosterone stimulates Na^+ reabsorption and K^+ secretion, there will be total-body retention of Na^+ and loss of K^+. Interestingly, the person in this situation actually retains very little Na^+ because urinary Na^+ excretion returns to normal after a few days despite the continued presence of the high aldosterone. One explanation for this is that *GFR* and atrial natriuretic factor both increase as a result of the initial Na^+ retention.

14.12 Sodium and water balance would become negative because of increased excretion of these substances in the urine. The person would also develop a decreased plasma bicarbonate ion concentration and metabolic acidosis because of increased bicarbonate ion excretion. The effects on acid–base status are explained by the fact that hydrogen ion secretion—blocked by the drug—is required both for HCO_3^- reabsorption and for the excretion of hydrogen ion (contribution of new HCO_3^- to the blood). The increased Na^+ excretion reflects the fact that much Na^+ reabsorption by the proximal tubule is achieved by Na^+/H^+ countertransport. By blocking hydrogen ion secretion, therefore, the drug also partially blocks Na^+ reabsorption. The increased water excretion occurs because the failure to reabsorb Na^+ and HCO_3^- decreases water reabsorption (remember that water reabsorption is secondary to solute reabsorption), resulting in an osmotic diuresis.

14.13 The overuse of diuretics can lead to significant hypovolemia, which leads to an increase in the release of renin from the kidney (see Figure 14.24). The resultant increase in angiotensin II and therefore aldosterone increases the distal tubular secretion of hydrogen ions (mostly in the form of NH_4^+), because of its exchange with sodium (see Figure 14.35). As you learned in Section B, 14.15, most diuretics not only increase sodium excretion (the desired effect) but increase potassium excretion. The resultant potassium depletion can weakly stimulate tubular hydrogen ion secretion. These two factors—increased aldosterone and potassium depletion—lead to an increase in the reabsorption of all the filtered bicarbonate as well as the generation of new bicarbonate from glutamine (see Figure 14.35). This can generate a marked metabolic alkalosis that can have profound effects on multiple organ systems.

General Principles Assessments

14.1 The anatomy of the renal corpuscle is ideally suited to filter the plasma. As you learned in Figure 14.3, the fenestrated capillaries of the glomerulus allow the filtration of plasma but prevent the loss of larger molecules (like albumin). The juxtaglomerular apparatus is ideally located to sense the amount of sodium in the distal tubule such that renin secretion can be appropriately regulated. The anatomical placement of the afferent and efferent arterioles allows the precise regulation of the blood pressure within the glomerulus, thus regulating glomerular filtration rate.

14.2 The appreciation of the physical forces—such as hydrostatic pressure—that determine net movement of plasma out of capillaries (Starling's forces; Figure 14.8) is vital to understand the ultimate glomerular filtration rate. The expression of the enzyme carbonic anhydrase in the tubular epithelial cells catalyzes the conversion of H_2O and CO_2 to H_2CO_3, which then breaks down to provide H^+ for secretion into the tubular lumen and HCO_3^- for reabsorption into the interstitial fluid. The equilibrium of this reaction obeys the chemical law known as mass action (see Chapter 3).

14.3 There are a variety of stimulatory and inhibitory inputs involved in the control of vasopressin (Figures 14.26, 14.27, and 14.28). For example, an increase in the osmolarity of the blood increases vasopressin by stimulation of the central osmoreceptor, whereas an increase in plasma volume decreases vasopressin by stimulation of the low-pressure baroreceptors in the heart. So, a person with an increased plasma osmolarity and plasma volume due to, for example, an extremely high salt intake, would demonstrate a smaller increase in vasopressin than a person with increased osmolarity but decreased plasma volume that may occur during dehydration.

CHAPTER 15

Test Questions

15.1 c When the stomach contents, which are very acidic, move into the small intestine, it stimulates the release of secretin, which circulates to the pancreas and stimulates the release of HCO_3^- into the small intestine. This neutralizes the acid and protects the small intestine.

15.2 d GIP release is a feedforward mechanism to signal the islet cells in the pancreas that the products of food digestion are on their way to the blood. This results in an augmented insulin response to a meal.

15.3 a Gastrin is a major controller of acid secretion by the stomach. When the stomach becomes very acidic, gastrin release is inhibited, preventing continued acid production.

15.4 b Cholecystokinin is the primary signal from the small intestine to the pancreas to increase digestive enzyme release into the small intestine.

15.5 d The enzyme pepsin is produced from pepsinogen in the presence of acid. This zymogen accelerates protein digestion.

15.6 b Because fat is insoluble in an aqueous environment, micelles keep fat droplets from re-aggregating and small enough to be absorbed.

15.7 c Distention of the duodenum signals the stomach that the meal has moved on and continued acid secretion in the stomach is not necessary until the next meal.

15.8 a HCO_3^- in the bile is secreted by the epithelial cells lining the bile ducts.

15.9 e Although the primary movement of chyme in segmentation is back and forth, the overall, net movement of chyme is from the small intestine to the large intestine.

15.10 a The active transport of Na^+ in the large intestine is the driving force for the osmotic absorption of water.

Quantitative and Thought Questions

15.1 If the salivary glands fail to secrete amylase, the undigested starch that reaches the small intestine will still be digested by the amylase the pancreas secretes. Thus, starch digestion is not significantly affected by the absence of salivary amylase.

15.2 Alcohol can be absorbed across the stomach wall, but absorption is much more rapid from the small intestine with its larger surface area. Ingestion of foods containing fat releases enterogastrones from the small intestine, and these hormones inhibit gastric emptying and thereby prolong the time alcohol spends in the stomach before reaching the small intestine. Milk, contrary to popular belief, does not "protect" the lining of the stomach from alcohol by coating it with a fatty layer. Rather, the fat content of milk decreases the rate of absorption of alcohol by decreasing the rate of gastric emptying.

15.3 Vomiting results in the loss of fluid and acid from the body. The fluid comes from the luminal contents of the stomach and duodenum, most of which was secreted by the gastric glands, pancreas, and liver and thus is derived from the blood. The cardiovascular symptoms of this patient are the result of the decrease in blood volume that accompanies vomiting.

The secretion of acid by the stomach produces an equal number of bicarbonate ions, which are released into the blood. Normally, these bicarbonate ions are neutralized by hydrogen ions released into the blood by the pancreas when this organ secretes bicarbonate ions. Because gastric acid is lost during vomiting, the pancreas is not stimulated to secrete HCO_3^- by the usual high-acidity signal from the duodenum, and no corresponding hydrogen ions are formed to neutralize the

HCO_3^- released into the blood by the stomach. As a result, the acidity of the blood decreases. Loss of K^+ from the loss of stomach contents can also lead to hypokalemia.

15.4 Fat can be digested and absorbed in the absence of bile salts, but in greatly decreased amounts. Without adequate emulsification of fat by bile salts and phospholipids, only the fat at the surface of large lipid droplets is available to pancreatic lipase, and the rate of fat digestion is very slow. Without the formation of micelles with the aid of bile salts, the products of fat digestion become dissolved in the large lipid droplets, where they are not readily available for diffusion into the epithelial cells. In the absence of bile salts, only about 50% of the ingested fat is digested and absorbed. The undigested fat is passed on to the large intestine, where bacteria produce compounds that increase colonic motility and promote the secretion of fluid into the lumen of the large intestine, leading to diarrhea.

15.5 Damage to the lower portion of the spinal cord produces a loss of voluntary control over defecation due to disruption of the somatic nerves to the skeletal muscle of the external anal sphincter. Damage to the somatic nerves leaves the external sphincter in a continuously relaxed state. Under these conditions, defecation occurs whenever the rectum becomes distended and the defecation reflex is initiated.

15.6 Vagotomy decreases the secretion of acid by the stomach. Impulses in the parasympathetic nerves directly stimulate acid secretion by the parietal cells and also cause the release of gastrin, which in turn stimulates acid secretion. Impulses in the vagus nerves are increased during both the cephalic and gastric phases of digestion. Vagotomy, by decreasing the amount of acid secreted, decreases irritation of existing ulcers, which promotes healing and decreases the probability of acid contributing to the production of new ulcers.

General Principles Assessments

15.1 The liver is ideally situated to process materials absorbed from the lumen of the small intestine that end up in the hepatic portal vein (Figure 15.32). One very important example of this is the detoxification of harmful substances that are ingested and absorbed. Notice in Figure 15.31 that the hepatocytes (liver cells) form sheets, thereby maximizing their contact with blood in the hepatic sinusoids. This ensures that most, if not all, of the toxic substances absorbed in the small intestine can be taken up from the blood in the branches of the portal vein and rendered harmless in the hepatocytes. Furthermore, contact with the bile canaliculi ensures the ability of the hepatocytes to rid the body of toxic metabolites by secretion into the bile.

15.2 (1) Figures 15.10, 15.11, 15.12, and 15.13 demonstrate the chemical property of polarity. That is, steroids are nonpolar rendering them relatively insoluble in water. Chemical additions to the basic structure of the steroid molecule (for example, hydroxyl groups) result in polar portions exposed on the surface of the molecule that are water soluble. This results in a molecule that is amphipathic enabling it to bind to lipids on the nonpolar regions and also to dissolve in water on the polar region, thereby emulsifying lipids for absorption. Interestingly, chemical emulsifiers are often added to salad dressing to allow the oil and the water portions to stay mixed after shaking. (2) Figure 15.19 demonstrates the ability of an enzyme—carbonic anhydrase—to catalyze the conversion of CO_2 and H_2O to H_2CO_3 which then breaks down to HCO_3^- and H^+; the secretion of the latter in the lumen of the stomach results in a very acidic environment ideal for the initial digestion of proteins as well as a way to kill most ingested bacteria. (3) Another interesting example of chemistry is shown in Figure 15.22 in which an inactive enzyme precursor (pepsinogen) is activated in the acidic environment of the gastric lumen to the active enzyme pepsin that catalyzes the breakdown of proteins to peptides. (Figure 15.28 gives another example of this concept for pancreatic enzymes.) In both cases, the secretion of an inactive form of the enzyme prevents self-destruction of the cells responsible for producing the enzyme.

15.3 Figure 15.14 illustrates in several ways the general principle that *information flow between cells, tissues, and organs is an essential feature of homeostasis and allows for integration of physiological processes.* How do you perceive the sensation of "fullness" when you have ingested a large meal? Afferent nerves from the upper GI tract "tell" the brain that you are full. How do emotions influence gastrointestinal motility? Efferent autonomic input to the GI tract can alter the activity of the enteric nervous system, thus altering smooth muscle activity in the GI tract.

CHAPTER 16

Test Questions

16.1 a Glucose can be converted to fat, but fatty acids cannot be converted to glucose.

16.2 b HSL is an intracellular enzyme that acts on triglycerides.

16.3 a Glucagon acts to prevent hypoglycemia from occurring.

16.4 c If untreated, type 1 DM causes an osmotic diuresis when the transport maximum for glucose is exceeded in the kidneys.

16.5 d Insulin stimulates lipogenesis, not lipolysis.

16.6 e Recall that vitamin deficiencies can occur even with normal dietary intake of vitamins, because the metabolic rate is increased in hyperthyroidism.

16.7 b

16.8 T

16.9 F Core temperature is generally kept fairly constant, but skin temperature can vary.

16.10 T

16.11 F As muscles begin contracting during exercise, they become partially insulin-independent.

16.12 F BMI equals body mass in kg divided by (height in meters)^2.

16.13 T

16.14 F Skin vessels dilate in such conditions in order to help dissipate heat by bringing warm blood close to the skin surface.

16.15 T

Quantitative and Thought Questions

16.1 The concentration in plasma would increase, and the amount stored in adipose tissue would decrease. Lipoprotein lipase cleaves plasma triglycerides, so its blockade would decrease the rate at which these molecules were cleared from plasma and would decrease the availability of the fatty acids in them for the synthesis of intracellular triglycerides. However, this would only reduce but not eliminate such synthesis, because the adipose-tissue cells could still synthesize their own fatty acids from glucose.

16.2 It will lower plasma cholesterol concentration. Bile salts are formed from cholesterol, and losses of these bile salts in the feces will be replaced by the synthesis of new ones from cholesterol. Chapter 15 describes how bile salts are normally absorbed from the small intestine so that very few of those secreted into the bile are normally lost from the body.

16.3 Plasma concentrations of HDL and LDL. It is the ratio of LDL cholesterol to HDL cholesterol that best correlates with the development of atherosclerosis (HDL cholesterol is "good" cholesterol). The answer to this question would have been the same regardless of whether the person was an athlete, but the question was phrased this way to emphasize that people who exercise generally have increased HDL cholesterol.

16.4 The person may have type 1 diabetes mellitus and require insulin, or may be a healthy fasting person; plasma glucose would be increased in the first case but decreased in the second. Plasma insulin concentration would be useful because it would be decreased in both cases. The fact that the person was resting and unstressed was specified because severe stress or strenuous exercise could also produce the plasma changes mentioned. Plasma glucose would increase during stress and decrease during strenuous exercise.

16.5 Glucagon, epinephrine, cortisol, and growth hormone. The insulin will produce hypoglycemia, which then induces reflexive increases in the secretion of all these hormones.

16.6 It may reduce it but not eliminate it. The sympathetic effects on organic metabolism during exercise are mediated not only by circulating epinephrine but also by sympathetic nerves to the liver (glycogenolysis and gluconeogenesis), to adipose tissue (lipolysis), and to the pancreatic islets (inhibition of insulin secretion and stimulation of glucagon secretion).

16.7 Heat loss from the head, mainly via convection and sweating, is the major route for loss under these conditions. The rest of the body is *gaining* heat by conduction, and sweating is of no value in the rest of the body because the water cannot evaporate. Heat is also lost via the expired air (insensible loss), and some people actually begin to pant under such conditions. The rapid, shallow breathing increases airflow and heat loss without causing hyperventilation.

16.8 They seek out warmer places, if available, so that their body temperature increases. That is, they use behavior to develop a fever.

General Principles Assessments

16.1 Insulin and glucagon are both secreted by the endocrine pancreas; they have opposite effects on plasma concentrations of glucose. They achieve these effects in part through opposite actions on key metabolic organs such as the liver. In the liver, insulin stimulates glycogen synthesis and inhibits gluconeogenesis, whereas glucagon stimulates glycogen breakdown and gluconeogenesis. Insulin and glucagon are always present in plasma; it is the ratio of the two hormones that determines the net effect that will be to either decrease (insulin) or increase (glucagon) the concentration of plasma glucose.

16.2 The factors that control hunger (appetite) are summarized in Figure 16.15. Neural and endocrine signals arising from the gastrointestinal tract and adipocytes appear to be very important regulators of appetite. Other factors, such as plasma glucose and insulin concentrations, body temperature, and behavioral mechanisms also play a role.

16.3 As described in the chapter, the first law of thermodynamics states that energy can neither be created nor destroyed but can be transformed from one type to another. This is demonstrated by the production of heat within cells during the breakdown of organic molecules such as glucose. Some of the energy from the chemical bonds in organic molecules is transferred to ATP, and some is released as heat. This heat contributes to body temperature. Maintaining body temperature in a homeostatic range also depends upon the properties of heat; for example, heat flows from a region of higher temperature to one of lower temperature. In Figure 16.17, for example, heat is shown entering the body by radiation from the sun and conduction from the hot water.

CHAPTER 17

Test Questions

17.1 e Without the presence of the Y chromosome in the testes and the local production of SRY protein, the undifferentiated gonads are programmed to differentiate into ovaries.

17.2 c Only females exhibit gonadal steroid (estrogen) positive feedback on GnRH release.

17.3 d The luteal phase of the ovary, when progesterone production is maximal, occurs after ovulation but before the end of the menstrual cycle.

17.4 c Estrogen stimulates LH release (positive feedback) just before the LH surge and ovulation (usually on day 14).

17.5 b One follicle becomes dominant early in the menstrual cycle.

17.6 e The death of the corpus luteum (in the absence of pregnancy and hCG) results in a dramatic decrease in ovarian progesterone and estrogen production.

17.7 a The loss of ovarian steroid production with the death of the corpus luteum releases the pituitary gland from negative feedback and allows FSH to increase. This stimulates the maturation of a small number of follicles for the next menstrual cycle.

17.8 c The primary function of the Leydig cell is the production of testosterone in response to stimulation with LH.

17.9 b Prolactin is produced by the maternal pituitary gland. It is homologous to but not the same peptide as human placental lactogen, which is produced by the placenta.

17.10 a The primary event in menopause is the loss of ovarian function. The decrease in estrogen leads to an increase in pituitary gland gonadotropin release (loss of negative feedback).

Quantitative and Thought Questions

17.1 Sterility due to lack of spermatogenesis would be the common finding. The Sertoli cells are essential for spermatogenesis, and so is testosterone produced by the Leydig cells. The person with Leydig cell destruction, but not the person with Sertoli cell destruction, would also have other symptoms of testosterone deficiency.

17.2 The androgens act on the hypothalamus and anterior pituitary gland to inhibit the secretion of the gonadotropins. Therefore, spermatogenesis is inhibited. Importantly, even if this man were given FSH, the sterility would probably remain because the lack of LH would cause deficient testosterone secretion, and *locally* produced testosterone is required for spermatogenesis (i.e., the exogenous androgen cannot do this job).

17.3 Impaired function of the seminiferous tubules, notably of the Sertoli cells. The increased plasma FSH concentration is due to the lack of negative feedback inhibition of FSH secretion by inhibin, itself secreted by the Sertoli cells. The Leydig cells seem to be functioning normally in this person because the lack of demasculinization and the normal plasma LH indicate normal testosterone secretion.

17.4 FSH secretion. FSH acts on the Sertoli cells and LH acts on the Leydig cells, so sterility would result in either case, but the loss of LH would also cause undesirable elimination of testosterone and its effects.

17.5 These findings are all due to testosterone deficiency. You would also expect to find that the testes and penis were small if the deficiency occurred before puberty.

17.6 They will be eliminated or become very irregular. The androgens act on the hypothalamus to inhibit the secretion of GnRH and on the pituitary gland to inhibit the response to GnRH. The result is inadequate secretion of gonadotropins and therefore inadequate stimulation of the ovaries. In addition to the loss of regular menstrual cycles, the woman may suffer some degree of masculinization of the secondary sex characteristics because of the combined effects of androgen excess and estrogen deficiency.

17.7 Such treatment may cause so much secretion of FSH that multiple follicles become dominant and have their eggs ovulated during the LH surge.

17.8 An increased plasma LH. The other two are due to increased plasma progesterone and so do not occur until *after* ovulation and formation of the corpus luteum.

17.9 The absence of sperm capacitation. When test-tube fertilization is performed, special techniques are used to induce capacitation.

17.10 The fetus is in difficulty. The placenta produces progesterone entirely on its own, whereas estriol secretion requires participation of the fetus, specifically, the fetal adrenal cortex.

17.11 Prostaglandin antagonists, oxytocin antagonists, and drugs that lower cytosolic Ca^{2+} concentration. You might not have thought of the last category because Ca^{2+} is not mentioned in this context in the chapter, but as in all muscle, Ca^{2+} is the immediate cause of contraction in the myometrium.

17.12 This person would have normal male external genitals and testes, although the testes might not have descended fully, but would also have some degree of development of uterine tubes, a uterus, and a vagina. These internal female structures would tend to develop because no MIS was present to cause degeneration of the Müllerian duct system.

17.13 No. These two hormones are already increased in menopause, and the problem is that the ovaries are unable to respond to them with estrogen secretion. Thus, the treatment must be with estrogen itself.

General Principles Assessments

17.1 Although several answers are possible, differentiation of the internal and external genitalia is a wonderful example of the general principle that *structure is a determinant of—and has coevolved with—function*. The male and female genitalia arise from the same primordial cluster of cells in the embryo. The reproductive structures diverge in early embryonic development to form organs suited for their function. For the male, it is the production of sperm and the development of a penis that evolved to fit into the vagina of the female. In the female, it is to produce ova and to receive sperm to allow fertilization of the ova. So even though they started the same, through differentiation, the male and female tracts develop into complementary structures ideally suited for their functions.

17.2 The amount of FSH and LH secreted from the gonadotrophs of the anterior pituitary at any one time in the male is determined by two opposing inputs. Stimulatory input is from GnRH released from hypophysiotropic nerves into the hypophyseal portal blood, and inhibitory negative feedback input is from the two different hormones released by the testes—inhibin and testosterone—that reach the anterior pituitary from the systemic circulation. The effect of inhibin at the anterior pituitary primarily reduces the release of FSH, whereas testosterone primarily reduces the release of LH.

17.3 The adaptation to pregnancy is one of the best examples of integration of multiple organ systems. Here are some examples that are listed in Table 17.9:

- Increase in maternal bone turnover to supply calcium and phosphorus to the placenta necessary for normal fetal bone development.
- Increase in maternal blood volume and red blood cell production. This allows the increase in cardiac output and perfusion of the rapidly growing placenta as well as increase in blood flow to, for example, the maternal kidneys to enable the excretion of the additional waste products produced by the fetus.
- Increase in maternal alveolar ventilation enables the mother to rid the body of the extra carbon dioxide produced by the fetus.
- Mobilization of maternal glucose meets the metabolic needs of the developing fetus.

As a test of your knowledge, you should be able to explain the mechanism of these and other adaptations to pregnancy listed in Table 17.9.

CHAPTER 18

Test Questions

18.1 c

18.2 a

18.3 b This is known as active immunity.

18.4 c IgA antibodies act in this way.

18.5 F Antibiotics are bactericidal. They are sometimes given in viral diseases to eliminate or prevent secondary infections caused by bacteria, however.

18.6 T For example, rheumatoid arthritis and inflammatory bowel disease are not associated with infection.

18.7 T Some lymphocytes are B cells.

18.8 F Edema is a consequence of inflammation and has no known adaptive value.

18.9 F These are the primary lymphoid organs. An example of a secondary organ is a lymph node.

Quantitative and Thought Questions

18.1 Both would be impaired because T cells would not differentiate. The absence of cytotoxic T cells would eliminate responses mediated by these cells. The absence of helper T cells would impair antibody-mediated responses because most B cells require cytokines from helper T cells to become activated.

18.2 Neutrophil deficiency would impair nonspecific (innate) inflammatory responses to bacteria. Monocyte deficiency, by causing macrophage deficiency, would impair both innate inflammation and adaptive immune responses.

18.3 The drug may reduce but would not eliminate the action of complement, because this system destroys cells directly (via the membrane attack complex) as well as by facilitating phagocytosis.

18.4 Antibodies would bind normally to antigen but may not be able to activate complement, act as opsonins, or recruit NK cells in ADCC. The reason for these defects is that the sites to which complement C1, phagocytes, and NK cells bind are all located in the Fc portion of antibodies.

18.5 They do develop fever, although often not to the same degree as normal. They can do so because IL-1 and other cytokines secreted by macrophages cause fever, whereas the defect in AIDS is failure of helper T-cell function.

General Principles Assessments

18.1 As shown in Figure 18.22, a wide range of changes occur in physiological variables following infection, including changes in plasma concentrations of minerals (iron, zinc), energy sources (fatty acids, amino acids), and hormones (cortisol). In each case, the respective variable is decreased or increased beyond its usual homeostatic range. Although these changes are adaptive to fight infection, they may come with a cost, as does any challenge to homeostasis. For example, elevated concentrations of cortisol may temporarily result in hyperglycemia, water retention, and potentiated actions of catecholamines on cardiovascular function. Other responses to infection, such as fever, accelerate the rate of chemical reactions in all cells (increase metabolism) and, if fever is sufficiently high, may damage neuronal function.

Appendix B INDEX OF CLINICAL TERMS

DISEASES AND DISORDERS

INFECTIOUS OR CAUSATIVE AGENTS

SIGNS AND SYMPTOMS

TREATMENTS, DIAGNOSTICS, AND THERAPEUTIC DRUGS

Glossary

A

A band one of the transverse bands making up repeated striations of cardiac and skeletal muscle; region of aligned myosin-containing thick filaments

abortion spontaneous or clinically-induced death of an embryo or fetus after implantation

absolute refractory period time during which an excitable membrane cannot generate an action potential in response to any stimulus

absorption movement of materials across an epithelial layer from body cavity or compartment toward the blood

absorptive state period during which nutrients enter bloodstream from gastrointestinal tract

accessory reproductive organ duct through which sperm or egg is transported, or a gland emptying into such a duct (in the female, the breasts are usually included)

acclimatization (ah-climb-ah-tih-ZAY-shun) environmentally induced improvement in functioning of a physiological system with no change in genetic endowment

accommodation adjustment of eye for viewing various distances by changing shape of lens

acetylcholine (ACh) (ass-ih-teel-KOH-leen) a neurotransmitter released by pre- and postganglionic parasympathetic neurons, preganglionic sympathetic neurons, somatic neurons, and some CNS neurons

acetylcholinesterase (ass-ih-teel-koh-lin-ES-ter-ase) enzyme that breaks down acetylcholine into acetic acid and choline

acetyl coenzyme A (acetyl CoA) (ASS-ih-teel koh-EN-zime A) metabolic intermediate that transfers acetyl groups to Krebs cycle and various synthetic pathways

acid molecule capable of releasing a hydrogen ion; solution having an H^+ concentration greater than that of pure water (that is, pH less than 7); *see also* strong acid, weak acid

acidic solution any solution with a pH less than 7.0

acidity concentration of free, unbound hydrogen ion in a solution; the higher the H^+ concentration, the greater the acidity

acquired reflex behaviors that appear to be stereotypical and automatic but that in fact result from considerable conscious effort to be learned; also called *learned reflex*

acrosome (AK-roh-sohm) cytoplasmic vesicle containing digestive enzymes and located at head of a sperm

acrosome reaction process that occurs in the sperm after it binds to the zona pellucida of the egg, exposing acrosomal enzymes

actin filaments polymers of G-actin that form part of the cell cytoskeleton and are part of the contractile apparatus of muscle cells; also called *microfilaments*

action potential electrical signal propagated by neurons and muscle cells; an all-or-none depolarization of membrane polarity; has a threshold and refractory period and is conducted without decrement

action potential propagation the movement of an action potential along an axon; in myelinated axons, it occurs via saltatory conduction

activated macrophage macrophage whose killing ability has been enhanced by cytokines, particularly IL-2 and interferon-gamma

activation energy energy necessary to disrupt existing chemical bonds during a chemical reaction

active hyperemia (hy-per-EE-me-ah) increased blood flow through a tissue associated with increased metabolic activity

active immunity resistance to reinfection acquired by contact with microorganisms, their toxins, or other antigenic material; *compare* passive immunity

active site region of enzyme to which substrate binds

active transport energy-requiring system that uses transporters to move ions or molecules across a membrane against an electrochemical difference; *see also* primary active transport, secondary active transport

active zone region within an axon terminal where neurotransmitter vesicles are clustered prior to secretion

acuity sharpness or keenness of perception

acute phase protein group of proteins secreted by liver during systemic response to injury or infection

acute phase response responses of tissues and organs distant from site of infection or immune response

adaptation (evolution) a biological characteristic that favors survival in a particular environment; (neural) decrease in action potential frequency in a neuron despite constant stimulus

adaptive immune response the specific response of the cells of the immune system to a particular pathogen; subsequent responses to the same pathogen are amplified

adenine one of the four bases making up DNA; also a breakdown product of ATP used as a neurotransmitter

adenoid lymphoid tissue; also known as *pharyngeal tonsil*

adenosine a nucleoside composed of adenine bound to a ribose sugar; building block for ATP; neurotransmitter in CNS

adenosine diphosphate (ADP) (ah-DEN-oh-seen dye-FOS-fate) two-phosphate product of ATP breakdown

adenosine triphosphate (ATP) nucleotide that transfers energy from metabolism to cell functions during its breakdown to ADP and release of P_i

adenylyl cyclase (ad-DEN-ah-lil SYE-klase) enzyme that catalyzes transformation of ATP to cyclic AMP

adequate stimulus the modality of stimulus to which a particular sensory receptor is most sensitive

adipocyte (ad-DIP-oh-site) cell specialized for triglyceride synthesis and storage; fat cell

adipose tissue (AD-ah-poze) tissue composed largely of fat-storing cells

adrenal cortex (ah-DREE-nal KORE-tex) endocrine gland that forms outer shell of each adrenal gland; secretes steroid hormones—mainly cortisol, aldosterone, and androgens; *compare* adrenal medulla

adrenal gland one of a pair of endocrine glands above each kidney; each gland consists of outer *adrenal cortex* and inner *adrenal medulla*

adrenal medulla (meh-DUL-ah or meh-DOOL-ah) endocrine gland that forms inner core of each adrenal gland; secretes amine hormones, mainly epinephrine; *compare* adrenal cortex

adrenergic (ad-ren-ER-jik) pertaining to norepinephrine or epinephrine; compound that acts like norepinephrine or epinephrine

adrenocorticotropic hormone (ACTH) (ad-ren-oh-kor-tih-koh-TROH-pik) polypeptide hormone secreted by anterior pituitary gland; stimulates adrenal cortex to secrete cortisol; also called *corticotropin*

aerobic (air-OH-bik) in presence of oxygen

afferent arteriole vessel in kidney that carries blood from artery to renal corpuscle

afferent division (of the peripheral nervous system) neurons in the peripheral nervous system that project to the central nervous system

afferent neuron neuron that carries information from sensory receptors at its peripheral endings to CNS; cell body lies outside CNS

afferent pathway component of reflex arc that transmits information from receptor to integrating center

affinity strength with which ligand binds to its binding site

afterbirth placenta and associated membranes expelled from uterus after delivery of infant

afterhyperpolarization decrease in membrane potential in neurons at the end of the action potential due to opened voltage-gated K^+ channels

afterload the work the heart does while ejecting blood; a function of the arterial blood pressure, as well as the diameter and thickness of the ventricles

agonist (AG-ah-nist) chemical messenger that binds to receptor and triggers cell's response; often refers to drug that mimics action of chemical normally in the body

airway tubes through which air flows between external environment and lung alveoli

albumin (al-BU-min or AL-bu-min) most abundant plasma protein

aldosterone (al-doh-STEER-own or al-DOS-stir-own) mineralocorticoid steroid hormone secreted by adrenal cortex; regulates electrolyte balance

alkaline solution any solution having H^+ concentration lower than that of pure water (that is, having a pH greater than 7)

all-or-none pertaining to event that occurs maximally or not at all

allosteric protein (al-low-STAIR-ik or al-low-STEER-ik) protein whose binding site characteristics are subject to allosteric modulation in which modulator molecules that bind to regions of the protein other than the binding site alter the protein's ligand-binding capacity

alpha-adrenergic receptor one type of plasma membrane receptor for epinephrine and norepinephrine; also called *alpha adrenoceptor; compare* beta-adrenergic receptor

alpha cell glucagon-secreting cell of pancreatic islets of Langerhans

alpha–gamma coactivation simultaneous firing of action potentials along alpha motor neurons to extrafusal fibers of a muscle and along gamma motor neurons to the contractile ends of intrafusal fibers within that muscle

α-glycerol phosphate three-carbon molecule that combines with fatty acids to form triglyceride; also called *glycerol 3-phosphate*

alpha helix coiled regions of proteins or DNA formed by hydrogen bonds

α-ketoacid (AL-fuh KEY-toh) molecule formed from amino acid metabolism and containing carbonyl (—CO—) and carboxyl (—COOH) groups

alpha motor neuron motor neuron that innervates extrafusal skeletal muscle fibers

alpha rhythm prominent 8 to 13 Hz oscillation on the electroencephalograms of awake, relaxed adults with their eyes closed

alternative complement pathway sequence for complement activation that bypasses first steps in classical pathway and is not antibody dependent

alveolar dead space (al-VEE-oh-lar) volume of fresh inspired air that reaches alveoli but does not undergo gas exchange with blood

alveolar pressure (P_{alv}) air pressure in pulmonary alveoli

alveolar ventilation ($\dot{V}_A$) volume of atmospheric air entering alveoli each minute

alveolus (al-VEE-oh-lus or al-vee-OH-lus) (lungs) thin-walled, air-filled "outpocketing" from terminal air passageways in lungs; (glands) cell cluster at end of duct in secretory gland

amacrine cell (AM-ah-krin) a specialized type of neuron found in the retina of the eye that integrates information between local photoreceptor cells

amine hormone (ah-MEEN) hormone derived from amino acid tyrosine; includes thyroid hormones, epinephrine, norepinephrine, and dopamine

amino acid (ah-MEEN-oh) molecule containing amino group, carboxyl group, and side chain attached to a carbon atom; molecular subunit of protein

amino acid side chain the variable portions of amino acids; may contain acidic or basic charged regions, or may be hydrophobic

amino group $—NH_2$; ionizes to $—NH_3^+$

aminopeptidase (ah-meen-oh-PEP-tih-dase) one of a family of enzymes located in the intestinal epithelial membrane; breaks peptide bond at amino end of polypeptide

amnion another term for amniotic sac

amniotic cavity (am-nee-AHT-ik) fluid-filled space surrounding the developing fetus enclosed by amniotic sac

amniotic fluid liquid within amniotic cavity that has a composition similar to extracellular fluid

amniotic sac membrane surrounding fetus in utero

AMPA receptor receptor protein found in the membrane of some brain neurons, named for its binding to alpha-amino-3 hydroxy-5 methyl-4 isoxazole proprionic acid

amphipathic (am-fuh-PATH-ik) a molecule containing polar or ionized groups at one end and nonpolar groups at the other

ampulla structure in the wall of the semicircular canals containing hair cells that respond to head movement

amylase (AM-ih-lase) enzyme that partially breaks down polysaccharides

anabolism (an-AB-oh-lizm) cellular synthesis of organic molecules

anaerobic (an-ih-ROH-bik) in the absence of oxygen

anatomical dead space (V_D) space in respiratory tract airways where gas exchange does not occur with blood

androgen (AN-dro-jen) any hormone with testosterone-like actions

androgen-binding protein (ABP) synthesized and secreted by Sertoli cell of the testes—binds to and increases local testosterone concentration in fluid in the seminiferous tubule

anemia (ah-NEE-me-ah) reduction in total blood hemoglobin

anemic hypoxia decrease in oxygen content of the blood due to a reduction in the amount of hemoglobin (usually due to a reduction in the number of erythrocytes)

angiogenesis (an-gee-oh-JEN-ah-sis) the development and growth of capillaries; stimulated by angiogenic factors

angiogenic factor chemical signal that induces the development and growth of blood vessels

angiotensin I small polypeptide generated in plasma by the action of the enzyme renin on angiotensinogen; inactive precursor of angiotensin II

angiotensin II hormone formed by action of angiotensin-converting enzyme on angiotensin I; stimulates aldosterone secretion from adrenal cortex, vascular smooth muscle contraction, and possibly thirst

angiotensin-converting enzyme (ACE) enzyme on capillary endothelial cells that catalyzes removal of two amino acids from angiotensin I to form angiotensin II

angiotensinogen (an-gee-oh-ten-SIN-oh-gen) plasma protein precursor of angiotensin I; produced by liver

anion (AN-eye-on) negatively charged ion; *compare* cation

antagonist (muscle) muscle whose action opposes intended movement; (drug) molecule that competes with another for a receptor and binds to the receptor but does not trigger the cell's response

anterior pituitary gland anterior portion of pituitary gland; synthesizes, stores, and releases ACTH, GH, TSH, PRL, FSH, and LH

anterograde (AN-ter-oh-grayd) movement of a substance or action potential in the forward direction from a neuron's dendrites and/or cell body toward the axon terminal

anterolateral pathway ascending neural pathway running in the anterolateral column of the spinal cord white matter; conveys information about pain and temperature

antibody (AN-tih-bah-dee) immunoglobulin secreted by plasma cell; combines with type of antigen that stimulated its production; directs attack against antigen or cell bearing it

antibody-dependent cellular cytotoxicity (ADCC) killing of target cells by toxic chemicals secreted by NK cells; the target cells are linked to the NK cells by antibodies

antibody-mediated response humoral immune response mediated by circulating antibodies; major defense against microbes and toxins in the extracellular fluid

anticodon (an-tie-KOH-don) three-nucleotide sequence in tRNA able to base-pair with complementary codon in mRNA during protein synthesis

antidiuretic hormone (ADH) (an-tye-dye-yoor-ET-ik or an-tee-dye-yoor-ET-ik) *see* vasopressin

antigen (AN-tih-jen) any molecule that stimulates a specific immune response

antigen-binding site one of the two variable "prongs" on an immunoglobulin capable of binding to a specific antigen

antigen presentation process by which an antigen-presenting cell, such as a macrophage, combines proteolytic fragments of a foreign antigen with host cell class II MHC proteins, which are transported to the host cell's surface

antigen-presenting cell (APC) cell that presents antigen, complexed with MHC proteins on its surface, to T cells

antithrombin III a plasma protein activated by heparin that limits clot formation by inactivating thrombin and other clotting factors

antrum (AN-trum) (gastric) lower portion of stomach (that is, region closest to pyloric sphincter); (ovarian) fluid-filled cavity in maturing ovarian follicle

anus lowest opening of the digestive tract through which fecal matter is extruded

aorta (a-OR-tah) largest artery in body; carries blood from left ventricle of heart to thorax and abdomen

aortic arch baroreceptor (a-OR-tik) *see* arterial baroreceptor

aortic body chemoreceptor located near aortic arch; sensitive to arterial blood O_2 content and H^+ concentration

aortic valve valve between left ventricle of heart and aorta

apical membrane the surface of an epithelial cell that faces a lumen, such as that of the intestines

apneustic center (ap-NOOS-tik) area in the lower pons in the brain with input to the medullary inspiratory neurons; helps to terminate inspiration

apoptosis (ay-pop-TOE-sis) programmed cell death that typically occurs during differentiation and development

appendix small fingerlike projection from cecum of large intestine

aprosodia (ay-proh-SO-dee-ah) neurological disorder involving the loss of ability to understand the emotional content of language

aquaporin (ah-qua-PORE-in) protein membrane channel through which water can diffuse

aqueous humor fluid filling the anterior chamber of the eye

arachidonic acid (ah-rak-ah-DON-ik) polyunsaturated fatty acid precursor of eicosanoids

arachnoid mater (ah-RAK-noid) the middle of three membranes (meninges) covering the brain

area postrema a circumventricular organ outside the blood–brain barrier

aromatase enzyme that converts androgens to estrogens; located predominantly in the ovaries, the placenta, the brain, and adipose tissue

arterial baroreceptor neuronal endings sensitive to stretch or distortion produced by arterial blood pressure changes; located in carotid sinus or aortic arch; also called *carotid sinus* and *aortic arch baroreceptor*

arteriole (ahr-TEER-ee-ole) blood vessel between artery and capillary, surrounded by smooth muscle; primary site of vascular resistance

arteriosclerosis (ahr-TEER-ee-oh-sklare-OH-sis) "hardening" of arterial walls that can have different causes, including deposition of collagenous fibers that occurs with aging

artery (AHR-ter-ee) thick-walled elastic vessel that carries blood away from heart to arterioles

ascending limb portion of Henle's loop of renal tubule leading to distal convoluted tubule

ascending pathway neural pathway that goes to the brain; also called *sensory pathway*

aspartate (ah-SPAR-tate) an excitatory neurotransmitter in CNS; ionized form of the amino acid aspartic acid

aspiration inhalation of liquid or a foreign body into the airways

astrocyte a form of glial cell that regulates composition of extracellular fluid around neurons and forms part of the blood–brain barrier

atmospheric pressure (P_{atm}) air pressure surrounding the body (760 mmHg at sea level); also called *barometric pressure*

atom smallest unit of matter that has unique chemical characteristics; has no net charge; combines with other atoms to form chemical substances

atomic mass (also called *atomic weight*) value that indicates an atom's mass relative to mass of other types of atoms based on the assignment of a value of 12 to carbon atom

atomic nucleus dense region, consisting of protons and neutrons, at center of atom

atomic number number of protons in nucleus of atom

ATP *see* adenosine triphosphate

ATP synthase the enzyme complex present in mitochondria responsible for the synthesis of ATP using the energy of an electrochemical gradient for hydrogen ions

atresia degeneration of nondominant follicles in the ovary

atrial natriuretic peptide (ANP) (nay-tree-yor-ET-ik) peptide hormone secreted by cardiac atrial cells in response to atrial distension; causes increased renal sodium excretion

atrioventricular (AV) node (ay-tree-oh-ven-TRIK-you-lar) region at base of right atrium near interventricular septum, containing specialized cardiac muscle cells through which electrical activity must pass to go from atria to ventricles

atrioventricular (AV) valve valve between atrium and ventricle of heart; AV valve on right side of heart is the *tricuspid valve*, and that on left side is the *mitral valve*

atrium (AY-tree-um) chamber of heart that receives blood from veins and passes it on to ventricle on same side of heart

atropine (AT-roh-peen) a drug that specifically blocks the binding of acetylcholine to muscarinic acetylcholine receptors

audition (aw-DIH-shun) sense of hearing

auditory cortex region of cerebral cortex that receives nerve fibers from auditory (hearing) pathways

autocrine substance (AW-toh-crin) chemical messenger secreted into extracellular fluid that acts upon the cell that secreted it; *compare* paracrine substance

automaticity (aw-toh-mah-TISS-ih-tee) capable of spontaneous, rhythmic self-excitation

autonomic ganglion group of neuron cell bodies in the peripheral nervous system

autonomic nervous system (aw-toh-NAHM-ik) component of efferent division of peripheral nervous system that consists of sympathetic and parasympathetic subdivisions; innervates cardiac muscle, smooth muscle, and glands; *compare* somatic nervous system

autoreceptor a receptor on a cell affected by a chemical messenger released from the same cell

autotransfusion shift of fluid from the interstitial space to the blood following a decrease in blood pressure

axo–axonic synapse presynaptic synapse where an axon stimulates the presynaptic terminal of another axon

axon (AX-ahn) extension from neuron cell body; propagates action potentials away from cell body; also called a *nerve fiber*

axon hillock part of the axon nearest the cell body where the action potential begins

axon terminal end of axon; forms synaptic or neuroeffector junction with postjunctional cell

axonal transport process involving intracellular filaments by which materials are moved from one end of axon to other

B

baroreceptor receptor sensitive to pressure and to rate of change in pressure; *see also* arterial baroreceptor, intrarenal baroreceptor

Barr body sex chromatin nuclear mass formed by the nonfunctional X chromosome in female cell nuclei

basal cell cell found within taste buds that can divide and differentiate to replace worn-out taste receptor cells

basal ganglia *see* basal nuclei

basal metabolic rate (BMR) metabolic rate when a person is at mental and physical rest but not sleeping, at comfortable temperature, and has fasted at least 12 h; also called *metabolic cost of living*

basal nuclei nuclei deep in cerebral hemispheres that code and relay information associated with control of body movements; specifically, caudate nucleus, globus pallidus, and putamen; also called *basal ganglia*

base (acid–base) any molecule that can combine with H^+; (nucleotide) molecular ring of carbon and nitrogen that, with a phosphate group and a sugar, constitutes a nucleotide

basement membrane thin layer of extracellular proteinaceous material upon which epithelial and endothelial cells sit

basic electrical rhythm spontaneous depolarization–repolarization cycles of pacemaker cells in longitudinal smooth muscle layer of stomach and intestines; coordinates repetitive muscular activity of GI tract

basilar membrane (BAS-ih-lar) membrane that separates cochlear duct and scala tympani in inner ear; supports organ of Corti

basolateral membrane (bay-zo-LAH-ter-al) sides of epithelial cell other than luminal surface; also called *serosal* or *blood side* of cell

basophil (BAY-zo-fill) polymorphonuclear granulocytic leukocyte whose granules stain with basic dyes; enters tissues and becomes mast cell

B cell (immune system) *see* B lymphocyte; (endocrine cell) *see* beta cell

beta-adrenergic receptor (BAY-ta ad-ren-ER-jik) a type of plasma membrane receptor for epinephrine and norepinephrine; *compare* alpha-adrenergic receptor; also called *beta adrenoceptor*

beta cell insulin-secreting cell in pancreatic islets of Langerhans; also called *B cell*

beta-endorphin putative hormone released from the anterior pituitary gland, believed to play a role in adaptation to stress and pain relief; also acts as a neurotransmitter

beta-lipotropin a protein formed from the proopiomelanocortin precursor in the anterior pituitary gland; further processing results in the putative hormone beta-endorphin

beta oxidation (ox-ih-DAY-shun) series of reactions that generate hydrogen atoms (for oxidative phosphorylation) from breakdown of fatty acids to acetyl CoA

beta pleated sheet a form of secondary protein structure determined by the relative hydrophobicity of amino acid side chains

beta rhythm low, fast EEG oscillations in alert, awake adults who are paying attention to (or thinking hard about) something

bicuspid valve another term for the left atrioventricular valve, also called the *mitral valve*

bile fluid secreted by liver into bile canaliculi; contains bicarbonate, bile salts, cholesterol, lecithin, bile pigments, metabolic end products, and certain trace metals

bile canaliculi (kan-al-IK-you-lee) small ducts adjacent to liver cells into which bile is secreted

bile pigment colored substance, derived from breakdown of heme group of hemoglobin, secreted in bile

bile salt one of a family of steroid molecules produced from cholesterol and secreted in bile by the liver; promotes solubilization and digestion of fat in small intestine

bilirubin (bil-eh-RUE-bin) yellow substance resulting from heme breakdown; excreted in bile as a bile pigment

binding site region of protein to which a specific ligand binds

binocular vision visual perception of overlapping fields from the two eyes

biogenic amine (by-oh-JEN-ik ah-MEEN) one of family of neurotransmitters having basic formula R—NH_2; includes dopamine, norepinephrine, epinephrine, serotonin, and histamine

bipolar cell type of neuron that has one input branch and one output branch

bivalent paired homologous chromosomes, each with two sister chromatids, that are produced during meiosis

bladder urinary bladder; thick-walled sac composed of smooth muscle; stores urine prior to urination

blastocyst (BLAS-toh-cyst) particular early embryonic stage consisting of ball of developing cells surrounding central cavity

block to polyspermy process that prevents more than one sperm cell from fertilizing an ovum

blood pressurized contents of the cardiovascular system composed of a liquid phase (plasma) and cellular phase (red and white blood cells, platelets)

blood–brain barrier group of anatomical barriers and transport systems in brain capillary endothelium that controls kinds of substances entering brain extracellular space from blood and their rates of entry

blood coagulation (koh-ag-you-LAY-shun) blood clotting

blood vessel tubular structures of various sizes that transport blood throughout the body

B lymphocyte lymphocyte that, upon activation, proliferates and differentiates into antibody-secreting plasma cell; also called *B cell*

body (of stomach) middle portion of the stomach; secretes mucus, pepsinogen, and hydrochloric acid

body mass index (BMI) method for assessing degree of obesity; calculated as weight in kilograms divided by square of height in meters

bone age an x-ray determination of the degree of bone development; often used in assessing reasons for unusual stature in children

bone marrow highly vascular, cellular substance in central cavity of some bones; site of erythrocyte, leukocyte, and platelet synthesis

Bowman's capsule blind sac at beginning of tubular component of kidney nephron

Bowman's space fluid-filled space within Bowman's capsule into which protein-free fluid filters from the glomerulus

Boyle's law pressure of a fixed amount of gas in a container is inversely proportional to container's volume

bradykinin (braid-ee-KYE-nin) protein formed by action of the enzyme kallikrein on precursor

brain self-stimulation phenomenon in which animals will press a bar to get electrical stimulation of certain parts of their brains

brainstem brain subdivision consisting of medulla oblongata, pons, and midbrain and located between spinal cord and forebrain

brainstem pathway descending motor pathway whose cells of origin are in the brainstem

Broca's area (BRO-kahz) region of left frontal lobe associated with speech production

bronchiole (BRON-key-ole) small airway distal to bronchus

bronchus (BRON-kus) large-diameter air passage that enters lung; located between trachea and bronchioles

brown adipose tissue type of adipose (fat) tissue found in newborns and in many mammals, with a higher heat-producing capacity than ordinary white fat; may be important in regulating body temperature in extreme conditions

brush border small projections (microvilli) of epithelial cells covering the villi of the small intestine; major absorptive surface of the small intestine

buffer weak acid or base that can exist in undissociated (H buffer) or dissociated (H^+ + buffer) form

bulbourethral gland (bul-bo-you-REETH-ral) one of paired glands in male that secretes fluid components of semen into the urethra

bulk flow movement of fluids or gases from region of higher pressure to one of lower pressure

bundle branches (right and left) pathway composed of cells that rapidly conduct electrical signals down the right and left sides of the interventricular septum; these pathways connect the bundle of His to the Purkinje network

bundle of His (HISS) nervelike structure composed of modified heart cells that carries electrical impulses from the atrioventricular node down the interventricular septum

C

cadherin protein that extends from a cell surface and links up with cadherins from other cells; important in the formation of tissues

calcitonin hormone from the thyroid gland that inhibits bone resorption, although physiological role in humans is minimal

caldesmon (kal-DEZ-mun) protein involved in regulating contraction in some smooth muscles and non-muscle tissue

calmodulin (kal-MADJ-you-lin) intracellular calcium-binding protein that mediates many of calcium's second-messenger functions

calmodulin-dependent protein kinase an intracellular enzyme that, when activated by calcium and the protein calmodulin, phosphorylates many protein substrates within cells; it is a component of many intracellular signaling mechanisms

calorie (cal) unit of heat–energy measurement; amount of heat needed to raise temperature of 1 g of water 1° C; *compare* kilocalorie

calorigenic effect (kah-lor-ih-JEN-ik) increase in metabolic rate caused by epinephrine or thyroid hormones

calyx (KAY-licks) funnel-shaped structure that drains urine into the ureter

cAMP-dependent protein kinase (KYE-nase) *see* cyclic AMP-dependent protein kinase

cAMP phosphodiesterase an enzyme in all cells that converts cAMP into an inactive molecule of AMP

canaliculus (parietal cell) thin canal formed by invagination of the cell membrane

capacitation process by which sperm in female reproductive tract gains ability to fertilize egg; also called *sperm capacitation*

capillary one of the smallest blood vessels across which most exchange of nutrients and wastes occurs with interstitial fluid

capillary filtration coefficient a measure of fluid flow across a capillary wall at a given hydrostatic pressure gradient; determined by porosity of the barrier

capsaicin (kap-SAY-sin) the molecule in chili peppers that causes sensations of heat and pain in the mouth and throat

capsule connective tissue surrounding an organ, such as the kidneys or adrenal glands

carbaminohemoglobin (kar-bah-MEEN-oh-HEE-ma-gloh-bin) compound resulting from combination of carbon dioxide and amino groups in hemoglobin

carbohydrate organic substance composed of carbon, hydrogen, and oxygen; includes mono-, di-, and polysaccharides

carbonic anhydrase (an-HYE-drase) enzyme that catalyzes the reaction $CO_2 + H_2O \leftrightarrow H_2CO_3$

carbon monoxide CO; gas that binds to hemoglobin; decreases blood oxygen-carrying capacity and shifts oxygen–hemoglobin dissociation curve to the left; also acts as an intracellular messenger in neurons

carboxyl group (kar-BOX-il) —COOH; ionizes to carboxyl ion ($—COO^-$)

carboxypeptidase (kar-box-ee-PEP-tih-dase) enzyme secreted into small intestine by exocrine pancreas as precursor, procarboxypeptidase; breaks peptide bond at carboxyl end of protein

cardiac cycle one contraction–relaxation sequence of heart

cardiac muscle heart muscle

cardiac output (CO) blood volume pumped by each ventricle per minute (not total output pumped by both ventricles)

cardiovascular system heart, blood, and blood vessels

carotid body chemoreceptor near main branching of carotid artery; sensitive to blood O_2 and CO_2 content and H^+ concentration

carotid sinus region of internal carotid artery just above main carotid branching; location of carotid baroreceptors

catabolism (kuh-TAB-oh-lizm) cellular breakdown of organic molecules

catalyst (KAT-ah-list) substance that accelerates chemical reactions but does not itself undergo any net chemical change during the reaction

catch-up growth a period of rapid growth during which a child attains his or her predicted height for a given age after a temporary period of slow growth due to illness or malnourishment

catecholamine (kat-eh-COLE-ah-meen) dopamine, epinephrine, or norepinephrine, all of which have similar chemical structures

cation (KAT-eye-on) ion having net positive charge; *compare* anion

caveolus (kav-ee-OH-lus) small invagination of the plasma membrane that pinches off and forms endocytotic vesicles that deliver their contents directly to the cytosol

cecum (SEE-come) dilated pouch at beginning of large intestine into which the ileum, colon, and appendix open

cell the functional unit of living organisms; four broad classes included epithelial, connective, nervous, and muscle

cell body in cells with long extensions, the part that contains the nucleus

cell differentiation process by which unspecialized cells acquire specialized structural and functional properties

cell organelle (or-guh-NEL) membrane-bound compartment, nonmembranous particle, or filament that performs specialized functions in cell

central chemoreceptor receptor in brainstem medulla oblongata that responds to changes in H^+ concentration of brain extracellular fluid

central command fatigue muscle fatigue due to failure of appropriate regions of cerebral cortex to excite motor neurons

central nervous system (CNS) brain and spinal cord

central sulcus a deep infolding on each half of the brain that separates the parietal and central lobes

central thermoreceptor temperature receptor in hypothalamus, spinal cord, abdominal organ, or other internal location

centriole (SEN-tree-ole) small cytoplasmic body having nine fused sets of microtubules; participates in nuclear and cell division

centrosome region of cell cytoplasm in which microtubule formation and elongation occur, particularly during cell division

cephalic phase (seh-FAL-ik) (of gastrointestinal control) initiation of the neural and hormonal reflexes regulating gastrointestinal functions by stimulation of receptors in head, that is, cephalic receptors—sight, smell, taste, and chewing—as well as by emotional states

cerebellum (ser-ah-BEL-um) brain subdivision lying behind forebrain and above brainstem; plays important role in skeletal muscle movement control

cerebral cortex (SER-ah-brul or sah-REE-brul) cellular layer covering the cerebrum

cerebral hemisphere either left or right half of the cerebral cortex

cerebral ventricle one of four interconnected spaces in the brain; filled with cerebrospinal fluid

cerebrospinal fluid (CSF) (sah-ree-broh-SPY-nal) fluid that fills cerebral ventricles and the subarachnoid space surrounding brain and spinal cord

cerebrum (SER-ah-brum or sah-REE-brum) part of the brain that, with diencephalon, forms the forebrain

cervix (SIR-vix) lower portion of uterus; cervical opening connects uterine and vaginal lumens

cGMP-dependent protein kinase (KYE-nase) enzyme that is activated by cyclic GMP and then phosphorylates specific proteins, thereby altering their activity

cGMP phosphodiesterase an enzyme in cells that converts cGMP into GMP

channel gating process of opening and closing ion channels

chemical element specific type of atom

chemical equilibrium state when rates of forward and reverse components of a chemical reaction are equal, and no net change in reactant or product concentration occurs

chemical specificity *see* specificity

chemical synapse (SIN-aps) synapse at which neurotransmitters released by one neuron diffuse across an extracellular gap to influence a second neuron's activity

chemiosmosis the mechanism by which ATP is formed during oxidative phosphorylation; the movement of protons across mitochondrial inner membranes is coupled with ATP production

chemoattractant any mediator that causes chemotaxis; also called *chemotaxin*

chemokine any cytokine that functions as a chemoattractant

chemoreceptor afferent neuron ending (or cell associated with it) sensitive to concentrations of certain chemicals

chemotaxin (kee-moh-TAX-in) *see* chemoattractant

chemotaxis (kee-moh-TAX-iss) movement of cells, particularly phagocytes, in a specific direction in response to a chemical stimulus

chief cell gastric gland cell that secretes pepsinogen, precursor of pepsin

cholecystokinin (CCK) (koh-lee-sis-toh-KYE-nin) peptide hormone secreted by duodenum that regulates gastric motility and secretion, gallbladder contraction, and pancreatic enzyme secretion; possible satiety signal

cholesterol particular steroid molecule; precursor of steroid hormones and bile salts and a component of plasma membranes

cholinergic (koh-lin-ER-jik) pertaining to acetylcholine; a compound that acts like acetylcholine or a neuron that contains acetylcholine

chondrocyte (KON-droh-site) cell types that form new cartilage

chordae tendineae (KORE-day TEN-den-ay) strong, fibrous cords that connect papillary muscles to the edges of atrioventricular valves; they prevent backward flow of blood during ventricular systole

chorion outermost fetal membrane derived from trophoblast cells; becomes part of the placenta

chorionic villi fingerlike projections of the trophoblast cells extending from the chorion into the endometrium of the uterus

choroid (KORE-oyd) pigmented layer of eye that lies next to retina

choroid plexus highly vascular epithelial structure lining portions of cerebral ventricles; responsible for much of cerebrospinal fluid formation

chromatin (KROM-ih-tin) combination of DNA and nuclear proteins; principal component of chromosomes

chromophore retinal light-sensitive component of a photopigment

chromosome highly coiled, condensed form of chromatin formed in cell nucleus during mitosis and meiosis

chylomicron (kye-loh-MYE-kron) small droplet consisting of lipids and protein released from intestinal epithelial cells into the lacteals during fat absorption

chyme (kyme) solution of partially digested food in stomach and intestinal lumens

chymotrypsin enzyme secreted by exocrine pancreas; breaks certain peptide bonds in proteins and polypeptides

cilia (SIL-ee-ah) hairlike projections from specialized epithelial cells that sweep back and forth in a synchronized way to propel material along epithelial surface

ciliary muscle involved in movement and shape of the lens during accommodation

circadian rhythm (sir-KAY-dee-an) occurring in an approximately 24 h cycle

circular muscle smooth muscle layer in stomach and intestinal walls that has muscle fibers circumferentially oriented around these organs

circulatory system (SIRK-you-la-tor-ee) the heart and system of vessels that deliver blood to all parts of the body

citric acid cycle *see* Krebs cycle

classical complement pathway antibody-dependent system for activating complement; begins with complement molecule Cl

class I MHC proteins form complexes with antigens on all cells except erythrocytes; required for T-cell recognition

class II MHC proteins form complexes with antigens on surface of macrophages, B lymphocytes, and dendritic cells; required for T-cell recognition

clathrin a cytosolic protein that binds to regions of the plasma membrane and helps initiate receptor-mediated endocytosis

clathrin-coated pits aggregations of ligand-bound receptors on a cell membrane that pinches off and is internalized into the cell

clearance volume of plasma from which a particular substance has been completely removed in a given time

cleavage mitotic cell division

clitoris (KLIT-or-iss) small body of erectile tissue in female external genitalia; homologous to penis

clonal deletion destruction by apoptosis in the thymus of those T cells that have receptors capable of binding to self proteins

clonal expansion lymphocyte cell divisions initiated by binding of an antigen to a lymphocyte cell membrane receptor

clonal inactivation process occurring in the periphery (that is, not in the thymus) that causes potentially self-reacting T cells to become nonresponsive

clone one of a set of genetically identical molecules, cells, or organisms

clot solid phase of blood, formed from platelets, trapped blood cells, and a polymer of the protein fibrin

clotting phase transition of blood from a liquid cell suspension into a solid, gel-like mass

cochlea (KOK-lee-ah) inner ear; fluid-filled spiral-shaped compartment that contains cochlear duct

cochlear duct (KOK-lee-er) fluid-filled membranous tube that extends length of inner ear, dividing it into compartments; contains organ of Corti

coding process by which neural signals from sensory receptors are converted into action potentials in the CNS

codon (KOH-don) three-base sequence in mRNA that determines the position of a specific amino acid during protein synthesis or that designates the end of the coded sequence of a protein

coenzyme (koh-EN-zime) organic cofactor; generally serves as a carrier that transfers atoms or small molecular fragments from one reaction to another; is not consumed in the reaction and can be reused

cofactor organic or inorganic substance that binds to a specific region of an enzyme and is necessary for the enzyme's activity

colipase protein secreted by pancreas that binds lipase, bringing it in contact with lipid droplets in the small intestine

collagen fiber (KOLL-ah-jen) strong, fibrous protein that functions as extracellular structural element in connective tissue

collateral branch of a neuron axon

collecting-duct system portion of renal tubules between distal convoluted tubules and renal pelvis; comprises *cortical collecting duct* and *medullary collecting duct*

colloid (KOLL-oid) large molecule, mainly protein, to which capillaries are relatively impermeable; also, part of the inner structure of the thyroid gland

colon (KOH-lun) a portion of the large intestine, specifically the part extending from cecum to rectum

colostrum watery, protein-rich liquid secreted by mother's breasts for first 24 to 48 hours after delivery of baby

commissure (KOM-ih-shur) bundle of nerve fibers linking right and left halves of the brain

common bile duct carries bile from gallbladder to small intestine

competition ability of similar molecules to combine with the same binding site or receptor

complement (KOM-plih-ment) one of a group of plasma proteins that, upon activation, kills microbes directly and facilitates the inflammatory process, including phagocytosis

compliance stretchability; *see also* lung compliance

concentration amount of solute per unit volume of solution

concentric contraction muscle activity that involves shortening of muscle length

conceptus collective term for the fertilized egg and everything derived from it

conducting system network of cardiac muscle fibers specialized to conduct electrical activity between different areas of heart

conducting zone air passages that extend from top of trachea to beginning of respiratory bronchioles and have walls too thick for gas exchange between air and blood

conduction (heat) transfer of thermal energy during collisions of adjacent molecules

cone one of two retinal receptor types for photic energy; gives rise to color vision

conformation three-dimensional shape of a molecule

congenital existing at birth; usually referring to a birth defect

connective tissue one of the four major categories of tissues in the body; major component of extracellular matrices, cartilage, and bone

connective-tissue cell cell specialized to form extracellular elements that connect, anchor, and support body structures

conscious experience things of which a person is aware; thoughts, feelings, perceptions, ideas, and reasoning during any state of consciousness

consolidation process by which short-term memories are converted into long-term memories

contractility (kon-trak-TIL-ity) force of heart contraction that is independent of sarcomere length

contraction operation of the force-generating process in a muscle

contraction time time between beginning of force development and peak twitch tension by the muscle

contralateral on the opposite side of the body

convection (kon-VEK-shun) process by which a fluid or gas next to a warm body is heated by conduction, moves away, and is replaced by colder fluid or gas that in turn follows the same cycle

convergence (neuronal) many presynaptic neurons synapsing upon one postsynaptic neuron; (of eyes) turning of eyes inward (that is, toward nose) to view near objects

cooperativity interaction between functional binding sites in a multimeric protein

core body temperature temperature of inner body

cornea (KOR-nee-ah) transparent structure covering front of eye; forms part of eye's optical system and helps focus an object's image on retina

coronary artery vessel delivering oxygenated blood to the muscular walls of the heart

coronary blood flow blood flow to heart muscle

corpus callosum (KOR-pus kal-LOH-sum) wide band of nerve fibers connecting the two cerebral hemispheres; a brain commissure

corpus luteum (KOR-pus LOO-tee-um) ovarian structure formed from the follicle after ovulation; secretes estrogen and progesterone

cortical association area region of cerebral cortex that receives input from various sensory types, memory stores, and so on, and performs further perceptual processing

cortical collecting duct primary site of sodium ion reabsorption at the distal end of a nephron

cortical (nephron) functional unit of the kidney contained in the renal cortex and with a small (or no) loop of Henle

cortical reaction release of factors by the ovum that hardens the zona pellucida

corticobulbar pathway (kor-tih-koh-BUL-bar) descending pathway having its neuron cell bodies in cerebral cortex; its axons pass without synapsing to region of brainstem motor neurons

corticospinal pathway descending pathway having its neuron cell bodies in cerebral cortex; its axons pass without synapsing to region of spinal motor neurons; also called the *pyramidal tract; compare* brainstem pathway, corticobulbar pathway

corticotropin-releasing hormone (CRH) (kor-tih-koh-TROH-pin) hypophysiotropic peptide hormone that stimulates ACTH (corticotropin) secretion by anterior pituitary gland

cortisol (KOR-tih-sol) main glucocorticoid steroid hormone secreted by adrenal cortex; regulates various aspects of organic metabolism

costameres clusters of structural proteins linking Z disks of sarcomeres to the sarcolemma of striated muscle cells

costimulus nonspecific interactions between proteins on the surface of antigen-presenting cells and helper T cells; required for T-cell activation

cotransmitter chemical messenger released with a neurotransmitter from synapse or neuroeffector junction

cotransport form of secondary active transport in which net movement of actively transported substance and "downhill" movement of molecule supplying the energy are in the same direction

countercurrent multiplier system mechanism associated with loops of Henle that creates a region having high interstitial fluid osmolarity in renal medulla

countertransport form of secondary active transport in which net movement of actively transported molecule is in direction opposite "downhill" movement of molecule supplying the energy

covalent bond (koh-VAY-lent) chemical bond between two atoms in which each atom shares one of its electrons with the other

covalent modulation alteration of a protein's shape, and therefore its function, by the covalent binding of various chemical groups to it

cranial nerve one of 24 peripheral nerves (12 pairs) that join brainstem or forebrain with structures outside CNS

C-reactive protein an acute phase protein that functions as a nonspecific opsonin

creatine phosphate (CP) (KREE-ah-tin) molecule that transfers phosphate and energy to ADP to generate ATP

creatinine (kree-AT-ih-nin) waste product derived from muscle creatine

creatinine clearance (C_{Cr}) plasma volume from which creatinine is removed by the kidneys per unit time; approximates glomerular filtration rate

cristae (mitochondrial) the inner membrane of mitochondria, which may assume sheetlike or tubular appearances; site containing cytochrome P450 enzymes involved in steroid hormone production

cross-bridge in muscle, myosin projection extending from thick filament and capable of exerting force on thin filament, causing the filaments to slide past each other

cross-bridge cycle sequence of events between binding of a cross-bridge to actin, its release, and reattachment during muscle contraction

crossed-extensor reflex increased activation of extensor muscles contralateral to limb flexion

crossing-over process in which segments of maternal and paternal chromosomes exchange with each other during chromosomal pairing in meiosis

crystalloid low-molecular-weight solute in plasma

C3b a complement molecule that attaches phagocytes to microbes; also amplifies complement cascade

cumulus oophorous layers of granulosa cells that surround the egg within the dominant follicle

cupula a gelatinous mass within the semicircular canals that contains stereocilia and responds to head movement

current movement of electrical charge; in biological systems, this is achieved by ion movement

cusp a flap or "leaflet" of a heart valve

cyclic AMP (cAMP) cyclic 3′,5′-adenosine monophosphate; cyclic nucleotide that serves as a second messenger for many "first" chemical messengers

cyclic AMP-dependent protein kinase (KYE-nase) enzyme that is activated by cyclic AMP and then phosphorylates specific proteins, thereby altering their activity; also called *protein kinase A*

cyclic endoperoxide eicosanoid formed from arachidonic acid by cyclooxygenase

cyclic GMP (cGMP) cyclic 3′,5′-guanosine monophosphate; cyclic nucleotide that acts as second messenger in some cells

cyclooxygenase (COX) (sye-klo-OX-ah-jen-ase) enzyme that acts on arachidonic acid and initiates production of cyclic endoperoxides, prostaglandins, and thromboxanes

cystic fibrosis transmembrane conductance regulator (CFTR) epithelial chloride channel; mutations in the *CFTR* gene can cause cystic fibrosis

cytochrome (SYE-toe-krom) one of a series of enzymes that couples energy to ATP formation during oxidative phosphorylation

cytokine (SYE-toh-kine) general term for protein extracellular messengers that regulate immune responses; secreted by macrophages, monocytes, lymphocytes, neutrophils, and several nonimmune cell types

cytoplasm (SYE-toh-plasm) region of cell interior outside the nucleus

cytosine (C) (SYE-toh-seen) pyrimidine base in DNA and RNA

cytoskeleton cytoplasmic filamentous network associated with cell shape and movement

cytosol (SYE-toh-sol) intracellular fluid that surrounds cell organelles and nucleus

cytotoxic T cell (SYE-toh-TOX-ik) T lymphocyte that, upon activation by specific antigen, directly attacks a cell bearing that type of antigen and destroys it; major killer of virus-infected and cancer cells

D

Dalton's law pressure exerted by each gas in a mixture of gases is independent of the pressure exerted by the other gases

dark adaptation process by which photoreceptors in the retina adjust to darkness

declarative memory memories of facts and events

decremental decreasing in amplitude

decussation (dek-uh-SAY-shun) crossover of neuronal pathways from one side of the body to the other

defecation (def-ih-KAY-shun) expulsion of feces from rectum

defecation reflex urge to extrude feces caused by sudden distension of the walls of the rectum

defensins (dee-FENS-ins) small peptides released by immune cells involved in destroying bacteria, fungi, and some viruses

dehydration type of chemical reaction in which two smaller molecules, such as amino acids, are joined to form a larger molecule; a single molecule of water is lost in the process

delta rhythm slow-wave, high-amplitude EEG waves associated with the deepest stages of slow-wave sleep

dendrite (DEN-drite) highly branched extension of neuron cell body; receives synaptic input from other neurons

dendritic cell a type of immune cell with phagocytic and antigen-presenting properties

dendritic spine a small protrusion from a dendrite that receives a synapse from an axon

dense body cytoplasmic structure to which thin filaments of a smooth muscle fiber are anchored

deoxyhemoglobin (Hb) (dee-ox-see-HEE-moh-gloh-bin) hemoglobin not combined with oxygen; reduced hemoglobin

deoxyribonucleic acid (DNA) (dee-ox-see-rye-boh-noo-KLAY-ik) nucleic acid that stores and transmits genetic information; consists of double strand of nucleotide subunits that contain deoxyribose

deoxyribose a ribose molecule with a single hydroxyl group removed; a component of DNA

depolarize to change membrane potential value toward zero so that cell interior becomes less negative than resting level

descending limb (of Henle's loop) segment of renal tubule into which proximal tubule drains

descending pathway neural pathways that go from the brain down to the spinal cord

desmosome (DEZ-moh-some) junction that holds two cells together; consists of plasma membranes of adjacent cells linked by fibers, yet separated by a 20 nm extracellular space filled with a cementing substance

detrusor muscle (duh-TRUSS-or) the smooth muscle that forms the wall of the urinary bladder

diacylglycerol (DAG) (dye-ace-ul-GLIS-er-ol) second messenger that activates protein kinase C, which then phosphorylates a large number of other proteins

diapedesis (dye-app-uh-DEE-suhs) passage of leukocytes out of the blood and into the surrounding tissue

diaphragm (DYE-ah-fram) dome-shaped skeletal muscle sheet that separates the abdominal and thoracic cavities; principal muscle of respiration

diastole (dye-ASS-toh-lee) period of cardiac cycle when ventricles are relaxing

diastolic pressure (DP) (dye-ah-STAL-ik) minimum blood pressure during cardiac cycle

dicrotic notch deflection of the arterial pressure wave associated with closing of the semilunar valve

diencephalon (dye-en-SEF-ah-lon) core of anterior part of brain; lies beneath cerebral hemispheres and contains *thalamus* and *hypothalamus*

diet-induced thermogenesis the creation of heat within the body following a meal, particularly one rich in protein; at least part of the heat is generated secondarily to the increased activity of the gastrointestinal tract

diffusion (dif-FU-shun) movement of molecules from one location to another because of random thermal molecular motion; net diffusion always occurs from a region of higher concentration to a region of lower concentration; *see* simple diffusion, facilitated diffusion

diffusion equilibrium state during which diffusion fluxes in opposite directions are equal; that is, the net flux equals zero

digestion process of breaking down large particles and high-molecular-weight substances into small molecules

digestive system the gastrointestinal tract and its accessory organs

dihydropyridine (DHP) receptor (dye-hydro-PEER-a-deen) nonconducting calcium channels in the T-tubule membranes of skeletal muscle cells, which act as voltage sensors in excitation–contraction coupling

dihydrotestosterone (DHT) (dye-hy-droh-tes-TOS-ter-own) steroid formed by enzyme-mediated alteration of testosterone; active form of testosterone in certain of its target cells

1,25-dihydroxyvitamin D [1,25-$(OH)_2D$] (1-25-dye-hy-DROX-ee-vy-tah-min DEE) hormone that is formed by kidneys and is the active form of vitamin D

diiodotyrosine (DIT) a doubly iodinated tyrosine molecule that is an intermediate in the formation of thyroid hormones

2,3-diphosphoglycerate (DPG) (2-3-dye-fos-foh-GLISS-er-ate) substance produced by erythrocytes during glycolysis; binds reversibly to hemoglobin, causing it to release oxygen

disaccharide (dye-SAK-er-ide) carbohydrate molecule composed of two monosaccharides

disc layer of membranes in outer segment of photoreceptor; contains photopigments

distal convoluted tubule portion of kidney tubule between loop of Henle and collecting-duct system

disulfide bond R—S—S—R bonds in a protein

diuresis (dye-uh-REE-sis) increased urine excretion

diuretic (dye-uh-RET-ik) substance that inhibits fluid reabsorption in renal tubule, thereby increasing urine excretion

divergence (dye-VER-gence) (neuronal) one presynaptic neuron synapsing upon many postsynaptic neurons; (of eyes) turning of eyes outward to view distant objects

dominant follicle most mature developing follicle in the ovary from which the mature egg is ovulated

dopamine (DA) (DOPE-ah-meen) biogenic amine (catecholamine) neurotransmitter and hormone; precursor of epinephrine and norepinephrine

dorsal column pathway ascending pathway for somatosensory information; runs through dorsal area of spinal white matter

dorsal horn region of gray matter in the spinal cord that receives sensory input and connects with motor neurons in ventral horn

dorsal respiratory group (DRG) neurons in the medullary respiratory center that fire during inspiration

dorsal root group of afferent nerve fibers that enters dorsal region of spinal cord

dorsal root ganglion group of sensory neuron cell bodies that have axons projecting to the dorsal horn of the spinal cord

down-regulation decrease in number of target-cell receptors for a given messenger in response to a chronic high concentration of that messenger; *compare* up-regulation

dual innervation (in-ner-VAY-shun) innervation of an organ or gland by both sympathetic and parasympathetic nerve fibers

duodenum (doo-oh-DEE-num or doo-ODD-en-um) first portion of small intestine (between stomach and jejunum)

dura mater thick, outermost membrane (meninges) covering the brain

dynamic constancy a way of describing homeostasis that includes the idea that a variable such as blood glucose may vary in the short term but is stable and predictable when averaged over the long term

dynein (DYE-neen) motor protein that uses the energy from ATP to transport attached cellular cargo molecules along microtubules

dynorphin (dye-NOR-fin) one of a group of endogenous opioid peptides that act as neuromodulators in the brain

dystrophin protein in muscle cells that links actin to proteins embedded in sarcolemma; stabilizes muscle cells during contractions

E

eccentric contraction muscle activity that is accompanied by lengthening of the muscle generally by an external load that exceeds muscle force

ECG lead combination of a reference electrode (designated negative) and a recording electrode (designated positive); this combination is placed on the surface of the body and provides a "view" of the electrical activity of the heart

edema (ed-DEE-mah) accumulation of excess fluid in interstitial space

EEG arousal transformation of EEG pattern from alpha to beta rhythm during increased levels of attention

effector (ee-FECK-tor) cell or cell collection whose change in activity constitutes the response in a control system

efferent arteriole renal vessel that conveys blood from glomerulus to peritubular capillaries

efferent division (of the peripheral nervous system) neurons in the peripheral nervous system that project out of the central nervous system

efferent neuron neuron that carries information away from CNS

efferent pathway component of reflex arc that transmits information from integrating center to effector

egg female germ cell at any of its stages of development

eicosanoid (eye-KOH-sah-noid) general term for modified fatty acids that are products of arachidonic acid metabolism (cyclic endoperoxides, prostaglandins, thromboxanes, and leukotrienes); function as paracrine or autocrine substances

ejaculation (ee-jak-you-LAY-shun) discharge of semen from penis

ejaculatory duct (ee-JAK-you-lah-tory) continuation of vas deferens after it is joined by seminal vesicle duct; joins urethra in prostate gland

ejection fraction (EF) the ratio of stroke volume to end-diastolic volume; EF = SV/EDV

elastic recoil tendency of an elastic structure to oppose stretching or distortion

elastin fiber a protein with elastic or springlike properties; found in large arteries and in the airways

electrical potential (*E*) (or electrical potential difference) *see* potential

electrical synapse (SIN-aps) synapse at which local currents resulting from electrical activity flow between two neurons through gap junctions joining them

electrocardiogram (ECG, *also abbreviated* EKG) (ee-lek-troh-KARD-ee-oh-gram) recording at skin surface of the electrical currents generated by cardiac muscle action potentials

electrochemical gradient the driving force across a plasma membrane that dictates whether an ion will move into or out of a cell; established by both the concentration difference and the electrical charge difference between the cytosolic and extracellular surfaces of the membrane

electroencephalogram (EEG) (eh-lek-troh-en-SEF-ah-loh-gram) recording of brain electrical activity from scalp

electrogenic pump (elec-troh-JEN-ik) active-transport system that directly separates electrical charge, thereby producing a potential difference

electrolyte (ee-LEK-troh-lite) substance that dissociates into ions when in aqueous solution

electron (ee-LEK-tron) subatomic particle that carries one unit of negative charge

electron-transport chain a series of metal-containing proteins within mitochondria that participate in the flow of electrons from proteins to molecular oxygen; they are key components of the energy-producing processes in all cells

electronegativity measure of an atom's ability to attract electrons in a covalent bond

embryo (EM-bree-oh) organism during early stages of development; in human beings, the first 2 months of intrauterine life

emission (ee-MISH-un) movement of male genital duct contents into urethra prior to ejaculation

emotional behavior outward expression and display of inner emotions

emulsification (eh-mul-suh-fah-KAY-shun) division of large lipid droplets into very small droplets that are prevented from coalescing through the action of amphipathic substances

end-diastolic volume (EDV) (dye-ah-STAH-lik) amount of blood in ventricle just prior to systole

endocrine gland (EN-doh-krin) group of epithelial cells that secrete into the extracellular space hormones that then diffuse into bloodstream; also called a *ductless gland*

endocrine system all the body's hormone-secreting glands

endocytosis (en-doh-sye-TOH-sis) process in which plasma membrane folds into the cell, forming small pockets that pinch off to produce intracellular, membrane-bound vesicles; *see also* phagocytosis

endogenous opioid (en-DAHJ-en-us OH-pee-oid) an example of certain neuropeptides—endorphin, dynorphin, or enkephalin

endogenous pyrogen (EP) (en-DAHJ-en-us PY-roh-jen) any of the cytokines (including interleukin 1 and interleukin 6) that act physiologically in the brain to cause fever

endolymph extracellular fluid found in the cochlea and vestibular apparatus

endometrium (en-doh-MEE-tree-um) glandular epithelium lining uterine cavity

endoplasmic reticulum (en-doh-PLAS-mik reh-TIK-you-lum) cell organelle that consists of interconnected network of membrane-bound branched tubules and flattened sacs; two types are distinguished: *rough*, with ribosomes attached, and *smooth*, which is smooth-surfaced (does not contain ribosomes)

endorphins (en-DOR-fins) endogenous opioid peptide neurotransmitters released during exercise and other active neurological states; involved in inhibition of pain pathways and creation of positive mood

endosome (EN-doh-some) intracellular vesicles and tubular elements between Golgi apparatus and plasma membrane; sorts and distributes vesicles during endocytosis and exocytosis

endothelial cell *see* endothelium

endothelin-1 (ET-1) (en-doh-THEE-lin) one member of a family of peptides secreted by many tissues that can act as a paracrine or hormonal signal; one major action is vasoconstriction

endothelium (en-doh-THEE-lee-um) thin layer of cells that lines heart cavities and blood vessels

endothelium-derived relaxing factor (EDRF) nitric oxide and possibly other substances; secreted by vascular endothelium, it relaxes vascular smooth muscle and causes arteriolar dilation

endotherm an animal that generates its own internal body heat without having to rely on the environment

end-plate potential (EPP) depolarization of motor end plate of skeletal muscle fiber in response to acetylcholine; initiates action potential in muscle plasma membrane

end-product inhibition inhibition of a metabolic pathway by final product's action upon allosteric site on an enzyme (usually the rate-limiting enzyme) in the pathway

end-systolic volume (ESV) (sis-TAH-lik) amount of blood remaining in ventricle after ejection

enkephalin (en-KEF-ah-lin) peptide neurotransmitter at some synapses activated by opiate drugs; an endogenous opioid

enteric nervous system (en-TAIR-ik) neural network residing in and innervating walls of gastrointestinal tract

enterochromaffin-like (ECL) cell histamine-secreting cell of the stomach

enteroendocrine cell cell located in the gastric gland in the stomach; secretes gastrin

enterogastrones (en-ter-oh-GAS-trones) collective term for hormones released by intestinal tract; inhibit stomach activity

enterohepatic circulation (en-ter-oh-hih-PAT-ik) reabsorption of bile salts (and other substances) from intestines, passage to liver (via hepatic portal vein), and secretion back to intestines (via bile)

enterokinase (en-ter-oh-KYE-nase) enzyme in luminal plasma membrane of intestinal epithelial cells; converts pancreatic trypsinogen to trypsin

entrainment (en-TRAIN-ment) adjusting biological rhythm to environmental cues

enzyme (EN-zime) protein catalyst that accelerates specific chemical reactions but does not itself undergo net chemical change during the reaction

enzyme activity rate at which enzyme converts reactant to product; may be measure of the properties of enzyme's active site as altered by allosteric or covalent modulation; affects rate of enzyme-mediated reaction

eosinophil (ee-oh-SIN-oh-fil) polymorphonuclear granulocytic leukocyte whose granules take up red dye eosin; involved in parasite destruction and allergic responses

ependymal cell (ep-END-ih-mel) type of glial cell that lines internal cavities of the brain and produces cerebrospinal fluid

epicardium (epp-ee-KAR-dee-um) layer of connective tissue closely affixed to outer surface of the heart

epididymis (ep-ih-DID-ih-mus) portion of male reproductive duct system located between seminiferous tubules and vas deferens

epiglottis (ep-ih-GLOT-iss) thin cartilage flap that folds down, covering trachea, during swallowing

epinephrine (ep-ih-NEF-rin) amine hormone secreted by adrenal medulla and involved in regulation of organic metabolism; a biogenic amine (catecholamine) neurotransmitter; also called *adrenaline*

epiphyseal closure (ep-ih-FIZ-ee-al) conversion of epiphyseal growth plate to bone

epiphyseal growth plate actively proliferating cartilage near bone ends; region of bone growth

epiphysis (eh-PIF-ih-sis) end of long bone

epithalamus a small portion of the dorsal posterior diencephalon containing the pineal gland

epithelial cell (ep-ih-THEE-lee-al) cell at surface of body or hollow organ; specialized to secrete or absorb ions and organic molecules; with other epithelial cells, forms an *epithelium*

epithelial tissue one of the four major tissue types in the body, comprised of aggregates of epithelial cells

epithelium (ep-ih-THEE-lee-um) tissue that covers all body surfaces, lines all body cavities, and forms most glands

epitope (EP-ih-tope) antigenic portion of a molecule complexed to the MHC protein and presented to the T cell; also called an *antigenic determinant*

equilibrium (ee-quah-LIB-ree-um) no net change occurs in a system; requires no energy

equilibrium potential voltage gradient across a membrane that is equal in force but opposite in direction to concentration force affecting a given ion species

erection penis or clitoris becoming stiff due to vascular congestion

erythrocyte (eh-RITH-roh-site) red blood cell

erythropoiesis (eh-rith-roh-poy-EE-sis) erythrocyte production

erythropoietin (eh-rith-roh-POY-ih-tin) peptide hormone secreted mainly by kidney cells; stimulates red blood cell production; one of the hematopoietic growth factors

esophagus (eh-SOF-uh-gus) portion of digestive tract that connects throat (pharynx) and stomach

essential amino acid amino acid that cannot be formed by the body at all (or at a rate adequate to meet metabolic requirements) and so must be obtained from diet

essential nutrient substance required for normal or optimal body function but synthesized by the body either not at all or in amounts inadequate to prevent disease

estradiol (es-tra-DYE-ol) steroid hormone of estrogen family; major female sex hormone

estriol (ES-tree-ol) estrogen present in pregnancy; produced primarily by the placenta

estrogen (ES-troh-jen) group of steroid hormones that have effects similar to estradiol on female reproductive tract

estrogen priming increase in responsiveness to progesterone caused by prior exposure to estrogen (e.g., in the uterus)

estrone estrogen that is less prominent than estradiol

eukaryotic cell cell containing a membrane-enclosed nucleus with genetic material; plant and animal cells

eustachian tube (yoo-STAY-shee-an) duct connecting the middle ear with the nasopharynx

evaporation the loss of body water by perspiration, resulting in cooling

excitability ability to produce electrical signals

excitable membrane membrane capable of producing action potentials

excitation–contraction coupling in muscle fibers, mechanism linking plasma membrane stimulation with cross-bridge force generation

excitatory amino acid amino acid that acts as an excitatory (depolarizing) neurotransmitter in the nervous system

excitatory postsynaptic potential (EPSP) (post-sin-NAP-tic) depolarizing graded potential in postsynaptic neuron in response to activation of excitatory synapse

excitatory synapse (SIN-aps) synapse that, when activated, increases likelihood that postsynaptic neuron will undergo action potentials or increases frequency of existing action potentials

excitotoxicity (eggs-SYE-toe-tocks-ih-city) spreading damage to brain cells due to release of glutamate from ruptured neurons

exocrine gland (EX-oh-krin) cluster of epithelial cells specialized for secretion and having ducts that lead to an epithelial surface

exocytosis (ex-oh-sye-TOE-sis) process in which intracellular vesicle fuses with plasma membrane, the vesicle opens, and its contents are liberated into the extracellular fluid

exon (EX-on) DNA gene region containing code words for a part of the amino acid sequence of a protein

expiration (ex-pur-AY-shun) movement of air out of lungs

expiratory reserve volume (ERV) (ex-PYE-ruh-tor-ee) volume of air that can be exhaled by maximal contraction of expiratory muscles after normal resting expiration

extension straightening a joint

external anal sphincter ring of skeletal muscle around lower end of rectum

external auditory canal outer canal of the ear between the pinna and the tympanic membrane

external environment environment surrounding external surface of an organism

external urethral sphincter ring of skeletal muscle that surrounds the urethra at base of bladder

external work movement of external objects by skeletal muscle contraction

extracellular fluid fluid outside cell; interstitial fluid and plasma

extracellular matrix (MAY-trix) a complex consisting of a mixture of proteins (and, in some cases, minerals) interspersed with extracellular fluid

extrafusal fiber primary muscle fiber in skeletal muscle, as opposed to modified (intrafusal) fiber in muscle spindle

extrapyramidal system *see* brainstem pathway

extrinsic pathway formation of fibrin clots by pathway using tissue factor on cells in interstitium; once activated, it also recruits the intrinsic clotting pathway beyond factor XII

F

facilitated diffusion (fah-SIL-ih-tay-ted) system using a transporter to move molecules from high to low concentration across a membrane; energy not required

F-actin the polymerized form of actin found in actin filaments

FAD flavin adenine dinucleotide, a coenzyme derived from the B-vitamin riboflavin that participates in transfer of hydrogen atoms during metabolism

fallopian tube one of two tubes that carries egg from ovary to uterus

fast fiber skeletal muscle fiber that contains myosin having high ATPase activity

fast-glycolytic fiber type of skeletal muscle fiber that has high intrinsic contraction speed and abundant capacity for production of ATP by anaerobic glycolysis

fast-oxidative-glycolytic fiber type of skeletal muscle fiber that has high intrinsic contraction speed and abundant capacity for production of ATP by aerobic oxidative phosphorylation

fat-soluble vitamin *see* vitamin

fatty acid carbon chain with carboxyl group at one end through which chain can be linked to glycerol to form triglyceride; *see also* polyunsaturated fatty acid, saturated fatty acid, unsaturated fatty acid

Fc "stem" part of antibody

feces (FEE-sees) material expelled from large intestine during defecation

feedforward aspect of some control systems that allows system to anticipate changes in a regulated variable

female external genitalia mons pubis, labia majora, labia minora, clitoris, outer vagina, and its glands

female internal genitalia (jen-ih-TALE-ee-ah) ovaries, uterine tubes, uterus, and vagina

ferritin (FERR-ih-tin) iron-binding protein that stores iron in body

fertilization union of sperm and egg

fetal hemoglobin oxygen-carrying molecule with high oxygen affinity

fetus (FEE-tus) human being from third month of intrauterine life until birth

fiber *see* muscle fiber, nerve fiber

fibrin (FYE-brin) protein polymer resulting from enzymatic cleavage of fibrinogen; can turn blood into gel (clot)

fibrinogen (fye-BRIN-oh-jen) plasma protein precursor of fibrin

fibrinolytic system (fye-brin-oh-LIT-ik) cascade of plasma enzymes that breaks down clots; also called *thrombolytic system*

fight-or-flight response activation of sympathetic nervous system during stress

filtered load amount of any substance filtered from renal glomerular capillaries into Bowman's capsule

fimbria (FIM-bree-ah) opening of the fallopian tube; it has fingerlike projections lined with ciliated epithelium through which the ovulated egg passes into the fallopian tube

first messenger extracellular chemical messenger such as a hormone

first polar body non-functional structure containing one of the two nuclei resulting from the first meiotic division of a primary oocyte in the ovary

5-α-reductase intracellular enzyme that converts testosterone to dihydrotestosterone

flatus (FLAY-tus) intestinal gas expelled through anus

flexion (FLEK-shun) bending a joint

flow autoregulation ability of individual arterioles to alter their resistance in response to changing blood pressure so that relatively constant blood flow is maintained

fluid endocytosis invagination of a plasma membrane by which a cell can engulf extracellular fluid

fluid-mosaic model (moh-ZAY-ik) cell membrane structure consists of proteins embedded in bimolecular lipid that has the physical properties of a fluid, allowing membrane proteins to move laterally within it

flux amount of a substance crossing a surface in a unit of time; *see also* net flux

folic acid (FOH-lik) vitamin of B-complex group; essential for formation of nucleotide thiamine

follicle (FOL-ih-kel) egg and its encasing follicular, granulosa, and theca cells at all stages prior to ovulation; also called *ovarian follicle*

follicle-stimulating hormone (FSH) protein hormone secreted by anterior pituitary gland in males and females that acts on gonads; a gonadotropin

follicular phase (fuh-LIK-you-lar) that portion of menstrual cycle during which follicle and egg develop to maturity prior to ovulation

foot process large extension of sarcoplasmic reticulum calcium channels (ryanodine receptors), which connect them to the T-tubule membrane and mediate excitation–contraction coupling in skeletal muscle; also known as *junctional feet*

forebrain large, anterior brain subdivision consisting of right and left cerebral hemispheres (the cerebrum) and diencephalon

formed element solid phase of blood, including cells (erythrocytes and leukocytes) and cell fragments (platelets)

fovea centralis (FOH-vee-ah) area near center of retina where cones are most concentrated; gives rise to most acute vision

Frank–Starling mechanism the relationship between stroke volume and end-diastolic volume such that stroke volume increases as end-diastolic volume increases; also called *Starling's law of the heart*

fraternal twins dizygotic twins that occur when two eggs are fertilized

free radical atom that has an unpaired electron in its outermost orbital; molecule containing such an atom

free-running rhythm cyclical activity driven by biological clock in absence of environmental cues

frequency number of times an event occurs per unit time

frontal lobe region of anterior cerebral cortex where motor areas, Broca's speech center, and some association cortex are located

F-type channel the "funny" sodium-conducting channel mainly responsible for the inward flow of positive current in autorhythmic cardiac cells

functional residual capacity lung volume after relaxed expiration

functional site binding site on allosteric protein that, when activated, carries out protein's physiological function; also called *active site*

functional unit one of a number of small structures within an organ that act similarly to carry out an organ's function; for example, nephrons are the functional units of the kidneys

fundus upper portion of the stomach; secretes mucus, pepsinogen, and hydrochloric acid

fused tetanus (TET-ah-nuss) skeletal muscle activation in which action potential frequency is sufficiently high to cause a smooth, sustained, maximal strength contraction

fused-vesicle channel endocytotic or exocytotic vesicles that have fused to form a continuous water-filled channel through capillary endothelial cell

G

GABA (gamma-aminobutyric acid) an amino acid neurotransmitter commonly occurring at inhibitory synapses in the central nervous system

G-actin a monomer of actin that polymerizes to form F-actin, that makes up actin filaments

gallbladder small sac under the liver; concentrates bile and stores it between meals; contraction of gallbladder ejects bile, which eventually flows into small intestine

gamete (GAM-eet) germ cell or reproductive cell; sperm in male and egg in female

gametogenesis (gah-mee-toh-JEN-ih-sis) gamete production

gamma globulin immunoglobulin G (IgG), most abundant class of plasma antibodies

gamma motor neuron small motor neuron that controls intrafusal muscle fibers in muscle spindles

gamma rhythm high-frequency (30–100 Hz) pattern detected on electroencephalogram associated with processing sensory inputs and other specific cognitive tasks

ganglion (GANG-lee-on) (plural, *ganglia*) generally reserved for cluster of neuron cell bodies outside CNS

ganglion cell retinal neuron that is postsynaptic to bipolar cells; axons of ganglion cells form optic nerves

gap junction protein channels linking cytosol of adjacent cells; allows ions and small molecules to flow between cytosols of the connected cells

gastric (GAS-trik) pertaining to the stomach

gastric phase (of gastrointestinal control) initiation of neural and hormonal gastrointestinal reflexes by stimulation of stomach wall

gastrin (GAS-trin) peptide hormone secreted by antral region of stomach; stimulates gastric acid secretion

gastroileal reflex (gas-troh-IL-ee-al) increase in contractions of ileum during gastric emptying

gastrointestinal (GI) tract mouth, pharynx, esophagus, stomach, small and large intestines, and anus

gene unit of hereditary information; portion of DNA containing information required to determine a protein's amino acid sequence

genome complete set of an organism's genes

genotype the set of alleles present in an individual; determines genetic sex (XX, female; XY, male)

germ cell cell that gives rise to male or female gametes (sperm and eggs)

gestation (jess-TAY-shun) length of time of intrauterine fetal development (usually about 9 months in humans)

ghrelin (GREH-lin) hormone released from cells of the stomach; stimulates hunger

glial cell (GLEE-al) nonneuronal cell in CNS; helps regulate extracellular environment of CNS; also called *neuroglia*

globin (GLOH-bin) collective term for the four polypeptide chains of the hemoglobin molecule

globulin (GLOB-you-lin) one of a family of proteins found in blood plasma

glomerular capillary very small blood vessel within the glomerulus of the kidney through which plasma is filtered

glomerular filtrate ultrafiltrate of plasma produced in the glomerulus that is usually free of cells and large proteins

glomerular filtration process by which components of plasma in the glomerular capillary are passed to the Bowman's space of the glomerulus; process is governed by net glomerular filtration pressure

glomerular filtration rate (GFR) volume of fluid filtered from renal glomerular capillaries into Bowman's capsule per unit time

glomerulus (gloh-MER-you-lus) tufts of glomerular capillaries at beginning of kidney nephron

glottis opening between vocal cords through which air passes, and surrounding area

glucagon (GLOO-kah-gahn) peptide hormone secreted by alpha cells of pancreatic islets of Langerhans; leads to rise in plasma glucose

glucagon-like peptide 1 (GLP-1) an incretin hormone secreted by cells of the small intestine following a meal; enhances the insulin response to glucose

glucocorticoid (gloo-koh-KOR-tih-koid) steroid hormone produced by adrenal cortex and having major effects on nutrient metabolism and the body's response to stress

gluconeogenesis (gloo-koh-nee-oh-JEN-ih-sis) formation of glucose by the liver or kidneys from pyruvate, lactate, glycerol, or amino acids

glucose major monosaccharide in the body; a six-carbon sugar, $C_6H_{12}O_6$; also called *blood sugar*

glucose-counterregulatory control neural or hormonal factors that oppose insulin's actions; includes glucagon, epinephrine, sympathetic nerves to liver and adipose tissue, cortisol, and growth hormone

glucose-dependent insulinotropic peptide (GIP) intestinal hormone; stimulates insulin secretion in response to glucose and fat in small intestine

glucose sparing switch from glucose to fat utilization by most cells during postabsorptive state

glutamate (GLU-tah-mate) anion formed from the amino acid glutamic acid; a major excitatory CNS neurotransmitter

gluten a collective term for several proteins found in wheat and other foods; some individuals develop autoimmunity to these proteins

glycerol (GLISS-er-ol) three-carbon carbohydrate; forms backbone of triglyceride

glycine (GLYE-seen) an amino acid; a neurotransmitter at some inhibitory synapses in CNS

glycocalyx (glye-koh-KAY-lix) fuzzy coating on extracellular surface of plasma membrane; consists of short, branched carbohydrate chains

glycogen (GLYE-koh-jen) highly branched polysaccharide composed of glucose subunits; major carbohydrate storage form in body

glycogenolysis (glye-koh-jen-NOL-ih-sis) glycogen breakdown to glucose

glycogen phosphorylase intracellular enzyme required to begin the process of breaking down glycogen into glucose; inhibited by insulin

glycogen synthase intracellular enzyme required to synthesize glycogen; stimulated by insulin

glycolysis (glye-KOL-ih-sis) metabolic pathway that breaks down glucose to two molecules of pyruvate (aerobically) or two molecules of lactate (anaerobically)

glycolytic fiber skeletal muscle fiber that has a high concentration of glycolytic enzymes and large glycogen stores; white muscle fiber

glycoprotein protein containing covalently linked carbohydrates

Goldman-Hodgkin-Katz (GHK) equation calculation for electrochemical equilibrium when a membrane is permeable to more than one ion

Golgi apparatus (GOAL-gee) cell organelle consisting of flattened membranous sacs; usually near nucleus; processes newly synthesized proteins for secretion or distribution to other organelles

Golgi tendon organ tension-sensitive mechanoreceptor ending of afferent nerve fiber; wrapped around collagen bundles in tendon

gonad (GOH-nad) gamete-producing reproductive organ—testes in male and ovaries in female

gonadal steroid hormone synthesized in the testes (testosterone) and ovaries (estrogen and progesterone)

gonadotropic hormone *see gonadotropin*

gonadotropin glycoprotein hormone secreted by anterior pituitary gland (LH, FSH) and placenta (hCG) that influence gonadal function

gonadotropin-releasing hormone (GnRH) hypophysiotropic hormone that stimulates LH and FSH secretion by anterior pituitary gland in males and females

G protein one protein from a family of regulatory proteins that reversibly bind guanosine nucleotides; plasma membrane G proteins interact with membrane ion channels or enzymes

G-protein-coupled receptor a cell membrane protein that binds an extracellular signal and then activates an associated G protein, leading to activation of another protein such as adenylyl cyclase

graafian follicle (GRAF-ee-un) mature follicle just before ovulation

graded potential membrane potential change of variable amplitude and duration that is conducted decrementally; has no threshold or refractory period

gram atomic mass amount of element in grams equal to the numerical value of its atomic weight

granulosa cell (gran-you-LOH-sah) cell that contributes to the layers surrounding egg and antrum in ovarian follicle; secretes estrogen, inhibin, and other messengers that influence the egg

gray matter area of brain and spinal cord that appears gray in unstained specimens and consists mainly of cell bodies and unmyelinated portions of nerve fibers

growth cone tip of developing axon

growth factor one of a group of peptides that is highly effective in stimulating cell division and/or differentiation of certain cell types

growth hormone (GH) peptide hormone secreted by anterior pituitary gland; stimulates insulin-like growth factor 1 release; enhances body growth by stimulating protein synthesis

growth hormone–releasing hormone (GHRH) hypothalamic peptide hormone that stimulates growth hormone secretion by anterior pituitary gland

guanine (G) (GWAH-neen) purine base in DNA and RNA

guanylyl cyclase (GUAN-ah-lil) enzyme that catalyzes transformation of GTP to cyclic GMP

gustation (gus-TAY-shun) the sense of taste

gustatory cortex (GUS-ta-toree) region of cerebral cortex receiving primary sensory inputs from the taste buds

gyrus (JYE-rus) sinuous raised ridges on the outer surface of the cerebral cortex

H

habituation (hab-bit-you-A-shun) reversible decrease in response strength upon repeatedly administered stimulation

hair cell mechanoreceptor cell in organ of Corti and vestibular apparatus characterized by stereocilia on cell surface

heart muscular pump that generates blood pressure and flow in the cardiovascular system

heart rate number of heart contractions per minute

heart sound noise that results from vibrations due to closure of atrioventricular valves (first heart sound) or pulmonary and aortic valves (second heart sound)

heavy chain pair of large, coiled polypeptides that makes up the rod and globular head of a myosin molecule

helicotrema outer point in the cochlea where the scala vestibuli and scala tympani meet

helper T cell T cell that, via secreted cytokines, enhances the activation of B cells and cytotoxic T cells

hematocrit (heh-MAT-oh-krit) percentage of total blood volume occupied by red blood cells

hematopoietic growth factor (HGF) (heh-MAT-oh-poi-ET-ik) group of protein hormones and paracrine agents that stimulate proliferation and differentiation of various types of blood cells

heme (heem) iron-containing organic complex bound to each of the four polypeptide chains of hemoglobin or to cytochromes

hemodynamics the factors describing what determines the movement of blood, in particular, pressure, flow, and resistance

hemoglobin (HEE-ma-gloh-bin) protein composed of four polypeptide chains, each attached to a heme; located in erythrocytes and transports most blood oxygen

hemostasis (hee-moh-STAY-sis) stopping blood loss from a damaged vessel

Henry's law amount of gas dissolved in a liquid is proportional to the partial pressure of gas with which the liquid is in equilibrium

heparin (HEP-ah-rin) anticlotting agent found on endothelial cell surfaces; binds antithrombin III to tissues; used as an anticoagulant drug

hepatic (hih-PAT-ik) pertaining to the liver

hepatic lobule functional unit of the liver

hepatic portal vein vein that conveys blood from capillaries in the intestines and portions of the stomach and pancreas to capillaries in the liver

hepatocyte parenchymal cell of the liver

Hering–Breuer reflex inflation of the lung stimulates afferent nerves, which inhibit the inspiratory nerves in the medulla and thereby help to terminate inspiration

hertz (Hz) (hurts) cycles per second; measure used for wave frequencies

hexose a six-carbon sugar, such as glucose

high-density lipoprotein (HDL) lipid-protein aggregate having low proportion of lipid; promotes removal of cholesterol from cells

hilum (HIGH-lum) indented surface of the kidney through which blood vessels enter and leave

hippocampus (hip-oh-KAM-pus) portion of limbic system associated with learning and emotions

histamine (HISS-tah-meen) inflammatory chemical messenger secreted mainly by mast cells; monoamine neurotransmitter

histone class of proteins that participate in the packaging of DNA within the nucleus; strands of DNA form coils around the histones

homeostasis (home-ee-oh-STAY-sis) relatively stable condition of internal environment that results from regulatory system actions

homeostatic control system (home-ee-oh-STAT-ik) collection of interconnected components that keeps a physical or chemical variable of internal environment within a predetermined normal range of values

homeotherm an animal that maintains a relatively narrow range of body temperature despite changes in ambient temperature

horizontal cell a specialized type of neuron found in the retina of the eye that integrates information from local photoreceptor cells

hormone chemical messenger synthesized by specific endocrine cells in response to certain stimuli and secreted into the blood, which carries it to target cells

hormone-sensitive lipase (HSL) an enzyme present in adipose tissue that acts to break down triglycerides into glycerol and fatty acids, which then enter the circulation; it is inhibited by insulin and stimulated by catecholamines

human chorionic gonadotropin (hCG) (kor-ee-ON-ik go-NAD-oh-troh-pin) glycoprotein hormone secreted by trophoblastic cells of embryo; maintains secretory activity of corpus luteum during first 3 months of pregnancy

human placental lactogen (plah-SEN-tal LAK-toh-jen) hormone produced by placenta that has effects similar to those of growth hormone and prolactin

hydrochloric acid (hy-droh-KLOR-ik) HCl; strong acid secreted into stomach lumen by parietal cells

hydrogen bond weak chemical bond between two molecules or parts of the same molecule in which negative region of one polarized substance is electrostatically attracted to a positively charged region of polarized hydrogen atom in the other

hydrogen peroxide H_2O_2; chemical produced by phagosome and highly destructive to macromolecules and pathogens

hydrogen sulfide a type of gas that sometimes functions as a neurotransmitter

hydrolysis (hye-DRAHL-ih-sis) breaking of chemical bond with addition of elements of water (—H and —OH) to the products formed; also called *hydrolytic reaction*

hydrophilic (hye-droh-FIL-ik) attracted to, and easily dissolved in, water

hydrophobic (hye-droh-FOH-bik) not attracted to, and insoluble in, water

hydrostatic pressure (hye-droh-STAT-ik) pressure exerted by fluid

hydroxyapatite crystals composed primarily of calcium and phosphate deposited in bone matrix (mineralization)

hydroxyl group (hye-DROX-il) —OH

hymen membrane that partially covers the opening to the vagina

hypercalcemia increased plasma calcium

hyperemia (hye-per-EE-me-ah) increased blood flow; *see also* active hyperemia

hyperosmotic (hye-per-oz-MAH-tik) having total solute concentration greater than normal extracellular fluid

hyperpolarize to change membrane potential so cell interior becomes more negative than its resting state

hypertension chronically increased arterial blood pressure

hypertonic (hye-per-TAH-nik) solutions containing a higher concentration of effectively membrane-impermeable solute particles than normal (isotonic) extracellular fluid

hypertrophy (hye-PER-troh-fee) enlargement of a tissue or organ due to increased cell size rather than increased cell number

hypnic jerk (HIP-nik) brief muscle twitches sometimes occurring at the beginning of sleep

hypocalcemia the condition of low blood (and interstitial) calcium concentration

hypocretins (high-poe-CREE-tins) *see* orexin

hypoglycemia (hye-poh-gly-SEE-me-ah) low blood glucose (sugar) concentration

hypoosmotic (hye-poh-oz-MAH-tik) having total solute concentration less than that of normal extracellular fluid

hypophysiotropic hormone (hye-poh-fiz-ee-oh-TROH-pik) any hormone secreted by hypothalamus that controls secretion of an anterior pituitary gland hormone

hypotension low blood pressure

hypothalamo–pituitary portal vessels small veins that link the capillaries of the median eminence at the base of the hypothalamus to capillaries that bathe the cells of the anterior pituitary gland; neurohormones are secreted from the hypothalamus into these vessels

hypothalamus (hye-poh-THAL-ah-mus) brain region below thalamus; responsible for integration of many basic neural, endocrine, and behavioral functions, especially those concerned with regulation of internal environment

hypotonic (hye-poh-TAH-nik) solutions containing a lower concentration of effectively nonpenetrating solute particles than normal (isotonic) extracellular fluid

H zone one of transverse bands making up striated pattern of cardiac and skeletal muscle; light region that bisects A band

I

I band one of transverse bands making up repeating striations of cardiac and skeletal muscle; located between A bands of adjacent sarcomeres and bisected by Z line

IgA class of antibodies secreted by, and acting locally in, lining of gastrointestinal, respiratory, and genitourinary tracts

IgD class of antibodies whose function is unknown

IgE class of antibodies that mediate immediate hypersensitivity and resistance to parasites

IgG gamma globulin; most abundant class of antibodies

IgM class of antibodies that, along with IgG, provide major specific humoral immunity against bacteria and viruses

ileocecal sphincter (il-ee-oh-SEE-kal) ring of smooth muscle separating small and large intestines (that is, ileum and cecum)

ileum (IL-ee-um) final, longest segment of small intestine; site of bile salt reabsorption

immune surveillance (sir-VAY-lence) recognition and destruction of cancer cells that arise in body

immune system widely dispersed cells and tissues that participate in the elimination of foreign cells, microbes, and toxins from the body

immune tolerance the lack of immune responses to self components

immunoglobulin (Ig) (im-mune-oh-GLOB-you-lin) proteins that are antibodies and antibody-like receptors on B cells (five classes are IgG, IgA, IgD, IgM, and IgE)

immunology the study of the defenses by which the body destroys or neutralizes foreign cells, microbes, and toxins

implantation (im-plan-TAY-shun) event during which fertilized egg becomes embedded in uterine wall

inactivation gate portion of the voltage-gated sodium or potassium channel that closes the channel

incretins gut hormones such as GLP-1 and GIP that amplify the insulin response to glucose

incus one of three bones in the inner ear that transmit movements of the tympanic membrane to the inner ear

inferior vena cava (VEE-nah KAY-vah) large vein that carries blood from lower parts of body to right atrium of heart

inflammation (in-flah-MAY-shun) local response to injury or infection characterized by swelling, pain, heat, and redness

infundibulum (in-fun-DIBB-yoo-lum) the stalk of tissue connecting the median eminence at the base of the hypothalamus with the pituitary gland

inhibin (in-HIB-in) protein hormone secreted by seminiferous-tubule Sertoli cells and ovarian granulosa cells; inhibits FSH secretion

inhibitory postsynaptic potential (IPSP) hyperpolarizing graded potential that arises in postsynaptic neuron in response to activation of inhibitory synaptic endings upon it

inhibitory synapse (SIN-aps) synapse that, when activated, decreases likelihood that postsynaptic neuron will fire an action potential (or decreases frequency of existing action potentials)

initial segment first portion of axon plus the part of the cell body where axon arises

initiation factor a protein required for ribosomal assembly and the establishment of an initiation complex that allows new protein synthesis to begin

innate immune response the nonspecific immune response to conserved molecular features of pathogens; response that nonselectively protects against foreign material without having to recognize its specific identity

inner cell mass portion of the blastocyst that becomes the embryo

inner ear cochlea; contains organ of Corti

inner emotion emotional feelings that are entirely within a person

inner hair cells cells of the cochlea with stereocilia that transduce pressure waves into electrical signals

inner segment portion of photoreceptor that contains cell organelles; synapses with bipolar cells of retina

inositol trisphosphate (IP_3) (in-OS-ih-tol-tris-FOS-fate) second messenger that causes release of calcium from endoplasmic reticulum into cytosol

insensible water loss water loss of which a person is unaware—that is, loss by evaporation from skin (excluding sweat) and respiratory passage lining

inspiration air movement from atmosphere into lungs

inspiratory reserve volume (IRV) maximal air volume that can be inspired above resting tidal volume

insulin (IN-suh-lin) peptide hormone secreted by beta cells of pancreatic islets of Langerhans; has metabolic and growth-promoting effects; stimulates glucose and amino acid uptake by most cells and stimulates protein, fat, and glycogen synthesis

insulin-like growth factor 1 (IGF-1) insulin-like growth factor that mediates mitosis-stimulating effect of growth hormone on bone and other tissues and has feedback effect on anterior pituitary gland

insulin-like growth factor 2 (IGF-2) mitogenic hormone active during fetal life; postnatal role, if any, is unknown

integral membrane protein protein embedded in membrane lipid layer; may span entire membrane or be located at only one side

integrating center *see* integrator

integrator brain region that compares the actual value of a variable such as body temperature to a set point

integrin (in-TEH-grin or IN-teh-grin) transmembrane protein in plasma membrane; binds to specific proteins in extracellular matrix and on adjacent cells to help organize cells into tissues

intercalated disk (in-TER-kuh-lay-tid) structure connecting adjacent cardiac myocytes, having components for tensile strength (desmosomes) and low-resistance electrical pathways (gap junctions)

intercellular cleft a narrow, water-filled space between capillary endothelial cells

intercostal muscle (in-ter-KOS-tal) skeletal muscle that lies between ribs and whose contraction causes rib cage movement during breathing

interferon (type I) (in-ter-FEER-on) family of proteins that nonspecifically inhibit viral replication inside host cells

interferon-gamma (type II interferon) stimulates the killing ability of macrophages and NK cells

interleukin 1 (IL-1) cytokine secreted by macrophages and other cells that activates helper T cells; exerts many inflammatory effects; mediates many of the systemic, acute phase responses, including fever

interleukin 2 (IL-2) cytokine secreted by activated helper T cells that causes antigen-activated helper T, cytotoxic T, and NK cells to proliferate; also causes activation of macrophages

interleukin 6 (IL-6) cytokine secreted by macrophages and other cells that exerts multiple effects on immune system cells, inflammation, and the acute phase response

intermediate filament actin-containing filament associated with desmosomes

internal anal sphincter smooth muscle ring around lower end of rectum

internal environment extracellular fluid (interstitial fluid and plasma)

internalization down-regulation of plasma membrane receptors by receptor-mediated endocytosis

internal urethral sphincter (you-REE-thrul) part of smooth muscle of urinary bladder wall that opens and closes the bladder outlet

internal work energy-requiring activities in body; *compare* external work

interneuron neuron whose cell body and axon lie entirely in CNS

internodal pathway (in-ter-NO-dal) low-resistance conducting-cell pathway connecting the sinoatrial and atrioventricular nodes of the heart

interstitial fluid extracellular fluid surrounding tissue cells; excludes plasma

interstitium (in-ter-STISH-um) interstitial space; fluid-filled space between tissue cells

interventricular septum the muscular wall separating the right and left ventricles of the heart

intestinal phase (of gastrointestinal control) initiation of neural and hormonal gastrointestinal reflexes by simulation of intestinal tract walls

intestino-intestinal reflex cessation of contractile activity in intestines in response to various stimuli in intestine

intracellular fluid fluid in cells; cytosol plus fluid in cell organelles, including nucleus

intrafusal fiber modified skeletal muscle fiber in muscle spindle

intrapleural fluid (in-trah-PLUR-al) thin fluid film in thoracic cavity between pleura lining the inner wall of thoracic cage and pleura covering lungs

intrapleural pressure (P_{ip}) pressure in pleural space; also called *intrathoracic pressure*

intrarenal baroreceptor pressure-sensitive juxtaglomerular cells of afferent arterioles, which respond to decreased renal arterial pressure by secreting more renin

intrinsic factor glycoprotein secreted by stomach epithelium and necessary for absorption of vitamin B_{12} in the ileum

intrinsic pathway intravascular sequence of fibrin clot formation initiated by factor XII or, more usually, by the initial thrombin generated by the extrinsic clotting pathway

intrinsic tone spontaneous low-level contraction of smooth muscle, independent of neural, hormonal, or paracrine input

intron (IN-trahn) regions of noncoding nucleotides in a gene

inulin polysaccharide that is filtered but not reabsorbed, secreted, or metabolized in the renal tubules; can be used to measure glomerular filtration rate

iodide trapping active transport of iodide from extracellular fluid across the thyroid follicular cell membrane, followed by diffusion of iodide into the colloid of the follicle

iodine chemical found in certain foods and as an additive to table salt; concentrated by the thyroid gland, where it is incorporated into the structure of thyroid hormone

ion (EYE-on) atom or small molecule containing unequal number of electrons and protons and therefore carrying a net positive or negative electrical charge

ion channel small passage in plasma membrane formed by integral membrane proteins and through which certain small-diameter molecules and ions can diffuse; *see also* ligand-gated channel, mechanically gated channel, voltage-gated channel

ionic bond (eye-ON-ik) strong electrical attraction between two oppositely charged ions

ionotropic receptor (eye-ohn-uh-TROPE-ik) membrane protein through which ionic current is controlled by the binding of extracellular signaling molecules

ipsilateral (ip-sih-LAT-er-al) on the same side of the body

iris ringlike structure surrounding and determining the diameter of the pupil of eye

iron an element that forms part of each subunit of hemoglobin and binds molecular oxygen

irreversible reaction chemical reaction that releases large quantities of energy and results in almost all the reactant molecules being converted to product; *compare* reversible reaction

ischemia (iss-KEE-me-ah) reduced blood supply to a region of the body

islet of Langerhans (EYE-let of LAN-ger-hans) cluster of pancreatic endocrine cells; distinct islet cells secrete insulin, glucagon, somatostatin, and pancreatic polypeptide

isometric contraction (eye-soh-MET-rik) contraction of muscle under conditions in which it develops tension but does not change length

isoosmotic (eye-soh-oz-MAH-tik) having the same total solute concentration as extracellular fluid

isotonic (eye-soh-TAH-nik) containing the same number of effectively nonpenetrating solute particles as normal extracellular fluid; *see also* isotonic contraction

isotonic contraction contraction of muscle under conditions in which load on the muscle remains constant but muscle changes length

isotope an atom consisting of one or more additional neutrons than protons in its nucleus

isovolumetric ventricular contraction (eye-soh-vol-you-MET-rik) early phase of systole when atrioventricular and aortic valves are closed and ventricular size remains constant

isovolumetric ventricular relaxation early phase of diastole when atrioventricular and aortic valves are closed and ventricular size remains constant

J

janus kinase (JAK) cytoplasmic kinase bound to a receptor but not intrinsic to it

jejunum (jeh-JU-num) middle segment of small intestine

J receptor receptor in the lung capillary walls or interstitium that responds to increased lung interstitial pressure

junctional feet *see* foot process

juxtaglomerular apparatus (JGA) (jux-tah-gloh-MER-you-lar) renal structure consisting of macula densa and juxtaglomerular cells; site of renin secretion and sensors for renin secretion and control of glomerular filtration rate

juxtaglomerular (JG) cell renin-secreting cells in the afferent arterioles of the renal nephron in contact with the macula densa

juxtamedullary (nephron) functional unit of the kidney with glomeruli in the deep cortex and a long loop of Henle, which plunges into the medulla

K

kallikrein (KAL-ih-cryn) an enzyme produced by gland cells that catalyzes the conversion of the circulating protein kininogen into the signaling molecule bradykinin

karyotype chromosome characteristics of a cell, usually visualized with a microscope

K complex large-amplitude waveform seen in the electroencephalogram during stage 2 sleep

keto acid a class of breakdown products formed from the deamination of amino acids

ketone (KEE-tone) product of fatty acid metabolism that accumulates in blood during starvation and in severe untreated diabetes mellitus; acetoacetic acid, acetone, or B-hydroxybutyric acid; also called *ketone body*

kilocalorie (kcal) (KIL-oh-kal-ah-ree) amount of heat energy required to raise the temperature of 1 kg water by 1°C; also called *Calorie* (capital *C*)

kinesin (kye-NEE-sin) motor protein that uses the energy from ATP to transport attached cellular cargo along microtubules

kinesthesia (kin-ess-THEE-zee-ah) sense of movement derived from movement at a joint

kininogen (kye-NIN-oh-jen) plasma protein from which kinins are generated in an inflamed area

kisspeptin peptide produced in neurons in the hypothalamus involved in the control of GnRH secretion

knee jerk reflex often used in clinical assessment of nerve and muscle function; striking the tendon just below the kneecap causes reflex contraction of anterior thigh muscles, which extends the knee

Korotkoff's sounds (Kor-OTT-koff) sounds caused by turbulent blood flow during determination of blood pressure with a pressurized cuff

Krebs cycle mitochondrial metabolic pathway that utilizes fragments derived from carbohydrate, protein, and fat breakdown and produces carbon dioxide, hydrogen (for oxidative phosphorylation), and small amounts of ATP; also called *tricarboxylic acid cycle* or *citric acid cycle*

L

labeled lines principle describing the idea that a unique anatomical pathway of neurons connects a given sensory receptor directly to the CNS neurons responsible for processing that modality and location on the body

labyrinth complicated bony structure that houses the cochlea and vestibular apparatus

lactase (LAK-tase) small intestine enzyme that breaks down lactose (milk sugar) into glucose and galactose

lactate ionized form of lactic acid, a three-carbon molecule formed by glycolytic pathway; production is increased in absence of oxygen

lactation (lak-TAY-shun) production and secretion of milk by mammary glands

lacteal (lak-TEEL) blind-ended lymph vessel in center of each intestinal villus

lactogenesis the synthesis of milk by the mammary glands

lamina propria layer of connective tissue under an epithelium

laminar flow (LAM-ih-ner) when a fluid (e.g., blood) flows smoothly through a tube in concentric layers, without any turbulence

large intestine part of the gastrointestinal tract between the small intestine and rectum; absorbs salts and water

larynx (LAR-inks) part of air passageway between pharynx and trachea; contains the vocal cords

latch state contractile state of some smooth muscles in which force can be maintained for prolonged periods with very little energy use; cross-bridge cycling slows to the point where thick and thin filaments are effectively "latched" together

latent period (LAY-tent) period lasting several milliseconds between action potential initiation in a muscle fiber and beginning of mechanical activity

lateral inhibition method of refining sensory information in afferent neurons and ascending pathways whereby fibers inhibit each other, the most active fibers causing the greatest inhibition of adjacent fibers

lateral sac (*see* terminal cisternae)

lateral traction force (in the lung) holding small airways open; exerted by elastic connective tissue linked to surrounding alveolar tissue

Law of Laplace (lah-PLAHS) transmural pressure difference = 2 × surface tension divided by the radius of a hollow ball (e.g., an alveolus)

law of mass action maxim that an increase in reactant concentration causes a chemical reaction to proceed in direction of product formation; the opposite occurs with decreased reactant concentration

L dopa L dihydroxyphenylalanine; precursor to dopamine formation; also called *levodopa*

leak K^+ channels potassium channels that are open when a membrane is at rest

learned reflex *see* acquired reflex

learning acquisition and storage of information as a result of experience

lengthening contraction contraction as an external force pulls a muscle to a longer length despite opposing forces generated by the active cross-bridges

lens adjustable part of eye's optical system, which helps focus object's image on retina

leptin adipose-derived hormone that acts within the brain to decrease appetite and increase metabolism

leukocyte (LOO-koh-site) white blood cell

leukotrienes (loo-koh-TRYE-eenz) type of eicosanoid that is generated by lipoxygenase pathway and functions as inflammatory mediator

Leydig cell (LYE-dig or LAY-dig) testosterone-secreting endocrine cell that lies between seminiferous tubules of testes; also called *interstitial cell*

LH surge large rise in luteinizing hormone secretion by anterior pituitary gland about day 14 of menstrual cycle

libido (luh-BEE-doh) sex drive

ligand (LYE-gand) any molecule or ion that binds to protein surface by noncovalent bonds

ligand-gated channel membrane channel operated by the binding of specific molecules to channel proteins

light adaptation process by which photoreceptors in the retina adjust to sudden bright light

light chain pair of small polypeptides bound to each globular head of a myosin molecule; function is to *modulate* contraction

limbic system (LIM-bik) interconnected brain structures in cerebrum; involved with emotions and learning

lingual papillae taste buds located on the tongue

lipase (LYE-pase) enzyme that hydrolyzes triglyceride to monoglyceride and fatty acids; *see also* lipoprotein lipase

lipid (LIP-id) molecule composed primarily of carbon and hydrogen and characterized by insolubility in water

lipid raft cholesterol-rich regions of reduced membrane fluidity that are believed to serve as organizing centers for the generation of complex intracellular signals

lipolysis (lye-POL-ih-sis) triglyceride breakdown

lipoprotein (lip-oh-PROH-teen or LYE-poh-proh-teen) lipid aggregate partially coated by protein; involved in lipid transport in blood

lipoprotein lipase capillary endothelial enzyme that hydrolyzes triglyceride in lipoprotein to monoglyceride and fatty acids

lipoxygenase (lye-POX-ih-jen-ase) enzyme that acts on arachidonic acid and leads to leukotriene formation

liver large organ located in the upper right portion of the abdomen with exocrine, endocrine, and metabolic functions

load external force acting on muscle

local control mechanism existing within tissues that modulates activity independent of neural or hormonal input (e.g., blood flow into a local vascular bed)

local homeostatic response (home-ee-oh-STAT-ik) response acting in immediate vicinity of a stimulus, without nerves or hormones, and having net effect of counteracting stimulus

longitudinal muscle thin outer layer of the intestine; contraction shortens the length of the tube

long-loop negative feedback inhibition of anterior pituitary gland and/or hypothalamus by hormone secreted by third endocrine gland in a sequence

long reflex neural loop from afferents in the gastrointestinal tract to the central nervous system and back to nerve plexuses and effector cells via the autonomic nervous system; involved in the control of motility and secretory activity

long-term depression condition in which nerves show reduced responses to stimuli after an earlier stimulation

long-term memory information stored in the brain for prolonged periods

long-term potentiation (LTP) process by which certain synapses undergo long-lasting increase in effectiveness when heavily used

loop of Henle (HEN-lee) hairpinlike segment of kidney nephron with *descending* and *ascending limbs;* situated between proximal and distal tubules

low-density lipoprotein (LDL) (lip-oh-PROH-teen) protein–lipid aggregate that is major carrier of plasma cholesterol to cells

lower esophageal sphincter smooth muscle of last portion of esophagus; can close off esophageal opening into the stomach

lower motor neurons neurons that synapse directly onto muscle cells and stimulate their contraction

L-type Ca^{2+} channel voltage-gated channel permitting calcium entry into heart cells during the action potential; L denotes the long-lasting open time that characterizes these channels

luminal membrane *see* apical membrane

lung compliance (C_L) (come-PLYE-ance) change in lung volume caused by a given change in transpulmonary pressure; the greater the lung compliance, the more readily the lungs are expanded

luteal phase (LOO-tee-al) last half of menstrual cycle following ovulation; corpus luteum is active ovarian structure

luteinizing hormone (LH) (LOO-tee-en-ize-ing) peptide gonadotropic hormone secreted by anterior pituitary gland; rapid increase in females at midmenstrual cycle initiates ovulation; stimulates Leydig cells in males

lymph (limf) fluid in lymphatic vessels

lymphatic capillary (lim-FAT-ik) smallest-diameter vessel type of the lymphatic system; site of entry of excess extracellular fluid

lymphatic system network of vessels that conveys lymph from tissues to blood and to lymph nodes along these vessels

lymphatic vessel any vessel of the lymphatic system in which excess interstitial fluid is transported and returned to the circulation; along the way, the fluid (lymph) passes through lymph nodes

lymph node small organ containing lymphocytes, located along lymph vessel; a site of lymphocyte cell division and initiation of adaptive immune responses

lymphocyte (LIMF-oh-site) type of leukocyte responsible for adaptive immune defenses; B cells, T cells, and NK cells

lymphocyte activation cell division and differentiation of lymphocytes following antigen binding

lymphoid organ (LIMF-oid) bone marrow, lymph node, spleen, thymus, tonsil, or aggregate of lymphoid follicles; *see also* primary lymphoid organ, secondary lymphoid organ

lysosome (LYE-soh-some) membrane-bound cell organelle containing digestive enzymes in a highly acid solution that break down bacteria, large molecules that have entered the cell, and damaged components of the cell

M

macromolecule large organic molecule composed of up to thousands of atoms, such as a protein or polysaccharide

macrophage (MAK-roh-fahje or MAK-roh-fayj) cell that phagocytizes foreign matter, processes it, presents antigen to lymphocytes, and secretes cytokines (monokines) involved in inflammation, activation of lymphocytes, and systemic acute phase response to infection or injury; *see also* activated macrophage

macula densa (MAK-you-lah DEN-sah) specialized sensor cells of renal tubule at end of loop of Henle; component of juxtaglomerular apparatus

macula lutea a region at the center of the retina that is relatively free of blood vessels and that is specialized for highly acute vision

major histocompatibility complex (MHC) group of genes that code for major histocompatibility complex proteins, which are important for specific immune function

malleus one of three bones in the inner ear that transmit movements of the tympanic membrane to the inner ear

mammary gland milk-secreting gland in breast

margination initial step in leukocyte action in inflamed tissues, in which leukocytes adhere to the endothelial cell

mass movement contraction of large segments of colon; propels fecal matter into rectum

mast cell tissue cell that releases histamine and other chemicals involved in inflammation

matrix (mitochondrial) the innermost mitochondrial compartment

maximal oxygen consumption ($\dot{V}_{O_2}$ max) peak rate of oxygen use as physical exertion is increased; increments in workload above this point must be fueled by anaerobic metabolism

mean arterial pressure (MAP) average blood pressure during cardiac cycle; approximately diastolic pressure plus one-third pulse pressure

mechanically gated channel membrane ion channel that is opened or closed by deformation or stretch of the plasma membrane

mechanoreceptor (meh-KAN-oh-ree-sep-tor or MEK-an-oh-ree-sep-tor) sensory neuron specialized to respond to mechanical stimuli such as touch receptors in the skin and stretch receptors in muscle

median eminence (EM-ih-nence) region at base of hypothalamus containing capillary tufts into which hypophysiotropic hormones are secreted

mediated transport movement of molecules across membrane by binding to protein transporter; characterized by specificity, competition, and saturation; includes facilitated diffusion and active transport

medulla oblongata (ob-long-GOT-ah) part of the brainstem closest to the spinal cord; controls many vegetative functions such as breathing, heart rate and others

medullary cardiovascular center neuron cluster in medulla oblongata that serves as major integrating center for reflexes affecting heart and blood vessels

medullary collecting duct terminal component of the nephron in which vasopressin-sensitive passive water reabsorption occurs

medullary respiratory center part of the medulla oblongata involved in the neural control of rhythmic breathing

megakaryocyte (meg-ah-KAR-ee-oh-site) large bone marrow cell that gives rise to platelets

meiosis (my-OH-sis) process of cell division leading to gamete (sperm or egg) formation; daughter cells receive only half the chromosomes present in original cell

meiotic arrest state of primary oocytes from fetal development until puberty, after which meiosis is completed

melatonin an amine derived from tryptophan produced in the pineal gland and that plays a role in circadian rhythms

membrane attack complex (MAC) group of complement proteins that form channels in microbe surface and destroy microbe

membrane potential voltage difference between inside and outside of cell

memory *see* declarative memory, procedural memory, working memory

memory cell B cell or T cell that differentiates during an initial infection and responds rapidly during subsequent exposure to same antigen

memory encoding processes by which an experience is transformed to a memory of that experience

menarche (MEN-ark-ee) onset, at puberty, of menstrual cycling in women

meninges (men-IN-jees) protective membranes that cover brain and spinal cord

menopause (MEN-ah-paws) cessation of menstrual cycling in middle age

menstrual cycle (MEN-stroo-al) cyclical rise and fall in female reproductive hormones and processes, beginning with menstruation

menstrual phase time during menstrual cycle in which menstrual blood is present

menstruation (men-stroo-AY-shun) flow of menstrual fluid from uterus; also called *menstrual period*

menthol an alcohol derived from mint oil that activates ion channels found in temperature receptors that sense cool temperatures

mesangial cell modified smooth muscle cell that surrounds renal glomerular capillary loops; they help to control glomerular filtration rate

mesolimbic dopamine pathway neural pathway through the limbic system that uses dopamine as its neurotransmitter and is involved in reward

messenger RNA (mRNA) ribonucleic acid that transfers genetic information for a protein's amino acid sequence from DNA to ribosome

metabolic pathway sequence of enzyme-mediated chemical reactions by which molecules are synthesized and broken down in cells

metabolic rate total-body energy expenditure per unit time

metabolism (meh-TAB-uhl-izm) chemical reactions that occur in a living organism

metabotropic receptor (meh-tab-oh-TRO-pik) membrane receptor in neurons that initiates formation of second messengers when bound with ligand

metarteriole (MET-are-teer-ee-ole) blood vessel that directly connects arteriole and venule

MHC protein (class I and class II) plasma membrane protein coded for by a major histocompatibility complex; restricts T-cell receptor's ability to combine with antigen on cell

micelle (MY-sell) soluble cluster of amphipathic molecules in which molecules' polar regions line surface and nonpolar regions orient toward center; formed from fatty acids, monoglycerides, and bile salts during fat digestion in small intestine

microcirculation blood circulation in arterioles, capillaries, and venules

microglia a type of glial cell that acts as a macrophage

microtubule tubular cytoplasmic filament composed of the protein tubulin; provides internal support for cells and allows change in cell shape and organelle movement in cell

microvillus (my-kroh-VIL-us) small fingerlike projection from epithelial-cell surface; microvilli greatly increase surface area of cell; characteristic of epithelium lining small intestine and kidney nephrons

micturition (mik-chur-RISH-un) urination

midbrain the most rostral section of the brainstem

middle ear air-filled space in temporal bone; contains three ear bones that conduct sound waves from tympanic membrane to cochlea

migrating myoelectrical complex (MMC) pattern of peristaltic waves that pass over small segments of intestine after absorption of meal

milk ejection reflex process by which milk is moved from mammary gland alveoli into ducts, from which it can be sucked; due to oxytocin

mineralization the process of calcifying bone collagen to form lamellar bone

mineralocorticoid (min-er-al-oh-KORT-ih-koid) steroid hormone produced by adrenal cortex; has major effect on sodium and potassium balance; major mineralocorticoid is aldosterone

minute ventilation ($\dot{V}_E$) total ventilation per minute; equals tidal volume times respiratory rate

mitochondrion (my-toh-KON-dree-un) rod-shaped or oval cytoplasmic organelle that produces most of cell's ATP; site of Krebs cycle and oxidative-phosphorylation enzymes

mitogen (MY-tuh-jen) chemical that stimulates cell division

mitosis (my-TOH-sis) process in cell division in which DNA is duplicated and copies of each chromosome are passed to daughter cells as the nucleus divides

mitral valve (MY-tral) valve between left atrium and left ventricle of heart

M line transverse stripe occurring at the center of the A band in cardiac and skeletal muscle; location of energy-generating enzymes and proteins connecting adjacent thick filaments

modality (moh-DAL-ih-tee) type of sensory stimulus

modulator molecule ligand that, by acting at an allosteric regulatory site, alters properties of other binding sites on a protein and thus regulates its functional activity

molecular weight sum of atomic weights of all atoms in molecule

molecule chemical substance formed by linking atoms together

monoamine oxidase (MAO) enzyme that breaks down catecholamines in axon terminal and synapse

monocular vision visual perception by a single eye

monocyte (MAH-noh-site) type of leukocyte; leaves bloodstream and is transformed into a macrophage

monoiodotyrosine (MIT) a singly iodinated tyrosine molecule that is an intermediate in the synthesis of thyroid hormones

monosaccharide (mah-noh-SAK-er-ide) carbohydrate consisting of one sugar molecule, which generally contains five or six carbon atoms

monosynaptic reflex (mah-noh-sih-NAP-tik) reflex in which the afferent neuron directly activates motor neurons

monounsaturated fatty acid a fatty acid, such as oleic acid, in which one carbon–carbon double bond is formed within the hydrocarbon chain due to the removal of two hydrogen atoms

mood a long-term inner emotion that affects how individuals perceive their environment

motilin (moh-TIL-in) intestinal hormone thought to initiate the migrating myoelectrical complex in the GI tract

motility movement of the gastrointestinal tract mediated by muscular contractions

motivation *see* primary motivated behavior

motor having to do with muscles and movement

motor cortex strip of cerebral cortex along posterior border of frontal lobe; gives rise to many axons descending in corticospinal and multineuronal pathways; also called *primary motor cortex*

motor end plate specialized region of muscle cell plasma membrane that lies directly under axon terminal of a motor neuron

motor neuron somatic efferent neuron, which innervates skeletal muscle

motor neuron pool all the motor neurons for a given muscle

motor program pattern of neural activity required to perform a certain movement

motor unit motor neuron plus the muscle fibers it innervates

mouth general term for the expanded uppermost portion of the digestive tract

mucosa (mew-KOH-sah) three layers of gastrointestinal tract wall nearest lumen—that is, *epithelium*, *lamina propria*, and *muscularis mucosa*

Müller cells (Myoo-ler) funnel-shaped glial cells that aid light transmission through the retina

Müllerian duct (mul-AIR-ee-an) part of embryo that, in a female, develops into reproductive system ducts, but in a male, degenerates

Müllerian-inhibiting substance (MIS) protein secreted by fetal testes that causes Müllerian ducts to degenerate

multimeric protein a protein in which two or more proteins are associated via hydrogen bonds, hydrophobic attractions, and other forces, to yield a single, larger protein

multiunit smooth muscle smooth muscle that exhibits little, if any, propagation of electrical activity from fiber to fiber and whose contractile activity is closely coupled to its neural input

muscarinic receptor (muss-kur-IN-ik) acetylcholine receptor that responds to the mushroom poison muscarine; located on smooth muscle, cardiac muscle, some CNS neurons, and glands

muscle number of muscle fibers bound together by connective tissue

muscle cell specialized cell containing actin and myosin filaments and capable of generating force and movement

muscle fatigue decrease in muscle tension with prolonged activity

muscle fiber muscle cell

muscle spindle a receptor organ, made up of specialized muscle fibers, that detects stretch of skeletal muscles

muscle-spindle stretch receptor capsule-enclosed arrangement of afferent nerve fiber endings around specialized skeletal muscle fibers; sensitive to stretch

muscle tissue one of the four major tissue types in the body, comprising smooth, cardiac, and skeletal muscle; can be under voluntary or involuntary control

muscle tone degree of resistance of muscle to passive stretch due to ongoing contractile activity; *see also* smooth muscle tone

muscularis externa two layers of muscle in the gastrointestinal tract consisting of circular and longitudinal muscle

muscularis mucosa layer of muscular tissue beneath the lamina propria of the gut

mutagen (MUTE-uh-jen) factor in the environment that increases mutation rate

mutation (mew-TAY-shun) any change in base sequence of DNA that changes genetic information

myelin (MYE-uh-lin) insulating material covering axons of many neurons; consists of layers of myelin-forming cell plasma membrane wrapped around axon

myenteric plexus (mye-en-TER-ik PLEX-us) nerve cell network between circular and longitudinal muscle layers in esophagus, stomach, and intestinal walls

myoblast (MYE-oh-blast) embryological cell that gives rise to muscle fibers

myocardium (mye-oh-KARD-ee-um) cardiac muscle, which forms heart walls

myoepithelial cell (mye-oh-ep-ih-THEE-lee-al) specialized contractile cell in certain exocrine glands; contraction forces gland's secretion through ducts

myofibril (mye-oh-FY-bril) bundle of thick and thin contractile filaments in cytoplasm of striated muscle; myofibrils exhibit a repeating sarcomere pattern along longitudinal axis of muscle

myogenic response (mye-oh-JEN-ik) response originating in muscle

myoglobin (mye-oh-GLOH-bin) muscle fiber protein that binds oxygen

myometrium (mye-oh-MEE-tree-um) uterine smooth muscle

myosin (MYE-oh-sin) contractile protein that forms thick filaments in muscle fibers

myosin ATPase enzymatic site on globular head of myosin that catalyzes ATP breakdown to ADP and P_i, releasing the chemical energy used to produce force of muscle contraction

myosin light-chain kinase smooth muscle protein kinase; when activated by Ca^{2+}–calmodulin, phosphorylates myosin light chain

myosin light-chain phosphatase enzyme that removes high-energy phosphate from myosin; important in the relaxation of smooth muscle cells

myostatin (my-oh-STAT-in) a protein secreted from skeletal muscle cells as a negative regulator of muscle growth

N

NAD^+ nicotinamide adenine dinucleotide; formed from the B-vitamin niacin and involved in transfer of hydrogens during metabolism

Na^+/K^+-ATPase pump primary active-transport protein that hydrolyzes ATP and releases energy used to transport sodium ions out of cell and potassium ions in

natriuresis significant increase in sodium excretion in the urine, which secondarily causes water loss

natural killer (NK) cell type of lymphocyte that binds to virus-infected and cancer cells without specific recognition and kills them directly; participates in antibody-dependent cellular cytotoxicity

natural selection the process whereby mutations in a gene lead to traits that favor survival of an organism

negative balance loss of substance from body exceeds gain, and total amount in body decreases; also used for physical parameters such as body temperature and energy; *compare* positive balance

negative feedback characteristic of control systems in which system's response opposes the original change in the system; *compare* positive feedback

nephron (NEF-ron) functional unit of kidney; has vascular and tubular components

Nernst equation calculation for electrochemical equilibrium across a membrane for any single ion

nerve group of many nerve fibers traveling together in peripheral nervous system

nerve fiber axon of a neuron

nervous tissue one of the four major tissue types in the body, responsible for coordinated control of muscle activity, reflexes, and conscious thought

net filtration pressure (NFP) algebraic sum of inward- and outward-directed forces that determine the direction and magnitude of fluid flow across a capillary wall

net flux difference between two one-way fluxes

net glomerular filtration pressure sum of the relevant forces resulting in glomerular filtration; it is the hydrostatic pressure within the glomerular capillary (P_{GC}) minus the hydrostatic pressure in Bowman's space (P_{BS}) and minus the osmotic force in the glomerular capillary (π_{GC})

neuromodulator chemical messenger that acts on neurons, usually by a second-messenger system, to alter response to a neurotransmitter

neuromuscular junction synapselike junction between an axon terminal of an efferent nerve fiber and a skeletal muscle fiber

neuron (NUR-ahn) cell in nervous system specialized to initiate, integrate, and conduct electrical signals

neuropeptide family of more than 50 neurotransmitters composed of 2 or more amino acids; often also functions as chemical messenger in nonneural tissues

neuropeptide Y a peptide found in the brain whose actions include control of reproduction, appetite, and metabolism

neurotransmitter chemical messenger used by neurons to communicate with each other or with effectors

neurotrophic factor (neur-oh-TRO-fic) protein that stimulates growth and differentiation of some neurons

neutral solution a solution that is neither basic nor acidic (pH 7.0)

neutron noncharged component of the nucleus of an atom

neutrophil (NOO-troh-fil) polymorphonuclear granulocytic leukocyte whose granules show preference for neither eosin nor basic dyes; functions as phagocyte and releases chemicals involved in inflammation

nicotinic receptor (nik-oh-TIN-ik) acetylcholine receptor that responds to nicotine; primarily, receptors at motor end plate and on postganglionic autonomic neurons

nitric oxide a gas that functions as intercellular messenger, including neurotransmitters; is endothelium-derived relaxing factor; destroys intracellular microbes

NMDA receptor (*N*-methyl-D-aspartate receptor) ionotropic glutamate receptor involved in learning and memory

nociceptor (NOH-sih-sep-tor) sensory receptor whose stimulation causes pain

node of Ranvier (RAHN-vee-ay) space between adjacent myelin-forming cells along myelinated axon where axonal plasma membrane is exposed to extracellular fluid; also called *neurofibril node*

nonpenetrating solute dissolved substance that does not passively diffuse across a plasma membrane

nonpolar covalent bond a bond between two atoms of similar electronegativities

nonpolar molecule any molecule with characteristics that favor solubility in oil and decreased solubility in water

nonshivering thermogenesis the creation of bodily heat by processes other than shivering; for example, certain hormones can stimulate metabolism in brown adipose tissue, resulting in heat production in infants (but this does not occur to any significant extent in adults)

nonspecific ascending pathway chain of synaptically connected neurons in CNS that are activated by sensory units of several different types; signals general information; *compare* specific ascending pathway

nonvolatile acid organic (e.g., lactic) or inorganic (e.g., phosphoric and sulfuric) acid not derived directly from carbon dioxide

norepinephrine (NE) (nor-ep-ih-NEF-rin) biogenic amine (catecholamine) neurotransmitter released at most sympathetic postganglionic endings, from adrenal medulla, and in many CNS regions

NREM sleep sleep state associated with large, slow EEG waves and considerable postural muscle tone but not dreaming; also called *slow-wave sleep*

nuclear bag fiber specialized stretch receptor in skeletal muscle spindles that responds to both the magnitude of muscle stretch and the speed at which it is stretched

nuclear chain fiber specialized stretch receptor in skeletal muscle spindles that responds in direct proportion to the length of a muscle

nuclear envelope double membrane surrounding cell nucleus

nuclear pore opening in nuclear envelope through which molecular messengers pass between nucleus and cytoplasm

nucleic acid (noo-KLAY-ik) nucleotide polymer in which phosphate of one nucleotide is linked to the sugar of the adjacent one; stores and transmits genetic information; includes DNA and RNA

nucleolus (noo-KLEE-oh-lus or noo-klee-OH-lus) densely staining nuclear region containing portions of DNA that code for ribosomal proteins

nucleosome (NOO-clee-oh-some) nuclear complexes of several histones and their associated coils of DNA

nucleotide (NOO-klee-oh-tide) molecular subunit of nucleic acid; purine or pyrimidine base, sugar, and phosphate

nucleus (NOO-klee-us) (plural, *nuclei*) (cell) large membrane-bound organelle that contains cell's DNA; (neural) cluster of neuron cell bodies in CNS

O

obligatory water loss minimal amount of water required to excrete waste products

occipital lobe (ok-SIP-ih-tul) posterior region of cerebral cortex where primary visual cortex is located

odorant molecule received by the olfactory system that induces a sensation of smell

Ohm's law current (*I*) is directly proportional to voltage (*V*) and inversely proportional to resistance (*R*) such that $I = V/R$

olfaction (ol-FAK-shun) sense of smell

olfactory bulb (ol-FAK-tor-ee) anterior protuberance of the brain containing cells that process odor inputs

olfactory cortex region on the inferior and medial surface of the frontal lobe of the cerebral cortex where information about the sense of smell is processed

olfactory epithelium mucous membrane in upper part of nasal cavity containing receptors for sense of smell

oligodendrocyte (oh-lih-goh-DEN-droh-site) type of glial cell; responsible for myelin formation in CNS

oogenesis (oh-oh-JEN-ih-sis) gamete production in female

oogonium (oh-oh-GOH-nee-um) primitive germ cell that gives rise to primary oocyte

opponent color cell ganglion cells in the retina that are inhibited by input from one type of cone photoreceptor but activated by another type of cone photoreceptor

opsin (OP-sin) protein component of photopigment

opsonin (op-SOH-nin or OP-soh-nin) any substance that binds a microbe to a phagocyte and promotes phagocytosis

optic chiasm (KYE-azm) place at base of brain at which optic nerves meet; some neurons cross here to other side of brain

optic disc region of the retina where neurons to the brain exit the eye; lack of photoreceptors here results in a "blind spot"

optic nerve bundle of neurons connecting the eye to the optic chiasm

optic tract bundle of neurons connecting the optic chiasm to the lateral geniculate nucleus of the thalamus

optimal length (L_0) sarcomere length at which muscle fiber develops maximal isometric tension

orexins (oh-REK-sins) peptide neurotransmitters involved in the regulation of wakefulness, food intake, and energy expenditure; also known as *hypocretins*

organ collection of tissues joined in structural unit to serve common function

organ of Corti (KOR-tee) structure in inner ear capable of transducing sound wave energy into action potentials

organ system organs that together serve an overall function

orgasm (OR-gazm) inner emotions and systemic physiological changes that mark apex of sexual intercourse, usually accompanied in the male by ejaculation

orienting response behavior in response to a novel stimulus; that is, the person stops what he or she is doing, looks around, listens intently, and turns toward stimulus

osmol (OZ-mole) 1 mole of solute ions and molecules

osmolarity (oz-moh-LAR-ih-tee) total solute concentration of a solution; measure of water concentration in that the higher the solution osmolarity, the lower the water concentration

osmoreceptor (OZ-moh-ree-sep-tor) receptor that responds to changes in osmolarity of surrounding fluid

osmosis (oz-MOH-sis) net diffusion of water across a selective barrier from region of higher water concentration (lower solute concentration) to region of lower water concentration (higher solute concentration)

osmotic diuresis increase in urine flow resulting from increased solute excretion (e.g., glucose in uncontrolled diabetes mellitus)

osmotic pressure (oz-MAH-tik) pressure that must be applied to a solution on one side of a membrane to prevent osmotic flow of water across the membrane from a compartment of pure water; a measure of the solution's osmolarity

osteoblast (OS-tee-oh-blast) cell type responsible for laying down protein matrix of bone; called osteocyte after calcified matrix has been set down

osteoclast (OS-tee-oh-clast) cell that breaks down previously formed bone

osteocyte cell transformed from osteoblast when surrounded by mineralized bone matrix

osteoid collagen matrix in bone that becomes mineralized

otolith (OH-toe-lith) calcium carbonate crystal embedded in the mucous covering of the auditory hair cell

outer hair cells cells of the cochlea with stereocilia that sharpen frequency tuning by modulating the movement of the tectorial membrane

outer segment light-sensitive portion of the photoreceptor containing photopigments

oval window membrane-covered opening between middle ear cavity and scala vestibuli of inner ear

ovary (OH-vah-ree) gonad in female

overshoot part of the action potential in which the membrane potential goes above zero

ovulation (ov-you-LAY-shun) release of egg, surrounded by its zona pellucida and granulosa cells, from ovary

ovum (plural, *ova*) gamete of female; egg

oxidative deamination (dee-am-ih-NAY-shun) reaction in which an amino group (—NH_2) from an amino acid is replaced by oxygen to form a keto acid

oxidative fiber muscle fiber that has numerous mitochondria and therefore a high capacity for oxidative phosphorylation; red muscle fiber

oxidative phosphorylation (fos-for-ih-LAY-shun) process by which energy derived from reaction between hydrogen and oxygen to form water is transferred to ATP during its formation

oxygen-carrying capacity maximum amount of oxygen the blood can carry; in general, proportional to the amount of hemoglobin per unit volume of blood

oxygen debt decrease in energy reserves during exercise that results in an increase in oxygen consumption and an increased production of ATP by oxidative phosphorylation following the exercise

oxygen–hemoglobin dissociation curve *S*-shaped (sigmoid) relationship between the gas pressure of oxygen (partial pressure of O_2) and amount of oxygen bound to hemoglobin per unit blood (hemoglobin saturation)

oxyhemoglobin (HbO_2) (ox-see-HEE-moh-gloh-bin) hemoglobin combined with oxygen

oxytocin (ox-see-TOE-sin) peptide hormone synthesized in hypothalamus and released from posterior pituitary; stimulates mammary glands to release milk and uterus to contract

P

pacemaker neurons that set rhythm of biological clocks independent of external cues; any neuron or muscle cell that has an inherent autorhythmicity and determines activity pattern of other cells

pacemaker potential spontaneous gradual depolarization to threshold of some neurons and muscle cells' plasma membrane

pancreas elongated gland behind the stomach with both exocrine (secretes digestive enzymes into the gastrointestinal tract) and endocrine (secretes insulin into the blood) functions

papilla (puh-PIL-ah) connection between the tip of the medulla and the calyx in the kidney

papillary muscle (PAP-ih-lair-ee) muscular projections from interior of ventricular chambers that connect to atrioventricular valves and prevent backward flow of blood during ventricular contraction

paracellular pathway the space between adjacent cells of an epithelium through which some molecules diffuse as they cross the epithelium

paracrine substance (PAR-ah-krin) chemical messenger that exerts its effects on cells near its secretion site; by convention, excludes neurotransmitters; *compare* autocrine substance

paradoxical sleep *see* REM sleep

parasympathetic division (of the autonomic nervous system) (par-ah-sim-pah-THET-ik) portion of autonomic nervous system whose preganglionic fibers leave CNS from brainstem and sacral portion of spinal cord; most of its postganglionic fibers release acetylcholine; *compare* sympathetic division

parathyroid gland one of four parathyroid-hormone-secreting glands on thyroid gland surface

parathyroid hormone (PTH) peptide hormone secreted by parathyroid glands; regulates calcium and phosphate concentrations of extracellular fluid

parietal cell (pah-RYE-ih-tal) gastric gland cell that secretes hydrochloric acid and intrinsic factor

parietal lobe region of cerebral cortex containing sensory cortex and some association cortex

parietal-lobe association cortex region of cerebrum involved in integrating inputs from primary sensory cortices, as well as higher-order cognitive processing and motor control

parietal pleura (pah-RYE-it-al ploor-ah) serous membranes covering the inside of the chest wall, the diaphragm, and the mediastinum

partial pressure that part of total gas pressure due to molecules of one gas species; measure of concentration of a gas in a gas mixture

parturition events leading to and including delivery of infant

passive immunity resistance to infection resulting from direct transfer of antibodies or sensitized T cells from one person (or animal) to another; *compare* active immunity

pathogen virus or microbe that elicits an immune response in the body, and which may cause disease

pathogen-associated molecular patterns (PAMPs) conserved molecular features common to many types of pathogens; they are recognized by cells mediating the innate immune response

pathophysiology the study of disease states

pathway series of connected neurons that move a particular type of information from one part of the brain to another part

pattern-recognition receptors (PRRs) a family of proteins that bind to ligands found in many types of pathogens; include the Toll-like receptors found on dendritic cells

pentose any five-carbon monosaccharide

pepsin (PEP-sin) family of several protein-digesting enzymes formed in the stomach; breaks protein down to peptide fragments

pepsinogen (pep-SIN-ah-jen) inactive precursor of pepsin; secreted by chief cells of gastric mucosa

peptide (PEP-tide) short polypeptide chain; by convention, having fewer than about 50 amino acids

peptide bond polar covalent chemical bond joining the amino and carboxyl groups of two amino acids; forms protein backbone

peptide hormone any of a family of hormones, like insulin, composed of approximately two to 50 amino acids; generally soluble in acid, unlike larger protein hormones, which are insoluble

peptidergic neuron that releases peptides

percent hemoglobin saturation the percentage of available hemoglobin subunits bound to molecular oxygen at any given time

perception understanding of objects and events of external world that we acquire from neural processing of sensory information

perforin protein secreted by cytotoxic T cells; may form channels in plasma membrane of target cell, which destroys it

pericardium (per-ee-KAR-dee-um) connective-tissue sac surrounding heart

perilymph fluid that fills the cochlear duct of the inner ear

perimenopause beginning period leading to cessation of menstruation

peripheral chemoreceptor carotid or aortic body; responds to changes in arterial blood P_{O_2} and H^+ concentration

peripheral membrane protein hydrophilic proteins associated with cytoplasmic surface of cell membrane

peripheral nervous system nerve fibers extending from CNS

peripheral thermoreceptor cold or warm receptor in skin or certain mucous membranes

peripheral vein blood vessel outside the chest cavity that returns blood from capillaries toward the heart

peristaltic wave (per-ih-STAL-tik) progressive wave of smooth muscle contraction and relaxation that proceeds along wall of a tube, compressing the tube and causing its contents to move

peritubular capillary capillary closely associated with renal tubule

permeability coefficient *P* number that defines the proportionality between a flux and a concentration gradient and depends on the properties of the membrane and the diffusing molecule

permissiveness the facilitation of the action of one hormone by another; for example, the effects of epinephrine are exacerbated by thyroid hormone and by cortisol

peroxisome (per-OX-ih-some) cell organelle that destroys certain toxic products by oxidative reactions

Peyer's patches lymphatic tissue located in the lamina propria of the ileum of the small intestine

pH expression of a solution's acidity; negative logarithm to base 10 of H^+ concentration; pH decreases as acidity increases

phagocyte (FA-go-site) any cell capable of phagocytosis

phagocytosis (fag-oh-sye-TOH-sis) engulfment of particles by a cell

phagolysosome an intracellular vesicle formed when a lysosome and a phagosome combine; the contents of the lysosome begin the process of destroying the contents of the phagosome

phagosome plasma-membrane-bound, intracellular sac formed when a phagocyte engulfs a microbe

pharynx (FA-rinks) throat; passage common to routes taken by food and air

phase-shift a resetting of the circadian clock due to altered environmental cues

phenotype (FEE-noh-type) gender based on physical appearance

phospholipase A_2 (fos-foh-LY-pase A-two) enzyme that splits arachidonic acid from plasma membrane phospholipid

phospholipase C receptor-controlled plasma membrane enzyme that catalyzes phosphatidylinositol bisphosphate breakdown to inositol trisphosphate and diacylglycerol

phospholipid (fos-foh-LIP-id) lipid subclass similar to triglyceride except that a phosphate group (—PO_4^{2-}) and small nitrogen-containing molecule are attached to third hydroxyl group of glycerol; major component of cell membranes

phosphoprotein phosphatase (FOS-fah-tase) enzyme that removes phosphate from protein

phosphorylation (fos-for-ah-LAY-shun) addition of phosphate group to an organic molecule

photopigment light-sensitive molecule altered by absorption of photic energy of certain wavelengths; consists of opsin bound to a chromophore

photoreceptor sensory cell specialized to respond to light; contains pigments that make it sensitive to different light wavelengths

phrenic nerves main motor nerves innervating the diaphragm and providing the impulses to inspire

physiological dead space sum of the anatomical and alveolar dead spaces; it is the part of the respiratory tree in which gas exchange with blood does not occur

physiology (fiz-ee-OL-uh-jee) branch of biology dealing with the mechanisms by which living organisms function

pia mater (PEE-ah MAH-ter) innermost of three membranes (meninges) covering the brain

pigment epithelium dark, innermost layer of the retina; absorbs light that bypasses photopigments

pineal gland part of the epithalamus of the brain; produces melatonin involved in circadian rhythms

pinocytosis (pin-oh-sye-TOH-sis or PYE-no-sye-toh-sis) endocytosis when the vesicle encloses extracellular fluid or specific molecules in the extracellular fluid that have bound to proteins on the extracellular surface of the plasma membrane

pituitary gland (pih-TOO-ih-tar-ee) endocrine gland that lies in bony pocket below hypothalamus; constitutes anterior pituitary gland and posterior pituitary gland

placenta (plah-SEN-tah) interlocking fetal and maternal tissues that serve as organ of molecular exchange between fetal and maternal circulations

plasma (PLAS-muh) liquid portion of blood; component of extracellular fluid

plasma cell cell that differentiates from activated B lymphocytes and secretes antibodies

plasma membrane membrane that forms outer surface of cell and separates cell's contents from extracellular fluid

plasma protein most are albumins, globulins, or fibrinogen

plasmin (PLAZ-min) proteolytic enzyme able to decompose fibrin and thereby to dissolve blood clots

plasminogen (plaz-MIN-oh-jen) inactive precursor of plasmin

plasminogen activator any plasma protein that activates proenzyme plasminogen

plasticity (plas-TISS-ih-tee) ability of neural tissue to change its responsiveness to stimulation because of its past history of activation

platelet (PLATE-let) cell fragment present in blood; plays several roles in blood clotting

platelet activation changes in the metabolism, shape, and surface proteins of platelets that begin the clotting process

platelet aggregation positive feedback process resulting in platelets sticking together

platelet factor (PF) phospholipid exposed in membranes of aggregated platelets; important in activation of several plasma factors in clot formation

platelet plug blockage of a vessel by activated, adherent platelets

pleura (PLOOR-ah) thin cellular sheet attached to thoracic cage interior (*parietal pleura*) and, folding back upon itself, attached to lung surface (*visceral pleura*); forms two enclosed *pleural sacs* in thoracic cage

pleural sac membrane enclosing each lung

pluripotent hematopoietic stem cells (plur-ih-POH-tent) single population of bone marrow cells from which all blood cells are descended

pneumotaxic center (noo-moh-TAK-sik) area of the upper pons in the brain that modulates activity of the apneustic center

podocyte epithelial cells lining Bowman's capsule, whose foot processes form filtration slits

polar covalent bond covalent chemical bond in which two electrons are shared unequally between two atoms of different electronegativities; atom to which the electrons are drawn becomes slightly negative, while other atom becomes slightly positive; also called *polar bond*

polar molecule pertaining to molecule or region of molecule containing polar covalent bonds or ionized groups; part of molecule to which electrons are drawn becomes slightly negative, and region from which electrons are drawn becomes slightly positive; molecule is soluble in water

polymer (POL-ih-mer) large molecule formed by linking together smaller similar subunits

polymodal neuron sensory neuron that responds to more than one type of stimulus

polymorphonuclear granulocyte (pol-ee-morf-oh-NUKE-lee-er GRAN-you-loh-site) subclass of leukocytes consisting of eosinophils, basophils, and neutrophils

polypeptide (pol-ee-PEP-tide) polymer consisting of amino acid subunits joined by peptide bonds

polysaccharide (pol-ee-SAK-er-ide) large carbohydrate formed by linking monosaccharide subunits together

polysynaptic a neuronal pathway such as occurs in some reflexes in which two or more synapses are present

polyunsaturated fatty acid fatty acid that contains more than one double bond

pons large area of the brainstem containing many neuron axons

pontine respiratory group neurons in the pons that modulate respiratory rhythms

pool the readily available quantity of a substance in the body; often equals amounts in extracellular fluid

portal system a type of circulation characterized by two capillary beds connected by veins called portal veins

portal triad structure in the liver composed of branches of the hepatic artery, the hepatic portal vein, and the bile duct

positive balance gain of substance exceeds loss, and amount of that substance in body increases; *compare* negative balance

positive feedback characteristic of control systems in which an initial disturbance sets off train of events that increases the disturbance even further; *compare* negative feedback

positive nitrogen balance a period in which there is net gain of nitrogen (amino acids) in the body

postabsorptive state period during which nutrients are not being absorbed by gastrointestinal tract and energy must be supplied by body's endogenous stores

posterior pituitary portion of pituitary gland from which oxytocin and vasopressin are released

postganglionic neuron (post-gang-glee-ON-ik) autonomic-nervous-system neuron or nerve fiber whose cell body lies in a ganglion; conducts impulses away from ganglion toward periphery; *compare* preganglionic neuron

postsynaptic density area in the postsynaptic cell membrane that contains neurotransmitter receptors and structural proteins important for synapse function

postsynaptic neuron (post-sin-NAP-tik) neuron that conducts information away from a synapse

postural reflex reflex that maintains or restores upright, stable posture

potential (or potential difference) voltage difference between two points; *see also* action potential, graded potential

potential difference a difference in charge between two points

potentiation (poh-ten-she-AY-shun) presence of one agent enhances response to a second such that final response is greater than sum of the two individual responses

potocytosis (poh-toe-si-toe-sis) a type of receptor-mediated endocytosis in which vesicle contents are delivered directly to the cytosol

power stroke the step of a cross-bridge cycle involving physical rotation of the globular head

preattentive processing neural processes that occur to direct our attention to a particular aspect of the environment

pre-Botzinger complex neurons of the ventral respiratory group in the medulla that are the respiratory rhythm generator

precapillary sphincter (SFINK-ter) smooth muscle ring around capillary where it exits from thoroughfare channel or arteriole

preganglionic neuron autonomic-nervous-system neuron or nerve fiber whose cell body lies in CNS and whose axon terminals lie in a ganglion; conducts action potentials from CNS to ganglion; *compare* postganglionic neuron

preinitiation complex a group of transcription factors and accessory proteins that associate with promoter regions of specific genes; the complex is required for gene transcription to commence

preload the amount of filling of ventricles just prior to contraction; the end-diastolic volume

premotor area region of the cerebral cortex found on the lateral sides of the brain in front of the primary motor cortex; involved in planning and enacting complex muscle movements

pre-mRNA *see* primary RNA transcript

pressure natriuresis increase in sodium excretion induced by a local action within the renal tubules due to an increase in the arterial pressure within the kidney

presynaptic facilitation (pre-sin-NAP-tik) excitatory input to neurons through synapses at the nerve terminal

presynaptic inhibition inhibitory input to neurons through synapses at the axon terminal

presynaptic neuron neuron that conducts action potentials toward a synapse

primary active transport active transport in which chemical energy is transferred directly from ATP to transporter protein

primary lymphoid organs organs that supply secondary lymphoid organs with mature lymphocytes; bone marrow and thymus

primary motivated behavior behavior related directly to achieving homeostasis

primary motor cortex *see* motor cortex

primary oocyte (OH-oh-site) female germ cell that undergoes first meiotic division to form secondary oocyte and polar body

primary RNA transcript an RNA molecule transcribed from a gene before intron removal and splicing

primary spermatocyte (sper-MAT-uh-site) male germ cell derived from spermatogonia; undergoes meiotic division to form two secondary spermatocytes

primary structure the amino acid sequence of a protein

primordial follicle (FAH-lik-el) an immature oocyte encased in a single layer of granulosa cells

procedural memory the memory of how to do things

process long extension from neuron cell body

progesterone (proh-JES-ter-own) steroid hormone secreted by corpus luteum and placenta; stimulates uterine gland secretion, inhibits uterine smooth muscle contraction, and stimulates breast growth

prohormone peptide precursor from which are cleaved one or more active peptide hormones

prokaryotic cell cell such as a bacterium that does not contain its genetic information within a membrane-enclosed nucleus

prolactin (pro-LAK-tin) peptide hormone secreted by anterior pituitary gland; stimulates milk synthesis by mammary glands

prolactin-releasing factor (PRF) putative hypothalamic factor that stimulates prolactin release

proliferative phase (pro-LIFF-er-ah-tive) stage of menstrual cycle between menstruation and ovulation during which endometrium repairs itself and grows

promoter specific nucleotide sequence at beginning of gene that controls the initiation of gene transcription; determines which of the paired strands of DNA is transcribed into RNA

proprioception (PROH-pree-oh-sep-shun) sense of posture and position; sensory information dealing with the position of the body in space and its parts relative to one another

prosody (PRO-so-dee) attributes of human speech that include rhythm, emphasis, and intonation

prostacyclin eicosanoid that inhibits platelet aggregation in blood clotting; also called *prostaglandin* I_2 *(*PGI_2*)*

prostaglandin (pross-tah-GLAN-din) one class of a group of modified unsaturated fatty acids (eicosanoids) that function mainly as paracrine or autocrine factors

prostaglandin I_2 **(**PGI_2**)** *see* prostacyclin

prostate gland (PROSS-tate) large gland encircling urethra in the male; secretes seminal fluid into urethra

protease (PROH-tee-ase) an enzyme capable of breaking peptide bonds in a protein

proteasome a complex of proteins capable of denaturing (unfolding) other proteins and assisting in protein degradation

protein large polymer consisting of one or more sequences of amino acid subunits joined by peptide bonds to form a functional molecule with multiple levels of structure

protein binding site *see* binding site

protein C plasma protein that inhibits clotting

protein kinase (KYE-nase) any enzyme that phosphorylates other proteins by transferring to them a phosphate group from ATP

protein kinase C enzyme that phosphorylates certain intracellular proteins when activated by diacylglycerol

proteolysis the process whereby peptides and proteins are cleaved into smaller molecules, by the actions of specific enzymes (proteases)

proteome all of the proteins expressed by a particular cell at a given time

prothrombin (proh-THROM-bin) inactive precursor of thrombin; produced by liver and normally present in plasma

proton (PROH-tahn) positively charged subatomic particle

proximal tubule first tubular component of a nephron after Bowman's capsule; comprises *convoluted* and *straight segments*

puberty attainment of sexual maturity when conception becomes possible; as commonly used, refers to 3 to 5 years of sexual development that culminates in sexual maturity

pulmonary (PUL-mah-nar-ee) pertaining to lungs

pulmonary artery large, branching vessel carrying oxygen-poor blood away from the heart toward the lungs

pulmonary circulation circulation through lungs; portion of cardiovascular system between pulmonary trunk, as it leaves the right ventricle, and pulmonary veins, as they enter the left atrium

pulmonary stretch receptor afferent neuron ending located in airway smooth muscle and activated by lung inflation

pulmonary trunk large artery that splits into the pulmonary arteries that carry blood from right ventricle of heart to lungs

pulmonary valve valve between right ventricle of heart and pulmonary trunk

pulmonary vein large, converging vessel that returns oxygen-rich blood toward the heart from the lungs

pulse pressure difference between systolic and diastolic arterial blood pressures

pupil opening in iris of eye through which light passes to reach retina

purine (PURE-ene) double-ring, nitrogen-containing subunit of nucleotide; adenine or guanine

Purkinje fiber (purr-KIN-jee) specialized myocardial cell that constitutes part of conducting system of heart; conveys excitation from bundle branches to ventricular muscle

P wave component of electrocardiogram reflecting atrial depolarization

pyloric sphincter (py-LOR-ik) ring of smooth muscle between stomach and small intestine

pyramidal cell large neuron with characteristic pyramid-shaped cell body and apical dendrite

pyramidal system descending nervous system pathways that originate in the cerebral cortex, cross over the midline in the medulla, and control fine movements of the distal extremities

pyramidal tract *see* corticospinal pathway

pyrimidine (pi-RIM-ih-deen) single-ring, nitrogen-containing subunit of nucleotide; cytosine, thymine, or uracil

pyrogen *see* endogenous pyrogen

pyruvate (PYE-roo-vayt or pye-ROO-vayt) anion formed when pyruvic acid loses a hydrogen ion

pyruvic acid (pye-ROO-vik) three-carbon intermediate in glycolysis that, in absence of oxygen, forms lactic acid or, in presence of oxygen, enters Krebs cycle

Q

QRS complex component of electrocardiogram corresponding to ventricular depolarization

quaternary structure formed when two or more proteins associate with each other by hydrogen bonds and other forces; the individual proteins are then termed *subunits*

R

radiation emission of heat from the surface of an object

rapid eye movement sleep *see* REM sleep

rapidly adapting receptor sensory receptor that fires for a brief period at the onset and/or offset of a stimulus

rate-limiting reaction slowest reaction in metabolic pathway; catalyzed by rate-limiting enzyme

reactive hyperemia (hye-per-EE-me-ah) transient increase in blood flow following release of occlusion of blood supply

receptive field (of neuron) area of body that, if stimulated, results in activity in that neuron

receptive relaxation relaxation of the smooth muscles of the stomach (fundus and body) when food is swallowed; mediated by parasympathetic nerves in the enteric nerve plexuses

receptor (for messengers) protein either on cell surface, in the cytosol, or in the nucleus that binds a chemical messenger such as a hormone or neurotransmitter and mediates its actions; (in sensory system) specialized peripheral ending of afferent neuron, or separate cell intimately associated with it, that detects changes in some aspect of environment

receptor activation change in receptor conformation caused by combination of messenger with receptor

receptor desensitization temporary inability of a receptor to respond to its ligand due to prior ligand binding

receptor-mediated endocytosis the specific uptake of ligands in the extracellular fluid by regions of the plasma membrane that invaginate and form intracellular vesicles

receptor potential graded potential that arises in afferent neuron ending, or a specialized cell intimately associated with it, in response to stimulation

receptor tyrosine kinase the major type of receptor protein that is itself an enzyme; these receptors are on plasma membranes and respond to many different water-soluble chemical messengers

reciprocal innervation inhibition of motor neurons activating muscles whose contraction would oppose an intended movement

recognition binding of antigen to receptor specific for that antigen on lymphocyte surface

recruitment activation of additional cells in response to increased stimulus strength; increasing the number of active motor units in a muscle

rectum short segment of large intestine between sigmoid colon and anus

red muscle fiber muscle fiber having high oxidative capacity and large amount of myoglobin

reflex (REE-flex) biological control system linking stimulus with response and mediated by a reflex arc

reflex arc neural or hormonal components that mediate a reflex; usually includes receptor, afferent pathway, integrating center, efferent pathway, and effector

refraction bending of light rays when passing between compartments of different density, as from air into the cornea of the eyes

refractory period (of cardiac muscle) (reh-FRAK-tor-ee) time during which an excitable membrane does not respond to a stimulus that normally causes response; *see also* absolute refractory period, relative refractory period

regulatory site site on protein that interacts with modulator molecule; alters functional site properties

regulatory T cell a type of immune (T) cell that is believed to suppress immune function and may minimize the likelihood of autoimmunity

relative refractory period time during which excitable membrane will produce action potential but only to a stimulus of greater strength than the usual threshold strength

relaxation return of muscle to a low force-generating state, caused by detachment of cross-bridges

relaxin hormone secreted by the ovary before parturition

REM sleep (rem) sleep state associated with small, rapid EEG oscillations, complete loss of tone in postural muscles, and dreaming; also called *rapid eye movement sleep, paradoxical sleep*

renal (REE-nal) pertaining to kidneys

renal artery high pressure vessel bringing blood to the kidney

renal corpuscle combination of glomerulus and Bowman's capsule

renal cortex outer portion of the kidney

renal medulla inner portion of the kidney

renal pelvis cavity at base of each kidney; receives urine from collecting-duct system and empties it into ureter

renal plasma flow the total amount of plasma (blood minus red cell volume) that passes through both kidneys per unit time

renal vein low pressure vessel draining blood from the kidney

renin (REE-nin) enzyme secreted by kidneys that catalyzes splitting off of angiotensin I from angiotensinogen in plasma

renin–angiotensin system hormonal system consisting of renin-stimulated angiotensin I production followed by conversion to angiotensin II by angiotensin-converting enzyme

repolarize return transmembrane potential to its resting level

residual volume (RV) air volume remaining in lungs after maximal expiration

resistance (R) hindrance to movement through a particular substance, tube, or opening

respiration (1) utilization of oxygen and production of carbon dioxide at the cellular level (i.e., cellular respiration); (2) exchange of oxygen and carbon dioxide between the organism and the environment via the lungs

respiratory bronchiole largest branch of the respiratory tree in which the units of gas exchange (alveoli) appear

respiratory cycle changes in the lung volumes from the beginning of an inspiration, including the expiration, to the beginning of the next inspiration

respiratory physiology the study of the respiratory system, including its structures and functions and regulation

respiratory pump mechanism whereby reductions in intrathoracic pressure during the breathing cycle tend to favor the return of blood to the heart from peripheral veins

respiratory quotient (RQ) ratio of carbon dioxide produced to oxygen consumed during metabolism

respiratory rate number of breaths per minute

respiratory rhythm generator neural network in the brainstem that generates output to the phrenic nerve

respiratory system the anatomical pathway of air from the atmosphere to the alveoli

respiratory zone portion of airways from beginning of respiratory bronchioles to alveoli; contains alveoli across which gas exchange occurs

resting membrane potential voltage difference between inside and outside of cell in absence of excitatory or inhibitory stimulation; also called *resting potential*

rest-or-digest state homeostatic state characteristic of parasympathetic nervous system activation

rete testes (REE-tee TES-teez) network of canals at the ends of the seminiferous tubules in the testes

reticular activating system (RAS) extensive neuron network extending through brainstem core; receives and integrates information from many afferent pathways and from other CNS regions; also called *reticular formation*

reticulocyte (ruh-TIK-you-low-site) name given to immature red blood cells that have a weblike pattern in the cytosol due to the persistence of ribosomes

retina thin layer of neural tissue lining back of eyeball; contains receptors for vision

retinal (ret-in-AL) form of vitamin A that forms chromophore component of photopigment

retrograde movement of a substance or action potential backward along a neuron, from axon terminals toward the cell body and dendrites

reuptake active process that recaptures excess secreted neurotransmitter back into the presynaptic cell; can be inhibited with drugs

reversible reaction chemical reaction in which energy release is small enough for reverse reaction to occur readily; *compare* irreversible reaction

Rh factor group of erythrocyte plasma membrane antigens that may (Rh^+) or may not (Rh^-) be present

rhodopsin (roh-DOP-sin) photopigment in rods

ribonucleic acid (RNA) (rye-boh-noo-KLAY-ik) single-stranded nucleic acid involved in transcription of genetic information and translation of that information into protein structure; contains the sugar ribose; *see also* messenger RNA, ribosomal RNA, transfer RNA

ribose the sugar backbone of RNA

ribosomal RNA (rRNA) (rye-boh-SOME-al) type of RNA used in ribosome assembly; becomes part of ribosome

ribosome (RYE-boh-some) cytoplasmic particle that mediates linking together of amino acids to form proteins; attached to endoplasmic reticulum as bound ribosome, or suspended in cytoplasm as free ribosome

rigor mortis (rig-or MOR-tiss) stiffness of skeletal muscles after death due to failure of cross-bridges to dissociate from actin because of the loss of ATP

RNA polymerase (poh-LIM-uh-rase) enzyme that forms RNA by joining together appropriate nucleotides after they have base-paired to DNA

rod one of two receptor types for photic energy; contains the photopigment rhodopsin

round window membrane-covered opening in the cochlea that responds to fluid movement in the scala tympani

ryanodine receptor calcium-release channel found in the lateral sacs of the sarcoplasmic reticulum in skeletal muscle cells

S

saccade (sah-KAAD) short, jerking eyeball movement

saccule structure in the semicircular canals that responds to changes in linear movement of the head by mechanical forces on otoliths located on its surface

saliva watery solution of salts and proteins, including mucins and amylase, secreted by salivary glands

salivary gland one of three pairs of exocrine glands around the mouth that produce saliva

salt appetite desire for salt, consisting of hedonistic and regulatory components

saltatory conduction propagation of action potentials along a myelinated axon such that the action potentials jump from one node of Ranvier in the myelin sheath to the next

sarcomere (SAR-kuh-meer) repeating structural unit of myofibril; composed of thick and thin filaments; extends between two adjacent Z lines

sarcolemma (sar-ko-LEM-uh) the plasma membrane surrounding muscle cells

sarcoplasmic reticulum (sar-koh-PLAZ-mik reh-TIK-you-lum) endoplasmic reticulum in muscle fiber; site of storage and release of calcium ions

satellite cell undifferentiated cell found within skeletal muscle tissue that can fuse and develop into new muscle fiber following muscle injury

satiety signal (sah-TYE-ih-tee) input to appetite-control centers that causes hunger to cease and sets time period before hunger returns

saturated fatty acid fatty acid whose carbon atoms are all linked by single covalent bonds

saturation occupation of all available binding sites by their ligand

scala tympani (SCALE-ah TIM-pah-nee) fluid-filled inner-ear compartment that receives sound waves from basilar membrane and transmits them to round window

scala vestibuli (ves-TIB-you-lee) fluid-filled inner-ear compartment that receives sound waves from oval window and transmits them to basilar membrane and cochlear duct

Schwann cell nonneural cell that forms myelin sheath in peripheral nervous system

sclera (SKLAIR-ah) the tough, outermost tissue layer of the eyeball

scrotum (SKROH-tum) sac that contains testes and epididymides

second polar body nonfunctional structure containing one of two nuclei resulting from the second meiotic division in the ovary

secondary active transport active transport in which energy released during transmembrane movement of one substance from higher to lower concentration is transferred to the simultaneous movement of another substance from lower to higher concentration

secondary lymphoid organ lymph node, spleen, tonsil, or lymphocyte accumulation in gastrointestinal, respiratory, urinary, or reproductive tract; site of stimulation of lymphocyte response

secondary oocyte daughter cell (23 chromosomes) retaining most cytoplasm resulting from first meiotic division in the ovary

secondary peristalsis (per-ih-STAL-sis) esophageal peristaltic waves not immediately preceded by pharyngeal phase of swallow

secondary sexual characteristic external difference between male and female not directly involved in reproduction

secondary spermatocyte a 23-chromosome cell resulting from the first meiotic division of the primary spermatocyte in the testes

secondary structure the alpha-helical and beta pleated sheet structures of a protein

second messenger intracellular substance that serves as relay from plasma membrane to intracellular biochemical machinery, where it alters some aspect of cell's function

secretin (SEEK-reh-tin) peptide hormone secreted by upper small intestine; stimulates pancreas to secrete bicarbonate into small intestine

secretion (sih-KREE-shun) elaboration and release of organic molecules, ions, and water by cells in response to specific stimuli

secretory phase (SEEK-rih-tor-ee) stage of menstrual cycle following ovulation during which secretory type of endometrium develops

secretory vesicle membrane-bound vesicle produced by Golgi apparatus; contains protein to be secreted by cell

segmentation (seg-men-TAY-shun) series of stationary rhythmic contractions and relaxations of rings of intestinal smooth muscle; mixes intestinal contents

selective attention paying attention to or focusing on a particular stimulus or event while ignoring other ongoing sources of information

semen (SEE-men) sperm-containing fluid of male ejaculate

semicircular canal passage in temporal bone; contains sense organs for equilibrium and movement

seminal vesicle exocrine glands (in males) that secrete fluid into vas deferens

seminiferous tubule (sem-ih-NIF-er-ous) tubule in testis in which sperm production occurs; lined with Sertoli cells

semipermeable membrane (sem-ee-PER-me-ah-bul) membrane permeable to some substances (usually water) but not to others (some solutes)

sensation the mental perception of a stimulus

sensorimotor cortex (sen-sor-ee-MOH-tor) all areas of cerebral cortex that play a role in skeletal muscle control

sensory information information that originates in stimulated sensory receptors

sensory pathway a group of neuron chains, each chain consisting of three or more neurons connected end to end by synapses; carries action potentials to those parts of the brain involved in conscious recognition of sensory information

sensory receptor a cell or portion of a cell that contains structures or chemical molecules sensitive to changes in an energy form in the outside world or internal environment; in response to activation by this energy, the sensory receptor initiates action potentials in that cell or an adjacent one

sensory system part of nervous system that receives, conducts, or processes information that leads to perception of a stimulus

sensory transduction neural process of changing a sensory stimulus into a change in neuronal function

sensory unit afferent neuron plus receptors it innervates

serosa (sir-OH-sah) connective-tissue layer surrounding outer surface of stomach and intestines

serotonin (sair-oh-TONE-in) biogenic amine neurotransmitter; paracrine agent in blood platelets and digestive tract; also called *5-hydroxytryptamine* or *5-HT*

Sertoli cell (sir-TOH-lee) cell intimately associated with developing germ cells in seminiferous tubule; creates blood–testis barrier, secretes fluid into seminiferous tubule, and mediates hormonal effects on tubule

Sertoli cell barrier barrier to the movement of chemicals from the blood into the lumen of the seminiferous tubules in the testes

serum (SEER-um) blood plasma from which fibrinogen and other clotting proteins have been removed as result of clotting

set point steady-state value maintained by homeostatic control system

sex chromatin (CHROM-ah-tin) nuclear mass not usually found in cells of males; condensed X chromosome

sex chromosome X or Y chromosome

sex determination genetic basis of individual's sex, XY determining male, and XX, female

sex differentiation development of male or female reproductive organs

sex hormone estrogen, progesterone, testosterone, or related hormones

sexual dimorphism sex-linked differences in appearance or form

shaft portion of bone between epiphyseal plates

shear stress force exerted perpendicular to a surface (e.g., force exerted on the walls of a vessel by fluid flowing past)

shivering thermogenesis neurally induced cycles of contraction and relaxation of skeletal muscle in response to decreased body temperature; little or no external work is performed, and thus the increased metabolism of muscle leads primarily to heat production

short-loop negative feedback influence of hypothalamus by an anterior pituitary gland hormone

short reflex local neural loop from gastrointestinal receptors to nerve plexuses

short-term memory storage of incoming neural information for seconds to minutes; may be converted into long-term memory

signal sequence initial portion of newly synthesized protein (if protein is destined for secretion)

signal transduction pathway sequence of mechanisms that relay information from plasma membrane receptor to cell's response mechanism

simple diffusion movement of solutes down a concentration gradient without a transporter or ATP hydrolysis

single-unit smooth muscle smooth muscle that responds to stimulation as single unit because gap junctions join muscle fibers, allowing electrical activity to pass from cell to cell

sinoatrial (SA) node (sye-noh-AY-tree-al) region in right atrium of heart containing specialized cardiac muscle cells that depolarize spontaneously faster than other cells in the conducting system; determines heart rate

sinus vascular channel for the passage of blood or lymph

skeletal muscle striated muscle attached to bone or skin and responsible for skeletal movements and facial expression; controlled by somatic nervous system

skeletal muscle pump pumping effect of contracting skeletal muscles on blood flow through underlying vessels

sleep spindles high-frequency waveforms seen in the electroencephalogram during stage 2 sleep

sliding-filament mechanism process of muscle contraction in which shortening occurs by thick and thin filaments sliding past each other

slow fiber muscle fiber whose myosin has low ATPase activity

slowly adapting receptor sensory receptor that fires repeatedly as long as a stimulus is ongoing

slow-oxidative fiber type of skeletal muscle fiber that has slow intrinsic contraction speed but fatigues very slowly due to abundant capacity for production of ATP by aerobic oxidative phosphorylation

slow wave slow, rhythmic oscillation of smooth muscle membrane potentials toward and away from threshold, due to regular fluctuations in ionic permeability

small intestine longest portion of the gastrointestinal tract; between the stomach and large intestine

smooth muscle nonstriated muscle that surrounds hollow organs and tubes; *see also* multiunit smooth muscle, single-unit smooth muscle

smooth muscle tone smooth muscle tension due to low-level cross-bridge activity in absence of external stimuli

SNARE protein soluble *N*-ethylmaleimide-sensitive fusion protein attachment protein receptor

solute (SOL-yoot) substances dissolved in a liquid

solution liquid (solvent) containing dissolved substances (solutes)

solvent liquid in which substances are dissolved

soma cell body of neuron

somatic nervous system component of efferent division of peripheral nervous system; innervates skeletal muscle; *compare* autonomic nervous system

somatic receptor neural receptor in the framework or outer wall of the body that responds to mechanical stimulation of skin or hairs and underlying tissues, rotation or bending of joints, temperature changes, or painful stimuli

somatic sensation feelings/perceptions coming from muscle, skin, and bones

somatosensory cortex (suh-mat-uh-SEN-suh-ree) strip of cerebral cortex in parietal lobe in which nerve fibers transmitting somatic sensory information synapse

somatostatin (SS) (suh-mat-uh-STAT-in) hypophysiotropic hormone that inhibits growth hormone secretion by anterior pituitary gland; possible neurotransmitter; also found in stomach and pancreatic islets

somatotopic map a representation of the different regions of the body formed by neurons of the cerebral cortex

spatial summation adding together effects of simultaneous inputs to different places on a neuron to produce potential change greater than that caused by single input

specific ascending pathway chain of synaptically connected neurons in CNS, all activated by sensory units of same type

specificity selectivity; ability of binding site to react with only one, or a limited number of, types of molecules

sperm *see* spermatozoan

spermatic cord structure including the vas deferens and blood vessels and nerves supplying the testes

spermatid (SPER-mah-tid) immature sperm

spermatogenesis (sper-mah-toh-JEN-ih-sis) sperm formation

spermatogonium (sper-mah-toh-GOH-nee-um) undifferentiated germ cell that gives rise to primary spermatocyte

spermatozoan (sper-ma-toh-ZOH-in) male gamete; also called *sperm*

sphincter (SFINK-ter) smooth muscle ring that surrounds a tube, closing tube as muscle contracts

sphincter of Oddi (OH-dye) smooth muscle ring surrounding common bile duct at its entrance into duodenum

spinal nerve one of 86 peripheral nerves (43 pairs) that join spinal cord

spleen largest lymphoid organ; located between stomach and diaphragm

spliceosome protein and nuclear RNA complex that removes introns and links exons together during gene transcription

***SRY* gene** gene on the Y chromosome that determines development of testes in genetic male

stable balance net loss of substance from body equals net gain, and amount of substance in body neither increases nor decreases; *compare* negative balance, positive balance

stapedius (stah-PEE-dee-us) skeletal muscle that attaches to the stapes and protects the auditory apparatus by dampening the movement of the ear ossicles during persistent, loud sounds

stapes one of three bones in the inner ear that transmit movements of the tympanic membrane to the inner ear

Starling force factor that determines direction and magnitude of fluid movement across capillary wall

state of consciousness degree of mental alertness—that is, whether awake, drowsy, asleep, and so on

steady state no net change; continual energy input to system is required, however, to prevent net change; *compare* equilibrium

stem cell undifferentiated cell that divides and forms supply of cells for differentiation into mature cells

stereocilia (ster-ee-oh-SIL-ee-ah) nonmotile cilia containing actin filaments

steroid (STER-oid) lipid subclass; molecule consists of four interconnected carbon rings to which polar groups may be attached

steroid hormone any of a family of hormones, like progesterone, whose structure is derived from cholesterol

steroid-hormone-receptor superfamily class of intracellular receptor proteins that bind steroid hormones and other lipophilic molecules and induce changes in gene transcription

stimulus detectable change in internal or external environment

stomach expandable, saclike structure in the gastrointestinal tract between the esophagus and small intestine; site of initial digestion of proteins

stop signal three-nucleotide sequence in mRNA that signifies end of protein-coding sequence

stress environmental change that must be adapted to if health and life are to be maintained; event that elicits increased cortisol secretion

stretch reflex monosynaptic reflex, mediated by muscle-spindle stretch receptor, in which muscle stretch causes contraction of that muscle

striated muscle (STRY-ay-ted) muscle having transverse banding pattern due to repeating sarcomere structure; *see also* cardiac muscle, skeletal muscle

stroke volume (SV) blood volume ejected by a ventricle during one heartbeat

strong acid acid that ionizes completely to form hydrogen ions and corresponding anions when dissolved in water; *compare* weak acid

strychnine an alkaloid nervous system poison that blocks the action of the inhibitory neurotransmitter, glycine

subarachnoid space space between the arachnoid and pia mater meninges containing cerebrospinal fluid

subcortical nuclei groups of cells in brain below the cerebral cortex

submucosa layer of tissue beneath the gastrointestinal mucosa

submucosal plexus (sub-mu-KOH-zal PLEX-us) neuronal network in submucosa of esophageal, stomach, and intestinal walls

substance P neuropeptide neurotransmitter released by afferent neurons in pain pathway as well as other sites

substantia nigra (sub-STAN-sha NIE-gra) a subcortical nucleus containing dark-staining neurons that release dopamine and are important for suppressing extraneous muscle activity

substrate (SUB-strate) reactant in enzyme-mediated reaction

substrate-level phosphorylation (fos-for-ih-LAY-shun) direct transfer of phosphate group from metabolic intermediate to ADP to form ATP

subthreshold potential depolarization less than threshold potential

subthreshold stimulus stimulus capable of depolarizing membrane but not by enough to reach threshold

sucrose (SOO-krose) disaccharide composed of glucose and fructose; also called *table sugar*

sulcus (plural, *sulci*) a deep groove between gyri on the surface of the cerebral cortex

summation (sum-MAY-shun) increase in muscle tension or shortening in response to rapid, repetitive stimulation relative to single twitch

superior vena cava (VEE-nah KAY-vah) large vein that carries blood from upper half of body to right atrium of heart

supplementary motor cortex region of the cerebral cortex found on the medial side of brain hemispheres in front of the primary motor cortex; involved in planning and enacting complex muscle movements

suprachiasmatic nucleus group of cells in the hypothalamus involved in production of circadian rhythms

surface tension attractive forces between water molecules at an air–water interface resulting in net force that acts to reduce surface area

surfactant (sir-FAK-tent) detergent-like phospholipid–protein mixture produced by pulmonary type II alveolar cells; reduces surface tension of fluid film lining alveoli

swallowing center area of the medulla oblongata in the central nervous system that receives afferent neural input from the mouth and sends efferent output to the muscles of the pharynx, esophagus, and respiratory system, coordinating swallowing

sweat gland gland beneath the skin that is capable of secreting a salty fluid through ducts to the surface of the skin in response to heat-induced neural signals from the autonomic nervous system

Sylvian fissure a large sulcus in both brain hemispheres that divides the temporal lobes from the frontal and parietal lobes

sympathetic division (of the autonomic nervous system) portion of autonomic nervous system whose preganglionic fibers leave CNS at thoracic and lumbar portions of spinal cord; *compare* parasympathetic division

sympathetic trunk one of paired chains of interconnected sympathetic ganglia that lie on either side of vertebral column

synapse (SIN-aps) anatomically specialized junction between two neurons where electrical activity in one neuron influences excitability of second; *see also* chemical synapse, electrical synapse, excitatory synapse, inhibitory synapse

synaptic cleft narrow extracellular space separating pre- and postsynaptic neurons at chemical synapse

synaptic delay length of time it takes for neurotransmitters to diffuse from the presynaptic to the postsynaptic membrane and initiate electrical changes in postsynaptic cell

synaptic vesicle cellular structure that holds and releases neurotransmitter at the synapse

synaptotagmin (sin-ap-toh-TAG-min) protein present in wall of synaptic vesicle that binds calcium and helps stimulate the process of exocytosis

synergistic muscle (sin-er-JIS-tik) muscle that exerts force to aid intended motion

systemic circulation (sis-TEM-ik) circulation from left ventricle through all organs except lungs and back to heart

systole (SIS-toh-lee) period of ventricular contraction

systolic pressure (SP) (sis-TAHL-ik) maximum arterial blood pressure during cardiac cycle

T

target cell cell influenced by a certain hormone

taste bud sense organ that contains chemoreceptors for taste

T cell *see* T lymphocyte

tectorial membrane (tek-TOR-ee-al) structure in organ of Corti in contact with receptor cell hairs

template strand the DNA strand with the correct orientation relative to a promoter to bind RNA polymerase

temporal lobe region of cerebral cortex where primary auditory cortex and Wernicke's speech center are located

temporal summation membrane potential produced as two or more inputs, occurring at different times, are added together; potential change is greater than that caused by single input

tendon (TEN-don) collagen fiber bundle that connects skeletal muscle to bone and transmits muscle contraction force to the bone

tension in muscle physiology, the force exerted by a contracting muscle on object

tensor tympani muscle skeletal muscle that attaches to the ear drum and protects the auditory apparatus from loud sounds by dampening the movement of the tympanum

terminal cisternae (ter-mih-null sys-TER-nay) expanded regions of sarcoplasmic reticulum, associated with T-tubules and involved in the storage and release of Ca^{2+} in skeletal muscle cells; also known as *lateral sacs*

tertiary structure the three-dimensional folded structure of a protein formed by hydrogen bonds, hydrophobic attractions, electrostatic interactions, and cysteine cross-bridges

testis (TES-tiss) (plural, *testes*) gonad in male

testosterone (test-TOS-ter-own) steroid hormone produced in interstitial cells of testes; major male sex hormone

tetanus (TET-ah-nus) maintained mechanical response of muscle to high-frequency stimulation; also the disease lockjaw

thalamus (THAL-ah-mus) subdivision of diencephalon; integrating center for sensory input on its way to cerebral cortex; also contains motor nuclei

theca (THEE-kah) cell layer that surrounds ovarian-follicle granulosa cells

thermoneutral zone temperature range over which changes in skin blood flow can regulate body temperature

thermoreceptor sensory receptor for temperature and temperature changes, particularly in low (cold receptor) or high (warm receptor) range

theta rhythm slow-frequency, high-amplitude waves of the EEG associated with early stages of slow-wave sleep

thick filament myosin filament in muscle cell

thin filament actin filament in muscle cell

thorax (THOR-aks) closed body cavity between neck and diaphragm; contains lung, heart, thymus, large vessels, and esophagus; also called the *chest*

threshold potential membrane potential above which an excitable cell fires an action potential

threshold stimulus stimulus capable of depolarizing membrane just to threshold

thrifty gene gene postulated to have evolved in order to increase the body's ability to store fat

thrombin (THROM-bin) enzyme that catalyzes conversion of fibrinogen to fibrin; has multiple other actions in blood clotting

thrombomodulin an endothelial receptor to which thrombin can bind, thereby eliminating thrombin's clot-producing effects and causing it to bind and activate protein C

thromboxane an eicosanoid derived from arachidonic acid by the action of cyclooxygenase; among other functions, thromboxanes are involved in platelet aggregation

thromboxane A_2 an eicosanoid formed in platelets that stimulates platelet aggregation and secretion of clotting factors

thrombus (THROM-bus) blood clot

thymine (T) (THIGH-meen) pyrimidine base in DNA but not RNA

thymus (THIGH-mus) lymphoid organ in upper part of chest; site of T-lymphocyte differentiation

thyroglobulin (thigh-roh-GLOB-you-lin) large protein precursor of thyroid hormones in colloid of follicles in thyroid gland; storage form of thyroid hormones

thyroid hormone collective term for amine hormones released from thyroid gland—that is, thyroxine (T_4) and triiodothyronine (T_3)

thyroid peroxidase enzyme within the thyroid gland that mediates many of the steps of thyroid hormone synthesis

thyroid-stimulating hormone (TSH) glycoprotein hormone secreted by anterior pituitary gland; induces secretion of thyroid hormone; also called *thyrotropin*

thyrotropin-releasing hormone (TRH) hypophysiotropic hormone that stimulates thyrotropin and prolactin secretion by anterior pituitary gland

thyroxine (T_4) (thigh-ROCKS-in) tetraiodothyronine; iodine-containing amine hormone secreted by thyroid gland

tidal volume (V_t) air volume entering or leaving lungs with single breath during any state of respiratory activity

tight junction cell junction in which extracellular surfaces of the plasma membrane of two adjacent cells are joined together; extends around epithelial cell and restricts molecule diffusion through space between cells

tip link small, extracellular fiber connecting adjacent stereocilia that activates ion channels when the cilia are bent

tissue aggregate of single type of specialized cell; also denotes general cellular fabric of a given organ

tissue factor protein involved in initiation of clotting via the extrinsic pathway; located on plasma membrane of subendothelial cells

tissue factor pathway inhibitor (TFPI) a plasma protein secreted by endothelial cells; one of several mechanisms for protecting against excessive blood coagulation

tissue plasminogen activator (t-PA) plasma protein produced by endothelial cells; after binding to fibrinogen, activates the proenzyme plasminogen

titin protein that extends from the Z line to the thick filaments and M line of skeletal muscle sarcomere

T lymphocyte (T cell) lymphocyte derived from precursor that differentiated in thymus; *see also* cytotoxic T cell, helper T cell

Toll-like receptors (TLRs) members of the pattern-recognition-receptor family that bind to ligands commonly found on many types of pathogens

tonsil one of several small lymphoid organs in pharynx

total-blood carbon dioxide sum total of dissolved carbon dioxide, bicarbonate, and carbamino-CO_2

total energy expenditure sum of external work done plus heat produced plus energy stored by body

total peripheral resistance (TPR) total resistance to flow in systemic blood vessels from beginning of aorta to ends of venae cavae

totipotent cells of the conceptus that have the capacity to develop into a normal, mature fetus

trace element mineral present in body in extremely small quantities

trachea (TRAY-kee-ah) single airway connecting larynx with bronchi; windpipe

tract large, myelinated nerve fiber bundle in CNS

transamination (trans-am-in-NAY-shun) reaction in which an amino acid amino group (—NH_2) is transferred to a keto acid, the keto acid thus becoming an amino acid

transcellular pathway crossing an epithelium by movement into an epithelial cell, diffusion through the cytosol of that cell, and exit across the opposite membrane

transcription formation of RNA containing, in linear sequence of its nucleotides, the genetic information of a specific gene; first stage of protein synthesis

transcription factor one of a class of proteins that act as gene switches, regulating the transcription of a particular gene by activating or repressing the initiation process

transducin (trans-DOO-sin) G protein in disc membranes of photoreceptor; initiates inactivation of cGMP

trans fatty acid an unsaturated fatty acid in which the hydrogen atoms around a carbon:carbon double bond are distributed in a trans orientation (on the same side); implicated in a variety of negative health consequences

transferrin (trans-FERR-in) iron-binding protein that carries iron in plasma

transfer RNA (tRNA) type of RNA; different tRNAs combine with different amino acids and with codon on mRNA specific for that amino acid, thus arranging amino acids in sequence to form specific protein

transient receptor potential (TRP) proteins family of ion channel proteins involved in sensing temperature

translation during protein synthesis, assembly of amino acids in correct order according to genetic instructions in mRNA; occurs on ribosomes

transmembrane protein a protein that spans the plasma membrane and contains both hydrophilic and hydrophobic regions; often acts as a receptor or an ion channel

transmural pressure pressure difference exerted on the two sides of a wall

transporter integral membrane protein that mediates passage of molecule through membrane; also called *carrier*

transport maximum (T_m) upper limit to amount of material that carrier-mediated transport can move across the renal tubule

transpulmonary pressure (P_{tp}) difference in pressure between the inside and outside of the lung (alveolar pressure minus the intrapleural pressure)

transverse tubule (T-tubule) tubule extending from striated muscle plasma membrane into the fiber, passing between opposed sarcoplasmic reticulum segments; conducts muscle action potential into muscle fiber

tricarboxylic acid cycle *see* Krebs cycle

tricuspid valve (try-CUSS-pid) valve between right atrium and right ventricle of heart

triglyceride subclass of lipids composed of glycerol and three fatty acids

triiodothyronine (T_3) (try-eye-oh-doh-THIGH-roh-neen) iodine-containing amine hormone secreted by thyroid gland

trophoblast (TROH-foh-blast) outer layer of blastocyst; gives rise to fetal portion of placental tissue

tropic hormone hormone that stimulates the secretion of another hormone

tropomyosin (troh-poh-MY-oh-sin) regulatory protein capable of reversibly converting binding sites on actin; associated with muscle thin filaments

troponin (troh-POH-nin) regulatory protein bound to actin and tropomyosin of striated muscle thin filaments; site of calcium binding that initiates contractile activity

trypsin (TRIP-sin) enzyme secreted into small intestine by exocrine pancreas as precursor trypsinogen; breaks certain peptide bonds in proteins and polypeptides

trypsinogen (trip-SIN-oh-jen) inactive precursor of trypsin; secreted by exocrine pancreas

T-type Ca^{2+} channel channel that carries inward calcium current that briefly supports diastolic depolarization of cardiac pacemaker cells (T: "transient")

tubular reabsorption transfer of materials from kidney tubule lumen to peritubular capillaries

tubular secretion transfer of materials from peritubular capillaries to kidney tubule lumen

tubule a hollow structure lined by epithelial cells, often involved in transport processes such as those in the kidney nephrons

tubulin (TOOB-you-lin) the major protein component of microtubules

tumor necrosis factor-alpha (TNF-α) (neh-KROH-sis) cytokine secreted by macrophages (and other cells); has many of the same functions as IL-1

T wave component of electrocardiogram corresponding to ventricular repolarization

twitch mechanical response of muscle to single action potential

tympanic membrane (tim-PAN-ik) membrane stretched across end of ear canal; also called *eardrum*

type I alveolar cell a flat epithelial cell that with others forms a continuous layer lining the air-facing surface of the pulmonary alveoli

type II alveolar cell pulmonary cell that produces surfactant

U

ubiquitin (you-BIK-wit-in) small intracellular peptide that attaches to proteins and directs them to proteasomes

ultrafiltrate (ul-tra-FIL-trate) protein-free fluid formed from plasma as it is forced through capillary walls by pressure gradient

umami (oo-MOM-ee) unique taste sensation roughly equivalent to "flavorfulness"

umbilical artery artery transporting blood from the fetus into the capillaries of the chorionic villi

umbilical cord (um-BIL-ih-kul) long, ropelike structure that connects the fetus to the placenta and contains umbilical arteries and vein

umbilical vein vein transporting blood from the chorionic villi capillaries back to the fetus

unfused tetanus stimulation of skeletal muscle at a low-to-moderate action potential frequency that results in oscillating, submaximal force

unsaturated fatty acid fatty acid containing one or more double bonds

upper airway part of the respiratory tree consisting of the nose, mouth, pharynx, and larynx

upper esophageal sphincter (ih-soff-ih-JEE-al SFINK-ter) skeletal muscle ring surrounding esophagus just below pharynx that, when contracted, closes entrance to esophagus

upper motor neuron neuron of the motor cortex and descending pathways involved in motor control; they are not technically "motor neurons" because they synapse on neurons, not muscle cells

up-regulation increase in number of target-cell receptors for given messenger in response to chronic low extracellular concentration of that messenger; *compare* down-regulation

uracil (U) (YOOR-ah-sil) pyrimidine base; present in RNA but not DNA

urea (you-REE-ah) major nitrogenous waste product of protein breakdown and amino acid catabolism

ureter (YOOR-ih-ter) tube that connects kidney to bladder

urethra (you-REE-thrah) tube that connects bladder to outside of body

uric acid (YOOR-ik) waste product derived from nucleic acid catabolism

uterus (YOU-ter-us) hollow organ in pelvic region of females; houses fetus during pregnancy; also called *womb*

utricle structure in the semicircular canals that responds to changes in linear movement of the head by mechanical forces on otoliths located on its surface

V

vagina (vah-JY-nah) canal leading from uterus to outside of body

vagus nerve (VAY-gus) cranial nerve X; major parasympathetic nerve

van der Waals forces (walls) weak forces between atoms and molecules due to transient electrical forces generated by the orbits of electrons in the outer energy shells of atoms

varicosity (vair-ih-KOS-ih-tee) swollen region of axon; contains neurotransmitter-filled vesicles; analogous to presynaptic ending

vasa recta (VAY-zuh REK-tah) blood vessels that form loops parallel to the loops of Henle in the renal medulla

vascular system closed system of blood vessels that includes all arteries, arterioles, capillaries, venules, and veins

vas deferens (vas DEF-er-enz) one of paired male reproductive ducts that connect epididymis of testis to urethra; also called *ductus deferens*

vasoconstriction (vayz-oh-kon-STRIK-shun) decrease in blood vessel diameter due to vascular smooth muscle contraction

vasodilation (vayz-oh-dy-LAY-shun) increase in blood vessel diameter due to vascular smooth muscle relaxation

vasopressin (vayz-oh-PRES-sin) peptide hormone synthesized in hypothalamus and released from posterior pituitary gland; increases water permeability of kidneys' collecting ducts and causes vasoconstriction; also called *antidiuretic hormone (ADH)*

vault recently discovered cytoplasmic structures composed of protein and RNA; their function is uncertain but may involve cytoplasmic-nuclear transport and modulation of a cell's sensitivity to certain drugs

vein any vessel that returns blood to heart

venous return (VR) blood volume flowing *to* heart per unit time

ventilation air exchange between atmosphere and alveoli; alveolar airflow

ventral horn the ventral gray matter of the spinal cord that contains cell bodies of motor neurons

ventral respiratory group (VRG) region of the brainstem containing expiratory neurons important during exercise

ventral root one of two groups of efferent fibers that leave ventral side of spinal cord

ventricle (VEN-trih-kul) cavity, as in cerebral ventricle or heart ventricle; lower chamber of heart

ventricular ejection phase of the cardiac pump cycle during ventricle contraction when blood exits through the semilunar valves

ventricular filling phase of the cardiac pump cycle during which the ventricles are resting and blood enters through the atrioventricular valves

ventricular-function curve relation of the increase in stroke volume as end-diastolic volume increases, all other factors being equal

venule (VEEN-ule) small vessel that carries blood from capillary network to vein

very-low-density lipoprotein (VLDL) (lip-oh-PROH-teen) lipid–protein aggregate having high proportion of fat

vestibular apparatus sense organ in temporal bone of skull; consists of three semicircular canals, a utricle, and a saccule; also called *sense organ of balance*, *vestibular system*

vestibulocochlear nerve (ves-tibb-yoo-loh-KOKE-lee-ar) eighth cranial nerve; transmits sensory information about sound and motion from the inner ear to the brain

villus (VIL-us) fingerlike projection from highly folded surface of small intestine; covered with single-layered epithelium

visceral pleura (VISS-er-al PLOO-rah) serous membranes covering the surface of the lung

viscosity (viss-KOS-ih-tee) measure of friction between adjacent layers of a flowing liquid; property of fluid that makes it resist flow

visible spectrum wavelengths of electromagnetic radiation capable of stimulating photoreceptors of the eye

vital capacity (VC) maximal amount of air that can be expired, regardless of time required, following maximal inspiration

vitamin organic molecule required in trace amounts for normal health and growth; usually not manufactured in the body and must be supplied by diet; classified as water-soluble (vitamins C and the B complex) and fat-soluble (vitamins A, D, E, and K)

vitamin B_{12} an essential vitamin found in animal products that plays an important role in the production of red blood cells

vitamin D secosteroid absorbed in the diet or released from the skin under UV light; there are two forms: D_2 is from plants and D_3 is from animals

vitamin D_2 (ergocalciferol) plant vitamin D

vitamin D_3 (cholecalciferol) animal vitamin D

vitamin K a lipid-soluble substance absorbed from the diet and manufactured by bacteria of the large intestine; required for production of numerous factors involved in blood clotting

vitreous humor jellylike fluid filling the posterior chamber of the eye

vocal cord one of two elastic-tissue bands stretched across laryngeal opening and caused to vibrate when air moves past them, producing sounds

volt (V) unit of measurement of electrical potential between two points

voltage measure of potential of separated electrical charges to do work; measure of electrical force between two points

voltage-gated channel cell membrane ion channel opened or closed by changes in membrane potential

voluntary movement consciously carried-out motions mediated by the somatic nervous system and skeletal muscle contraction

vomiting center neurons in brainstem medulla oblongata that coordinate vomiting reflex

von Willebrand factor (vWF) (von-VILL-ih-brant) plasma protein secreted by endothelial cells; facilitates adherence of platelets to damaged vessel wall

vulva (VUL-vah) female external genitalia; mons pubis, labia majora and minora, clitoris, vestibule of vagina, and vestibular glands

W

water diuresis increase in urine flow due to increased fluid output (usually due to decreased secretion or action of vasopressin)

water-soluble vitamin *see* vitamin

wavelength distance between two successive wave peaks in oscillating medium

weak acid acid whose molecules do not completely ionize to form hydrogen ions when dissolved in water; *compare* strong acid

Wernicke's area brain area involved in language comprehension

white matter portion of CNS that appears white in unstained specimens and contains primarily myelinated nerve fibers

white muscle fiber muscle fiber lacking appreciable amounts of myoglobin

withdrawal reflex bending of those joints that withdraw an injured part away from a painful stimulus

Wolffian duct (WOLF-ee-an) part of embryonic duct system that, in male, remains and develops into reproductive system ducts, but in female, degenerates

working memory short-term memory storage process serving as initial depository of information

X

X chromosome one of the two sex chromosomes; found in females and males

Y

Y chromosome one of the two sex chromosomes; found only in males

Z

Z line structure running across myofibril at each end of striated muscle sarcomere; anchors one end of thin filaments and titin

zona pellucida (ZOH-nah peh-LOO-sih-dah) thick, clear layer separating egg from surrounding granulosa cells

zonular fiber connecting the ciliary muscles with the lens of the eye

zygote (ZYE-goat) a newly fertilized egg

zymogen (ZYE-moh-jen) enzyme precursor requiring some change to become active

Photo Credits

Chapter 1
Opener: © Photodisc Red/Getty Images.

Chapter 2
Opener: © Drs. Ali Yazdani& Daniel J. Hornbaker/Photo Researchers, Inc.;2.2: © Living Art Enterprises/Photo Researchers, Inc.

Chapter 3
Opener: © Professors P. Motta & T. Naguro/ Science Photo Library/Photo Researchers, Inc.;3.2: © Don W. Fawcett/Photo Researchers, Inc.;3.5a: From "Unit Membranes" J. D. Robertson in Michael Locke (ed.), "Cell Membranes in Development," © 1964 by Academic Press;3.9c: Reproduced from The Journal of Cell Biology, 1963, 17:375-412 by copyright permission of The Rockefeller University Press;3.10 (left): Courtesy of the Keith Porter Endowment Fund for Cell Biology;3.11: Electron micrograph from D. W. Fawcett, The Cell, An Atlas of Fine Structure, W. B. Saunders Company, Philadelphia, 1966;3.12 (left): © Dr. Dennis Kunkel/Visuals Unlimited;3.13 (left): Courtesy of the Keith Porter Endowment Fund for Cell Biology;3.14: Courtesy of Hans Hoppeler.

Chapter 4
Opener: © VVG/Science Photo Library/Photo Researchers, Inc.

Chapter 5
Opener: © Pr. Lavery, Laboratory of Biochemical Theory/Eurelios/Phototake.

Chapter 6
Opener: © Su-Chun Zhang, MD, PhD;6.2c: © C. Raines/Science VU/Visuals Unlimited.

Chapter 7
Opener: © Getty Images/Brand X;7.22c: © Lisa Klancher;7.27: Courtesy of Beckman Vision Center at UCSF School of Medicine/D. Copenhagen, S. Mittman and M. Maglio;7.41a: From C.M. Hackney and D.N. Furness (1995) "Mechanotransduction in vertebrate hair cells: the structure and function of the stereocillary bundle" in American Journal Physiology, 268: (Cell Physiol. 37): CA-C13. Micrograph by C.M. Hackney and D. N. Furness.;7.47c: © Ed Reschke.

Chapter 8
Opener: © Richard T. Nowitz/Photo Researchers, Inc.;8.12, 8.16: Courtesy Marcus E. Raichle, MD, Washington University School of Medicine;8.17 (both): © Shaywitz, et al., 1995 NMR Research/ Yale Medical School;8.18: Courtesy of Lee Faucher, MD, University of Wisconsin SMPH.

Chapter 9
Opener: © Steve Gschmeissner/Photo Researchers, Inc.;9.1a, 9.1b: © Ed Reschke;9.1c: © McGraw-Hill Higher Education;9.4a: © Marion L. Greaser, University of Wisconsin;9.5a: From H.E. Huxley, Journal of Molecular Biology, 37:507-520, 1968;9.8a: © Don W. Fawcett/Photo Researchers, Inc.;9.24: © Dr. Gladden Willis/ Visuals Unlimited;9.32, 9.39a: © Ed Reschke.

Chapter 10
Opener: © USA-Stock Inc/Alamy;10.14 (both): © Kevin Strang.

Chapter 11
Opener: © ISM/Phototake;11.20b: © Biophoto Assoicates/Photo Researchers, Inc.;11.23: © CNRI/Phototake;11.25 (both): Source: From H.G. Turney of London, "Discussion on Disease of the Pituitary Body" in Proceedings of the Royal Society of Medicine, 1913.;11.33: © Marcelo Sayao/epa/Corbis.

Chapter 12
Opener: © Lunagrafix, Inc./Photo Researchers, Inc.;12.28: © Carolina Biological Supply/ Phototake;12.37b: © Michael Noel Hart, M.D., Dept. of Pathology, University of Wisconsin, Madison;12.48: © R. UmeshChandran, TDR, WHO/SPL/Photo Researchers, Inc.;12.66 (all): © Matthew R. Wolff, M.D., University of Wisconsin, Madison;12.68: © Dr. Dennis Kunkel/ Visuals Unlimited;12.71: © Dr. Stanley Flegler/ Visuals Unlimited/Corbis;12.75: © Science Photo Library RF/Getty Images.

Chapter 13
Opener: © SPL/Photo Researchers, Inc.

Chapter 14
Opener: © Dennis Kunkel Microscopy, Inc./ Visuals Unlimited.

Chapter 15
Opener: © SPL/Photo Researchers, Inc.;15.5: © Science Photo Library RF/Getty Images;15.36c: Courtesy Fernando Carballo, M.D.;15.37: Courtesy of Dr. David Olson.

Chapter 16
Opener: AP Photo/The Rockefeller University.

Chapter 17
Opener: © David M. Phillips/Photo Researchers, Inc.;17.16: © Glenn D. Braunstein, M.D., Cedars-Sinai Medical Center, Los Angeles, CA.

Chapter 18
Opener: © Superstock;18.1: © Biophoto Associates/Photo Researchers, Inc.;18.3: © Eye of Science/Photo Researchers, Inc.;18.9b: © Dr. GopalMurti/SPL/Photo Researchers, Inc.;18.12b: Courtesy of Mike Clark, Cambridge University;18.23b: © Dr. Fred Hossler/Visuals Unlimited;18.24: © agencyby/iStockphoto.

Chapter 19
Opener: © Comstock/Jupiter Images;19.1 (both): © Custom Medical Stock;19.3 (both): From Lawrence M. Tierney, Current Medical Diagnosis and Treatment, 2006;19.4 (both): © Dr. David Schwartz, New York University School of Medicine from Schwartz DT, Reisdorff EJ Emergency Radiology, McGraw-Hill 2000;19.7 (both): Courtesy of Dr. Douglas Woo/Medical College of Wisconsin;Clinical Case Studies Boxes: © Comstock/Jupiter Images.

Index

Page numbers followed by f or t indicate figures or tables respectively.